medical

immerse yourself

language

susan turley

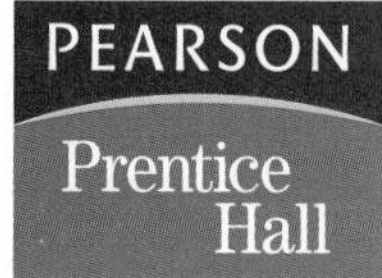

Upper Saddle River,
New Jersey 07458

Library of Congress Cataloging-in-Publication Data

Turley, Susan M.
Medical language / Susan Turley.
p. ; cm.
Includes index.
ISBN 0-13-094009-7
1. Medicine—Terminology I. Title
[DNLM: 1. Terminology—Problems and Exercises.
W 18.2 T941m 2007]
R123.T87 2007
610'.1'4—dc22

2005023235

Notice:
The author and the publisher of this volume have taken care that the information and technical recommendations contained herein are based on research and expert consultation, and are accurate and compatible with the standards generally accepted at the time of publication. Nevertheless, as new information becomes available, changes in clinical and technical practices become necessary. The reader is advised to carefully consult manufacturers' instructions and information material for all supplies and equipment before use, and to consult with a health care professional as necessary. This advice is especially important when using new supplies or equipment for clinical purposes. The author and publisher disclaim all responsibility for any liability, loss, injury, or damage incurred as a consequence, directly or indirectly, of the use and application of any of the contents of this volume.

Publisher: Julie Levin Alexander
Assistant to Publisher: Regina Bruno
Executive Editor: Mark Cohen
Associate Editor: Melissa Kerian
Editorial Assistant: Karen DePodwin
Media Product Manager: John J. Jordan
Development Editor: Cathy Wein
Director of Production and Manufacturing: Bruce Johnson
Managing Production Editor: Patrick Walsh
Production Liaison: Christina Zingone
Production Editor: Jessica Balch, Pine Tree Composition
Manufacturing Manager: Ilene Sanford
Manufacturing Buyer: Pat Brown
Design Director: Cheryl Asherman
Design Coordinator: Mary Siener
Interior Design: Mary Siener
Medical Illustrator: Anita Impagliazzo
Cover Design: Blair Brown
Cover Photo: Getty Images, Inc./Allsport Photography
Director of Marketing: Karen Allman
Executive Marketing Manager: Katrin Beacom
Manager of Media Production: Amy Peltier
New Media Project Manager: Stephen Hartner
Composition: Pine Tree Composition, Inc.
Printer/Binder: Courier Kendallville
Cover Printer: Phoenix Color Corporation

Pearson Education Ltd., *London*
Pearson Education Australia Pty. Limited, *Sydney*
Pearson Education Singapore, Pte. Ltd.
Pearson Education North Asia Ltd., *Hong Kong*
Pearson Education Canada, Ltd., *Toronto*
Pearson Educación de Mexico, S.A. de C.V.
Pearson Education—Japan, *Tokyo*
Pearson Education Malaysia, Pte. Ltd.
Pearson Education, Upper Saddle River, New Jersey

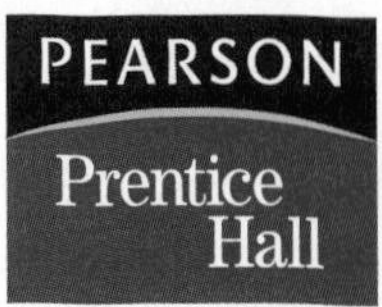

10 9 8 7 6 5 4 3 2 1
ISBN 0-13-094009-7

Dedication

To my husband Al
for his support and love

To my children, Daniel,
Minh, and Lien.

Contents in Brief

PART I INTRODUCTION TO MEDICAL LANGUAGE 3

CHAPTER 1 The Structure of Medical Language 3

CHAPTER 2 The Body in Health and Disease 33

PART II MEDICAL SPECIALTIES AND BODY SYSTEMS 87

CHAPTER 3 Gastroenterology • Gastrointestinal System 87

CHAPTER 4 Pulmonology • Respiratory System 153

CHAPTER 5 Cardiology • Cardiovascular System 205

CHAPTER 6 Hematology and Immunology • Blood and Lymphatic System 275

CHAPTER 7 Dermatology • Integumentary System 337

CHAPTER 8 Orthopedics • Skeletal System 395

CHAPTER 9 Orthopedics • Muscular System 457

CHAPTER 10 Neurology • Nervous System 511

CHAPTER 11 Urology • Urinary System 581

CHAPTER 12 Male Reproductive Medicine • Male Genitourinary System 635

CHAPTER 13 Gynecology and Obstetrics • Female Reproductive System 673

CHAPTER 14 Endocrinology • Endocrine System 751

CHAPTER 15 Ophthalmology • Eyes 805

CHAPTER 16 Otolaryngology • Ears, Nose, and Throat 853

PART III OTHER MEDICAL SPECIALTIES 901

CHAPTER 17 Psychiatry 901

CHAPTER 18 Oncology 943

CHAPTER 19 Radiology and Nuclear Medicine 991

APPENDICES A-1

APPENDIX A Glossary of Medical Word Parts: Combining Forms, Prefixes, and Suffixes A-1

APPENDIX B Abbreviations Glossary A-17

ANSWER KEY AK-1

PHOTO CREDITS PC-1

INDEX I-1

Two Journeys

In August 2000, I began two journeys—the adoption of children into our family and the writing of this textbook. Although very different, these two journeys shared a common thread of language and communication!

The first journey was the adoption of two beautiful children, Minh and Lien (ages 8 and 9), who joined our family from an orphanage in Vietnam in 2001. This journey of adoption involved completing much paperwork and research, learning a new language and culture, and traveling to an exotic land.

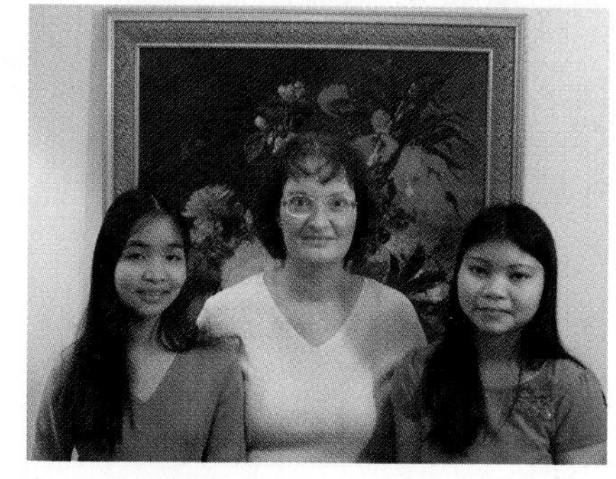

For many months prior to the adoption, nearly everything I did on a day-to-day basis was, in some way, affected by the decision to adopt. I purchased a Vietnamese dictionary, an English/Vietnamese dictionary, and a Vietnamese language CD-ROM and began to spend at least an hour each day studying the Vietnamese language. A Vietnamese-American friend tutored me, teaching me Vietnamese phrases and laughing with me when I unknowingly said something I didn't intend to say. My studies were rewarded, however, when I was able to communicate with my new daughters in their own language, even as they quickly learned to speak English. As I write this page now in late 2005, our family is preparing to adopt again, and I am ever-mindful of the many children who remain, waiting for adoption.

The second journey was the process of writing this textbook. This journey also involved paperwork and research, but I did not need to learn a new language or culture. Because of my many years of experience in the healthcare field, I already understood medical language and culture.

I did, however, need to determine the best way to convey that knowledge to each student who studies this textbook. And so, as I wrote, I drew on my own efforts and struggles to learn a new language during the adoption process. Those insights helped me identify with students who are learning medical language for the first time and enabled me to include textbook features that would support and strengthen students' efforts as they learned!

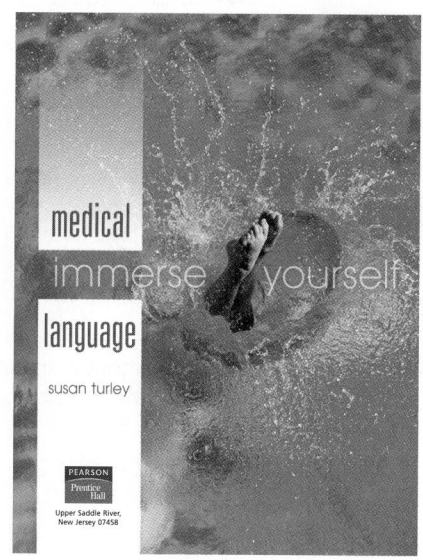

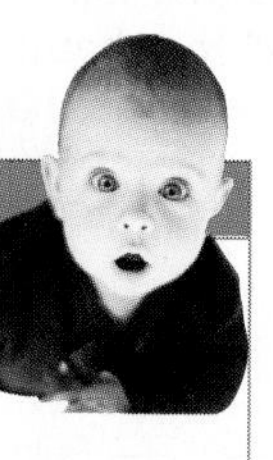

Did You Know?

All of the royalties from this textbook are being used for adoption-related expenses and to provide ongoing financial support to orphanages and programs for orphans and street children in various countries around the world.

Dive Into Something Different

This is your book! We created ***Medical Language*** to meet your needs as students and educators. In order to accomplish this, we asked our development team (reviewers, focus groups, and students) at each stage to not only critique our ideas but to offer their suggestions and recommendations for features that would enhance the teaching and learning process. The result has been an integration of features that "you," the customer, have asked for and will not find in other books.

CHAPTER FORMAT

Each medical specialty chapter follows a consistent organization that is designed for student success.

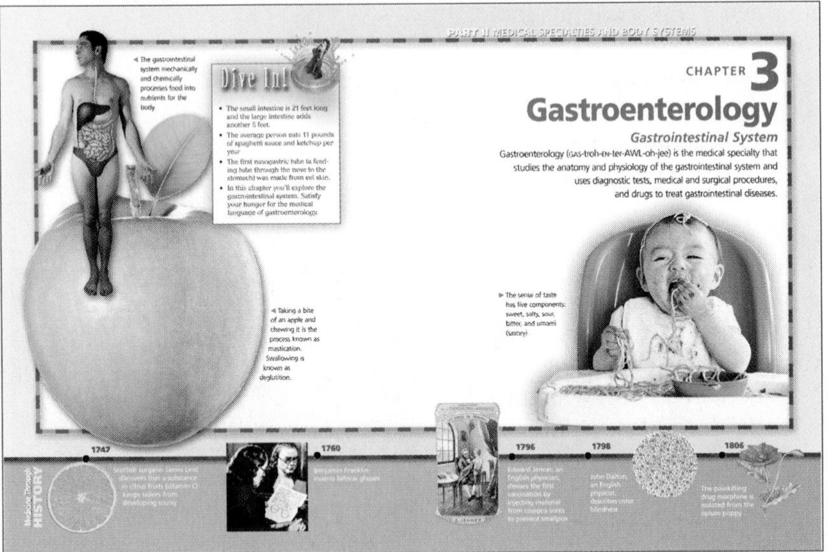

1 **Visual Introduction**—Engages readers with a stimulating collection of fun facts and images that help "launch" the chapter. These sections paint a visual portrait of what is to come in the pages that follow.

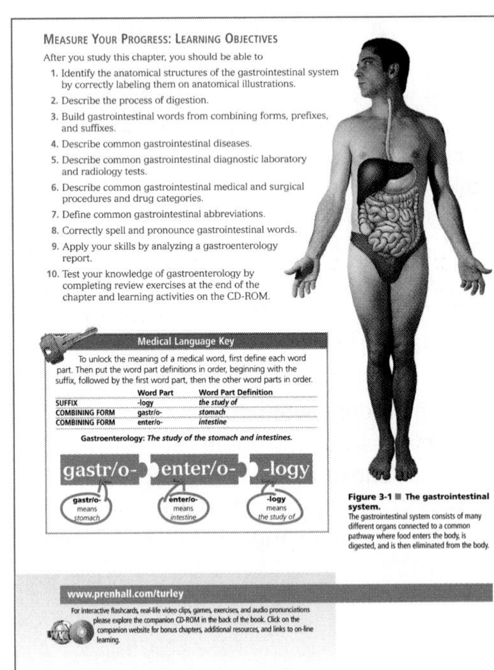

MEASURE YOUR PROGRESS: LEARNING OBJECTIVES

After you study this chapter, you should be able to

1. Identify the anatomical structures of the gastrointestinal system by correctly labeling them on anatomical illustrations.
2. Describe the process of digestion.
3. Build gastrointestinal words from combining forms, prefixes, and suffixes.
4. Describe common gastrointestinal diseases.
5. Describe common gastrointestinal diagnostic laboratory and radiology tests.
6. Describe common gastrointestinal medical and surgical procedures and drug categories.
7. Define common gastrointestinal abbreviations.
8. Correctly spell and pronounce gastrointestinal words.
9. Apply your skills by analyzing a gastroenterology report.
10. Test your knowledge of gastroenterology by completing review exercises at the end of the chapter and learning activities on the CD-ROM.

Medical Language Key

To unlock the meaning of a medical word, first define each word part. Then put the word part definitions in order, beginning with the suffix, followed by the first word part, then the other word parts in order.

	Word Part	Word Part Definition
SUFFIX	-logy	*the study of*
COMBINING FORM	gastr/o-	*stomach*
COMBINING FORM	enter/o-	*intestine*

Gastroenterology: ***The study of the stomach and intestines.***

Figure 3-1 ■ The gastrointestinal system.
The gastrointestinal system consists of many different organs connected to a common pathway where food enters the body, is digested, and is then eliminated from the body.

www.prenhall.com/turley

For interactive flashcards, real-life video clips, games, exercises, and audio pronunciations please explore the companion CD-ROM in the back of the book. Click on the companion website for bonus chapters, additional resources, and links to on-line learning.

2 **Objectives and Medical Language Key**—Focuses readers on the goals of each chapter and provides a word analysis of the chapter title, demonstrating the importance and utility of word part analysis.

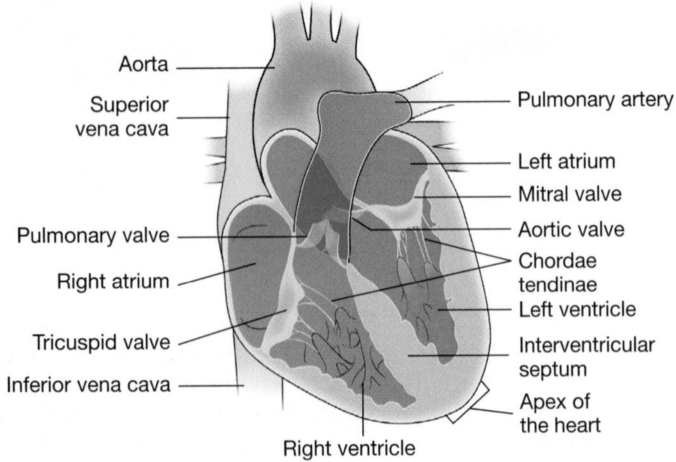

3 **Anatomy and Physiology**—Illustrates fundamental information about relevant body systems. This section is thorough, but not exhaustive, and reflects the level of detail that the vast majority of educators told us they need. Key words are analyzed as soon as they are introduced, thus reinforcing the continual importance of wordbuilding.

Vocabulary Review

Anatomy and Physiology

Now that you have studied the anatomy and physiology of the gastrointestinal system, take time to review those new words and descriptions. Memorize the combining forms and their definitions before going on to the next section.

Word or Phrase	Combining Form and Definition	Description
abdominopelvic cavity	abdomin/o- *abdomen* pelv/o- *pelvis (hip bone; renal pelvis)* cav/o- *hollow space*	Continuous cavity within the abdomen and pelvis that contains the largest organs of the gastrointestinal system
absorption	absorpt/o- *absorb or take in*	Process by which digested food nutrients move through villi of the small intestine into the blood
alimentary canal	aliment/o- *food, nourishment*	Alternate name for the gastrointestinal system
amylase	amyl/o- *carbohydrate, starch*	Digestive enzyme from the pancreas. It breaks down carbohydrates and starch in the duodenum into simple sugars and food fibers
antrum		Transition between the body of the stomach and the narrowing channel of the pylorus
anus	an/o- *anus*	External opening of the rectum. The external anal sphincter is under voluntary control. The perianal area is around the anus.

Labeling Exercise

A. Match each anatomy word or phrase to its numbered structure in Figure 5-15. Write that word or phrase on the blank line next to its number. Use the Answer Key at the end of the book to check your answers.

aorta	inferior vena cava	mitral valve	right ventricle
aortic valve	interventricular septum	pulmonary artery	superior vena cava
apex	left atrium	pulmonary valve	tricuspid valve
chordae tendineae	left ventricle	right atrium	

1. ______
2. ______
3. ______
4. ______
5. ______
6. ______
7. ______
8. ______
9. ______
10. ______
11. ______
12. ______
13. ______

4 Vocabulary Review—Reinforces reader understanding by providing an at-a-glance format of every key word, an analysis of its word parts, and a description. A comprehensive interactive quiz section follows.

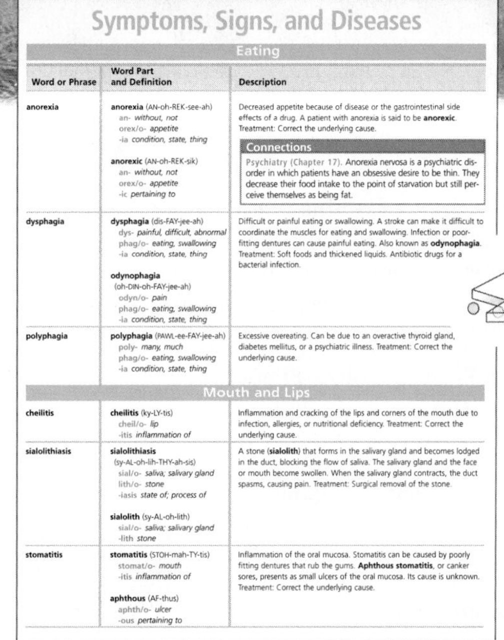

Symptoms, Signs, and Diseases

Eating

Word or Phrase	Word Part and Definition	Description
anorexia	anorexia (AN-oh-REK-see-ah) an- *without, not* orex/o- *appetite* -ia *condition, state, thing*; anorexic (AN-oh-REK-sik) an- *without, not* orex/o- *appetite* -ic *pertaining to*	Decreased appetite because of disease or the gastrointestinal side effects of a drug. A patient with anorexia is said to be **anorexic**. Treatment: Correct the underlying cause. Connections: Psychiatry (Chapter 17). Anorexia nervosa is a psychiatric disorder in which patients have an obsessive desire to be thin. They decrease their food intake to the point of starvation but still perceive themselves as being fat.
dysphagia	dysphagia (dis-FAY-jee-ah) dys- *painful, difficult, abnormal* phag/o- *eating, swallowing* -ia *condition, state, thing*; odynophagia (oh-DIN-oh-FAY-jee-ah) odyn/o- *pain* phag/o- *eating, swallowing* -ia *condition, state, thing*	Difficult or painful eating or swallowing. A stroke can make it difficult to coordinate the muscles for eating and swallowing. Infection or poor-fitting dentures can cause painful eating. Also known as **odynophagia**. Treatment: Soft foods and thickened liquids. Antibiotic drugs for a bacterial infection.
polyphagia	polyphagia (PAWL-ee-FAY-jee-ah) poly- *many, much* phag/o- *eating, swallowing* -ia *condition, state, thing*	Excessive overeating. Can be due to an overactive thyroid gland, diabetes mellitus, or a psychiatric illness. Treatment: Correct the underlying cause.

Mouth and Lips

Word or Phrase	Word Part and Definition	Description
cheilitis	cheilitis (ky-LY-tis) cheil/o- *lip* -itis *inflammation of*	Inflammation and cracking of the lips and corners of the mouth due to infection, allergies, or nutritional deficiency. Treatment: Correct the underlying cause.
sialolithiasis	sialolithiasis (sy-AL-oh-lih-THY-ah-sis) sial/o- *saliva; salivary gland* lith/o- *stone* -iasis *state of; process of*; sialolith (sy-AL-oh-lith) sial/o- *saliva; salivary gland* -lith *stone*	A stone (**sialolith**) that forms in the salivary gland and becomes lodged in the duct, blocking the flow of saliva. The salivary gland and the face or mouth become swollen. When the salivary gland contracts, the duct spasms, causing pain. Treatment: Surgical removal of the stone.
stomatitis	stomatitis (STOH-mah-TY-tis) stomat/o- *mouth* -itis *inflammation of*; aphthous (AF-thus) aphth/o- *ulcer* -ous *pertaining to*	Inflammation of the oral mucosa. Stomatitis can be caused by poorly fitting dentures that rub the gums. **Aphthous stomatitis**, or canker sores, presents as small ulcers of the oral mucosa. Its cause is unknown. Treatment: Correct the underlying cause.

5 Symptoms, Signs, and Diseases Diagnostic Procedures Medical and Surgical Procedures—Word analysis and description of pathologies and conditions, diagnostic procedures, medical procedures, and surgeries.

Drug Categories

Several different categories of drugs are used to treat the symptoms, signs, and diseases of the gastrointestinal system. The most common drugs in each category are listed.

Category	Word Part and Definition	Description	Examples
antacid drugs	antacid (ant-AS-id) Antacid is a combination of anti- (against) and the word acid. The *i* in anti- is deleted.	Treat heartburn and peptic ulcer disease by neutralizing acid in the stomach	Maalox, Mylanta, Tums
antibiotic drugs	antibiotic (AN-tee-by-AWT-ik) anti- *against* bi/o- *life; living organisms; living tissue* -tic *pertaining to*	Treat bacterial gastrointestinal infections, including acute *Helicobacter pylori*. Antibiotic drugs are not effective against viral gastrointestinal infections.	amoxicillin, Biaxin, Flagyl, tetracycline
antidiarrheal drugs	antidiarrheal (AN-tee-DY-ah-REE-al) anti- *against* dia- *complete; completely through* -rrhe/o- *flow; discharge* -al *pertaining to*	Treat diarrhea. They slow peristalsis and this increases water absorption from the feces.	Imodium, Lomotil
antiemetic drugs	antiemetic (AN-tee-eh-MET-ik) anti- *against* emet/o- *to vomit* -ic *pertaining to*	Treat nausea and vomiting and motion sickness	Antivert, Compazine, Phenergan
chemotherapy	chemotherapy	Kill rapidly dividing cancer cells of tumors in	Adriamycin, Taxol, VePesid

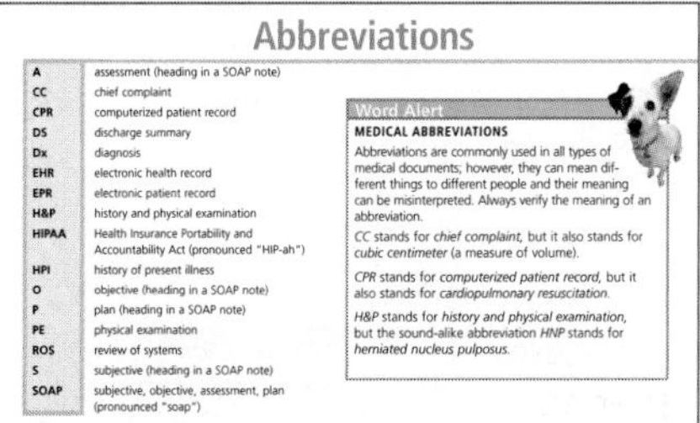

Abbreviations

A	assessment (heading in a SOAP note)
CC	chief complaint
CPR	computerized patient record
DS	discharge summary
Dx	diagnosis
EHR	electronic health record
EPR	electronic patient record
H&P	history and physical examination
HIPAA	Health Insurance Portability and Accountability Act (pronounced "HIP-ah")
HPI	history of present illness
O	objective (heading in a SOAP note)
P	plan (heading in a SOAP note)
PE	physical examination
ROS	review of systems
S	subjective (heading in a SOAP note)
SOAP	subjective, objective, assessment, plan (pronounced "soap")

Word Alert

MEDICAL ABBREVIATIONS

Abbreviations are commonly used in all types of medical documents; however, they can mean different things to different people and their meaning can be misinterpreted. Always verify the meaning of an abbreviation.

CC stands for *chief complaint*, but it also stands for *cubic centimeter* (a measure of volume).

CPR stands for *computerized patient record*, but it also stands for *cardiopulmonary resuscitation*.

H&P stands for *history and physical examination*, but the sound-alike abbreviation *HNP* stands for *herniated nucleus pulposus*.

6 Drug Categories and Abbreviations—Rounds out chapter content with current, useful material.

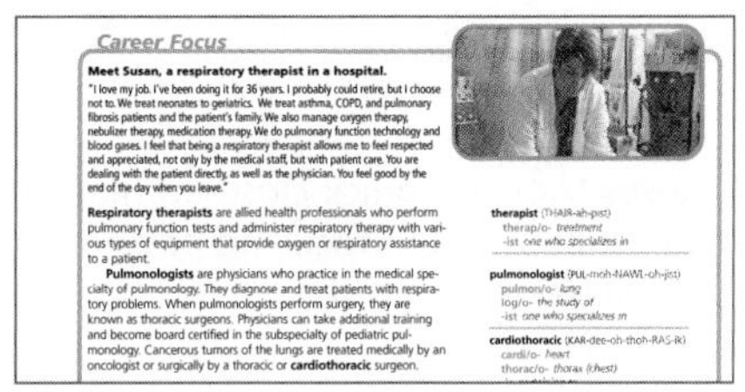

Career Focus

Meet Susan, a respiratory therapist in a hospital.

"I love my job. I've been doing it for 36 years. I probably could retire, but I choose not to. We treat neonates to geriatrics. We treat asthma, COPD, and pulmonary fibrosis patients and the patient's family. We also manage oxygen therapy, nebulizer therapy, medication therapy. We do pulmonary function technology and blood gases. I feel that being a respiratory therapist allows me to feel respected and appreciated, not only by the medical staff, but with patient care. You are dealing with the patient directly, as well as the physician. You feel good by the end of the day when you leave."

Respiratory therapists are allied health professionals who perform pulmonary function tests and administer respiratory therapy with various types of equipment that provide oxygen or respiratory assistance to a patient.

Pulmonologists are physicians who practice in the medical specialty of pulmonology. They diagnose and treat patients with respiratory problems. When pulmonologists perform surgery, they are known as thoracic surgeons. Physicians can take additional training and become board certified in the subspecialty of pediatric pulmonology. Cancerous tumors of the lungs are treated medically by an oncologist or surgically by a thoracic or **cardiothoracic** surgeon.

therapist (THAIR-ah-pist) therap/o- *treatment* -ist *one who specializes in*

pulmonologist (PUL-moh-NAWL-oh-jist) pulmon/o- *lung* log/o- *the study of* -ist *one who specializes in*

cardiothoracic (KAR-dee-oh-thoh-RAS-ik) cardi/o- *heart* thorac/o- *thorax (chest)*

7 Career Focus—Orients readers to a career option in each medical specialty. Instructors have access to the *Real People, Real Medicine* video library.

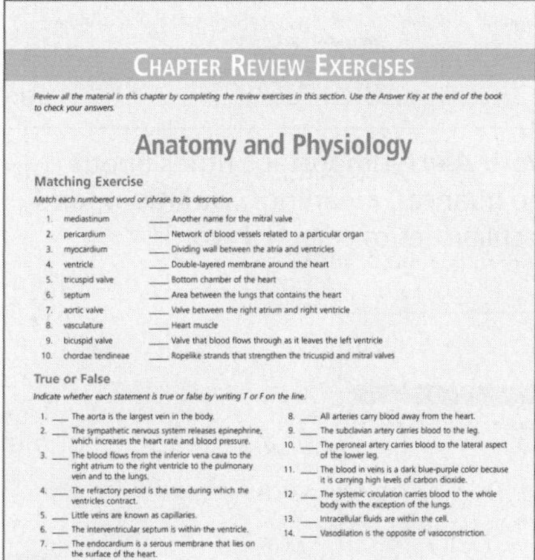

Chapter Review Exercises

Review all the material in this chapter by completing the review exercises in this section. Use the Answer Key at the end of the book to check your answers.

Anatomy and Physiology

Matching Exercise

Match each numbered word or phrase to its description.

1. mediastinum ___ Another name for the mitral valve
2. pericardium ___ Network of blood vessels related to a particular organ
3. myocardium ___ Dividing wall between the atria and ventricles
4. ventricle ___ Double-layered membrane around the heart
5. tricuspid valve ___ Bottom chamber of the heart
6. septum ___ Area between the lungs that contains the heart
7. aortic valve ___ Valve between the right atrium and right ventricle
8. vasculature ___ Heart muscle
9. bicuspid valve ___ Valve that blood flows through as it leaves the left ventricle
10. chordae tendineae ___ Ropelike strands that strengthen the tricuspid and mitral valves

True or False

Indicate whether each statement is true or false by writing T or F on the line.

1. ___ The aorta is the largest vein in the body.
2. ___ The sympathetic nervous system releases epinephrine, which increases the heart rate and blood pressure.
3. ___ The blood flows from the inferior vena cava to the right atrium to the right ventricle to the pulmonary vein and to the lungs.
4. ___ The refractory period is the time during which the ventricles contract.
5. ___ Little veins are known as capillaries.
6. ___ The interventricular septum is within the ventricle.
7. ___ The endocardium is a serous membrane that lies on the surface of the heart.
8. ___ All arteries carry blood away from the heart.
9. ___ The subclavian artery carries blood to the leg.
10. ___ The peroneal artery carries blood to the lateral aspect of the lower leg.
11. ___ The blood in veins is a dark blue-purple color because it is carrying high levels of carbon dioxide.
12. ___ The systemic circulation carries blood to the whole body with the exception of the lungs.
13. ___ Intracellular fluids are within the cell.
14. ___ Vasodilation is the opposite of vasoconstriction.

8 Chapter Review—Fortifies the reader's understanding with a fun and extensive variety of quizzes designed for a range of learning styles.

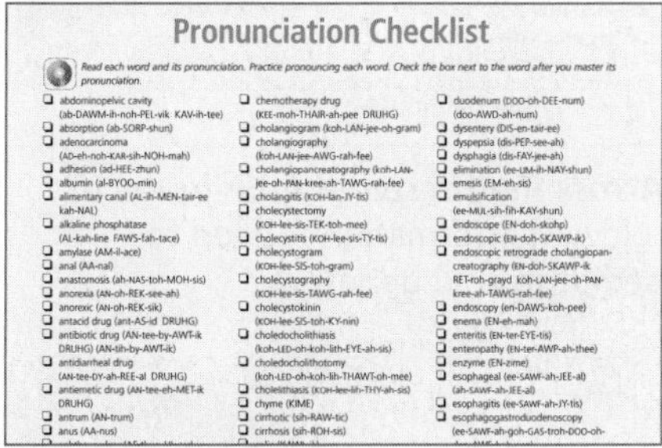

Pronunciation Checklist

Read each word and its pronunciation. Practice pronouncing each word. Check the box next to the word after you master its pronunciation.

- abdominopelvic cavity (ab-DAWM-ih-noh-PEL-vik KAV-ih-tee)
- absorption (ab-SORP-shun)
- adenocarcinoma (AD-eh-noh-KAR-sih-NOH-mah)
- adhesion (ad-HEE-zhun)
- albumin (al-BYOO-min)
- alimentary canal (AL-ih-MEN-tair-ee kah-NAL)
- alkaline phosphatase (AL-kah-line FAWS-fah-tace)
- amylase (AM-ih-ace)
- anal (AA-nal)
- anastomosis (ah-NAS-toh-MOH-sis)
- anorexia (AN-oh-REK-see-ah)
- anorexic (AN-oh-REK-sik)
- antacid drug (ant-AS-id DRUHG)
- antibiotic drug (AN-tee-by-AWT-ik DRUHG)
- antidiarrheal drug (AN-tee-DY-ah-REE-al DRUHG)
- antiemetic drug (AN-tee-eh-MET-ik DRUHG)
- antrum (AN-trum)
- anus (AA-nus)
- chemotherapy drug (KEE-moh-THAIR-ah-pee DRUHG)
- cholangiogram (koh-LAN-jee-oh-gram)
- cholangiography (koh-LAN-jee-AWG-rah-fee)
- cholangiopancreatography (koh-LAN-jee-oh-PAN-kree-ah-TAWG-rah-fee)
- cholangitis (KOH-lan-JY-tis)
- cholecystectomy (KOH-lee-sis-TEK-toh-mee)
- cholecystitis (KOH-lee-sis-TY-tis)
- cholecystogram (KOH-lee-SIS-toh-gram)
- cholecystography (KOH-lee-sis-TAWG-rah-fee)
- cholecystokinin (KOH-lee-SIS-toh-KY-nin)
- choledocholithiasis (koh-LED-oh-koh-lih-THY-ah-sis)
- choledocholithotomy (koh-LED-oh-koh-lih-THAWT-oh-mee)
- cholelithiasis (KOH-lee-lih-THY-ah-sis)
- chyme (KIME)
- cirrhotic (sih-RAW-tic)
- cirrhosis (sih-ROH-sis)
- duodenum (DOO-oh-DEE-num) (doo-AWD-eh-num)
- dysentery (DIS-en-tair-ee)
- dyspepsia (dis-PEP-see-ah)
- dysphagia (dis-FAY-jee-ah)
- elimination (ee-LIM-ih-NAY-shun)
- emesis (EM-eh-sis)
- emulsification (ee-MUL-sih-fih-KAY-shun)
- endoscope (EN-doh-skohp)
- endoscopic (EN-doh-SKAWP-ik)
- endoscopic retrograde cholangiopancreatography (EN-doh-SKAWP-ik RET-roh-grayd koh-LAN-jee-oh-PAN-kree-ah-TAWG-rah-fee)
- endoscopy (en-DAWS-koh-pee)
- enema (EN-eh-mah)
- enteritis (EN-ter-EYE-tis)
- enteropathy (EN-ter-AWP-ah-thee)
- enzyme (EN-zime)
- esophageal (ee-SAWF-ah-JEE-al) (ah-SAWF-ah-JEE-al)
- esophagitis (ee-SAWF-ah-JY-tis)
- esophagogastroduodenoscopy (ee-SAWF-ah-goh-GAS-troh-DOO-oh-

9 Pronuciation Checklist—Reinforces the importance of correct pronunciation by providing readers with an all-in-one list for quick review. Readers may also listen to each word pronounced on the accompanying CD-ROM and website.

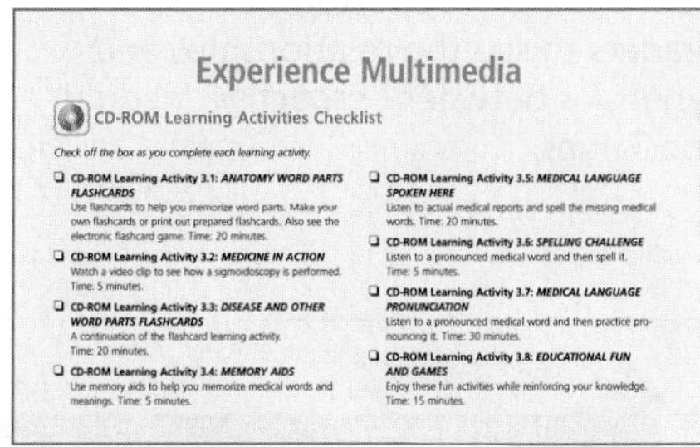

Experience Multimedia

CD-ROM Learning Activities Checklist

Check off the box as you complete each learning activity.

- **CD-ROM Learning Activity 3.1: *ANATOMY WORD PARTS FLASHCARDS*** Use flashcards to help you memorize word parts. Make your own flashcards or print out prepared flashcards. Also see the electronic flashcard game. Time: 20 minutes.
- **CD-ROM Learning Activity 3.2: *MEDICINE IN ACTION*** Watch a video clip to see how a sigmoidoscopy is performed. Time: 5 minutes.
- **CD-ROM Learning Activity 3.3: *DISEASE AND OTHER WORD PARTS FLASHCARDS*** A continuation of the flashcard learning activity. Time: 20 minutes.
- **CD-ROM Learning Activity 3.4: *MEMORY AIDS*** Use memory aids to help you memorize medical words and meanings. Time: 5 minutes.
- **CD-ROM Learning Activity 3.5: *MEDICAL LANGUAGE SPOKEN HERE*** Listen to actual medical reports and spell the missing medical words. Time: 20 minutes.
- **CD-ROM Learning Activity 3.6: *SPELLING CHALLENGE*** Listen to a pronounced medical word and then spell it. Time: 5 minutes.
- **CD-ROM Learning Activity 3.7: *MEDICAL LANGUAGE PRONUNCIATION*** Listen to a pronounced medical word and then practice pronouncing it. Time: 30 minutes.
- **CD-ROM Learning Activity 3.8: *EDUCATIONAL FUN AND GAMES*** Enjoy these fun activities while reinforcing your knowledge. Time: 15 minutes.

10 Experience Multimedia—Challenges readers to extend their exploration of medical language by completing the CD-ROM activities that accompany each chapter. This checklist provides a description and estimated time for completion of each learning activity.

SPECIAL FEATURES

Here is a summary of the items that make this book unique. These features were crafted in tandem with our development team of students and instructors, whom we challenged to answer the question: "How would you describe the ideal medical terminology textbook?"

Highly Visual Illustrations and Photographs—Brings medical language to life and stimulates understanding, especially for visual learners.

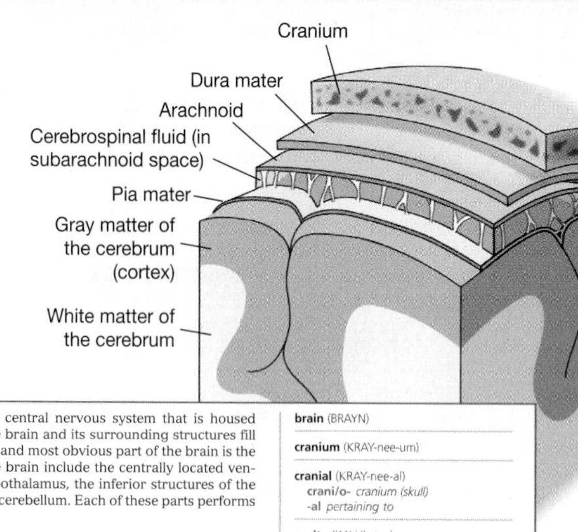

Word Analysis—A section in the margins and within various tables throughout, this appears whenever a new word is introduced—not tucked away in the back of each chapter. This provides readers with the wordbuilding tools to understand unfamiliar words on their own, reinforcing that wordbuilding is an ongoing process.

The **brain** is the part of the central nervous system that is housed within the bony **cranium.** The brain and its surrounding structures fill the **cranial cavity.** The largest and most obvious part of the brain is the cerebrum. Other parts of the brain include the centrally located ventricles, the thalamus and hypothalamus, the inferior structures of the brainstem, and the posterior cerebellum. Each of these parts performs several specialized functions.	**brain** (BRAYN) **cranium** (KRAY-nee-um) **cranial** (KRAY-nee-al) **crani/o-** *cranium (skull)* **-al** *pertaining to* **cavity** (KAV-ih-tee) **cav/o-** *hollow space* **-ity** *state; condition*

Special Boxes—Spark reader interest with key details that relate the material to the real world of medicine.

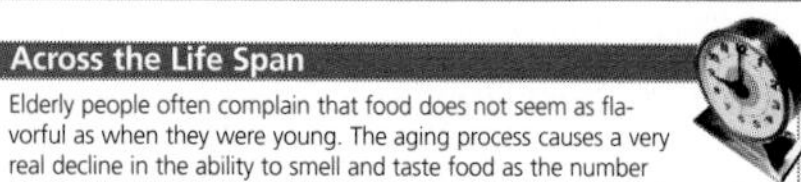

Across the Life Span

Elderly people often complain that food does not seem as flavorful as when they were young. The aging process causes a very real decline in the ability to smell and taste food as the number of receptors in the nose and tongue decreases.

Across the Lifespan—An infusion of relevant information related to pediatrics and geriatrics.

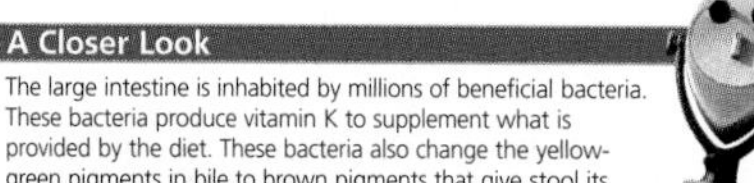

A Closer Look

The large intestine is inhabited by millions of beneficial bacteria. These bacteria produce vitamin K to supplement what is provided by the diet. These bacteria also change the yellow-green pigments in bile to brown pigments that give stool its characteristic color. Bacteria in the large intestine feed on undigested food fiber, producing intestinal gas or **flatus.**

A Closer Look—A quick close-up glance at a pertinent detail focusing on the material being covered.

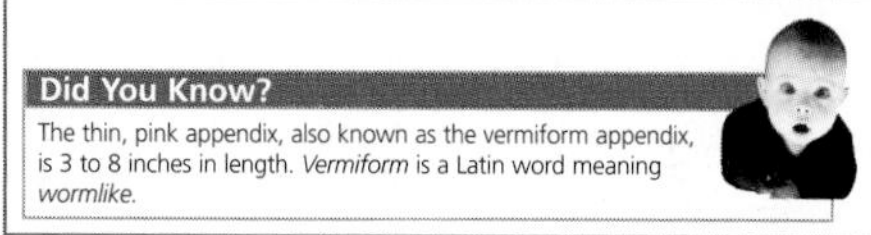

Did You Know?

The thin, pink appendix, also known as the vermiform appendix, is 3 to 8 inches in length. *Vermiform* is a Latin word meaning *wormlike.*

Did You Know?—Fun, interesting information designed to stimulate reader curiosity about the material being covered.

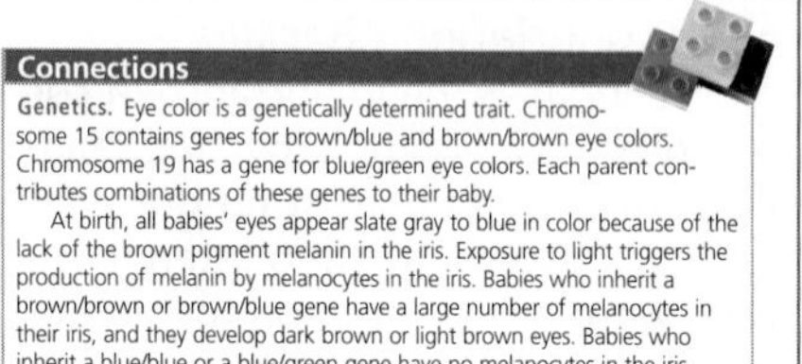

Connections

Genetics. Eye color is a genetically determined trait. Chromosome 15 contains genes for brown/blue and brown/brown eye colors. Chromosome 19 has a gene for blue/green eye colors. Each parent contributes combinations of these genes to their baby.

At birth, all babies' eyes appear slate gray to blue in color because of the lack of the brown pigment melanin in the iris. Exposure to light triggers the production of melanin by melanocytes in the iris. Babies who inherit a brown/brown or brown/blue gene have a large number of melanocytes in their iris, and they develop dark brown or light brown eyes. Babies who inherit a blue/blue or a blue/green gene have no melanocytes in the iris.

Connections—Opportunities for readers to see the relationships and synergies between respective medical specialties.

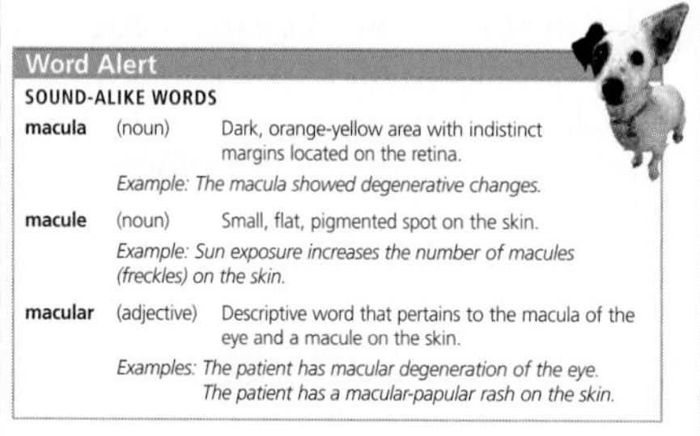

Word Alert

SOUND-ALIKE WORDS

macula (noun) Dark, orange-yellow area with indistinct margins located on the retina.
Example: The macula showed degenerative changes.

macule (noun) Small, flat, pigmented spot on the skin.
Example: Sun exposure increases the number of macules (freckles) on the skin.

macular (adjective) Descriptive word that pertains to the macula of the eye and a macule on the skin.
Examples: The patient has macular degeneration of the eye. The patient has a macular-papular rash on the skin.

Word Alert—Important notes about the nuances, meanings, variations, and peculiarities of selected words.

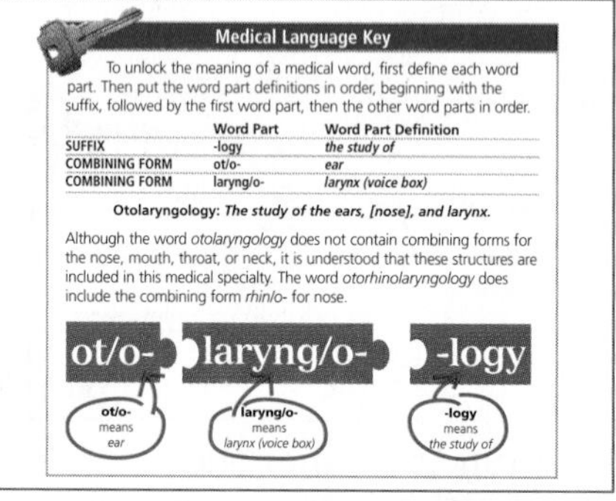

Medical Language Key

To unlock the meaning of a medical word, first define each word part. Then put the word part definitions in order, beginning with the suffix, followed by the first word part, then the other word parts in order.

	Word Part	Word Part Definition
SUFFIX	-logy	*the study of*
COMBINING FORM	ot/o-	*ear*
COMBINING FORM	laryng/o-	*larynx (voice box)*

Otolaryngology: ***The study of the ears, [nose], and larynx.***

Although the word *otolaryngology* does not contain combining forms for the nose, mouth, throat, or neck, it is understood that these structures are included in this medical specialty. The word *otorhinolaryngology* does include the combining form *rhin/o-* for nose.

Medical Language Key—A practical hint related to the construction of word parts that builds readers' grasp of word building concepts.

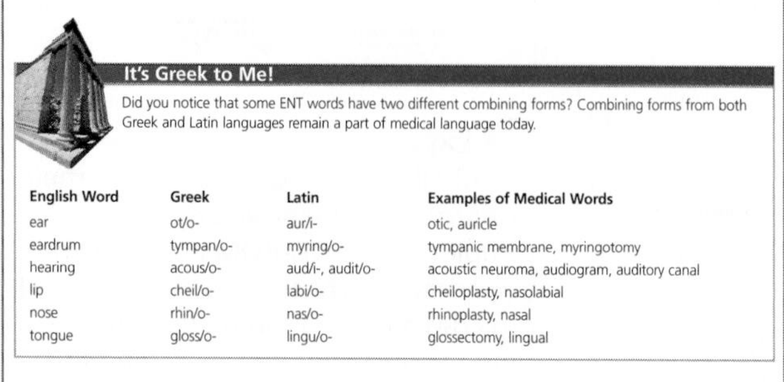

It's Greek to Me!

Did you notice that some ENT words have two different combining forms? Combining forms from both Greek and Latin languages remain a part of medical language today.

English Word	Greek	Latin	Examples of Medical Words
ear	ot/o-	aur/i-	otic, auricle
eardrum	tympan/o-	myring/o-	tympanic membrane, myringotomy
hearing	acous/o-	aud/i-, audit/o-	acoustic neuroma, audiogram, auditory canal
lip	cheil/o-	labi/o-	cheiloplasty, nasolabial
nose	rhin/o-	nas/o-	rhinoplasty, nasal
tongue	gloss/o-	lingu/o-	glossectomy, lingual

It's Greek to Me!—Useful reminders about how Greek and Latin combining forms remain part of medical language today.

STUDENT CD-ROM

Packaged with every copy of the textbook this revolutionary CD-ROM maximizes readers' opportunity to reinforce concepts and practice what they have learned in each chapter.

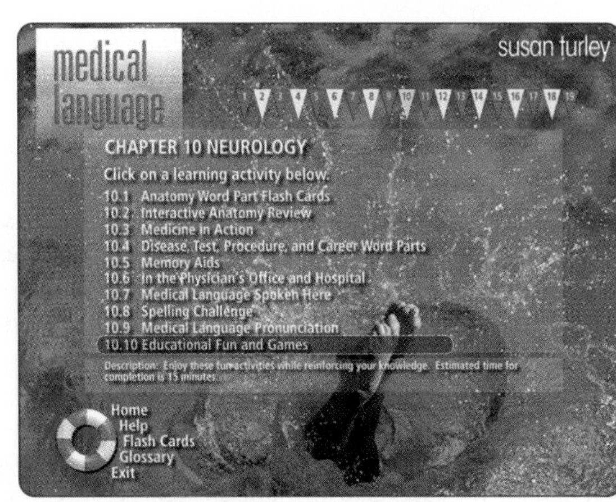

The CD-ROM is organized in eight primary learning modules—

1. ***Anatomy Word Parts Flashcards***—A unique program that invites students to create and edit their own flashcards or to select a preprogrammed collection.

2. ***Medicine in Action***—Dynamic videos and animations that highlight a condition, disease, or disorder discussed in the chapter, bringing the content to life.

3. ***Disease and Other Word Parts Flashcards***—Using the same system as the anatomy flashcards, this is a specific set that focuses on diseases, tests, procedures, surgeries, and careers.

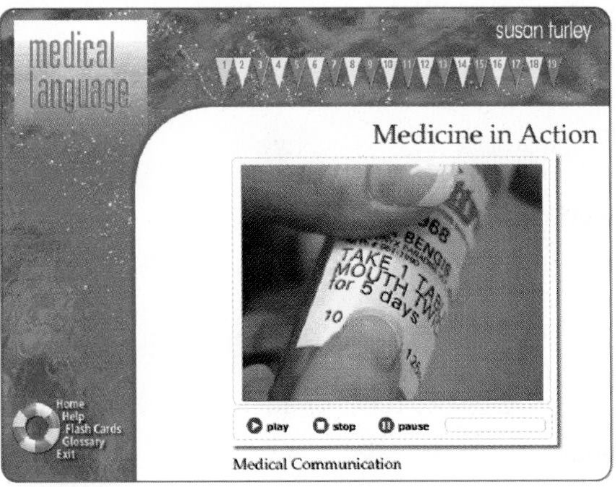

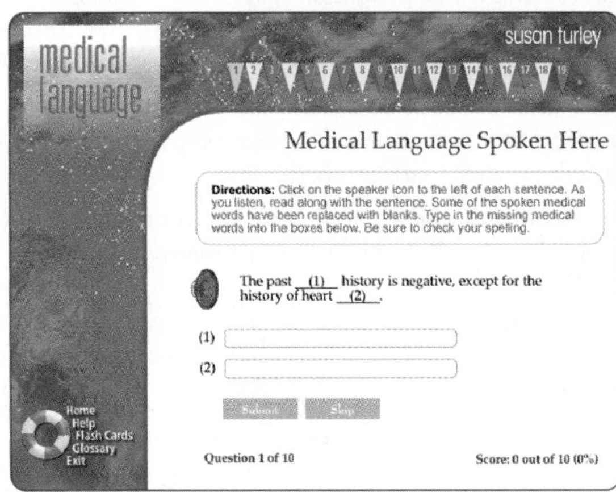

4. ***Memory Aids***—An array of tips and suggestions designed to help students remember medical words in a fun and engaging way.

5. ***Medical Language Spoken Here***—A spelling exercise that prompts users to complete a medical report by listening to authentic physician dictation.

6. ***Spelling Challenge***—A collection of the 20 most difficult words in each chapter is presented to build students' listening and spelling skills.

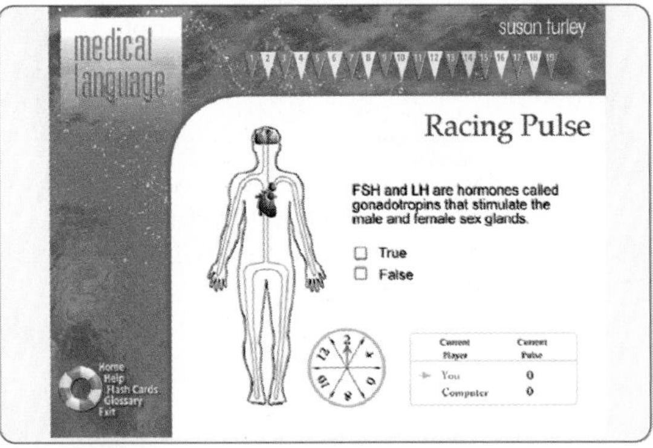

7. ***Medical Language Pronunciation***—A complete audio glossary with pronunciations of key words in each chapter. Students are encouraged to pronounce the words and check off their progress.

8. ***Educational Fun & Games***—An array of fun challenges such as Beat the Clock, Quest for a Million, Racing Pulse, Crossword, Strikeout, and more.

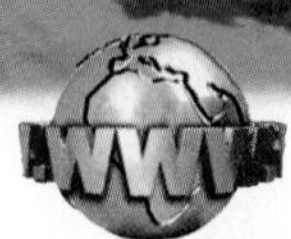

ONLINE LEARNING

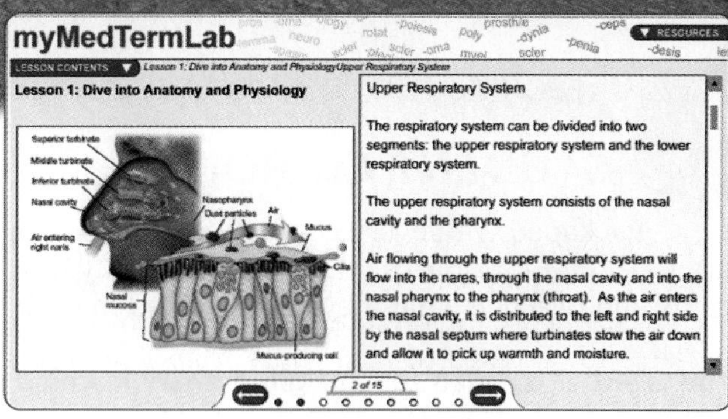

To foster an active approach to learning we have created a dynamic array of interactive applications on the website.

MyMedTermLab—The most robust, dynamic online medical terminology course available today! Compatible within BlackBoard and WebCT learning environments, this revolutionary, self-paced program engages students in activities, assessments, and rich media that is unmatched in the market. Features include:

- *Integrated e-Book*—This provides a one-to-one match with the text and a wide variety of options to integrate links to media and assessment directly onto the text page.
- *Flexible organization*—Each lesson is broken into small chunks that can be re-ordered, deleted, and customized by instructors using Blackboard or WebCT. This allows the course to be optimally tailored to specific course needs.
- *Tracking and progress report functions*—These tools allow instructors and students alike to monitor and assess progress. A special "Progress Report" feature allows students to print, save, and e-mail results. While other comparable courses only allow tracking of results for one chapter at a time, MyMedTermLab provides several mid-chapter progress-tracking opportunities.
- *An active, media-rich, and visual approach* that prompts students to employ multiple learning styles rather than simply reading from the screen.

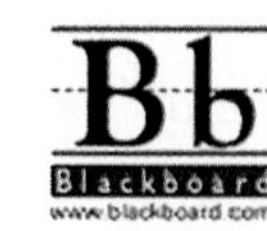

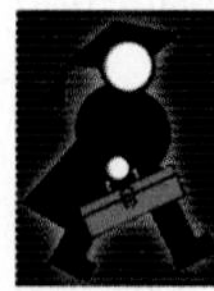

MyMedTermLab is a one-of-a-kind learning tool and a perfect compliment to traditional instruction. For a demo of this exciting program, visit **www.prenhall.com/turley**.

Companion Website—Students and faculty will both benefit from the **free** Companion Website at **www.prenhall.com/turley**. This website serves as a text-specific, interactive online workbook to ***Medical Language***. The Companion Website includes:

- Two bonus chapters, Dentistry and Dietetics. These are ideal for supplemental assignments in programs that cover these medical specialties in their curricula.
- Audio glossary in which key words in the book are pronounced.
- **Syllabus Manager™**. Faculty adopting this textbook have free access to the online Syllabus Manager feature of the Companion Website. It offers a host of features that facilitate the students' use of the Companion Website, and allows faculty to post syllabi and course information online for their students. For more information or a demonstration of Syllabus Manager, please visit **www.prenhall.com/demo**, click Companion Website then Syllabus Manager Tour.
- Drug Updates that allow users to search for current drug information and updates for the drugs discussed in each chapter.
- Links to updates on health care news items from the ***New York Times***.

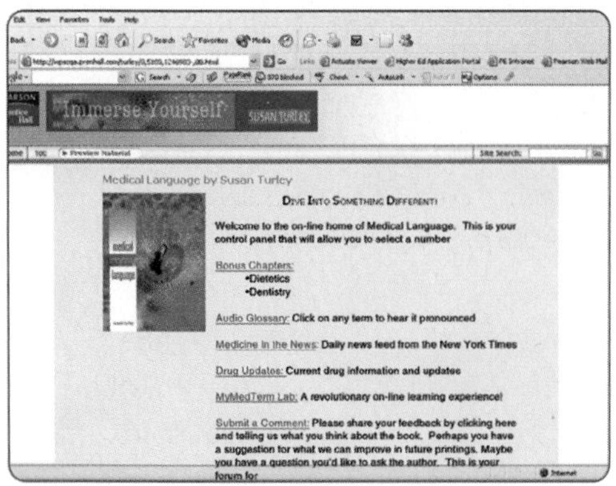

COMPREHENSIVE LEARNING PACKAGE

Medical Language offers a rich array of ancillary materials to benefit instructors and help infuse a spark in the classroom. The full complement of supplemental teaching materials is available to all qualified instructors from your Prentice Hall Health sales representative (www.prenhall.com/replocator).

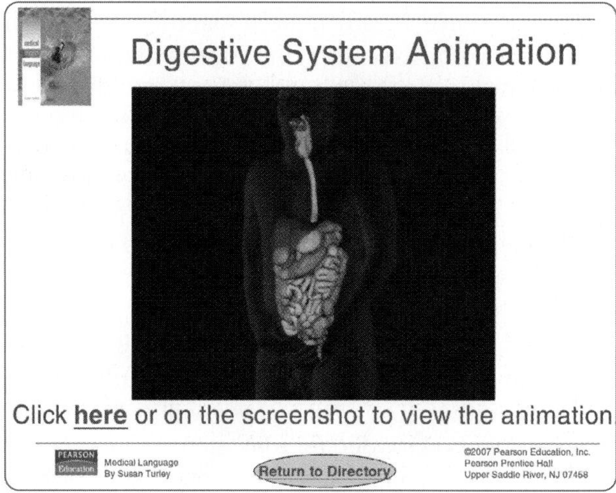

PowerPoint Slides

Instructor's Resource Manual (IRM)—This manual contains a wealth of material to help faculty plan and manage the medical terminology course. It includes:

- Educational articles with useful ideas for classroom management, information on how to construct test questions, and how to put students at ease on the first day of class.
- Step-by-step lecture suggestions, outlines, learning objectives, and interesting facts and anecdotes.
- A wealth of extra "Did You Know" teaching pearls.
- A complete 2500-question test bank.
- A sample course syllabus.

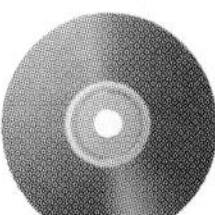

Instructor's Resource CD-ROM—Packaged along with the Instructor's Resource Manual, this cross-platform CD-ROM provides many resources in an electronic format. It includes the following:

- The complete 2500-question test bank that allows instructors to generate customized exams and quizzes
- A comprehensive, turn-key lecture package in PowerPoint format containing discussion points, along with embedded color images from the textbook as well as bonus illustrations, animations, and videos to help infuse an extra spark into the classroom experience.
- A collection of 22 *Real People, Real Medicine* career video profiles correlated with chapter content that can be presented in class.
- PowerPoint content to support instructors who wish to use Personal Response Systems. For more information visit www.prenhall.com/prs.
- Complete image library that includes every photograph and illustration contained in the textbook.

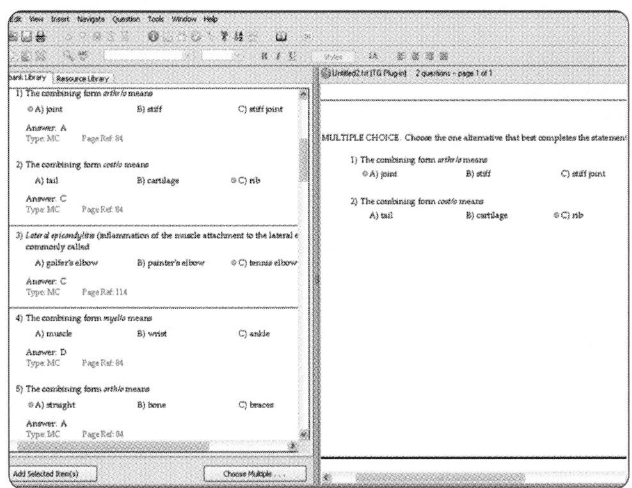

TestGen Software

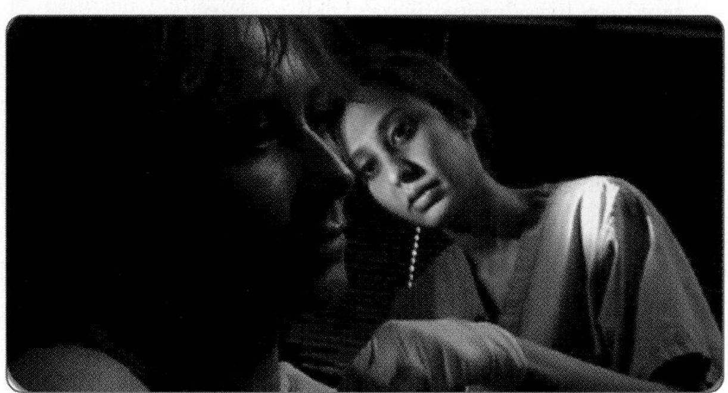

***Real People, Real Medicine* videos**

Preface

SOMETHING DIFFERENT

You may have already noticed that there is something different about this book. Perhaps by examining the cover and thumbing through the pages, you have taken note of the abundance of real-world images. Maybe you have discovered some of the practice exercises that abound within these pages, placing you in the hypothetical role of an actual healthcare provider. Or perhaps you have already begun exploring the revolutionary CD-ROM that is packaged inside the back cover, rich with highly engaging and interactive activities that add a unique dimension to your learning. As you begin this exciting and important journey into the world of medicine we offer you a single promise—that you will soon become immersed in a new, exciting experience. And therefore we feel it is fitting for this textbook to follow suit.

As a healthcare professional you will never be sitting on the sidelines. Your hard work, knowledge, competence, and interpersonal skills will have a direct impact on patient services throughout your career. Therefore it is with this spirit that we wish to empower you to affect others with the fruits of your learning. And thus, we encourage you to immerse yourself in the language and culture of health care as presented in this book.

THE TITLE OF THIS BOOK

As part of your experience, you will learn how to construct and deconstruct medical words using their basic elements, called word parts. So let us start at the beginning by examining the title of this book, ***Medical Language.***

Medical

Medicine is the drama of life and death, and few subjects are as compelling, profound, or worthy of study. This book is about real medicine. As you know, real medicine affects real patients—their lives, their families, and their futures. As a healthcare professional, no matter which aspect of patient care you touch, you will have great responsibilities. Therefore, we feel it is our responsibility to provide you with as realistic a view as possible of medicine today. Here are some examples of how we have done this:

- The majority of the images in this book incorporate medical illustrations and photographs that include a diverse array of real people, instead of cartoon-like illustrations.
- Among the many features on the accompanying CD-ROM, you will find an exercise called *Medical Language Spoken Here* that challenges you to listen to and interpret authentic physician dictation courtesy of Health Professions Institute, creator of the SUM program and the leader in medical transcription education.
- Instructors who assign this book will have access to the video library *Real People, Real Medicine* that was filmed in association with this book to profile a variety of healthcare workers on the job.
- As part of our respect for real medicine, and the importance of getting it right the first time, we have made a commitment to accuracy. The author draws on her 30 years of experience as a nurse, medical transcriptionist, health information manager, and educator to provide accurate and complete information throughout. We have also engaged the technical editing services of four physician specialists who have carefully reviewed the chapters that correspond to their respective practices.

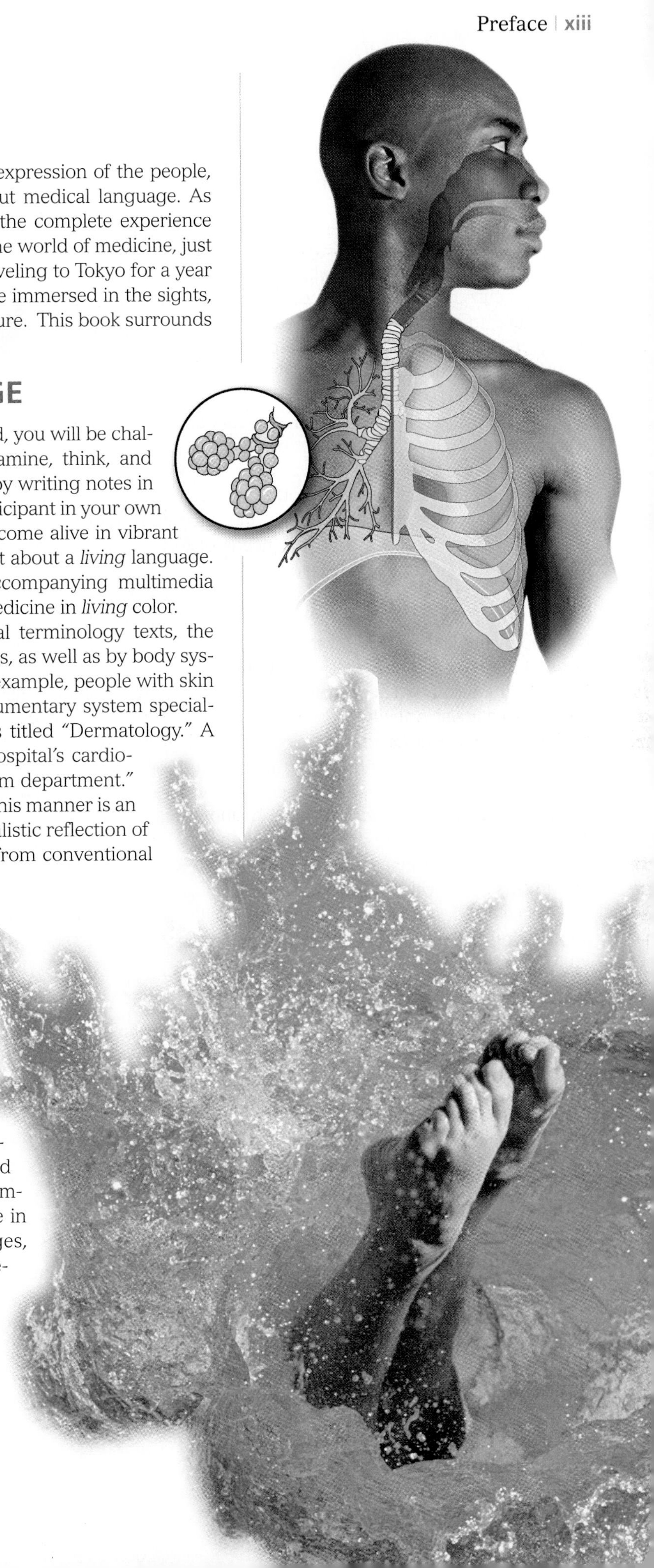

Language

A language is a method of communicating and an expression of the people, events, and culture it represents. This book is about medical language. As opposed to simply memorizing vocabulary words, the complete experience that this book offers is the opportunity to embrace the world of medicine, just as if you were learning a foreign language. Like traveling to Tokyo for a year to learn Japanese, the goal here is for you to become immersed in the sights, sounds, and even the tastes and smells of a new culture. This book surrounds you with context that brings the words to life.

A LIVING LANGUAGE

You will not be a passive reader of this book. Instead, you will be challenged to listen, speak, write, watch, respond, examine, think, and make connections. You should consume this book by writing notes in it and filling in your answers. By being an active participant in your own learning process, the concepts presented here will come alive in vibrant color and full texture. This book is a *living* document about a *living* language. Throughout the features of this book and the accompanying multimedia resources you will get a true taste of the world of medicine in *living* color.

You will notice that, unlike most other medical terminology texts, the chapters in this book are titled by medical specialties, as well as by body systems. This reflects the real world of medicine. For example, people with skin conditions will visit a dermatologist, not an "integumentary system specialist." That's why the related chapter in our book is titled "Dermatology." A patient with heart problems will be treated in a hospital's cardiology department and not in a "cardiovascular system department." Our decision to present the chapters of the book in this manner is an example of our commitment to make this book a realistic reflection of actual medicine in the real world. This distinction from conventional texts was tested extensively during development of this book and we are gratified by the overwhelming support for this chapter presentation.

IMMERSE YOURSELF!

You are about to begin an interactive learning experience between you, this book, and your instructor—one that will equip you with a vital tool and inspire you to become a true consumer of medical language. The goal of this book is to connect with you, to engage your visual, auditory, and kinesthetic senses, to stimulate you, and fuel your complete understanding of the topic. So as you engage in this multisensory experience within these pages, remember that we are not encouraging you to merely *discover, learn, know,* or even *understand,* the information. Instead we want you to ***live it!*** So dig in, dive in, and immerse yourself!

What makes this book different

WE LISTENED

In creating this book, we immersed ourselves in the perspective of you, our readers. We strove to make ***Medical Language*** a customer-driven text by aggressively and comprehensively researching the needs and desires of current medical terminology students and instructors. We wanted to guarantee that we were "speaking the same language" as the people who would ultimately be using this book. To this end, we formed a highly qualified development team of 148 educators, with a collective 1,921 years of teaching experience, four physician specialists, as well as 11 students across the United States whom we called upon to help steer us toward success.

Over a three-year span we sat down together in classrooms, hosted focus groups, and conducted thorough manuscript reviews. We asked for blunt and uncompromising opinions and insights regarding (1) the challenges posed by the course, (2) the needs of today's ever-changing student population, and (3) the ideas and features we were proposing in order to provide a more effective teaching and learning tool. We also commissioned dozens of detailed manuscript reviews from instructors, asking them to analyze and evaluate each draft of the manuscript. These reviewers not only told us what they did and didn't like about our approach, but they identified, page by page, numerous ways in which we could refine and enhance our key features. Their invaluable feedback was compiled, analyzed, and incorporated throughout ***Medical Language***.

The text you are seeing is truly the product of a successful partnership between the author, the publisher, and our development team of students and educators. We asked our team to imagine and visualize their ideal medical terminology book—what it should include, how it should look. We asked the author to meet personally with several members of our development team to discuss the specifics of the book's organization, layout, format and features. We worked with our team to assess the quality and accuracy of the design, manuscript, and pictures. We asked question after question. We listened.

AND WE LEARNED

Here are some of the recommendations that we heard from our team and responded to as we created this book:

- **Design** Students and instructors alike told us they wanted an appealing, uncluttered design with lots of rich images and enough white space to allow for notetaking.
- **Exercises** Both students and instructors suggested that we provide a greater quantity and variety of exercises than any other book, thus providing maximum opportunities to reinforce learning.
- **Illustrations** Students and instructors alike suggested that we display colorful and interesting illustrations as large as possible on the page, with various opportunities to label those images as practice opportunities.
- **Special Boxed Features** Students asked for highlight boxes that would help break up the reading and also provide them with opportunities to learn something new or interesting about a word—thereby providing additional context.

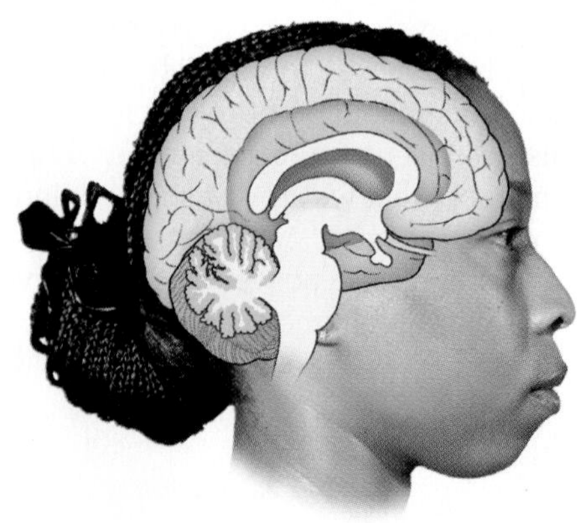

- **Medical Specialties Approach** A substantial majority (75%) of instructors told us that they prefer a medical specialties approach, rather than just an anatomical body systems organization.
- **Focus on Wordbuilding** Another substantial majority of instructors (over 70%) asked for a focus on wordbuilding and suggested that we present the analysis of combining forms, suffixes, and prefixes throughout each chapter and not simply at the end of each chapter or in isolated boxes.

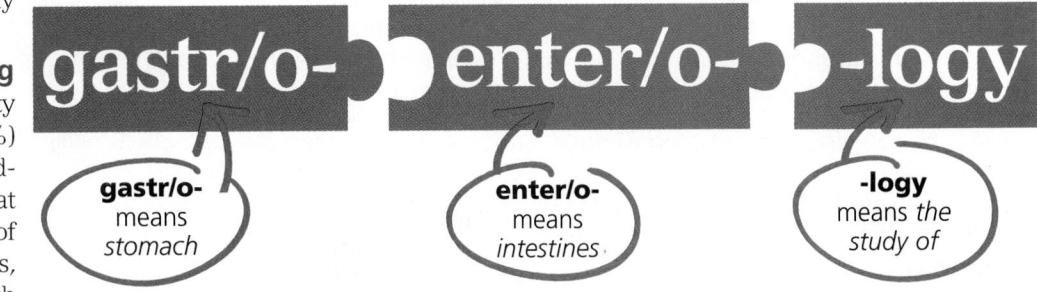

gastr/o- means *stomach*
enter/o- means *intestines*

- **Medical Report Activities** Instructors suggested that we include an activity in each chapter that challenges students to analyze an actual medical report.
- **Lecture Support Materials** Instructors told us about the increased challenge of creating interesting, dynamic lectures and suggested that we create a fully-loaded PowerPoint presentation system that is complete with ready-to-use lectures that include a multitude of illustrations, photographs, plus animations, and real-world videos.
- **Tools for Testing** Instructors asked for a complete testing package that is customizable to fit their needs. Additionally, they asked for these test items to be available in online course formats such as Blackboard and WebCT.
- **A Commitment to Accuracy** Finally, we were repeatedly reminded about the importance of ensuring complete accuracy in the content of the book and all ancillary resources. It was important to us to attain the highest level of accuracy possible throughout this educational program in order to match the requirement for precision in today's healthcare environment. To this end, our thorough manuscript review process charged members of our development team to read every page, every test question, and every vocabulary word. No less than 12 content experts have read each chapter for accuracy and analyzed every bit of content that comprises the ancillary resources. While our intent and actions have been directed at creating an error-free text, it is still possible for some mistakes to occur. Prentice Hall takes this issue seriously and therefore welcomes any and all feedback that you can provide along the lines of helping us enhance the accuracy of this text. If you identify any errors that need to be corrected in a subsequent printing, please send them to:

  Prentice Hall Health Editorial; Medical Terminology Corrections; 1 Lake St.; Upper Saddle River, NJ 07458.

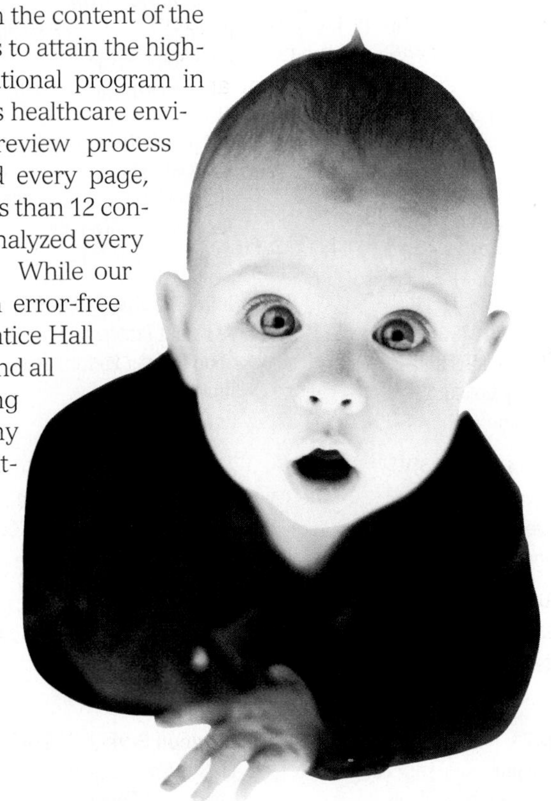

Our Development Team

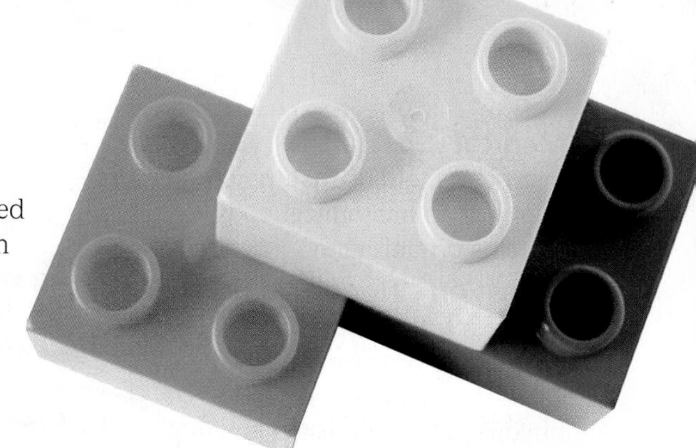

We can truly say that each individual on our development team has infused this book with ideas, vision, and passion for medical language. Our team crafted the blueprints for this book and has contributed to the birth of a landmark educational tool. Their influence will continue to have an impact for decades to come. Let us introduce the members of our team.

Physician Specialist Consultants

Stephen Caldwell, M.D.
Director of Hepatology
Digestive Health Center of Excellence
Charlottesville, Virginia

John H. Dirckx, M.D.
Former Medical Director
University of Dayton
Student Health Center
Dayton, Ohio

Joseph Gibbons, M.D.
Internal Medicine Physician
Centennial Medical Group
Elkridge, Maryland

James Michelson, M.D.
Professor of Orthopedic Surgery
George Washington University
School of Medicine
Washington, D.C.

Manuscript Reviewers
(*Reviewer conference attendee)

Denise M. Abrams, PT, MASS
Professor, Physical Therapy Assisting
SUNY Broome Community College
Appalachian, New York

Betsy Adams, AAS, BS, MSBE
Instructor, Office Systems Technology
Alamance Community College
Graham, North Carolina

Diana Alagna, RN, AHI, CPT
Program Director, Medical Assisting
Branford Hall Career Institute
Southington, Connecticut

Mercedes Alafriz-Gordon, BS
Surgical Technology Program
High Tech Institute
Phoenix, Arizona

Jana Allen, BS, MT*
Instructor, Allied Health
Volunteer State Community College
Gallatin, Tennessee

Ellen Anderson, RHIA
Instructor, Health Information Technology
College of Lake County
Northfield, Illinois

Judy Anderson, MEd
Instructor, Medical Office Administration
Coastal Carolina Community College
Jacksonville, North Carolina

Lori Andreucci, MEd, CMT, CMA
Medical Assistant & Medical Transcription Programs
Gateway Technical College
Racine, Wisconsin

Debbie Bedford, CMA, AAS
Program Coordinator, Medical Assisting
North Seattle Community College
Seattle, Washington

Tricia Berry, OTR/L
Program Coordinator, Medical Program
Hamilton College
Urbandale, Iowa

Sue Biederman, MSHP, RHIA
Associate Professor and Chair, Health Information Management
Texas State University
San Marcos, Texas

Julie E. Boles, MS, RHIA
Assistant Professor, School of Health Science and Human Performance
Ithaca College
Ithaca, New York

Annie M. Boster, PT
Instructor, Physical Therapist Assistant Program
Bishop State Community College
Mobile, Alabama

Susan A. Boulden, RN
Coordinator, Medical Assistant Program
Mt. Hood Community College
Aloha, Oregon

Shannon Bruley, BAS, AEMT-IC
EMS & Fire Program Manager
Henry Ford Community College
Dearborn, Michigan

Juanita R. Bryant, CMA-A/C
Instructor, Medical Assisting
Sierra College
Penn Valley, California

Thomas Bubar, BA, MS
Associate Professor, Medical Laboratory Technology
Erie Community College
Williamsville, New York

Susan Buboltz, RN, MS, CMA
Instructor, Medical Assisting
Madison Area Technical College
Madison, Wisconsin

Mary Butler, BS
Associate Faculty
Collin County Community College
McKinney, Texas

Patricia Bufalino, MA, MN, RN, FNP
Chair, Health, Human, and Public Services
Riverside Community College
Moreno Valley, California

Toni Cade, MBA, RHIA, CCS, FAHIMA
Associate Professor, Health Information Management
University of Louisiana at Lafayette
Lafayette, Louisiana

Cara L. Carreon, BS, RRT, CMA, CPC
Instructor, Medical Assisting
Ivy Tech Community College
Lafayette, Indiana

Rafael Castilla, MD
Dean of Academics
Ho Ho Kus School
Ramsey, New Jersey

Julia I. Chapman, BS
Instructor, Sciences
Stark State College of Technology
North Canton, Ohio

Kim Christmon, BS, RRT
Director, Clinical Education
Volunteer State Community College
Gallatin, Tennessee

Paula-Beth Ciolek
Lead Instructor, Allied Health
National College of Business and Technology
Richmond, Kentucky

Ronald Coleman, EdD
Dean of Allied Health
Volunteer State Community College
Gallatin, Tennessee

Mike Cochran, BA, RT(R)(CT), ARRT, VSRT, SWDSRT
Assistant Professor, Radiologic Technology
Southwest Virginia Community College
Richlands, Virginia

Cathleen Currie, RN, BS
Instructor/Program Manager, Allied Health
College of Southern Idaho
Twin Falls, Idaho

Denise J. DeDeaux, AAS, BS, MBA*
Chair, Medical Office Administration
Fayetteville Technical Community College
Fayetteville, North Carolina

Anita Denson, BS, CMA
Director, Health Care Education
National College of Business and Technology
Danville, Kentucky

Susan D. Dooley, CMT*
Chair, Health Professions and Early Childhood Education
Professor, Medical Transcription and Allied Health
Seminole Community College
Sorrento, Florida

Vickie Findley, MPA, RHIA
Associate Professor, Health Information Technology
Fairmont State College
Fairmont, West Virginia

Kathie Folsom, MS, BSN, RN
Chair, Health Occupations
Skagit Valley College—Whidbley Island Campus
Oak Harbor, Washington

Joyce Foster
Instructor, Allied Health
State Fair Community College
Sedalia, Missouri

Elaine Garcia, RHIT
Instructor, Health Information Technology
Spokane Community College
Spokane, Washington

Barbara E. Geary, RN, MA
Instructor, Health and Human Services
North Seattle Community College
Seattle, Washington

Patricia Goshorn, MA, RN, CMA-AC
Professor Emeritus, Career and Technology
Cosumnes River College
Sacramento, California

Paula Hagstrom, MM, RHIA
Associate Professor, Health Management
Ferris State University
Big Rapids, Michigan

Dotty Hall, RN, MSN, CST
Associate Professor, Surgical Technology
Ivy Tech Community College
Lafayette, Indiana

Karen Hardney, MSEd, RT
Associate Professor, Health Sciences
Chicago State University
Chicago, Illinois

Barbara L. Henry, RN, BSN
Instructor, Health Careers
Gateway Technical College
Racine, Wisconsin

Cathy Hess, RHIA
Lecturer, Health Information Management
Texas State University
San Marcos, Texas

Jan C. Hess, MA
Program Coordinator, Health Information Management Systems
Metropolitan Community College
Omaha, Nebraska

Denise M. Hightower, RHIA
Lead Instructor, Medical Transcription
Cape Fear Community College
Wilmington, North Carolina

Valentina Holder, MA.Ed, RHIA
Instructor, Medical Office Administration
Pitt Community College
Winterville, North Carolina

Beulah A. Hofmann, RN, MSN, CMA
Assistant Professor/Director, Nursing
Ivy Tech Community College
Greencastle, Indiana

James E. Hudacek, MSEd*
Instructor, Allied Health & Nursing
Loraine County Community College
Amherst, Ohio

Pamela S. Huber, MS, MT(ASCP)
Professor, Medical Laboratory Technology
Medical Office Assisting
Erie Community College
Williamsville, New York

Bud W. Hunton, MA, RT (R) (QM)
Instructor, Allied Health Technologies
Sinclair Community College
Dayton, Ohio

Karen Jackson, NR-CMA
Program Director, Medical Assisting
Department of General Education
Remington College
Garland, Texas

Kathleen Kearney, BS, MED, EMT-P
Instructor, Health Education
Kent State University
Kent, Ohio

Cathy Kelley-Arney, CMA, MLTC, BSHS, AS
Institutional Director, Health Care Education
National College of Business and Technology
Bluefield, Virginia

Winifred Khalil, RN, MS
Professor, Humanities
San Diego Mesa College
San Diego, California

Marsha Lalley, BSM, MSM
Instructor, Medical Administrative Assisting
Minneapolis Community and Technical College
Minneapolis, Minnesota

Carol A. Lehman, ART
Instructor, Allied Health and Nursing
Hocking College
Nelsonville, Ohio

Sandra Lehrke, MS, RN
Instructor, Medical Assisting
Anoka Technical Community College
Anoka, Minnesota

Maria Teresa Lopez-Hill, MS
Instructor, Allied Health
Laredo Community College
Laredo, Texas

Instructor, Continuing Education
Bow Valley College
Calgary, Alberta

Instructor, Office Systems Technology
Collin County Community College
McKinney, Texas

Patricia McLane, RHIA, MA
Instructor, Health Information Technology
Henry Ford Community College
Dearborn, Michigan

Michael C. McMinn, MA, RRT
Professor, Division of Health Sciences
Mott Community College
Flint, Michigan

Michelle G. Miller, M.Ed. CMA, COMT
Professor, Medical Assisting
Lakeland Community College
Kirtland, Ohio

Ann Minks, FAAMT
Instructor, Medical Assisting/Medical Transcription
Lake Washington Technical College
Kirkland, Washington

Barbara S. Moffet, PhD, RN
Assistant Professor, Nursing
Southeastern Louisiana University
Hammond, Louisiana

Suzanne Moe, RN
Instructor, Health Division
Northwest Technical College
Bemidji, Minnesota

Karen Myers, CPC
Instructor, Office Technology
Pierce College Puyallup
Puyallup, Washington

Gloria Newton, MA-ED
Instructor, Center for Human Development
Shasta College
Redding, California

Erin Nixon, RN
Instructor, Health Information Management
Bakersfield College
Bakersfield, California

Alice M. Noblin, MBA, RHIA, LHRM
Instructor, Health Information Management
University of Central Florida
Orlando, Florida

Kerry Openshaw, PhD
Professor, Biology
Bemidji State University
Bemidji, Minnesotta

Tina Peer, MS, RN
Assistant Professor, Nursing Department
The College of Southern Idaho
Twin Falls, Idaho

Mary Rahr, MS, RN, CMA
Instructor, Health Sciences
Northeast Wisconsin Technical College
Madison, Wisconsin

Sheila G. Rockoff, EdD, MSN, BSN, AS, RN
Professor and Chair, Medical Assisting
Santa Ana College
Santa Ana, California

Mary Sayles, RN, MSN
Instructor, Medical Terminology
Sierra College—Nevada County Campus
Rocklin, California

Jody E. Scheller, MS, RHIA
Associate Professor, Health Information Technology
Schoolcraft College
Garden City, Michigan

Patricia Schrull, MSN, MBA, MEd, RN
Assistant Professor, Allied Health & Nursing
Lorain County Community College
Elyria, Ohio

Theresa R. Schuldt, MEd, HT/HTL (ASCP)
Associate Dean/Professor, Health Sciences
Rose State College
Midwest City, Oklahoma

Jan Sesser, BS, RMA (AMT), CMA
Corporate Director of Education, Allied Health
High Tech Institute
Phoenix, Arizona

Donna Sue Shellman, MA, CPC
Instructor, Office Systems Technology
Gaston College
Dallas, North Carolina

Karin Sherrill, BSN
Instructor, Nursing Department
Mesa Community College
Gilbert, Arizona

Erin Sitterley
Instructor, Allied Health
North Seattle Community College
Seattle, Washington

Tim J. Skaife, RT(R), MA
Director, Radiography Program
National Park Community College
Hot Springs, Arizona

Lynn G. Slack, CMA
Medical Programs Director
ICM School of Business and Medical Careers
Pittsburgh, Pennsylvania

Ellie Smith, RN, MSN
Instructor, Nursing Division
Cuesta College
San Luis Obispo, California

Darla K. Sparacino, MED, RHIA
Associate Professor
Health Information Management Program
Arkansas Tech University
Russelville, Arkansas

Sherman K. Sowby, PhD, CHES
Professor/Chair, Health Science
California State—Fresno
Fresno, California

Carolyn Stariha, BS, RHIA
Clinical Coordinator, Health & Science Center
Houston Community College—Coleman Campus
Houston, Texas

Kathy Stau, CPhT
Program Director, Pharmacy Technician
Medix School
Smyrna, Georgia

Deb Stockberger, MSN, RN
Instructor, Division of Business
North Iowa Community College
Mason City, Iowa

J. David Taylor, PhD, PT, CSCS
Assistant Professor, Physical Therapy
University of Central Arkansas
Conway, Arkansas

Sylvia Taylor, CMA, CPCA
Medical Office Administration
Cleveland State Community College
Cleveland, Tennessee

Jean Ternus, RN, MS
Professor/Clinical Coordinator, Nursing
Kansas City Community College
Kansas City, Kansas

Cindy B. Thompson, BSRT, MA*
Instructor, Medical Assisting
Alamance Community College
Graham, North Carolina

Margaret A. Tiemann, RN, BS
Instructor, Health Information Technology
St. Charles Community College
Cottleville, Missouri

Mary Jane Tremethick, PhD, RN, CHES
Instructor, Health/Physical Education and Recreation
Northern Michigan University
Marquette, Michican

Valeria D. Truitt, BS, MAEd
Instructor, Medical Office Administration
Craven Community College
New Bern, North Carolina

Patricia Von Knorring
Program Coordinator, Medical Transcription
Tacoma Community College
Gig Harbor, Washington

Mary Warren-Oliver, BA
Clinical Coordinator, Medical Assisting
Gibbs College
Vienna, Virginia

Kim Webb, RN, MN
Chair, Nursing Program
Northern Oklahoma College
Tonkawa, Oklahoma

Bonnie Welniak, RN, MSN
Assistant Professor, Nursing
Monroe County Community College
Monroe, Michigan

Richard Weidman, RHIA, CCS-P
Instructor, Health Information Technology
Tacoma Community College
Tacoma, Washington

Victoria Lee Wetle, RN, EdD
Chair, Health Services Management
Chemeketa Community College
Salem, Oregon

Connie Werner, MS, RHIA
Assistant Professor, Health Care Coding
York College of Pennsylvania
York, Pennsylvania

Jay W. Wilborn, MEd, MT(ASCP)
Program Director of Medical Laboratory Technology
National Park Community College
Hot Springs, Arkansas

Tammy L. Wilder, RN, MSN, CMSRN
Assistant Professor, Nursing Program
Ivy Tech Community College
Evansville, Indiana

Scott Zimmer, MS
Instructor, Biology
Metropolitan Community College
Omaha, Nebraska

Focus Group Participants

Kim Anthony Aaronson, BS, DC
Instructor, Biology
Harry S. Truman College
Chicago, Ilinois
Instructor
Harold Washington College
Chicago, Ilinois

Kendra J. Allen, LPN
Program Manager and Instructor, Office Technology
Ohio Institute of Health Careers
Columbus, Ohio

Delena Kay Austin, BTIS, CMA
Program Director, Medical Assisting
Macomb Community College
Clinton Township, Michigan

Molly Baxter
Dean of Health Sciences
Baker College—Port Huron
Port Huron, Michigan

Joan Berry, RN, MSN, CNS
Program Director, Nursing Careers
Lansing Community College
Lansing, Michigan

Kenneth Bretl, MA, RRT
Professor Emeritus, Health, Social, Behavioral Science
College of DuPage
Glen Ellyn, Ilinois

Carole Bretscher
Former Director, Allied Health
Southwestern College
Bellbrook, Ohio

Adrienne L. Carter, MEd, NRMA,
Instructor, Medical Assisting
Riverside Community College
Moreno Valley, California

Mary Dudash-White, MA, RHIA, CCS
Professor, Health Information Management
Sinclair Community College
Dayton, Ohio

Cathy Flite, MEd, RHIA
Assistant Professor, Health Information Technology
Temple University
Philadelphia, Pennsylvania

Sherry Gamble, RN, CNS, MSN, CNOR
Director/Assistant Professor, Surgical Technology
University of Akron
Akron, Ohio

Mary Garcia, BA, AD, RN
Instructor, Allied Health
Northwestern Business College
Northeastern Illinois University
Truman College
Chicago, Ilinois

Joyce Garozzo, MS, RHIA, CCS
Director, Health Information Technology
Community College of Philadelphia
Philadelphia, Pennsylvania

Patsy Gehring, PhD, RN, CS
Professor, Nursing
Lakeland Community College
Kirkland, Ohio

Michelle Heller, CMA, RMA
Program Director, Medical Assisting
Ohio Institute of Health Careers
Columbus, Ohio

Janet Hossli
Instructor, Allied Health
Northwestern Business College
Chicago, Illinois

Trudi James-Parks, RT, BS,
Instructor, Radiologic Technology
Lorain County Community College
Elyria, Ohio

Sherry L. Jones, RN, ASN
Instructor, Medical Assisting
Western School of Health and Business
Community College of Allegheny County
Pittsburgh, Pennsylvania

Esther H. Kim
Instructor, Health Sciences
Chicago State University
Chicago, Illinois

Richelle S. Laipply, PhD, CMA
Associate Professor, Medical Assisting Technology
University of Akron
Akron, Ohio

Andrea M. Lane, CMA-C, BAS RN, MS
Instructor, Healthcare Professions
Brookdale Community College
Lincroft, New Jersey

Mary Lou Liebal, BS, RTR, MA
Associate Professor, Radiologic Technology
Cuyahoga Community College
Cleveland, Ohio

Stacey Long, BS
Assistant Director, Massage Therapy
Miami Jacobs Career College
Dayton, Ohio

Anne Loochtan, MEd
Assistant Dean, Health and Public Safety
Columbus State Community College
Cincinnati, Ohio

Anne M. Lunde, BS, CMT
Instructor, Business and Information Systems
Waubonsee Community College
Sugar Grove, Ilinois

Janice Manning, MA, PCP
Chair, Health Care Administration
Baker College
Jackson, Michigan

Sandy Marks, RN, MS(HCA)
Associate Professor, Health Occupations
Cerritos College
Norwalk, California

Kathleen Masters, MS, RN
Assistant Professor, Nursing
Monroe County Community College
Monroe, Michigan

Mary Morgan, MS, CNMT
Instructor, Nuclear Medicine Technology
Columbus State Community College
Columbus, Ohio

Andrew Muniz, OT, BBA, MBA
Instructor, Allied Health
Baker College
Auburn Hills, Michigan

Michael Murphy, AAS, CMA, CLP
Instructor, Allied Health
Berdan Institute
Union, New Jersey

Stephen Nardozzi, BA
Assistant Professor, Emergency Medical Services Academy EMT-P
SUNY- Westchester Community College
Valhalla, New York

Ruth Ann O'Brien, MHA, RRT
Director, Allied Health Department
Miami Jacobs Career College
Dayton, Ohio

Donna Schnepp, MHA, RHIA
Professor, Health Information Technology
Moraine Valley Community College
Palos Hills, Ilinois

Ann M. Smith, MS
Associate Professor, Natural Science
Joliet Junior College
Joliet, Ilinois

Mark Velderrain
Instructor, Medical Assisting
Cerritos College
Norwalk, California

Barbara Wiggins, MT(ASCP)
Chair, Medical Laboratory Technology
Delaware Technical & Community College
Georgetown, Delaware

Gail S. Williams, Ph.D., MT(ASCP)SBB, CLS(NCA)
Assistant Professor, Clinical Laboratory Science
School of Allied Health Professions
Northern Illinois University
DeKalb, Ilinois

Karen Wright, RHIA, MHA
Coordinator, Health Information Technology
Hocking College
Nelsonville, Ohio

Student Advisors

Tobi Burch
Community College of Philadelphia
Philadelphia, Pennsylvania

Calvin Byrd
Temple University
Philadelphia, Pennsylvania

Kimberly Clark
Community College of Philadelphia
Philadelphia, Pennsylvania

Susan DiMaria
Brookdale Community College
Lincroft, New Jersey

Avelina Elam
Thomas Jefferson University
Philadelphia, Pennsylvania

Michael Flores
Berdan Institute
Union, New Jersey

Frederick Herbert
Temple University
Philadelphia, Pennsylvania

Brenda Merlino
Thomas Jefferson University
Philadelphia, Pennsylvania

Megan Milos
Ocean County College
Toms River, New Jersey

Payam Mohadjeri
Temple University
Philadelphia, Pennsylvania

Monica Narang
Westchester Community College
Valhalla, New York

About the Author

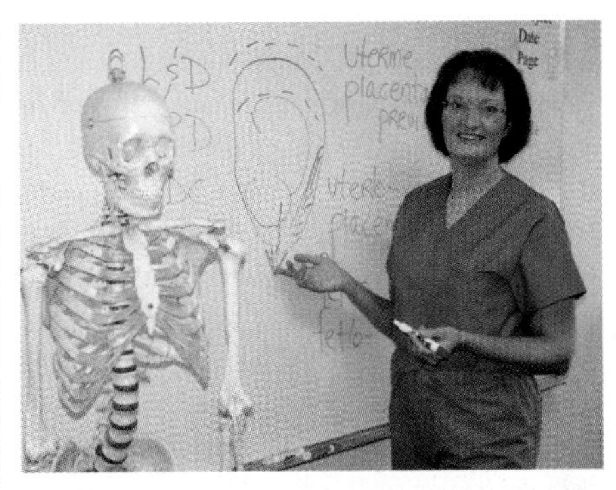

Susan M. Turley, MA (Educ), BSN, RN, RHIT, CMT, is an adjunct professor in the School of Health Professions, Wellness, and Physical Education at Anne Arundel Community College in Arnold, Maryland, where she teaches medical terminology and medical transcription courses. In the past, she was instrumental in gaining accreditation for the college's medical assisting program and has also taught courses in pharmacology, pathophysiology, and medical office procedures. She is an instructor and accreditation director for the International Institute of Original Medicine in Maryland. She is also a medical editor and author for Health Professions Institute in Modesto, California, and a curriculum consultant for The Andrews School for Medical Transcription and Medical Coding in Oklahoma City, Oklahoma.

As a healthcare professional, Susan has worked in a variety of healthcare settings over the past 30 years: acute care, long-term care, physicians' offices, and managed care. She has held positions as an intensive care nurse, plasmapheresis nurse, infection control officer, medical transcriptionist, medical grant writer, manager of the Medic Alert national difficult airway database, medical record coder, director of education, and director of quality management and corporate compliance.

Susan is the author of *Understanding Pharmacology for Health Professionals* (Prentice Hall), and of more than 40 articles published in medical transcription and health information management journals. She is a co-developer of The SUM Medical Transcription Training Program and reference books for Health Professions Institute. With a physician co-author, she has written two nationally funded grants and a chapter in a physician's anesthesiology textbook.

She has been a guest speaker at national seminars for accreditation of utilization management programs, medical transcription teacher training, and health information management certification exam review.

Susan holds a Master of Arts degree in adult education from Norwich University in Vermont, a Bachelor of Science degree in nursing from the Pennsylvania State University, state licensure as an RN, as well as national certification in medical transcription from the American Association for Medical Transcription and national certification in health information management from the American Health Information Management Association.

About the Illustrator

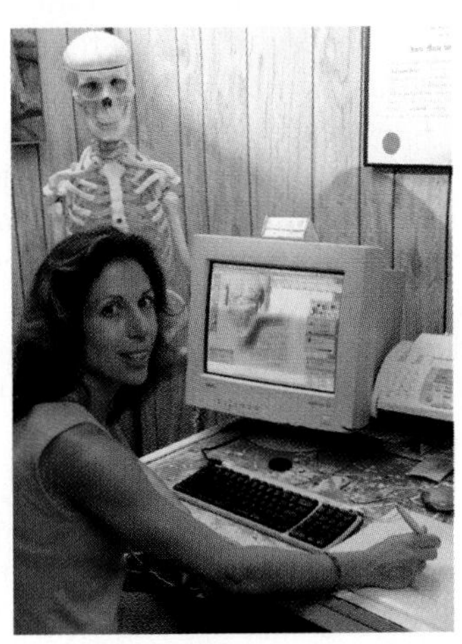

The illustrations throughout this book were carefully coordinated through a close collaborative effort between the author and artist. Every figure was custom developed specifically for this text, and refined to be precise, unique, and fresh. From a pedagogical point of view, it was important that all of the art be consistent throughout, rather than presenting a conglomeration of styles and levels of detail.

Anita Impagliazzo is a medical illustrator and designer in Charlottesville, Virginia. A graduate of the University of Virginia, she went on to complete the Biomedical Illustration Graduate Program at the University of Texas Southwestern Medical Center at Dallas and spent several years specializing in illustrating for medical malpractice litigation. She is currently self-employed, creating artwork for researchers and physicians at the University of Virginia Health System, basic science and surgical textbooks, medical journals, the courtroom, and presentations. She is a member of the Association of Medical Illustrators and has received several awards in its annual juried salons. She never tires of using medical language to learn new things about the human body: how it works, how it fails, how it is fixed, and how the fixing fails.

Acknowledgments

My thanks go to Mark Cohen, Executive Editor for Health Professions at Prentice Hall and my editor for ***Medical Language.*** We have worked together on various projects since 1997, and his responsiveness, creative insights, and professionalism make him a delight to work with. His vision of this textbook was one with mine, but he also envisioned the next level of excellence and continually moved the textbook toward that goal. His support and enthusiasm have been constant and invaluable as he expertly managed a complexity of details and guided this textbook from idea to reality.

My thanks go to Anita Impagliazzo, my medical illustrator. She embraced much more than her original role and quickly became a creative collaborator and advisor on this project. She is a wonderfully talented medical illustrator whose efforts made this textbook medically accurate, artistically unique, and without equal. My thanks, too, to the many models who appear in the real-life photographs throughout the textbook.

My thanks go to Cathy Wein, my development editor. She coordinated communication, manuscript copyediting review, and deadlines for everyone involved. She embraced this project, and it would never have been completed without her expert, professional, and timely editorial assistance and personal support.

My thanks go to the Prentice Hall design team. Their inspired work created a strikingly beautiful textbook. Cheryl Asherman applied her strong aesthetic and editorial sensibilities, laying the foundation for a clear vision of how the textbook should look. Mary Siener built upon that plan and executed it to perfection. She spent hundreds of hours doing image research and graphic design to create a dynamic textbook cover, fantastic chapter-opening spreads, as well as ingenious feature icons that appear throughout the textbook.

My thanks go to Melissa Kerian, Associate Editor at Prentice Hall, who has been involved in so many details—small and large. She directed the entire editorial development and quality management program for each of the ancillary materials that accompany this textbook. Instructors who appreciate complete, high-quality supplemental materials will have her to thank for her tireless, precise, and impassioned work.

My thanks go to Karen Allman and Katrin Beacom, my marketing team, for truly embracing the concept of developing a customer-driven textbook. They were committed to listening to the needs of the market and then consulting with me to help me shape the textbook around those needs.

My thanks go to the talented team at Pine Tree Composition, led by Jessica Balch who oversaw the extensive editing, layout, and indexing of my textbook. In light of the monumental complexity of the textbook, I especially appreciated her professionalism, flexibility, concentration, creative insights, and can-do approach. My thanks also go to Leanne Binette, the pager, who successfully navigated the formatting complexities for this textbook.

My thanks go to Patrick Walsh and Christina Zingone, who managed the complete production of this textbook from image research to page layout to the coordination of ancillary material content. They were masters at handling the complex and ever-evolving details of this huge project while maintaining a close watch over budgets and schedules.

My thanks go to the amazing media team at Prentice Hall that designed and produced a spectacular array of multimedia learning applications to support my textbook. John Jordan, Stephen Hartner, and

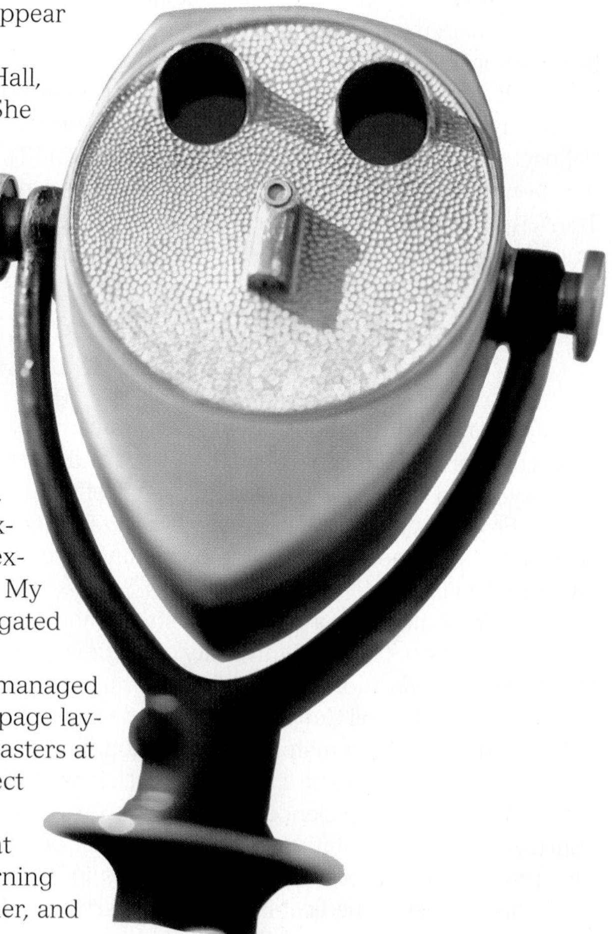

Amy Peltier managed the development of websites, test generator software, CD-ROM technology, animations, videos, and PowerPoint lectures. Dave and Georgia Green deserve credit for their development of the technological aspects of the CD-ROM. Chip Price, Amy McCorkle, Carrie Donohue, Richard Benton, and Brenda Boyce created the revolutionary MyMedTermLab online course. The creativity and expertise of each of these individuals helped set this textbook apart as the new standard in this field.

My thanks go to Dan Frank, the video producer, and his video team who coordinated the filming of 22 healthcare professionals on location across the United States for our *Real People, Real Medicine* video series. This is presented individually in the Career Focus section in each chapter and in its entirety in the instructional support package.

My thanks go to Prentice Hall President and CEO Tim Bozik, along with Division President Robin Baliszewski and Prentice Hall Health Vice President and Publisher Julie Alexander. Their understanding of and support for my vision allowed the entire Prentice Hall team to put forth maximum effort toward a landmark result.

My thanks go Meg and Glenn Turner and their team at Burrston House, who embraced my textbook as part of an extensive market development program that included focus groups, market reviews, and detailed analyses that helped me to truly understand our customers' needs.

My special thanks go to Sally Pitman and Linda Campbell of Health Professions Institute for granting permission and giving assistance in obtaining authentic medical dictation from The SUM Program for Training Medical Transcriptionists as exercises on the CD-ROM. I have worked with them for many years, and their dedication to medical language and innovative educational approaches was and still is inspiring.

My thanks go to the many classes of students who motivated me to continually research and present medical language clearly and thoroughly. It was their warm reception to my teaching methods and materials that encouraged me to keep improving.

My thanks go to the many teachers and practitioners who have overwhelmingly validated my efforts to write about medical language with a uniquely interesting, lively, and fresh approach. Each and every person listed on pages xvi–xx played an important role in the development of this textbook, and I hope they share my sense of pride in the end result.

Contents

PART I INTRODUCTION TO MEDICAL LANGUAGE 3

CHAPTER 1
The Structure of Medical Language 3
- Welcome to Medical Language 5
  - Communication and Medical Language 6
  - Medical Words and Word Parts 7
  - Medical Language Origins 20
  - Medical Word Singular and Plural Nouns 21
  - The Health Record 22
- Abbreviations 25
- Chapter Review Exercises 26

CHAPTER 2
The Body in Health and Disease 33
- The Body in Health 35
  - Body Planes and Body Directions Approach 35
  - Body Cavities Approach 42
  - Quadrants and Regions Approach 43
  - Anatomy and Physiology Approach 44
  - Microscopic-to-Macroscopic Approach 45
  - Body Systems Approach 45
  - Medical Specialties Approach 46
- Vocabulary Review 52
- The Body in Disease 62
  - Disease Categories 62
  - Onset, Course, and Outcome of Disease 63
- Healthcare Professionals and Healthcare Settings 66
  - Healthcare Professionals 66
  - Healthcare Settings 67
- Vocabulary Review 69
- Abbreviations 74
- Chapter Review Exercises 76

PART II MEDICAL SPECIALTIES AND BODY SYSTEMS 87

CHAPTER 3
Gastroenterology • Gastrointestinal System 87
- Anatomy and Physiology 89
  - Anatomy of the Gastrointestinal System 89
  - Physiology of Digestion 96
- Vocabulary Review 99
- Symptoms, Signs, and Diseases 107
- Diagnostic Procedures 123
- Medical and Surgical Procedures 127
- Drug Categories 133
- Abbreviations 134
- Chapter Review Exercises 136

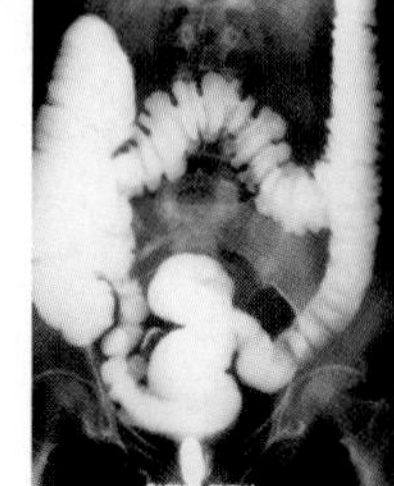

CHAPTER 4
Pulmonology • Respiratory System 153
- Anatomy and Physiology 155
  - Anatomy of the Respiratory System 155
  - Physiology of Respiration 160
- Vocabulary Review 163
- Symptoms, Signs, and Diseases 169
- Diagnostic Procedures 180
- Medical and Surgical Procedures 182
- Drug Categories 187
- Abbreviations 189
- Chapter Review Exercises 191

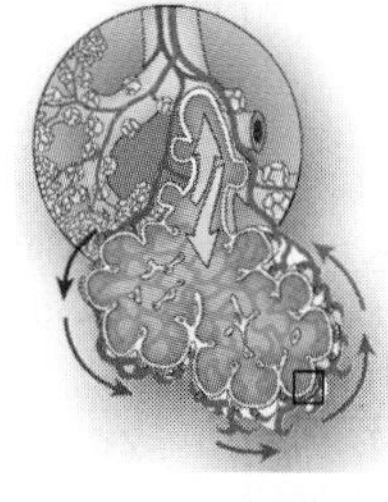

CHAPTER 5
Cardiology • Cardiovascular System 205
- Anatomy and Physiology 207
  - Anatomy of the Cardiovascular System 207
  - Physiology of a Heartbeat 217
- Vocabulary Review 219
- Symptoms, Signs, and Diseases 229
- Diagnostic Procedures 241
- Medical and Surgical Procedures 248
- Drug Categories 254
- Abbreviations 257
- Chapter Review Exercises 259

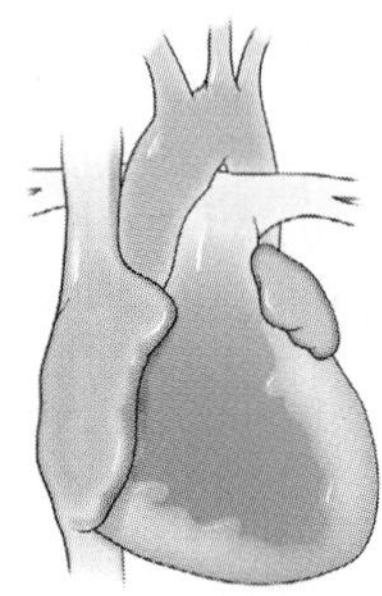

CHAPTER 6
Hematology and Immunology • Blood and Lymphatic System 275
- Anatomy and Physiology 277
  - Anatomy of the Blood 277
  - Physiology of Blood Clotting 286
  - Anatomy of the Lymphatic System 287
  - Physiology of the Immune Response 289
- Vocabulary Review 292
- Symptoms, Signs, and Diseases 300
- Diagnostic Procedures 310
- Medical and Surgical Procedures 315
- Drug Categories 318
- Abbreviations 320
- Chapter Review Exercises 321

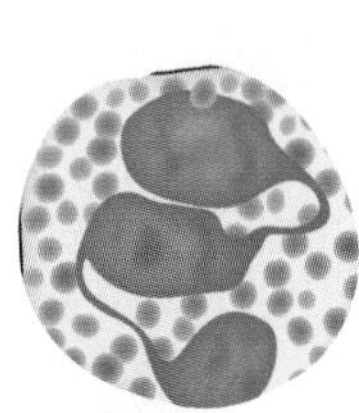

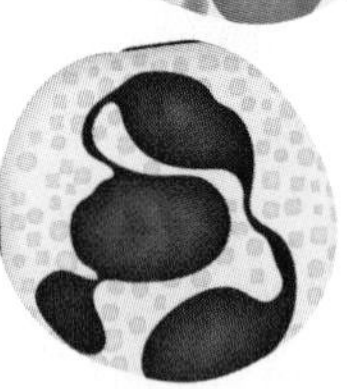

CHAPTER 7
Dermatology • Integumentary System 337
Anatomy and Physiology 339
Anatomy of the Integumentary System 339
Physiology of an Allergic Reaction 344
Vocabulary Review 345
Symptoms, Signs, and Diseases 350
Diagnostic Procedures 369
Medical and Surgical Procedures 370
Drug Categories 376
Abbreviations 377
Chapter Review Exercises 380

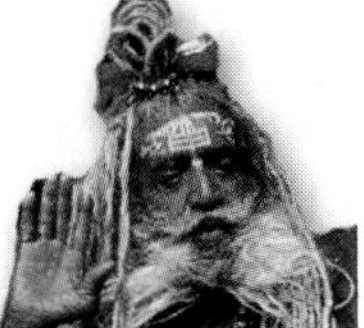

CHAPTER 8
Orthopedics • Skeletal System 395
Anatomy and Physiology 397
Anatomy of the Skeletal System 397
The Structure of Bone 411
Physiology of Bone Growth 419
Vocabulary Review 415
Symptoms, Signs, and Diseases 424
Diagnostic Procedures 434
Medical and Surgical Procedures 436
Drug Categories 440
Abbreviations 442
Chapter Review Exercises 444

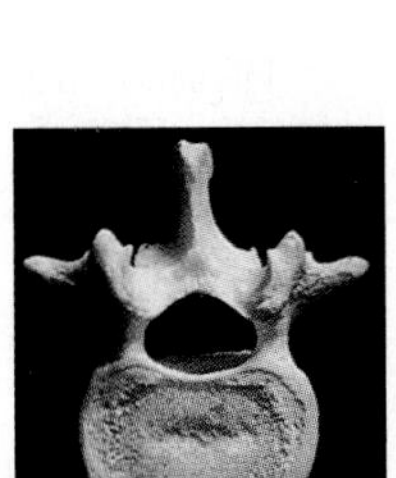

CHAPTER 9
Orthopedics • Muscular System 457
Anatomy and Physiology 459
Anatomy of the Muscular System 459
Physiology of a Muscle Contraction 472
Vocabulary Review 474
Symptoms, Signs, and Diseases 482
Diagnostic Procedures 489
Medical and Surgical Procedures 490
Drug Categories 493
Abbreviations 495
Chapter Review Exercises 497

CHAPTER 10
Neurology • Nervous System 511
Anatomy and Physiology 513
Anatomy of the Nervous System 513
Physiology of a Nerve Transmission 524
Vocabulary Review 526
Symptoms, Signs, and Diseases 536
Diagnostic Procedures 553
Medical and Surgical Procedures 556
Drug Categories 560
Abbreviations 562
Chapter Review Exercises 564

CHAPTER 11
Urology • Urinary System 581
Anatomy and Physiology 583
Anatomy of the Urinary System 583
Physiology of the Formation of Urine 588
Physiology of Other Functions of the Kidneys 590
Vocabulary Review 591
Symptoms, Signs, and Diseases 597
Diagnostic Procedures 606
Medical and Surgical Procedures 612
Drug Categories 618
Abbreviations 619
Chapter Review Exercises 621

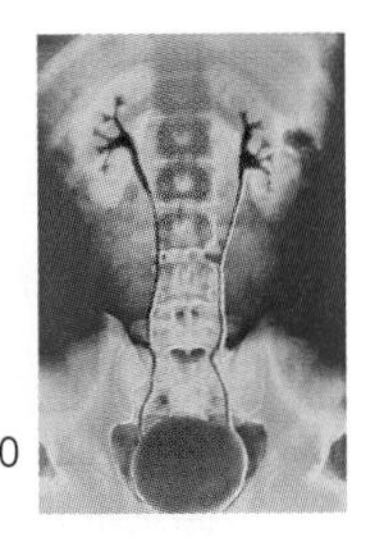

CHAPTER 12
Male Reproductive Medicine • Male Genitourinary System 635
Anatomy and Physiology 637
Anatomy of the Male Genitourinary System 637
Physiology of Spermatogenesis and Ejaculation 642
Vocabulary Review 644
Symptoms, Signs, and Diseases 649
Diagnostic Procedures 653
Medical and Surgical Procedures 655
Drug Categories 657
Abbreviations 658
Chapter Review Exercises 660

CHAPTER 13
Gynecology and Obstetrics • Female Reproductive System 673
Anatomy and Physiology 675
Anatomy of the Female Genital and Reproductive System 676
Physiology of Menstruation and Conception 683
Physiology of Labor and Delivery 687
The Newborn 690
Vocabulary Review 691
Symptoms, Signs, and Diseases 701
Diagnostic Procedures 714
Medical and Surgical Procedures 720
Drug Categories 729
Abbreviations 731
Chapter Review Exercises 734

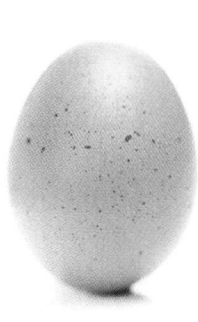

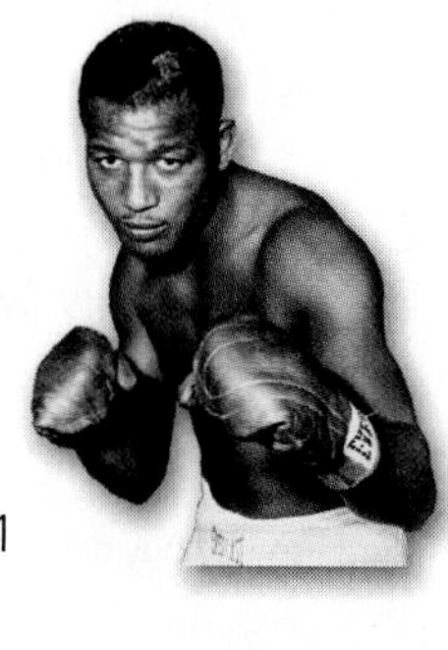

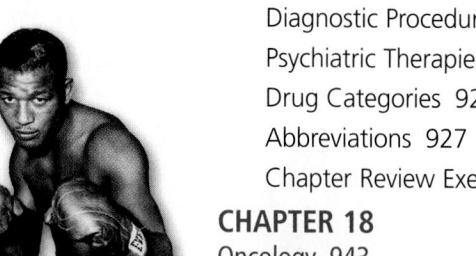

CHAPTER 14
Endocrinology • Endocrine System 751
Anatomy and Physiology 753
Anatomy of the Endocrine System 754
Physiology of Hormone Response and Feedback 762
Vocabulary Review 764
Symptoms, Signs, and Diseases 771
Diagnostic Procedures 784
Medical and Surgical Procedures 786
Drug Categories 787
Abbreviations 789
Chapter Review Exercises 791

CHAPTER 15
Ophthalmology • Eyes 805
Anatomy and Physiology 807
Anatomy of the Eye 807
Physiology of Vision 814
Vocabulary Review 816
Symptoms, Signs, and Diseases 821
Diagnostic Procedures 829
Medical and Surgical Procedures 831
Drug Categories 838
Abbreviations 839
Chapter Review Exercises 841

CHAPTER 16
Otolaryngology • Ears, Nose, and Throat 853
Anatomy and Physiology 855
Anatomy of the ENT System 855
Physiology of the Sense of Hearing 864
Vocabulary Review 865
Symptoms, Signs, and Diseases 871
Diagnostic Procedures 879
Medical and Surgical Procedures 882
Drug Categories 885
Abbreviations 887
Chapter Review Exercises 889

Part III OTHER MEDICAL SPECIALTIES 901

CHAPTER 17
Psychiatry 901
Anatomy and Physiology 903
Anatomy Related to Psychiatry 903
Physiology of Emotion and Behavior 905
Vocabulary Review 906
Symptoms, Signs, and Mental Disorders 908
Diagnostic Procedures 922
Psychiatric Therapies 924
Drug Categories 926
Abbreviations 927
Chapter Review Exercises 929

CHAPTER 18
Oncology 943
Anatomy and Physiology 945
Anatomy Related to Oncology 945
Physiology of Cellular Division and Cancer 947
Vocabulary Review 951
Symptoms, Signs, and Types of Cancer 955
Diagnostic Procedures 963
Medical, Surgical and Radiation Therapy Procedures 967
Drug Categories 974
Abbreviations 976
Chapter Review Exercises 978

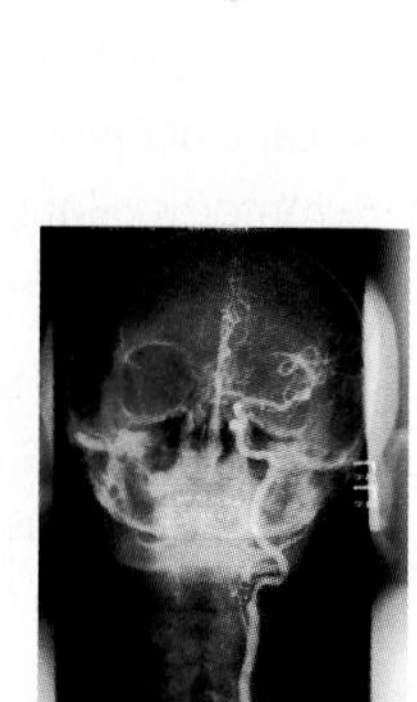

CHAPTER 19
Radiology and Nuclear Medicine 991
Anatomy and Physiology 993
Radiology 993
Nuclear Medicine 1007
Vocabulary Review 1012
Drug Categories 1019
Abbreviations 1020
Chapter Review Exercises 1021

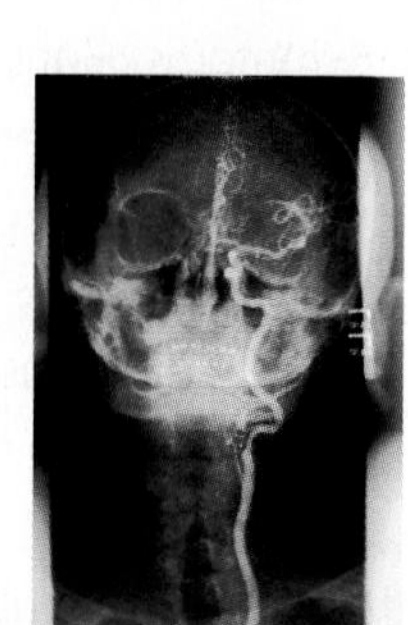

APPENDICES
APPENDIX A Glossary of Medical Word Parts: Combining Forms, Prefixes, and Suffixes A-1
APPENDIX B Abbreviations Glossary A-17

ANSWER KEY AK-1
PHOTO CREDITS PC-1
INDEX I-1

medical

immerse yourself

language

Dive In!

- With 19 letters, otorhinolaryngology is the longest word in this textbook, but soon you'll be able to analyze and understand it.
- Some medical words are actual Latin and Greek words that were used centuries ago.
- In this chapter you'll explore medical language communication in all its forms. The pieces will all fall into place when you master this chapter!

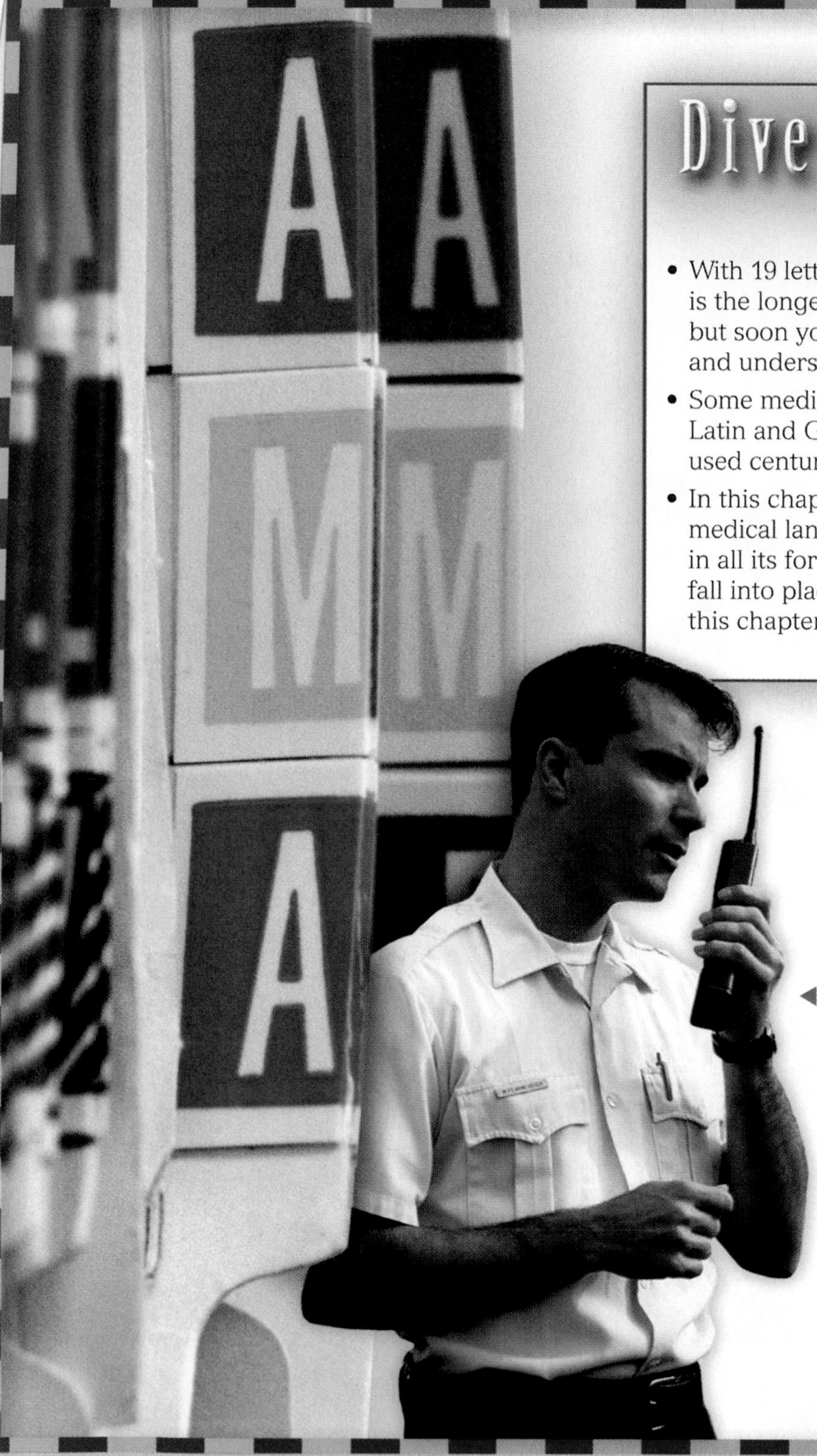

◀ Medical language is the key to a successful career in health care. If you want to "walk the walk," then you have to "talk the talk" of medical language.

Medicine Through HISTORY

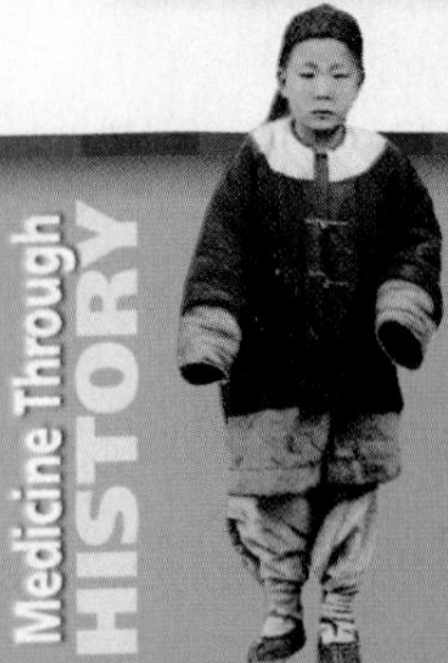

475 B.C.

The Chinese write a textbook on acupuncture and the treatment of disease

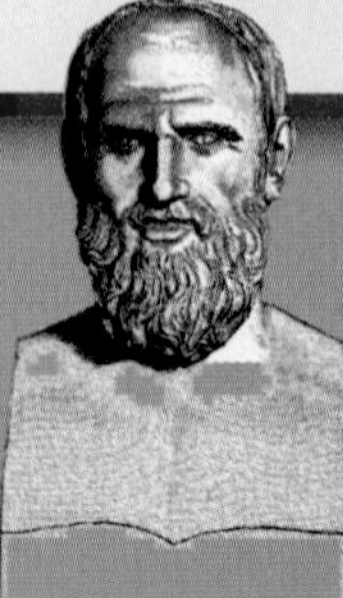

377 B.C.

Hippocrates is born, a Greek physician and the father of modern medicine

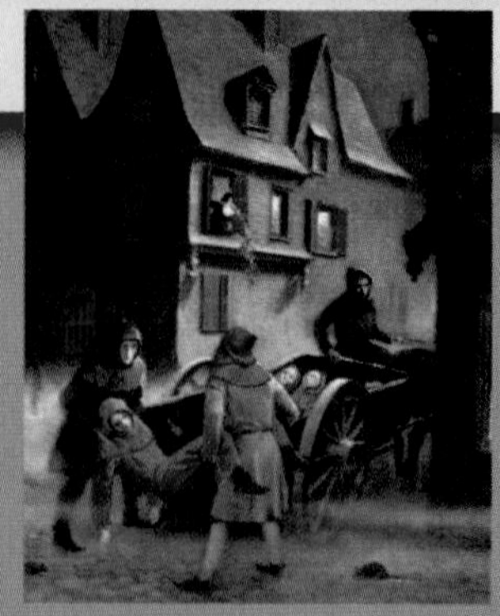

1347

The Black Death plague ravages Europe, killing one third of the population. It is transmitted by fleas carried by black rats

CHAPTER 1

The Structure of Medical Language

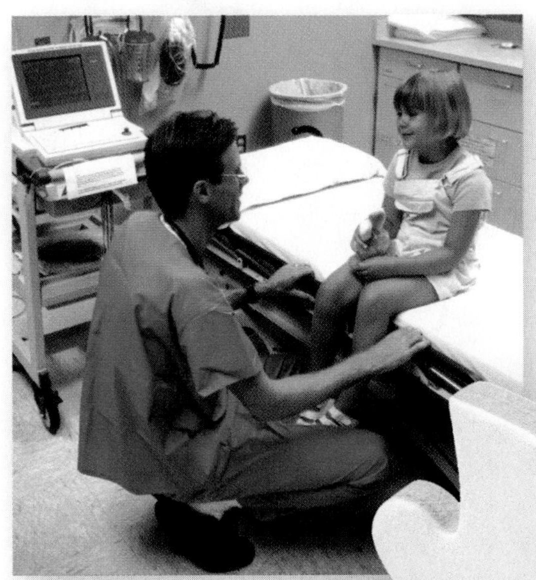

Medical language (MED-ih-kal LANG-gwij) is the framework on which the practice of medicine is built. Healthcare professionals use medical language every day to communicate with each other.

▶ Medical words are like puzzles, and their word parts are like the pieces. If you put them together correctly, you can understand the meaning of the medical word.

1500

The Chinese invent the toothbrush

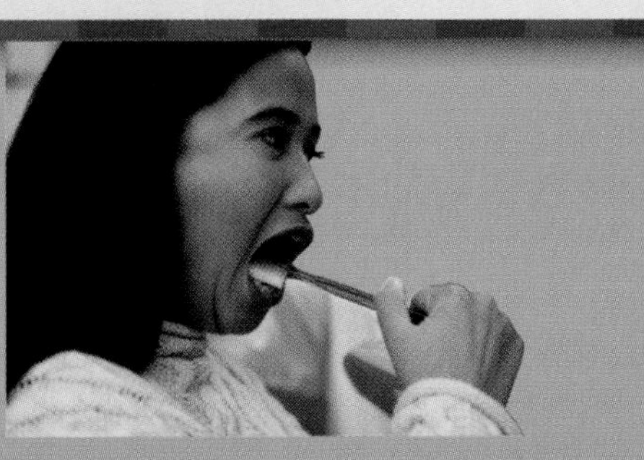

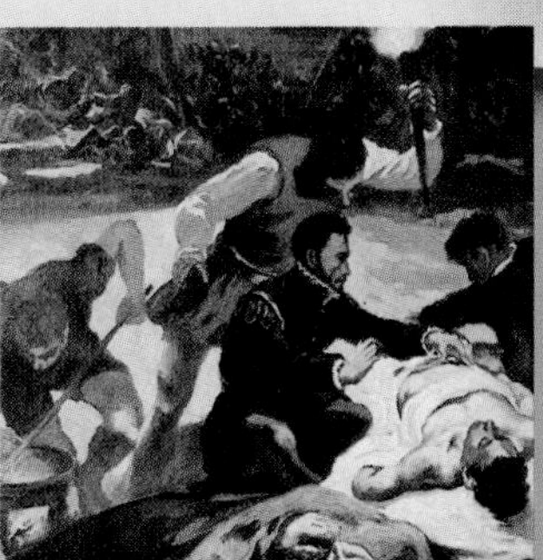

1529

French physician Ambroïse Paré devises amputation to save lives and also creates the first artificial leg. He is shown here working with wounded soldiers on the battlefield

Measure Your Progress: Learning Objectives

After you study this chapter, you should be able to

1. Identify the five skills that make up medical language communication.
2. Describe three characteristics of each of these word parts: combining form, suffix, prefix.
3. Give the medical meaning of common combining forms, suffixes, and prefixes.
4. Demonstrate how to combine word parts to build a medical word.
5. Demonstrate how to define and analyze medical words by dividing them into word parts.
6. Give six examples of common medical words derived from Latin, Greek, or other languages.
7. Describe how to form the plural of common Latin and Greek singular nouns.
8. Contrast the medical record with the health record, computerized patient record, and electronic patient record.
9. Correctly spell and pronounce medical words presented in this chapter.
10. Test your knowledge of medical word structure by completing review exercises at the end of the chapter and learning activities on the CD-ROM.

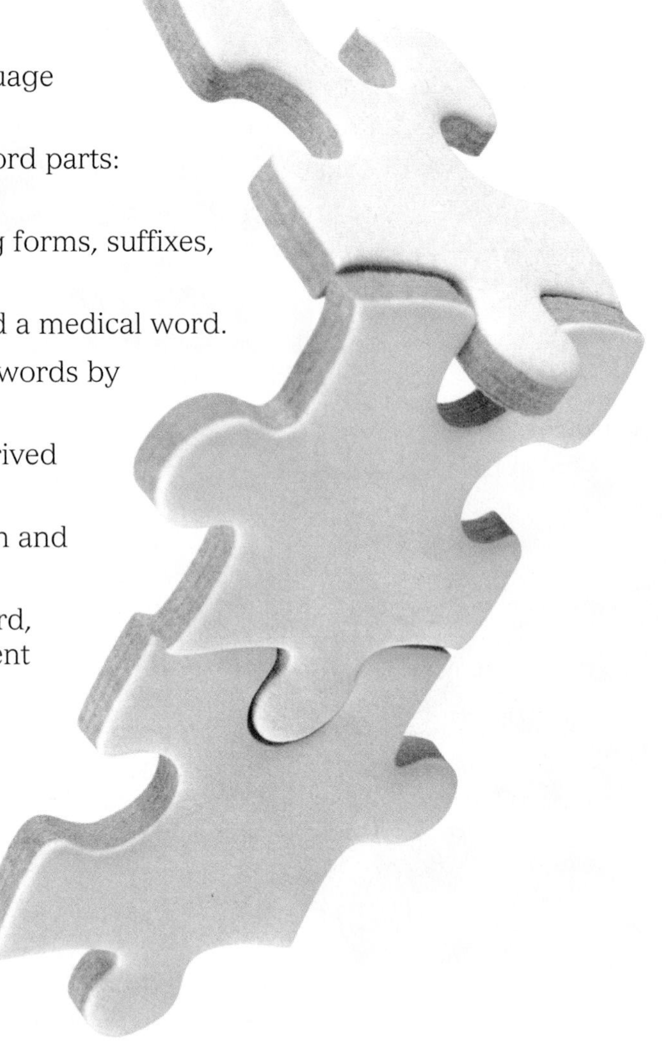

www.prenhall.com/turley

For interactive flashcards, real-life video clips, games, exercises, and audio pronunciations please explore the companion CD-ROM in the back of the book. Click on the companion website for bonus chapters, additional resources, and links to on-line learning.

Welcome to Medical Language

You are about to begin a study of medical language. This will involve time and effort on your part. What can you expect in return? What benefits come from learning medical language? To find out, read Scenario 1 that follows and contrast it with Scenario 2.

Scenario 1

Imagine that you just made an important decision that will affect the rest of your life: You decided to move to a foreign country. You are excited and anxious to get going! When you arrive, you are thrilled to be in this new, exotic environment. It is fascinating to you! You want to absorb everything you can. There are so many new sights and sounds. You want to join in and participate. You want to embrace this new culture and become part of it, but your first attempts at interacting are awkward because you do not know the language. You can't seem to make anyone understand you. All around you, people are engaged in interesting activities and important conversations, but you can't join in because you can't understand them. You feel confused and helpless. Your future in this country now seems uncertain, and you wonder if you will ever be anything more than just a spectator here. What went wrong?

Scenario 2

Imagine that you just made an important decision that will affect the rest of your life: You decided to pursue a career in the healthcare field. You are excited and anxious to get going! When you walk into a physician's office, clinic, or hospital, you are thrilled to be in this new, fast-paced, exotic environment. It is fascinating to you! You want to absorb everything you can. There are so many new sights and sounds. You want to join in and participate. You want to embrace the medical culture and become part of it. Your first attempts at interacting with other healthcare professionals are successful because you know medical language. Immediately, you are immersed in interesting medical activities and important conversations, and you understand what is going on. You feel excited and empowered! Your future in the healthcare field is certain because you took the time to study medical language.

Healthcare professionals know that there is no substitute for a thorough, working knowledge of medical language (see Figure 1-1 ■). Medical language is your key to a successful career in the healthcare field.

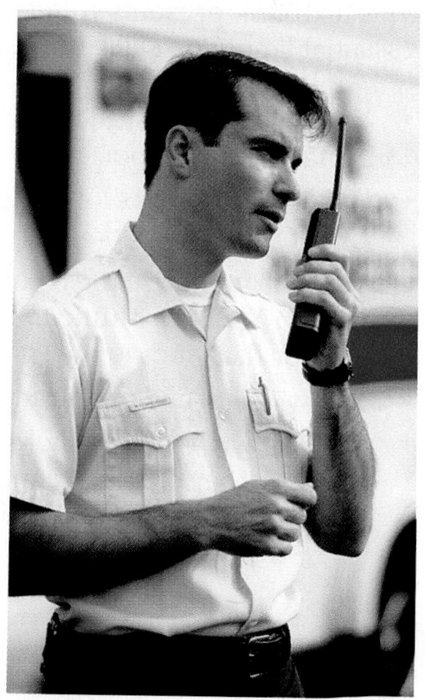

Figure 1-1 ■ Medical language.

This paramedic is using medical language to communicate with healthcare professionals in the emergency department of the hospital. He is describing the condition of the patient in the ambulance. How important do you think it is for this paramedic to have a thorough, working knowledge of medical language?

Communication and Medical Language

Communication in any language consists of five language skills:

1. Reading
2. Listening
3. Thinking and analyzing
4. Speaking
5. Writing

communication (koh-MYOO-nih-KAY-shun)
communicat/o- *impart, transmit*
-ion *action; condition*

These same five language skills are important in **medical language.** You need to be fluent in all five medical language skills in order to communicate with other healthcare professionals (see Figure 1-2■).

The first two skills involve receiving medical language: you read a medical document or listen to someone speak medical language. The third skill involves processing medical language: you think about what you see or hear. This involves memorizing, categorizing, analyzing, and understanding information. The last two skills involve relaying medical language: you speak medical language or write or type a medical document.

medical (MED-ih-kal)
medic/o- *physician; medicine*
-al *pertaining to*

language (LANG-gwij)

All five skills are critical in the communication of medical language. This textbook presents numerous opportunities to practice these five essential language skills until you have mastered all of them.

- You will **read** medical words in each chapter. You will also read many actual medical reports.
- You will **hear** real physicians speak medical language on the CD-ROM.
- You will memorize the meanings of word parts and **analyze** medical words. You will **think** about medical reports you have read and answer fact-finding as well as critical-thinking questions.
- You will practice **pronouncing** medical words.
- You will **write** medical words and word parts. You will type medical words in the context of a medical sentence in the CD-ROM exercises. You will correctly spell medical words.

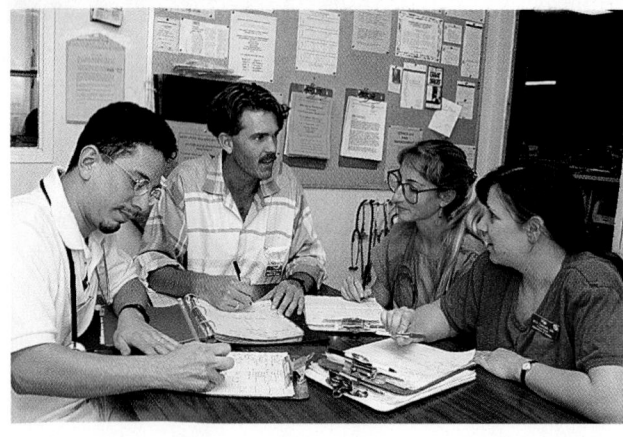

Figure 1-2 ■ Medical language communication.
These healthcare professionals are using all five medical language skills in order to communicate successfully. They are speaking medical language, listening to medical language, thinking about medical language, reading medical language, and writing medical language.

Even though the field of medicine is complex and there are many medical words to learn, that doesn't mean that everything about medical language is complex and hard to understand. Let's begin our study by looking at word parts and how they are used to build medical words.

Medical Words and Word Parts

Medical language is composed of medical words. Each medical word is composed of word parts. Word parts are the puzzle pieces that make up medical words.

There are only three different kinds of word parts: combining forms, suffixes, and prefixes. It is good to memorize the meanings of as many word parts as you can because the same word part appears again and again in different medical words, and its meaning remains the same. Let's look more closely at each of the three kinds of word parts.

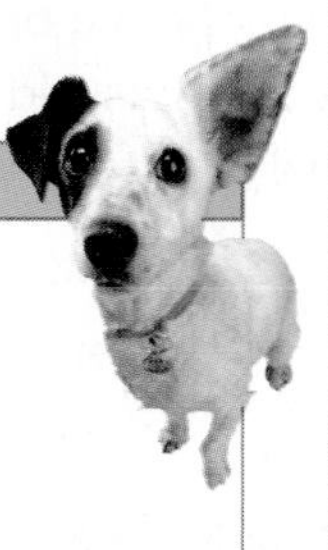

Word Alert

MEDICAL WORD PARTS

Word Part	Meaning
prefix	an optional word beginning
combining form	the foundation of the word
suffix	the word ending

Combining Forms

A combining form contains two parts: a root and a combining vowel (see Figure 1-3 ■). The root contains the medical meaning. The combining vowel allows the combining form to join with another word part. The root is separated from the combining vowel by a forward slash. The combining vowel (usually an *o,* occasionally an *i*) is at the end of the combining form.

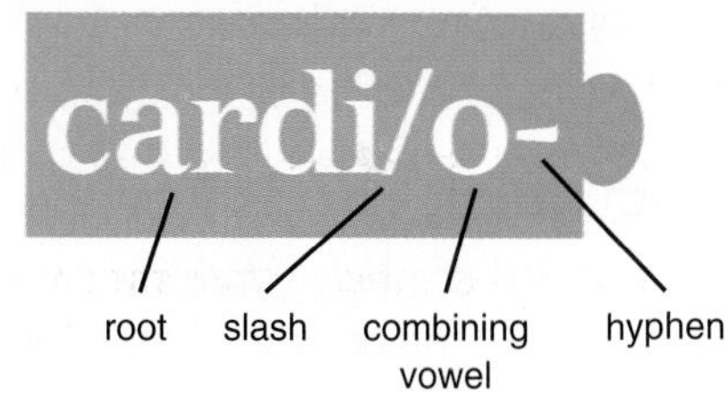

Figure 1-3 ■ Combining form.

A combining form is the foundation of a medical word. A combining form contains a root, a combining vowel, a forward slash that separates the root from the combining vowel, and a hyphen at the end to show that the combining form is a word part, not a complete word. The combining form *cardi/o-* means *heart.*

Characteristics of a Combining Form

- Every medical word contains a combining form.
- A combining form is the foundation of a medical word and gives the word its medical meaning.
- Sometimes a medical word contains two or more combining forms, one right after the other.
- Prefixes and suffixes modify the meaning of the combining form.
- A combining form is the first word part if there is no prefix. Otherwise, the combining form is positioned in the middle of a medical word between the prefix and the suffix.
- A combining form always ends with a hyphen to show that it is a word part, not a complete word. The hyphen is deleted when the combining form joins with a suffix.

Here are examples of some common combining forms that you will ncounter as you study the chapters in this book. Take a moment to udy these combining forms and memorize their meanings so that ou will be ready to use them to build medical words.

ome Common Combining Forms

Combining Form	Medical Meaning
appendic/o-	appendix
arthr/o-	joint
cardi/o-	heart
cutane/o-	skin
esthes/o-	sensation, feeling
gastr/o-	stomach
hemat/o-	blood
hepat/o-	liver
laryng/o-	larynx (voice box)
mast/o-	breast; mastoid process
nas/o-	nose
nat/o-	birth
neur/o-	nerve
pneumon/o-	lung; air
psych/o-	mind
retin/o-	retina (of the eye)
tonsill/o-	tonsil
trache/o-	trachea (windpipe)
urin/o-	urine; urinary system
ven/o-	vein

Combining Forms Review

Here are the combining forms you have learned so far. Next to each combining form, write its meaning. Use the Answer Key at the end of the book to check your answers. The first one has been done for you.

	Combining Form	Medical Meaning		Combining Form	Medical Meaning
1.	pneumon/o-	lung	11.	mast/o-	
2.	appendic/o-		12.	nas/o-	
3.	arthr/o-		13.	nat/o-	
4.	cardi/o-		14.	neur/o-	
5.	cutane/o-		15.	psych/o-	
6.	esthes/o-		16.	retin/o-	
7.	gastr/o-		17.	tonsill/o-	
8.	hemat/o-		18.	trache/o-	
9.	hepat/o-		19.	urin/o-	
10.	laryng/o-		20.	ven/o-	

Suffixes

Characteristics of a Suffix

- Every medical word contains a suffix.
- A suffix can be a single letter or a group of letters.
- A suffix cannot be the foundation of a medical word.
- A suffix is always positioned at the end of a medical word. Occasionally, a medical word contains two suffixes, one right after the other.
- A suffix attaches to the end of a combining form and modifies its meaning.
- A suffix always begins with a hyphen to show that it is a word part, not a complete word. The hyphen is deleted when the suffix joins the combining form.

Here are examples of some common suffixes. Take a moment to study these suffixes and memorize their meanings so that you will be ready to use them to build medical words.

Some Common Suffixes

Suffix	*Medical Meaning*	*Example and Definition*
-ac	pertaining to	cardiac (pertaining to the heart)
-al	pertaining to	nasal (pertaining to the nose)
-ar	pertaining to	muscular (pertaining to the muscle)
-ary	pertaining to	urinary (pertaining to urine)
-ation	a process; being or having	urination (a process of making urine)
-ous	pertaining to	venous (pertaining to the vein)
-tic	pertaining to	dietetic (pertaining to the diet)

Some Common Suffixes that Describe Diseases

Suffix	*Medical Meaning*	*Example and Definition*
-ia	condition, state, thing	pneumonia (condition of the lung)
-ion	action; condition	digestion (action of digesting food)
-ism	process; disease from a specific cause	alcoholism (disease caused by alcohol)
-itis	inflammation of	tonsillitis (inflammation of the tonsil)
-megaly	enlargement	hepatomegaly (enlargement of the liver)
-oma	tumor, mass	neuroma (tumor of the nerve)
-osis	condition; abnormal condition; process	psychosis (abnormal condition of the mind)
-pathy	disease, suffering	retinopathy (disease of the retina of the eye)

Some Common Suffixes that Describe Procedures or Instruments

Suffix	*Medical Meaning*	*Example and Definition*
-ectomy	surgical excision	appendectomy (surgical excision [removal] of the appendix)
-graphy	process of recording	electrocardiography (process of recording the electrical activity of the heart)
-scopy	process of using an instrument to examine	gastroscopy (process of using an instrument to examine the stomach)

Some Common Suffixes that Describe Medical Specialties or Specialists

Suffix	*Medical Meaning*	*Example and Definition*
-iatry	medical treatment	psychiatry (medical treatment for the mind)
-itian	a skilled professional or expert	dietitian (a skilled professional or expert in foods and diet)
-logy	the study of	urology (the study of the urinary system)

Suffixes Review

Here are the suffixes you have learned so far. Next to each suffix, write its meaning. Use the Answer Key at the end of the book to check your answers. The first one has been done for you.

Suffix	Medical Meaning	Suffix	Medical Meaning
1. -ac	pertaining to	11. -ion	
2. -al		12. -ism	
3. -ar		13. -itis	
4. -ary		14. -logy	
5. -ation		15. -megaly	
6. -ectomy		16. -oma	
7. -graphy		17. -osis	
8. -ia		18. -ous	
9. -iatry		19. -pathy	
10. -itian		20. -scopy	

Building Medical Words: Combining Forms and Suffixes

Medical words are like puzzles, and their word parts are like the pieces of the puzzle. To build a medical word, you must put the word part puzzle pieces together in the correct way.

Follow these two simple rules for joining a combining form to a suffix to make a medical word.

1. If the suffix begins with a vowel, delete the combining vowel from the combining form. Delete the slash and hyphen from the combining form, delete the hyphen from the suffix, and then join the two word parts (see Figure 1-4 ■).
2. If the suffix begins with a consonant, keep the combining vowel on the combining form (see Figure 1-5 ■).

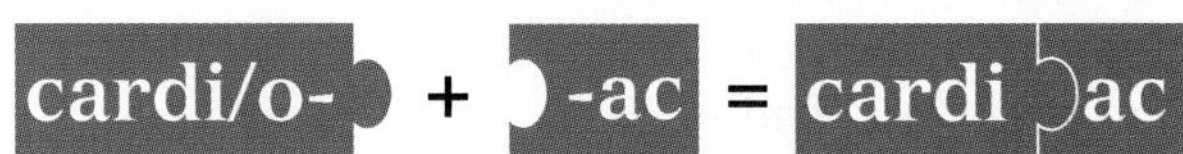

Figure 1-4 ■ Combining form plus a suffix that begins with a vowel.

The combining form *cardi/o-* plus the suffix *-ac* equals the medical word *cardiac. Cardiac* means *pertaining to the heart.*

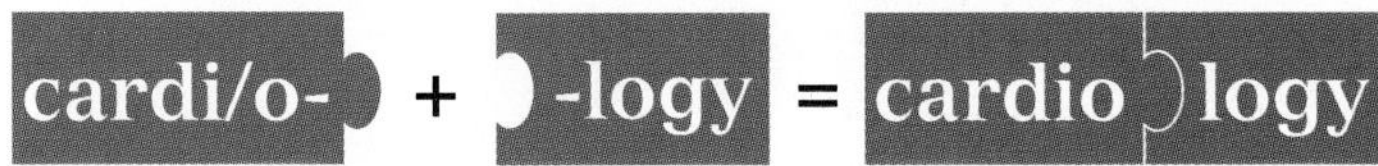

Figure 1-5 ■ Combining form plus a suffix that begins with a consonant.

The combining form *cardi/o-* plus the suffix *-logy* equals the medical word *cardiology. Cardiology* means *the study of the heart.*

Building Medical Words Exercise

Correctly join these combining forms and suffixes to make a medical word. Use the Answer Key at the end of the book to check your answers. The first one has been done for you.

	Combining Form	Suffix	Medical Word		Combining Form	Suffix	Medical Word
1.	hepat/o-	-ic	hepatic	14.	appendic/o-	-itis	
2.	nas/o-	-al		15.	laryng/o-	-itis	
3.	tonsill/o-	-ar		16.	hepat/o-	-itis	
4.	trache/o-	-al		17.	gastr/o-	-itis	
5.	cardi/o-	-ac		18.	tonsill/o-	-itis	
6.	cutane/o-	-ous		19.	mast/o-	-itis	
7.	gastr/o-	-ic		20.	arthr/o-	-itis	
8.	neur/o-	-al		21.	hepat/o-	-megaly	
9.	urin/o-	-ary		22.	hemat/o-	-oma	
10.	retin/o-	-al		23.	psych/o-	-osis	
11.	ven/o-	-ous		24.	retin/o-	-pathy	
12.	urin/o-	-ation		25.	neur/o-	-pathy	
13.	pneumon/o-	-ia		26.	append/o-	-ectomy	

	Combining Form	Suffix	Medical Word		Combining Form	Suffix	Medical Word
27.	mast/o-	-ectomy	________	32.	psych/o-	-iatry	________
28.	tonsill/o-	-ectomy	________	33.	cardi/o-	-logy	________
29.	laryng/o-	-ectomy	________	34.	hemat/o-	-logy	________
30.	gastr/o-	-scopy	________	35.	neur/o-	-logy	________
31.	arthr/o-	-scopy	________	36.	psych/o-	-logy	________

Analyzing and Defining Medical Words: Combining Forms and Suffixes

When you analyze something, you break it into smaller pieces that are easier to understand. When you analyze a medical word, you break it into its component word parts. In order to define a medical word, you must first define each word part by giving its medical meaning. The meanings of all the word parts are then combined to give the definition of the entire medical word.

Follow these three simple rules to define a medical word that contains a combining form and a suffix.

1. To unlock the meaning of a medical word with two word parts (combining form and suffix), define each word part.
2. Then put the definitions of the word parts in order, beginning with the definition of the suffix, followed by the definition of the combining form.
3. Add small connecting words to make a correct and complete definition.

Analyzing and Defining Medical Words Exercise

Look at the medical word that is given. On the first line, write the suffix and its definition. On the second line, write the combining form and its definition. On the third line, write the complete definition of the medical word. Use the Answer Key at the end of the book to check your answers. The first one has been done for you.

	Medical Word		Word Part	Word Part Meaning
1.	laryngitis	SUFFIX	-itis	inflammation of
	(LAIR-in-JY-tis)	COMBINING FORM	laryng/o-	larynx (voice box)
		MEDICAL WORD DEFINITION	inflammation of the larynx	
	When you have laryngitis, you often lose your voice.			
2.	cardiac	SUFFIX	________	________
	(KAR-dee-ak)	COMBINING FORM	________	________
		MEDICAL WORD DEFINITION	________	
	Patients with cardiac disease may have an abnormal heart rhythm or a weakened heart muscle.			
3.	neurology	SUFFIX	________	________
	(nyoo-RAWL-oh-jee)	COMBINING FORM	________	________
		MEDICAL WORD DEFINITION	________	
	Patients with diseases like multiple sclerosis and Parkinson's disease are treated in the neurology clinic.			

Medical Word		Word Part	Word Part Meaning
4. mastectomy	SUFFIX	________	______________
(mas-TEK-toh-mee)	COMBINING FORM	________	______________
	MEDICAL WORD DEFINITION	______________________	
A patient with cancer of the breast may have to have a mastectomy.			
5. tonsillar	SUFFIX	________	______________
(TAWN-sih-lar)	COMBINING FORM	________	______________
	MEDICAL WORD DEFINITION	______________________	
The tonsillar area in the back of the throat is a frequent site of infections.			
6. gastroscopy	SUFFIX	________	______________
(gas-TRAWS-koh-pee)	COMBINING FORM	________	______________
	MEDICAL WORD DEFINITION	______________________	
A patient with constant stomach pain may need to have a gastroscopy to look for ulcers or bleeding.			
7. hematoma	SUFFIX	________	______________
(HEE-mah-TOH-mah)	COMBINING FORM	________	______________
	MEDICAL WORD DEFINITION	______________________	
After an injury, a hematoma may form under the skin.			
8. hepatic	SUFFIX	________	______________
(heh-PAT-ik)	COMBINING FORM	________	______________
	MEDICAL WORD DEFINITION	______________________	
Hepatic diseases that affect the liver include hepatitis and liver cancer.			
9. psychology	SUFFIX	________	______________
(sy-KAWL-oh-jee)	COMBINING FORM	________	______________
	MEDICAL WORD DEFINITION	______________________	
An understanding of psychology enables healthcare professionals to deal with difficult patients.			
10. pneumonia	SUFFIX	________	______________
(noo-MOH-nee-ah)	COMBINING FORM	________	______________
	MEDICAL WORD DEFINITION	______________________	
An infection of the lungs like pneumonia causes hazy, white areas on a chest x-ray.			
11. venous	SUFFIX	________	______________
(VEE-nus)	COMBINING FORM	________	______________
	MEDICAL WORD DEFINITION	______________________	
Venous blood is dark blue-purple because it does not contain much oxygen.			
12. arthritis	SUFFIX	________	______________
(ar-THRY-tis)	COMBINING FORM	________	______________
	MEDICAL WORD DEFINITION	______________________	
Arthritis in the hip joints can make walking very painful.			

Pronouncing Medical Words: Combining Forms and Suffixes

Knowing the meaning of a medical word is important, but being able to pronounce the word correctly is equally important. Because medical word pronunciation is such a vital skill, you need to start practicing it right now. Each chapter in this textbook includes pronunciation guides for the medical words presented. These are "see and say" pronunciation guides. They are straightforward and easy to use. The syllables are separated by hyphens. Just say each syllable by following the phonetic spelling. Accented syllables are in all capital letters; secondary accented syllables are in smaller capital letters. When you look at a medical word and use the pronunciation guide to help you say the word correctly, you are forming a complete and accurate word memory. Now use the "see and say" pronunciation guides to help you practice the correct pronunciation of the medical words you have built.

Pronouncing Medical Words Exercise

Look at each medical word and its pronunciation guide. Practice pronouncing the word several times until you have mastered its pronunciation.

	Medical Word	Pronunciation		Medical Word	Pronunciation
1.	appendectomy	(AP-pen-DEK-toh-mee)	19.	mastitis	(mas-TY-tis)
2.	appendicitis	(ah-PEN-dih-SY-tis)	20.	nasal	(NAY-zal)
3.	arthritis	(ar-THRY-tis)	21.	neural	(NYOOR-al)
4.	arthroscopy	(ar-THRAWS-koh-pee)	22.	neurology	(nyoo-RAWL-oh-jee)
5.	cardiac	(KAR-dee-ak)	23.	neuropathy	(nyoo-RAWP-ah-thee)
6.	cardiology	(KAR-dee-AWL-oh-jee)	24.	pneumonia	(nyoo-MOH-nee-ah)
7.	cutaneous	(kyoo-TAY-nee-us)	25.	psychiatry	(sy-KY-ah-tree)
8.	gastric	(GAS-trik)	26.	psychology	(sy-KAWL-oh-jee)
9.	gastritis	(gas-TRY-tis)	27.	psychosis	(sy-KOH-sis)
10.	gastroscopy	(gas-TRAWS-koh-pee)	28.	retinal	(RET-ih-nal)
11.	hematology	(HEE-mah-TAWL-oh-jee)	29.	retinopathy	(RET-ih-NAWP-ah-thee)
12.	hematoma	(HEE-mah-TOH-mah)	30.	tonsillar	(TAWN-sih-lar)
13.	hepatic	(heh-PAT-ik)	31.	tonsillectomy	(TAWN-sih-LEK-toh-mee)
14.	hepatitis	(HEP-ah-TY-tis)	32.	tonsillitis	(TAWN-sih-LY-tis)
15.	hepatomegaly	(HEP-ah-toh-MEG-ah-lee)	33.	tracheal	(TRAY-kee-al)
16.	laryngectomy	(LAIR-in-JEK-toh-mee)	34.	urinary	(YOO-rih-nair-ee)
17.	laryngitis	(LAIR-in-JY-tis)	35.	urination	(YOO-rih-NAY-shun)
18.	mastectomy	(mas-TEK-toh-mee)	36.	venous	(VEE-nus)

Prefixes

Characteristics of a Prefix

- Not every medical word contains a prefix. It is an optional word part.
- A prefix can be a single letter or a group of letters.
- A prefix cannot be the foundation of a medical word.
- When present, a prefix is always positioned at the beginning of a medical word. Occasionally, a medical word has two prefixes, one right after the other.
- A prefix attaches to the beginning of a combining form and modifies its meaning.
- A prefix always ends with a hyphen to show that it is a word part, not a complete word. The hyphen is deleted when the prefix joins the combining form.

Here are examples of some common prefixes. Take a moment to study these prefixes and memorize their meanings so that you will be ready to use them to build medical words.

Some Common Prefixes that Describe Location or Direction

Prefix	*Medical Meaning*	*Example and Definition*
endo-	innermost, within	endotracheal (pertaining to within the trachea)
intra-	within	intravenous (pertaining to within the vein)
peri-	around	perinatal (pertaining to around the time of birth)
sub-	below; underneath; less than	subcutaneous (pertaining to underneath the skin)

Some Common Prefixes that Describe Amount or Size

Prefix	*Medical Meaning*	*Example and Definition*
an-	without, not	anesthesia (condition of not feeling)
hyper-	above; more than normal	hyperactive (pertaining to more than normal activity)
hypo-	below; deficient	hypothyroidism (disease from a specific cause of below-normal functioning of the thyroid gland)
poly-	many, much	polyuria (condition of much urine)

Some Common Prefixes that Describe Time or Speed

Prefix	*Medical Meaning*	*Example and Definition*
brady-	slow	bradycardia (condition of a slow heart rate)
pre-	before, in front of	prenatal (pertaining to before birth)
post-	after, behind	postnatal (pertaining to after birth)
tachy-	fast	tachycardia (condition of a fast heart rate)

Some Common Prefixes that Describe a Characteristic

Prefix	*Medical Meaning*	*Example and Definition*
anti-	against	antipsychotic (pertaining to a drug that is against psychosis)
dys-	painful, difficult, abnormal	dysfunctional (pertaining to abnormal function)

Prefixes Review

Here are the prefixes you have learned so far. Next to each prefix, write its medical meaning. Use the Answer Key at the end of the book to check your answers. The first one has been done for you.

Prefix	Medical Meaning	Prefix	Meaning
1. an-	without, not	8. intra-	______
2. anti-	______	9. peri-	______
3. brady-	______	10. poly-	______
4. dys-	______	11. post-	______
5. endo-	______	12. pre-	______
6. hyper-	______	13. sub-	______
7. hypo-	______	14. tachy-	______

Building Medical Words: Prefixes, Combining Forms, and Suffixes

Follow these two simple rules for joining a prefix to a combining form with suffix to make a medical word.

1. Delete the hyphen from the prefix (see Figure 1-6 ■). (Note: Some medical words, but not all, keep the hyphen if the last letter of the prefix is the same as the first letter of the combining form.)
2. Join the prefix to the beginning of the combining form.

intra- + cardi/o- + -ac = intra cardi ac

Figure 1-6 ■ Prefix plus a combining form plus a suffix.

The prefix *intra-* plus the combining form *cardi/o-* plus the suffix *-ac* equals the medical word *intracardiac. Intracardiac* means *pertaining to within the heart.*

Building Medical Words Exercise

Correctly join these prefixes, combining forms, and suffixes to make a medical word. Use the Answer Key at the end of the book to check your answers. The first one has been done for you.

Prefix	Combining Form	Suffix	Medical Word
1. post-	nat/o-	-al	postnatal
2. peri-	tonsill/o-	-ar	________
3. intra-	nas/o-	-al	________
4. an-	esthes/o-	-ia	________
5. anti-	psych/o-	-tic	________
6. sub-	cutane/o-	-ous	________
7. tachy-	cardi/o-	-ia	________
8. poly-	neur/o-	-pathy	________
9. endo-	trache/o-	-al	________
10. intra-	ven/o-	-ous	________

Analyzing and Defining Medical Words: Prefixes, Combining Forms, and Suffixes

In order to define a medical word, you must first define each word part by giving its medical meaning. The meanings of all the word parts are then combined to give the definition of the entire medical word.

Follow these three simple rules to define a medical word that contains a prefix, combining form, and a suffix.

1. Define each word part.
2. Put the definitions of the word parts in order, beginning with the suffix, followed by the prefix, and then the combining form.
3. Add small connecting words to make a correct and complete definition.

Analyzing and Defining Medical Words Exercise

Look at the medical word that is given. On the first line, write the suffix and its definition. On the second line, write the prefix and its definition. On the third line, write the combining form and its definition. On the fourth line, write the complete definition of the medical word. Use the Answer Key at the end of the book to check your answers. The first one has been done for you.

Medical Word		Word Part	Word Part Meaning
1. postnatal	SUFFIX	-al	pertaining to
(post-NAY-tal)	PREFIX	post-	after, behind
	COMBINING FORM	nat/o-	birth
	MEDICAL WORD DEFINITION	pertaining to after birth	

After birth, the newborn baby enters the postnatal period.

Medical Word		Word Part	Word Part Meaning
2. anesthesia	SUFFIX	________	____________
(AN-es-THEE-zee-ah)	PREFIX	________	____________
	COMBINING FORM	________	____________
	MEDICAL WORD DEFINITION	____________________	

Drugs are used to numb the skin and produce anesthesia prior to a procedure.

3. intranasal	SUFFIX	________	____________
(IN-trah-NAY-zal)	PREFIX	________	____________
	COMBINING FORM	________	____________
	MEDICAL WORD DEFINITION	____________________	

An intranasal gauze pad is placed in the nostril to control bleeding from the nose.

4. polyneuropathy	SUFFIX	________	____________
(PAWL-ee-nyoo-RAWP-ah-thee)	PREFIX	________	____________
	COMBINING FORM	________	____________
	MEDICAL WORD DEFINITION	____________________	

Polyneuropathy is a disease condition that affects many nerves.

5. peritonsillar	SUFFIX	________	____________
(PAIR-ee-TAWN-sih-lar)	PREFIX	________	____________
	COMBINING FORM	________	____________
	MEDICAL WORD DEFINITION	____________________	

A peritonsillar abscess can form in the area around an infected tonsil.

6. subcutaneous	SUFFIX	________	____________
(SUB-kyoo-TAY-nee-us)	PREFIX	________	____________
	COMBINING FORM	________	____________
	MEDICAL WORD DEFINITION	____________________	

Diabetic patients give themselves insulin injections under the skin into the fatty subcutaneous tissue.

7. tachycardia	SUFFIX	________	____________
(TAK-ih-KAR-dee-ah)	PREFIX	________	____________
	COMBINING FORM	________	____________
	MEDICAL WORD DEFINITION	____________________	

Tachycardia is a medical condition in which the heart has an abnormally fast rhythm.

Medical Word		Word Part	Word Part Meaning
8. intravenous	SUFFIX	________	________________
(IN-trah-VEE-nus)	PREFIX	________	________________
	COMBINING FORM	________	________________
	MEDICAL WORD DEFINITION	________________________	

Patients who are unable to eat are given fluids through an intravenous line into a vein.

Medical Word		Word Part	Word Part Meaning
9. endotracheal	SUFFIX	________	________________
(EN-doh-TRAY-kee-al)	PREFIX	________	________________
	COMBINING FORM	________	________________
	MEDICAL WORD DEFINITION	________________________	

An endotracheal tube is inserted through the mouth and into the trachea to help a patient breathe.

Word Alert

Some medical words contain more than one combining form. When joining two combining forms, keep the combining vowel on the first combining form and delete the slashes and hyphens.

Example: gastr/o- + intestin/o- + -al = gastrointestinal

Occasionally a medical word has two suffixes. Join the two suffixes by deleting the hyphens. The same is true for two prefixes.

Example: neur/o- + log/o- + -ic + -al = neurological

Pronouncing Medical Words: Prefixes, Combining Forms, and Suffixes

Use the "see and say" pronunciation guides to help you practice the correct pronunciation of the medical words you built.

Pronouncing Medical Words Exercise

Look at each medical word and its pronunciation guide. Practice pronouncing the word several times until you have mastered its pronunciation.

Medical Word	Pronunciation	Medical Word	Pronunciation
1. anesthesia	(AN-es-THEE-zee-ah)	6. subcutaneous	(SUB-kyoo-TAY-nee-us)
2. intranasal	(IN-trah-NAY-zal)	7. tachycardia	(TAK-ih-KAR-dee-ah)
3. polyneuropathy	(PAWL-ee-nyoo-RAWP-ah-thee)	8. intravenous	(IN-trah-VEE-nus)
4. peritonsillar	(PAIR-ee-TAWN-sih-lar)	9. endotracheal	(EN-doh-TRAY-kee-al)
5. postnatal	(post-NAY-tal)		

Medical Language Origins

Now let's briefly look at how medical language began. By doing this, you will begin to see some underlying patterns that will make it easier for you to learn medical language.

Etymology is the study of word origins and derivations. In medical language, as in the English language, many words have been taken (derived) from other languages, particularly Latin and Greek. Why? Because in ancient times both the Greeks and Romans advanced the study and practice of medicine. They named anatomic structures, diseases, and treatments in their own languages, and these Latin and Greek words remain a part of medical language today. Some medical words are the actual Latin or Greek words that were used centuries ago. You'll be surprised to see how many of these words are familiar to you.

etymology (ET-ih-MAWL-oh-jee)
etym/o- *word origin*
-logy *the study of*

Word Alert

Medical Word	Language of Origin	Definition	Pronunciation
nucleus	Latin *nucleus*	the command center of a cell	**nucleus** (NOO-klee-us)
pelvis	Latin *pelvis*	the hip bones	**pelvis** (PEL-vis)
sinus	Latin *sinus*	hollow cavity in the cranial bone	**sinus** (SY-nus)
thorax	Greek *thorax*	the chest and chest cavity	**thorax** (THOR-aks)

Medical words are also derived from similar (but not identical) Latin or Greek words.

Medical Word	Language of Origin	Definition	Pronunciation
artery	Latin *arteria*	blood vessel that carries blood away from the heart	**artery** (AR-ter-ee)
cell	Latin *cella*	smallest independent part of the body	**cell** (SELL)
muscle	Latin *musculus*	structure that contracts and enables the body to move	**muscle** (MUS-el)
phobia	Greek *phobos*	an irrational fear	**phobia** (FOH-bee-ah)
sperm	Greek *sperma*	male sex cell that fertilizes the female's egg	**sperm** (SPERM)
vein	Latin *vena*	blood vessel that carries blood back to the heart	**vein** (VAYN)

Medical words are also derived from other ancient languages: English, Dutch, and French.

Medical Word	Language of Origin	Description	Pronunciation
bladder	English *blaedre*	hollow sac that holds urine	**bladder** (BLAD-er)
drug	Dutch *droog*	medicine	**drug** (DRUHG)
heart	English *heorte*	muscle that pumps the blood	**heart** (HART)
physician	French *physicien*	doctor	**physician** (fih-ZISH-un)

Medical Word Singular and Plural Nouns

Because medical language contains so many Latin and Greek words, it is important to know how to make the plural forms of Latin and Greek words. The Latin and Greek languages had rules that governed how plural nouns were formed, and those rules still apply today.

Singular and Plural Noun Endings

Category	*Singular Ending*	*How to Form the Plural*	*Example*
Latin noun (feminine)	*-a*	Change *-a* to *-ae*	vertebra → vertebrae
Latin noun (masculine)	*-us*	Change *-us* to *-i*	nucleus → nuclei
Latin noun (neuter)	*-um*	Change *-um* to -a	atrium → atria bacterium → bacteria
Latin noun (other)	*-is*	Change *-is* to *-es*	diagnosis → diagnoses testis → testes
	-ex, -ix	Change *-ex* or *-ix* to *-ices*	helix → helices apex → apices
Greek noun	*-nx*	Change *-nx* to *-nges*	phalanx → phalanges
	-on	Change *-on* to *-a*	ganglion → ganglia
	-oma	Change *-oma* to *-omata*	carcinoma → carcinomata

Pronunciation Guide for Latin Singular and Plural Nouns

Latin feminine, masculine, and neuter nouns have rules that govern the pronunciation of their singular and plural forms.

Latin Feminine Singular	*Latin Feminine Plural*	*Medical Meaning*
bursa (BER-sah)	bursae (BER-see)	fluid-filled sac under a tendon
scapula (SKAP-yoo-lah)	scapulae (SKAP-yoo-lee)	shoulder blade
vertebra (VER-teh-brah)	vertebrae (VER-teh-bree)	bone in the spinal column

Latin Masculine Singular	*Latin Masculine Plural*	*Medical Meaning*
bronchus (BRONG-kus)	bronchi (BRONG-kigh)	air tube leading to the lung
musculus (MUS-kyoo-lus)	musculi (MUS-kyoo-lie)	Latin word for *muscle*

Latin Neuter Singular	*Latin Neuter Plural*	*Medical Meaning*
atrium (AA-tree-um)	atria (AA-tree-ah)	upper chamber of the heart
bacterium (bak-TEER-ee-um)	bacteria (bak-TEER-ee-ah)	microscopic disease-causing cell

The Health Record

Three of the six medical language skills necessary for communication are needed to understand medical documents: reading, thinking, and writing (or typing). Let's briefly look at some of the more common types of medical documents and how they are used.

The **medical record** is where healthcare professionals document all care provided to a patient. More recently, the medical record has become known as the **health record,** a reflection of the emphasis on preventive medicine. Most physician office records include a preventive medicine checklist that documents preventive care given to the patient (immunizations, routine physical exams, and so forth), as well as things the patient should do (limit sun exposure and apply sunscreen, have smoke detectors in the home, use seat belts, do monthly examination of the breasts or testicles, secure any firearms kept in the house, and so forth).

medical (MED-ih-kal)
medic/o- *physician; medicine*
-al *pertaining to*

health (HELTH)
Health is derived from an Old English word meaning *whole.*

The paper medical record has been the traditional form of patient medical record. Its disadvantages are that only one person can access it at a time, it can become lost or damaged, and it can take hours or even days to retrieve a patient's past medical records, particularly if they are stored off-site. This delay can compromise the delivery of quality care.

Recently, however, more and more offices, hospitals, and other healthcare facilities are converting some or all of their paper medical records into **computerized patient records (CPRs)** (see Figure 1-7 ■). In these facilities, healthcare professionals can have immediate access to both current and previous medical records.

In the future, it is hoped that an all-encompassing **electronic patient record (EPR)** or an **electronic health record (EHR)** will provide seamless and immediate access by many healthcare professionals to all parts of a patient's record regardless of where those parts were created or stored.

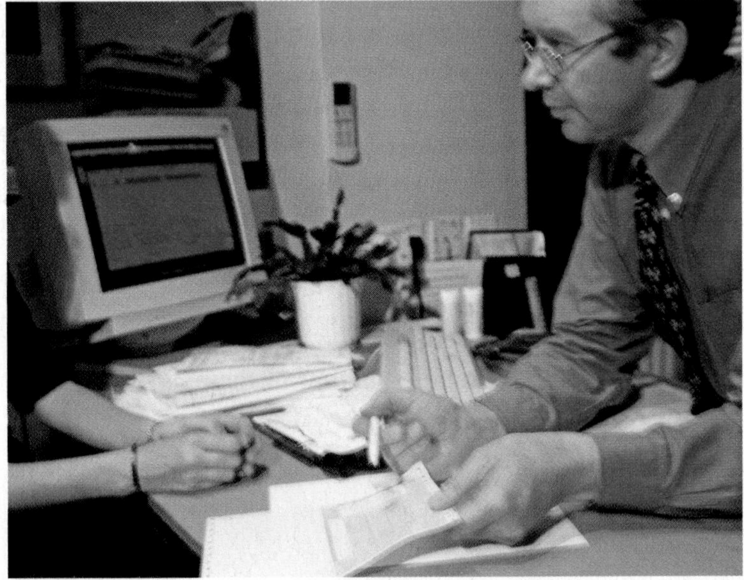

Figure 1-7 ■ Computerized patient record (CPR).

The computerized patient record can provide immediate access to a patient's current and previous medical records from one facility, although it has not entirely replaced the paper record.

Types of Documents in the Health Record

The health record is a medicolegal record. This means that the documents in it contain medical information but are also legal documents.

Before patients can be treated at any type of healthcare facility, they must sign **consent to treatment** forms that give physicians and other healthcare professionals the right to treat them. Treatment without consent is against the law and is considered to be battery (touching another person without his or her consent). For patients who are minors, the parent or legal guardian signs the consent to treatment. In an emergency situation, care is provided until the appropriate person is able to sign. A patient must sign another consent form before surgery can be performed. First, the physician describes the purpose of the proposed surgery and informs the patient of alternatives, risks, and possible complications. Then the patient signs a consent to surgery. This is known as giving **informed consent.**

Patients must also sign a form that allows the facility to contact their insurance companies to obtain payment for health care provided. Under the federal regulations of **HIPAA (the Health Insurance Portability and Accountability Act of 1996),** all healthcare settings must provide patients with a statement verifying that their health record information is kept secure and that it is only released to authorized inquiries from other healthcare providers, insurance companies or healthcare quality monitoring organizations.

The health record varies in format and content from one facility to the next. Short narrative notes and checklists are used in many physicians' offices and clinics. These notes usually contain a brief history of the present illness, pertinent past medical or surgical history, a physical examination, a diagnosis, treatments given, and a follow-up plan. Alternatively, the physician office note may use the **SOAP format** with its headings of subjective, objective, assessment, and plan. Subjective (S) is for the patient's symptoms, objective (O) is for the results of the physical examination by the physician, assessment (A) is for the diagnosis, and plan (P) is for the plan for follow-up care.

SOAP NOTE

Johnson, Roberta C.

11/19/20xx

S: Patient is here today for a routine gynecologic examination. She is currently on Ortho-Novum and reports no difficulty with this oral contraceptive.

O: Breasts reveal no masses or tenderness. Abdomen negative. Pelvic exam was entirely negative. Pap smear taken.

A: Normal gynecologic examination.

P: Reminded to use alternative forms of contraceptive if she misses a pill. Given a prescription for a refill of Ortho-Novum 1/35. To return in 9 months.

Elizabeth R. Lawrence, M.D.

Elizabeth R. Lawrence, M.D.

ERL: btg
D: 11/19/xx
T: 11/19/xx

Hospitals use more extensive documentation than physicians' offices. Common documents for a hospitalized patient include the Admission History and Physical Examination (H&P), Operative Report, and Discharge Summary (DS). These documents include standard headings, as described below. In addition, physicians write orders and progress notes, nurses write nurses' notes, therapists write therapy notes, and other departments contribute their own patient care notes and forms.

Standard Headings in Hospital Documents

- Chief Complaint (CC)
- History of Present Illness (HPI)
- Past Medical and Surgical History
- Review of Systems (ROS)
- Physical Examination (PE)
- Laboratory and X-Ray Data
- Diagnosis (Dx)
- Disposition

Career Focus

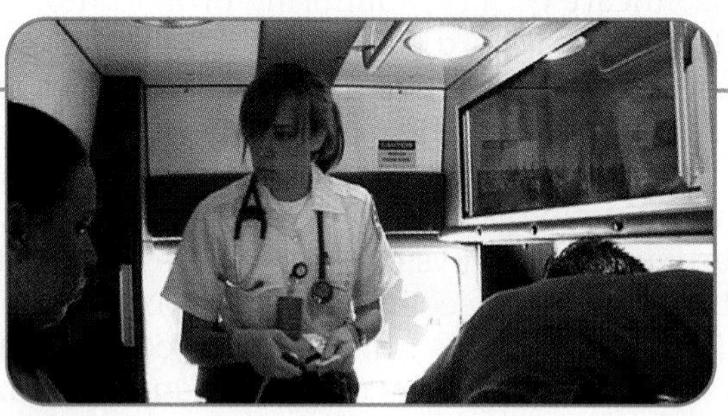

Meet Erica, a paramedic.

"I was always interested in health care. EMTs give basic life support. They can do things such as back boarding a patient, splinting, giving oxygen, taking vital signs, and transporting to the hospital. Paramedics give advanced life support. We can start IVs, give medications. We can defibrillate, give electrocardiotherapy. It's hard to describe a typical day, because no day is like the other. We do a lot of patients with chest pains, shortness of breath, diabetes, seizures, traumas, obviously auto accidents, and industrial accidents. I use medical terminology mostly when I'm writing my run reports, because those are legal documents and they can be looked at by lawyers in the future."

Paramedics are allied health professionals who respond to emergency calls from the community, treat patients in ambulances, and transport them to the emergency department of the hospital. The paramedic provides medical care in a setting that is apart from a hospital or physician's office.

paramedic (PAIR-ah-MED-ik)
para- *beside or apart from*
medic *a shortened form of medical*

Abbreviations

A	assessment (heading in a SOAP note)
CC	chief complaint
CPR	computerized patient record
DS	discharge summary
Dx	diagnosis
EHR	electronic health record
EPR	electronic patient record
H&P	history and physical examination
HIPAA	Health Insurance Portability and Accountability Act (pronounced "HIP-ah")
HPI	history of present illness
O	objective (heading in a SOAP note)
P	plan (heading in a SOAP note)
PE	physical examination
ROS	review of systems
S	subjective (heading in a SOAP note)
SOAP	subjective, objective, assessment, plan (pronounced "soap")

Word Alert

MEDICAL ABBREVIATIONS

Abbreviations are commonly used in all types of medical documents; however, they can mean different things to different people and their meaning can be misinterpreted. Always verify the meaning of an abbreviation.

CC stands for *chief complaint,* but it also stands for *cubic centimeter* (a measure of volume).

CPR stands for *computerized patient record,* but it also stands for *cardiopulmonary resuscitation.*

H&P stands for *history and physical examination,* but the sound-alike abbreviation *HNP* stands for *herniated nucleus pulposus.*

Chapter Review Exercises

Matching Exercise

Match each word part to its description. The word parts may be used more than once.

1. combining form
2. suffix
3. prefix

_____ Begins with a hyphen

_____ Gives the medical meaning of the word

_____ Ends with a combining vowel

_____ Sometimes a medical word doesn't have one

_____ Always positioned at the end of a word

_____ Always positioned at the beginning of a word

_____ When there is no prefix, this is the first part of the word

Definition of Prefix Exercise

Given the definition of a prefix, write the prefix on the line provided. Also write a medical word from this chapter that includes that prefix. The first one has been done for you.

Definition	Prefix	Example	Definition	Prefix	Example
1. within	intra-	intravenous	5. many, much	_____	_____
2. slow	_____	_____	6. against	_____	_____
3. without, not	_____	_____	7. after, behind	_____	_____
4. below, underneath	_____	_____	8. innermost, within	_____	_____

True or False Exercise

Indicate whether each statement is true or false by writing T or F on the line provided.

1. _____ Before you can begin the study of medical language, it is necessary to first memorize many chapters of combining forms, prefixes, and suffixes.
2. _____ Every medical word contains a prefix.
3. _____ The suffix is the end or foundation of a medical word.
4. _____ The plural of a Latin singular feminine noun is formed by changing *-a* to *-ae*.
5. _____ A root and a combining vowel together form a medical word.
6. _____ The suffixes *-ac* and *-al* mean *pertaining to.*
7. _____ All medical words are derived from Latin words.
8. _____ You can increase your chance of success in a healthcare career by learning medical language.

Naming Exercise

1. Name the three word parts that can be used to build a medical word.

   ____

   ____

   ____

2. The ______________________ is the grammatical link that allows a combining form to join with a suffix.

3. Name the five medical language skills needed for successful communication.

____

____

____

____

____

Singular and Plural Forms Exercise

Given the definition of a medical word, write the singular and plural forms of that medical word on the line provided. The first one has been done for you.

Definition	Singular Form	Plural Form
1. Upper chamber of the heart	atrium	atria
2. Bone of the spinal column	______	______
3. The command center of a cell	______	______
4. Tube that carries air to the lungs	______	______
5. Abbreviated as *Dx*	______	______
6. Shoulder blade	______	______

Word-Building Exercise

Read the definition of the medical word. Look at the list of combining forms and the list of suffixes and select a combining form and suffix to create a medical word to match the definition. Write that medical word on the line provided. Remember to remove the hyphens and the combining vowel (if necessary) before combining the word parts. The first one has been done for you.

Combining Forms		Suffixes	
appendic/o- (appendix)	neur/o- (nerve)	-ectomy (surgical excision)	-pathy (disease, suffering)
cardi/o- (heart)	retin/o- (retina)	-itis (inflammation of)	-scopy (process of using an instrument to examine)
gastr/o- (stomach)	tonsill/o- (tonsil)	-logy (the study of)	
hepat/o- (liver)		-oma (tumor, mass)	

Definition	Medical Word	Definition	Medical Word
1. The study of the heart	cardiology	6. Surgical excision of the tonsils	______
2. Surgical excision of the appendix	______	7. Inflammation of the tonsils	______
3. Process that uses an instrument to examine the stomach	______	8. Inflammation of the liver	______
4. Tumor or mass of the liver	______	9. Disease of the nerves	______
5. Disease of the retina of the eye	______	10. Inflammation of the appendix	______

Matching Exercise

Match each numbered word or word part to its description.

1.	arthr/o-	_____ A tube that assists with breathing
2.	endo-	_____ Plural noun for the command centers in cells
3.	retinopathy	_____ Adjective meaning *pertaining to the heart*
4.	endotracheal	_____ Combining form meaning *skin*
5.	intranasal	_____ Within the nose
6.	cutane/o-	_____ Suffix meaning *inflammation of*
7.	-ectomy	_____ Prefix meaning *innermost, within*
8.	nuclei	_____ Way to get fluids when not eating
9.	-itis	_____ Combining form meaning *joint*
10.	intravenous	_____ Combining form meaning *muscle*
11.	muscul/o-	_____ Medical word for *disease of the retina of the eye*
12.	cardiac	_____ Suffix meaning surgical excision

Circle Exercise

Circle the correct word from the choices given.

1. Daniel Frist broke his left middle (**phalanges, phalanx**) while playing baseball.
2. Baby Phong Nyugen's mother took him to the doctor when she noticed that his left (**testes, testis**) was not present in the scrotum.
3. On the x-ray, Leona Calvin's spine shows several (**vertebra, vertebrae**) that are misaligned.
4. Dr. James Gibbons treated Al Smith's (**gastric, gastroscopy**) ulcer with an antacid.
5. The physical examination at the walk-in clinic revealed that Jose Rodriguez had (**tonsillectomy, tonsillitis**).
6. The laboratory identified several (**bacteria, bacterium**) that were present in the patient's wound.
7. Alan Witherspoon underwent a (**cardiac, hematology**) stress test to evaluate his chest pain.
8. Alicyn Smart experienced sharp right lower abdominal pain, and the emergency department physician ordered that she have an (**appendectomy, appendicitis**).
9. Dr. Matthew Cohen decided to specialize in treating the (**tonsillectomy, urinary**) system.
10. When Briana Charles had severe pain, she made an appointment in the (**anesthesia, subcutaneous**) department to get a numbing shot in the area of her pain.

Abbreviation Exercise

Write the definition for each abbreviation on the line.

1. CPR ______________________________
2. DS ______________________________
3. SOAP ______________________________
4. H&P ______________________________
5. Dx ______________________________
6. ROS ______________________________

Word Analysis Exercise

These are the two longest words you will study in this textbook. See if you can analyze each word, define the word parts, and then define the entire medical word. Some of the word parts will be familiar to you; others will not. Use the Glossary in Appendix A to look up the meanings of any word parts that you do not know.

1. gastroduodenoscopy

	Word Part	Word Part Meaning
SUFFIX	____________	____________
COMBINING FORM	____________	____________
COMBINING FORM	____________	____________
WORD DEFINITION	____________	

2. otorhinolaryngology

	Word Part	Word Part Meaning
SUFFIX	____________	____________
COMBINING FORM	____________	____________
COMBINING FORM	____________	____________
COMBINING FORM	____________	____________
WORD DEFINITION	____________	

Pronunciation Checklist

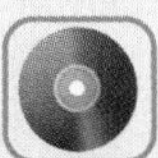

Read each word and its pronunciation. Practice pronouncing each word. Verify your pronunciation by listening to the Pronunciation List on the CD-ROM. Check the box next to the word after you master its pronunciation.

- ❑ alcoholism (AL-koh-hawl-izm)
- ❑ anesthesia (AN-es-THEE-zee-ah)
- ❑ antipsychotic (AN-tee-sy-KAWT-ik)
- ❑ apex (AA-peks)
- ❑ apices (AP-ah-seez)
- ❑ appendectomy (AP-pen-DEK-toh-mee)
- ❑ appendicitis (ah-PEN-dih-SY-tis)
- ❑ artery (AR-ter-ee)
- ❑ arthritis (ar-THRY-tis)
- ❑ arthroscopy (ar-THRAWS-koh-pee)
- ❑ atria (AA-tree-ah)
- ❑ atrium (AA-tree-um)
- ❑ bacteria (bak-TEER-ee-ah)
- ❑ bacterium (bak-TEER-ee-um)
- ❑ bladder (BLAD-er)
- ❑ bradycardia (BRAD-ee-KAR-dee-ah)
- ❑ bronchi (BRONG-kigh)
- ❑ bronchus (BRONG-kus)
- ❑ bursa (BER-sah)
- ❑ bursae (BER-see)
- ❑ carcinoma (KAR-sih-NOH-mah)
- ❑ carcinomata (KAR-sih-NOH-mah-tah)
- ❑ cardiac (KAR-dee-ak)
- ❑ cardiology (KAR-dee-AWL-oh-jee)
- ❑ cell (SELL)
- ❑ communication (koh-MYOO-nih-KAY-shun)
- ❑ cutaneous (kyoo-TAY-nee-us)
- ❑ diagnosis (DY-ag-NOH-sis)
- ❑ diagnoses (DY-ag-NOH-seez)
- ❑ dietitian (DY-ah-TISH-un)
- ❑ digestion (dy-JES-chun)
- ❑ drug (DRUHG)
- ❑ dysfunctional (dis-FUNK-shun-al)
- ❑ electrocardiography (ee-LEK-troh-KAR-dee-AWG-rah-fee)
- ❑ endotracheal (EN-doh-TRAY-kee-al)
- ❑ etymology (ET-ih-MAWL-oh-jee)
- ❑ ganglia (GANG-glee-ah)
- ❑ ganglion (GANG-glee-on)
- ❑ gastric (GAS-trik)
- ❑ gastritis (gas-TRY-tis)
- ❑ gastroscopy (gas-TRAWS-koh-pee)
- ❑ health (HELTH)
- ❑ heart (HART)
- ❑ helix (HEE-liks)
- ❑ helices (HEE-lih-seez)
- ❑ hematology (HEE-mah-TAWL-oh-jee)
- ❑ hematoma (HEE-mah-TOH-mah)
- ❑ hepatic (heh-PAT-ik)
- ❑ hepatitis (HEP-ah-TY-tis)
- ❑ hepatomegaly (HEP-ah-toh-MEG-ah-lee)
- ❑ hyperactive (HY-per-AK-tiv)
- ❑ hyperthyroidism (HY-per-THY-roy-dizm)
- ❑ intranasal (IN-trah-NAY-zal)
- ❑ intravenous (IN-trah-VEE-nus)
- ❑ language (LANG-gwij)
- ❑ laryngectomy (LAIR-in-JEK-toh-mee)
- ❑ laryngitis (LAIR-in-JY-tis)
- ❑ mastectomy (mas-TEK-toh-mee)
- ❑ mastitis (mas-TY-tis)
- ❑ medical (MED-ih-kal)
- ❑ muscular (MUS-kyoo-lar)
- ❑ muscle (MUS-el)
- ❑ musculi (MUS-kyoo-lie)
- ❑ musculus (MUS-kyoo-lus)
- ❑ nasal (NAY-zal)
- ❑ neural (NYOOR-al)
- ❑ neurology (nyoo-RAWL-oh-jee)
- ❑ neuroma (nyoor-OH-mah)
- ❑ neuropathy (nyoo-RAWP-ah-thee)
- ❑ nuclei (NOO-klee-eye)
- ❑ nucleus (NOO-klee-us)
- ❑ paramedic (PAIR-ah-MED-ik)
- ❑ pelvis (PEL-vis)
- ❑ perinatal (PAIR-ee-NAY-tal)
- ❑ peritonsillar (PAIR-ee-TAWN-sih-lar)
- ❑ phalanges (fah-LAN-jeez)
- ❑ phalanx (FAY-langks)
- ❑ phobia (FOH-bee-ah)
- ❑ physician (fih-ZISH-un)
- ❑ pneumonia (noo-MOH-nee-ah)
- ❑ polyneuropathy (PAWL-ee-nyoo-RAWP-ah-thee)
- ❑ polyuria (PAWL-ee-YOOR-ee-ah)
- ❑ postnatal (post-NAY-tal)
- ❑ prenatal (pree-NAY-tal)
- ❑ psychiatry (sy-KY-ah-tree)
- ❑ psychology (sy-KAWL-oh-jee)
- ❑ psychosis (sy-KOH-sis)
- ❑ retinal (RET-ih-nal)
- ❑ retinopathy (RET-ih-NAWP-ah-thee)
- ❑ scapula (SKAP-yoo-lah)
- ❑ scapulae (SKAP-yoo-lee)
- ❑ sinus (SY-nus)
- ❑ sperm (SPERM)
- ❑ subcutaneous (SUB-kyoo-TAY-nee-us)
- ❑ tachycardia (TAK-ih-KAR-dee-ah)
- ❑ testes (TES-teez)
- ❑ testis (TES-tis)
- ❑ thorax (THOR-aks)
- ❑ tonsillar (TAWN-sih-lar)
- ❑ tonsillectomy (TAWN-sih-LEK-toh-mee)
- ❑ tonsillitis (TAWN-sih-LY-tis)
- ❑ tracheal (TRAY-kee-al)
- ❑ urinary (YOO-rih-nair-ee)
- ❑ urination (YOO-rih-NAY-shun)
- ❑ urology (yoo-RAWL-oh-jee)
- ❑ vein (VAYN)
- ❑ venous (VEE-nus)
- ❑ vertebra (VER-teh-brah)
- ❑ vertebrae (VER-teh-bree)

Experience Multimedia

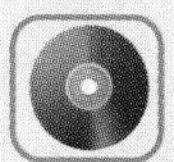

CD-ROM Learning Activities Checklist

Check off the box as you complete each learning activity.

- ❑ **CD-ROM Learning Activity 1.1: WORD PARTS FLASHCARDS**
  Use flashcards to help you memorize word parts. Make your own flashcards or print out prepared flashcards. Time: 20 minutes.
- ❑ **CD-ROM Learning Activity 1.2: MEDICINE IN ACTION**
  Watch a video clip of healthcare professionals using medical language to communicate. Time: 5 minutes.
- ❑ **CD-ROM Learning Activity 1.3: MEMORY AIDS**
  Use memory aids to help you memorize medical words and meanings. Time: 5 minutes.
- ❑ **CD-ROM Learning Activity 1.4: MEDICAL LANGUAGE SPOKEN HERE**
  Listen to medical sentences and spell the missing medical words. Time: 5 minutes.
- ❑ **CD-ROM Learning Activity 1.5: SPELLING CHALLENGE**
  Listen to a pronounced medical word and then spell it. Time: 5 minutes.
- ❑ **CD-ROM Learning Activity 1.6: MEDICAL LANGUAGE PRONUNCIATION**
  Listen to a pronounced medical word or phrase and then practice pronouncing it. Time: 5 minutes.
- ❑ **CD-ROM Learning Activity 1.7: EDUCATIONAL FUN AND GAMES**
  Enjoy these fun activities while reinforcing your knowledge. Time: 15 minutes.

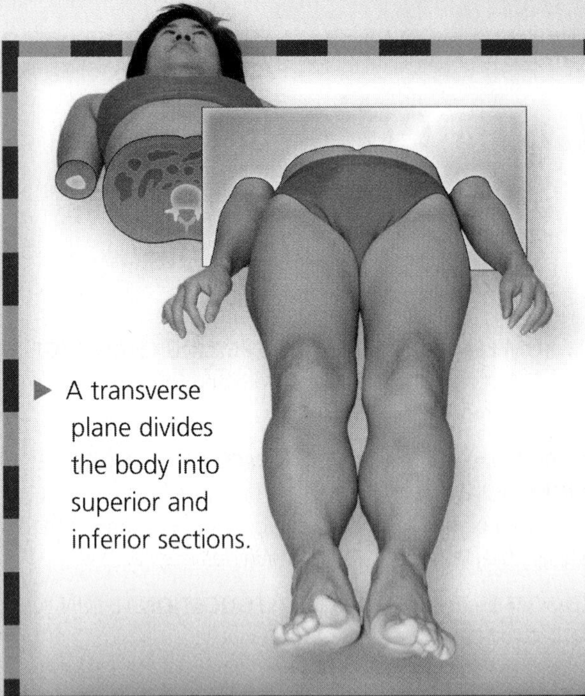

A transverse plane divides the body into superior and inferior sections.

Dive In!

- Attention! Stand up! Arms at your sides and palms forward. Look straight ahead. Now you are in anatomical position.
- The first human dissection was performed about 2,500 years ago in Greece.
- In this chapter you'll explore body positions, cavities, systems, and medical specialties. Then you'll be in a position to master the language of the body as a whole!

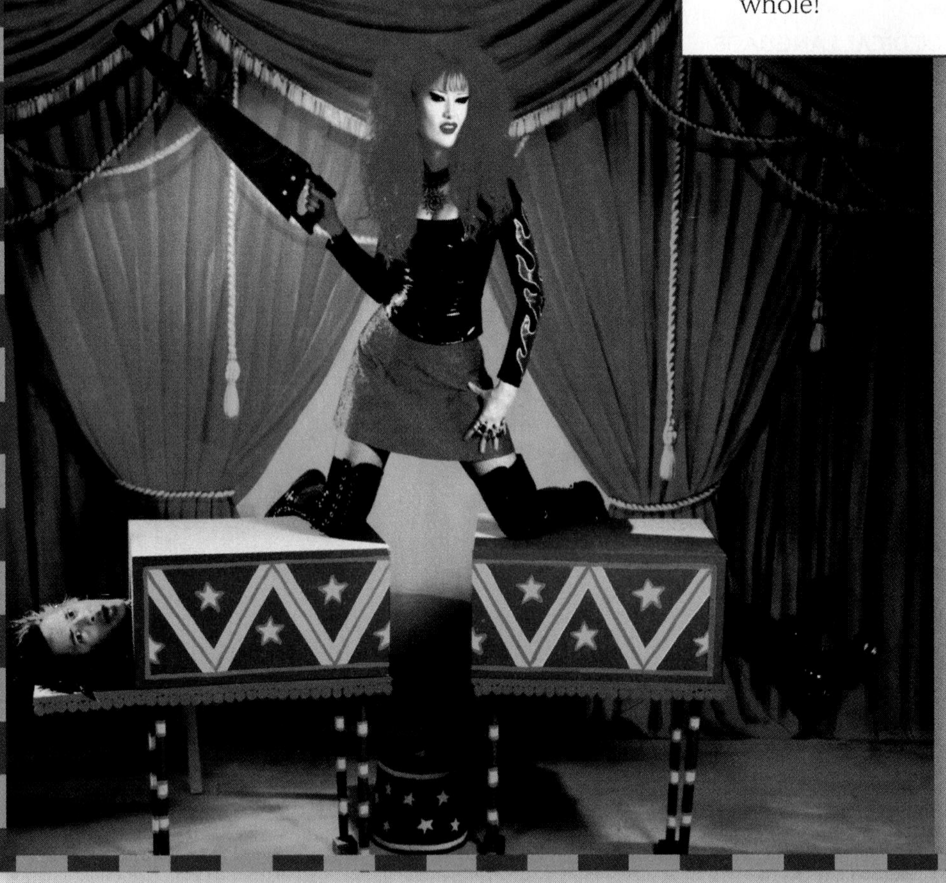

The magic of advanced medical imaging techniques allows healthcare professionals to divide and view the body in various ways.

Medicine Through HISTORY

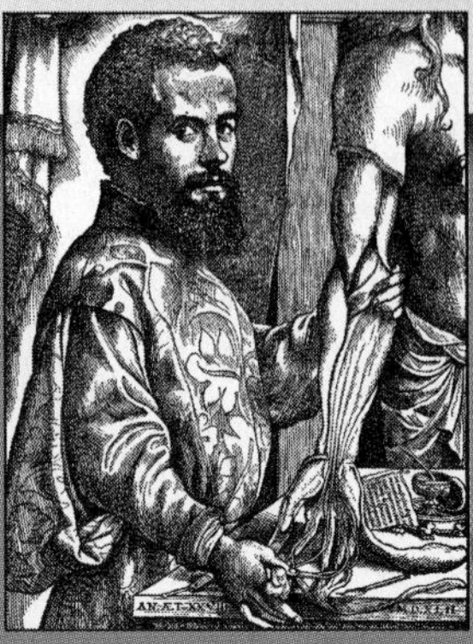

1543

The first complete anatomy textbook is written and illustrated by Andreas Vesalius of Brussels, Belgium

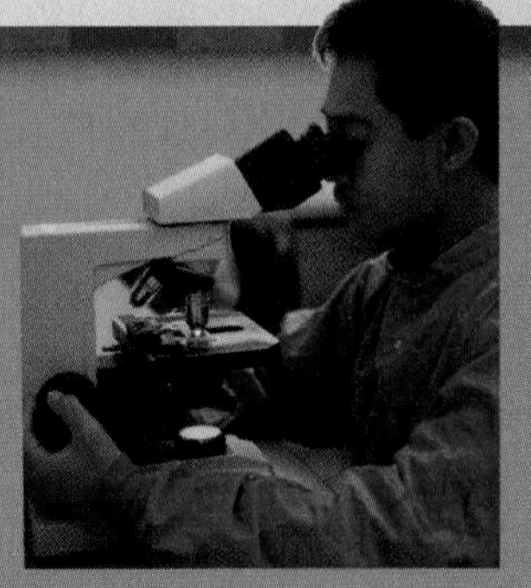

1609

Galileo invents a microscope that includes a magnifying lens and focusing mechanism

CHAPTER 2

The Body in Health and Disease

The human body is a marvelous, intricate creation that can be organized and studied in different ways. When functioning properly, the body operates in a state of health; when it fails, it experiences disease.

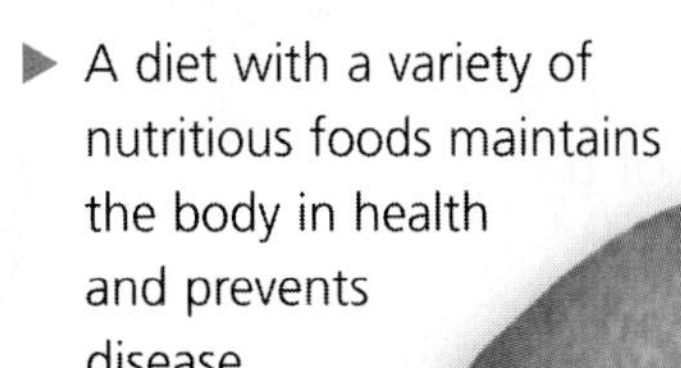

▶ A diet with a variety of nutritious foods maintains the body in health and prevents disease.

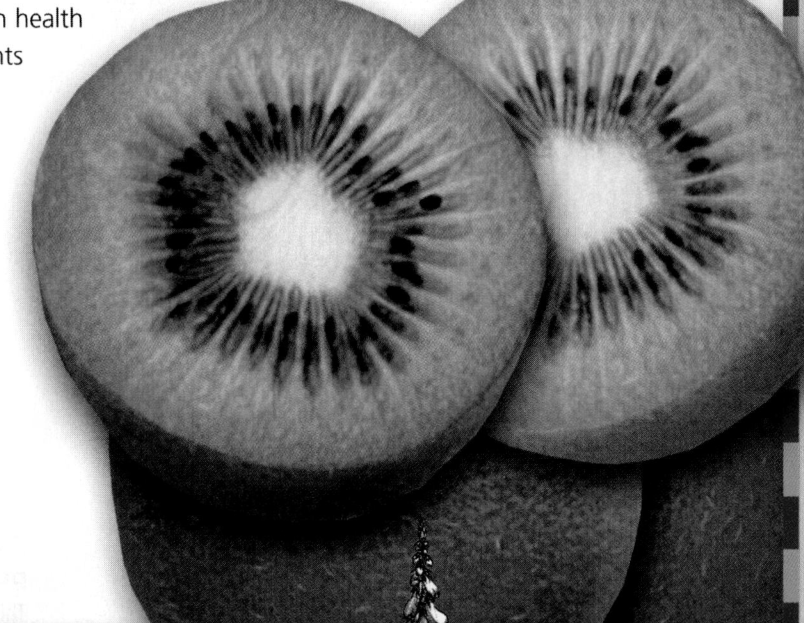

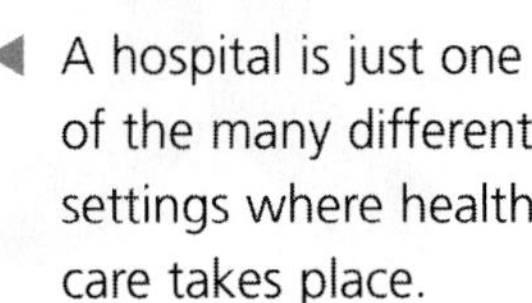

◀ A hospital is just one of the many different settings where health care takes place.

1616

William Harvey, an English physician, describes the circulation of the blood throughout the body

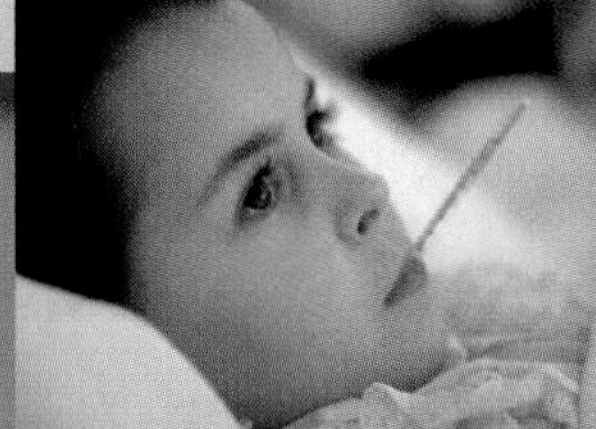

1714

German physicist Gabriel Fahrenheit invents the mercury thermometer

1741

Dr. William Wuthering, an English physician, introduces the use of the foxglove plant as a drug for the heart. It contains the modern drug digitalis

Measure Your Progress: Learning Objectives

After you study this chapter, you should be able to

1. Describe seven approaches used to organize information about the human body.
2. Identify body directions, body cavities, body systems, and medical specialties by correctly labeling them on anatomical illustrations.
3. Define ten categories of diseases.
4. Describe four techniques used to perform a physical examination.
5. Describe three types of healthcare professionals.
6. Describe seven settings where health care is provided.
7. Build medical words from combining forms, prefixes, and suffixes.
8. Define common abbreviations for body systems, medical specialties, and healthcare professionals.
9. Correctly spell and pronounce medical words presented in this chapter.
10. Test your knowledge of the body in health and disease by completing review exercises at the end of the chapter and learning activities on the CD-ROM.

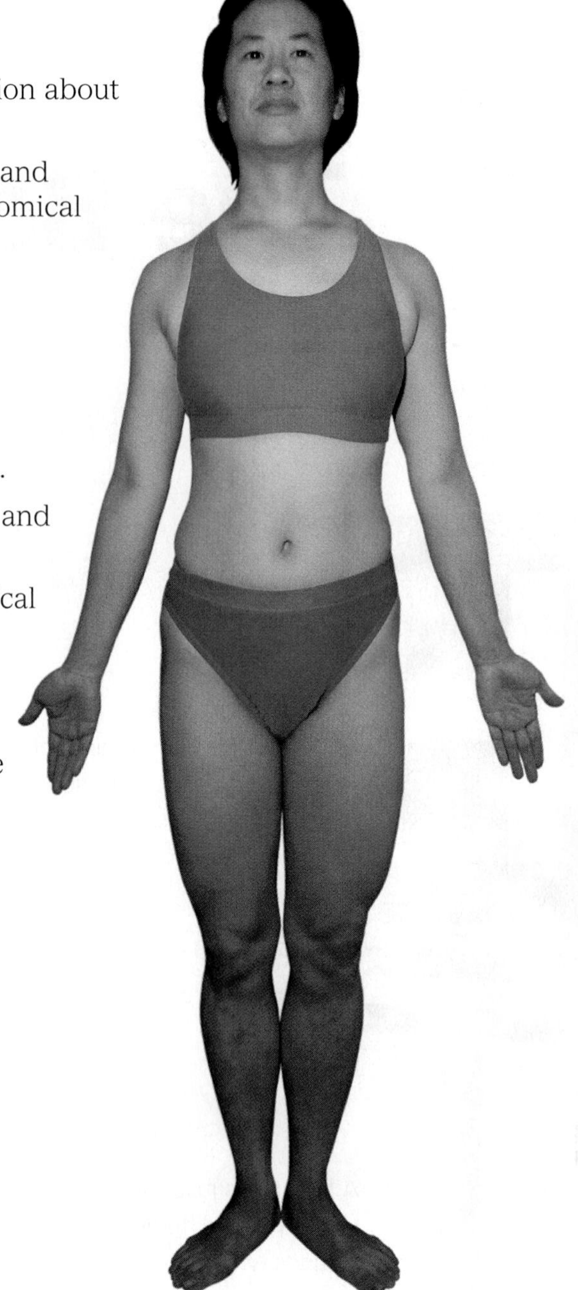

Figure 2-1 ■ The human body in anatomical position.

This is a standard position in which the body is standing erect, the head is up with the eyes looking forward, the arms are by the sides with the palms facing forward, and the legs are straight with the toes pointing forward.

www.prenhall.com/turley

For interactive flashcards, real-life video clips, games, exercises, and audio pronunciations please explore the companion CD-ROM in the back of the book. Click on the companion website for bonus chapters, additional resources, and links to on-line learning.

The Body in Health

When the human body's countless parts function correctly, the body is in a state of **health** or optimum wellness. The study of the healthy human body can be done in several different ways. Each way approaches the body from a specific standpoint and provides unique information about the body. Each approach divides and organizes complex information about the body in a logical way. These approaches include the following:

1. Body planes and body directions approach
2. Body cavities approach
3. Quadrant and regions approach
4. Anatomy and physiology approach
5. Microscopic-to-macroscopic approach
6. Body systems approach
7. Medical specialty approach

health (HELTH)
Health is derived from an Old English word meaning *robust and sound.*

Body Planes and Body Directions Approach

Once the human body is in **anatomical position** (see Figure 2-1■), it can be studied by dividing it with planes. A **plane** is an imaginary flat surface, like a plate of glass. There are three body planes: the coronal plane, the midsagittal plane, and the transverse plane. These body planes divide the body into front and back, right and left, and top and bottom sections. Body directions represent movement away from or toward those planes.

anatomical (AN-ah-TAWM-ih-kal)
ana- *apart from; excessive*
tom/o- *a cut, slice, or layer*
-ical *pertaining to*

plane (PLAYN)
Plane is derived from a Latin word meaning *flat.*

The Coronal Plane and Body Directions

The **coronal plane** (or **frontal plane**) is an imaginary vertical plane that divides the entire body into front and back sections (see Figure 2-2■). The coronal plane is named for the coronal suture where the anterior and posterior cranial bones meet (see Figure 2-3■).

coronal (kor-OH-nal)
coron/o- *encircling structure*
-al *pertaining to*
Coronal is derived from a Latin word meaning *crown.*

frontal (FRUN-tal)
front/o- *front*
-al *pertaining to*

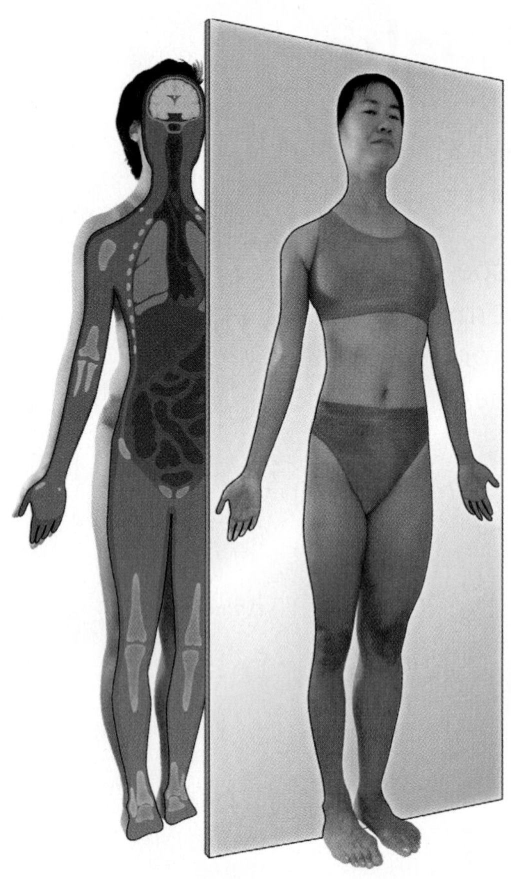

Figure 2-2 ■ The coronal plane.

The coronal or frontal plane divides the body into anterior (front) and posterior (back) sections.

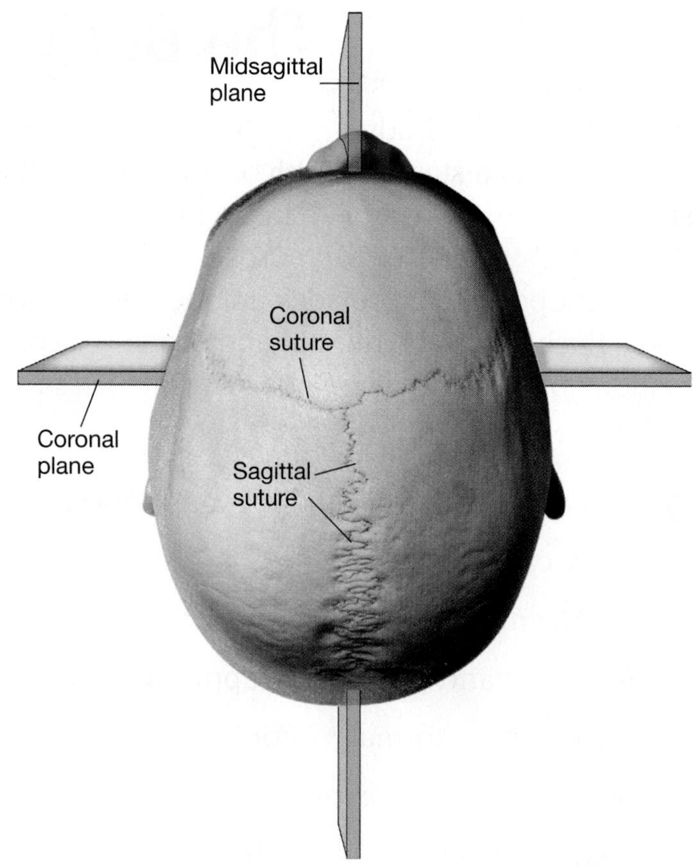

Figure 2-3 ■ The coronal and midsagittal sutures of the cranium.

The coronal and midsagittal planes are named for the coronal and sagittal sutures that join the bones of the cranium together. Each plane is oriented in the same direction as the suture for which it is named.

The front of the body is known as the **anterior** or **ventral** section. The back of the body is known as the **posterior** or **dorsal** section. Lying with the anterior section of the body down is known as the **prone** position. Lying with the posterior section of the body down is known as the **dorsal supine** position.

anterior (an-TEER-ee-or)
anter/o- *before; front part*
-ior *pertaining to*

ventral (VEN-tral)
ventr/o- *front; abdomen*
-al *pertaining to*

posterior (pohs-TEER-ee-or)
poster/o- *back part*
-ior *pertaining to*

dorsal (DOR-sal)
dors/o- *back; dorsum; uppermost part*
-al *pertaining to*

prone (PROHN)
Prone is derived from a Latin word meaning *inclined downward.*

supine (soo-PINE) (SOO-pine)
Supine is derived from a Latin word meaning *lying on the back.*

Moving toward the front of the body is moving in an **anterior direction** or **anteriorly.** Moving toward the back of the body is moving in a posterior direction or **posteriorly** (see Figure 2-4■). The directions anterior and posterior can be combined to form **anteroposterior (AP)** or **posteroanterior (PA).** Anteroposterior means moving from outside the body through the anterior section and then through the posterior section. Posteroanterior means moving from outside the body through the posterior section and then through the anterior section (see Figure 2-5■).

anteriorly (an-TEER-ee-or-lee)
anter/o- *before; front part*
-ior *pertaining to*
-ly *going toward*

posteriorly (pohs-TEER-ee-or-lee)
poster/o- *back part*
-ior *pertaining to*
-ly *going toward*

anteroposterior
(AN-ter-oh-pohs-TEER-ee-or)
anter/o- *before; front part*
poster/o- *back part*
-ior *pertaining to*

posteroanterior
(POHS-ter-oh-an-TEER-ee-or)
poster/o- *back part*
anter/o- *before; front part*
-ior *pertaining to*

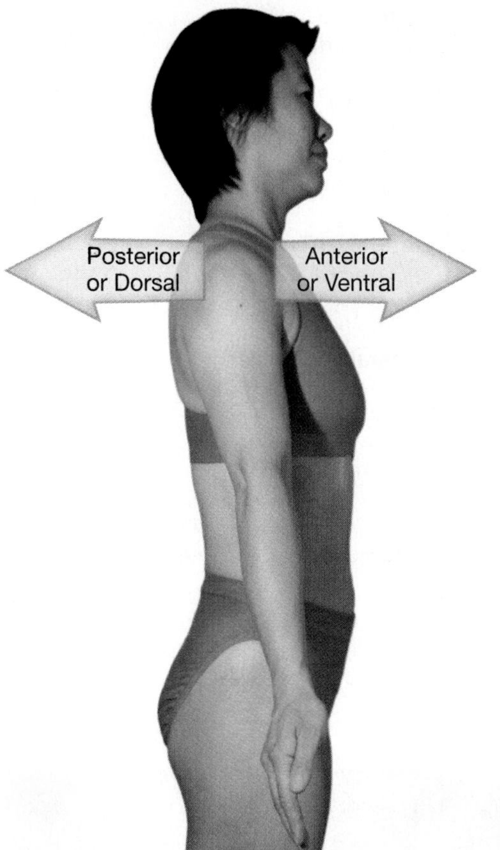

Figure 2-4 ■ Anterior and posterior are directional opposites.

Moving in an anterior direction is moving toward the front of the body. Moving in a posterior direction is moving toward the back of the body.

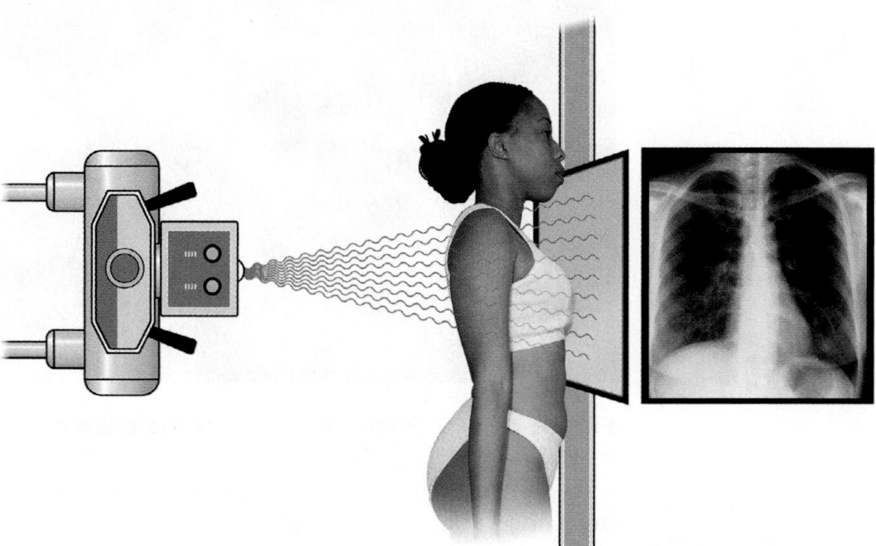

Figure 2-5 ■ Posteroanterior direction.

For a posteroanterior (PA) chest x-ray, the x-ray beam enters the posterior chest, moves anteriorly, goes through the anterior chest wall, and then exposes the x-ray plate to produce an image.

The Midsagittal Plane and Body Directions

The **midsagittal plane** is an imaginary vertical plane that divides the entire body into right and left sections (see Figures 2-6■ and 2-7■). The midsagittal plane is named for the sagittal suture of the skull (see Figure 2-3).

Moving from the side of the body toward the midline is moving in a **medial** direction or **medially.** Moving from the midline toward the side of the body is moving in a **lateral** direction or **laterally** (see Figure 2-8■).

midsagittal (mid-SAJ-ih-tal)
mid- *middle*
sagitt/o- *going from front to back*
-al *pertaining to*
Sagittal is derived from a Latin word meaning *an arrow,* implying the path of an arrow that goes through the body from front to back.

medial (MEE-dee-al)
medi/o- *middle*
-al *pertaining to*

medially (MEE-dee-ah-lee)
medi/o- *middle*
-al *pertaining to*
-ly *going toward*

lateral (LAT-er-al)
later/o- *side*
-al *pertaining to*

laterally (LAT-er-ah-lee)
later/o- *side*
-al *pertaining to*
-ly *going toward*

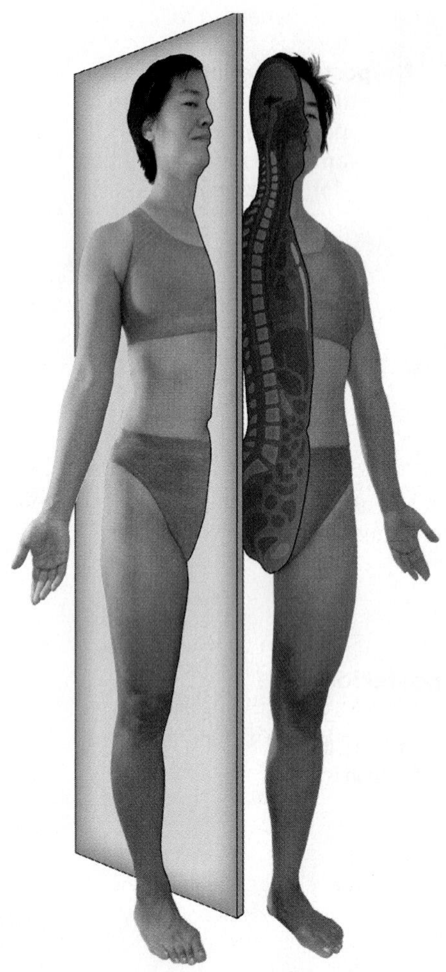

Figure 2-6 ■ The midsagittal plane.
The midsagittal plane divides the body into right and left sides and creates a midline.

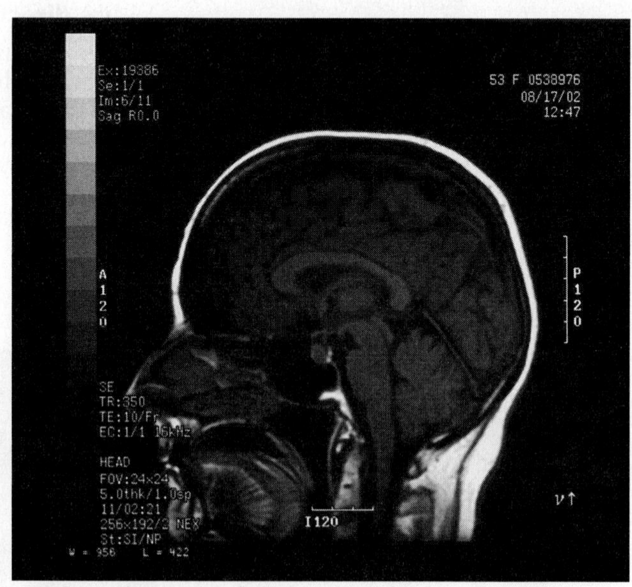

Figure 2-7 ■ Midsagittal view of the head on an MRI scan.
A magnetic resonance imaging (MRI) scan uses a magnetic field to create images of the body in "slices."

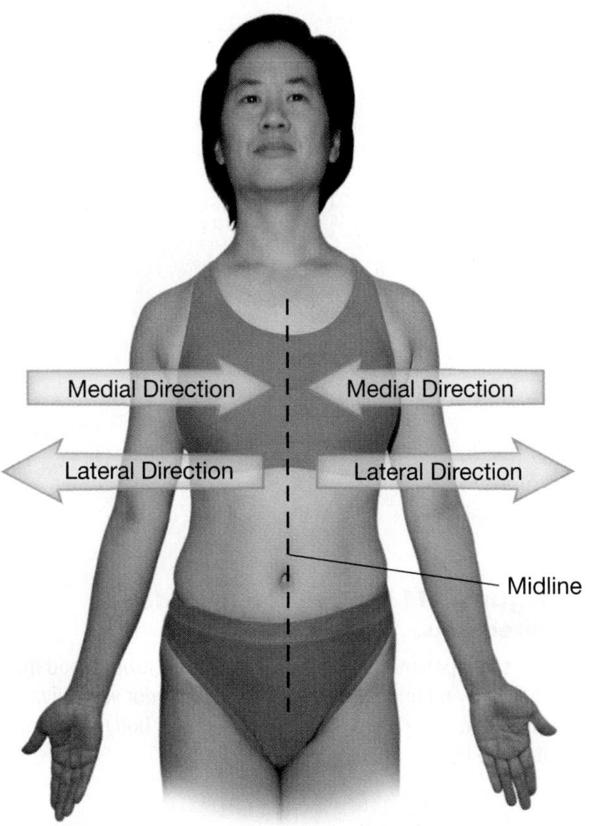

Figure 2-8 ■ Medial and lateral are directional opposites.

Moving in a medial direction is moving toward the midline of the body. Moving in a lateral direction is moving away from the midline of the body.

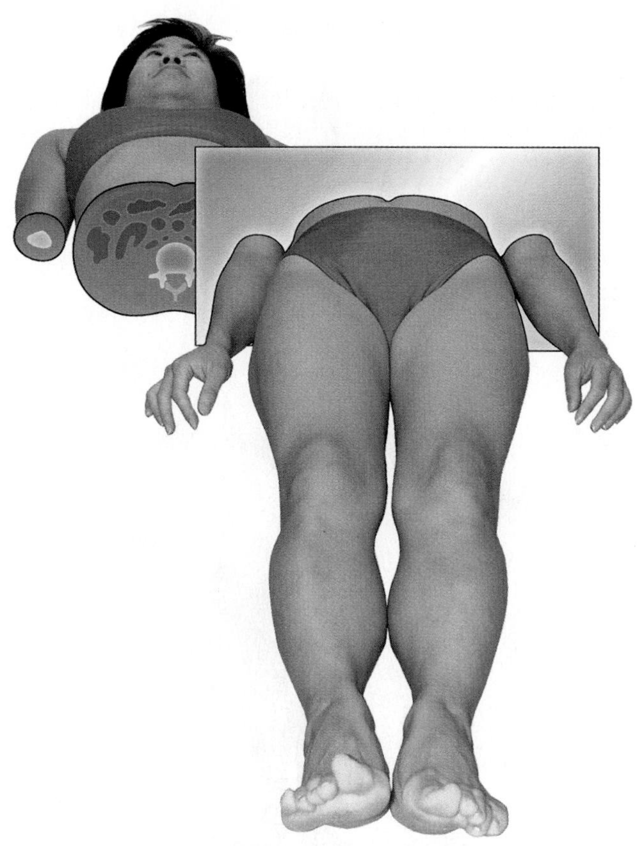

Figure 2-9 ■ The transverse plane.

The transverse or horizontal plane divides the body into superior (top) and inferior (bottom) sections.

The Transverse Plane and Body Directions

The **transverse plane** (or **horizontal plane**) is an imaginary horizontal plane that divides the entire body into top and bottom sections (see Figure 2-9■).

The upper half of the body is known as the **superior** section, and the lower half is known as the **inferior** section.

transverse (trans-VERS)
trans- *across, through*
-verse *to turn; to travel*
Every medical word must contain a combining form. The medical word *transverse* looks like it only contains a prefix and a suffix, but the suffix actually contains the combining form (*vers/o-*) plus a one-letter suffix (-*e*).

horizontal (HOR-ih-ZAWN-tal)
horizont/o- *boundary between the earth and sky*
-al *pertaining to*

superior (soo-PEER-ee-or)
super/o- *above*
-ior *pertaining to*

inferior (in-FEER-ee-or)
infer/o- *below*
-ior *pertaining to*

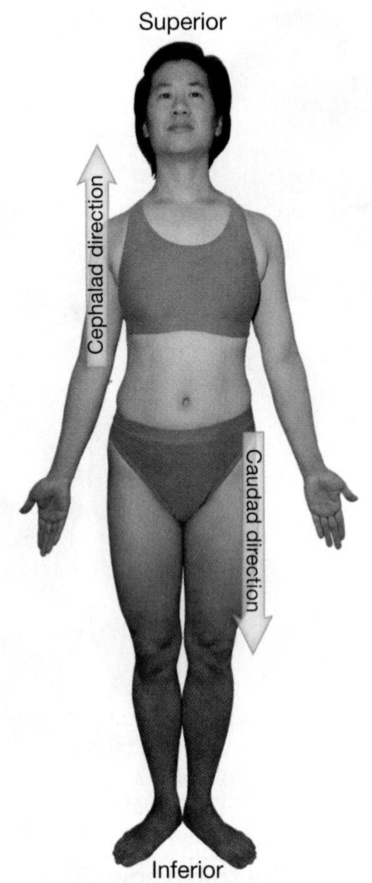

Figure 2-10 ■ Cephalad and caudad are directional opposites.

Moving in a cephalad direction is moving toward the head. Moving in a caudad direction is moving toward the tailbone or lower parts of the body.

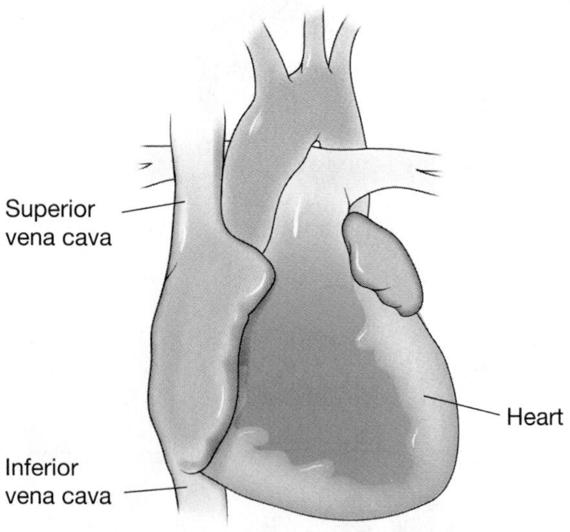

Figure 2-11 ■ Superior and inferior directions.

The superior vena cava is a large vein that carries blood from the head and brings it to the heart. The inferior vena cava is a large vein that carries blood from the lower body and brings it to the heart.

Moving toward the head is moving in a superior direction or **superiorly.** This is also known as the **cephalad** direction. Moving toward the tail bone or the feet is moving in an inferior direction or **inferiorly.** This is also known as the **caudad** direction (see Figures 2-10■ and 2-11■).

superiorly (soo-PEER-ee-or-lee)
super/o- *above*
-ior *pertaining to*
-ly *going toward*

cephalad (SEF-ah-lad)
cephal/o- *head*
-ad *toward, in the direction of*

inferiorly (in-FEER-ee-or-lee)
infer/o- *below*
-ior *pertaining to*
-ly *going toward*

caudad (KAW-dad)
caud/o- *tailbone; lower part of the body*
-ad *toward, in the direction of*
Caudad means *toward or in the direction of the tail,* but the human body does not have a tail! It does have a tailbone, however. *Caud/o-* also means the *lower part of the body.*

Other Body Directions and Positions

Moving from the body toward the end of a limb (arm or leg) is moving in a **distal** direction or **distally.** Moving from the end of a limb toward where it is attached to the body is moving in a **proximal** direction or **proximally** (see Figure 2-12■).

Structures on the surface of the body are **superficial** or **external** structures. Structures below the surface and inside the body are deep or **internal** structures (see Figure 2-13■).

distal (DIS-tal)
dist/o- *away from the center or point of origin*
-al *pertaining to*

distally (DIS-tah-lee)
dist/o- *away from the center or point of origin*
-al *pertaining to*
-ly *going toward*

proximal (PRAWK-sih-mal)
proxim/o- *near the center or point of origin*
-al *pertaining to*

proximally (PRAWK-sih-mah-lee)
proxim/o- *near the center or point of origin*
-al *pertaining to*
-ly *going toward*

superficial (SOO-per-FISH-al)
superfici/o- *on or near the surface*
-al *pertaining to*

external (eks-TER-nal)
extern/o- *outside*
-al *pertaining to*

internal (in-TER-nal)
intern/o- *inside*
-al *pertaining to*

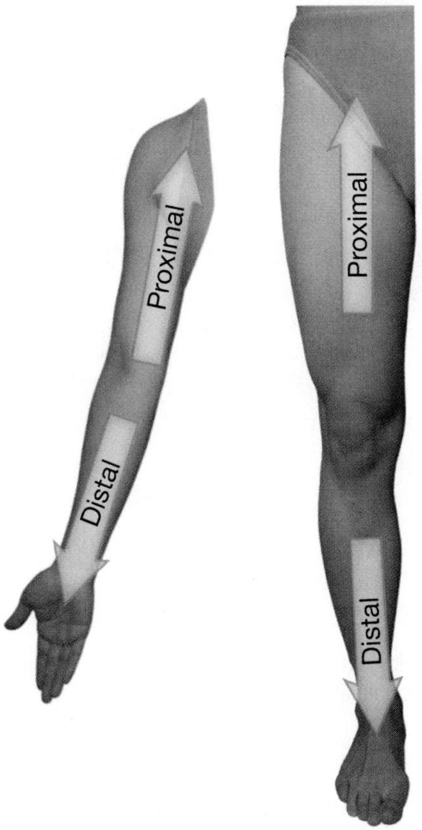

Figure 2-12 ■ Distal and proximal are directional opposites.

Moving in a distal direction is moving from where the limb is attached to the body toward the fingers or toes (end of the limb). Moving in a proximal direction is moving from the fingers or toes toward where the limb is attached to the body.

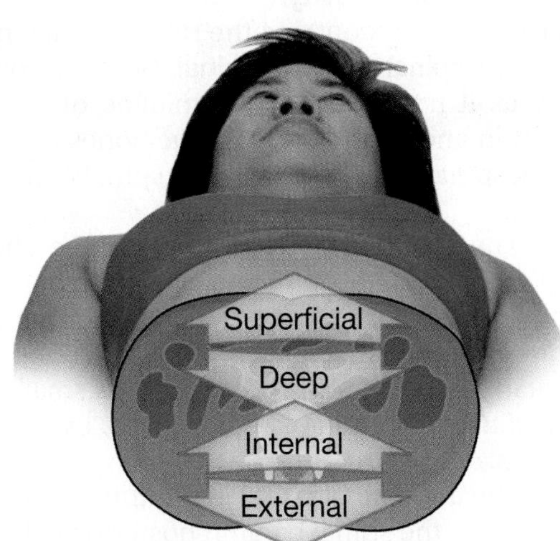

Figure 2-13 ■ Superficial and deep are directional opposites.

Moving from the deep or internal structures of the body toward the body's external surface is moving in a superficial direction.

Body Cavities Approach

The human body can be studied according to its body cavities and their internal organs (see Figure 2-14■). A **cavity** is a hollow space that is surrounded by bones or muscles. The bones or muscles support and protect the organs and structures within the cavity.

cavity (KAV-ih-tee)
cav/o- *hollow space*
-ity *state; condition*

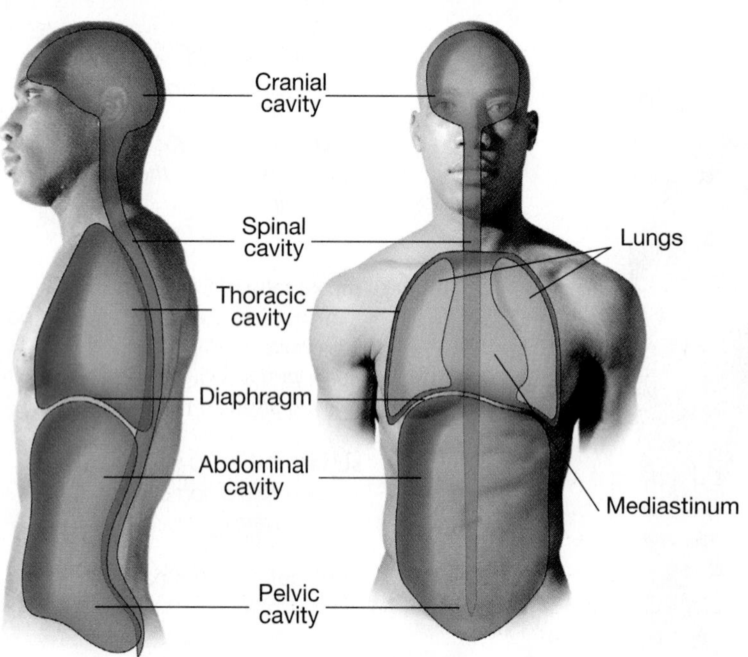

Figure 2-14 ■ The five body cavities.
The cranial and spinal cavities are continuous with each other. The thoracic cavity is separated from the abdominal cavity by the muscular diaphragm. The abdominal cavity is continuous with the pelvic cavity.

The **cranial cavity** lies within and is protected by the cranium. The cranial cavity contains the brain, cranial nerves, and other structures.

The **spinal cavity** or **spinal canal** is a continuation of the cranial cavity as it travels down the midline of the back. The spinal cavity lies within and is protected by the bones (vertebrae) of the spinal column. The spinal cavity contains the spinal cord, the spinal nerves, and spinal fluid.

The **thoracic cavity** lies within the chest and is protected by the breast bone (sternum) anteriorly, the bony ribs laterally, and the spinal column posteriorly. The inferior border of the thoracic cavity is the large, muscular diaphram that functions during respiration. The thoracic cavity contains both lungs. A smaller, central area known as the **mediastinum** contains the trachea, esophagus, heart, and other structures.

The **abdominal cavity** lies within the abdomen. It is protected by the bones of the spinal column posteriorly. The abdominal muscles anteriorly provide support. The **pelvic cavity** is a continuation of the abdominal cavity inferiorly. The pelvic cavity lies within and is protected by the pelvic bones anteriorly and laterally. It is also protected by the base of the spinal column posteriorly. These two cavities are often referred

cranial (KRAY-nee-al)
crani/o- *cranium (skull)*
-al *pertaining to*

spinal (SPY-nal)
spin/o- *spine; backbone*
-al *pertaining to*

thoracic (thoh-RAS-ik)
thorac/o- *thorax (chest)*
-ic *pertaining to*

mediastinum (MEE-dee-as-TY-num)
Mediastinum is derived from a Latin word meaning *middle.*

abdominal (ab-DAWM-ih-nal)
abdomin/o- *abdomen*
-al *pertaining to*

pelvic (PEL-vik)
pelv/o- *pelvis (hip bone; renal pelvis)*
-ic *pertaining to*

to as the **abdominopelvic cavity** because they form one continuous cavity that has no dividing structure in it. The abdominopelvic cavity contains many of the structures of the gastrointestinal, reproductive, and urinary systems.

The internal organs of all of these body cavities are collectively known as the **viscera.**

abdominopelvic
(ab-DAWM-ih-noh-PEL-vik)
abdomin/o- *abdomen*
pelv/o- *pelvis (hip bone; renal pelvis)*
-ic *pertaining to*

viscera (VIS-er-ah)
Viscera is a Latin word meaning *soft internal organs.* Because there are many internal organs in the body, the singular form *viscus* is seldom used.

Quadrants and Regions Approach

The human body can be studied according to its quadrants and regions.

The anterior surface of the abdominopelvic area can be divided into four **quadrants** or nine regions, either of which is helpful as a reference during a physical examination of the internal organs. The four quadrants include the right upper quadrant (RUQ), left upper quadrant (LUQ), left lower quadrant (LLQ), and right lower quadrant (RLQ). The nine regions include the right **hypochondriac** region, the **epigastric** region, the left hypochondriac region, the right **lumbar** region, the **umbilical** region, the left lumbar region, the right **inguinal** or **iliac** region, the **hypogastric** region, and the left inguinal region (see Figures 2-15■ and 2-16■).

Did You Know?

The Greeks considered the hypochondriac regions to be the seat of melancholy (sad feelings) because they contained the liver and spleen, and they thought these organs released humors that caused different moods. This is the basis for the word *hypochondriac,* a person who is depressed, worried, and talks excessively about imaginary illnesses.

quadrant (KWAH-drant)
Quadrant is derived from a Latin word meaning *pertaining to four parts.*

hypochondriac (HY-poh-CON-dree-ak)
hypo- *below; deficient*
chondr/o- *cartilage*
-iac *pertaining to*
Hypochondrium is a Greek word for the area below the cartilage of the ribs on either side of the abdomen.

epigastric (EP-ih-GAS-trik)
epi- *upon, above*
gastr/o- *stomach*
-ic *pertaining to*

lumbar (LUM-bar)
lumb/o- *lower back; area between the ribs and pelvis*
-ar *pertaining to*

umbilicus (um-BIL-ih-kus) (um-bih-LIE-kus)
Umbilicus is a Latin word meaning *the navel.*

umbilical (um-BIL-ih-kal)
umbilic/o- *umbilicus, navel*
-al *pertaining to*

inguinal (ING-gwih-nal)
inguin/o- *groin*
-al *pertaining to*

iliac (IL-ee-ak)
ili/o- *ilium (hip bone)*
-ac pertaining to

hypogastric (HY-poh-GAS-trik)
hypo- *below; deficient*
gastr/o- *stomach*
-ic *pertaining to*

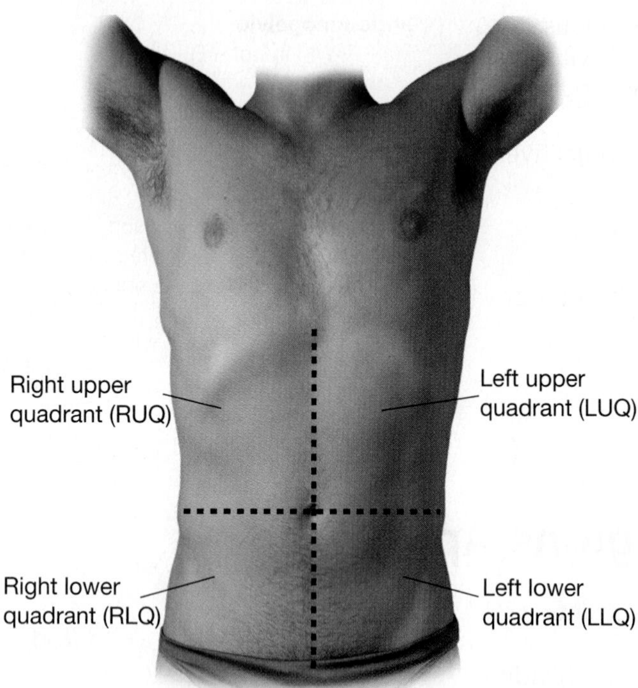

Figure 2-15 ■ Quadrants of the abdominopelvic area.

The four quadrants are formed by an imaginary grid of one horizontal line and one vertical line that cross at the umbilicus (navel). Remember, when you are facing the patient (as in this illustration), the patient's right side (right upper and lower quadrants) are on your left.

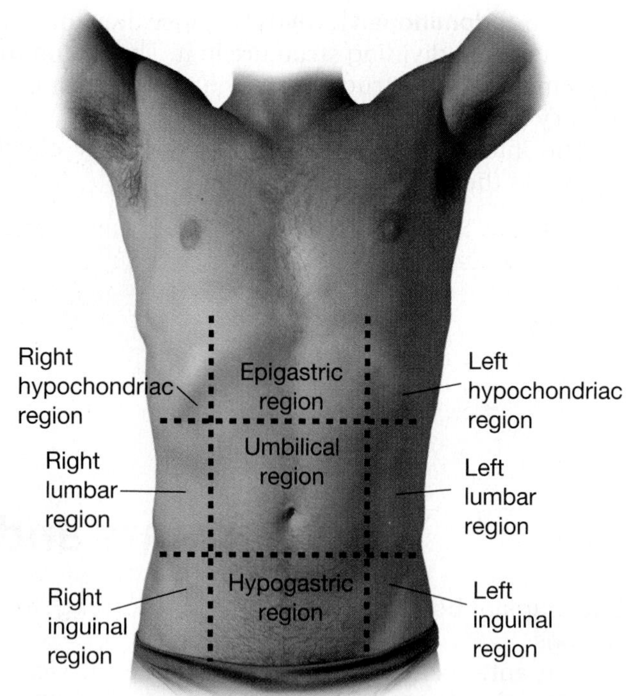

Figure 2-16 ■ Regions of the abdominopelvic area.

The nine regions are formed by an imaginary grid of two horizontal lines and two vertical lines that cross to form the four sides of a square around the umbilicus.

Anatomy and Physiology Approach

The human body can be studied according to its structures and the functions of those structures. **Anatomy** is the study of the structures of the human body. **Physiology** is the study of the function and workings of those structures.

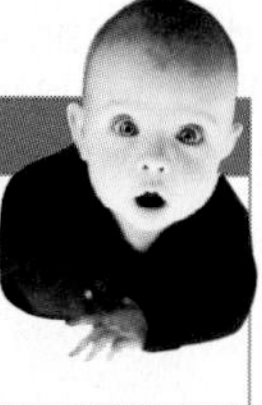

Did You Know?

The anatomy of the human body was first studied by doctors who secretly carried away and dissected the unclaimed dead bodies of criminals.

anatomy (ah-NAT-oh-mee)
ana- *apart from; excessive*
-tomy *process of cutting or making an incision*
Every medical word must contain a combining form. The suffix of *anatomy* contains the combining form *tom/o-*.

physiology (FIZ-ee-AWL-oh-jee)
physi/o- *physical function*
-logy *the study of*

Microscopic-to-Macroscopic Approach

The human body can be studied according to its smallest parts and how they combine to make larger and more complex structures and systems.

Cells and cellular structures are **microscopic** in size; they can only be seen through a **microscope** (see Figure 2-17 ■). Cells combine to form tissues, and tissues combine to form organs. Organs are **macroscopic,** that is, they can be seen with the unaided eye. Organs combine to form a body system. The human body contains several different body systems.

microscopic (MY-kroh-SKAWP-ik)
micr/o- *small*
scop/o- *examine with an instrument*
-ic *pertaining to*

microscope (MY-kroh-skohp)
micr/o- *small*
-scope *instrument used to examine*
A microscope is not a small instrument used to examine things. It is an instrument that is used to examine small things.

macroscopic (MAK-roh-SKAWP-ik)
macr/o- *large*
scop/o- *examine with an instrument*
-ic *pertaining to*
There is no such instrument as a macroscope. A macroscopic examination uses the eye itself as the examining "instrument."

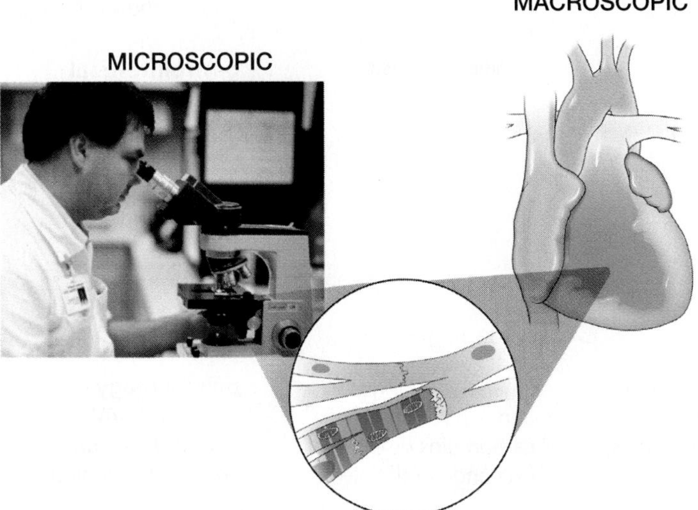

Figure 2-17 ■ Using a microscope to study the human body.

A microscope enhances our ability to understand the human body because it allows us to see anatomic structures not visible to the unaided eye. With the help of its magnification, we can see cells and even tiny structures within the cells.

Body Systems Approach

The human body can be studied according to its various organs and how they function together in a **body system.** The following is a list of those body systems.

- Gastrointestinal (GI) system
- Respiratory system
- Cardiovascular (CV) system
- Blood
- Lymphatic system
- Integumentary system
- Skeletal system
- Muscular system
- Nervous system
- Urinary system
- Male genital and reproductive system
- Female genital and reproductive system
- Endocrine system
- Eyes
- Ears, nose, and throat (ENT) system

system (SIS-tem)
System is derived from a Greek word meaning *combination of parts to make an organized whole.*

Medical Specialties Approach

The human body can be studied according to the **medical specialties** that make up the practice of medicine. The medical specialty approach organizes the anatomy, physiology, diseases, diagnostic tests, medical and surgical procedures, and drugs for each body system.

medical (MED-ih-kal)
medic/o- *physician; medicine*
-al *pertaining to*

Medical Specialty/Body System	Structure	Function	Word Part
Gastroenterology Gastrointestinal System (Chapter 3)	Mouth, teeth, tongue, salivary glands, pharynx (throat), esophagus, stomach, small intestine, large intestine, liver, gallbladder, pancreas	Digestion of food by breaking it down mechanically and chemically. Perception of taste stimuli. Absorption of nutrients into the blood. Excretion of undigested waste materials.	**gastroenterology** (GAS-troh-EN-ter-AWL-oh-jee) **gastr/o-** *stomach* **enter/o-** *intestine* **-logy** *the study of* **gastrointestinal** (GAS-troh-in-TES-tih-nal) **gastr/o-** *stomach* **intestin/o-** *intestine* **-al** *pertaining to*
Pulmonology Respiratory System (Chapter 4)	Nose, pharynx (throat), larynx (voice box), trachea, bronchi, lungs, alveoli	Inhalation of oxygen and exhalation of carbon dioxide and gas exchange in the alveoli	**pulmonology** (PUL-moh-NAWL-oh-jee) **pulmon/o-** *lung* **-logy** *the study of* **respiratory** (RES-pih-rah-TOR-ee) (reh-SPYR-ah-tor-ee) **re-** *again and again; backward; unable to* **spir/o-** *breathe* **-atory** *pertaining to* Some word parts have more than one definition. The best definition of *respiratory is pertaining to again and again breathing.*
Cardiology Cardiovascular System (Chapter 5)	Heart, arteries, veins, capillaries	Circulates the blood throughout the body	**cardiology** (KAR-dee-AWL-oh-jee) **cardi/o-** *heart* **-logy** *the study of* **cardiovascular** (KAR-dee-oh-VAS-kyoo-lar) **cardi/o-** *heart* **vascul/o-** *blood vessel* **-ar** *pertaining to*

Medical Specialty/Body System	Structure	Function	Word Part
Hematology Blood (Chapter 6)	Blood cells and plasma (liquid portion of blood)	Transportation of oxygen and nutrients to the body. Transportation of carbon dioxide to the lungs and waste products to the kidneys.	**hematology** (HEE-mah-TAWL-oh-jee) **hemat/o-** *blood* **-logy** *the study of* **blood** (BLUD)
Immunology Blood, Lymphatic System (Chapter 6)	Lymphatic vessels, lymph nodes, lymph, spleen, thymus, white blood cells	Recognition and destruction of disease-causing organisms and abnormal cells	**immunology** (IM-yoo-NAWL-oh-jee) **immun/o-** *immune response* **-logy** *the study of* **lymphatic** (lim-FAT-ik) **lymph/o-** *lymph; lymphatic system* **-atic** *pertaining to*
Dermatology Integumentary System (Chapter 7)	Skin, hair, nails, sweat glands, oil glands	Perception of pain, touch, and temperature stimuli. Protection of the internal organs from infection and trauma. Regulation of the body temperature by sweating.	**dermatology** (DER-mah-TAWL-oh-jee) **dermat/o-** *skin* **-logy** *the study of* **integumentary** (in-TEG-yoo-MEN-tair-ee) **integument/o-** *skin* **-ary** *pertaining to*
Orthopedics Skeletal System (Chapter 8)	Bones, cartilage, ligaments, joints	Maintenance of body support	**orthopedics** (OR-thoh-PEE-diks) **orth/o-** *straight* **ped/o-** *child* **-ics** *knowledge, practice* Add words to make a correct and complete definition of *orthopedics: Knowledge and practice [of producing] straight[ness in a] child [or an adult].* **skeletal** (SKEL-eh-tal) **skelet/o-** *skeleton* **-al** *pertaining to*

Medical Specialty/Body System	Structure	Function	Word Part
Orthopedics Muscular System (Chapter 9)	Muscles, tendons	Production of body movement	**muscular** (MUS-kyoo-lar) **muscul/o-** *muscle* **-ar** *pertaining to*
Neurology Nervous System (Chapter 10)	Brain, cranial nerves, spinal cord, spinal nerves, neurons	Perception and interpretation of pain, touch, temperature, body position, taste, visual, smell, and auditory stimuli. Coordination of movement. Maintenance and interpretation of memory and emotion.	**neurology** (nyoo-RAWL-oh-jee) **neur/o-** *nerve* **-logy-** *the study of* **nervous** (NER-vus) **nerv/o-** *nerve* **-ous** *pertaining to*
Urology Urinary System (Chapter 11)	Kidneys, ureters, bladder, urethra, nephrons Male: Urethra, penis	Excretion of urine and waste products from the body	**urology** (yoo-RAWL-oh-jee) **ur/o-** *urine; urinary system* **-logy** *the study of* **urinary** (YOO-rih-nair-ee) **urin/o-** *urine; urinary system* **-ary** *pertaining to*

Medical Specialty/Body System	Structure	Function	Word Part
Male Reproductive Medicine Male Genital and Reproductive System (Chapter 12)	Scrotum, testes, epididymides, vas deferens, seminal vesicles, prostate gland, urethra, penis	Production of sperm and sex hormones. Delivery of sperm to the female reproductive system.	**reproductive** (REE-proh-DUK-tiv) **re-** *again and again; backward; unable to* **product/o-** *produce* **-ive** *pertaining to* Some word parts have more than one definition. The best definition of *reproductive* is *pertaining to again and again producing [children].* **genital** (JEN-ih-tal) **genit/o-** *genitalia* **-al** *pertaining to*
Gynecology (GYN) and Obstetrics (OB) Female Genital and Reproductive System (Chapter 13)	Breasts, ovaries, fallopian tubes, uterus, vagina, external genitalia	Production of eggs and sex hormones. Regulation of menstruation and pregnancy. Acceptance of sperm from the male reproductive system.Milk production after childbirth.	**gynecology** (GY-neh-KAWL-oh-jee) **gynec/o-** *female, woman* **-logy** *the study of* **obstetrics** (awb-STET-riks) **obstetr/o-** *pregnancy and childbirth* **-ics** *knowledge, practice* **genital** (JEN-ih-tal) **genit/o-** *genitalia* **-al** *pertaining to*

Medical Specialty/Body System	Structure	Function	Word Part
Endocrinology Endocrine System (Chapter 14)	Testes, ovaries, pancreas, adrenal glands, thymus, thyroid gland, parathyroid glands, pituitary gland, pineal gland	Production and release of hormones. Direction of activities of other body organs.	**endocrinology** (EN-doh-krih-NAWL-oh-jee) **endo-** *innermost, within* **crin/o-** *secrete* **-logy** *the study of* **endocrine** (EN-doh-krin) (EN-doh-krine) **endo-** *innermost, within* **-crine** *a thing that secretes* Add words to make a correct and complete definition of *endocrine: A thing [organ or gland] that secretes [hormones] internally within [the body].* Every medical word must contain a combining form. The suffix of *endocrine* contains the combining form *crin/o-*.
Ophthalmology Eyes (Chapter 15)	Eyes	Perception of visual stimuli	**ophthalmology** (OFF-thal-MAWL-oh-jee) **ophthalm/o-** *eye* **-logy** *the study of*
Otolaryngology Ears, Nose, and Throat System (Chapter 16)	Ears, nose, sinuses, pharynx (throat), larynx (voice box)	Perception of smell and auditory stimuli. Production of speech.	**otolaryngology** (OH-toh-LAIR-ing-GAWL-oh-jee) **ot/o-** *ear* **laryng/o-** *larynx (voice box)* **-logy** *the study of*

Other Medical Specialties

Other medical specialties that are not directly related to a body system are included in this textbook. These include the following:

Medical Specialty	Chapter	Description	Word Part and Definition
Psychiatry	17	Study and treatment of the mind	**psychiatry** (sy-KY-ah-tree) **psych/o-** *mind* **-iatry** *medical treatment*
Oncology	18	Study and treatment of cancer	**oncology** (ong-KAWL-oh-jee) **onc/o-** *tumor, mass* **-logy** *the study of*
Radiology and Nuclear Medicine	19	Use of x-rays, sound waves, and other forms of radiation and energy to diagnose disease	**radiology** (RAY-dee-AWL-oh-jee) **radi/o-** *radius (forearm bone); x-rays; radiation* **-logy** *the study of* **nuclear** (NOO-klee-ar) **nucle/o-** *nucleus* **-ar** *pertaining to* **medicine** (MED-ih-sin) **medic/o-** *physician; medicine* **-ine** *pertaining to*
Dentistry	*	Study and treatment of the teeth and gums	**dentistry** (DEN-tis-tree) **dent/o-** *tooth* **-istry** *process related to the specialty of*
Dietetics	*	Study and use of nutrition, nutrients, and diet	**dietetics** (DY-eh-TET-iks) **dietet/o-** *foods, diet* **-ics** *knowledge, practice*
Pharmacology	*	Study and use of drugs as medicines	**pharmacology** (FAR-mah-KAWL-oh-jee) **pharmac/o-** *medicine, drug* **-logy** *the study of*
Neonatology	*	Study and treatment of newborns	**neonatology** (NEE-oh-nay-TAWL-oh-jee) **ne/o-** *new* **nat/o-** *birth* **-logy** *the study of*
Pediatrics	*	Study and treatment of infants and children	**pediatrics** (PEE-dee-AT-riks) **ped/o-** *child* **iatr/o-** *physician; medical treatment* **-ics** *knowledge, practice*
Geriatrics	*	Study and treatment of the elderly	**geriatrics** (JAIR-ee-AT-riks) **ger/o-** *old age* **iatr/o-** *physician; medical treatment* **-ics** *knowledge, practice*

*These medical specialties are mentioned in Across the Lifespan and Connections boxes scattered throughout the textbook.

Vocabulary Review

Anatomy and Physiology

Now that you have been introduced to ways to study the human body and its structures, take time to review those new words and descriptions. Memorize the combining forms and their definitions before going on to the next section.

Word or Phrase	Combining Form and Definition	Description
abdominal cavity	**abdomin/o-** *abdomen*	Cavity that is surrounded by the diaphragm superiorly, the abdominal wall anteriorly, and the spinal column posteriorly
abdominopelvic cavity	**abdomin/o-** *abdomen* **pelv/o-** *pelvis (hip bones; renal pelvis)*	Continuous cavity that includes the abdominal cavity superiorly and the pelvic cavity inferiorly
anatomical position	**tom/o-** *a cut, slice, or layer*	Standard position of the body for the purpose of studying it. The body is erect, head up, hands by the side with palms facing forward, and the legs are straight with toes pointing forward.
anatomy	**tom/o-** *a cut, slice, or layer*	The study of the structure of the human body and its parts
anterior	**anter/o-** *before; front part*	Pertaining to the front of the body or the front part of an organ or structure. *Anteroposterior* means *moving from the front to the back*.
cardiology	**cardi/o-** *heart*	Medical specialty that deals with the cardiovascular system
cardiovascular system	**cardi/o-** *heart* **vascul/o-** *blood vessel*	Body system that includes the heart, arteries, veins, and capillaries. It circulates the blood throughout the body.
caudad	**caud/o-** *tail bone; lower part of the body*	Toward the tail bone, feet, or lower part of the body
cavity	**cav/o-** *hollow space*	Hollow space surrounded by bones or muscles and containing organs and structures
cephalad	**cephal/o-** *head*	Toward the head of the body
coronal plane	**coron/o-** *encircling structure*	Plane that divides the body into front and back sections, anterior and posterior. Also known as the frontal plane.
cranial cavity	**crani/o-** *cranium (skull)*	Cavity in the head that is surrounded by the cranium and contains the brain, cranial nerves, and other structures
dentistry	**dent/o-** *tooth*	Medical specialty that deals with the teeth and gums
dermatology	**dermat/o-** *skin*	Medical specialty that deals with the integumentary system
dietetics	**dietet/o-** *foods, diet*	Medical specialty that deals with nutrition, nutrients, and diet

Word or Phrase	Combining Form and Definition	Description
distal	dist/o- *away from the center or point of origin*	Pertaining to away from the point of origin, particularly of an arm or leg
dorsal	dors/o- *back; dorsum*	Pertaining to the posterior of the body, particularly the back
endocrine system	crin/o- *a thing that secretes*	Body system that includes the testes, ovaries, pancreas, adrenal glands, thymus, thyroid gland, parathyroid glands, pituitary gland, and pineal gland. It produces and releases hormones that direct other body organs.
endocrinology	crin/o- *a thing that secretes*	Medical specialty that deals with the endocrine system
epigastric region	gastr/o- *stomach*	One of the nine regions of the surface of the abdominopelvic area. It is centered and superior to the umbilical region.
external	extern/o- *outside*	Pertaining to near or on the outside surface of the body or an organ
frontal plane	front/o- *front*	Another name for the coronal plane
gastroenterology	gastr/o- *stomach* enter/o- *intestine*	Medical specialty that deals with the gastrointestinal system
gastrointestinal system	gastr/o- *stomach* intestin/o- *intestine*	Body system that includes the mouth, teeth, tongue, salivary glands, pharynx (throat), esophagus, stomach, small intestine, large intestine, liver, gallbladder, and pancreas. It digests food, absorbs nutrients into the blood, and excretes undigested waste materials.
gynecology	gynec/o- *female, woman*	Medical specialty that deals with the female genital system
health		Optimum state of physical, mental, spiritual, and social well-being
hematology	hemat/o- *blood*	Medical specialty that deals with the blood
horizontal plane	horizont/o- *boundary between the earth and sky*	Another name for the transverse plane
hypochondriac region	chondr/o- *cartilage*	Two of the nine regions of the surface of the abdominopelvic area. The right and left hypochondriac regions are inferior to the lower edges of the anterior right and left ribs.
hypogastric region	gastr/o- *stomach*	One of the nine regions of the surface of the abdominopelvic area. It is centered on and inferior to the umbilical region.
immunology	immun/o- *immune response*	Medical specialty that deals with the lymphatic system and the immune response
inferior	infer/o- *below*	Pertaining to the lower half of the body or a position below an organ or structure
inguinal region	inguin/o- *groin* ili/o- *ilium (hip bone)*	Two of the nine regions of the surface of the abdominopelvic area. The right and left inguinal regions are inferior to the right and left lumbar regions. Also known as the iliac region.

Word or Phrase	Combining Form and Definition	Description
integumentary system	**integument/o-** *skin*	Body system that includes the skin, hair, nails, sweat glands, and oil glands. It perceives pain, touch, and temperature. It protects the internal organs from infection and trauma. It regulates body temperature by sweating.
internal	**intern/o-** *inside*	Within the body or an organ
lateral	**later/o-** *side*	Pertaining to the side of the body or the side of an organ or structure
lumbar region	**lumb/o-** *lower back; area between the ribs and pelvis*	Two of the nine regions of the surface of the abdominopelvic area. The right and left lumbar regions are positioned at the same level as the lumbar area of the back and to either side of the umbilical region.
lymphatic system	**lymph/o-** *lymph; lymphatic system*	Body system that includes the lymphatic vessels, lymph nodes, lymph, spleen, thymus, and white blood cells
macroscopic	**macr/o-** *large* **scop/o-** *examine with an instrument*	Large. Pertaining to structures that can be seen with the unaided eye.
medial	**medi/o-** *middle*	Pertaining to the middle of the body or the middle of an organ or structure
mediastinum		Central area within the thoracic cavity. It contains the trachea, esophagus, heart, and other structures.
microscopic	**micr/o-** *small* **scop/o-** *examine with an instrument*	Very small in size. Pertaining to tissues, cells, and structures within a cell that cannot be seen with the unaided eye.
microscope	**micr/o-** *small* **scop/o-** *examine with an instrument*	Instrument used to examine very small structures
midsagittal plane	**sagitt/o-** *going from front to back*	Plane that divides the body into right and left sections and creates a midline
muscular system	**muscul/o-** *muscle*	Body system that includes the muscles and tendons. It produces body movement.
neurology	**neur/o-** *nerve*	Medical specialty that deals with the nervous system
nervous system	**nerv/o-** *nerve*	Body system that includes the brain, cranial nerves, spinal cord, spinal nerves, and neurons. It receives signals from parts of the body and interprets them as pain, touch, temperature, body position, taste, sight, smell, or hearing. It coordinates body movement. It maintains and interprets memory and emotion.
obstetrics	**obstetr/o-** *pregnancy and childbirth*	Medical specialty that deals with the female reproductive system
oncology	**onc/o-**	Medical specialty that deals with the prevention, diagnosis, and
	tumor, mass	treatment of cancer

Word or Phrase	Combining Form and Definition	Description
ophthalmology	**ophthalm/o-** *eye*	Medical specialty that deals with the eyes
orthopedics	**orth/o-** *straight* **ped/o-** *child*	Medical specialty that deals with the skeletal system and muscular system
otolaryngology	**ot/o-** *ear* **laryng/o-** *larynx (voice box)*	Medical specialty that deals with the ears, nose, and throat
pelvic cavity	**pelv/o-** *pelvis (hip bone; renal pelvis)*	Cavity that is the inferior continuation of the abdominal cavity. It is surrounded by the pelvic bones and the base of the spinal column.
pharmacology	**pharmac/o-** *medicine, drug*	Medical specialty that deals with the use of drugs as medicines
physiology	**physi/o-** *physical function*	The study of the function of the human body and its parts
plane		An imaginary flat surface, like a plate of glass, that divides the body into parts. There are three planes: the coronal plane, midsagittal plane, and transverse plane.
posterior	**poster/o-** *back part*	Pertaining to the back of the body or the back part of an organ or structure. *Posteroanterior* means *moving from the back to the front.*
prone		Position of lying on the anterior part of the body
proximal	**proxim/o-** *near the center or point of origin*	Pertaining to near the point of origin, particularly of an arm or leg
psychiatry	**psych/o-** *mind*	Medical specialty that deals with the mind, mental health, and mental illness
pulmonology	**pulmon/o-** *lung*	Medical specialty that deals with the respiratory system
quadrant		One-quarter of an area that has been divided into four parts by an imaginary grid. The four quadrants of the surface of the abdominopelvic area are the right upper quadrant (RUQ), the left upper quadrant (LUQ), the left lower quadrant (LLQ), and the right lower quadrant (RLQ).
radiology	**radi/o-** *radius (forearm bone); x-rays; radiation*	Medical specialty that deals with the use of x-rays, sound waves, and other forms of radiation and energy to diagnose disease
reproductive system	**product/o-** *produce*	Body system that includes the breasts, ovaries, fallopian tubes, uterus, vagina, external genitalia for the female and the scrotum, testes, epididymides, vas deferens, seminal vesicles, prostate gland, urethra, and penis for the male. It produces eggs and sex hormones in the female and regulates menstruation, pregnancy, and milk production from the breasts. It produces sperm and sex hormones in the male.
respiratory system	**spir/o-** *breathe*	Body system that includes the nose, pharynx (throat), larynx (voice box), trachea, bronchi, lungs, and alveoli. It inhales oxygen, exhales carbon dioxide, and exchanges gases in the alveoli.

Word or Phrase	Combining Form and Definition	Description
skeletal system	**skelet/o-** *skeleton*	Body system that includes the bones, cartilage, ligaments, and joints. It supports the body.
spinal cavity	**spin/o-** *spine; backbone*	Cavity that is surrounded by the spinal column and contains the spinal cord, spinal nerves, and spinal fluid
superficial	**superfici/o-** *on or near the surface*	On or near the surface of the body or the surface of an organ or structure
superior	**super/o-** *above*	Pertaining to the upper half of the body or a position above an organ or structure
supine		Position of lying on the posterior part of the body. Also known as the dorsal supine position.
thoracic cavity	**thorac/o-** *thorax (chest)*	Cavity that is surrounded by the breast bone (sternum), ribs, and spinal column. The diaphragm makes up the inferior side of the cavity. The thoracic cavity contains the lungs. Within the thoracic cavity is the mediastinum.
transverse plane	**vers/o-** *to turn; to travel*	Plane that divides the body into top and bottom sections, superior and inferior
umbilical region	**umbilic/o-** *umbilicus, navel*	One of the nine regions of the surface of the abdominopelvic area. The centered umbilical region is located around the umbilicus.
urinary system	**urin/o-** *urine; urinary system*	Body system that includes the kidneys, ureters, bladder, urethra, and nephrons. It excretes urine and waste products.
urology	**ur/o-** *urine; urinary system*	Medical specialty that deals with the urinary system
ventral	**ventr/o-** *front; abdomen*	Pertaining to the anterior of the body, particularly the abdomen
viscera		All of the internal organs in every body cavity

Labeling Exercise

A. *Match each directional word to its number in the illustration (see Figure 2-18 ■). Write the directional word on the blank line next to its number. Use the Answer Key at the end of the book to check your answers.*

anterior (ventral)	lateral	posterior (dorsal)
distal	medial	proximal
dorsal		

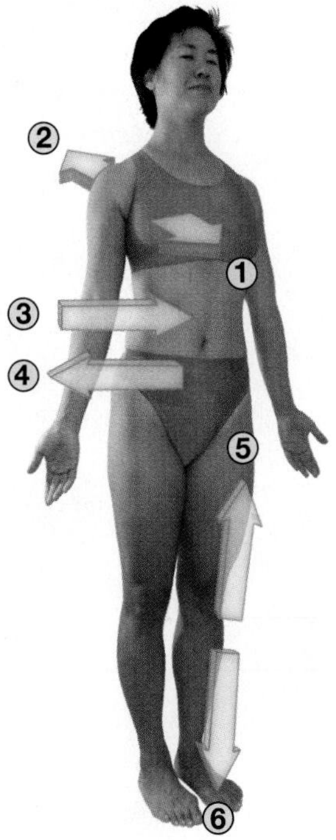

1. ______________________
2. ______________________
3. ______________________
4. ______________________
5. ______________________
6. ______________________

Figure 2-18 ■

B. *Match each body cavity to its number in the illustration (see Figure 2-19 ■). Write the name of the body cavity on the blank line next to its number.*

abdominal cavity	pelvic cavity	thoracic cavity
cranial cavity	spinal cavity	

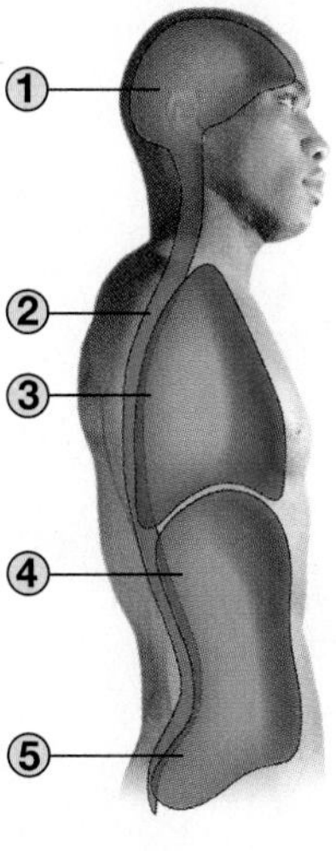

1. ______________________
2. ______________________
3. ______________________
4. ______________________
5. ______________________

Figure 2-19 ■

C. *Write the name of the body system and its medical specialty under each illustration (see Figures 2-20 ■ through 2-23 ■).*

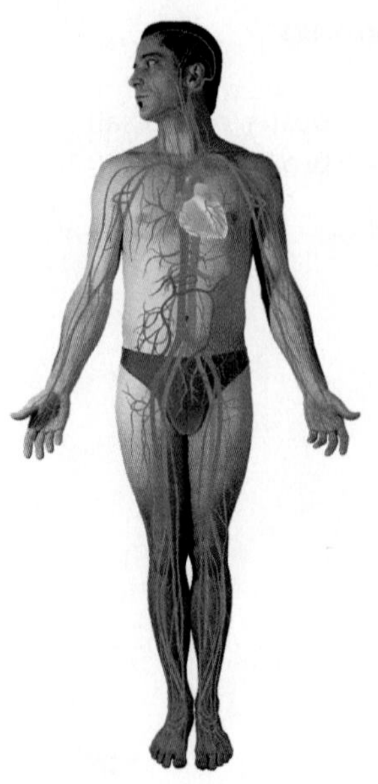

Figure 2-20 ■

1. ______________________________
2. ______________________________

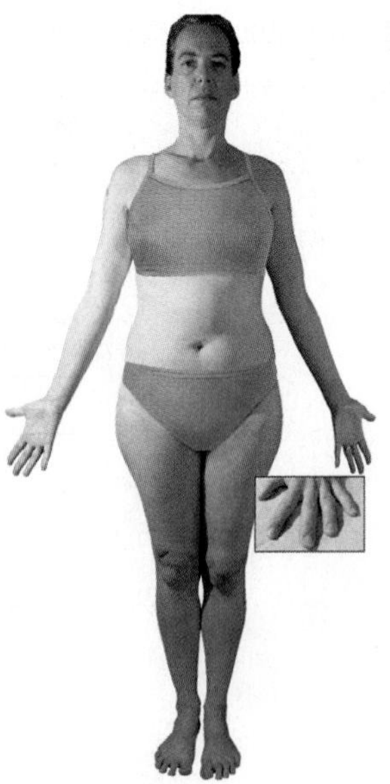

Figure 2-21 ■

1. ______________________________
2. ______________________________

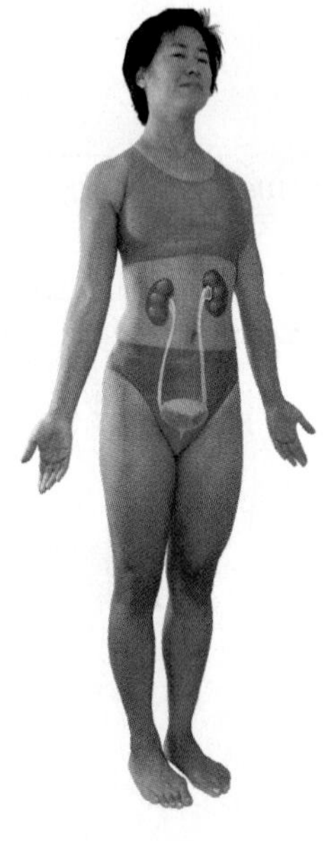

Figure 2-22 ■

1. ______________________________
2. ______________________________

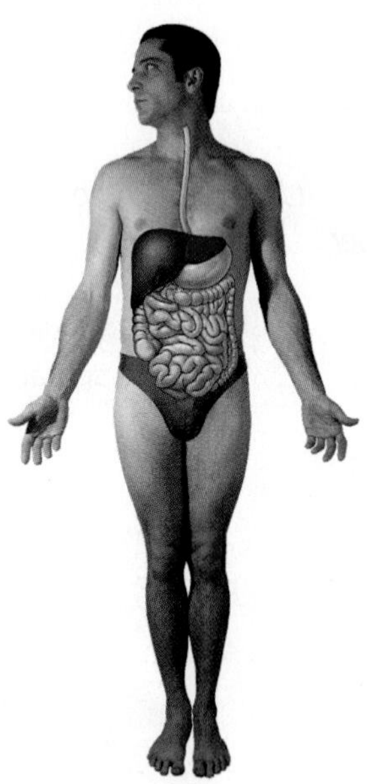

Figure 2-23 ■

1. ______________________________
2. ______________________________

Building Medical Words

Combining Forms

Here are the combining forms you have learned so far. Next to each combining form, write its meaning. Use the Answer Key at the end of the book to check your answers. The first one has been done for you.

	Combining Form	Medical Meaning		Combining Form	Medical Meaning
1.	dors/o-	back; dorsum	39.	medi/o-	
2.	abdomin/o-		40.	micr/o-	
3.	anter/o-		41.	muscul/o-	
4.	cardi/o-		42.	nat/o-	
5.	caud/o-		43.	ne/o-	
6.	cav/o-		44.	nerv/o-	
7.	cephal/o-		45.	neur/o-	
8.	chondr/o-		46.	nucle/o-	
9.	coron/o-		47.	obstetr/o-	
10.	crani/o-		48.	onc/o-	
11.	crin/o-		49.	ophthalm/o-	
12.	dent/o-		50.	orth/o-	
13.	dermat/o-		51.	ot/o-	
14.	dietet/o-		52.	ped/o-	
15.	dist/o-		53.	pelv/o-	
16.	enter/o-		54.	pharmac/o-	
17.	extern/o-		55.	physi/o-	
18.	front/o-		56.	poster/o-	
19.	gastr/o-		57.	product/o-	
20.	genit/o-		58.	proxim/o-	
21.	ger/o-		59.	psych/o-	
22.	gynec/o-		60.	pulmon/o-	
23.	hemat/o-		61.	radi/o-	
24.	horizont/o-		62.	sagitt/o-	
25.	iatr/o-		63.	scop/o-	
26.	ili/o-		64.	skelet/o-	
27.	immun/o-		65.	spin/o-	
28.	infer/o-		66.	spir/o-	
29.	inguin/o-		67.	superfici/o-	
30.	integument/o-		68.	super/o-	
31.	intern/o-		69.	thorac/o-	
32.	intestin/o-		70.	tom/o-	
33.	laryng/o-		71.	umbilic/o-	
34.	later/o-		72.	urin/o-	
35.	lumb/o-		73.	ur/o-	
36.	lymph/o-		74.	vascul/o-	
37.	macr/o-		75.	ventr/o-	
38.	medic/o-				

Combining Forms and Suffixes

Read the definition hint for the medical word you are to build. Look at the combining form that is given. Write the correct suffix on the blank line. Then write the medical word. (Remember: You may need to remove the combining vowel. Always remove the hyphens and slash.) Use the Answer Key at the end of the book to check your answers. The first one has been done for you.

SUFFIX LIST

-ac (pertaining to)	-ary (pertaining to)	-ics (knowledge, practice)
-ad (toward, in the direction of)	-atic (pertaining to)	-ior (pertaining to)
-al (pertaining to)	-iatry (medical treatment)	-logy (the study of)
-ar (pertaining to)	-ic (pertaining to)	-ous (pertaining to)

Definition Hint	Combining Form	Suffix	Write the Medical Word
1. Pertaining to the abdomen	abdomin/o-	-al	abdominal
2. The study of the physical functioning of the body	physi/o-	______	__________
3. Pertaining to the lower back	lumb/o-	______	__________
4. In the direction of the head	cephal/o-	______	__________
5. Pertaining to away from the point of origin	dist/o-	______	__________
6. Pertaining to the chest	thorac/o-	______	__________
7. Pertaining to the skull	crani/o-	______	__________
8. Pertaining to the back part	poster/o-	______	__________
9. The study of the skin	dermat/o-	______	__________
10. Pertaining to lymph system	lymph/o-	______	__________
11. Pertaining to the side	later/o-	______	__________
12. Pertaining to inside	intern/o-	______	__________
13. The study of the heart	cardi/o-	______	__________
14. The practice of pregnancy and childbirth	obstetr/o-	______	__________
15. The study of the urine and urinary system	ur/o-	______	__________
16. The study of the lungs	pulmon/o-	______	__________
17. The study of the eye	ophthalm/o-	______	__________
18. Pertaining to the skin	integument/o-	______	__________
19. The study of females	gynec/o-	______	__________
20. Medical treatment of the mind	psych/o-	______	__________
21. Pertaining to the nerves	nerv/o-	______	__________
22. Pertaining to the urine	urin/o-	______	__________
23. The study of tumors	onc/o-	______	__________

Combining Forms and Prefixes

Read the definition hint for the medical word you are to build. Look at the medical word or word part that is given. It already contains a combining form and a suffix. Write the correct prefix on the blank line. Then write the medical word. (Remember: You may need to remove the combining vowel. Always remove the hyphens and slash.) Use the Answer Key at the end of the book to check your answers. The first one has been done for you.

PREFIX LIST		
ana- (apart from; excessive)	epi- (upon, above)	mid- (middle)
endo- (innermost, within)	hypo- (below; deficient)	re- (again and again; backward; unable to)

Definition Hint	Prefix	Medical Word or Word Part	Write the Medical Word
1. Secretes hormones within the body	endo-	-crine	*endocrine*
2. Pertaining to cut apart or slice through	________	tomical	________
3. Pertaining to in the middle, going front to back	________	sagittal	________
4. Pertaining to below the cartilage [of the ribs]	________	chondriac	________
5. Pertaining to above the stomach	________	gastric	________
6. Pertaining to breathing again and again	________	spiratory	________
7. Pertaining to produce again and again	________	productive	________

The Body in Disease

Preventive medicine is the healthcare specialty whose goal it is to keep a person in a state of health and prevent the occurrence of disease. But despite the best efforts of modern medicine, the human body does not always remain in a state of health. A significant portion of medical language deals with diseases and how they are diagnosed and treated. **Disease** is any change in the normal structure or function of the body. This change might be slight and short lived or severe and life threatening. The cause or origin of a disease is known as its **etiology.** In most cases, the cause of a disease is known or can be discovered through medical testing. In some cases, however, the exact cause of a disease can never be completely explained.

preventive (pree-VEN-tiv)
prevent/o- *prevent*
-ive *pertaining to*

medicine (MED-ih-sin)
medic/o- *physician; medicine*
-ine *pertaining to*

disease (dih-ZEEZ)
Disease is a combination of the prefix *dis-* (*apart from*) and the English word *ease* (*freedom from pain or discomfort*).

etiology (ee-tee-AWL-oh-jee)
eti/o- *cause of disease*
-logy *the study of*

Disease Categories

Diseases can be divided into several different categories based on their etiologies:

Disease Type	Etiology	Word Part and Definition
congenital	Caused by an abnormality as the fetus develops or one that occurs during the birth process Examples: Cleft lip and palate, cerebral palsy	**congenital** (con-JEN-ih-tal) **congenit/o-** *present at birth* **-al** *pertaining to*
degenerative	Caused by the progressive destruction of cells due to disease or the aging process Examples: Multiple sclerosis, loss of hearing	**degenerative** (dee-JEN-er-ah-tiv) **de-** *reversal of; without* **gener/o-** *production; creation* **-ative** *pertaining to*
environmental	Caused by exposure to external substances Examples: Allergies to pollen, skin cancer from the sun	**environmental** (en-VY-rawn-MEN-tal)
hereditary	Caused by an inherited or spontaneous mutation in the genetic material of a cell Examples: Down syndrome, sickle cell disease	**hereditary** (heh-RED-ih-tair-ee) **heredit/o-** *genetic inheritance* **-ary** *pertaining to*
iatrogenic	Caused by medicine or treatment given to the patient Examples: Wrong drug given to a patient, surgery performed on the wrong leg	**iatrogenic** (eye-AT-roh-JEN-ik) **iatr/o-** *physician; medical treatment* **gen/o-** *arising from; produced by* **-ic** *pertaining to*
idiopathic	Having no identifiable cause	**idiopathic** (ID-ee-oh-PATH-ik) **idi/o-** *unknown; individual* **path/o-** *disease, suffering* **-ic** *pertaining to*

Disease Type	Etiology	Word Part and Definition
infectious	Caused by a **pathogen** (disease-causing microorganism such as a bacterium, virus, fungus, and so forth). A **communicable** disease is an infectious disease that is transmitted by direct contact with another infected person, animal, or insect. Examples: Gonorrhea (a sexually transmitted disease), rabies from an animal bite	**infectious** (in-FEK-shus) **infect/o-** *disease within* **-ious** *pertaining to* Add words to make a correct and complete definition of *infectious: pertaining to disease[-causing organisms] within the body.* **pathogen** (PATH-oh-jen) **path/o-** *disease, suffering* **-gen** *that which produces* **communicable** (koh-MYOON-ih-kah-bl) **communic/o-** *impart, transmit* **-able** *able to be*
neoplastic	Caused by the growth of benign or malignant tumors Examples: Benign cyst, cancerous tumor of the skin	**neoplastic** (NEE-oh-PLAS-tik) **ne/o-** *new* **plas/o-** *growth, formation* **-tic** *pertaining to* A neoplasm is a new growth or formation. It can be either benign (not cancerous) or malignant (cancerous).
nosocomial	Caused by exposure to infection while the patient is in the hospital Examples: Surgical wound infection	**nosocomial** (NOS-oh-KOH-mee-al) *Nosocomial* is derived from a Greek word meaning *hospital.*
nutritional	Caused by a lack of nutritious food, insufficient amounts of food, or an inability to utilize nutrients in the food Examples: Malnutrition, pernicious anemia caused by lack of intrinsic factor production in the stomach	**nutritional** (noo-TRISH-un-al) **nutri/o-** *nourishment* **-tion** *a process; being or having* **-al** *pertaining to*

Onset, Course, and Outcome of Disease

The onset of a disease is made evident by symptoms and/or signs. A **symptom** is any deviation from health that can only be perceived or felt by the **patient.** When a symptom has a physical manifestation that can be detected by others, it is known as a sign. An elevated temperature (as measured by a thermometer), coughing, tremors, paleness, vomiting, and a palpable lump are all signs of disease. **Symptomatology** is the clinical picture of all the patient's symptoms and signs. A **syndrome** is a set of symptoms and signs associated with and characteristic of one particular disease. Patients who are **asymptomatic** (showing no symptoms or signs) can still have a disease, but it can only be detected by medical tests.

To fully understand the patient's symptoms, the physician takes a history and performs a physical examination. For the history of the present illness, the physician asks the patient in detail about the location, onset, duration, and severity of the symptoms. The physician also asks about the patient's past medical history, past surgical history, family history, social history, and history of allergies to drugs.

After taking the patient's history, the physician performs a physical examination to look for signs of disease. The physician uses the following techniques (as needed) during the physical examination (see Figures 2-24■ and 2-25■).

symptom (SIMP-tom)
Symptom is derived from a Greek word meaning *something that has happened to someone.*

patient (PAY-shent)
Patient is derived from a Latin word meaning *to suffer.*

symptomatology
(SIMP-toh-mah-TAWL-oh-jee)
symptomat/o- *collection of symptoms*
-logy *the study of*

syndrome (SIN-drohm)
syn- *together*
-drome *a running*
Every medical word must contain a combining form. The suffix of *syndrome* contains the combining form *drom/o-*.

asymptomatic (AA-simp-toh-MAT-ik)
a- *away from; without*
symptomat/o- *collection of symptoms*
-ic *pertaining to*

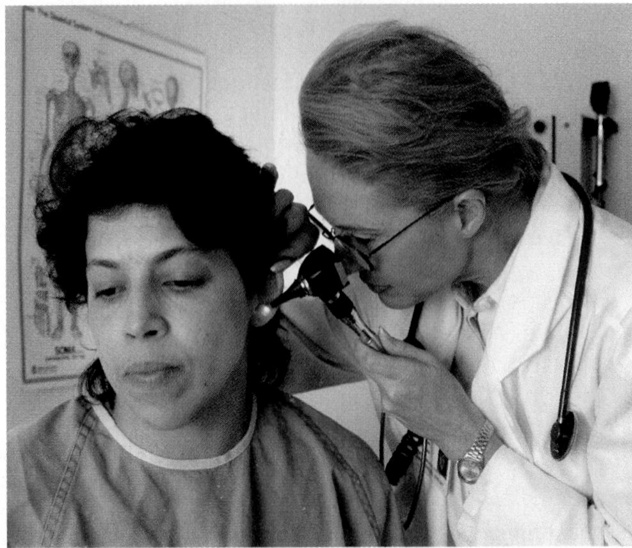

Figure 2-24 ■ Inspection.
This physician is using a lighted instrument to illuminate the patient's internal ear canal.

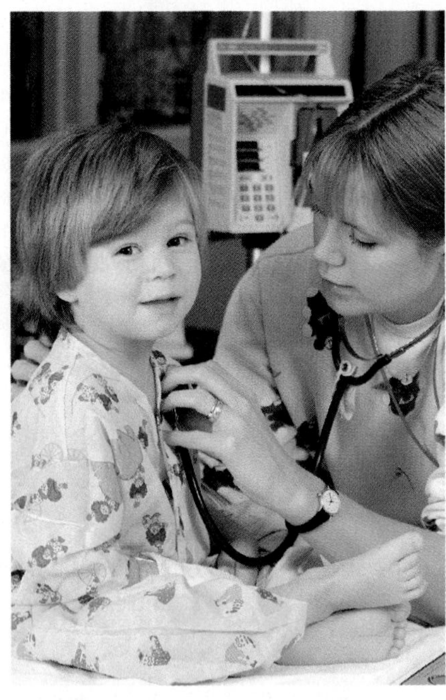

Figure 2-25 ■ Auscultation.
This nurse is using a stethoscope to listen to this child's breathing.

- **Inspection:** using the eyes to examine the external surfaces or internal cavities of the body
- **Palpation:** using the fingers to press on the body to feel masses or enlarged organs or to detect tenderness
- **Auscultation:** using a **stethoscope** to listen to the sounds of the heart, lungs, or intestines
- **Percussion:** Using the finger of one hand to tap on the finger of the other hand while that hand is spread over a large body cavity. After a few taps, the hand is moved to another location, and the variation in sound is compared.

After taking the patient's history and performing the physical examination, the physician may be able to make a **diagnosis** or determination as to the cause of the patient's symptoms and signs. The patient may have several different problems and therefore several diagnoses. If the physician cannot make a diagnosis, the patient is scheduled to undergo **diagnostic** tests or referred to an appropriate physician specialist.

The course of a disease includes all events from the onset of the disease until its final outcome. During the course of a disease, the symptoms and signs may be **acute** (sudden in its nature and severe in

inspection (in-SPEK-shun)
inspect/o- *looking at*
-ion *action; condition*

palpation (pal-PAY-shun)
palpat/o- *touching, feeling*
-ion *action; condition*

auscultation (AWS-kul-TAY-shun)
auscult/o- *listening*
-ation *a process; being or having*

stethoscope (STETH-oh-skohp)
steth/o- *chest*
-scope *instrument used to examine*

percussion (per-KUSH-un)
percuss/o- *tapping*
-ion *action; condition*

diagnosis (DY-ag-NOH-sis)
dia- *complete; completely through*
gnos/o- *knowledge*
-osis *condition; abnormal condition; process*
Diagnosis is a Greek word meaning *a deciding.* Form the plural (*diagnoses*) by changing *-is* to *-es.*

diagnostic (DY-ag-NAWS-tik)
dia- *complete; completely through*
gnos/o- *knowledge*
-tic *pertaining to*

acute (ah-KYOOT)
Acute is derived from a Latin word meaning *sharp.*

intensity), **subacute** (less severe in intensity), or **chronic** in nature (continuing for three months or more). An **exacerbation** is a sudden worsening in the severity of the symptoms or signs. A **sequela** is an abnormal condition or complication that arises because of the original disease and remains after the original disease has resolved. **Remission** is a temporary improvement in the symptoms and signs of a disease without the underlying disease being cured. A relapse or recurrence is a return of the original symptoms and signs of the disease.

The course and outcome of a disease can be affected by treatment: the physician prescribes drugs or orders **therapy** for the patient. The disease improves if the treatment is **therapeutic** and causes improvement in the symptoms or signs. A disease that is **refractory** to treatment is one that does not respond well to treatment. Certain diseases that cannot be treated with drugs or therapy may require **surgery.**

The predicted outcome of a disease is known as the **prognosis.** The natures of many diseases are so well known that the physician can predict with a great deal of accuracy what the patient's prognosis will be. The course of a disease can have one of three outcomes. **Recuperation** or recovery is a return to a normal state of health. When recuperation is not complete, residual chronic disease or disability remains. A **disability** is a permanent inability to perform certain activities or function in a given way. A **terminal** illness is one from which the patient cannot recover and which eventually results in death.

subacute (SUB-ah-KYOOT)
Subacute is a combination of the prefix *sub-* (*below, underneath, less than*) and the word *acute.*

chronic (KRAW-nik)
chron/o- *time*
-ic *pertaining to*

exacerbation (eg-ZAS-er-BAY-shun)
exacerb/o- *increase; provoke*
-ation *a process; being or having*

sequela (see-KWEL-ah)
sequelae (see-KWEL-ee)
Sequela is a Latin singular feminine noun meaning *something that follows*. Form the plural by changing *-a* to *-ae.*

remission (ree-MISH-un)
remiss/o- *send back*
-ion *action; condition*

therapy (THAIR-ah-pee)

therapeutic (THAIR-ah-PYOO-tik)
therapeut/o- *treatment*
-ic *pertaining to*

refractory (ree-FRAK-tor-ee)
re- *again and again; backward; unable to*
fract/o- *break up*
-ory *having the function of*
Add words to make a complete and correct definition of *refractory*: *pertaining to [a disease that treatment is] unable to break up, [treat, or cure].*

surgery (SER-jer-ee)
surg/o- *operative procedure*
-ery *process of*
Surgery is derived from a Latin word meaning *hand work.*

prognosis (prawg-NOH-sis)
pro- *before*
gnos/o- *knowledge*
-osis *condition; abnormal condition; process*

recuperation (ree-KOO-per-AA-shun)
recuper/o- *recover*
-ation *a process; being or having*

disability (DIS-ah-BIL-ah-tee)
Disability is a combination of the prefix *dis-* (*away from*) and the English word *ability* (*competence*).

terminal (TER-mih-nal)
termin/o- *end; boundary*
-al *pertaining to*

Healthcare Professionals and Healthcare Settings

Healthcare Professionals

Physicians

A **physician** or **doctor** is the leader of the healthcare team. The physician orders tests, diagnoses diseases, and treats diseases by prescribing drugs or therapy or by performing surgery. When physicians perform surgery, they are known as surgeons. Physicians who graduate from medical school receive a Doctor of Medicine (M.D.) degree. Physicians who graduate from a school of osteopathy receive a Doctor of Osteopathy (D.O.) degree. After graduation, physicians select a specialized area (family practice, pediatrics, psychiatry, and so forth) in which to continue their studies. **Surgeons** are physicians who complete additional training in surgery.

Some doctors graduate from schools that focus their training on just one part of the body. Chiropracters have a Doctor of Chiropractic (D.C.) degree and only treat the alignment of the bones, muscles, and nerves. Optometrists have a Doctor of Optometry (O.D.) degree and treat only the eyes. Podiatrists have a Doctor of Podiatric Medicine (D.P.M.) degree and treat only the feet. Dentists have a Doctor of Dental Surgery (D.D.S.) degree and treat only the teeth. Pharmacists have a Doctor of Pharmacy (Pharm.D.) degree and only fill prescriptions for medicines.

Primary care physicians (PCPs) specialize in family practice or pediatrics. They see the majority of patients on a day-to-day basis. A physician who is on the medical staff of a hospital and admits a patient to the hospital is known as the attending physician.

physician (fih-ZISH-un)
physi/o- *physical function*
-ician *a skilled professional or expert*
Delete the duplicate *i*.
Physician is derived from a Latin word, but it also came to mean *philosopher in* French.

doctor (DAWK-ter)
Doctor is derived from a Latin word meaning *teacher.*

surgeon (SER-jun)
surg/o- *operative procedure*
-eon *one who performs*

Physician Extenders

Physician extenders are healthcare professionals who perform some of the duties of a physician. They examine, diagnose, and treat patients and prescribe medications.

They give care under the supervision of a physician (M.D. or D.O). Physician extenders include physicians' assistants (PAs), nurse practitioners (NPs), certified nurse midwives (CNMs), and certified registered nurse anesthetists (CRNAs).

Allied Health Professionals

Nurses are allied health professionals who examine patients, make nursing diagnoses, and administer treatments or drugs ordered by the physician. Nurses often given hands-on care and focus on the physical as well as emotional needs of the patient and the family.

Other allied health professionals include **technologists, technicians, therapists,** as well as dieticians, medical assistants, phlebotomists, dental hygienists, and audiologists.

nurse (NERS)
Nurse is derived from a French word meaning *to tend.*

technologist (tek-NAWL-oh-jist)
techn/o- *technical skill*
log/o- *the study of*
-ist *one who specializes in*

technician (tek-NISH-un)
techn/o- *technical skill*
-ician *a skilled professional or expert*

therapist (THAIR-ah-pist)
therap/o- *treatment*
-ist *one who specializes in*

Healthcare Settings

Health care is provided in many different settings, depending on the healthcare needs of the patient and which setting can most cost-effectively meet those needs.

Hospital

A **hospital** is a healthcare facility that is the traditional setting for providing care for patients who are acutely ill and require medical or surgical care for longer than 24 hours. Each hospital stay begins with an admission to the hospital and ends with a discharge from the hospital. A physician must write an order in the patient's medical record to admit or discharge the patient. The physician also monitors the patient's care and orders diagnostic tests, treatments, therapies, drugs, and surgeries as needed. A patient in the hospital is known as an **inpatient.**

A hospital is divided into areas that provide care for specific types of patients. These areas are known as floors or nursing units. There are also specialty care units such as the intensive care unit. **Ancillary** departments in the hospital provide additional types of services. Ancillary departments include the radiology department, the clinical laboratory, the physical therapy (PT) department, dietary department, pharmacy, and the emergency department (ED). Nonmedical departments provide other services such as health information management (medical records), finances and billing, housekeeping, and so forth.

hospital (HAWS-pih-tal)
Hospital is derived from a Latin word meaning *receiving guests and strangers* and is related to the English word *hospitable.*

inpatient (IN-pay-shent)
Inpatient is a combination of the English word *in* (in a facility) and the medical word *patient.*

ancillary (AN-sih-lair-ee)
ancill/o- *servant, accessory*
-ary *pertaining to*

Physician's Office

The physician's office or doctor's office is the most frequently used healthcare setting. A single physician or group of physicians (a group practice) maintains an office where patients are seen, diagnosed, treated, and counseled. Some offices have their own laboratory and x-ray equipment for performing diagnostic tests. Seriously ill patients who cannot be quickly diagnosed or adequately treated in the office are sent to a hospital.

Clinic

A **clinic** provides healthcare services similar to that of a physician's office but for just one type of patient or one type of disease. For example, a methadone clinic treats former drug addicts, and a well-baby clinic provides care to newborn infants. Clinics that are located in a hospital are known as outpatient clinics and their patients are known as **outpatients.** Outpatients are never formally admitted to the hospital and do not stay overnight at the clinic.

clinic (KLIN-ik)
Clinic is derived from a Greek word meaning *bed.* Clinics no longer have beds because the patients do not stay overnight.

outpatient (OUT-pay-shent)
Outpatient is a combination of the English word *out* (of a facility) and the word *patient.*

Ambulatory Surgery Center (ASC)

An **ambulatory** surgery center is a facility where minor surgery is performed and the patient does not stay overnight. The patients are known as outpatients.

ambulatory (AM-byoo-lah-TOR-ee)
ambulat/o- *walking*
-ory *having the function of*
An ambulatory facility is one in which the outpatients are able leave the facility shortly after surgery.

Long-Term Care Facility

A **long-term care facility**, previously known as a nursing home, is primarily a residential facility for elderly or disabled persons who are unable to care for themselves. Long-term care facilities provide 24-hour nursing care. Persons in long-term care facilities are known as **residents** rather than patients. Facilities that have a special nursing unit that provides a high level of medical and nursing care for patients discharged from the hospital are designated as skilled nursing facilities (SNFs). Many long-term care facilities also provide **rehabilitation** services to transition a patient from hospital to home.

rehabilitation (REE-hah-BIL-ih-TAY-shun)
re- *again and again; backward; unable to*
habilitat/o- *give ability*
-ion *action; condition*

Home Health Agency

A **home health agency** provides a range of healthcare services to persons in their homes. These services are particularly useful to those who are unable to come to a physician's office or clinic and do not want to live in a long-term care facility. Home health patients are known as **clients.**

Hospice

A **hospice** is a facility for patients who are dying. Patients are admitted to a hospice only if a physician certifies that they have less than six months to live. A hospice patient has a terminal illness from which there is no hope of recovery. Hospice services include **palliative** care (supportive medical and nursing care to keep the patient comfortable), counseling, and emotional support for the patient and family.

hospice (HAWS-pis)
Hospice is derived from a Latin word meaning *receiving guests and strangers.*

palliative (PAL-ee-ah-tiv)
palliat/o- *reduce the severity of*
-ive *pertaining to*
Palliative care alleviates the patient's suffering as much as possible but cannot cure the underlying terminal illness.

Vocabulary Review

Now that you have studied about healthcare settings and healthcare personnel, take time to review those new words and descriptions. Memorize the combining forms and their definitions.

Word or Phrase	Combining Form and Definition	Description
acute		Symptoms and signs that occur suddenly and are severe in nature
allied health professionals		Healthcare professionals who support the work of physicians and perform specific services ordered by the physician. Allied health professionals include technologists, technicians, therapists, and others.
ambulatory	**ambulat/o-** *walking*	Any healthcare facility for medical or surgical care where patients arrive at the time of their appointments, leave within a few minutes or hours, do not occupy a bed, and are not admitted to the facility
ambulatory surgery center (ASC)	**ambulat/o-** *walking* **surg/o-** *operative procedure*	Facility where minor surgical procedures are performed. Patients are known as **outpatients.** They do not stay overnight and are not admitted.
ancillary department	**ancill/o-** *servant, accessory*	Department that provides services that support the medical and surgical care given in the hospital. Examples: radiology department, physical therapy department, dietary department, pharmacy, emergency department.
asymptomatic	**symptomat/o-** *collection of symptoms*	Showing no symptoms or signs
attending physician	**physi/o-** *physical function*	Physician on the medical staff of a hospital who admits patients and directs their care
auscultation	**auscult/o-** *listening*	Using a stethoscope to listen to heart, lung, or intestinal sounds
chronic	**chron/o-** *time*	Symptoms or signs that continue for three months or more
clinic		An ambulatory facility that provides physician office–type healthcare services for just one type of patient or one type of disease. Example: Well-baby checkups for newborns. Clinic patients are known as **outpatients** and the facility is an outpatient clinic.
congenital	**congenit/o-** *present at birth*	Disease caused by an abnormality in fetal development or one that occurs during birth
degenerative	**gener/o-** *production; creation*	Disease caused by progressive destruction of cells due to disease or the aging process
diagnosis	**gnos/o-** *knowledge*	A determination as to the cause of the patient's symptoms and signs
disability		Permanent inability to perform certain activities or function in a given way
discharge		Release by a hospital of a patient who no longer needs hospital-level care. The patient can be discharged to home or transferred to another healthcare facility.
disease		Any change in the normal structure or function of the body

Word or Phrase	Combining Form and Definition	Description
environmental		Disease caused by exposure to substances in the environment (smoke, pollen, sun rays, and so forth)
etiology	**eti/o-** *cause of disease*	The cause or origin of a disease
exacerbation	**exacerb/o-** *increase; provoke*	Sudden worsening in the severity of symptoms or signs
hereditary	**heredit/o-** *genetic inheritance*	Disease caused by an inherited or spontaneous mutation in the genetic material of a cell
home health agency		Agency that provides nursing and non-nursing services to patients in their homes. These patients are known as **clients.**
hospice		Facility for patients who have a terminal illness and require palliative supportive care, counseling, and emotional support for themselves and their families.
hospital		Healthcare facility that provides care for acutely ill medical and surgical patients for longer than 24 hours. The person being treated is known as an **inpatient.** The patient is admitted, occupies a bed in the hospital, and is discharged.
iatrogenic	**iatr/o-** *physician; medical treatment* **gen/o-** *arising from; produced by*	Disease caused by medicine or treatment given to the patient
idiopathic	**idi/o-** *unknown; individual* **path/o-** *disease, suffering*	Disease having no identifiable cause
infectious	**infect/o-** *disease within* **communic/o-** *impart, transmit*	Disease caused by a pathogen. A **communicable** disease is an infectious disease that is transmitted by direct contact with another infected person or with an infected animal or insect
inpatient		A patient in a hospital
inspection	**inspect/o-** *looking at*	Using the eyes or an instrument to examine the body
long-term care facility		Residential facility for persons who are unable to care for themselves. Long-term care facilities, formerly known as nursing homes, provide 24-hour nursing care. Persons in this facility are known as **residents.**
neoplastic	**plas/o-** *growth, formation*	Disease caused by the growth of a benign (not cancerous) or malignant (cancerous) tumor or mass
nosocomial		Disease caused by exposure to an infection while the patient is in the hospital
nutritional	**nutri/o-** *nourishment*	Disease caused by lack of nutritious food, too little food, or an inability to utilize the food that is eaten

Word or Phrase	Combining Form and Definition	Description
palliative care	palliat/o- *reduce the severity of*	Supportive medical and nursing care that keeps the patient comfortable but does not cure the disease
palpation	palpat/o- *touching, feeling*	Using the fingers to press on a body part to detect a mass, enlarged organs, or tenderness
pathogen	path/o- *disease, suffering*	Disease-causing microorganism like a bacterium, virus, fungus, and so forth
percussion	percuss/o- *tapping*	Tapping one finger on another finger of a hand that is spread across the chest or abdomen to listen for differences in sound that would indicate the presence of fluid
physician	physi/o- *physical function*	Healthcare professional who directs the activities of the healthcare team. The physician orders tests, diagnoses, and treats patients. Also known as a **doctor.** A primary care physician (PCP) is a general practitioner who specializes in family practice or pediatrics.
physician extender		Healthcare professionals who perform some of the duties of a physician such as examining, diagnosing, ordering treatments, and prescribing medicines. These include physicians' assistants, nurse practitioners, certified nurse midwives, and certififed registered nurse anesthetists.
physician's office		Ambulatory facility where a physician or a group of physicians (group practice) maintains an office. The patients are known as outpatients. They are seen for a short period of time to diagnose and prescribe treatment for diseases that do not require hospital-level care.
preventive medicine	prevent/o- *prevent*	Keeps a person in a state of health and prevents the occurrence of disease
prognosis	gnos/o- *knowledge*	Predicted outcome of a disease.
recuperation	recuper/o- *recover*	Return to a normal state of health
refractory	fract/o- *break up*	A disease that does not respond well to treatment
remission	remiss/o- *send back*	Temporary improvement in the symptoms and signs of a disease without the underlying disease being cured
sequela		Abnormal condition or complication that is caused by the original disease and remains after the original disease has resolved
skilled nursing facility (SNF)		Long-term care facility with a special nursing unit that can admit patients directly from a hospital and provide a high level of medical and nursing care. Persons in this facility are known as **residents.**
symptom		A deviation from health that can only be perceived by the patient
symptomatology	symptomat/o- *collection of symptoms*	The clinical picture of all the patient's symptoms and signs
syndrome	drom/o- *a running*	Set of symptoms and signs associated with one particular disease
surgeon		Physician or doctor who performs surgery

Word or Phrase	Combining Form and Definition	Description
subacute		Symptoms and signs that are less severe in intensity than acute symptoms
surgery	**surg/o-** *operative procedure*	A treatment that involves invading the patient's body, often by cutting
technician	**techn/o-** *technical skill*	A trained professional who has technical skill in a particular field of medicine
technologist	**techn/o-** *technical skill* **log/o-** *the study of*	A trained professional who specializes in a technical area of a field of medicine and performs technical tests
terminal illness	**termin/o-** *end; boundary*	A disease from which there is no hope of recovery and one which will eventually result in the patient's death
therapeutic	**therapeut/o-** *treatment*	Pertaining to an action (from therapy or medicines) that results in improvement in the symptoms or signs of a disease
therapist	**therap/o-** *treatment*	A trained health professional who performs therapy on patients to treat a specific disease

Building Medical Words

Combining Forms

Here are the combining forms you have learned so far. Next to each combining form, write its meaning. Use the Answer Key at the end of the book to check your answers. The first one has been done for you.

Combining Form	Medical Meaning	Combining Form	Medical Meaning
1. termin/o-	end; boundary	20. log/o-	
2. ambulat/o-		21. medic/o-	
3. ancill/o-		22. ne/o-	
4. auscult/o-		23. nutri/o-	
5. chron/o-		24. palliat/o-	
6. communic/o-		25. palpat/o-	
7. congenit/o-		26. path/o-	
8. eti/o-		27. percuss/o-	
9. exacerb/o-		28. physi/o-	
10. fract/o-		29. plas/o-	
11. gener/o-		30. prevent/o-	
12. gen/o-		31. recuper/o-	
13. gnos/o-		32. remiss/o-	
14. habilitat/o-		33. steth/o-	
15. heredit/o-		34. surg/o-	
16. iatr/o-		35. symptomat/o-	
17. idi/o-		36. techn/o-	
18. infect/o-		37. therapeut/o-	
19. inspect/o-		38. therap/o-	

Combining Forms and Suffixes

Read the definition hint for the medical word you are to build. Look at the combining form that is given. Write the correct suffix on the blank line. Then write the medical word. (Remember: You may need to remove the combining vowel. Always remove the hyphens and slash.) Use the Answer Key at the end of the book to check your answers. The first one has been done for you.

SUFFIX LIST

-al (pertaining to)	-gen (that which produces)	-ist (one who specializes in)
-ary (pertaining to)	-ic (pertaining to)	-ive (pertaining to)
-ation (a process; being or having)	-ician (a skilled professional or expert)	-logy (the study of)
-eon (one who performs)	-ion (action; condition)	-ory (having the function of)
-ery (process of)	-ious (pertaining to)	

	Definition Hint	Combining Form	Suffix	Write the Medical Word
1.	One who performs operative procedures	surg/o-	-eon	surgeon
2.	Pertaining to an end of life	termin/o-	______	______
3.	One who specializes in treatment	therap/o-	______	______
4.	Having the function of walking	ambulat/o-	______	______
5.	Pertaining to reducing the severity	palliat/o-	______	______
6.	Skilled professional or expert with technical skills	techn/o-	______	______
7.	Pertaining to genetic inheritance	heredit/o-	______	______
8.	That which produces disease or suffering	path/o-	______	______
9.	The study of the collection of all symptoms	symptomat/o-	______	______
10.	Action of touching or feeling	palpat/o-	______	______
11.	The process of listening	auscult/o-	______	______
12.	Pertaining to disease-causing organisms in the body	infect/o-	______	______
13.	Pertaining to treatment	therapeut/o-	______	______
14.	The process of an operative procedure	surg/o-	______	______
15.	The action of tapping	percuss/o-	______	______
16.	Pertaining to continuing over time	chron/o-	______	______
17.	Pertaining to being present at birth	congenit/o-	______	______
18.	The study of the cause of a disease	eti/o-	______	______

Prefixes and Combining Forms

Read the definition hint for the medical word you are to build. Look at the word or word part that is given. It already contains a combining form and a suffix. Write the correct prefix on the blank line. Then write the medical word. (Remember: You may need to remove the combining vowel. Always remove the hyphens and slash.) Use the Answer Key at the end of the book to check your answers. The first one has been done for you.

PREFIX LIST

a- (without)	dia- (complete, completely through)	re- (again and again; backward; unable to)
de- (reversal of, without)	pro- (before)	

	Definition Hint	Prefix	Medical Word or Word Part	Write the Medical Word
1.	Condition of complete knowledge	dia-	gnosis	diagnosis
2.	Pertaining to the reversal of production	________	generative	________________
3.	Pertaining to without symptoms	________	symptomatic	________________
4.	Condition of before knowledge	________	gnosis	________________
5.	Pertaining to being unable to break up	________	fractory	________________

Abbreviations

A&P	anatomy and physiology
AP	anteroposterior
ASC	ambulatory surgery center
CNM	certified nurse midwife
CRNA	certified registered nurse anesthetist
CV	cardiovascular
D.C.	Doctor of Chiropractic
D.D.S.	Doctor of Dental Surgery
D.O.	Doctor of Osteopathy
D.P.M.	Doctor of Podiatric Medicine
Dr.	doctor
Dx	diagnosis
ED	emergency department
ENT	ears, nose, and throat
GI	gastrointestinal
GYN	gynecology
H&P	history and physical examination
Hx	history
LPN	licensed practical nurse
M.D.	Doctor of Medicine
NP	nurse practitioner
OB	obstetrics
O.D.	Doctor of Optometry
PA	physician's assistant
PA	posteroanterior
PCP	primary care physician
PE	physical examination
Pharm.D.	Doctor of Pharmacy
PT	physical therapy
RN	registered nurse
SNF	skilled nursing facility (pronounced "sniff")
Sx	symptoms
Tx	treatment

Word Alert

MEDICAL ABBREVIATIONS

Abbreviations are commonly used in all types of medical documents; however, they can mean different things to different people and their meaning can be misinterpreted. Always verify the meaning of an abbreviation.

PA stands for *physician's assistant,* but it also stands for *posteroanterior.*

PCP stands for *primary care physician,* but it also stands for *Pneumocystis carinii pneumonia* and *phencyclidine* (the street drug known as *angel dust*).

Career Focus

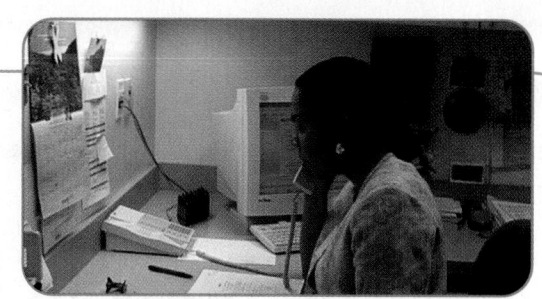

Meet April, a health information manager.

"My title is Applications Manager for our Patient Information Management Department. I've moved from straight health information management to really managing software and how we use the software to gather information. For anything that is done to the patient, there would be documentation, and all of it comes to the medical record department to be stored. We end up interacting with every single clinical department. Since we hold the information, we also help to disseminate it. You get to know a whole lot about medicine without actually being the person who takes care of a patient. You definitely have to have a strong background in medical terminology in order to be really effective in this kind of setting. You're looking at records and trying to make sure that things are correct, and a misunderstood word can change the meaning. Not only for transcription, but for coding, for analysis of the record—there's almost no place that it's not important. The tasks that we perform really help make health care run smoothly for the people who are delivering the care."

Health information management staff work in physician group practices, clinics, hospitals, nursing homes, and for transcription and coding companies.

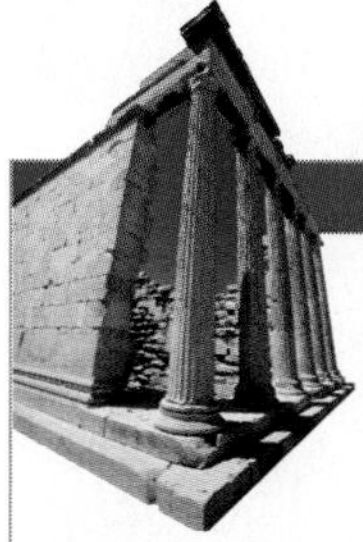

It's Greek to Me!

Did you notice that some words have two different combining forms? In ancient times, the Greeks and the Romans independently advanced the study and practice of medicine, naming many things in their own languages. Combining forms from both Greek and Latin languages remain a part of medical language today.

English Word	Greek	Latin	Example of Medical Words
intestine	enter/o-	intestin/o-	gastroenterology, gastrointestinal
nerve	neur/o	nerv/o-	neurology, nervous system
skin	dermat/o-	integument/o-	dermatology, integumentary system

CHAPTER REVIEW EXERCISES

Review all the material in this chapter by completing the review exercises in this section. Use the Answer Key at the end of the book to check your answers.

The Body in Health and Disease

Matching Exercise

Match each numbered word to its description.

1. anatomy	____ Medical specialty that diagnoses and treats mental illness
2. cephalad	____ Body system that supports the body and produces motion
3. cranial	____ The study of the human body and its parts
4. midsagittal	____ The front of the body
5. muscular	____ Divides the body into right and left sections
6. physiology	____ Moving towards the head from a lower area of the body
7. psychiatry	____ The study of the body and its functions
8. superficial	____ Structures that are on the surface of the body
9. ventral	____ Body cavity that contains the brain

Circle Exercise

Circle the correct word or phrase from the choices given.

1. Hematology is the study of the (**blood, brain, muscles**).
2. Which of the following is related to a body cavity? (**endocrine, thoracic, ventral**)
3. The microscopic approach to the human body helps us gain knowledge about (**body systems, cavities, cells**).
4. The medical specialty of (**gastroenterology, immunology, obstetrics**) studies the stomach, intestines, and related organs.
5. The (**anatomical, anatomy, plane**) position is a standard position of the body for study purposes.
6. There are superior and inferior parts to this anatomical structure: (**cartilage in the knee, pituitary gland, vena cavae**).
7. If you move your arm and point to something ahead of you, you have moved it in a/an (**anterior, lateral, superficial**) direction.
8. The (**cranial, pelvic, thoracic**) cavity contains the lungs.
9. The (**endocrine, reproductive, respiratory**) system provides oxygen to the body and rids the body of carbon dioxide.
10. The tips of the fingers are (**anterior, distal, proximal**) to the elbow.

English and Medical Word Equivalents

For each English word, write its equivalent medical word. The first one has been done for you.

English Word	Medical Word
1. front	anterior or ______
2. back	______ or ______
3. side	______
4. midline	______
5. lying on the back	______
6. lying on the stomach	______
7. upper half	______
8. lower half	______
9. going toward the head	______
10. going toward the feet	______

True or False Exercise

Indicate whether the statement is true or false by writing T or F on the line.

1. ____ The lymphatic system contains the lymph nodes.
2. ____ Things on the macroscopic level cannot be seen with the naked eye.
3. ____ The coronal plane is also known as the horizontal plane.
4. ____ When you lie on your back, you are in the dorsal supine position.
5. ____ The abdominopelvic cavity contains the heart and the lungs.
6. ____ The integumentary system consists of the skin and other related structures.
7. ____ The medical specialty of orthopedics includes the skeletal system and the muscular system.
8. ____ Dermatology and the integumentary system both pertain to the skin.
9. ____ Something in a lateral position is located toward the side.
10. ____ Going from your waist toward your head, would be moving in a caudad direction.

Fill in the Blank Exercise

Read these scenarios and then fill in the blank with the correct medical specialty. The first one has been done for you.

1. Diseases of the female genital system are studied in the medical specialty of gynecology.
2. Mrs. Claire English is four months pregnant. It is time for her to see a physician who specializes in ______.
3. Bobby McCollum seems to constantly have a runny nose, a sore throat, and repeated ear infections. His regular physician may refer him to a specialist in the field of ______ for possible surgery on his ears.
4. ______ is the medical specialty that helps patients who have diseases of the nervous system.
5. County road worker Jeremy Walker accidentally touched poison ivy while clearing some brush. He has severe itching and redness on the skin of his hands and arms, right greater than left. He has an appointment this afternoon in the ______ clinic.
6. Alfred Dunley has a chronic lung condition and is seen annually for pulmonary function tests that are performed in the ______ department of Allegheny General Hospital.
7. Sarah Gibbs was born four weeks prematurely, but is going home today after being cared for by the nurses and doctors who specialize in ______.
8. When Chris Sutton fell down the steps, she went to the emergency room, and a physician in the medical specialty of ______ read her x-rays and found she had fractured her little toe.
9. The team physician for the Baltimore Ravens football team is a specialist in the field of ______, because team members have so many bone and muscle injuries during the season.

True or False Exercise

Indicate whether each statement is true or false by writing T or F on the line.

1. ____ Doctors and therapists form the core of the health-care team.
2. ____ A hospital stay begins with the physician's order to admit the patient.
3. ____ Lung disease caused by smoking would be an example of an environmental exposure that caused disease.
4. ____ The predicted outcome of a disease is known as the diagnosis.
5. ____ A pathogen is a microorganism that produces disease in the body.
6. ____ A nurse orders therapy for a patient.
7. ____ A Doctor of Chiropractic treats only the eyes.
8. ____ A dietitian is an example of a technologist.

Circle Exercise

Circle the correct word or phrase from the choices given.

1. The (**clinic, hospital, physician's office**) is the most frequently used healthcare setting.
2. The cause of a disease is the (**etiology, sequela, syndrome**).
3. A disease that does not respond well to treatment is said to be (**acute, refractory, therapeutic**).
4. A/an (**exacerbation, remission, sequela**) is a temporary improvement in the symptoms and signs of a disease.
5. A disease that is inherited from one's parents is (**congenital, hereditary, nutritional**).

Fill in the Blank Exercise

Fill in the blank with the correct word from the word list.

auscultation	palpation	symptomatology
clinic	subacute	syndrome
idiopathic		

1. ____________________ symptoms are slightly less severe than acute symptoms.
2. ____________________ is performed by pressing the fingers on the abdomen.
3. ____________________ is using a stethoscope to listen to the heart sounds.
4. A/an ____________________ is a set of symptoms and signs associated with one particular disease.
5. A/an ____________________ disease has no known cause.
6. ____________________ is all of the patient's symptoms and signs.
7. A healthcare facility that sees just one type of outpatient is called a/an ____________________.

Medical Language Word Parts

Name that Word Part

Identify each of the word parts given here by writing in the correct letter (P, C, or S) on the line beside it. Then write the definition of the word part on the blank line. The first one has been done for you.

Prefix = P **Combining Form = C** **Suffix = S**

		Word Part	Definition			Word Part	Definition
1.	dors/o-	C	back, dorsum	37.	endo-		
2.	a-			38.	enter/o-		
3.	abdomin/o-			39.	-eon		
4.	-able			40.	epi-		
5.	-ad			41.	-ery		
6.	-al			42.	eti/o-		
7.	ambulat/o-			43.	exacerb/o-		
8.	ana-			44.	extern/o-		
9.	ancill/o-			45.	fract/o-		
10.	anter/o-			46.	front/o-		
11.	-ar			47.	gastr/o-		
12.	-ary			48.	-gen		
13.	-atic			49.	gener/o-		
14.	-ation			50.	gen/o-		
15.	-ative			51.	ger/o-		
16.	-atory			52.	gnos/o-		
17.	auscult/o-			53.	gynec/o-		
18.	cardi/o-			54.	habilitat/o-		
19.	caud/o-			55.	hemat/o-		
20.	cav/o-			56.	heredit/o-		
21.	cephal/o-			57.	horizont/o-		
22.	chondr/o-			58.	hypo-		
23.	chron/o-			59.	-iac		
24.	communic/o-			60.	iatr/o-		
25.	congenit/o-			61.	-iatry		
26.	coron/o-			62.	-ic		
27.	crani/o-			63.	-ical		
28.	-crine			64.	-ician		
29.	chrin/o-			65.	-ics		
30.	de-			66.	idi/o-		
31.	dent/o-			67.	immun/o-		
32.	dermat/o-			68.	infect/o-		
33.	dia-			69.	infer/o-		
34.	dietet/o-			70.	inguin/o-		
35.	dist/o-			71.	inspect/o-		
36.	-drome			72.	integument/o-		

		Word Part	Definition
73.	intern/o-		
74.	intestin/o-		
75.	-ion		
76.	-ior		
77.	-ious		
78.	-ist		
79.	-istry		
80.	-ity		
81.	-ive		
82.	laryng/o-		
83.	later/o-		
84.	log/o-		
85.	-logy		
86.	lumb/o-		
87.	lymph/o-		
88.	macr/o-		
89.	medi/o-		
90.	medic/o-		
91.	micr/o-		
92.	mid-		
93.	muscul/o-		
94.	nat/o-		
95.	ne/o-		
96.	neur/o-		
97.	nerv/o-		
98.	nucle/o-		
99.	nutri/o-		
100.	obstetr/o-		
101.	onc/o-		
102.	ophthalm/o-		
103.	orth/o-		
104.	-ory		
105.	-osis		
106.	ot/o-		
107.	-ous		
108.	palliat/o-		
109.	palpat/o-		
110.	path/o-		
111.	ped/o-		
112.	pelv/o-		
113.	percuss/o-		
114.	pharmac/o-		
115.	physi/o-		
116.	plas/o-		
117.	poster/o-		
118.	prevent/o-		
119.	pro-		
120.	product/o-		
121.	proxim/o-		
122.	psych/o-		
123.	pulmon/o-		
124.	radi/o-		
125.	re-		
126.	recuper/o-		
127.	remiss/o-		
128.	sagitt/o-		
129.	-scope		
130.	scop/o-		
131.	skelet/o-		
132.	spin/o-		
133.	spir/o-		
134.	steth/o-		
135.	superfici/o-		
136.	super/o-		
137.	surg/o-		
138.	symptomat/o-		
139.	syn-		
140.	techn/o-		
141.	termin/o-		
142.	therapeut/o-		
143.	therap/o-		
144.	thorac/o-		
145.	-tic		
146.	-tion		
147.	tom/o-		
148.	-tomy		
149.	trans-		
150.	umbilic/o-		
151.	urin/o-		
152.	ur/o-		
153.	vascul/o-		
154.	ventr/o-		
155.	-verse		

Word-Building Exercise

Use the combining forms, prefixes, and suffixes given here to build medical words that match the definitions given. Write the word you build in the blank provided. Some word parts may be used more than once. The first one has been done for you.

WORD PARTS

abdomin/o- (abdomen)	interno- (inside)	pulmon/o- (lung)
-al (pertaining to)	intestin/o- (intestine)	re- (again and again; backward; unable to)
anter/o- (front part)	-ior (pertaining to)	
cardi/o- (heart)	-ive (pertaining to)	-scope (instrument used to examine)
dermat/o- (skin)	-logy (the study of)	super/o- (above)
gastr/o- (stomach)	micr/o- (small)	thorac/o- (thorax, chest)
-iatr/o- (physician; medical treatment)	neur/o (nerve)	trans- (across, through)
-ic (pertaining to)	ped/o- (child)	-verse (to turn; to travel)
-ics (knowledge, practice)	product/o- (produce)	

1. The study of the nerves (You think *neur/o-* + *-logy.*) You write neurology ______
2. Pertaining to the front part ______
3. Instrument used to examine small things ______
4. Pertaining to the abdomen ______
5. The study of the heart ______
6. To turn across; lying crosswise ______
7. Pertaining to above ______
8. Pertaining to the chest cavity ______
9. The study of the lungs ______
10. Pertaining to inside ______
11. Pertaining to the stomach and intestines ______
12. The study of the skin ______
13. Pertaining to producing again and again ______
14. Medical treatment of children ______

Divide and Conquer

Separate these words into their component parts (prefix, combining form, suffix). Note: Some words do not contain all three word parts. The first one has been done for you.

Medical Word	Prefix	Combining Form	Suffix	Medical Word	Prefix	Combining Form	Suffix
1. anatomical	*ana-*	*tom/o-*	*-ical*	7. ophthalmology	___	___	___
2. cavity	___	___	___	8. pharmacology	___	___	___
3. cephalad	___	___	___	9. posterior	___	___	___
4. endocrinology	___	___	___	10. reproductive	___	___	___
5. gynecology	___	___	___	11. thoracic	___	___	___
6. midsagittal	___	___	___	12. urinary	___	___	___

Matching Exercise

Match each numbered word part to its definition.

1. cardi/o-	10. onc/o-	_____ x-rays, radiation	_____ head
2. cephal/o-	11. ot/o-	_____ lung	_____ thorax (chest)
3. dietet/o-	12. pulmon/o-	_____ skin	_____ ear
4. enter/o-	13. radi/o-	_____ middle	_____ above
5. extern/o-	14. super/o-	_____ blood	_____ heart
6. hemat/o-	15. thorac/o-	_____ intestines	_____ outside
7. integument/o-	16. tom/o-	_____ a cut, slice, or layer	_____ the study of
8. -logy	17. ventr/o-	_____ tumor	_____ foods, diet
9. medi/o-		_____ front; abdomen	

Abbreviations

Matching Exercise

Match each abbreviation to its description.

1. M.D.	____ Minor outpatient surgery is performed here
2. NP	____ Physician extender who delivers babies
3. SNF	____ Doctor who treats the feet
4. ASC	____ Female reproductive system
5. CNM	____ Physician who graduated from a medical school
6. D.P.M.	____ Registered nurse
7. GI	____ Acts as a physician extender
8. RN	____ Patients here are known as *residents*
9. D.D.S.	____ Ancillary department within a hospital
10. ED	____ Doctor who treats the teeth
11. GYN	____ Has to do with the stomach and intestines

Applied Skills

Proofreading and Spelling Exercise

Read this paragraph and identify any misspelled medical words. Write the correct spelling of the word in the blank at the right.

Beginning with the body in anetomical position is a good way to study the human body. Traveling posteriorily from the breast bone to the spine takes you through the tharacic cavty that holds the heart, the main organ of the kardiovascular system. The study of the eye is known as ophthamology, While the study of the ears, nose, and throat is as otolarngology. The study of the lungs, which are in the thoracic cavity, is known as pulmonawlogy. However, most students like gyenecology the best because it has interesting anatomy and fisiology.

1. ______________________________
2. ______________________________
3. ______________________________
4. ______________________________
5. ______________________________
6. ______________________________
7. ______________________________
8. ______________________________
9. ______________________________
10. ______________________________

Pronunciation Checklist

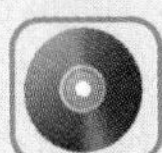

Read each word and its pronunciation. Practice pronouncing each word. Verify your pronunciation by listening to the Pronunciation List on the CD-ROM. Check the box next to the word after you master its pronunciation.

- ❑ abdominal cavity (ab-DAWM-ih-nal KAV-ih-tee)
- ❑ abdominopelvic cavity (ab-DAWM-ih-noh-PEL-vik KAV-ih-tee)
- ❑ acute (ah-KYOOT)
- ❑ ambulatory (AM-byoo-lah-TOR-ee)
- ❑ anatomical (AN-ah-TAWM-ih-kal)
- ❑ anatomy (ah-NAT-oh-mee)
- ❑ ancillary (AN-sih-lair-ee)
- ❑ anterior (an-TEER-ee-or)
- ❑ anteriorly (an-TEER-ee-or-lee)
- ❑ anteroposterior (AN-ter-oh-pohs-TEER-ee-or)
- ❑ asymptomatic (AA-simp-toh-MAT-ik)
- ❑ auscultation (AWS-kul-TAY-shun)
- ❑ cardiology (KAR-dee-AWL-oh-jee)
- ❑ cardiovascular (KAR-dee-oh-VAS-kyoo-lar)
- ❑ caudad (KAW-dad)
- ❑ cavity (KAV-ih-tee)
- ❑ cephalad (SEF-ah-lad)
- ❑ chronic (KRAW-nik)
- ❑ communicable disease (koh-MYOON-ih-kah-bl dih-ZEEZ)
- ❑ congenital disease (con-JEN-ih-tal dih-ZEEZ)
- ❑ coronal plane (kor-OH-nal PLAYN)
- ❑ cranial cavity (KRAY-nee-al KAV-ih-tee)
- ❑ degenerative disease (dee-JEN-er-ah-tiv dih-ZEEZ)
- ❑ dentistry (DEN-tis-tree)
- ❑ dermatology (DER-mah-TAWL-oh-jee)
- ❑ diagnosis (DY-ag-NOH-sis)
- ❑ diagnostic (DY-ag-NAWS-tik)
- ❑ dietetics (DY-eh-TET-iks)
- ❑ disability (DIS-ah-BIL-ah-tee)
- ❑ disease (dih-ZEEZ)
- ❑ distal (DIS-tal)
- ❑ distally (DIS-tah-lee)
- ❑ dorsal (DOR-sal)
- ❑ endocrine (EN-doh-krin) (EN-doh-krine)
- ❑ endocrinology (EN-doh-krih-NAWL-oh-jee)
- ❑ environmental (en-VY-rawn-MEN-tal)
- ❑ epigastric (EP-ih-GAS-trk)
- ❑ etiology (ee-tee-AWL-oh-jee)
- ❑ exacerbation (eg-ZAS-er-BAY-shun)
- ❑ external (eks-TER-nal)
- ❑ frontal plane (FRUN-tal PLAYN)
- ❑ gastroenterology (GAS-troh-en-ter-AWL-oh-jee)
- ❑ gastrointestinal system (GAS-troh-in-TES-tih-nal SIS-tem)
- ❑ geriatrics (JAIR-ee-AT-riks)
- ❑ gynecology (GY-neh-KAWL-oh-jee)
- ❑ health (HELTH)
- ❑ health information technician (HELTH IN-for-MAY-shun tek-NISH-un)
- ❑ hematology (HEE-mah-TAWL-oh-jee)
- ❑ hereditary disease (heh-RED-ih-tair-ee dih-ZEEZ)
- ❑ horizontal plane (HOR-ih-ZAWN-tal PLAYN)
- ❑ hospice (HAWS-pis)
- ❑ hypochondriac (HY-poh-KAWN-dree-ak)
- ❑ hypogastric (HY-poh-GAS-trik)
- ❑ iatrogenic disease (eye-AT-roh-JEN-ik dih-ZEEZ)
- ❑ idiopathic disease (ID-ee-oh-PATH-ik dih-ZEEZ)
- ❑ iliac (IL-ee-ak)
- ❑ immunology (IM-yoo-NAWL-oh-jee)
- ❑ infectious disease (in-FEK-shus dih-ZEEZ)
- ❑ inferior (in-FEER-ee-or)
- ❑ inferiorly (in-FEER-ee-or-lee)
- ❑ inguinal (ING-gwih-nal)
- ❑ inspection (in-SPEK-shun)
- ❑ integumentary system (in-TEG-yoo-MEN-tair-ee SIS-tem)
- ❑ internal (in-TER-nal)
- ❑ lateral (LAT-er-al)
- ❑ laterally (LAT-er-ah-lee)
- ❑ lumbar (LUM-bar)
- ❑ lymphatic system (lim-FAT-ik SIS-tem)
- ❑ macroscopic (MAK-roh-SKAWP-ik)
- ❑ medial (MEE-dee-al)
- ❑ medially (MEE-dee-ah-lee)
- ❑ mediastinum (MEE-dee-as-TY-num)
- ❑ medicine (MED-ih-sin)
- ❑ microscope (MY-kroh-skohp)
- ❑ microscopic (MY-kroh-SKAWP-ik)
- ❑ midsagittal plane (mid-SAJ-ih-tal PLAYN)
- ❑ muscular system (MUS-kyoo-lar SIS-tem)
- ❑ neoplastic disease (NEE-oh-PLAS-tik dih-ZEEZ)
- ❑ nervous system (NER-vus SIS-tem)
- ❑ neurology (nyoo-RAWL-oh-jee)
- ❑ nosocomial disease (NOS-oh-KOH-mee-al dih-ZEEZ)
- ❑ nutritional disease (noo-TRISH-un-al dih-ZEEZ)
- ❑ obstetrics (awb-STET-riks)
- ❑ oncology (ong-KAWL-oh-jee)
- ❑ ophthalmology (OFF-thal-MAWL-oh-jee)
- ❑ orthopedics (OR-thoh-PEE-diks)
- ❑ otolaryngology (OH-toh-LAIR-ing-GAWL-oh-jee)
- ❑ palliative (PAL-ee-ah-tiv)
- ❑ palpation (pal-PAY-shun)
- ❑ pathogen (PATH-oh-jen)
- ❑ pediatrics (PEE-dee-AT-riks)
- ❑ pelvic cavity (PEL-vik KAV-ih-tee)
- ❑ percussion (per-KUSH-un)
- ❑ pharmacology (FAR-mah-KAWL-oh-jee)
- ❑ physician (fih-ZISH-un)
- ❑ physiology (FIZ-ee-AWL-oh-jee)
- ❑ plane (PLAYN)
- ❑ posterior (pohs-TEER-ee-or)
- ❑ posteriorly (pohs-TEER-ee-or-lee)
- ❑ posteroanterior (POHS-ter-oh-an-TEER-ee-or)
- ❑ preventive (pree-VEN-tiv)
- ❑ prognosis (prawg-NOH-sis)
- ❑ prone (PROHN)
- ❑ proximal (PRAWK-sih-mal)
- ❑ proximally (PRAWK-sih-mah-lee)
- ❑ psychiatry (sy-KY-ah-tree)
- ❑ pulmonology (PUL-moh-NAWL-oh-jee)
- ❑ quadrant (KWAH-drant)
- ❑ radiology (RAY-dee-AWL-oh-jee)
- ❑ recuperation (ree-KOO-per-AA-shun)
- ❑ refractory (ree-FRAK-tor-ee)
- ❑ rehabilitation (REE-hah-BIL-ih-TAY-shun)
- ❑ remission (ree-MISH-un)
- ❑ reproductive system (REE-proh-DUK-tiv SIS-tem)
- ❑ respiratory system (RES-pih-rah-TOR-ee SIS-tem) (reh-SPYR-ah-tor-ee)
- ❑ sequela (see-KWEL-ah)
- ❑ sequelae (see-KWEL-ee)
- ❑ skeletal system (SKEL-eh-tal SIS-tem)
- ❑ spinal cavity (SPY-nal KAV-ih-tee)

- ❑ stethoscope (STETH-oh-skohp)
- ❑ subacute (SUB-ah-KYOOT)
- ❑ superficial (SOO-per-FISH-al)
- ❑ superior (soo-PEER-ee-or)
- ❑ superiorly (soo-PEER-ee-or-lee)
- ❑ supine (soo-PINE) (SOO-pine)
- ❑ surgeon (SER-jun)
- ❑ surgery (SER-jer-ee)
- ❑ symptom (SIMP-tom)
- ❑ symptomatology (SIMP-toh-mah-TAWL-oh-jee)
- ❑ syndrome (SIN-drohm)
- ❑ technician (tek-NISH-un)
- ❑ technologist (tek-NAWL-oh-jist)
- ❑ terminal (TER-mih-nal)
- ❑ therapeutic (THAIR-ah-PYOO-tik)
- ❑ therapist (THAIR-ah-pist)
- ❑ therapy (THAIR-ah-pee)
- ❑ thoracic cavity (thoh-RAS-ik KAV-ih-tee)
- ❑ transverse plane (trans-VERS PLAYN)
- ❑ umbilical (um-BIL-ih-kal)
- ❑ umbilicus (um-BIL-ih-kus) (um-bih-LIE-kus)
- ❑ urinary system (YOO-rih-nair-ee SIS-tem)
- ❑ urology (yoo-RAWL-oh-jee)
- ❑ ventral (VEN-tral)
- ❑ viscera (VIS-er-ah)

Experience Multimedia

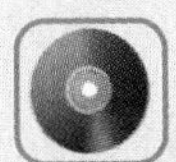

CD-ROM Learning Activities Checklist

Check off the box as you complete each learning activity.

- ❑ **CD-ROM Learning Activity 2.1: *ANATOMY WORD PARTS FLASHCARDS***
  Use flashcards to help you memorize word parts. Make your own flashcards or print out prepared flashcards. Also see the electronic flashcard game. Time: 20 minutes.
- ❑ **CD-ROM Learning Activity 2.2: *MEDICINE IN ACTION***
  Watch a video clip of healthcare professionals using physical examination techniques. TIme: 20 minutes.
- ❑ **CD-ROM Learning Activity 2.3: *DISEASE AND OTHER WORD PARTS FLASHCARDS***
  A continuation of the flashcard learning activity. Time: 20 minutes.
- ❑ **CD-ROM Learning Activity 2.4: *MEMORY AIDS***
  Use memory aids to help you memorize medical words and meanings. Time: 5 minutes.
- ❑ **CD-ROM Learning Activity 2.5: *MEDICAL LANGUAGE SPOKEN HERE***
  Listen to actual medical reports and spell the missing medical words. Time: 5 minutes.
- ❑ **CD-ROM Learning Activity 2.6: *SPELLING CHALLENGE***
  Listen to a pronounced medical word and then spell it. Time: 5 minutes.
- ❑ **CD-ROM Learning Activity 2.7: *MEDICAL LANGUAGE PRONUNCIATION***
  Listen to a pronounced medical word and then practice pronouncing it. Time: 30 minutes.
- ❑ **CD-ROM Learning Activity 2.8: *EDUCATIONAL FUN AND GAMES***
  Enjoy these fun activities while reinforcing your knowledge. Time: 15 minutes.

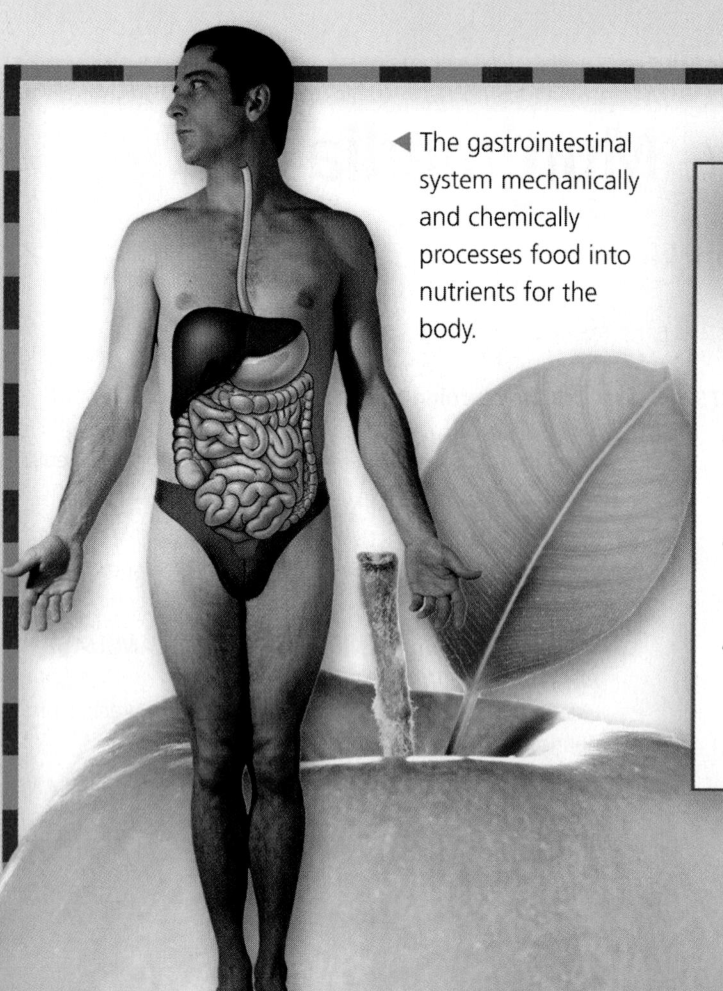

◀ The gastrointestinal system mechanically and chemically processes food into nutrients for the body.

Dive In!

- The small intestine is 21 feet long and the large intestine adds another 5 feet.
- The average person eats 11 pounds of spaghetti sauce and ketchup per year.
- The first nasogastric tube (a feeding tube through the nose to the stomach) was made from eel skin.
- In this chapter you'll explore the gastrointestinal system. Satisfy your hunger for the medical language of gastroenterology.

◀ Taking a bite of an apple and chewing it is the process known as mastication. Swallowing is known as deglutition.

Medicine Through HISTORY

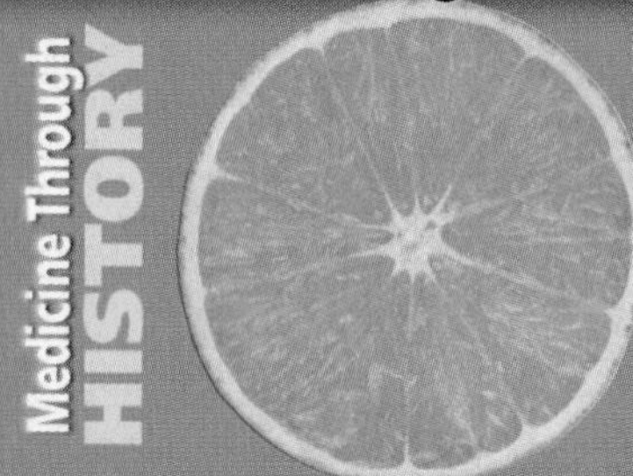

1747

Scottish surgeon James Lind discovers that a substance in citrus fruits (vitamin C) keeps sailors from developing scurvy

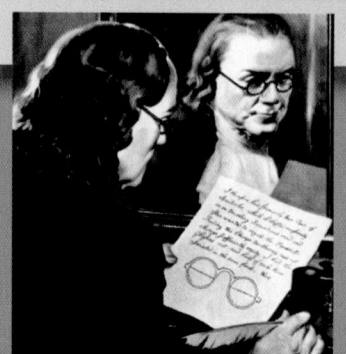

1760

Benjamin Franklin invents bifocal glasses

CHAPTER 3

Gastroenterology

Gastrointestinal System

Gastroenterology (GAS-troh-EN-ter-AWL-oh-jee) is the medical specialty that studies the anatomy and physiology of the gastrointestinal system and uses diagnostic tests, medical and surgical procedures, and drugs to treat gastrointestinal diseases.

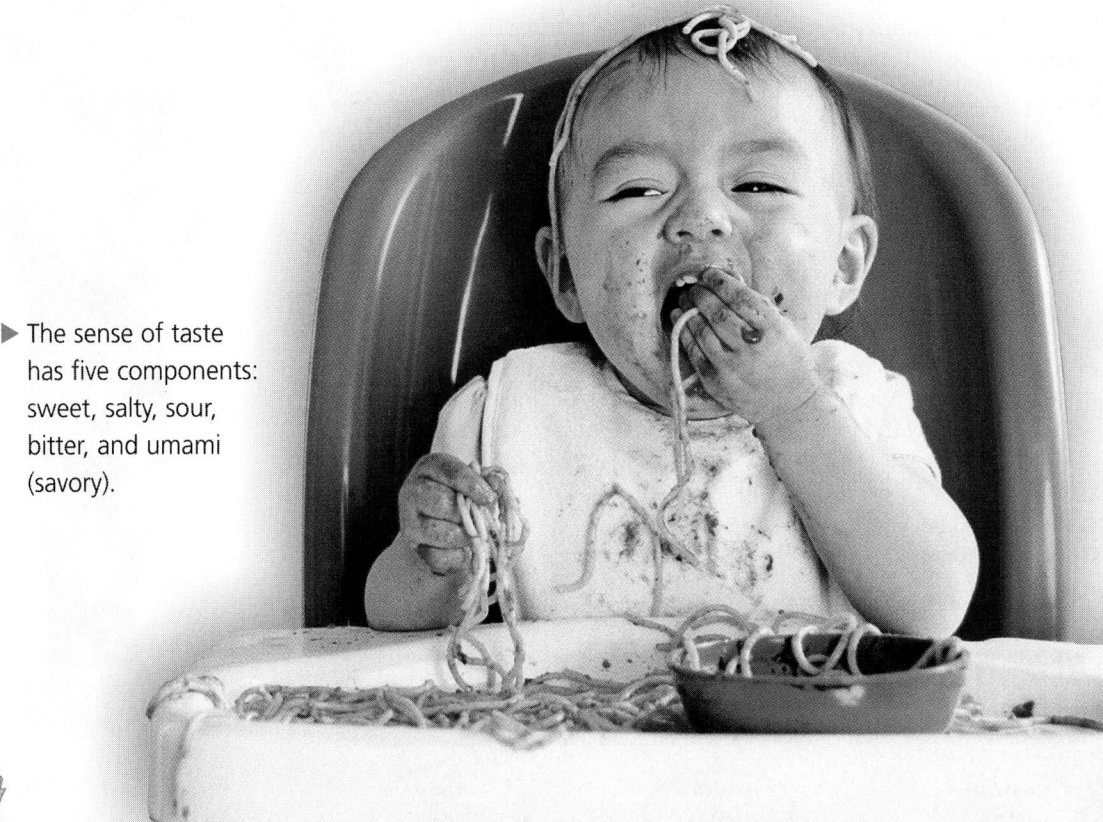

▶ The sense of taste has five components: sweet, salty, sour, bitter, and umami (savory).

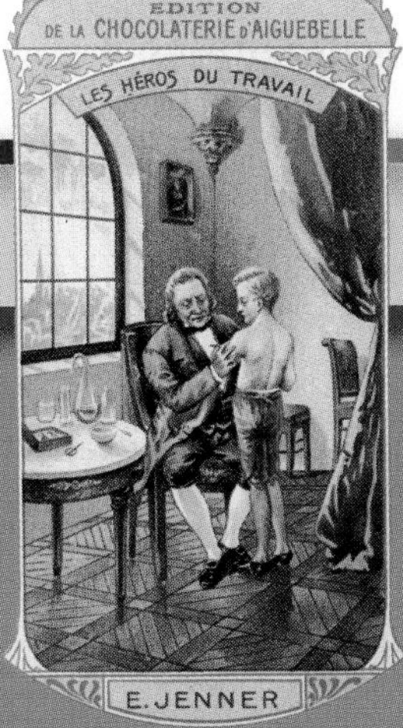

1796
Edward Jenner, an English physician, devises the first vaccination by injecting material from cowpox sores to prevent smallpox

1798
John Dalton, an English physicist, describes color blindness

1806
The painkilling drug morphine is isolated from the opium poppy

Measure Your Progress: Learning Objectives

After you study this chapter, you should be able to

1. Identify the anatomical structures of the gastrointestinal system by correctly labeling them on anatomical illustrations.
2. Describe the process of digestion.
3. Build gastrointestinal words from combining forms, prefixes, and suffixes.
4. Describe common gastrointestinal diseases.
5. Describe common gastrointestinal diagnostic laboratory and radiology tests.
6. Describe common gastrointestinal medical and surgical procedures and drug categories.
7. Define common gastrointestinal abbreviations.
8. Correctly spell and pronounce gastrointestinal words.
9. Apply your skills by analyzing a gastroenterology report.
10. Test your knowledge of gastroenterology by completing review exercises at the end of the chapter and learning activities on the CD-ROM.

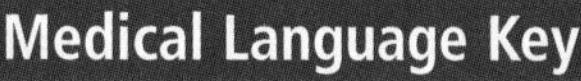

Medical Language Key

To unlock the meaning of a medical word, first define each word part. Then put the word part definitions in order, beginning with the suffix, followed by the first word part, then the other word parts in order.

	Word Part	Word Part Definition
SUFFIX	-logy	*the study of*
COMBINING FORM	gastr/o-	*stomach*
COMBINING FORM	enter/o-	*intestine*

Gastroenterology: ***The study of the stomach and intestines.***

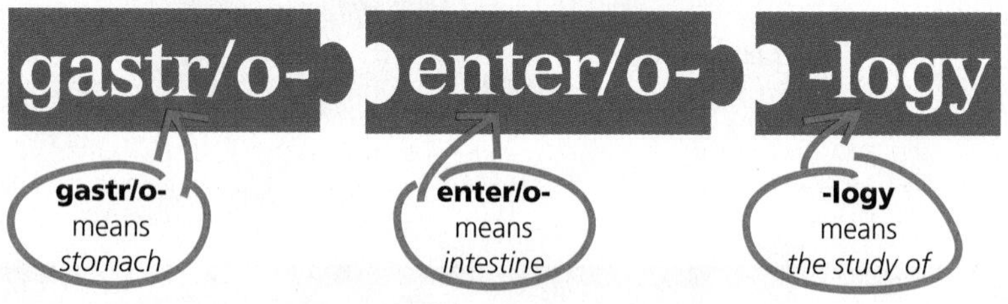

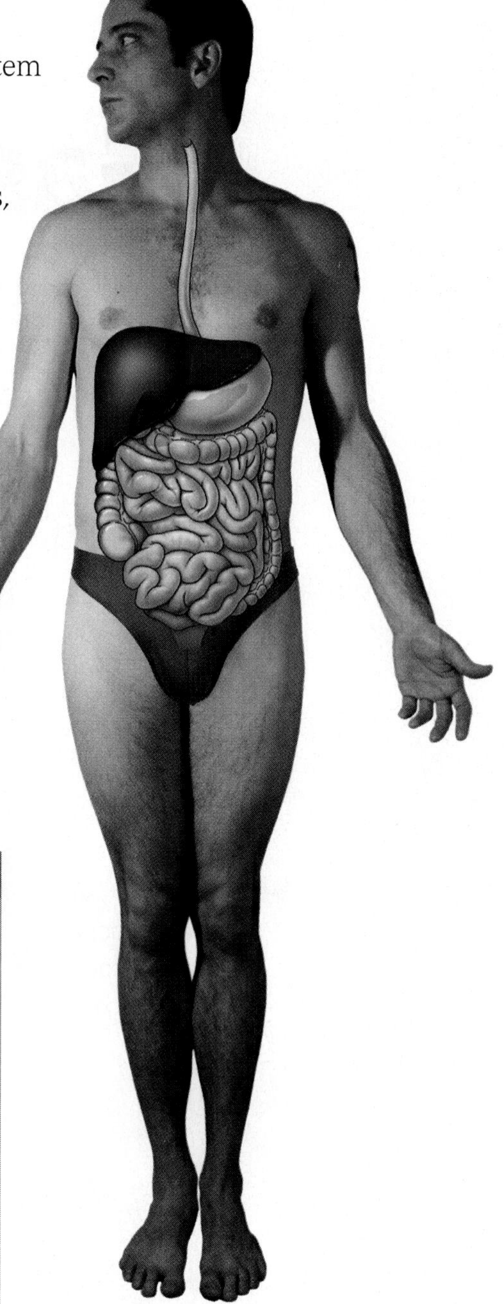

Figure 3-1 ■ The gastrointestinal system.
The gastrointestinal system consists of many different organs connected to a common pathway where food enters the body, is digested, and is then eliminated from the body.

www.prenhall.com/turley

For interactive flashcards, real-life video clips, games, exercises, and audio pronunciations please explore the companion CD-ROM in the back of the book. Click on the companion website for bonus chapters, additional resources, and links to on-line learning.

Anatomy and Physiology

The **gastrointestinal system** is an elongated body system that begins at the mouth, continues through the thoracic cavity of the chest, and fills most of the abdominal cavity (see Figure 3-1■). The upper gastrointestinal system includes the structures from the mouth to the stomach. The lower gastro-intestinal system includes the small and large intestines. The function of the gastrointestinal system is to digest food and remove undigested matter from the body. The body's sense of taste is associated with the gastrointestinal system.

gastrointestinal (GAS-troh-in-TES-tih-nal)
gastr/o- *stomach*
intestin/o- *intestine*
-al *pertaining to*

system (SIS-tem)
System is derived from a Greek word meaning *combination of parts to make an organized whole.*

Anatomy of the Gastrointestinal System

Oral Cavity and Pharynx

The gastrointestinal system begins in the mouth or **oral cavity.** The oral cavity contains the teeth, tongue, the bony hard **palate,** the soft palate, and the fleshy, hanging **uvula** (see Figure 3-2■). The uvula initiates the gag reflex if food touches it. The sense of taste begins with taste receptors on the tongue. They relay information to the **gustatory** cortex in the brain. The oral cavity is lined with **mucosa,** a mucous membrane that produces thin mucus.

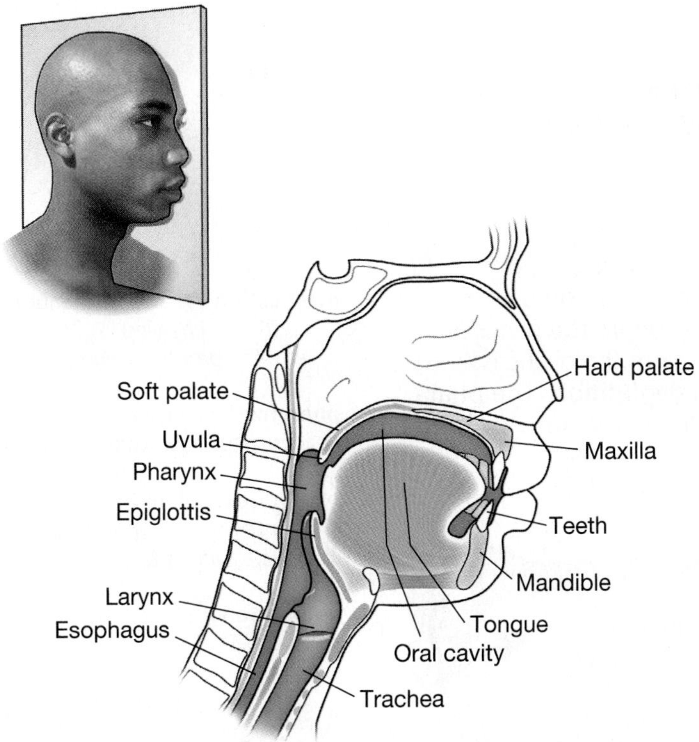

Figure 3-2 ■ The oral cavity and pharynx.
The hard and soft palates form the roof of the oral cavity. The muscular tongue is attached to the lower jaw bone and nearly fills the oral cavity. Food passes from the oral cavity into the pharynx and then the esophagus.

oral (OR-al)
or/o- *mouth*
-al *pertaining to*
Oral is the adjective form for *mouth.*

cavity (KAV-ih-tee)
cav/o- *hollow space*
-ity *state; condition*

palate (PAL-at)
Palate is derived from a Latin word meaning *roof of the mouth.*

uvula (YOO-vyoo-lah)
Uvula is derived from a Latin word meaning *little grape.* The uvula looks like a little grape hanging in the oral cavity.

lingual (LING-gwal)
lingu/o- *tongue*
-al *pertaining to*

glossal (GLAWS-al)
gloss/o- *tongue*
-al *pertaining to*
Lingual and *glossal* are the adjective forms for *tongue.*

gustatory (GUS-tah-tor-ee)
gustat/o- *the sense of taste*
-ory *having the function of*

mucosa (myoo-KOH-sah)
Mucosa is a Latin word meaning *mucus.*

mucosal (myoo-KOH-sal)
mucos/o- *mucous membrane*
-al *pertaining to*

The sight, smell, and taste of food cause the salivary glands to release **saliva** into the mouth. Saliva is a lubricant that moistens food so that it can be easily swallowed. It also contains an enzyme that begins the process of digestion. There are three pairs of **salivary glands:** the **parotid** glands, the **submandibular** glands, and the **sublingual** glands (see Figure 3-3■).

saliva (sah-LY-vah)

salivary (SAL-ih-vair-ee)
saliv/o- *saliva*
-ary *pertaining to*

gland (GLAND)

parotid (pah-ROT-id)
par- *beside*
ot/o- *ear*
-id *resembling; source or origin*

submandibular (SUB-man-DIB-yoo-lar)
sub- *below; underneath; less than*
mandibul/o- *mandible (lower jaw)*
-ar *pertaining to*

sublingual (sub-LING-gwal)
sub- *below; underneath; less than*
lingu/o- *tongue*
-al *pertaining to*

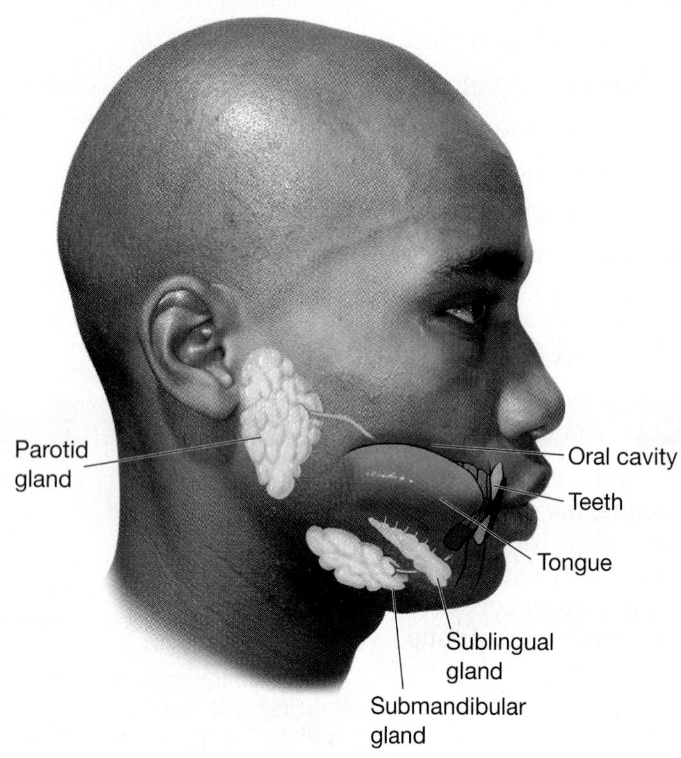

Figure 3-3 ■ The salivary glands.
The parotid glands are large and flat and cover part of the cheek in front of the ear. The sublingular glands are located under the tongue. The submandibular glands are located under the lower jaw bone (mandible). Ducts from these glands bring saliva into the oral cavity.

The teeth tear, chew, and grind the food, a process known as **mastication.** The tongue mixes the food with saliva to begin the process of digestion. The food is then swallowed, moving from the oral cavity to the throat or **pharynx.** This movement is called **deglutition.** The pharynx acts as a passageway for food as well as for inhaled and exhaled air.

mastication (MAS-tih-KAY-shun)
mastic/o- *chewing*
-ation *a process; being or having*

pharynx (FAIR-ingks)
Pharynx is a Greek word meaning *throat.*

pharyngeal (fah-RIN-jee-al)
pharyng/o- *pharynx (throat)*
-eal *pertaining to*

deglutition (DEE-gloo-TISH-un) (DEG-loo-TISH-un)
degluti/o- *swallowing*
-tion *a process; being or having*

Across the Life Span

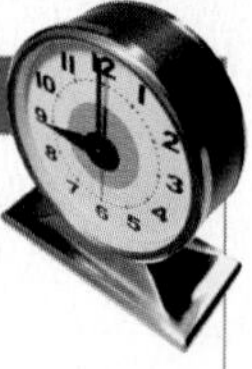

Elderly people often complain that food does not seem as flavorful as when they were young. The aging process causes a very real decline in the ability to smell and taste food as the number of receptors in the nose and tongue decreases.

Esophagus

The **esophagus** is a flexible, muscular tube in the thoracic cavity that connects the pharynx to the stomach (see Figure 3-4■). It is lined with mucosa that produces mucus to lubricate its walls. A layer of smooth muscle in the wall moves food with a series of strong, coordinated contractions. This process is known as **peristalsis.**

esophagus (ee-SAWF-ah-gus) (ah-SAWF-ah-gus)

esophageal (ee-SAWF-ah-JEE-al) (ah-SAWF-ah-JEE-al)
esophag/o- *esophagus*
-eal *pertaining to*

peristalsis (PAIR-ih-STAL-sis)
peri- *around*
-stalsis *process of contraction*
Every medical word must contain a combining form. The suffix of *peristalsis* contains the combining form *stal/o-* (*contraction*).

Stomach

The stomach is a large, elongated sac in the upper abdominal cavity that receives food from the esophagus. The stomach is divided into five areas: the **cardia, fundus,** body, **antrum,** and **pylorus** (see Figure 3-4). The **gastric** mucosa is arranged in thick, deep folds known as **rugae** that expand as the stomach fills with food. The mucosa produces mucus that protects the stomach from acid. It also produces a digestive enzyme secreted by stomach glands. Two sphincters (muscular rings) keep food in the stomach. The lower esophageal sphincter (LES) or **cardiac sphincter** is at the inferior end of the esophagus. The

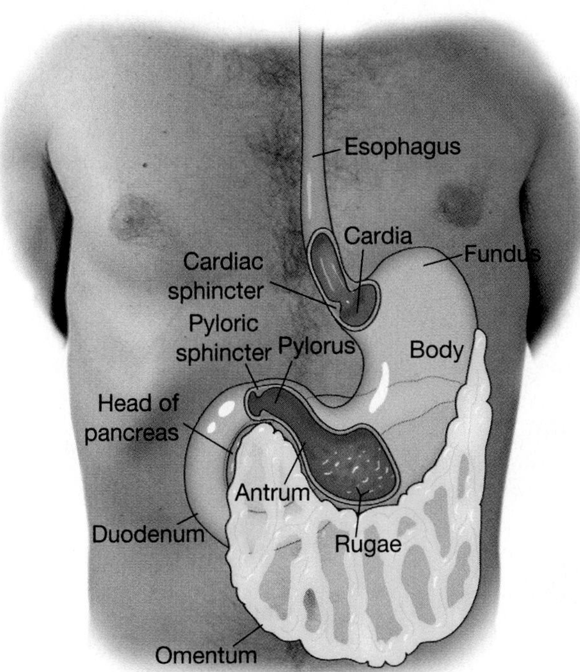

Figure 3-4 ■ The stomach.

The stomach can be divided into five regions. The cardia is a small area where the esophagus connects to the stomach. The fundus is the rounded top of the stomach. The largest, curved part of the stomach is the body. The antrum is the transition between the body of the stomach and the narrow canal that is the pylorus.

cardia (KAR-dee-ah)
Cardia is derived from a Greek word meaning *heart.* The cardia of the stomach and the cardiac sphincter of the esophagus are near, but not part of, the heart.

fundus (FUN-dus)
Fundus is a Latin word meaning *the part of a hollow organ that is the farthest from the opening.*

antrum (AN-trum)
Antrum is a Latin word meaning *cave.*

pylorus (py-LOR-us)
Pylorus is derived from a Greek word meaning *gatekeeper.* The pyloric sphincter acts as a gatekeeper, keeping food in the stomach and then opening to let food into the duodenum.

gastric (GAS-trik)
gastr/o- *stomach*
-ic *pertaining to*
Gastric is the adjective form for *stomach.*

rugae (ROO-gee)
Ruga is a Latin singular feminine noun meaning *a wrinkle.* Form the plural by changing the *-a* to *-ae.* Because there are so many rugae in the stomach, the singular form is seldom used.

cardiac (KAR-dee-ak)
cardi/o- *heart*
-ac *pertaining to*

sphincter (SFINGK-ter)
Sphincter is derived from a Greek word meaning *bind up tightly.*

pyloric sphincter at the inferior end of the stomach keeps food from leaving the stomach. **Chyme** is the semisolid mixture of partially digested food, saliva, and digestive juices in the stomach. An hour or so after eating, the pyloric sphincter opens and waves of peristalsis propel the chyme into the small intestine.

pyloric (py-LOR-ik)
pylor/o- *pylorus*
-ic *pertaining to*

chyme (KIME)
Chyme is derived from a Greek word meaning *juice.*

Small Intestine

The **small intestine** or **small bowel** is a long, hollow tube that receives partially digested food from the stomach. The small intestine is divided into three parts: the duodenum, jejunum, and ileum (see Figure 3-5■). The **duodenum** is a 10-inch, C-shaped segment that curves around the pancreas and connects with the jejunum. The mucosa of the duodenum produces mucus to protect itself from stomach acid. Digestive enzymes from the gallbladder and pancreas enter the duodenum through ducts. The **jejunum,** the second part of the small intestine, is an 8-foot segment that repeatedly twists and turns in the abdominal cavity. Digestion continues in the jejunum. Peristalsis slowly moves the chyme along for several hours until it reaches the ileum, the final part of the small intestine. The **ileum** is a 12-foot segment where digestion is completed and absorption of digested food begins. There, thousands of small, thin structures known as **villi** project into the **lumen** of the intestine. The villi increase the amount of surface area that can actively absorb food nutrients and water. These are absorbed through the intestinal wall and into the blood. The remaining undigested food fibers and water move into the large intestine.

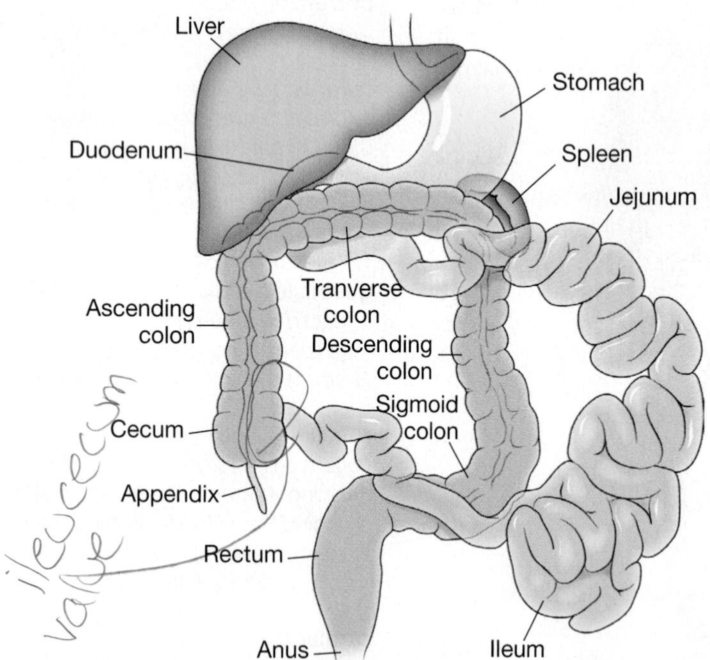

Figure 3-5 ■ The small and large intestines.

The small intestine consists of the duodenum, jejunum, and ileum. The large intestine consists of the cecum (and appendix), colon, rectum, and anus. The colon can be further divided into the ascending colon, the transverse colon, the descending colon, and the sigmoid colon. The bends or flexures of the colon are important landmarks that are mentioned in x-ray reports. The bend in the ascending colon as it approaches the liver is known as the hepatic flexure. The bend in the transverse colon as it approaches the spleen is known as the splenic flexure.

intestine (in-TES-tin)

intestinal (in-TES-tih-nal)
intestin/o- *intestine*
-al *pertaining to*

bowel (BAH-ool)
Bowel is derived from a Latin word meaning *sausage.* The loops and sections of intestine can look like a string of sausages.

duodenum (DOO-oh-DEE-num) (doo-AWD-ah-num)
Duodenum is derived from a Latin word meaning *twelve.* Ancient Roman physicians measured the duodenum as being 12 fingerbreadths in length.

duodenal (DOO-oh-DEE-nal) (doo-AWD-ah-nal)
duoden/o- *duodenum*
-al *pertaining to*

jejunum (jeh-JOO-num)
Jejunum is derived from a Latin word meaning *empty.* When ancient Roman physicians dissected dead bodies, they often found that the jejunum had no food in it.

jejunal (jeh-JOO-nal)
jejun/o- *jejunum*
-al *pertaining to*

ileum (IL-ee-um)
Ileum is derived from a Latin word meaning *to twist or roll up tightly.*

ileal (IL-ee-al)
ile/o- *ileum*
-al *pertaining to*

villi (VIL-eye)
Villus is a Latin singular masculine noun meaning *shaggy hairs.* Form the plural by changing the *-us* to *-i.* Because there are so many villi in the small intestine, the singular form is seldom used.

lumen (LOO-men)
Lumen is a Latin word meaning *window.*

Large Intestine

The large intestine or large bowel is a large tube whose walls contain many **haustra** or puckered pouches that can expand to hold large amounts of undigested food fibers and water. The mucosa produces mucus to lubricate the walls of the large intestine. Waves of peristalsis slowly move undigested food fibers through the large intestine as water is absorbed through the intestinal wall and into the blood.

The large intestine is divided into several parts: the cecum, colon, rectum, and anus (see Figure 3-5). The **cecum** is a short sac. Hanging from the external wall of the cecum is the **appendix,** a thin tube that is closed at its distal end. The appendix plays no role in the digestive process. It contains lymphoid tissue and is part of the lymphatic system and the immune response. This is discussed in Immunology (Chapter 6).

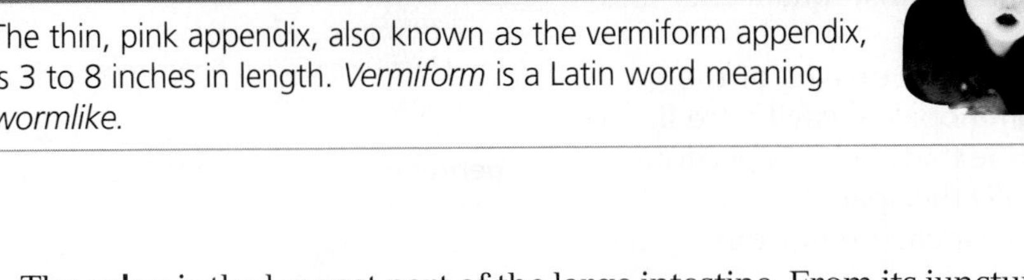

Did You Know?

The thin, pink appendix, also known as the vermiform appendix, is 3 to 8 inches in length. *Vermiform* is a Latin word meaning *wormlike.*

The **colon** is the longest part of the large intestine. From its juncture with the cecum, it proceeds through all four quadrants of the abdomen, roughly forming three sides of a square as it ascends, travels horizontally, and then descends. When the ascending colon nears the liver, it bends at a right angle known as the hepatic flexure. Then it continues horizontally as the transverse colon. Near the spleen it bends in the right angle of the splenic flexure and becomes the descending colon. Its final segment, the **sigmoid colon,** bends toward the midline in a gentle, S-shaped curve and then joins the rectum. The **rectum** is a short, straight segment that connects the sigmoid colon to the outside of the body. The **anus,** the external circular opening of the rectum, is located between the buttocks. The anal sphincter is a muscular ring around the anus, whose opening and closing is under conscious, voluntary control. The external skin around the anus is known as the **perianal area.**

Connections

Immunology (Chapter 6). Some parts of the gastrointestinal system function as part of the immune response. Saliva contains antibodies that destroy microorganisms in the food we eat. Small areas on the walls of the intestines (Peyer's patches), as well as the appendix, contain white blood cells that destroy microorganisms. However, overwhelming numbers of microorganisms present in spoiled food can still cause gastrointestinal illness.

haustra (HAW-strah)
Haustrum is a Latin singular neuter noun meaning *little drawer.* Form the plural by changing *-um* to *-a.* Because there are so many haustra in the large intestine, the singular form is seldom used.

cecum (SEE-kum)
Cecum is a Latin word meaning *cul-de-sac.*

cecal (SEE-kal)
cec/o- *cecum*
-al *pertaining to*

appendix (ah-PEN-diks)
append/o- *small structure hanging from a larger structure; appendix*
-ix *a structure*

appendiceal (AH-pen-DIS-ee-al)
appendic/o- *appendix*
-eal *pertaining to*

colon (KOH-lon)

colonic (koh-LAWN-ik)
colon/o- *colon*
-ic *pertaining to*

sigmoid (SIG-moyd)
Sigmoid is a combination of the Greek word *sigma* (the letter S) and the suffix *-oid* (resembling). The curving shape of the sigmoid colon resembles the letter *S.*

rectum (REK-tum)
Rectum is derived from a Latin word meaning *straight.* The rectum is the straight segment after the curving sigmoid colon.

rectal (REK-tal)
rect/o- *rectum*
-al *pertaining to*

anus (AA-nus)
Anus is a Latin word meaning *circle.*

anal (AA-nal)
an/o- *anus*
-al *pertaining to*

perianal (PAIR-ee-AA-nal)
peri- *around*
an/o- *anus*
-al *pertaining to*

Word Alert

ALTERNATE NAMES

The gastrointestinal (GI) system is known by several different names: the **gastrointestinal (GI) tract,** the **digestive system** or digestive tract, and the **alimentary canal**. Each name highlights a different characteristic of this body system.

1. Tract: a continuous pathway.
2. Digestive: describes the purpose of the system (to digest food).
3. Alimentary: refers to the nourishment of food. Canal: a tubular channel.

tract (TRAKT)

digestive (dy-JES-tiv)
diges/to- *break down food; digest*
-ive *pertaining to*

alimentary (AL-ih-MEN-tair-ee)
aliment/o- *food, nourishment*
-ary *pertaining to*

canal (kah-NAL)

Abdomen and Abdominopelvic Cavity

The anterior abdominal wall can be divided into four quadrants or nine regions, as previously described. Review those quadrants and regions now, as shown in Figures 2-15 and 2-16.

The **abdominopelvic cavity** contains the largest organs of the gastrointestinal system. The walls of the abdominopelvic cavity are lined with **peritoneum,** a double-layered membrane that secretes peritoneal fluid. **Peritoneal fluid** is a watery fluid that fills the spaces between the organs and allows them to smoothly slide past each other during the movements of digestion.

The peritoneum extends from the wall of the abdominopelvic cavity as a broad fatty pouch known as the omentum. The **omentum** supports the stomach in position within the abdominopelvic cavity and hangs down like an apron over the small intestine to protect and cushion it (see Figure 3-4). The peritoneum also forms a thick, fan-shaped sheet known as the **mesentery** that is attached to the posterior wall of the abdominal cavity and supports the jejunum and ileum.

The blood supply to the stomach, small intestine, liver, gallbladder, and pancreas comes from the **celiac** trunk of the aorta, the largest artery in the body.

abdominopelvic (ab-DAWM-ih-noh-PEL-vik)
abdomin/o- *abdomen*
pelv/o- *pelvis (hip bone; renal pelvis)*
-ic *pertaining to*

peritoneum (PAIR-ih-toh-NEE-um)
Peritoneum is a Latin word meaning *stretched around.*

peritoneal (PAIR-ih-toh-NEE-al)
peritone/o- *peritoneum*
-al *pertaining to*

omentum (oh-MEN-tum)
Omentum is a Latin word meaning *membrane that encloses the bowels.*

mesentery (MEZ-en-tair-ee)

mesenteric (mez-en-TAIR-ik)
meso- *middle*
enter/o- *intestine*
-ic *pertaining to*
The mesentery is only attached to the jejunum and ileum, the middle parts of the small intestine.

celiac (SEE-lee-ak)
celi/o- *abdomen*
-ac *pertaining to*

Liver

The **liver** is an accessory organ of digestion; it contributes to but is not physically involved in the process of digestion. The liver, a dark red-brown organ, is the largest solid organ in the body (see Figure 3-6 ■). It is located in the upper right abdominal cavity. Liver cells (**hepatocytes**) continuously produce **bile,** a yellow-brown or yellow-green, bitter-tasting, thick fluid. Bile is a combination of bile acids, mucus, fluid, and two pigments: the green pigment **biliverdin** and the yellow pigment **bilirubin.** Bile produced by the liver flows through the **hepatic ducts** to the gallbladder.

liver (LIV-er)

hepatocyte (HEP-ah-toh-site)
hepat/o- *liver*
-cyte *cell*

bile (BILE)

biliary (BIL-ee-air-ee)
bil/i- *bile, gall*
-ary *pertaining to*

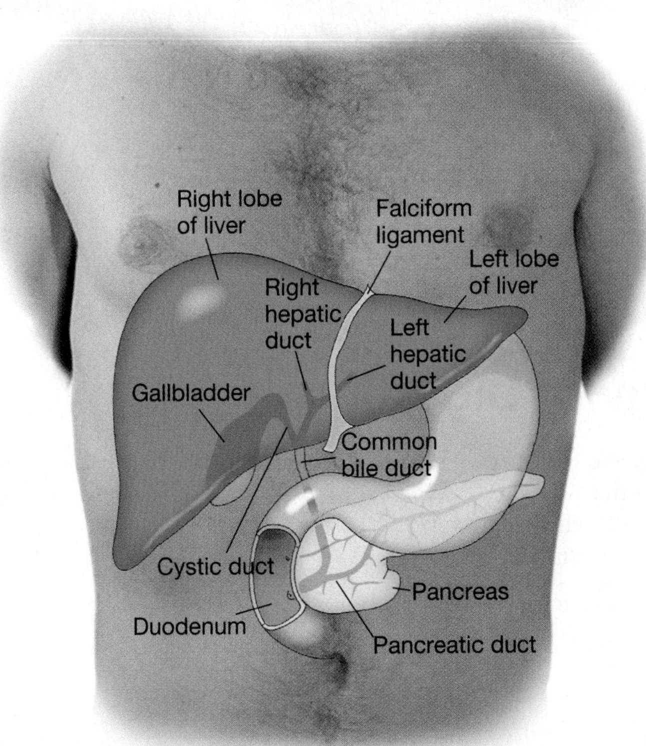

Figure 3-6 ■ The biliary tree.

In the liver, bile flows through the hepatic ducts, which then merge to form the common hepatic duct. The common hepatic duct joins the cystic duct from the gallbladder and together they form the common bile duct. Because these ducts look like the branches and trunk of a tree, they are known as the biliary tree. The pancreatic duct joins the common bile duct just before it enters the duodenum.

biliverdin (BIL-ih-VER-din)
bil/i- *bile, gall*
verd/o- *green*
-in *a substance*

bilirubin (BIL-ih-ROO-bin)
bil/i- *bile, gall*
rub/o- *red*
-in *a substance*
Bilirubin is not a red pigment. The combining form *rub/o-* indicates that bilirubin comes from the breakdown of old red blood cells.

hepatic (heh-PAT-ik)
hepat/o- *liver*
-ic *pertaining to*
Hepatic is the adjective form for *liver.*

duct (DUKT)
Duct is derived from a Latin word meaning *to lead through.*

Gallbladder

The **gallbladder** is an accessory organ of digestion. It is a teardrop-shaped, dark green sac posterior to the liver (see Figure 3-6). It concentrates and stores bile from the liver. The presence of food in the duodenum causes the gallbladder to contract, sending bile down the **cystic duct,** into the **common bile duct** and then into the duodenum. All of the bile ducts are collectively known as the **biliary tree.**

gallbladder (GAWL-blad-er)
Gall is an Old English word meaning *bitter* (the taste of bile). *Bladder* is an Old English word meaning *a fluid-filled sac.*

cholecystic (KOH-lee-SIS-tik)
chol/e- *bile, gall*
cyst/o- *bladder; fluid-filled sac; semisolid cyst*
-ic *pertaining to*
Cholecystic is the adjective form for *gallbladder.*

cystic (SIS-tik)
The combining form *cyst/o-* can be used by itself to designate the gallbladder or cystic duct.

Cholangi/o- means *bile duct,* and *choledoch/o-* means *common bile duct.*

biliary (BIL-ee-air-ee)
bil/i- *bile, gall*
-ary *pertaining to*

Pancreas

The **pancreas** is an accessory organ of digestion. It is a yellow, somewhat lumpy gland shaped like an elongated triangle (see Figure 3-6). It is located posterior to the stomach. The presence of food in the duodenum causes the pancreas to release several digestive enzymes through the pancreatic duct into the duodenum. The pancreas also functions as an organ of the endocrine system, as discussed in Endocrinology (Chapter 14).

pancreas (PAN-kree-as)
Pancreas is derived from a Greek word meaning *sweetbread.* The pancreas of a large animal was considered a culinary delicacy.

pancreatic (PAN-kree-AT-ik)
pancreat/o- *pancreas*
-ic *pertaining to*

Physiology of Digestion

The process of **digestion** begins in the oral cavity (see Figure 3-7 ■). There are two parts to digestion: mechanical and chemical.

Mechanical digestion consists of mastication (tearing, crushing, and grinding of food in the mouth), deglutition (swallowing), and peristalsis in the esophagus, stomach, and intestines (mixing and moving of food).

digestion (dy-JES-chun) (dih-JES-chun)
digest/o- *break down food; digest*
-ion *action; condition*

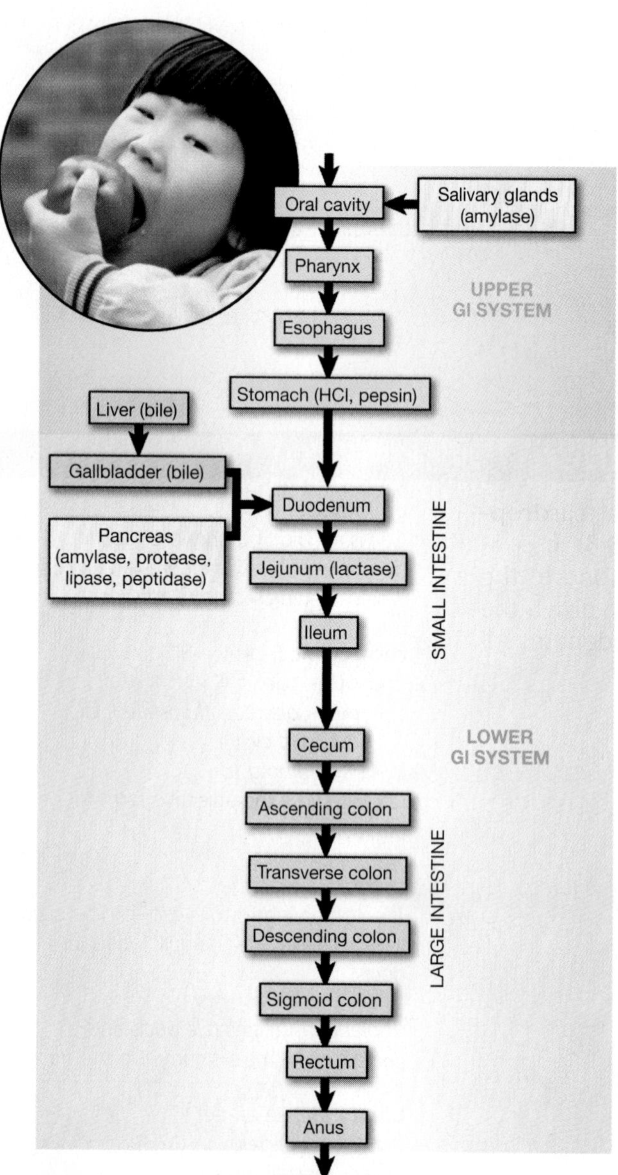

Figure 3-7 ■ The gastrointestinal system.

These structures and organs are connected to each other to make up the organized whole known as the gastrointestinal system.

Chemical digestion consists of the action of **enzymes** and acid that break down foods into molecules of nutrients that can be absorbed and used by the body. In the oral cavity, the enzyme amylase in the saliva begins to break down carbohydrates in the food. The stomach secretes the following substances that continue the process of chemical digestion.

- **Hydrochloric acid.** This strong acid kills microorganisms on ingested food, breaks down food fibers, and converts pepsinogen to the digestive enzyme pepsin.
- **Pepsinogen.** This inactive substance is converted to **pepsin**, a digestive enzyme that breaks protein-containing foods into protein molecules.
- **Gastrin.** This hormone stimulates the release of more hydrochloric acid and pepsinogen.

Connections

Hematology (Chapter 6). The stomach plays a supporting role in the production of red blood cells. The stomach secretes intrinsic factor, which helps vitamin B_{12} (one of the building blocks of red blood cells) be absorbed from the intestine into the blood. When the stomach does not produce enough intrinsic factor, there is not enough vitamin B_{12}, and the red blood cells are too small; this disease is known as pernicious anemia.

Mechanical digestion also involves breaking apart fats in the duodenum. Fatty foods in the chyme stimulate the duodenum to secrete the hormone **cholecystokinin,** which stimulates the gallbladder to contract and release bile. Bile breaks apart large globules of fat in the duodenum, a process known as **emulsification.**

Chemical digestion is completed in the small intestine. Cholecystokinin stimulates the pancreas to secrete four digestive enzymes into the duodenum, and the villi of the small intestine produce a digestive enzyme (lactase).

- **Amylase** continues the digestion of carbohydrates and starches that was begun by amylase in the saliva. It breaks down carbohydrates and starches into simple sugars and food fibers.
- **Lipase** breaks down small fat globules into fatty acids.
- **Protease** breaks down large protein molecules into smaller ones.
- **Peptidase** breaks down small protein molecules into amino acids.
- **Lactase** breaks down the sugar molecules in milk.

Absorption takes place in the ileum as food nutrients and water move through the intestinal wall into the blood. Absorption of water continues in the large intestine. Absorbed food nutrients are carried by blood in the **portal vein** directly to the liver. The liver plays an important role in regulating food nutrients like sugar and amino acids. Extra amounts of sugar are stored in the liver as glycogen and then released when the blood sugar is low. The liver uses amino acids to build plasma proteins and clotting factors.

enzyme (EN-zime)
Enzyme is a Greek word meaning *leaven*. Enzymes speed up chemical reactions just as leaven speeds up the rising of bread.

hydrochloric acid
(HY-droh-KLOR-ik AS-id)
hydr/o- *water; fluid*
chlor/o- *chloride*
-ic *pertaining to*

pepsinogen (pep-SIN-oh-jen)
pepsin/o- *pepsin*
-gen *that which produces*

pepsin (PEP-sin)
peps/o- *digestion*
-in *a substance*

gastrin (GAS-trin)
gastr/o- *stomach*
-in *a substance*

cholecystokinin (KOH-lee-SIS-toh-KY-nin)
cholecyst/o- *gallbladder*
kin/o- *movement*
-in *a substance*
Cholecystokinin moves (stimulates) the gallbladder and pancreas.

emulsification (ee-MUL-sih-fih-KAY-shun)
emulsific/o- *droplets of fat suspended in a liquid*
-ation *a process; being or having*

amylase (AM-il-ace)
amyl/o- *carbohydrate, starch*
-ase *enzyme*

lipase (LIP-ace)
lip/o- *lipid (fat)*
-ase *enzyme*

protease (PROH-tee-ace)
prote/o- *protein*
-ase *enzyme*

peptidase (PEP-tih-dace)
peptid/o- *peptide (two amino acids)*
-ase *enzyme*

lactase (LAK-tace)
lact/o- *milk*
-ase *enzyme*

absorption (ab-SORP-shun)
absorpt/o- *absorb or take in*
-ion *action; condition*

portal (POR-tal)
port/o- *point of entry*
-al *pertaining to*
Porta hepatis is the Latin name for the point of entry of this vein into the liver.

Elimination occurs when undigested food fibers and a small amount of remaining water are eliminated from the body in the form of a solid waste known as **feces** or **stool.** The process of elimination is also known as a bowel movement or **defecation.**

A Closer Look

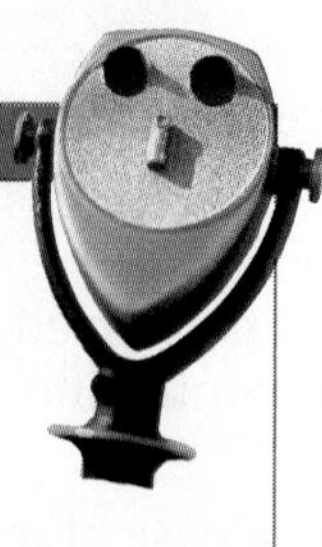

The large intestine is inhabited by millions of beneficial bacteria. These bacteria produce vitamin K to supplement what is provided by the diet. These bacteria also change the yellow-green pigments in bile to brown pigments that give stool its characteristic color. Bacteria in the large intestine feed on undigested food fiber, producing intestinal gas or **flatus.**

Across the Life Span

Stool forms in the intestines of the fetus while it is still in the uterus. The fetus swallows amniotic fluid, which contains sloughed-off cells from the fetal skin. The fluid and cells, plus mucus and bile from the fetal gastrointestinal tract, form **meconium,** a thick, sticky, green-to-black substance that is passed as the first stool.

elimination (ee-LIM-ih-NAY-shun)
elimin/o- *expel, remove*
-ation *a process; being or having*
Elimination is derived from a Latin word meaning *to throw something out the door.*

feces (FEE-seez)
Feces is derived from a Latin word meaning *the dregs.*

fecal (FEE-kal)
fec/o- *feces, stool*
-al *pertaining to*

stool (STOOL)
Stool is derived from an Old English word meaning *a seat with legs but no arms or back.* It then came to mean *a toilet* and then *waste expelled from the body.*

defecation (DEF-eh-KAY-shun)
de- *reversal of; without*
fec/o- *feces, stool*
-ation *a process; being or having*

flatus (FLAY-tus)
Flatus is a Latin word meaning *blowing.*

meconium (meh-KOH-nee-um)
Meconium is a Latin word meaning *waste from a newborn child.*

Vocabulary Review

Anatomy and Physiology

Now that you have studied the anatomy and physiology of the gastrointestinal system, take time to review those new words and descriptions. Memorize the combining forms and their definitions before going on to the next section.

Word or Phrase	Combining Form and Definition	Description
abdominopelvic cavity	abdomin/o- *abdomen* pelv/o- *pelvis (hip bone; renal pelvis)* cav/o- *hollow space*	Continuous cavity within the abdomen and pelvis that contains the largest organs of the gastrointestinal system
absorption	absorpt/o- *absorb or take in*	Process by which digested food nutrients move through villi of the small intestine into the blood
alimentary canal	aliment/o- *food, nourishment*	Alternate name for the gastrointestinal system
amylase	amyl/o- *carbohydrate, starch*	Digestive enzyme from the pancreas. It breaks down carbohydrates and starch in the duodenum into simple sugars and food fibers
antrum		Transition between the body of the stomach and the narrowing channel of the pylorus
anus	an/o- *anus*	External opening of the rectum. The external anal sphincter is under voluntary control. The perianal area is around the anus.
appendix	appendic/o- *appendix*	Long, thin pouch on the exterior wall of the cecum. It does not play a role in digestion. It contains lymphatic tissue and is active in the body's immune response.
bile	chol/e- *bile, gall*	Yellow-green, bitter fluid produced by the liver and stored in the gallbladder. It is released into the duodenum to digest the fat in foods.
bile ducts	cholangi/o- *bile duct* choledoch/o- *common bile duct*	Bile produced by the liver flows into the right and left hepatic ducts. Bile leaves the gallbladder through the cystic duct, which joins the hepatic duct to form the common bile duct. All of these ducts form a treelike structure known as the biliary tree.
cardia	cardi/o- *heart*	Small area of the stomach where the esophagus enters. It is the part of the stomach that is nearest the heart.
cardiac sphincter	cardi/o- *heart*	Muscular ring in the esophagus that keeps food in the stomach from going back into the esophagus. Also known as the lower esophageal sphincter (LES).
celiac trunk	celi/o- *abdomen*	Part of the abdominal aorta from which arteries arise to take blood to the stomach, small intestine, liver, gallbladder, and pancreas
cecum	cec/o- *cecum*	First part of the large intestine. A short, pouchlike area. The appendix is attached to its external wall.

Word or Phrase	Combining Form and Definition	Description
cholecystokinin	cholecyst/o- *gallbladder* kin/o- *movement*	Hormone released by the duodenum when it receives food from the stomach. Cholecystokinin causes the gallbladder to release bile and the pancreas to release its digestive enzymes.
chyme		Mixed food and digestive enzymes in the stomach and small intestine
colon	colon/o- *colon*	The longest part of the large intestine. It has four parts: the ascending colon, the transverse colon, the descending colon, and the S-shaped sigmoid colon.
defecation	fec/o- *feces, stool*	Process by which undigested food fiber and water are removed from the body in the form of a bowel movement
deglutition	degluti/o- *swallowing*	Process of swallowing food
digestion	digest/o- *break down food; digest*	Process of mechanically and chemically breaking down food into nutrients that can be used by the body
digestive system	digest/o- *break down food; digest*	Alternate name for the gastrointestinal system
duodenum	duoden/o- *duodenum*	First part of the small intestine. It secretes cholecystokinin, a hormone that stimulates the gallbladder and pancreas to release bile and digestive enzymes.
elimination	elimin/o- *expel, remove*	Process by which undigested food fibers and water are eliminated from the body
emulsification	emulsific/o- *droplets of fat suspended in a liquid*	Process performed by bile of breaking down large fat droplets into smaller droplets with more surface area
enzyme		Substance that breaks the chemical bonds that hold food molecules together. The name of an enzyme usually ends in *-ase.* The action of an enzyme in breaking down food is known as chemical digestion.
epiglottis		Lidlike structure that seals the larynx when food is swallowed and directs food into the esophagus
esophagus	esophag/o- *esophagus*	Flexible, muscular tube that moves food from the pharynx to the stomach
feces	fec/o- *feces, stool*	Formed, solid waste composed of undigested food fibers and water that is eliminated from the body. Also known as **stool.**
flatus		Gas produced by bacteria that inhabit the large intestine
fundus		Rounded, most superior part of the stomach
gallbladder	cholecyst/o- *gallbladder*	Small, dark green sac posterior to the liver that stores and concentrates bile. When stimulated by cholecystokinin from the duodenum, it contracts and releases bile into the common bile duct to the duodenum.
gastrin	gastr/o- *stomach*	Hormone produced by the stomach that stimulates the release of hydrochloric acid and pepsinogen in the stomach
gastrointestinal system	gastr/o- *stomach* intestin/o- *intestine*	Body system that includes the oral cavity, pharynx, esophagus, stomach, small and large intestines, and the accessory organs of the liver, gallbladder, and pancreas. Its function is to digest food and remove undigested wastes from the body. Also known as the gastrointestinal tract, digestive system, digestive tract, and the alimentary canal.

Word or Phrase	Combining Form and Definition	Description
haustra		Pouches in the wall of the large intestine that expand or contract to accommodate varying amounts of food
hepatocyte	hepat/o- *liver*	Liver cell
hydrochloric acid	hydr/o- *water; fluid*	Strong acid produced by the stomach. It breaks down food, kills microorganisms on food, and converts pepsinogen to pepsin.
ileum	ile/o- *ileum*	Third and last part of the small intestine. It connects to the cecum of the large intestine.
jejunum	jejun/o- *jejunum*	Second part of the small intestine
lactase	lact/o- *milk*	Digestive enzyme from villi in the small intestine. It breaks down lactose, the sugar in milk.
large intestine	intestin/o- *intestine*	Organ of absorption between the small intestine and the anal opening to the outside of the body. The large intestine includes the cecum, appendix, colon, rectum, and anus. Also known as the large bowel.
lipase	lip/o- *lipid (fat)*	Digestive enzyme from the pancreas. It breaks down fat globules in the duodenum into fatty acids.
liver	hepat/o- *liver*	Largest organ in the body. It produces bile.
lumen		Open channel inside the tubular structures of the gastrointestinal tract, like the esophagus, small intestine, and large intestine
mastication	mastic/o- *chewing*	Process of chewing, during which the teeth and tongue work together to tear, crush, and grind food. This is the first part of the process of mechanical digestion.
meconium		Thick, sticky, greenish-black stool that is the first stool passed by a newborn baby
mesentery	enter/o- *intestine*	Thick sheet of peritoneum that supports the jejunum and ileum
mucosa	mucos/o- *mucous membrane*	Mucous membrane lining throughout the gastrointestinal system. It produces mucus.
omentum		Broad, fatty pouch of peritoneum that supports the stomach and hangs down over the small intestine to protect and cushion it
oral cavity	or/o- *mouth* cav/o- *hollow space*	Mouth. Hollow area that contains the hard palate, soft palate, uvula, tongue, and teeth.
palate		The hard bone and soft, fleshy area that form the roof of the mouth
pancreas	pancreat/o- *pancreas*	Triangular organ located in the retroperitoneal cavity. It produces digestive enzymes (amylase, lipase, protease, peptidase) and releases them into the duodenum.
pepsin	peps/o- *digestion*	Digestive enzyme from the stomach. It breaks down food protein into large protein molecules.

Word or Phrase	Combining Form and Definition	Description
pepsinogen	**pepsin/o-** *pepsin*	Substance produced by the stomach. It is converted by hydrochloric acid to the digestive enzyme pepsin.
peptidase	**peptid/o-** *peptide (two amino acids)*	Digestive enzyme from the pancreas. It breaks down small protein molecules in the duodenum into amino acids.
peristalsis	**stal/o-** *contraction*	Contractions of the smooth muscle of the gastrointestinal tract that propel food through it
peritoneum	**peritone/o-** *peritoneum*	Membrane that lines the abdominopelvic cavity and secretes peritoneal fluid to fill the spaces between the organs
pharynx	**pharyng/o-** *pharynx (throat)*	Throat. It is a passageway for food and for inhaled and exhaled air.
portal vein	**port/o-** *point of entry*	Vein whose blood carries food nutrients from the intestines to the liver
protease	**prote/o-** *protein*	Digestive enzyme from the pancreas. It breaks down large protein molecules in the duodenum into smaller ones.
pyloric sphincter	**pylor/o-** *pylorus*	Muscular ring that closes to keep food in the stomach and opens to let food go into the duodenum
pylorus	**pylor/o-** *pylorus*	Narrowing channel of the stomach just before it joins the duodenum. It contains the pyloric sphincter.
rectum	**rect/o-** *rectum*	Final part of the large intestine. It is a short, straight segment that lies between the sigmoid colon and the outside of the body.
rugae		Deep folds in the gastric mucosa that expand or contract to accomodate varying amounts of food
saliva	**saliv/o-** *saliva*	Watery substance secreted by the salivary glands. It contains amylase, a digestive enzyme that begins the process of digestion in the mouth.
salivary gland	**saliv/o-** *saliva*	Three pairs of glands (parotid, submandibular, and sublingual) that produce and release saliva
small intestine	**intestin/o-** *intestine*	Organ of digestion between the stomach and the large intestine. The duodenum, jejunum, and ileum are the three parts of the small intestine. Also known as the small bowel.
stomach	**gastr/o-** *stomach*	Organ of digestion between the esophagus and the small intestine. Areas of the stomach: cardia, fundus, body, antrum, and pylorus. The stomach secretes hydrochloric acid, pepsinogen, and gastrin. The stomach secretes intrinsic factor needed to absorb vitamin B_{12}.
tongue	**lingu/o-** *tongue* **gloss/o-** *tongue*	Large muscle that fills the oral cavity and assists with eating and talking. It contains taste buds and receptors for the sense of taste.
uvula		Fleshy hanging part of the soft palate that activates the gag reflex when food touches it
villi		Microscopic projections of the mucosa within the lumen of the small intestine. The site where nutrients are absorbed into the blood.

Labeling Exercise

A. *Match each anatomy word or phrase to its numbered structure in Figure 3-8■. Write that word or phrase on the blank line next to its number. Use the Answer Key at the end of the book to check your answers.*

esophagus	parotid gland	sublingual gland	teeth
oral cavity	pharynx	submandibular gland	tongue

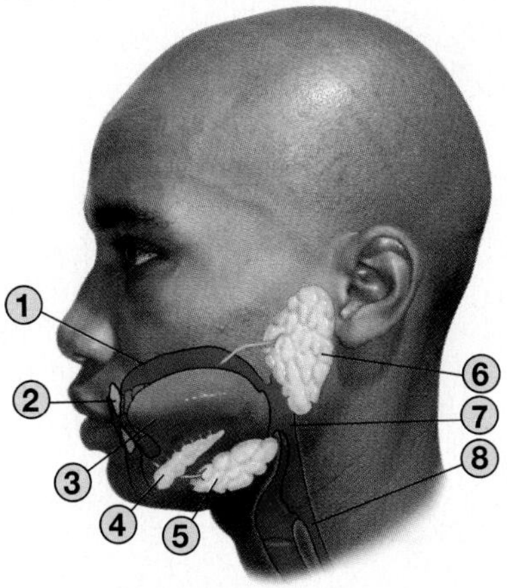

1. ______________________
2. ______________________
3. ______________________
4. ______________________
5. ______________________
6. ______________________
7. ______________________
8. ______________________

Figure 3-8 ■

B. *Match each anatomy word or phrase to its numbered structure in Figure 3-9■. Write that word or phrase on the blank line next to its number.*

antrum	cardiac sphincter	fundus	pyloric sphincter
body of stomach	duodenum	omentum	pylorus
cardia	esophagus	pancreas	rugae

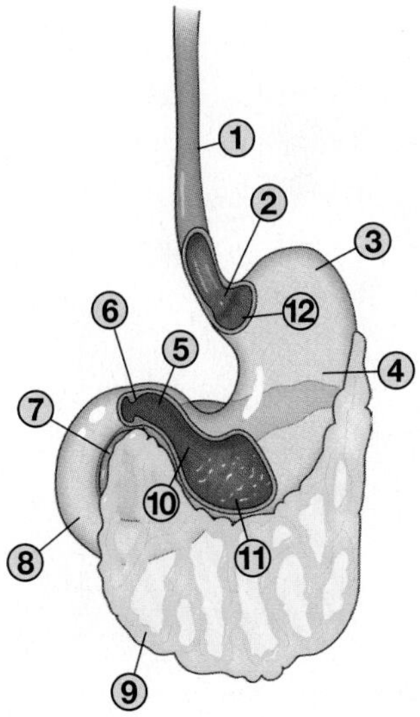

1. ______________________
2. ______________________
3. ______________________
4. ______________________
5. ______________________
6. ______________________
7. ______________________
8. ______________________
9. ______________________
10. ______________________
11. ______________________
12. ______________________

Figure 3-9 ■

C. *Match each anatomy word or phrase to its numbered structure in Figure 3-10 ■. Write that word or phrase on the blank line next to its number.*

anus	descending colon	liver	spleen
appendix	duodenum	rectum	stomach
ascending colon	ileum	sigmoid colon	transverse colon
cecum	jejunum		

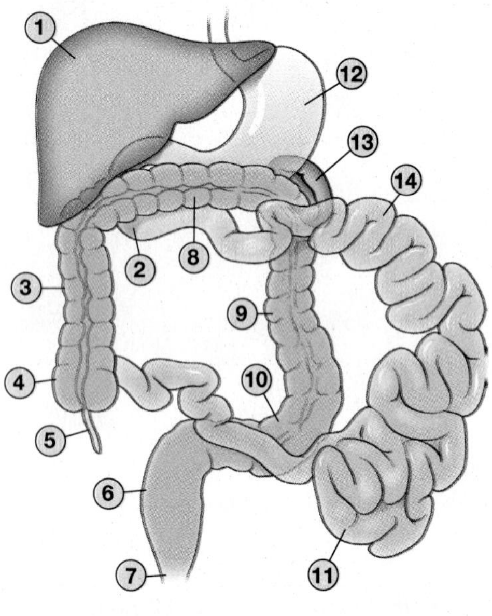

1. ______________________
2. ______________________
3. ______________________
4. ______________________
5. ______________________
6. ______________________
7. ______________________
8. ______________________
9. ______________________
10. ______________________
11. ______________________
12. ______________________
13. ______________________
14. ______________________

Figure 3-10 ■

Building Medical Words

Combining Forms

Here are the gastrointestinal combining forms you have learned so far. Next to each combining form, write its meaning. Use the Answer Key at the end of the book to check your answers. The first one has been done for you.

	Combining Form	Medical Meaning		Combining Form	Medical Meaning
1.	hydr/o-	water	30.	gloss/o-	
2.	abdomin/o-		31.	gustat/o-	
3.	absorpt/o-		32.	hepat/o-	
4.	aliment/o-		33.	ile/o-	
5.	amyl/o-		34.	intestin/o-	
6.	an/o-		35.	jejun/o-	
7.	appendic/o-		36.	kin/o-	
8.	append/o-		37.	lact/o-	
9.	bil/i-		38.	lingu/o-	
10.	cardi/o-		39.	lip/o-	
11.	cav/o-		40.	mandibul/o-	
12.	cec/o-		41.	mastic/o-	
13.	celi/o-		42.	mucos/o-	
14.	chlor/o-		43.	or/o-	
15.	cholangi/o-		44.	ot/o-	
16.	chol/e-		45.	pancreat/o-	
17.	cholecyst/o-		46.	pelv/o-	
18.	choledoch/o-		47.	peps/o-	
19.	colon/o-		48.	pepsin/o-	
20.	cyst/o-		49.	peptid/o-	
21.	degluti/o-		50.	peritone/o-	
22.	digest/o-		51.	pharyng/o-	
23.	duoden/o-		52.	port/o-	
24.	elimin/o-		53.	prote/o-	
25.	emulsific/o-		54.	pylor/o-	
26.	enter/o-		55.	rect/o-	
27.	esophag/o-		56.	rub/o-	
28.	fec/o-		57.	saliv/o-	
29.	gastr/o-		58.	verd/o-	

Combining Forms and Suffixes

Read the definition hint for the medical word you are to build. Look at the combining form that is given. Write the correct suffix on the blank line. Then write the medical word. (Remember: You may need to remove the combining vowel. Always remove the hyphens and slash.) Use the Answer Key at the end of the book to check your answers. The first one has been done for you.

SUFFIX LIST

-al (pertaining to)	-cyte (cell)	-ion (action; condition)
-ary (pertaining to)	-eal (pertaining to)	-ive (pertaining to)
-ase (enzyme)	-gen (that which produces)	-ix (a structure)
-ation (a process; being or having)	-ic (pertaining to)	-tion (a process; being or having)

Definition Hint	Combining Form	Suffix	Write the Medical Word
1. Pertaining to the abdomen	abdomin/o-	-al	abdominal
2. Pertaining to the stomach	gastr/o-	______	______
3. Liver cell	hepat/o-	______	______
4. Pertaining to the mouth	or/o-	______	______
5. Pertaining to the gland that makes saliva	saliv/o-	______	______
6. Pertaining to the tongue	lingu/o-	______	______
7. Process of chewing	mastic/o-	______	______
8. Pertaining to the rectum	rect/o-	______	______
9. Enzyme that digests fat	lip/o-	______	______
10. Pertaining to the appendix	appendic/o-	______	______
11. Thing that hangs on a larger structure	append/o-	______	______
12. Pertaining to the colon	colon/o-	______	______
13. Pertaining to digestion	digest/o-	______	______
14. Pertaining to the esophagus	esophag/o-	______	______
15. Process of swallowing	degluti/o-	______	______
16. Pertaining to the ileum	ile/o-	______	______
17. That which produces pepsin	pepsin/o-	______	______
18. Pertaining to the pancreas	pancreat/o-	______	______
19. Pertaining to a bile duct	bil/i-	______	______
20. Pertaining to the duodenum	duoden/o-	______	______

Symptoms, Signs, and Diseases

Eating

Word or Phrase	Word Part and Definition	Description
anorexia	**anorexia** (AN-oh-REK-see-ah) an- *without, not* orex/o- *appetite* -ia *condition, state, thing* **anorexic** (AN-oh-REK-sik) an- *without, not* orex/o- *appetite* -ic *pertaining to*	Decreased appetite because of disease or the gastrointestinal side effects of a drug. A patient with anorexia is said to be **anorexic**. Treatment: Correct the underlying cause. **Connections** **Psychiatry (Chapter 17).** Anorexia nervosa is a psychiatric disorder in which patients have an obsessive desire to be thin. They decrease their food intake to the point of starvation but still perceive themselves as being fat.
dysphagia	**dysphagia** (dis-FAY-jee-ah) dys- *painful, difficult, abnormal* phag/o- *eating, swallowing* -ia *condition, state, thing* **odynophagia** (oh-DIN-oh-FAY-jee-ah) odyn/o- *pain* phag/o- *eating, swallowing* -ia *condition, state, thing*	Difficult or painful eating or swallowing. A stroke can make it difficult to coordinate the muscles for eating and swallowing. Infection or poor-fitting dentures can cause painful eating. Also known as **odynophagia**. Treatment: Soft foods and thickened liquids. Antibiotic drugs for a bacterial infection.
polyphagia	**polyphagia** (PAWL-ee-FAY-jee-ah) poly- *many, much* phag/o- *eating, swallowing* -ia *condition, state, thing*	Excessive overeating. Can be due to an overactive thyroid gland, diabetes mellitus, or a psychiatric illness. Treatment: Correct the underlying cause.

Mouth and Lips

Word or Phrase	Word Part and Definition	Description
cheilitis	**cheilitis** (ky-LY-tis) cheil/o- *lip* -itis *inflammation of*	Inflammation and cracking of the lips and corners of the mouth due to infection, allergies, or nutritional deficiency. Treatment: Correct the underlying cause.
sialolithiasis	**sialolithiasis** (sy-AL-oh-lih-THY-ah-sis) sial/o- *saliva; salivary gland* lith/o- *stone* -iasis *state of; process of* **sialolith** (sy-AL-oh-lith) sial/o- *saliva; salivary gland* -lith *stone*	A stone (**sialolith**) that forms in the salivary gland and becomes lodged in the duct, blocking the flow of saliva. The salivary gland and the face or mouth become swollen. When the salivary gland contracts, the duct spasms, causing pain. Treatment: Surgical removal of the stone.
stomatitis	**stomatitis** (STOH-mah-TY-tis) stomat/o- *mouth* -itis *inflammation of* **aphthous** (AF-thus) aphth/o- *ulcer* -ous *pertaining to*	Inflammation of the oral mucosa. Stomatitis can be caused by poorly fitting dentures that rub the gums. **Aphthous stomatitis**, or canker sores, presents as small ulcers of the oral mucosa. Its cause is unknown. Treatment: Correct the underlying cause.

Esophagus and Stomach

Word or Phrase	Word Part and Definition	Description
dyspepsia	**dyspepsia** (dis-PEP-see-ah) **dys-** *painful, difficult, abnormal* **peps/o-** *digestion* **-ia** *condition, state, thing* **indigestion** (IN-dy-JES-chun) **in-** *in; within; not* **digest/o-** *break down food; digest* **-ion** *action; condition*	**Indigestion** or epigastric pain that may be accompanied by gas or nausea. It can be caused by excess secretion of stomach acid, overeating, spicy foods, or stress. Treatment: Antacid drugs. Avoid those things that cause it.
varices	**varix** (VAR-iks) **varices** (VAR-ih-seez) *Varix* is a Latin singular word meaning *dilated vein.* Form the plural by changing *-ix* to *-ices.*	Swollen, protruding veins in the mucosa of the lower esophagus or stomach. Liver disease causes blood to back up in the portal vein (from the intestines to the liver). This backed-up blood uses the gastroesophageal veins as another route, but eventually these veins become engorged. Esophageal and gastric varices are easily irritated by passing food. They can hemorrhage suddenly, causing death. Treatment: Correct the underlying liver disease. Drug injected into the varix to harden it and block the blood flow.
gastritis	**gastritis** (gas-TRY-tis) **gastr/o-** *stomach* **-itis** *inflammation of*	Acute or chronic inflammation of the stomach due to eating spicy foods, excess acid production, or a bacterial infection. Treatment: Antacid drugs; antibiotic drugs for a bacterial infection.
gastroenteritis	**gastroenteritis** (GAS-troh-EN-ter-EYE-tis) **gastr/o-** *stomach* **enter/o-** *intestine* **-itis** *inflammation of*	Acute inflammation or infection of the stomach and intestines. Gastroenteritis is due to a virus (intestinal flu) or bacterium (contaminated food). Symptoms include abdominal pain, nausea, vomiting, and diarrhea. Treatment: Antiemetic drugs, antidiarrheal drugs; antibiotic drugs for a bacterial infection.
gastroesophageal reflux disease (GERD)	**gastroesophageal** (GAS-troh-ee-SAWF-ah-JEE-al) **gastr/o-** *stomach* **esophag/o-** *esophagus* **-eal** *pertaining to* **reflux** (REE-fluks) *Reflux* is derived from a Latin word meaning *a backward flow.* **esophagitis** (ee-SAWF-ah-JY-tis) **esophag/o-** *esophagus* **-itis** *inflammation of*	Chronic inflammation and irritation of the esophagus due to **reflux** of stomach acid back into the esophagus. This occurs because the lower esophageal sphincter does not close tightly. Symptoms include sore throat, belching, and **esophagitis** (chronic inflammation of the esophagus). This inflammation can progress to esophageal ulcers or cancer of the esophagus. Treatment: Elevate the head of the bed while sleeping. Avoid alcohol and foods that stimulate acid secretion. Antacids, drugs that decrease the production of acid.
heartburn	**pyrosis** (py-ROH-sis) **pyr/o-** *fire; burning* **-osis** *condition; abnormal condition; process*	Temporary inflammation of the esophagus due to reflux of stomach acid. Also known as **pyrosis**. Treatment: Antacid drugs.
hematemesis	**hematemesis** (HEE-mah-TEM-ah-sis) **hemat/o-** *blood* **-emesis** *vomiting*	Vomiting of new or old blood from bleeding in the stomach or esophagus. Can be caused by an esophageal ulcer, esophageal varices, or a gastric ulcer. Coffee-grounds emesis contains old, dark blood that has been partially digested by the stomach. Treatment: Correct the underlying cause.

Word or Phrase	Word Part and Definition	Description
hiatal hernia	**hiatal** (hy-AA-tal) **hiatus** (hy-AA-tus) *Hiatal and hiatus* are Latin words meaning *an opening.* **hernia** (HER-nee-ah) *Hernia* is a Latin word meaning *a rupture or protrusion.*	Weakness in the diaphragm, the muscular wall between the thoracic and abdominopelvic cavities that allows the esophagus or stomach to slide through and balloon into the thoracic cavity. Also known as a **hiatus hernia**. Treatment: Elevate the head of the bed while sleeping. Surgery (herniorrhaphy) to close the defect.
nausea and vomiting (N&V)	**nausea** (NAW-see-ah) (NAW-zha) *Nausea* is derived from a Greek word meaning *seasick.* **nauseated** (NAW-zee-aa-ted) **nause/o-** *nausea* **-ated** *pertaining to a condition; composed of* **emesis** (EM-eh-sis) *Vomitus* is a Latin word and *emesis* is a Greek word meaning *ejected contents.* **vomit** (VAWM-mit) **vomitus** (VAWM-ih-tus) **regurgitation** (ree-GER-jih-TAY-shun) **regurgitat/o-** *flow backward* **-ion** *action; condition*	Nausea is an unpleasant, queasy feeling in the stomach that precedes the urge to vomit. A patient with nausea is said to be **nauseated**. Can be caused by inflammation or infection in the stomach or by motion sickness. Vomiting is the expelling of food from the stomach through the mouth. It is triggered when impulses from the stomach or inner ear stimulate the vomiting center in the brain. Also known as **emesis**. **Vomit** or **vomitus** is the expelled food or chyme. Projectile vomiting is when vomitus is expelled with force and projected a distance from the patient. Continual vomiting when there is no longer any food in the stomach is known as retching or dry heaves. **Regurgitation** is the reflux of small amounts of food and acid back into the mouth. Treatment: Antiemetic drugs.

Connections

hyperemesis (HY-per-EM-eh-sis)
hyper- *above; more than normal*
-emesis *vomiting*

gravidarum (GRAV-ih-DAIR-rum)
Gravidarum is a Latin word meaning *of pregnancy.*

Obstetrics (Chapter 13). Excessive vomiting during the first few months of pregnancy is known as **hyperemesis gravidarum**. This is thought to be caused by the change in hormone levels that occurs during pregnancy.

Word or Phrase	Word Part and Definition	Description
peptic ulcer disease (PUD)	**peptic** (PEP-tik) **pept/o-** *digestion* **-ic** *pertaining to* **ulcer** (UL-ser) *Ulcer* is derived from a Latin word meaning *a sore.*	Chronic irritation, burning pain, and erosion of the mucosa to the point of forming an ulcer. An esophageal ulcer, a gastric ulcer in the stomach, and a duodenal ulcer are all classified as peptic ulcers. Gastric ulcers are most commonly caused by the bacterium *Helicobacter pylori* (see Figure 3-11■). Ulcers can also be caused by excessive hydrochloric acid, stress, and by drugs like aspirin that irritate the mucosa. Treatment: Drugs to treat *H. pylori* infection. Drugs to decrease acid production. Antacid drugs. Avoid spicy foods, smoking, alcohol, caffeine, and aspirin-type drugs. **Figure 3-11 ■ Gastric ulcer.** As seen through an endoscope, the gastric mucosa is raw and irritated with a large central ulcer crater. The large blood clot indicates a recent episode of bleeding from the ulcer.
stomach cancer	**cancer** (KAN-ser) *Cancer* is a Latin word meaning *a crab.* Cancer spreads in all directions like the legs of a crab spread out from its body. **adenocarcinoma** (AD-eh-noh-KAR-sih-NOH-mah) **aden/o-** *gland* **carcin/o-** *cancer* **-oma** *tumor, mass*	Cancerous tumor of the stomach that most often arises from the glands in the mucosa of the stomach. Also known as **gastric adenocarcinoma**. It can develop following chronic irritation from a *Helicobacter pylori* infection. Treatment: Antibiotic drugs to eliminate *H. pylori* infection. Surgery to remove the cancerous tumor and part of the stomach (gastrectomy).
Duodenum, Jejunum, Ileum		
ileus	**ileus** (IL-ee-us) *Ileus* is a Latin word meaning *rolled up tightly, obstructed.* **postoperative** (post-AWP-er-ah-tiv) **post-** *after, behind* **operat/o-** *perform a procedure; surgery* **-ive** *pertaining to*	Abnormal absence of peristalsis in the small and large intestines. Can be caused by a tumor, adhesions, a hernia, severe infection in the bowel or abdominopelvic cavity, trauma, shock, or drugs. **Postoperative ileus** occurs after the intestines are manipulated during abdominal surgery and peristalsis is slow to return to normal. Treatment: Intravenous fluids for temporary nutritional support. Surgery (bowel resection and anastomosis) may be needed to correct the cause.

Word or Phrase	Word Part and Definition	Description
intussusception	**intussusception** (IN-tus-suh-SEP-shun) **intussuscep/o-** *to receive within* **-tion** *a process; being or having*	Telescoping of one segment of intestine into the lumen of an adjacent segment (see Figure 3-12■). Symptoms include vomiting and abdominal pain. The cause is unknown. Treatment: Surgery (bowel resection and anastomosis). **Figure 3-12 ■ Intussusception of the intestine.** The intestinal wall folds back on itself in the same way that one part of a telescope slides into the other. This causes inflammation, stops peristalsis, and can lead to tissue death if the blood flow is blocked in the arteries.
volvulus	**volvulus** (VAWL-vyoo-lus) *Volvulus* is a Latin word meaning *to roll.* **malrotation** (MAL-roh-TAY-shun) **mal-** *bad, inadequate* **rotat/o-** *rotate* **-ion** *action; condition*	Twisting of a loop of intestine around itself or around another segment of intestine because of a structural abnormality of the mesentery. Symptoms include vomiting and abdominal pain. Blood vessels to the intestines can also be twisted, decreasing the blood supply and causing the tissues to die. Also known as **malrotation** of the intestines. Treatment: Surgery (bowel resection and anastomosis).
Cecum and Colon		
appendicitis	**appendicitis** (ah-PEN-dih-SY-tis) **appendic/o-** *appendix* **-itis** *inflammation of*	Inflammation and infection of the appendix. Undigested food fibers become trapped in the narrow lumen of the appendix. Symptoms include steadily increasing abdominal pain that finally localizes to the right lower quadrant. The patient complains of rebound tenderness if the physician presses down on the lower right quadrant and then suddenly removes the hand, releasing the pressure. An inflamed appendix can rupture (burst), spilling infection into the abdominopelvic cavity and causing peritonitis (see Figure 3-16). Treatment: Surgery to remove the appendix (appendectomy).
colic	**colic** (KAWL-ik) **col/o-** *colon* **-ic** *pertaining to*	Common disorder in babies. Symptoms include crampy abdominal pain that occurs soon after eating. Can be caused by overfeeding, feeding too quickly, inadequate burping, or food allergies to milk. Treatment: Correct the underlying cause. Change to soy-based infant formula.
colon cancer	**colorectal** (KOH-loh-REK-tal) **col/o-** *colon* **rect/o-** *rectum* **-al** *pertaining to* **adenocarcinoma** (AD-eh-noh-KAR-sih-NOH-mah) **aden/o-** *gland* **carcin/o-** *cancer* **-oma** *tumor, mass*	Cancerous tumor of the colon. Caused by colonic polyps or ulcerative colitis that becomes cancerous. Also linked to a high-fat diet. Symptoms include blood in the stool. Also known as **colorectal adenocarcinoma**. Treatment: Preventative surgery to remove multiple polyps before they become cancerous. Surgery to remove the cancerous tumor and the affected segment of intestine (bowel resection) and temporarily reroute the colon to a new opening in the outside abdominal wall (colostomy).

Word or Phrase	Word Part and Definition	Description
diverticulum	**diverticulum** (DY-ver-TIK-yoo-lum) **diverticula** (DY-ver-TIK-yoo-lah) *Diverticulum* is a Latin singular neuter noun meaning *a by-road.* Form the plural by changing *-um to -a.* **diverticulosis** (DY-ver-TIK-yoo-LOH-sis) **diverticul/o-** *diverticulum* **-osis** *condition; abnormal condition; process* **diverticular** (DY-ver-TIK-yoo-lar) **diverticul/o-** *diverticulum* **-ar** *pertaining to* **diverticulitis** (DY-ver-TIK-yoo-LY-tis) **diverticul/o-** *diverticulum* **-itis** *inflammation of*	Area where the mucosa has been forced out through small defects in the wall of the colon. Diverticula can be in the shape of a pouch or a tube. Diverticula are not hereditary. They are thought to be caused by eating a low-fiber diet that forms small, compact stools. Increased intra-abdominal pressure from straining to pass these stools eventually creates diverticula. **Diverticulosis** or **diverticular disease** is the condition of having multiple diverticula (see Figure 3-13■). If feces become trapped inside a diverticular sac, this causes inflammation and infection, abdominal pain, and fever, a condition known as **diverticulitis** (see Figure 3-14■). Prevention: High-fiber diet. Treatment: Antibiotic drugs to treat diverticulitis. Surgery (bowel resection and anastomosis) to remove the affected segment of intestine. **Connections** **Dietetics.** Diverticular disease was unknown until the early 1900s, when refined flour began to replace whole wheat flour. Diverticular disease is common in industrialized countries where people eat a low-fiber diet, but it is uncommon in third-world countries where people eat a high-fiber diet with lots of roughage. Fiber adds bulk to the stools and holds in water to keep stools soft.

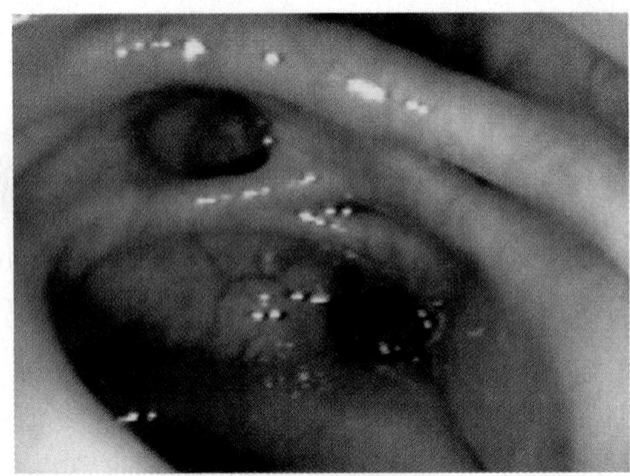

Figure 3-13 ■ Diverticula.
There are multiple openings in the wall of the colon, each of which leads to a diverticulum.

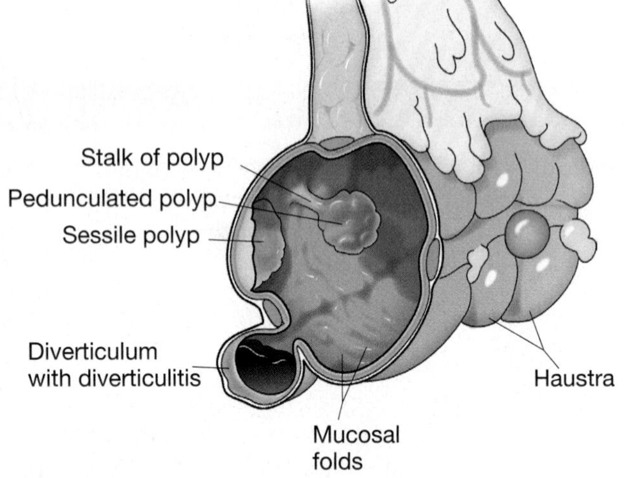

Figure 3-14 ■ Diverticulitis and polyposis.
A diverticulum becomes infected when feces and bacteria become trapped inside it. Polyps are irritated by the passage of feces, and they can eventually become cancerous.

Word or Phrase	Word Part and Definition	Description
dysentery	**dysentery** (DIS-en-tair-ee) **dys-** *painful, difficult, abnormal* **-entery** *condition of the intestine* Every medical word must contain a combining form. The suffix of *dysentery* contains the combining form *enter/o-*.	Bacterial infection caused by an unusual strain of *E. coli,* a common bacterium in the large intestine. Symptoms include watery diarrhea mixed with blood and mucus. Treatment: Antibiotic drugs.
gluten enteropathy	**gluten** (GLOO-ten) **enteropathy** (EN-ter-AWP-ah-thee) **enter/o-** *intestine* **-pathy** *disease, suffering* **celiac** (SEE-lee-ak) **celi/o-** *abdomen* **-ac** *pertaining to*	A food allergy to the gluten in wheat causes gluten enteropathy, in which the tissues of the small intestine are damaged by the allergic response. This is also known as **celiac disease.** Treatment: Avoid eating wheat.
inflammatory bowel disease (IBD)	**inflammatory** (in-FLAM-ah-tor-ee) **inflammat/o-** *redness and warmth* **-ory** *having the function of* **Crohn** (KROHN) **enteritis** (EN-ter-EYE-tis) **enter/o-** *intestine* **-itis** *inflammation of* **ulcerative** (UL-ser-ah-tiv) **ulcerat/o-** *ulcer* **-ive** *pertaining to* **colitis** (koh-LY-tis) **col/o-** *colon* **-itis** *inflammation of*	Chronic inflammation of various parts of the small and large intestine. The cause is not known. Symptoms include diarrhea, bloody stools, abdominal cramps, and fever. There are two types of inflammatory bowel disease: **Crohn's disease** affects the ileum and colon with areas of inflammation followed by areas of normal mucosa. Also known as **regional enteritis. Ulcerative colitis** affects the colon and rectum and causes inflammation and ulcers. Treatment: Steroid drugs to decrease inflammation. Surgery (bowel resection) to remove the affected segment of intestine and temporarily reroute the intestine to a new opening in the outside abdominal wall (ileostomy, colostomy).
irritable bowel syndrome (IBS)	**syndrome** (SIN-drohm) **syn-** *together* **-drome** *a running together* Every medical word must contain a combining form. The suffix of *syndrome* contains the combining form *drom/o-*. **spasm** (SPAZM) **spastic** (SPAS-tik) **spast/o-** *spasm* **-ic** *pertaining to* **colitis** (koh-LY-tis) **col/o-** *colon* **-itis** *inflammation of*	Disorder of the function of the colon, although the mucosa of the colon never shows any visible signs of inflammation. A syndrome consists of many interrelated symptoms and signs: severe **spasms** of cramping abdominal pain, diarrhea, and bloating alternating with constipation. There is also an excessive secretion of mucus from the colon. The cause is not known but may be related to lactose intolerance and emotional stress. Also known as **spastic colon** or **mucous colitis.** Treatment: Antidiarrheal and antispasmodic drugs. High-fiber diet and laxatives to prevent constipation.

Word or Phrase	Word Part and Definition	Description
polyps	**polyp** (PAW-lip) *Polyp* is derived from a Latin word meaning *many-footed.* The base or stalk (foot) of a polyp comes in different shapes and sizes. **pedunculated** (peh-DUNG-kyoo-lay-ted) *Peduncle* is derived from a Latin word meaning *a stalk with a little foot.* **sessile** (SES-il) *Sessile* is derived from a Latin word meaning *low growing with a broad base.* **benign** (bee-NINE) *Benign* is derived from a Latin word meaning *kind, not harmful.* **polyposis** (PAWL-ee-POH-sis) **polyp/o-** *polyp* **-osis** *condition; abnormal condition; process*	Small, fleshy, benign or precancerous growths that arise from the mucosa of the colon. A **pedunculated polyp** has a thin stalk that supports a ball-shaped, irregular top (see Figure 3-14). A **sessile polyp** is shaped like a mound with a broad, rounded base (see Figure 3-15■). **Benign familial polyposis** is an inherited condition in which many family members have multiple colon polyps. Although all polyps are benign, they can become cancerous. Treatment: Surgery to remove the polyps (polypectomy). **Figure 3-15 ■ Colonic polyps.** This patient has multiple sessile polyps of the colon. Note the many folds of haustra in the wall of the colon.

Rectum and Anus

Word or Phrase	Word Part and Definition	Description
hemorrhoids	**hemorrhoid** (HEM-oh-royd) **hemorrh/o-** *a flowing of blood* **-oid** *resembling*	Swollen, protruding veins in the rectum (internal hemorrhoids) or on the perianal skin (external hemorrhoids). Caused by increased intra-abdominal pressure from straining to pass hard stools. This repeatedly dilates the veins until they permanently protrude. Hemorrhoids are irritated as stool passes through the rectum and their surfaces bleed easily. Also known as **piles.** Treatment: Topical steroid drugs to decrease itching and irritation. Surgery to remove the hemorrhoids (hemorrhoidectomy).
rectocele	**rectocele** (REK-toh-seel) **rect/o-** *rectum* **-cele** *hernia*	Protruding wall of the rectum pushes on the adjacent wall of the vagina, causing it to collapse and partially block the vaginal canal. Treatment: Surgery to repair the defect.

Across the Life Span

patent (PAY-tent)
Patent is derived from a Latin word meaning *to lie open.*

imperforate (im-PER-for-ate)
im- *not*
perfor/o- *to have an opening*
-ate *composed of; pertaining to*

In the newborn nursery, the nurse always takes a rectal temperature on a newborn infant. This not only gives the most accurate body temperature, but also verifies that the rectum is **patent.** Occasionally, a newborn will have an **imperforate anus,** a congenital (present at birth) abnormality in which the rectum is closed. Treatment: Immediate surgery to open the rectum and connect it to the outside of the body.

Defecation and Feces

Word or Phrase	Word Part and Definition	Description
constipation	**constipation** (CON-stih-PAY-shun) **constip/o-** *compacted stool* **-ation** *a process; being or having* **obstipation** (AWB-stih-PAY-shun) **obstip/o-** *severe constipation* **-ation** *a process; being or having* **obstipated** (AWB-stih-PAY-ted) **obstip/o-** *severe constipation* **-ated** *pertaining to a condition; composed of*	Failure to have regular, soft bowel movements. Can be due to lack of dietary fiber, inadequate water intake, or the side effect of a drug. **Obstipation** is severe, unrelieved constipation. The patient is said to be **obstipated.** Treatment: Laxative drugs, high-fiber diet, enemas. **Across the Life Span** Constipation is a common complaint in the elderly. A diet of refined foods and low fiber, lack of water intake, and inactivity contribute to the formation of small, hard stools. Narcotic drugs used to treat pain are notorious for causing constipation and can actually cause bowel obstruction in elderly, inactive patients.
diarrhea	**diarrhea** (DY-ah-REE-ah) **dia-** *complete; completely through* **-rrhea** *flow, discharge* Every medical word must contain a combining form. The suffix of *diarrhea* contains the combining form *rrhe/o-*.	Abnormally frequent and loose, watery stools. Caused by an infection (bacteria, viruses), irritable bowel syndrome, ulcerative colitis, lactose intolerance, or a drug side effect. There is increased peristalsis, and the feces do not stay long enough in the large intestine for the water to be completely absorbed. Treatment: Antidiarrheal drugs, lactase supplements. Antibiotic drugs to treat bacterial infections.
fecalith	**fecalith** (FEE-kah-lith) **fec/a-** *feces, stool* **-lith** *stone*	Hardened feces that become a stonelike mass. This can form in the appendix or a diverticulum. Treatment: None, unless associated with inflammation or infection.
flatulence	**flatulence** (FLAT-yoo-lens) **flatul/o-** *flatus* **-ence** *state of* **flatus** (FLAY-tus)	Presence of excessive amounts of **flatus** (gas) in the stomach or intestines. Can be caused by milk (lactose) intolerance or indigestion. Treatment: Lactase supplements, antigas drugs.
hematochezia	**hematochezia** (hee-MAH-toh-KEE-zee-ah) **hemat/o-** *blood* **chez/o-** *to pass stool* **-ia** *condition, state, thing*	Blood in the stool. The source of bleeding can be an ulcer, cancer, Crohn's disease, polyp, diverticulum, or hemorrhoid. Bright red blood indicates active bleeding in the lower gastrointestinal system. Treatment: Correct the underlying cause.
incontinence	**incontinence** (in-CON-tih-nens) **in-** *in; within, not* **contin/o-** *hold together* **-ence** *state of* For *incontinence,* the best meaning of the prefix *in-* is *not.* Incontinence is a state of not holding in stool. **incontinent** (in-CON-tih-nent) **in-** *in; within; not* **contin/o-** *hold together* **-ent** *pertaining to*	Inability to voluntarily control bowel movements. Patients with paralysis of the lower extremities lack sensation and motor control of the external anal sphincter and are said to be **incontinent.** Patients with dementia are unaware of a bowel movement occurring. Treatment: None.

Word or Phrase	Word Part and Definition	Description
melena	**melena** (meh-LEE-nah) *Melena* is derived from a Greek word meaning *black*. **melenic** (meh-LEH-nik) **melen/o-** *black* **-ic** *pertaining to*	Dark, tarry stools that contain digested blood due to bleeding in the esophagus or stomach. These stools are said to be **melenic.** Treatment: Correct the underlying cause of bleeding.
steatorrhea	**steatorrhea** (stee-AT-oh-REE-ah) **steat/o-** *fat* **-rrhea** *flow, discharge*	Greasy, frothy, and foul-smelling stools that contain undigested fats. Caused by too little lipase due to pancreatic disease or cystic fibrosis. Treatment: Correct the underlying cause.

Abdominal Wall and Abdominal Cavity

Word or Phrase	Word Part and Definition	Description
adhesions	**adhesion** (ad-HEE-zhun) **adhes/o-** *to stick to* **-ion** *action; condition*	Abnormal fibrous bands of tissue that form after abdominal surgery. They connect the intestines to each other or to another organ in the abdominopelvic cavity. They can bind so tightly that peristalsis and intestinal function are affected. Treatment: Surgery to cut the adhesions (lysis of adhesions).
hernia	**hernia** (HER-nee-ah) *Hernia* is a Latin word meaning *a rupture.* **umbilical** (um-BIL-ih-kal) **umbilic/o-** *umbilicus, navel* **-al** *pertaining to* **ventral** (VEN-tral) **ventr/o-** *front; abdomen* **-al** *pertaining to* **inguinal** (ING-gwih-nal) **inguin/o-** *groin* **-al** *pertaining to* **incisional** (in-SIZH-un-al) **incis/o-** *to cut into* **-ion** *action; condition* **-al** *pertaining to* **omphalocele** (OM-fal-oh-seel) **omphal/o-** *umbilicus, navel* **-cele** *hernia* **incarcerated** (in-KAR-seh-ray-ted) **incarcer/o-** *to imprison* **-ate** *composed of; pertaining to*	A weakness in the muscles of the abdominal wall that allows loops of intestine to balloon outward. Symptoms include swelling and pain. There is an inherited tendency to hernias, but hernias can also be caused by pregnancy, obesity, or heavy lifting. Treatment: Surgery to correct the hernia (herniorrhaphy). 1. Hernias are named according to their location. An **umbilical hernia** occurs next to the umbilicus. A **ventral hernia** occurs anywhere on the anterior abdominal wall except at the umbilicus. An **inguinal hernia** occurs in the groin region. In a male patient with an inguinal hernia, the intestines travel through the inguinal canal and into the scrotum. An **incisional hernia** occurs along the suture line of a prior surgical incision. An **omphalocele** is an umbilical hernia that is present at birth and only has a thin covering of peritoneum rather than skin. 2. Hernias are named according to how freely the intestines can move back into their normal position. A sliding hernia moves back and forth between the hernia sac and the abdominopelvic cavity. Also known as a reducible hernia. An **incarcerated hernia** is one in which there is swelling and the intestines can no longer be pushed back into the abdominopelvic cavity. Also known as an irreducible hernia. A strangulated hernia is an incarcerated hernia whose blood supply has been cut off. This leads to tissue death.

Word or Phrase	Word Part and Definition	Description
peritonitis	**peritonitis** (PAIR-ih-toh-NY-tis) **periton/o-** *peritoneum* **-itis** *inflammation of*	Inflammation and infection of the peritoneum (see Figure 3-16■). Peritonitis occurs when an ulcer, diverticulum, or cancerous tumor penetrates into the abdominopelvic cavity. It also occurs when an inflamed appendix ruptures. The contents and its bacteria spill out and inflame and infect the peritoneum. Treatment: Correct the underlying cause. Antibiotic drugs for bacterial infection. **Figure 3-16 ■ Peritonitis.** This patient has a perforated duodenal ulcer that has spilled green bile, chyme, and bacteria into the abdominopelvic cavity. The areas of white are collections of pus that contain large numbers of white blood cells that are fighting this massive infection.
Liver		
ascites	**ascites** (ah-SY-teez) *Ascites* is derived from a Greek word meaning *a bag.* **ascitic** (ah-SIT-ik) **ascit/o-** *ascites* **-ic** *pertaining to* **portal** (POR-tal) **port/o-** *point of entry* **-al** *pertaining to* **hypertension** (HY-per-TEN-shun) **hyper-** *above; more than normal* **tens/o-** *pressure, tension* **-ion** *action; condition*	Accumulation of **ascitic** fluid in the abdominopelvic cavity, because of underlying liver disease. There is **portal hypertension,** an increased blood pressure in the portal vein. This causes fluid in the blood to move from the portal vein into the abdominopelvic cavity. Treatment: Removal of ascitic fluid from the abdomen by using a needle and syringe. Surgery: Permanent drainage of excess fluid via an implanted tube (shunt) from the portal vein to the inferior vena cava (vein). **Word Alert** **SOUND-ALIKE WORDS** **acidic** (adjective) Pertaining to an acid, having a low pH *Example: Hydrochloric acid makes a low pH environment in the stomach.* **ascitic** (adjective) Pertaining to ascites *Example: Ascitic fluid accumulates and causes the abdominal wall to bulge outward.*

Word or Phrase	Word Part and Definition	Description
cirrhosis	**cirrhosis** (sih-ROH-sis) **cirrh/o-** *yellow* **-osis** *condition; abnormal condition; process* **cirrhotic** (sih-RAW-tik) **cirrh/o-** *yellow* **-tic** *pertaining to*	Chronic, progressive inflammation and finally irreversible degeneration of liver tissue, characterized by nodules and scarring (see Figure 3-17■). The liver becomes enlarged, and many of its functions are severely impaired. The liver is said to be **cirrhotic.** Other symptoms include nausea and vomiting, weakness, and jaundice. Cirrhosis can be caused by alcoholism, viral hepatitis, or chronic obstruction of the bile ducts. Severe cirrhosis can progress to liver failure. Treatment: Correct the underlying cause. **Figure 3-17 ■ Cirrhosis of the liver.** The normally smooth surface of the liver becomes deformed with multiple nodules and scar tissue. The internal tissue is also affected, disrupting liver function.
hepatitis	**hepatitis** (HEP-ah-TY-tis) **hepat/o-** *liver* **-itis** *inflammation of* **viral** (VY-ral) **vir/o-** *virus* **-al** *pertaining to*	Inflammation and infection of the liver caused by the hepatitis virus. Symptoms include weakness, anorexia, nausea, fever, dark urine, and jaundice. Also known as **viral hepatitis.**

A Closer Look

Hepatitis is the most common chronic liver disease. There are five types of hepatitis: hepatitis A, hepatitis B, hepatitis C, hepatitis D, and hepatitis E.

- **Hepatitis A** is an acute but short-lived infection and most persons completely recover. There is no chronic form. Hepatitis A is caused by exposure to water or food that is contaminated with feces from a person who is already infected with the hepatitis A virus (HAV). Also known as **infectious hepatitis**. Treatment: There is a vaccination to prevent hepatitis A.
- **Hepatitis B** is an acute infection, and many persons completely recover from it. When it does become a chronic infection, it causes no symptoms for 20 years or more. During that time, however, the infected person is a carrier and can infect others. Hepatitis B is caused by exposure to the blood of a person who is already infected with the hepatitis B virus (HBV). Exposure can occur during blood transfusions or contact with contaminated instruments or

infectious (in-FEK-shus)
infect/o- *disease within*
-ous *pertaining to*

Word or Phrase	Word Part and Definition	Description
hepatitis *(continued)*	**serum** (SEER-um) *Serum* is the fluid portion of the blood without the blood cells. **delta** (DEL-tah) *Delta* (Δ) is a letter in the Greek alphabet. It also means *a change*.	needles. Drug addicts who share needles can contract hepatitis B. It is also spread during sexual activity by contact with saliva and vaginal secretions. An infected mother can pass hepatitis B to her fetus before birth or when breastfeeding. Also known as **serum hepatitis.** Treatment: There is a vaccination to prevent hepatitis B. Healthcare workers get vaccinated because of their constant exposure to blood and body fluids. • **Hepatitis C** is an acute infection that continues as a chronic infection. It is caused by exposure to the blood of a person who is already infected with the hepatitis C virus (HCV). Drug addicts who share needles account for most of the new cases of hepatitis C. Hepatitis C is not readily transmitted by sexual activity or from a mother to her fetus. Chronic hepatitis C is the most important cause of chronic liver disease, cirrhosis, and liver cancer. Treatment: Antiviral drugs. • **Hepatitis D** is a secondary infection by a mutated (changed) hepatitis virus that develops only in patients who already have hepatitis B. Also known as **delta hepatitis.** • **Hepatitis E** is similar to hepatitis A, but rarely occurs in the United States.
hepatomegaly	**hepatomegaly** (HEP-ah-toh-MEG-ah-lee) **hepat/o-** *liver* **-megaly** *enlargement* **hepatosplenomegaly** (HEP-ah-toh-splen-oh-MEG-ah-lee) **hepat/o-** *liver* **splen/o-** *spleen* **-megaly** *enlargement*	Enlargement of the liver due to liver damage from cirrhosis, hepatitis, or cancer. The enlarged liver can be felt on palpation of the abdomen. The degree of enlargement is measured as the number of fingerbreadths from the edge of the right rib cage to the inferior edge of the liver. Enlargement of both the liver and the spleen is known as **hepatosplenomegaly.** Treatment: Correct the underlying cause.

Word or Phrase	Word Part and Definition	Description
jaundice	**jaundice** (JAWN-dis) *Jaundice* is derived from a French word meaning *yellow.* **obstructive** (awb-STRUK-tiv) **obstruct/o-** *blocked by a barrier* **-ive** *pertaining to*	Yellowish discoloration of the skin and whites of the eyes (see Figure 3-18■). There are increased levels of unconjugated bilirubin in the blood. The bilirubin enters the tissues, giving them a yellow color. Jaundice occurs: 1. If the liver is too diseased to conjugate bilirubin. 2. If a gallstone is obstructing the flow of bile in the bile ducts. This is known as **obstructive jaundice.** 3. If the liver is too immature to conjugate bilirubin. This occurs in premature newborns. 4. If there is an excessive amount of unconjugated bilirubin in the blood because of the destruction of large numbers of red blood cells. Treatment: Correct the underlying disease.

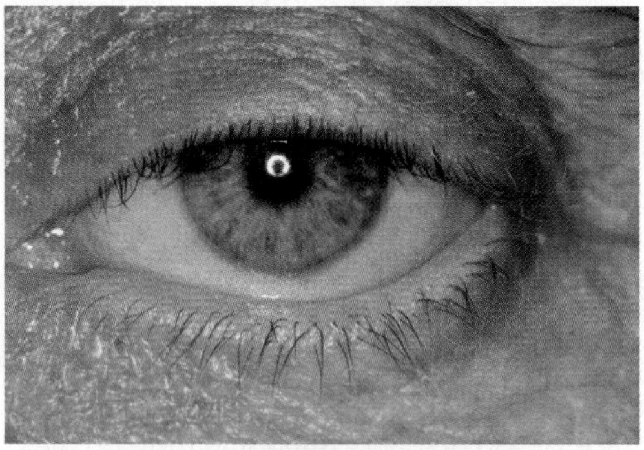

Figure 3-18 ■ Jaundice.

Jaundice is most easily observed as a yellow discoloration of the whites of the eyes. The skin also takes on a yellow cast, but normal skin pigmentation can mask this to varying degrees.

A Closer Look

Bilirubin is produced when old red blood cells are broken down by the spleen. This bilirubin is unconjugated (unjoined) bilirubin. The liver joins this bilirubin to another substance to make conjugated (joined) bilirubin, which is used to make bile. When the liver is damaged, it is unable to conjugate all the bilirubin produced by the spleen, and the level of unconjugated bilirubin rises in the blood. When gallstones obstruct the flow of bile, conjugated bilirubin leaves the bile and moves into the blood.

Word or Phrase	Word Part and Definition	Description
liver cancer	**hepatoma** (HEP-ah-TOH-mah) **hepat/o-** *liver* **-oma** *tumor, mass* **hepatocellular** (HEP-ah-toh-SEL-yoo-lar) **hepat/o-** *liver* **cellul/o-** *cell* **-ar** *pertaining to* **carcinoma** (KAR-sih-NOH-mah) **carcin/o-** *cancer* **-oma** *tumor, mass*	Cancerous tumor of the liver. This is usually a secondary cancer that arises from another site in the body and spreads (metastasizes) to the liver. Also known as **hepatoma** or **hepatocellular carcinoma.** Treatment: Surgery to remove the tumor, if possible. Chemotherapy.

Gallbladder and Bile Ducts

Word or Phrase	Word Part and Definition	Description
cholangitis	**cholangitis** (KOH-lan-JY-tis) cholangi/o- *bile duct* -itis *inflammation of*	Acute or chronic inflammation of the bile ducts because of cirrhosis or gallstones. Treatment: Correct the underlying disease.
cholecystitis	**cholecystitis** (KOH-lee-sis-TY-tis) cholecyst/o- *gallbladder* -itis *inflammation of*	Acute or chronic inflammation of the gallbladder because of gallstones. Acute cholecystitis occurs when a large gallstone blocks the cystic duct of the gallbladder. When the gallbladder contracts, the duct spasms, causing severe pain (biliary colic). Chronic inflammation occurs when stones partially block the cystic duct, causing backup of bile and thickening of the gallbladder wall. Treatment: Avoid fatty foods that cause the gallbladder to contract. Surgery to remove the gallbladder (cholecystectomy).
cholelithiasis	**cholelithiasis** (KOH-lee-lih-THY-ah-sis) chol/e- *bile, gall* lith/o- *stone* -iasis *state of; process of* **choledocholithiasis** (koh-LED-oh-koh-lith-EYE-ah-sis) choledoch/o- *common bile duct* lith/o- *stone* -iasis *state of; process of*	One or more gallstones in the gallbladder (see Figure 3-19■). When the bile is too concentrated, it forms a thick sediment (sludge) that begins to form small crystals that gradually grow into gallstones. Cholelithiasis can cause mild symptoms or severe biliary colic when the gallbladder contracts or a gallstone becomes lodged in a bile duct. **Choledocholithiasis** occurs when a gallstone becomes lodged in the common bile duct (see Figure 3-20■). Treatment: Avoid fatty foods that cause the gallbladder to contract. Surgery to remove the gallbladder (cholecystectomy) or surgery to remove a gallstone from the common bile duct (choledocholithotomy).

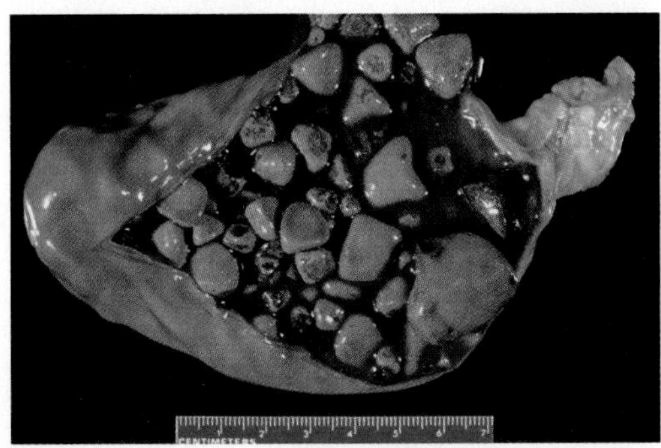

Figure 3-19 ■ Cholelithiasis.

This patient's gallbladder was removed during surgery. A cut section performed in the pathology department shows multiple small and large gallstones.

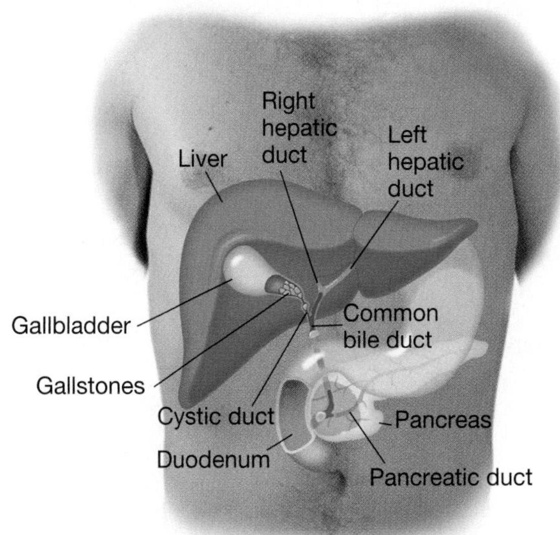

Figure 3-20 ■ Gallstones in the biliary ducts.

A gallstone lodged in the cystic duct causes bile to back up into the gallbladder. A gallstone lodged in the common bile duct causes bile to back up into the gallbladder and the liver. A gallstone lodged in the common bile duct just before the entrance to the duodenum causes pancreatic digestive enzymes to back up into the pancreatic duct.

Pancreas

Word or Phrase	Word Part and Definition	Description
pancreatic cancer	**pancreatic** (PAN-kree-AT-ik) **pancreat/o-** *pancreas* **-ic** *pertaining to* **adenocarcinoma** (AD-eh-noh-KAR-sih-NOH-mah) **aden/o-** *gland* **carcin/o-** *cancer* **-oma** *tumor, mass*	Cancerous tumor of the pancreas. Often an **adenocarcinoma** that arises from the pancreas. Most cases are advanced when they are diagnosed and so survival is usually less than one year. Treatment: Chemotherapy. Surgery to remove the tumor.
pancreatitis	**pancreatitis** (PAN-kree-ah-TY-tis) **pancreat/o-** *pancreas* **-itis** *inflammation of*	Inflammation or infection of the pancreas. Symptoms include abdominal pain, nausea, and vomiting. Inflammation occurs when a gallstone blocks the lower common bile duct and pancreatic enzymes back up into the pancreas. Inflammation can also be caused by chronic alcoholism. Infection is due to bacteria or viruses. A lack of pancreatic lipase causes incomplete digestion of fats and results in steatorrhea (fatty stools). Treatment: Stop drinking. Antibiotic drugs to treat a bacterial infection. Surgery to remove a gallstone (choledocholithotomy).

Diagnostic Procedures

Blood Tests

Word or Phrase	Word Part and Definition	Description
albumin	**albumin** (al-BYOO-min)	Blood test for albumin, the major protein molecule in the blood. Albumin is produced by the liver. Liver disease causes albumin levels to be low. Albumin levels are also low in patients with malnutrition from poor protein intake.
alkaline phosphatase	**alkaline phosphatase** (AL-kah-line FAWS-fah-tace)	Blood test for the enzyme alkaline phosphatase that is found in both liver cells and bone cells. Elevated blood levels suggest the presence of liver disease or bone disease.
ALT and AST		Blood test for the enzymes alanine transaminase (ALT) and aspartate transaminase (AST). These enzymes are mainly found in the liver. Elevated blood levels suggest damaged liver cells released these enzymes into the blood. Formerly known as **SGPT** and **SGOT.**
bilirubin	**bilirubin** (BIL-ih-ROO-bin)	Blood test for unconjugated, conjugated, and total bilirubin levels. These levels are abnormal when there is liver disease or gallstones. Conjugated bilirubin is also known as **direct bilirubin** because it reacts directly with the reagent used to perform the laboratory test. Unconjugated bilirubin is also known as **indirect bilirubin** because it only reacts when another substance is added to the reagent.
GGT		Blood test for the enzyme gamma-glutamyl transpeptidase (GGT). This enzyme is found mainly in the liver. Elevated blood levels suggest damaged liver cells released this enzyme into the blood. Also known as **GGTP**.
liver function tests (LFTs)		Panel of individual blood tests performed at the same time to give a comprehensive picture of liver function. Includes albumin, bilirubin, ALT, AST, GGT, as well as prothrombin time (to evaluate blood clotting factors produced by the liver).

Gastric and Stool Specimen Tests

Word or Phrase	Word Part and Definition	Description
CLO test	**CLO** (kloh)	Rapid screening test to detect the presence of the bacterium *Helicobacter pylori.* A biopsy of gastric mucosa is placed in contact with the substance urea. If *H. pylori* bacteria are present, they will metabolize the urea to ammonia, and ammonia changes the color of the test pad. CLO test stands for Campylobacter-like organism. This bacterium used to be classified with the genus Campylobacter but was reclassified to the genus Helicobacter.
fecal occult blood test	**occult** (oh-KULT) *Occult* is derived from a Latin word meaning *to hide.* **guaiac** (GWY-ak) *Guaiac* is a resin or gum derived from the tropical plant *Guaiacum.*	Diagnostic test to detect occult blood in the feces. A sample of feces is placed on paper and mixed with the chemical reagent **guaiac.** If blood is present, the guaiac will turn the paper blue (guaiac-positive stool). Hemoccult and Coloscreen cards can be purchased by consumers for home testing. These tests use guaiac-impregnated paper.

Word or Phrase	Word Part and Definition	Description
gastric analysis		Diagnostic test to determine the amount of hydrochloric acid in the stomach. An NG tube is inserted, and a sample of gastric juices is collected. Then a drug is given to stimulate acid production, and another sample is collected.
ova and parasites (O&P)	**ovum** (OH-vum) **ova** (OH-va) *Ovum* is a Latin singular neuter noun meaning *egg.* Form the plural by changing *-um* to *-a.* **parasite** (PAIR-ah-site) *Parasite* is derived from a Greek word meaning *a guest.*	Diagnostic test to determine if there is a parasitic infection of the gastrointestinal tract. Ova are the eggs of parasitic worms. They can be seen in the stool or by examining a sample of stool under a microscope.
stool culture and sensitivity (C&S)	**sensitivity** (SEN-sih-TIV-ih-tee) **sensitiv/o-** *affected by; sensitive to* **-ity** *state; condition*	Diagnostic test that determines which bacterium is causing an intestinal infection and which antibiotic drugs it is sensitive to. A stool specimen is swabbed on a culture dish that contains a nutrient medium for growing bacteria. After the bacterium grows, it can be identified by the appearance of the colonies. Then disks containing various antibiotic drugs are placed in the culture dish. An antibiotic drug that can kill that bacterium will have a ring of no growth around its disk.
Radiologic Procedures		
barium enema	**barium** (BAH-ree-um) **enema** (EN-eh-mah) *Enema* is derived from a Greek word meaning *to throw into.*	Radiologic procedure that uses a liquid radiopaque contrast dye (barium) introduced through the rectum (see Figure 3-21■). Barium outlines and coats the walls of the rectum and colon. An x-ray is then taken. Used to identify polyps, diverticula, ulcerative colitis, and colon cancer.

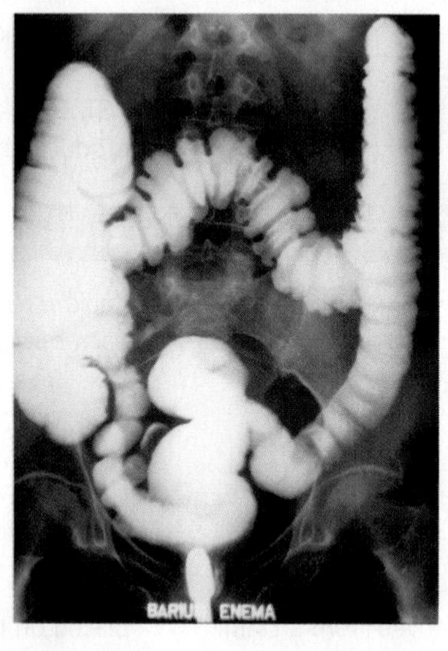

Figure 3-21 ■ Barium enema.

Barium contrast dye and air fill the cecum, ascending colon, transverse colon, sigmoid colon, and rectum on this x-ray.

Word or Phrase	Word Part and Definition	Description
cholangiography	**cholangiography** (koh-LAN-jee-AWG-rah-fee) **cholangi/o-** *bile duct* **-graphy** *process of recording* **cholangiogram** (koh-LAN-jee-oh-gram) **cholangi/o-** *bile duct* **-gram** *a record or picture* **intravenous** (IN-trah-VEE-nus) **intra-** *within* **ven/o-** *vein* **-ous** *pertaining to* **percutaneous** (PER-kyoo-TAY-nee-us) **per-** *through, throughout* **cutane/o-** *skin* **-ous** *pertaining to* **transhepatic** (TRANS-heh-PAT-ik) **trans-** *across, through* **hepat/o-** *liver* **-ic** *pertaining to* **endoscopic** (EN-doh-SKAW-pik) **endo-** *innermost, within* **scop/o-** *examine with an instrument* **-ic** *pertaining to* **retrograde** (RET-roh-grayd) **retro-** *behind, backward* **-grade** *going* **cholangiopancreatography** (koh-LAN-jee-oh-PAN-kree-ah-TAWG-rah-fee) **cholangi/o-** *bile duct* **pancreat/o-** *pancreas* **-graphy** *process of recording*	Radiologic procedure that uses a contrast dye to outline the bile ducts. An x-ray is taken to identify stones in the gallbladder and biliary ducts or thickening of the gallbladder wall. The x-ray image is known as a **cholangiogram**. In **intravenous cholangiography (IVC),** the contrast dye is injected intravenously, travels through the blood to the liver, and is excreted with bile into the gallbladder. In **percutaneous transhepatic cholangiography (PTC),** a needle is passed through the abdominal wall, and the contrast dye is injected into the liver. In **endoscopic retrograde cholangiopancreatography (ERCP),** an endoscope is passed through the mouth and into the duodenum. A catheter is passed through the endoscope, and the contrast dye is injected into the lower end of the common bile duct. The pancreatic duct is also visualized.
computerized axial tomography (CAT, CT scan)	**tomography** (toh-MAWG-rah-fee) **tom/o-** *a cut, slice, or layer* **-graphy** *process of recording*	Radiologic procedure that uses x-rays to create an image of many thin, successive slices of the abdomen and its organs.
flat plate of the abdomen		Radiologic procedure that uses x-rays (without contrast dye). The patient lies flat on the x-ray table for a plain x-ray of the abdomen.

Word or Phrase	Word Part and Definition	Description
gallbladder ultrasound	**ultrasound** (UL-trah-sound) *Ultrasound* is a combination of the prefix *ultra-* (beyond, higher) and the word *sound.* **sonogram** (SAWN-oh-gram) **son/o-** *sound* **-gram** *a record or picture*	Radiologic procedure that uses ultra high-frequency sound waves to create an image of the gallbladder. Used to identify gallstones and thickening of the gallbladder wall. Also known as a **gallbladder sonogram.**
magnetic resonance imaging (MRI scan)	**magnetic** (mag-NET-ik) **magnet/o-** *magnet* **-ic** *pertaining to*	Radiologic procedure that uses a strong magnetic field to align protons in the atoms of the patient's body. The protons emit signals to form images as thin, successive slices of the abdomen and its organs.
oral cholecystography (OCG)	**cholecystography** (KOH-lee-sis-TAWG-rah-fee) **cholecyst/o-** *gallbladder* **-graphy** *process of recording* **cholecystogram** (KOH-lee-SIS-toh-gram) **cholecyst/o-** *gallbladder* **-gram** *a record or picture*	Radiologic procedure that uses tablets of radiopaque contrast dye taken orally. The tablets dissolve in the intestine. The contrast dye is absorbed into the blood, travels to the liver, and is excreted with bile into the gallbladder. An x-ray is taken to identify stones in the gallbladder and biliary ducts or thickening of the gallbladder wall. The x-ray image is known as a **cholecystogram.**
upper gastrointestinal series (UGI)		Radiologic procedure that uses a liquid radiopaque contrast dye (barium) that is swallowed (a barium meal). Barium coats and outlines the walls of the esophagus, stomach, and duodenum. Also known as a **barium swallow.** Fluoroscopy (continuously moving x-ray image on a screen) is used to follow the barium through the small intestine. This is known as a **small bowel follow-through.** Individual x-rays are taken at specific times throughout the procedure. Used to identify ulcers, tumors, or obstruction.

Medical and Surgical Procedures

Medical Procedures

Word or Phrase	Word Part and Definition	Description
insertion of nasogastric tube (NG tube)	**nasogastric** (NAY-zoh-GAS-trik) **nas/o-** *nose* **gastr/o-** *stomach* **-ic** *pertaining to*	Medical procedure to insert a **nasogastric tube,** a long, flexible tube through the nostril to the stomach. It is used to drain secretions from the stomach or give feedings to the patient on a temporary basis (see Figure 3-22■).

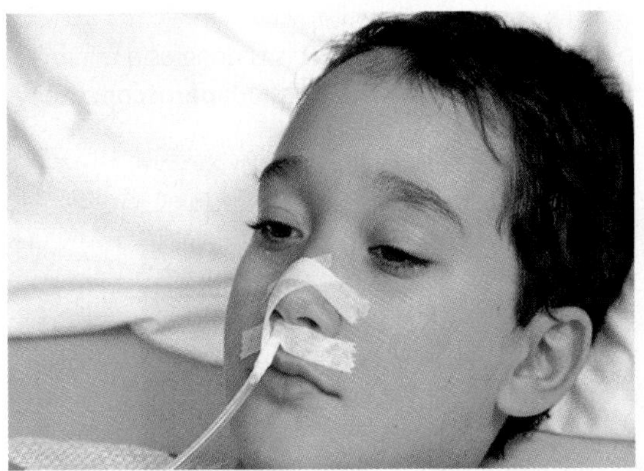

Figure 3-22 ■ Nasogastric tube.
This patient has a nasogastric tube that was inserted in one nostril and, as he swallowed, advanced through the esophagus and into the stomach. Only liquid feedings or drugs in a liquid form can be given through an NG tube.

Did You Know?

The first nasogastric tube, developed in the late 1700s, was constructed from eel skin. It was used for several weeks to feed a patient who could not eat.

Surgical Procedures

Word or Phrase	Word Part and Definition	Description
appendectomy	**appendectomy** (AP-pen-DEK-toh-mee) **append/o-** *small structure hanging from a larger structure; appendix* **-ectomy** *surgical excision*	Surgical procedure to remove the appendix because of appendicitis
biopsy	**biopsy** (BY-awp-see) **bi/o-** *life; living organism; living tissue* **-opsy** *process of viewing*	Surgical procedure to remove a small piece of tissue from an ulcer, polyp, mass, or tumor to look for abnormal or cancerous cells.

Word or Phrase	Word Part and Definition	Description
bowel resection and anastomosis	**resection** (ree-SEK-shun) **resect/o-** *to cut out and remove* **-ion** *action; condition* **anastomosis** (ah-NAS-toh-MOH-sis) **anastom/o-** *unite two tubular structures* **-osis** *condition; abnormal condition; process*	Surgical procedure to remove a section of diseased intestine and rejoin the intestine. An end-to-end anastomosis sutures the two cut ends together. An end-to-side anastomosis sutures the end of one segment to the side of the other segment.
cholecystectomy	**cholecystectomy** (KOH-lee-sis-TEK-toh-mee) **cholecyst/o-** *gallbladder* **-ectomy** *surgical excision* **laparoscopic** (LAP-ah-roh-SKAWP-ik) **lapar/o-** *abdomen* **scop/o-** *examine with an instrument* **-ic** *pertaining to* **laparoscope** (LAP-ah-roh-skohp) **lapar/o-** *abdomen* **-scope** *instrument used to examine*	Surgical procedure to remove the gallbladder. This is done as a minimally invasive **laparoscopic cholecystectomy** that uses a **laparoscope** (see Figure 3-23■). **Figure 3-23 ■ Laparoscopic cholecystectomy.** Carbon dioxide gas is used to inflate the abdominal cavity and separate the organs. A laparoscope is inserted through one of several small incisions to visualize the gallbladder, while other instruments grasp and remove the gallbladder. **Did You Know?** At one time, a cholecystectomy to remove the gallbladder required a 5- to 7-inch abdominal incision, followed by a painful 6-week recovery. The first minimally invasive surgical procedure ever performed was done in 1989 to remove a gallbladder. Minimally invasive surgery is done with instruments inserted through several tiny incisions at various places on the abdominal wall.

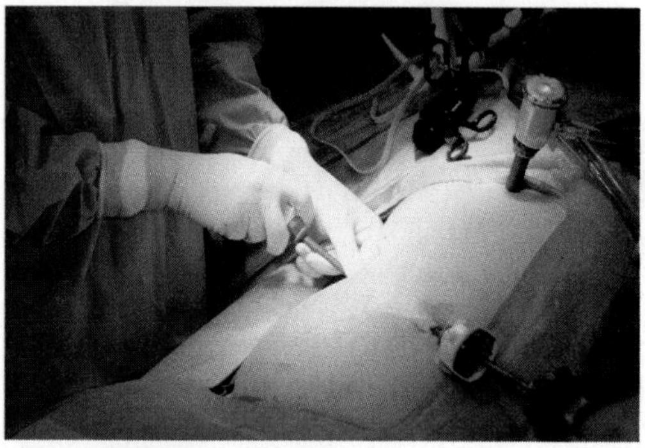

Word or Phrase	Word Part and Definition	Description
choledocholithotomy	**choledocholithotomy** (koh-LED-oh-koh-lih-THAWT-oh-mee) **choledoch/o-** *common bile duct* **lith/o-** *stone* **-tomy** *process of cutting or making an incision*	Surgical procedure to make an incision in the common bile duct to remove a gallstone
colostomy	**colostomy** (koh-LAWS-toh-mee) **col/o-** *colon* **-stomy** *surgically created opening* **stoma** (STOH-mah) *Stoma* is a Greek word meaning *a mouth.* **ileostomy** (IL-ee-AWS-toh-mee) **ile/o-** *ileum* **-stomy** *surgically created opening*	Surgical procedure to remove the diseased part of the colon and create a new opening in the abdominal wall where feces can leave the body. The colon is brought out through the abdominal wall. The edges of the wall of the colon are rolled to make a mouth (**stoma**) that is then sutured to the abdominal wall. The patient wears a plastic disposable pouch that adheres to the abdominal wall to collect feces (see Figure 3-24■). If part of the ileum and colon are removed and a stoma created, the procedure is known as an **ileostomy.**

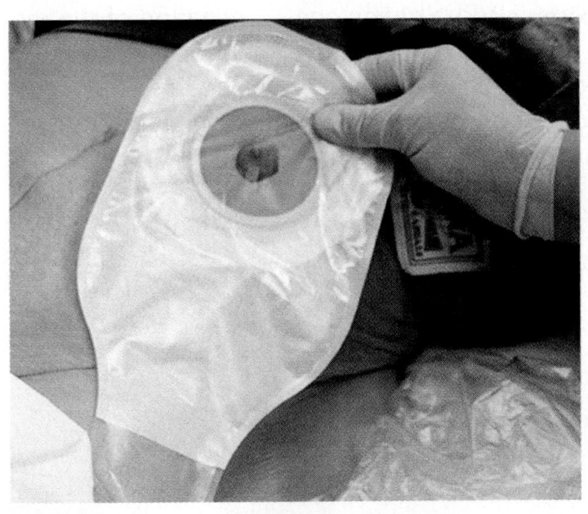

Figure 3-24 ■ Colostomy stoma.

A stoma is a surgically created, artificial opening on the outside of the body. The red mucosa of the colon is rolled back on itself to make the edges of the stoma. A plastic disposable bag for collecting feces is fitted over the stoma. Skin adhesive is used to provide a tight seal between the bag and the skin.

Word Alert

SOUND-ALIKE WORDS

stoma (noun) A surgically created opening like a mouth

Example: The colostomy patient wears a disposable pouch around the stoma on his abdominal wall.

stomach (noun) Organ of digestion between the esophagus and small intestine.

Example: The stomach releases gastric enzymes to aid in the digestion of food.

stomatitis (noun) Inflammation of the oral mucosa of the mouth.

Example: The patient was losing weight because of a painful stomatitis that prevented him from chewing his food.

Word or Phrase	Word Part and Definition	Description
endoscopy	**endoscopy** (en-DAWS-koh-pee) **endo-** *innermost, within* **-scopy** *process of using an instrument to examine* **endoscope** (EN-doh-skohp) **endo-** *innermost, within* **-scope** *instrument used to examine* Every medical word must contain a combining form. The suffixes of *endoscopy* and *endoscope* contain the combining form *scop/o-*. **endoscopic** (EN-doh-SKAWP-ik) **endo-** *innermost, within* **scop/o-** *examine with an instrument* **-ic** *pertaining to* **esophagoscopy** (ee-SAWF-ah-GAWS-koh-pee) **esophag/o-** *esophagus* **-scopy** *process of using an instrument to examine* **gastroscopy** (gas-TRAWS-koh-pee) **gastr/o-** *stomach* **-scopy** *process of using an instrument to examine* **esophagogastro-duodenoscopy** (ee-SAWF-ah-goh-GAS-troh-DOO-oh-den-AWS-koh-pee) **esophag/o-** *esophagus* **gastr/o-** *stomach* **duoden/o-** *duodenum* **-scopy** *process of using an instrument to examine* **sigmoidoscopy** (SIG-moy-DAWS-koh-pee) **sigmoid/o-** *sigmoid colon* **-scopy** *process of using an instrument to examine* **colonoscopy** (KOH-lon-AWS-koh-pee) **colon/o-** *colon* **-scopy** *process of using an instrument to examine*	Surgical procedure that uses an **endoscope** (a flexible, fiber optic scope with a magnifying lens and a light source) to internally examine the gastrointestinal tract. Endoscopy can be coupled with another procedure like a biopsy or removal of a polyp. **A Closer Look** These procedures use an endoscope inserted through the nose or mouth. • **esophagoscopy:** Visualization and examination of the esophagus • **gastroscopy:** Visualization and examination of the stomach • **esophagogastroduodenoscopy:** Visualization and examination of the esophagus, stomach, and duodenum The jejunum, ileum, cecum, and ascending colon cannot be visualized with endoscopy. Instead, the patient swallows a capsule that contains a small camera. It uses wireless technology to transmit pictures of the intestine until it is excreted in the feces after 24 hours. These procedures use an endoscope inserted through the rectum. • **sigmoidoscopy**: Visualization and examination of the rectum and sigmoid colon using a sigmoidoscope. • **colonoscopy**: Visualization and examination of the rectum, sigmoid colon, and parts of the descending and transverse colon using a colonoscope.

Word or Phrase	Word Part and Definition	Description
exploratory laparotomy	**laparotomy** (LAP-ah-ROT-ah-mee) **lapar/o-** *abdomen* **-tomy** *process of cutting or making an incision*	Surgical procedure that uses an abdominal incision to widely open the abdominopelvic cavity so that it can be explored
gastrectomy	**gastrectomy** (gas-TREK-toh-mee) **gastr/o-** *stomach* **-ectomy** *surgical excision*	Surgical procedure to remove part of the stomach because of a cancerous tumor
gastrostomy	**gastrostomy** (gas-TRAWS-toh-mee) **gastr/o-** *stomach* **-stomy** *surgically created opening* **percutaneous** (PER-kyoo-TAY-nee-us) **per-** *through, throughout* **cutane/o-** *skin* **-ous** *pertaining to* **endoscopic** (EN-doh-SKAW-pik) **endo-** *innermost, within* **scop/o-** *examine with an instrument* **-ic** *pertaining to*	Surgical procedure to create a permanent opening from the abdominal wall into the stomach to insert a **gastrostomy tube**. This is a permanent feeding tube. For a **percutaneous endoscopic gastrostomy (PEG)**, a PEG tube is inserted through the abdominal wall. Then under visual guidance from an endoscope that was previously passed through the mouth into the stomach, a catheter inside the PEG tube is positioned in the stomach (see Figure 3-25■). 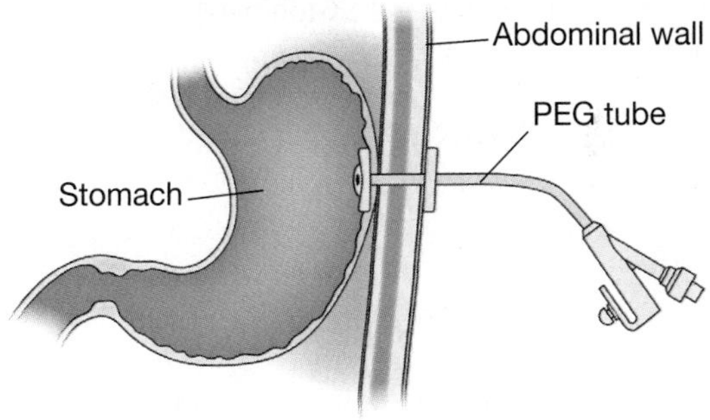 **Figure 3-25 ■ PEG tube.** This permanent feeding tube is inserted during a percutaneous endoscopic gastrostomy.
hemorrhoidectomy	**hemorrhoidectomy** (HEM-oh-roy-DEK-toh-mee) **hemorrhoid/o-** *hemorrhoid* **-ectomy** *surgical excision*	Surgical procedure to remove hemorrhoids from the rectum or around the anus.
herniorrhaphy	**herniorrhaphy** (HER-nee-OR-ah-fee) **herni/o-** *hernia* **-rrhaphy** *procedure of suturing*	Surgical procedure that uses sutures to close a defect in a muscle wall where there is a hernia.
jejunostomy	**jejunostomy** (JEH-joo-NAWS-toh-mee) **jejun/o-** *jejunum* **-stomy** *surgically created opening*	Surgical procedure to create a permanent opening from the abdominal wall into the jejunum through which to insert a **jejunostomy tube.** This is a permanent feeding tube. For a percutaneous endoscopic jejunostomy (PEJ), a PEJ tube is inserted through the abdominal wall. Then under visual guidance from an endoscope that was previously passed through the mouth, a catheter inside the PEJ tube is positioned in the jejunum.

Word or Phrase	Word Part and Definition	Description
liver transplantation	**transplantation** (TRANS-plan-TAY-shun) **transplant/o-** *move something to another place* **-ation** *a process; being or having* **donor** (DOH-nor) *Donor* is derived from a Latin word meaning *one who gives.*	Surgical procedure to remove a severely damaged liver from a patient with end-stage liver disease and insert a new liver from a **donor.** The patient (the recipient) is matched by blood type and tissue type to the donor. Liver transplant patients must take immunosuppressant drugs for the rest of their lives to keep their bodies from rejecting the foreign tissue that is their new liver.
gastroplasty	**gastroplasty** (GAS-troh-PLAS-tee) **gastr/o-** *stomach* **-plasty** *process of reshaping by surgery*	Surgical procedure to treat severely obese patients. Staples are placed in the stomach to make a small stomach pouch. A gastroplasty can be combined with an intestinal bypass in which the stapled stomach pouch is anastomosed (connected) to the cut end of the jejunum. This bypasses the duodenum where most fats are absorbed. Also known as a gastric stapling or gastric bypass.
polypectomy	**polypectomy** (PAWL-ih-PEK-toh-mee) **polyp/o-** *polyp* **-ectomy** *surgical excision*	Surgical excision of polyps from the colon using forceps or a snare.

Drug Categories

Several different categories of drugs are used to treat the symptoms, signs, and diseases of the gastrointestinal system. The most common drugs in each category are listed.

Category	Word Part and Definition	Description	Examples
antacid drugs	**antacid** (ant-AS-id) *Antacid* is a combination of *anti-* (*against*) and the word *acid.* The *i* in *anti-* is deleted.	Treat heartburn and peptic ulcer disease by neutralizing acid in the stomach	Maalox, Mylanta, Tums
antibiotic drugs	**antibiotic** (AN-tee-by-AWT-ik) (AN-tih-by-AWT-ik) **anti-** *against* **bi/o-** *life; living organisms; living tissue* **-tic** *pertaining to*	Treat bacterial gastrointestinal infections, including acute *Helicobacter pylori.* Antibiotic drugs are not effective against viral gastrontestinal infections.	amoxicillin, Biaxin, Flagyl, tetracycline
antidiarrheal drugs	**antidiarrheal** (AN-tee-DY-ah-REE-al) **anti-** *against* **dia-** *complete; completely through* **-rrhe/o-** *flow discharge* **-al** *pertaining to*	Treat diarrhea. They slow peristalsis and this increases water absorption from the feces.	Imodium, Lomotil
antiemetic drugs	**antiemetic** (AN-tee-eh-MET-ik) **anti-** *against* **emet/o-** *to vomit* **-ic** *pertaining to*	Treat nausea and vomiting and motion sickness	Antivert, Compazine, Phenergan
chemotherapy drugs	**chemotherapy** (KEE-moh-THAIR-ah-pee) **chem/o-** *chemical, drug* **-therapy** *treatment*	Kill rapidly dividing cancer cells of tumors in the GI tract	Adriamycin, Taxol, VePesid
H_2 blocker drugs		Treat peptic ulcers by blocking H_2 (histamine 2) receptors in the stomach that trigger the release of hydrochloric acid	Axid, Pepcid, Tagamet, Zantac
laxative drugs	**laxative** (LAK-sah-tiv) *Laxative* is derived from a Latin word meaning *to relax.*	Treat constipation	Colace, Ex-Lax, Metamucil, Surfak
proton pump inhibitor drugs		Treat peptic ulcers or gastroesophageal reflux disease (GERD) by blocking the final step in the production of hydrochloric acid	Nexium, Prevacid, Prilosec

Did You Know?

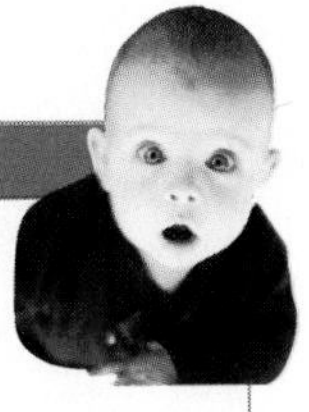

A **suppository** is a formed, bullet-shaped capsule that contains a drug. It is inserted into the rectum, where it melts and releases the drug.

suppository (soo-PAWZ-ih-tohr-ee)
supposit/o- *placed beneath*
-ory *having the function of*

Abbreviations

ABD	abdomen
ALT	alanine aminotransferase
AST	aspartate aminotransferase
BE	barium enema
BM	bowel movement
BRBPR	bright red blood per rectum
BS	bowel sounds
CBD	common bile duct
EGD	esophagogastroduodenoscopy
ERCP	endoscopic retrograde cholangiopancreatography
GERD	gastroesophageal reflux disease
GI	gastrointestinal
HAV	hepatitis A virus
HBV	hepatitis B virus
HCV	hepatitis C virus
IBD	inflammatory bowel disease
IBS	irritable bowel syndrome
IVC	intravenous cholangiography
LES	lower esophageal sphincter
LFTs	liver function tests
LLQ	left lower quadrant
LUQ	left upper quadrant
N&V	nausea and vomiting
NG	nasogastric
NPO (n.p.o.)	nothing by mouth (nil per os)
OCG	oral cholecystography
O&P	ova and parasites
PEG	percutaneous endoscopic gastrostomy
PEJ	percutaneous endoscopic jejunostomy
P.O. (p.o.)	by mouth (per os)
PTC	percutaneous transhepatic cholangiography
PUD	peptic ulcer disease
RLQ	right lower quadrant
RUQ	right upper quadrant
SGOT	serum glutamic-oxaloacetic transaminase
SGPT	serum glutamic-pyruvic transaminase
UGI	upper gastrointestinal (series)

Word Alert

ABBREVIATIONS

Abbreviations are commonly used in all types of medical documents; however, they can mean different things to different people and their meaning can be misinterpreted. Always verify the meaning of an abbreviation.

BS stands for *bowel sounds,* but it also stand for *breath sounds.*

PUD stands for *peptic ulcer disease,* but when handwritten the *U* can look like a *V; PVD* stands for *peripheral vascular disease.*

Career Focus

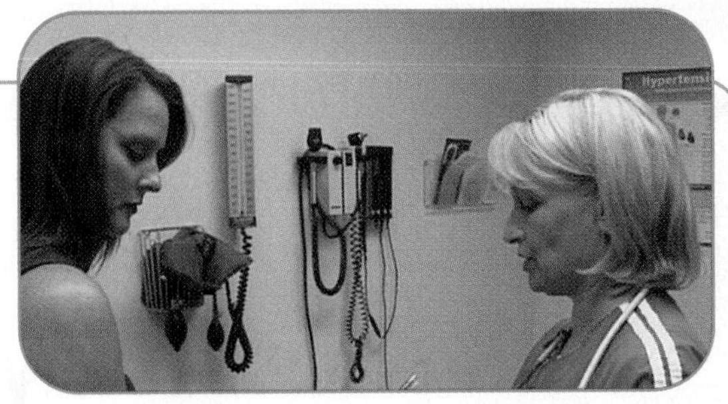

Meet Patricia, a medical assistant.

"The best part of my job as a medical assistant is dealing with the patients. I love coming to work and doing it every day. It just very fulfilling to me. I love helping people. I love talking to them. I love learning about their families, and that's what you find in this kind of practice. This is a huge clinic. It has internal medicine, pediatrics, OB/GYN, and plastic surgery. We have a specialty department with ears, nose, and throat doctors. We have optometry; we have physical therapy. I work with patients. I bring them in, I weigh them, take their blood pressure, find out what their problem is, write down their problem, go to the hysician and tell them why the patient is here. I definitely think medical asistants are the first line of defense for the doctor. I bring everything to the doctor. We work as a team. We have a great rapport together, with our patients."

Medical assistants are allied health professionals who perform and document a variety of clinical and laboratory procedures and assist the physician during medical procedures in the office or clinic.

Gastroenterologists are physicians who practice in the medical specialty of gastroenterology. They diagnose and treat patients with diseases of the gastrointestinal system. Physicians can take additional training and become board certified in the subspecialty of pediatric gastroenterology. Cancerous tumors of the gastrointestinal system are treated medically by an **oncologist** or surgically by a general **surgeon.**

gastroenterologist
(GAS-troh-EN-ter-AWL-oh-jist)
gastr/o- *stomach*
enter/o- *intestine*
log/o- *the study of*
-ist *one who specializes in*

oncologist (ong-KAWL-oh-jist)
onc/o- tumor, mass
log/o- *the study of*
-ist *one who specializes in*

surgeon (SER-jun)
surg/o- *operative procedure*
-eon *one who performs*
Surgeon is derived from a Latin word meaning *hand work*.

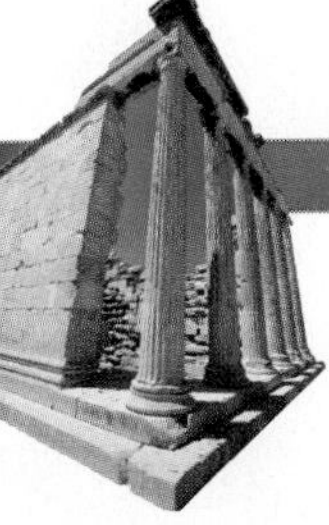

It's Greek to Me!

Did you notice that some gastrointestinal structures have two different combining forms? Combining forms from both Greek and Latin languages remain a part of medical language today.

English Word	Greek	Latin	Examples of Medical Words
abdomen	celi/o- lapar/o-	abdomin/o-	celiac trunk, celiac disease, abdominal laparoscopy, laparotomy
bile duct	cholangi/o- cholecyst/o- choledoch/o-	bil/i-	cholangitis, cholangiography, biliary cholecystitis choledocholithiasis, choledocholithotomy
digest	peps/o- pept/o-	digest/o-	pepsin, pepsinogen, digestive, digestion peptic
fats	steat/o-	lip/o-	steatorrhea, lipase
intestine	enter/o-	intestin/o-	enteropathy, gastroenteritis, gastroenterologist, gastroenterology, intestinal, gastrointestinal
mouth	stomat/o-	or/o-	stomatitis, oral
pass stool, stool	chez/o-	fec/o-	hematochezia, defecation
saliva	sial/o-	saliv/o-	sialolith, sialolithiasis, salivary
tongue	gloss/o-	lingu/o-	glossal, lingual, sublingual
umbilicus, navel	omphal/o-	umbilic/o-	omphalocele, umbilical

Chapter Review Exercises

Review all the material in this chapter by completing the review exercises in this section. Use the Answer Key at the end of the book to check your answers.

Anatomy and Physiology

Matching Exercise

Match each numbered word or phrase to its description.

1.	cholecystokinin	_____ Enzyme that breaks apart fats
2.	chyme	_____ The act of chewing
3.	deglutition	_____ One of the three salivary glands
4.	enzyme	_____ Hormone from the duodenum that stimulates the gallbladder to contract
5.	epiglottis	_____ Fatty sheet of peritoneum that supports the stomach
6.	haustra	_____ Lidlike structure that seals the larynx during eating
7.	jejunum	_____ Last part of the large intestine
8.	lipase	_____ First stool of newborn infants
9.	mastication	_____ Second part of the small intestine
10.	meconium	_____ Substance that breaks the chemical bonds between molecules of food
11.	omentum	_____ Pouches in the mucosa of the large intestine
12.	parotid gland	_____ The act of swallowing
13.	rectum	_____ Open channel inside the intestines
14.	lumen	_____ Food and digestive juices mixed in the stomach

Circle Exercise

Circle the correct word from the choices given.

1. The first part of the small intestine is the (**cecum, colon, duodenum**).
2. The process of having a bowel movement is known as (**defecation, emulsification, mastication**).
3. The part of the stomach that is closest to the esophagus is the (**body, cardia, pylorus**).
4. This structure secretes a digestive enzyme: (**esophagus, pharynx, salivary gland**).
5. The pancreas secretes all of these digestive enzymes EXCEPT (**amylase, hydrochloric acid, lipase**).
6. The S-shaped segment of colon is the (**jejunum, sigmoid, transverse**).
7. Emulsification of fat globules in food is done by (**bile, flatus, lactase**).

True or False Exercise

Indicate whether each statement is true or false by writing T or F on the line.

1. ____ The stomach is located superior to the small intestine.
2. ____ The salivary glands and pancreas both secrete amylase.
3. ____ The structure that comes after the duodenum is the ileum.
4. ____ The colon is the longest part of the large intestine.
5. ____ The appendix is considered to be part of the gastrointestinal system and the endocrine system.
6. ____ Mucosa lines the gastrointestinal tract.
7. ____ You can find villi in the large intestine.
8. ____ If food touches the uvula, it initiates the gag reflex.
9. ____ Deglutition is waves of contractions that propel food through the GI tract.
10. ____ The pancreas is located in the retroperitoneal cavity.
11. ____ The portal vein carries food nutrients from the intestines to the liver.
12. ____ The word part *stomat/o-* means *stomach.*

Sequencing Exercise

Beginning with food entering the mouth, write each structure of the gastrointestinal system in the order in which food moves through it. Use the list of anatomical structures to help you sequence the structures of the gastrointestinal tract in their correct order.

Structure	**Correct Order**
anus	1. ____________
cecum	2. ____________
colon	3. ____________
duodenum	4. ____________
esophagus	5. ____________
ileum	6. ____________
jejunum	7. ____________
oral cavity	8. ____________
pharynx	9. ____________
rectum	10. ____________
stomach	11. ____________

Medical Language Word Parts

Name That Word Part

Identify each of the word parts given here by writing in the correct letter (P, C, or S) on the line beside it. Then write the definition of the word part on the blank line. The first one has been done for you.

Prefix = P **Combining Form = C** **Suffix = S**

		Word Part	Definition			Word Part	Definition
1.	-al	S	pertaining to	36.	colon/o-		
2.	abdomin/o-			37.	constip/o-		
3.	absorpt/o-			38.	cyst/o-		
4.	-ac			39.	-cyte		
5.	aden/o-			40.	de-		
6.	adhes/o-			41.	degluti/o-		
7.	aliment/o-			42.	dia-		
8.	amyl/o-			43.	digest/o-		
9.	an-			44.	diverticul/o-		
10.	anastom/o-			45.	duoden/o-		
11.	an/o-			46.	dys-		
12.	anti-			47.	-eal		
13.	aphth/o-			48.	-ectomy		
14.	appendic/o-			49.	elimin/o-		
15.	append/o-			50.	-emesis		
16.	-ar			51.	emet./o-		
17.	-ary			52.	endo-		
18.	-ase			53.	-ent		
19.	-ation			54.	enter/o-		
20.	bil/i-			55.	-entery		
21.	bi/o-			56.	epi-		
22.	carcin/o-			57.	esophag/o-		
23.	cav/o-			58.	fec/a-		
24.	cec/o-			59.	fec/o-		
25.	-cele			60.	flatul/o-		
26.	celi/o-			61.	gastr/o-		
27.	cellul/o-			62.	-gen		
28.	cheil/o-			63.	gloss/o-		
29.	chez/o-			64.	-gram		
30.	cholangi/o-			65.	-graphy		
31.	chol/e-			66.	gustat/o-		
32.	cholecyst/o-			67.	hemat/o-		
33.	choledoch/o-			68.	hemorrhoid/o-		
34.	cirrh/o-			69.	hepat/o-		
35.	col/o-			70.	herni/o-		

		Word Part	Definition
71.	hyper-	______	______
72.	-ia	______	______
73.	-iasis	______	______
74.	-ic	______	______
75.	ile/o-	______	______
76.	-in	______	______
77.	incis/o-	______	______
78.	inguin/o-	______	______
79.	intestin/o-	______	______
80.	intussuscep/o-	______	______
81.	-ion	______	______
82.	-itis	______	______
83.	-ity	______	______
84.	-ive	______	______
85.	-ix	______	______
86.	lapar/o-	______	______
87.	lact/o-	______	______
88.	lingu/o-	______	______
89.	lip/o-	______	______
90.	-lith	______	______
91.	lith/o-	______	______
92.	-logy	______	______
93.	mal-	______	______
94.	mastic/o-	______	______
95.	medic/o-	______	______
96.	-megaly	______	______
97.	meleno-	______	______
98.	meso-	______	______
99.	mucos/o-	______	______
100.	nause/o-	______	______
101.	obstip/o-	______	______
102.	odyn/o-	______	______
103.	-oid	______	______
104.	-oma	______	______
105.	omphal/o-	______	______
106.	-opsy	______	______
107.	orex/o-	______	______
108.	or/o-	______	______
109.	-ory	______	______
110.	-osis	______	______
111.	-ous	______	______
112.	pancreat/o-	______	______

		Word Part	Definition
113.	-pathy	______	______
114.	pelv/o-	______	______
115.	peps/o-	______	______
116.	pept/o-	______	______
117.	peri-	______	______
118.	peritone/o-	______	______
119.	periton/o-	______	______
120.	phag/o-	______	______
121.	pharyng/o-	______	______
122.	-plasty	______	______
123.	poly-	______	______
124.	polyp/o-	______	______
125.	port/o-	______	______
126.	prote/o-	______	______
127.	pylor/o-	______	______
128.	pyr/o-	______	______
129.	rect/o-	______	______
130.	regurgit/o-	______	______
131.	resect/o-	______	______
132.	retro-	______	______
133.	rotat/o-	______	______
134.	-rrhaphy	______	______
135.	-rrhea	______	______
136.	rrhe/o-	______	______
137.	saliv/o-	______	______
138.	-scope	______	______
139.	scop/o-	______	______
140.	-scopy	______	______
141.	sensitiv/o-	______	______
142.	sial/o-	______	______
143.	son/o-	______	______
144.	splen/o-	______	______
145.	stalsis	______	______
146.	steat/o-	______	______
147.	stomat/o-	______	______
148.	-stomy	______	______
149.	sub-	______	______
150.	suppsit/o-	______	______
151.	-tion	______	______
152.	-tomy	______	______
153.	ulcerat/o-	______	______
154.	umbilic/o-	______	______

Word-Building Exercise

Use the combining forms, prefixes, and suffixes given here to build medical words that match the definitions given. Write the word that you build on the blank line. Some word parts may be used more than once. The first one has been done for you.

WORD PARTS

-al (pertaining to)
an- (without, not)
an/o- (anus)
chez/o- (to pass stool)
choledoch/o- (common bile duct)
col/o- (colon)
-cyte (cell)
duoden/o- (duodenum)
dys- (painful, difficult, abnormal)
-emesis (vomiting)
enter/o- (intestine)
epi- (upon, above)
esophag/o- (esophagus)
gastr/o- (stomach)
gloss/o- (tongue)
hemat/o- (blood)
hepat/o- (liver)
-ia (condition, state, thing)
-ic (pertaining to)
-itis (inflammation of)
lingu/o- (tongue)
-lith (stone)
lith/o- (stone)
-megaly (enlargement)
-orex/o- (appetite)
peri- (around)
peritone/o- (peritoneum)
phag/o- (eating, swallowing)
rect/o- (rectum)
retr/o- (behind, backward)
-scopy (process of using an instrument to examine)
sial/o- (saliva)
sub- (below; underneath; less than)
-tomy (process of cutting or making an incision)

1. Pertaining to the mouth (You think *or/o-* + *-al*.) You write oral ____
2. Pertaining to above the stomach ____
3. Condition of being without an appetite ____
4. Condition of difficult or painful eating ____
5. Pertaining to under the tongue ____
6. Inflammation of the stomach and intestine ____
7. Vomiting of blood ____
8. Pertaining to the colon and rectum ____
9. Condition of blood passed in the stool ____
10. Enlargement of the liver ____
11. Salivary gland stone ____
12. Process of using an instrument to examine the esophagus, stomach, and duodenum ____
13. Process of making an incision into the common bile duct to remove a stone ____
14. Liver cell ____
15. Pertaining to around the anus ____
16. Pertaining to behind the peritoneum ____

Symptoms, Signs, and Diseases

True or False

Indicate whether each statement is true or false by writing T or F on the line.

1. ____ Indigestion is known by the medical name *dyspepsia*.
2. ____ A hiatal hernia occurs in the groin.
3. ____ A peptic ulcer is any ulcer in the esophagus, stomach, or duodenum.
4. ____ An ileus is an abnormal fibrous band that forms between two organs following abdominal surgery.
5. ____ Newborn babies frequently get biliary colic.
6. ____ A ruptured appendix can cause diverticulosis.
7. ____ Hepatoma is another name for liver cancer.
8. ____ Pancreatitis can occur when a gallstone blocks the common bile duct near the duodenum.

Matching Exercise

Match each numbered word phrase to its description.

Word	Description
1. hematochezia	_____ Chronic liver disease with nodular liver
2. choledocholithiasis	_____ Dark, tarry stools that contain old blood
3. incontinence	_____ Gallstones in the common bile duct
4. hematemesis	_____ Inflammation of the lips
5. obstipation	_____ Enlargement of the liver and spleen
6. cheilitis	_____ Fatty stools and malabsorption of dietary fat
7. hepatosplenomegaly	_____ A type of stomach cancer
8. steatorrhea	_____ Blood in the stool
9. melena	_____ Excessive vomiting of pregnancy
10. varices	_____ Severe constipation
11. hyperemesis gravidarum	_____ Inability to control bowel movements
12. adenocarcinoma	_____ Vomiting blood
13. cirrhosis	_____ Swollen veins in the esophagus

Laboratory, Radiology, Surgery, and Drugs

Fill in the Blank Exercise

Fill in the blank with the correct word from the word list.

albumin	**cholangiography**	**nasogastric tube**	**sonogram**
antiemetic	**herniorrhaphy**	**ova and parasites**	**stoma**
barium swallow	**laxative**	**peristalsis**	

1. Surgically created opening like a mouth ____________________
2. A medicine used to treat vomiting ____________________
3. Major protein molecule in the blood ____________________
4. Eggs and worms in the GI tract ____________________
5. Radiologic procedure that uses contrast dye to show the bile ducts ____________________
6. An ultrasound is also known as a ____________________
7. Another name for an upper GI series ____________________
8. Provides temporary way to feed a patient ____________________
9. Procedure that sutures a weak area in the abdominal wall where the intestine protrudes through ____________________
10. A medicine used to treat constipation ____________________

Circle Exercise

Circle the correct word from the choices given.

1. The words *donor* and *recipient* are associated with this operative procedure: (**gastroplasty, organ transplantation, polypectomy**)
2. A gallbladder ultrasound is also known as a/an (**amylase test, ERCP, sonogram**).
3. Surgical removal of the gallbladder is known as a (**colectomy, cholecystectomy, colostomy**).
4. All of these are types of feedings tubes EXCEPT (**colostomy, gastrostromy, jejunostomy**).
5. Gastroplasty is a popular surgery to treat (**colon polyps, heartburn, obesity**).
6. ALT is the newer name for the lab test (**albumin, CBD, SGPT**).
7. *Helicobacter pylori* causes this test to be positive (**CLO, colonoscopy, gastric analysis**).
8. A/an (**anastomosis, endoscopy, laparotomy**) uses a long abdominal incision to explore the abdominal cavity.
9. The surgical procedure done to treat stomach cancer is a (**gastrectomy, gastroplasty, gastroscopy**).

Abbreviations

Matching Exercise

Match each abbreviation to its description.

1.	NG	_____ Also known as a barium swallow
2.	CLO test	_____ SGPT was its former name
3.	O&P	_____ A duct that bile flows through
4.	C&S	_____ Screening test for *Helicobacter pylori*
5.	ALT	_____ Feeding tube from nose to stomach
6.	N&V	_____ Stomach acid irritates the esophagus
7.	NPO	_____ Blood tests for hepatic function
8.	UGI	_____ Tells which antibiotic a bacterium is sensitive to
9.	RUQ	_____ Feeding tube surgically inserted in the stomach
10.	CBD	_____ Upset stomach and emesis
11.	GERD	_____ One of four abdominal quadrants
12.	LFTs	_____ Nothing by mouth
13.	PEG	_____ Test for worms and eggs of parasites in the stool

Applied Skills

Plural Noun and Adjective Spelling

Fill in the blanks with the correct word form. Be sure to check your spelling. The first one has been done for you.

Singular Noun	Plural Noun	Adjective
1. abdomen		abdominal
2. mouth		________
3. tongue		________ ________
4. mucosa		________
5. pharynx		________
6. esophagus		________
7. stomach		________
8. pylorus		________
9. duodenum		________
10. jejunum		________
11. ileum		________
12. villus	________	
13. cecum		________
14. appendix		________
15. colon		________
16. rectum		________
17. anus		________
18. peritoneum		________
19. liver		________
20. pancreas		________

Proofreading and Spelling Exercise

Read the following paragraph and identify any misspelled medical words. Write the correct spelling of the word in the blank at the right.

Gastrointerology is the study of the digestive	1. ________
organs. Food moves into the pharinxy from	2. ________
mouth and then down the esophogus.	3. ________
You won't develop diverticulee or	4. ________
hemorrhoids if you eat a high-fiber diet,	5. ________
but cholelithasis could still be a problem.	6. ________
If the lumin of your bowel is filled with	7. ________
polips, then you may need to have surgery.	8. ________
A rectoseel can affect the vagina in women.	9. ________
If you do not eat enough protein, the albumen	10. ________
level in your blood will be low.	

English and Medical Word Equivalents

For each English word, write its equivalent medical word. The first one has been done for you.

English Word	Medical Word
1. belly	*abdomen*
2. belly button	
3. bowel, gut	
4. bowel movement	
5. chewing	
6. gas	
7. heartburn	
8. indigestion	
9. mouth	
10. piles	
11. swallowing	
12. throat	
13. throwing up	

Dictionary Challenge

On the job, you will often encounter new medical words. Practice your medical dictionary skills by looking up the medical words in bold and writing their definitions on the blank lines.

Office Chart Note

This is a 68-year-old white female with episodic abdominal pain, some headaches, heartburn symptoms, **aerophagia** and **eructation,** obstipation, and **tenesmus.** The patient presented with a 3-day history of **singultus,** unrelieved by any over-the-counter medications or home remedies. The patient was in distress, having been unable to sleep normally for several days. Her physical examination revealed **borborygmus** and a slightly tender abdomen, but no evidence of rebound.

1. aerophagia ______
2. eructation ______
3. tenesmus ______
4. singultus ______
5. borborygmus ______

Analysis of a Medical Report

This exercise contains two related reports: a hospital Admission History and Physical Examination and a Pathology Report. Read both reports and answer the questions.

ADMISSION HISTORY AND PHYSICAL EXAMINATION

PATIENT NAME: MARTINEZ, JAVIER

HOSPITAL NUMBER: 138-524-7193

DATE OF ADMISSION: November 19, 20xx

HISTORY OF PRESENT ILLNESS

This is a 20-year-old Hispanic male who experienced severe abdominal pain beginning on the morning of admission. He was awakened at 6 a.m. by sharp pains in the stomach. Drinking a glass of milk, which usually helps this type of pain, was not effective. He also took his customary antacid, but with no relief. He went to college and ate lunch there and then developed nausea and vomiting. An hour later, he developed watery diarrhea with approximately 3–4 bowel movements over the next few hours. He denies any history of ulcerative colitis or Crohn's disease. By this evening, his pain was so severe that he came to the emergency room to be seen.

PHYSICAL EXAMINATION

Temperature 100.2, pulse 84, respiratory rate 30, blood pressure 132/88. He is alert and oriented, lying uncomfortably in bed. Abdominal examination: Abdomen is soft. There is tenderness at McBurney's point, and there is positive rebound.

LABORATORY DATA

Labs drawn in the emergency room showed an elevated white blood cell count of 14.6. Bilirubin and amylase were within normal limits. Urinalysis was unremarkable.

IMPRESSION

Acute appendicitis.

DISCUSSION

A detailed discussion was carried out with the patient and his parents. The dangers of waiting and observing his condition were discussed as well as the indications, possible risks, complications, and alternatives to an appendectomy. They agree with the plan to perform an appendectomy, and the patient will be taken to the operating room shortly.

James R. Rodgers, M.D.

James R. Rodgers, M.D.

JRR/bjg
D: 11/19/xx
T: 11/19/xx

PATHOLOGY REPORT

PATIENT NAME: MARTINEZ, JAVIER

HOSPITAL NUMBER: 138-524-7193

DATE OF REPORT: November 19, 20xx

SPECIMEN: Appendix

GROSS EXAMINATION
The specimen identified as "appendix" is an inflamed, vermiform appendix with an attached piece of the mesoappendix. The appendix measures 6.5 cm in length and up to 1.3 cm in diameter. There is a yellow-gray exudate noted inside with marked hemorrhage of the mucosa. There is no evidence of tumor or fecalith.

PATHOLOGICAL DIAGNOSIS
Acute appendicitis.

Leona T. Parkins, M.D.

Leona T. Parkins, M.D.

LTP:rrg
D: 11/19/xx
T: 11/19/xx

WORD ANALYSIS QUESTIONS

1. The patient had sharp pains in his stomach. If you wanted to use the adjective form of *stomach,* you would say, "He had sharp ________________ pains."
2. Divide *appendicitis* into its two word parts and define each word part.

   Word Part **Definition**

   ________________ ________________________________

   ________________ ________________________________

3. Divide *fecalith* into its two word parts and define each word part.

   Word Part **Definition**

   ________________ ________________________________

   ________________ ________________________________

4. The pathology specimen showed marked hemorrhage of the mucosa. If you wanted to use the adjective form of *mucosa,* you would say, "The pathology specimen showed marked ________________ hemorrhage.
5. What is the abbreviation for *nausea and vomiting*? ________________

FACT FINDING QUESTIONS

1. What is the name of the category of drug that neutralizes acid in the stomach?
   ____
2. What is another medical name for *vomiting*?
   ____
3. Ulcerative colitis and Crohn's disease both affect which part of the gastrointestinal system?
   ____
4. What does *vermiform* mean?
   ____
5. What is the medical word that means *surgical excision of the appendix*?
   ____
6. According to the pathology report on the specimen removed during surgery, what was the patient's diagnosis?
   ____

CRITICAL THINKING QUESTIONS

1. The patient has taken milk and an antacid in the past for his stomach pains. This suggests he has a previous history of what disease condition? Circle the correct answer.

   pyrosis **colon cancer** **hemorrhoids**

2. Acute symptoms of nausea and vomiting with diarrhea might lead you to think that the patient has what disease. Circle the correct answer.

   jaundice **hematochezia** **gastroenteritis**

3. An elevated white blood cell count is associated with an infection. Where was the site of this patient's infection?
   ____

4. The danger in waiting and observing the patient's condition was that he could develop a ruptured appendix that would lead to what condition. Circle the correct answer.

   peritonitis **gastritis** **cholecystitis**

5. The patient had a finding of "positive rebound" on the physical examination. Describe what the physician did to check for rebound.____

6. The patient's bilirubin was within normal limits. This tells you that he is not having any problems with which of these organs?

   stomach **liver** **pancreas**

7. The patient's amylase was within normal limits. This tells you that he is not having any problems with which of these organs?

   pancreas **colon** **esophagus**

Pronunciation Checklist

Read each word and its pronunciation. Practice pronouncing each word. Verify your pronunciation by listening to the Pronunciation List on the CD-ROM. Check the box next to the word after you master its pronunciation.

- ❑ abdominopelvic cavity (ab-DAWM-ih-noh-PEL-vik KAV-ih-tee)
- ❑ absorption (ab-SORP-shun)
- ❑ adenocarcinoma (AD-eh-noh-KAR-sih-NOH-mah)
- ❑ adhesion (ad-HEE-zhun)
- ❑ albumin (al-BYOO-min)
- ❑ alimentary canal (AL-ih-MEN-tair-ee kah-NAL)
- ❑ alkaline phosphatase (AL-kah-line FAWS-fah-tace)
- ❑ amylase (AM-il-ace)
- ❑ anal (AA-nal)
- ❑ anastomosis (ah-NAS-toh-MOH-sis)
- ❑ anorexia (AN-oh-REK-see-ah)
- ❑ anorexic (AN-oh-REK-sik)
- ❑ antacid drug (ant-AS-id DRUHG)
- ❑ antibiotic drug (AN-tee-by-AWT-ik DRUHG) (AN-tih-by-AWT-ik)
- ❑ antidiarrheal drug (AN-tee-DY-ah-REE-al DRUHG)
- ❑ antiemetic drug (AN-tee-eh-MET-ik DRUHG)
- ❑ antrum (AN-trum)
- ❑ anus (AA-nus)
- ❑ aphthous ulcer (AF-thus UL-ser)
- ❑ appendectomy (AP-pen-DEK-toh-mee)
- ❑ appendiceal (AH-pen-DIS-ee-al)
- ❑ appendicitis (ah-PEN-dih-SY-tis)
- ❑ appendix (ah-PEN-diks)
- ❑ ascites (ah-SY-teez)
- ❑ ascitic (ah-SIT-ik)
- ❑ barium (BAH-ree-um)
- ❑ benign (bee-NINE)
- ❑ bile (BILE)
- ❑ biliary (BIL-ee-air-ee)
- ❑ bilirubin (bil-ih-ROO-bin)
- ❑ biliverdin (BIL-ih-VER-din)
- ❑ biopsy (BY-awp-see)
- ❑ bowel (BAH-ool)
- ❑ canal (kah-NAL)
- ❑ cancer (KAN-ser)
- ❑ carcinoma (KAR-sih-NOH-mah)
- ❑ cardia (KAR-dee-ah)
- ❑ cardiac sphincter (KAR-dee-ak SFINGK-ter)
- ❑ cavity (KAV-ih-tee)
- ❑ cecal (SEE-kal)
- ❑ cecum (SEE-kum)
- ❑ celiac (SEE-lee-ak)
- ❑ cheilitis (ky-LY-tis)
- ❑ chemotherapy drug (KEE-moh-THAIR-ah-pee DRUHG)
- ❑ cholangiogram (koh-LAN-jee-oh-gram)
- ❑ cholangiography (koh-LAN-jee-AWG-rah-fee)
- ❑ cholangiopancreatography (koh-LAN-jee-oh-PAN-kree-ah-TAWG-rah-fee)
- ❑ cholangitis (KOH-lan-JY-tis)
- ❑ cholecystectomy (KOH-lee-sis-TEK-toh-mee)
- ❑ cholecystitis (KOH-lee-sis-TY-tis)
- ❑ cholecystogram (KOH-lee-SIS-toh-gram)
- ❑ cholecystography (KOH-lee-sis-TAWG-rah-fee)
- ❑ cholecystokinin (KOH-lee-SIS-toh-KY-nin)
- ❑ choledocholithiasis (koh-LED-oh-koh-lith-EYE-ah-sis)
- ❑ choledocholithotomy (koh-LED-oh-koh-lih-THAWT-oh-mee)
- ❑ cholelithiasis (KOH-lee-lih-THY-ah-sis)
- ❑ chyme (KIME)
- ❑ cirrhotic (sih-RAW-tic)
- ❑ cirrhosis (sih-ROH-sis)
- ❑ colic (KAWL-ik)
- ❑ colitis (koh-LY-tis)
- ❑ colon (KOH-lon)
- ❑ colonic (koh-LAWN-ik)
- ❑ colonoscope (koh-LAWN-oh-skohp)
- ❑ colonoscopy (KOH-lon-AWS-koh-pee)
- ❑ colorectal (KOH-loh-REK-tal)
- ❑ colostomy (koh-LAWS-toh-mee)
- ❑ constipation (CON-stih-PAY-shun)
- ❑ Crohn's disease (KROHNZ dih-ZEEZ)
- ❑ cystic duct (SIS-tik DUKT)
- ❑ defecation (DEF-eh-KAY-shun)
- ❑ deglutition (DEE-gloo-TISH-un) (DEG-loo-TISH-un)
- ❑ diarrhea (DY-ah-REE-ah)
- ❑ digestion (dy-JES-chun) (dih-JES-chun)
- ❑ digestive system (dy-JES-tiv SIS-tem)
- ❑ diverticula (DY-ver-TIK-yoo-lah)
- ❑ diverticular (DY-ver-TIK-yoo-lar)
- ❑ diverticulitis (DY-ver-TIK-yoo-LY-tis)
- ❑ diverticulosis (DY-ver-TIK-yoo-LOH-sis)
- ❑ diverticulum (DY-ver-TIK-yoo-lum)
- ❑ donor (DOH-nor)
- ❑ duct (DUKT)
- ❑ duodenal (DOO-oh-DEE-nal) (doo-AWD-ah-nal)
- ❑ duodenum (DOO-oh-DEE-num) (doo-AWD-ah-num)
- ❑ dysentery (DIS-en-tair-ee)
- ❑ dyspepsia (dis-PEP-see-ah)
- ❑ dysphagia (dis-FAY-jee-ah)
- ❑ elimination (ee-LIM-ih-NAY-shun)
- ❑ emesis (EM-eh-sis)
- ❑ emulsification (ee-MUL-sih-fih-KAY-shun)
- ❑ endoscope (EN-doh-skohp)
- ❑ endoscopic (EN-doh-SKAWP-ik)
- ❑ endoscopic retrograde cholangiopancreatography (EN-doh-SKAWP-ik RET-roh-grayd koh-LAN-jee-oh-PAN-kree-ah-TAWG-rah-fee)
- ❑ endoscopy (en-DAWS-koh-pee)
- ❑ enema (EN-eh-mah)
- ❑ enteritis (EN-ter-EYE-tis)
- ❑ enteropathy (EN-ter-AWP-ah-thee)
- ❑ enzyme (EN-zime)
- ❑ esophageal (ee-SAWF-ah-JEE-al) (ah-SAWF-ah-JEE-al)
- ❑ esophagitis (ee-SAWF-ah-JY-tis)
- ❑ esophagogastroduodenoscopy (ee-SAWF-ah-goh-GAS-troh-DOO-oh-den-AWS-koh-pee)
- ❑ esophagoscope (ee-SAWF-ah-goh-skohp)
- ❑ esophagoscopy (ee-SAWF-ah-GAWS-koh-pee)
- ❑ esophagus (ee-SAWF-ah-gus) (ah-SAWF-ah-gus)
- ❑ exploratory laparotomy (eks-PLOR-ah-TOHR-ee LAP-ah-ROT-ah-mee)
- ❑ fecal (FEE-kal)
- ❑ fecalith (FEE-kah-lith)
- ❑ feces (FEE-seez)
- ❑ flatulence (FLAT-yoo-lens)
- ❑ flatus (FLAY-tus)
- ❑ fundus (FUN-dus)
- ❑ gallbladder (GAWL-blad-er)
- ❑ gastrectomy (gas-TREK-toh-mee)
- ❑ gastric (GAS-trik)
- ❑ gastrin (GAS-trin)
- ❑ gastritis (gas-TRY-tis)
- ❑ gastroenteritis (GAS-troh-EN-ter-EYE-tis)
- ❑ gastroenterologist (GAS-troh-EN-ter-AWL-oh-jist)

- ❏ gastroenterology (GAS-troh-EN-ter-AWL-oh-jee)
- ❏ gastroesophageal (GAS-troh-ee-SAWF-ah-JEE-al)
- ❏ gastrointestinal system (GAS-troh-in-TES-tih-nal SIS-tem)
- ❏ gastroplasty (GAS-troh-PLAS-tee)
- ❏ gastroscope (GAS-troh-skohp)
- ❏ gastroscopy (gas-TRAWS-koh-pee)
- ❏ gastrostomy (gas-TRAWS-toh-mee)
- ❏ gland (GLAND)
- ❏ glossal (GLAWS-al)
- ❏ gluten (GLOO-ten)
- ❏ gluten enteropathy (GLOO-ten EN-ter-AWP-ah-thee)
- ❏ guaiac (GWY-ak)
- ❏ haustra (HAW-strah)
- ❏ hematemesis (HEE-mah-TEM-ah-sis)
- ❏ hematochezia (hee-MAH-toh-KEE-zee-ah)
- ❏ hemorrhoid (HEM-oh-royd)
- ❏ hemorrhoidectomy (HEM-oh-roy-DEK-toh-mee)
- ❏ hepatic (heh-PAT-ik)
- ❏ hepatitis (HEP-ah-TY-tis)
- ❏ hepatocellular (HEP-ah-toh-SEL-yoo-lar)
- ❏ hepatocyte (HEP-ah-toh-site)
- ❏ hepatoma (HEP-ah-TOH-mah)
- ❏ hepatomegaly (HEP-ah-toh-MEG-ah-lee)
- ❏ hernia (HER-nee-ah)
- ❏ herniorrhaphy (HER-nee-OR-ah-fee)
- ❏ hiatal hernia (hy-AA-tal HER-nee-ah)
- ❏ hiatus hernia (hy-AA-tus HER-nee-ah)
- ❏ hydrochloric acid (HY-droh-KLOR-ik AS-id)
- ❏ hyperemesis gravidarum (HY-per-EM-eh-sis GRAV-ih-DAIR-um)
- ❏ hypochondriac (HY-poh-CON-dree-ak)
- ❏ hypogastric (HY-poh-GAS-trik)
- ❏ ileal (IL-ee-al)
- ❏ ileostomy (IL-ee-AWS-toh-mee)
- ❏ ileum (IL-ee-um)
- ❏ ileus (IL-ee-us)
- ❏ imperforate anus (im-PER-for-ate AA-nus)
- ❏ incarcerated hernia (in-KAR-seh-ray-ted HER-nee-ah)
- ❏ incisional hernia (in-SIZH-un-al HER-nee-ah)
- ❏ incontinence (in-CON-tih-nens)
- ❏ incontinent (in-CON-tih-nent)
- ❏ indigestion (IN-dy-JES-chun)
- ❏ inflammatory (in-FLAM-ah-tor-ee)
- ❏ inguinal (ING-gwih-nal)
- ❏ intestinal (in-TES-tih-nal)
- ❏ intestine (in-TES-tin)
- ❏ intravenous (IN-trah-VEE-nus)
- ❏ intussusception (IN-tus-suh-SEP-shun)
- ❏ jaundice (JAWN-dis)
- ❏ jejunal (jeh-JOO-nal)
- ❏ jejunostomy (JEH-joo-NAWS-toh-mee)
- ❏ jejunum (jeh-JOO-num)
- ❏ lactase (LAK-tace)
- ❏ laparoscope (LAP-ah-roh-skohp)
- ❏ laparoscopic (LAP-ah-roh-SKAWP-ik)
- ❏ laparoscopy (LAP-ah-RAWS-koh-pee)
- ❏ laparotomy (LAP-ah-ROT-ah-mee)
- ❏ laxative (LAK-sah-tiv)
- ❏ lingual (LING-gwal)
- ❏ lipase (LIP-ace)
- ❏ liver (LIV-er)
- ❏ liver transplantation (LIV-er TRANS-plan-TAY-shun)
- ❏ lumen (LOO-men)
- ❏ malrotation (MAL-roh-TAY-shun)
- ❏ mastication (MAS-tih-KAY-shun)
- ❏ meconium (meh-KOH-nee-um)
- ❏ medical assistant (MED-ih-kal ah-SIS-tant)
- ❏ melena (meh-LEE-nah)
- ❏ melenic (meh-LEH-nik)
- ❏ mesenteric (MEZ-en-TAIR-ik)
- ❏ mesentery (MEZ-en-tair-ee)
- ❏ mucosa (myoo-KOH-sah)
- ❏ mucosal (myoo-KOH-sal)
- ❏ mucous (MYOO-kus)
- ❏ nasogastric (NAY-zoh-GAS-trik)
- ❏ nausea (NAW-see-ah) (NAW-zha)
- ❏ nauseated (NAW-zee-aa-ted)
- ❏ obstipation (AWB-stih-PAY-shun)
- ❏ obstructive (awb-STRUK-tiv)
- ❏ occult (oh-KULT)
- ❏ odynophagia (oh-DIN-oh-FAY-jee-ah)
- ❏ omentum (oh-MEN-tum)
- ❏ omphalocele (OM-fal-oh-seel)
- ❏ oncologist (ong-KAWL-oh-jist)
- ❏ oral (OR-al)
- ❏ ova and parasites (OH-vah and PAIR-ah-sites)
- ❏ palate (PAL-at)
- ❏ pancreas (PAN-kree-as)
- ❏ pancreatic (PAN-kree-AT-ik)
- ❏ pancreatitis (PAN-kree-ah-TY-tis)
- ❏ parotid (pah-ROT-id)
- ❏ patent (PAY-tent)
- ❏ pedunculated (peh-DUNG-kyoo-lay-ted)
- ❏ pepsin (PEP-sin)
- ❏ pepsinogen (pep-SIN-oh-jen)
- ❏ peptic (PEP-tik)
- ❏ peptic ulcer (PEP-ik UL-ser)
- ❏ peptidase (PEP-tih-dace)
- ❏ percutaneous transhepatic cholangiography (PER-kyoo-TAY-nee-us TRANS-heh-PAT-ik KOH-lan-jee-AWG-rah-fee)
- ❏ perianal (PAIR-ee-AA-nal)
- ❏ peristalsis (PAIR-ih-STAL-sis)
- ❏ peritoneal (PAIR-ih-toh-NEE-al)
- ❏ peritoneum (PAIR-ih-toh-NEE-um)
- ❏ peritonitis (PAIR-ih-toh-NY-tis)
- ❏ pharyngeal (fah-RIN-jee-al)
- ❏ pharynx (FAIR-ingks)
- ❏ polyp (PAW-lip)
- ❏ polypectomy (PAWL-ih-PEK-toh-mee)
- ❏ polyphagia (PAWL-ee-FAY-jee-ah)
- ❏ polyposis (PAWL-ee-POH-sis)
- ❏ portal (POR-tal)
- ❏ portal hypertension (POR-tal HY-per-TEN-shun)
- ❏ postoperative (post-AWP-er-ah-tiv)
- ❏ protease (PROH-tee-ace)
- ❏ pyloric (py-LOR-ik)
- ❏ pyloric sphincter (py-LOR-ik SFINGK-ter)
- ❏ pylorus (py-LOR-us)
- ❏ pyrosis (py-ROH-sis)
- ❏ rectal (REK-tal)
- ❏ rectum (REK-tum)
- ❏ rectocele (REK-toh-seel)
- ❏ reflux (REE-fluks)
- ❏ regurgitation (ree-GER-jih-TAY-shun)
- ❏ resection (ree-SEK-shun)
- ❏ retroperitoneal (REH-troh-PAIR-ih-toh-NEE-al)
- ❏ rugae (ROO-gee)
- ❏ saliva (sah-LY-vah)
- ❏ salivary (SAL-ih-vair-ee)
- ❏ sessile (SES-il)
- ❏ sialolith (sy-AL-oh-lith)
- ❏ sialolithiasis (sy-AL-oh-lih-THY-ah-sis)
- ❏ sigmoid colon (SIG-moyd KOH-lon)
- ❏ sigmoidoscope (sig-MOY-doh-skohp)
- ❏ sigmoidoscopy (SIG-moy-DAWS-koh-pee)
- ❏ sonogram (SAWN-oh-gram)
- ❏ spasm (SPAZM)
- ❏ spastic (SPAS-tik)
- ❏ sphincter (SFINGK-ter)
- ❏ steatorrhea (stee-AT-oh-REE-ah)
- ❏ stoma (STOH-mah)
- ❏ stomach (STUM-uk)
- ❏ stomatitis (STOH-mah-TY-tis)
- ❏ stool (STOOL)
- ❏ strangulated hernia (STRANG-gyoo-lay-ted HER-nee-ah)
- ❏ sublingual (sub-LING-gwal)
- ❏ submandibular (SUB-man-DIB-yoo-lar)

- ❑ suppository (soo-PAWZ-ih-tohr-ee)
- ❑ surgeon (SER-jun)
- ❑ syndrome (SIN-drohm)
- ❑ tomography (toh-MAWG-rah-fee)
- ❑ tract (TRAKT)
- ❑ transplantation (TRANS-plan-TAY-shun)
- ❑ ulcer (UL-ser)
- ❑ ulcerative (UL-ser-ah-tiv)
- ❑ ultrasound (UL-trah-sound)
- ❑ umbilical (um-BIL-ih-kal)
- ❑ umbilicus (um-BIL-ih-kus) (um-bih-LIE-kus)
- ❑ uvula (YOO-vyoo-lah)
- ❑ varices (VAR-ih-seez)
- ❑ varix (VAR-iks)
- ❑ ventral (VEN-tral)
- ❑ villi (VIL-eye)
- ❑ volvulus (VAWL-vyoo-lus)
- ❑ vomit (VAWM-it)
- ❑ vomitus (VAWM-ih-tus)

Experience Multimedia

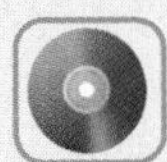

CD-ROM Learning Activities Checklist

Check off the box as you complete each learning activity.

- ❑ **CD-ROM Learning Activity 3.1: *ANATOMY WORD PARTS FLASHCARDS***
  Use flashcards to help you memorize word parts. Make your own flashcards or print out prepared flashcards. Also see the electronic flashcard game. Time: 20 minutes.
- ❑ **CD-ROM Learning Activity 3.2: *MEDICINE IN ACTION***
  Watch a video clip to see how a sigmoidoscopy is performed. Time: 5 minutes.
- ❑ **CD-ROM Learning Activity 3.3: *DISEASE AND OTHER WORD PARTS FLASHCARDS***
  A continuation of the flashcard learning activity. Time: 20 minutes.
- ❑ **CD-ROM Learning Activity 3.4: *MEMORY AIDS***
  Use memory aids to help you memorize medical words and meanings. Time: 5 minutes.
- ❑ **CD-ROM Learning Activity 3.5: *MEDICAL LANGUAGE SPOKEN HERE***
  Listen to actual medical reports and spell the missing medical words. Time: 20 minutes.
- ❑ **CD-ROM Learning Activity 3.6: *SPELLING CHALLENGE***
  Listen to a pronounced medical word and then spell it. Time: 5 minutes.
- ❑ **CD-ROM Learning Activity 3.7: *MEDICAL LANGUAGE PRONUNCIATION***
  Listen to a pronounced medical word and then practice pronouncing it. Time: 30 minutes.
- ❑ **CD-ROM Learning Activity 3.8: *EDUCATIONAL FUN AND GAMES***
  Enjoy these fun activities while reinforcing your knowledge. Time: 15 minutes.

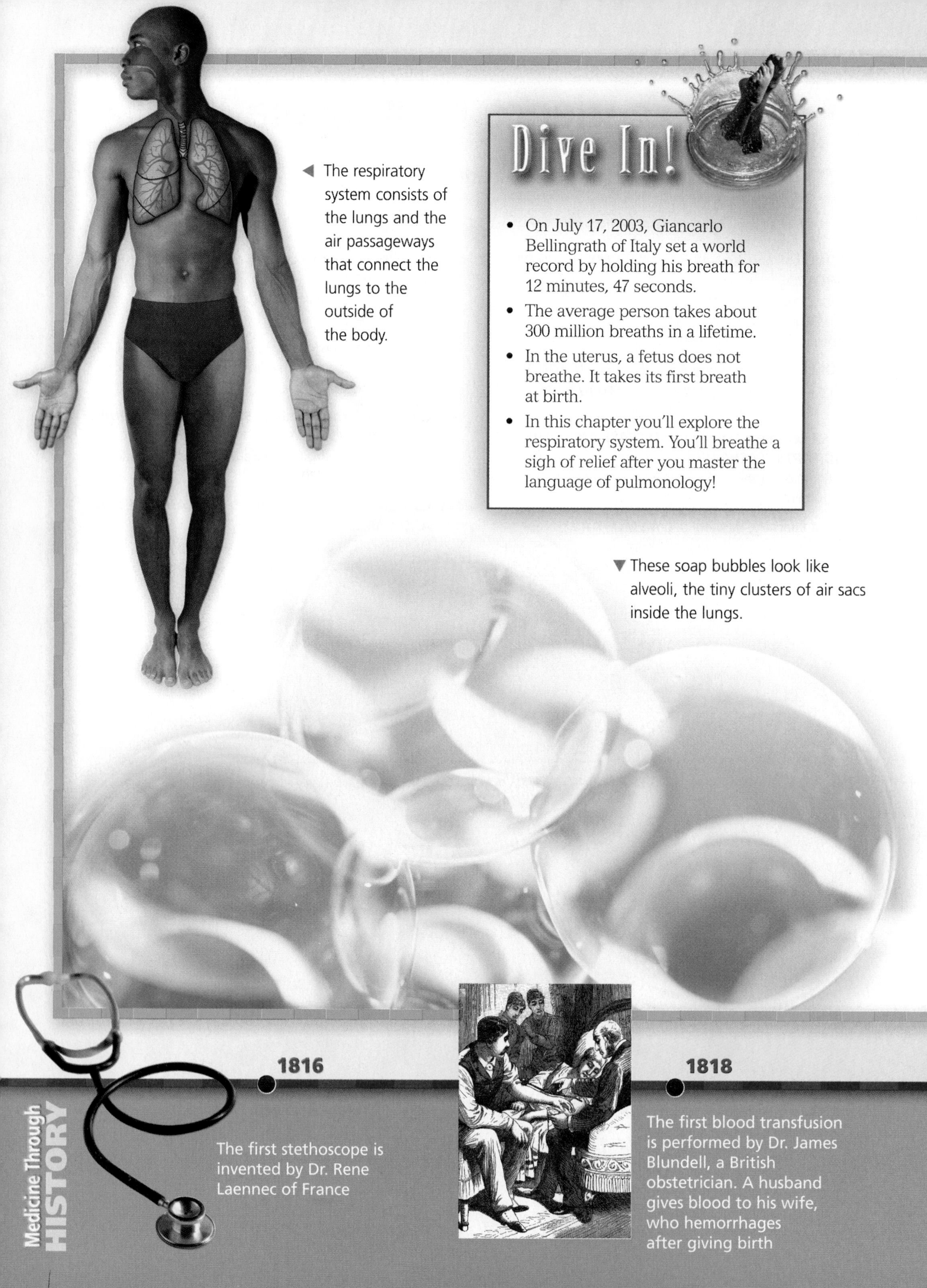

The respiratory system consists of the lungs and the air passageways that connect the lungs to the outside of the body.

Dive In!

- On July 17, 2003, Giancarlo Bellingrath of Italy set a world record by holding his breath for 12 minutes, 47 seconds.
- The average person takes about 300 million breaths in a lifetime.
- In the uterus, a fetus does not breathe. It takes its first breath at birth.
- In this chapter you'll explore the respiratory system. You'll breathe a sigh of relief after you master the language of pulmonology!

These soap bubbles look like alveoli, the tiny clusters of air sacs inside the lungs.

Medicine Through HISTORY

1816

The first stethoscope is invented by Dr. Rene Laennec of France

1818

The first blood transfusion is performed by Dr. James Blundell, a British obstetrician. A husband gives blood to his wife, who hemorrhages after giving birth

CHAPTER 4

Pulmonology

Respiratory System

Pulmonology (PUL-moh-NAWL-oh-jee) is the medical specialty that studies the anatomy and physiology of the respiratory system and uses diagnostic tests, medical and surgical procedures, and drugs to treat respiratory diseases.

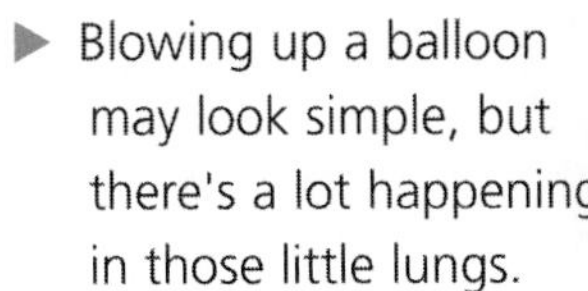

▶ Blowing up a balloon may look simple, but there's a lot happening in those little lungs.

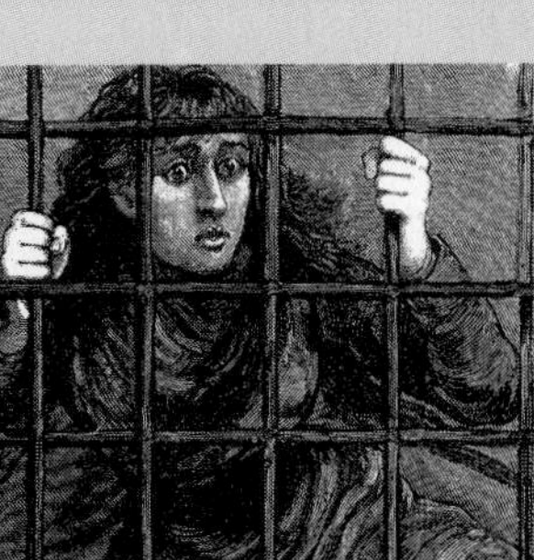

1841

Dorthea Dix advocates for the mentally ill and better conditions in mental hospitals

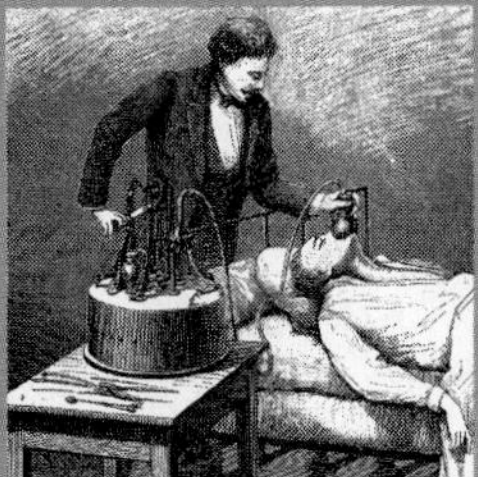

1846

Dr. William Morton uses ether gas to perform the first surgery under general anesthesia

1847

The American Medical Association (AMA) is founded

Measure Your Progress: Learning Objectives

After you study this chapter, you should be able to

1. Identify the anatomical structures of the respiratory system by correctly labeling them on anatomical illustrations.
2. Describe the process of respiration.
3. Build respiratory words from combining forms, prefixes, and suffixes.
4. Describe common respiratory diseases.
5. Describe common respiratory diagnostic laboratory and radiology tests.
6. Describe common respiratory medical and surgical procedures and drug categories.
7. Define common respiratory abbreviations.
8. Correctly spell and pronounce respiratory words.
9. Apply your skills by analyzing a pulmonology report.
10. Test your knowledge of pulmonology by completing review exercises at the end of the chapter and learning activities on the CD-ROM.

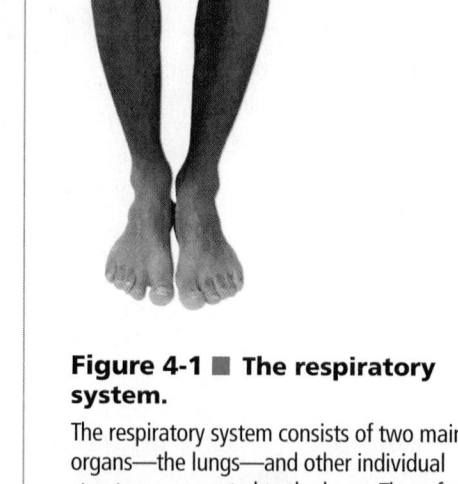

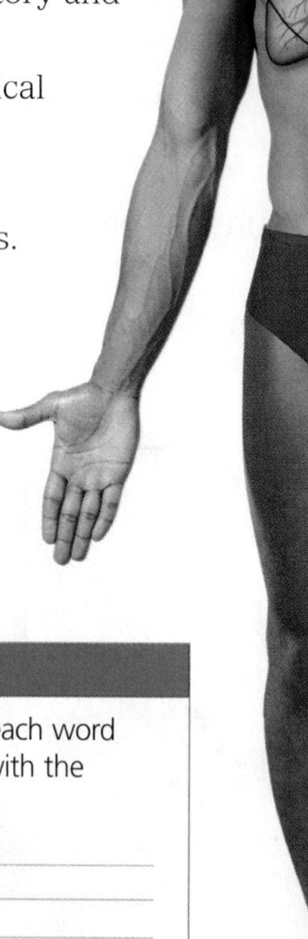

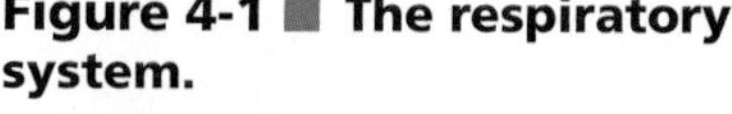

Figure 4-1 ■ The respiratory system.

The respiratory system consists of two main organs—the lungs—and other individual structures connected to the lungs. These form a pathway through which air flows into and out of the body.

Medical Language Key

To unlock the meaning of a medical word, first define each word part. Then put the word part definitions in order, beginning with the suffix, followed by the first word part.

	Word Part	Word Part Definition
SUFFIX	**-logy**	***the study of***
COMBINING FORM	**pulmon/o-**	***lung***

Pulmonology: ***The study of the lungs.***

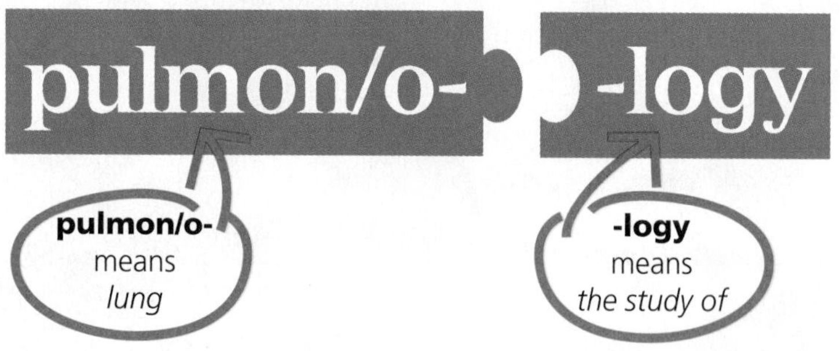

www.prenhall.com/turley

For interactive flashcards, real-life video clips, games, exercises, and audio pronunciations please explore the companion CD-ROM in the back of the book. Click on the companion website for bonus chapters, additional resources, and links to on-line learning.

Anatomy and Physiology

The **respiratory system** is a body system that consists of the right and left lungs and the air passageways that connect the lungs to the outside of the body (see Figure 4-1■). The respiratory system begins in the nose and throat and continues as the pharynx and trachea (windpipe). In the thoracic cavity, the trachea divides into bronchi that enter the right and left lungs. The lungs themselves fill much of the thoracic cavity.

The upper respiratory system is located in the head and neck and includes the nose, nasal cavity, and pharynx (throat). The upper respiratory system shares structures with the ENT (ears, nose, and throat) system, discussed in Otolaryngology (Chapter 16). The lower respiratory system is located in the neck and thoracic cavity and includes the larynx (voice box), trachea (windpipe), bronchi, lungs, and diaphragm. The purpose of the respiratory system is to bring oxygen into the body and expel the waste product carbon dioxide.

respiratory (RES-pih-rah-TOR-ee) (reh-SPYR-ah-tor-ee)
re- *again and again; backward; unable to*
spir/o- *breathe*
-atory *pertaining to*
Some word parts have more than one definition. The best definition of *respiratory* is *pertaining to again and again breathing.*

system (SIS-tem)
System is derived from a Greek word meaning *combination of parts to make an organized whole.*

Anatomy of the Respiratory System

Nose and Nasal Cavity

The nose contains the **nasal cavity,** which is divided internally by the **nasal septum** into right and left sides. On each side of the nasal septum, there are three elongated, bony projections known as the superior, middle, and inferior **turbinates** or **nasal conchae.** These jut out into the nasal cavity and act as barriers that divide and slow down inhaled air so that it can pick up warmth and moisture (see Figure 4-2■). The nasal cavity is lined with nasal **mucosa,** a moist **mucous membrane** that continuously humidifies the air and produces **mucus** to trap inhaled particles of dust, pollen, smoke, and bacteria before they can enter the lungs. Mast cells are special cells in the connective tissue of the respiratory system. In response to foreign particles, they release histamine. **Histamine** dilates blood vessels and allows fluid to leak through the blood vessel wall. This causes swelling and redness (edema) and itching.

nasal (NAY-zal)
nas/o- *nose*
-al *pertaining to*
Nasal is the adjective form for *nose.*

cavity (KAV-ih-tee)
cav/o- *hollow space*
-ity *state; condition*

septum (SEP-tum)
Septum is derived from a Latin word meaning *a partition.*

septal (SEP-tal)
sept/o- *septum (dividing wall)*
-al *pertaining to*

turbinate (TER-bih-nayt)
turbin/o- *scroll-like structure; turbinate*
-ate *composed of; pertaining to*
Turbinate is derived from a Latin word meaning *something that spins like a top.* The bone of each turbinate is rolled around itself, like a turban or a scroll.

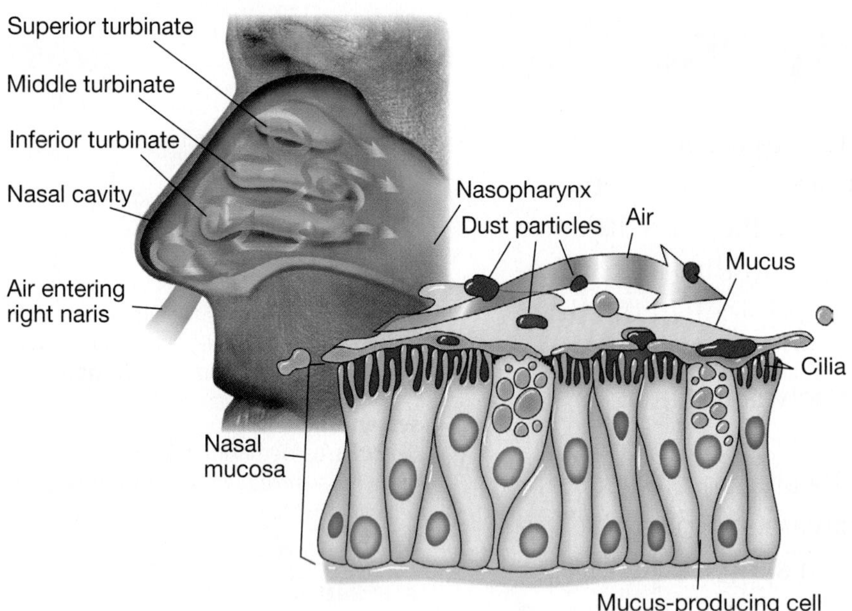

Figure 4-2 ■ The nasal cavity.

Visualize how air entering the nose and nasal cavity slowly swirls around the turbinates, allowing the nasal mucosa to moisten and warm it before it goes to the lungs. Prewarmed air helps the body maintain its core temperature, and the moisture keeps the delicate tissues of the lungs from becoming dehydrated. The mucosa also produces mucus to trap inhaled particles and bacteria before they can enter the lungs.

concha (CON-kah)
conchae (CON-kee)
Concha is derived from a Latin word meaning *a spiral seashell.*

mucosa (myoo-KOH-sah)
Mucosa is a Latin word meaning *mucus.*

mucosal (myoo-KOH-sal)
mucos/o- *mucous membrane*
-al *pertaining to*

mucous (MYOO-kus)
muc/o- *mucus*
-ous *pertaining to*

mucus (MYOO-kus)

histamine (HIS-tah-meen)

Pharynx

As the nasal cavity continues posteriorly, it merges with the upper part of the throat or **pharynx.** The mucous membranes of the pharynx also warm and moisten the inhaled air and trap inhaled particles. The pharynx acts as a common passageway for inhaled air, exhaled air, and ingested food.

pharynx (FAIR-ingks)
Pharynx is a Greek word meaning *throat.*

pharyngeal (fah-RIN-jee-al)
pharyng/o- *pharynx (throat)*
-eal *pertaining to*

Larynx

At its inferior end, the pharynx divides into two parts: the larynx that leads to the trachea and the esophagus that leads to the stomach. The **larynx** or voice box is a passageway for inhaled and exhaled air. The larynx remains open during respiration and speech, allowing air to pass through the vocal cords. During swallowing, muscles in the neck pull the larynx up to meet the **epiglottis,** a lidlike structure that seals off the larynx, so that food moves across the top of the epiglottis and into the esophagus, not into the larynx.

larynx (LAIR-ingks)
Larynx is a Greek word meaning *voice box.*

laryngeal (lah-RIN-jee-al)
laryng/o- *larynx (voice box)*
-eal *pertaining to*

epiglottis (EP-ih-GLAWT-is)
Glottis is a Greek word meaning *opening of the larynx.*

epiglottic (EP-ih-GLAWT-ik)
epi- *upon, above*
glott/o- *glottis (of the larynx)*
-ic *pertaining to*

Trachea

Below the vocal cords, the larynx merges into the trachea. The **trachea** or windpipe, a muscular tube about 1 inch in diameter and 4 inches in length, is a passageway for inhaled and exhaled air (see Figure 4-3■). On the anterior surface of the trachea is a column of C-shaped rings of cartilage that provide support to the trachea. On the posterior surface where there is no cartilage, the trachea is flexible and can flatten to make room when food passes through the esophagus.

trachea (TRAY-kee-ah)

tracheal (TRAY-kee-al)
trache/o- *trachea (windpipe)*
-al *pertaining to*

Bronchi

The trachea ends as it divides into an inverted *Y,* forming the right and left mainstem **bronchi** (see Figure 4-3). The tubular bronchi are encircled with cartilage rings that provide support. Each bronchus enters a lung and then further divides into many smaller passageways known as **bronchioles.** The bronchioles are composed of smooth muscle rather than cartilage. The **lumen** is the central opening in the bronchi and bronchioles through which air passes. **Bronchopulmonary** refers to the bronchi and the lungs.

Because the trachea, mainstem bronchi, and bronchioles look like the trunk and branches of an upside-down tree, they are known as the **tracheobronchial tree** or **bronchial tree** (see Figure 4-3). The tracheobronchial tree contains **cilia,** small hairs that move in coordinated waves and carry mucus and trapped particles toward the throat where they can be expelled.

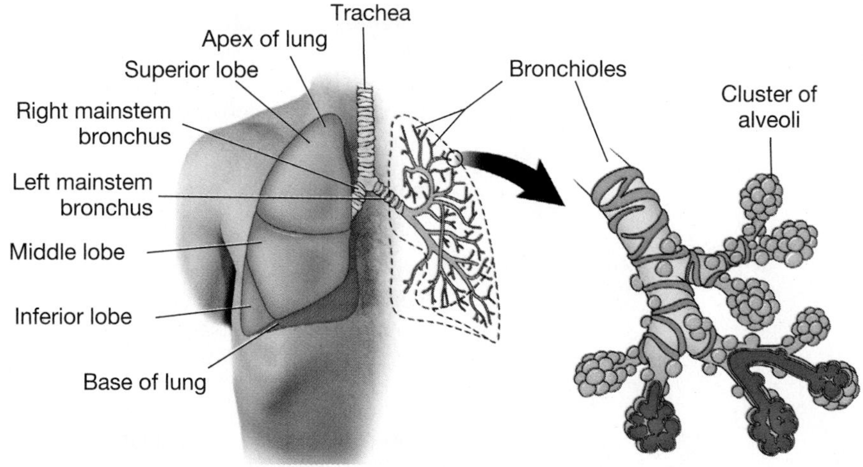

Figure 4-3 ■ The lungs and bronchi.

The larger right lung has three lobes. The left lung has two lobes. This left lung shows the many branches of the bronchioles. Remember when you are facing a patient, your right side corresponds to the patient's left side (left lung). Alveoli are microscopic air sacs at the end of each bronchiole where oxygen from the air and carbon dioxide from the body are exchanged.

bronchus (BRONG-kus)
bronchi (BRONG-kigh)
Bronchus is a Latin singular masculine noun. Form the plural by changing the *-us* to *-i.*

bronchial (BRONG-kee-al)
bronchi/o- *bronchus*
-al *pertaining to*

bronchiole (BRONG-kee-ohl)
bronchi/o- *bronchus*
-ole *little, small*

bronchiolar (BRONG-kee-OH-lar)
bronchiol/o- *bronchiole*
-ar *pertaining to*

lumen (LOO-men)
Lumen is a Latin word meaning *window.*

bronchopulmonary (BRONG-koh-PUL-moh-nair-ee)
bronch/o- *bronchus*
pulmon/o- *lung*
-ary *pertaining to*

tracheobronchial (TRAY-kee-oh-BRONG-kee-al)
trache/o- *trachea (windpipe)*
bronchi/o- *bronchus*
-al *pertaining to*

cilium (SIL-ee-um)
cilia (SIL-ee-ah)
Cilium is a Latin singular neuter noun meaning *an eyelash.* Form the plural by changing *-um* to *-a.* Because there are so many cilia in the respiratory system, the singular form is seldom used.

Did You Know?

Smoking immobilizes and eventually destroys the cilia lining the respiratory tract. This allows cigarette smoke particles to freely enter the lung and be deposited there permanently. The lung tissue of smokers is gray in color with speckles of black rather than the normal pink color.

Lungs

The lungs are spongy, air-filled structures that fill both sides of the thoracic cavity. Each lung contains large divisions known as **lobes.** The dividing lines between the lobes are visible on the outer surface of the lung. The right lung, which is larger, has three lobes: the right upper lobe (RUL), the right middle lobe (RML), and the right lower lobe (RLL). The left lung has only two lobes: the left upper lobe (LUL) and the left lower lobe (LLL). The rounded top of each lung is known as the **apex.** The bottom or base of each lung lies along the diaphragm (see Figure 4-3). Each bronchi enters a lung at the **hilum** (an indentation on the medial surface of the lung). The **pulmonary** artery and pulmonary veins also enter and exit there.

Within each lung, the bronchioles end in clusters of air sacs or **alveoli.** The **alveolus** is a hollow sphere of cells that expands and contracts with each breath (see Figure 4-3). Oxygen and carbon dioxide are exchanged between the alveoli and a nearby small blood vessel (capillary). The alveoli secrete **surfactant,** a protein-fat compound that creates surface tension and keeps the walls of the alveolus from collapsing with each exhalation. All the alveoli are collectively known as the **pulmonary parenchyma,** the functional part of the lung, as opposed to the connective tissue framework that surrounds and supports the alveoli.

lobe (LOHB)

lobar (LOH-bar)
lob/o- *lobe of an organ*
-ar *pertaining to*

apex (AA-peks)
apices (AA-pih-sees)
Apex is a Latin singular noun meaning *tip.* Form the plural by changing *-ex* to *-ices.*

apical (AP-ih-kal)
apic/o- *apex (tip)*
-al *pertaining to*

hilum (HY-lum)
hila (HY-lah)
Hilum is a Latin singular neuter noun meaning *a little mark.* Form the plural by changing *-um* to *-a.*

hilar (HY-lar)
hil/o- *hilum (indentation in an organ)*
-ar *pertaining to*

pulmonary (PUL-moh-nair-ee)
pulmon/o- *lung*
-ary *pertaining to*
Pulmonary is the adjective form for *lung.*

alveolus (al-VEE-oh-lus)
alveoli (al-VEE-oh-ligh)
Alveolus is a Latin singular masculine noun meaning *a small hollow cell or cavity.* Form the plural by changing *-us* to *-i.*

alveolar (al-VEE-oh-lar)
alveol/o- *alveolus (air sac)*
-ar *pertaining to*

surfactant (ser-FAK-tant)
Surfactant is a combination of the words *surface* and *active* plus the suffix *-ant* (pertaining to).

parenchyma (pah-RENG-kih-mah)

parenchymal (pah-RENG-kih-mal)
parenchym/o- *parenchyma (functional cells of an organ)*
-al *pertaining to*

Thoracic Cavity

The **thorax** is a bony cage that consists of the **sternum** (breast bone) anteriorly, the ribs laterally, and the spinal column posteriorly. It surrounds and protects the **thoracic cavity.** The lungs occupy most of the area on each side of the thoracic cavity. The **mediastinum,** an irregularly shaped area between the two lungs, contains the trachea. The inferior aspect of the thoracic cavity is covered by the **diaphragm,** a muscular sheet that contracts to enlarge the thoracic cavity and draw in air. The **intercostal muscles** between the ribs contract to pull the ribs together, decrease the size of the thoracic cavity, and forcefully expel air from the lungs. Other muscles in the neck, chest, and abdomen, known as the accessory muscles of respiration, are sometimes needed to help expand the thoracic cavity.

Each lung is surrounded by a double-layered **serous membrane** known as the **pleura** (see Figure 4-4■). The membrane that covers the surface of the lung is known as the **visceral pleura,** while the membrane that covers the wall of the thoracic cavity is known as the **parietal pleura.** The pleura secretes **pleural fluid,** a slippery, watery fluid that allows the two membranes to slide smoothly past one another as the lungs expand and contract during respiration.

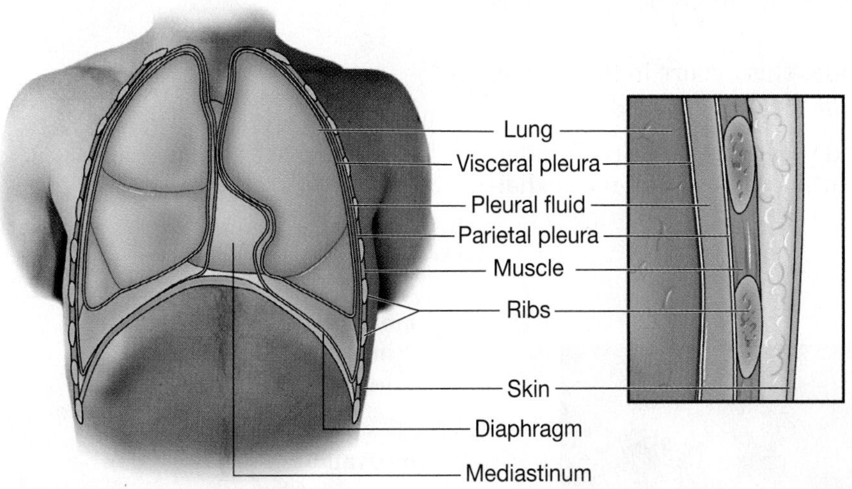

Figure 4-4 ■ The pleura.

The pleura folds back on itself to make two layers that are in nearly direct contact with each other. The visceral pleura covers the surface of the lungs. The parietal pleura lines the sides and floor of the thoracic cavity. The space between the two layers is filled with pleural fluid.

thorax (THOR-aks)
Thorax is a Greek word meaning *breastplate.*

sternum (STER-num)

sternal (STER-nal)
stern/o- *sternum (breast bone)*
-al *pertaining to*

thoracic (thoh-RAS-ik)
thorac/o- *thorax (chest)*
-ic *pertaining to*

cavity (KAV-ih-tee)
cav/o- *hollow space*
-ity *state; condition*

mediastinum (MEE-dee-as-TY-num)
Mediastinum is derived from a Latin word meaning *a lower servant who performs routine duties.* Perhaps the mediastinum seemed like a smaller, less important area compared to the larger, active thorax.

mediastinal (MEE-dee-as-TY-nal)
mediastin/o- *mediastinum*
-al *pertaining to*

diaphragm (DY-ah-fram)

diaphragmatic (DY-ah-frag-MAT-ik)
diaphragmat/o- *diaphragm*
-ic *pertaining to*

intercostal (IN-ter-KAWS-tal)
inter- *between*
cost/o- *rib*
-al *pertaining to*

serous (SEER-us)
ser/o- *serum of the blood; serumlike fluid*
-ous *pertaining to*
The serous membrane secretes a watery fluid that is like the clear, liquid serum of the blood.

pleura (PLOOR-ah)
Pleura is a Greek word meaning *rib or side.*

pleural (PLOOR-al)
pleur/o- *pleura (lung membrane)*
-al *pertaining to*

visceral (VIS-eh-ral)
viscer/o- *viscera (internal organs)*
-al *pertaining to*

parietal (pah-RY-eh-tal)
pariet/o- *wall of a cavity*
-al *pertaining to*

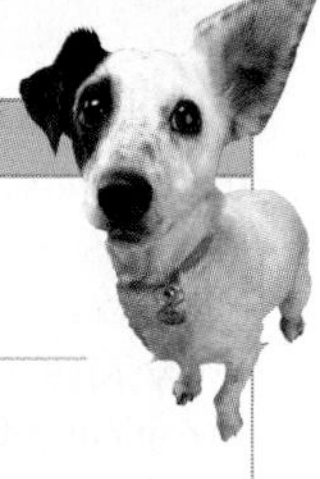

Word Alert

ALTERNATE NAMES

The respiratory system is also known as the **respiratory tract**. A tract is a pathway. The adjective **cardiopulmonary** reflects the close connection between the heart and the respiratory system. Without the heart, oxygen brought into the lungs would never reach the rest of the body, and carbon dioxide produced by the cells would never reach the lungs to be exhaled.

tract (TRAKT)

cardiopulmonary (KAR-dee-oh-PUL-moh-nair-ee)
cardi/o- *heart*
pulmon/o- *lung*
-ary *pertaining to*

Physiology of Respiration

The respiratory system has five basic functions:

1. It serves as a passageway through which air can enter and leave the body.
2. It mechanically causes air to flow into the lungs.
3. It warms and moistens incoming air.
4. It traps and expels foreign particles, bacteria, and other pathogens in the incoming air.
5. It exchanges oxygen for carbon dioxide. This occurs in the alveoli. (It also occurs in the rest of the body at the cellular level.)

Respiration consists of breathing in and breathing out. Breathing in is known as **inhalation** or **inspiration.** Breathing out is known as **exhalation** or **expiration** (see Figure 4-5■).

respiration (RES-pih-RAY-shun)
re- *again and again; backward; unable to*
spir/o- *breathe*
-ation *a process; being or having*

inhalation (IN-hah-LAY-shun)
in- *in; within; not*
hal/o- *breathe*
-ation *a process; being or having*

inspiration (IN-spih-RAY-shun)
in- *in; within; not*
spir/o- *breathe*
-ation *a process; being or having*

exhalation (EKS-hah-LAY-shun)
ex- *out, away from*
hal/o- *breathe*
-ation *a process; being or having*

expiration (EKS-pih-RAY-shun)
ex- *out, away from*
spir/o- *breathe*
-ation *a process; being or having*
The *s* is deleted from *spir/o-* because the prefix *ex-* already provides an *s* sound. *Expire* also means *to die* or *to take a last breath.*

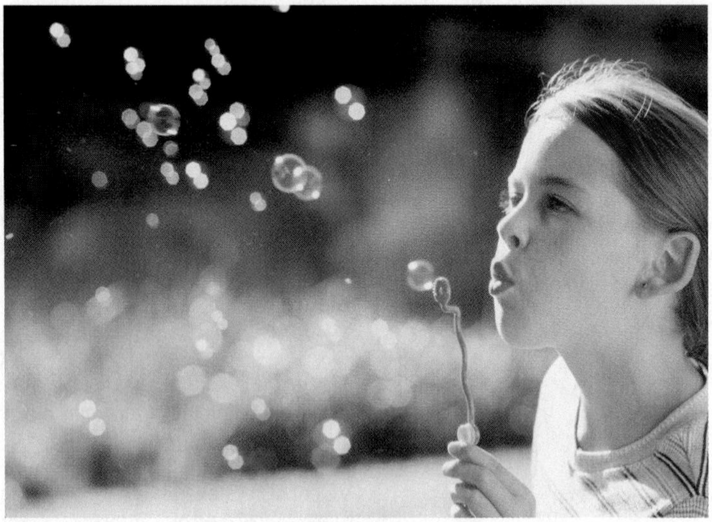

Figure 4-5 ■ Exhalation.

As the diaphragm relaxes, the thoracic cavity decreases in size and air slowly flows out of the nose. This occurs without conscious thought. However, if the intercostal muscles are consciously contracted, this quickly decreases the size of the thoracic cavity and expels a large volume of air in a few seconds.

Breathing is normally an involuntary process that occurs without any conscious effort. The respiratory control center in the brain regulates the depth and rate of respiration. It receives information from receptors on large arteries in the chest and neck that sense the levels of oxygen and carbon dioxide in the blood. The respiratory control center sends nerve impulses to the **phrenic nerve,** causing the diaphragm to contract and initiate inspiration. A normal depth and rate of respiration is known as **eupnea.** You can voluntarily control your respirations (when you hold your breath), but eventually involuntary control takes over, forcing you to breathe.

The two components of breathing are external respiration and internal respiration. **External respiration** includes the physical process of inhalation and exhalation and what happens to the inhaled and exhaled air. In the lungs, **oxygen** in the inhaled air moves from the alveoli into the blood (see Figure 4-6■). At the same time, **carbon dioxide** (a gaseous waste product of metabolism) is exhaled by the lungs. The oxygen molecules combine with the hemoglobin in red blood cells in the blood to form the compound oxyhemoglobin. **Oxyhemoglobin** is the form in which oxygen travels in the blood. **Oxygenated** blood travels from the lungs to the heart where it is pumped throughout the body to reach every cell.

phrenic (FREN-ik)
phren/o- *diaphragm; mind*
-ic *pertaining to*
Some word parts have more than one definition. The best definition of *phrenic* (in *phrenic nerve*) is *pertaining to the diaphragm.*

eupnea (YOOP-nee-ah)
eu- *normal, good*
-pnea *breathing*

eupneic (YOOP-nik)
eu- *normal, good*
pne/o- *breathing*
-ic *pertaining to*

external (eks-TER-nal)
extern/o- *outside*
-al *pertaining to*

oxygen (AWK-seh-jen)
Oxygen is derived from a French word meaning *acid.* It was thought that oxygen was an essential chemical component in the formation of acids.

carbon dioxide (KAR-bun dy-AWK-side)
Carbon dioxide is a description of the chemical content of the molecule; it contains one carbon atom and two oxygen atoms. *Di-* is a Greek prefix meaning *two.*

oxyhemoglobin
(AWK-see-HEE-moh-GLOH-bin)
ox/y- *oxygen*
hem/o- *blood*
glob/o- *shaped like a globe; comprehensive*
-in *a substance*
The hemoglobin molecule is shaped like a globe.

oxygenated (AWK-see-jen-aa-ted)
ox/y- *oxygen*
gen/o- *arising from; produced by*
-ated *pertaining to a condition; composed of*

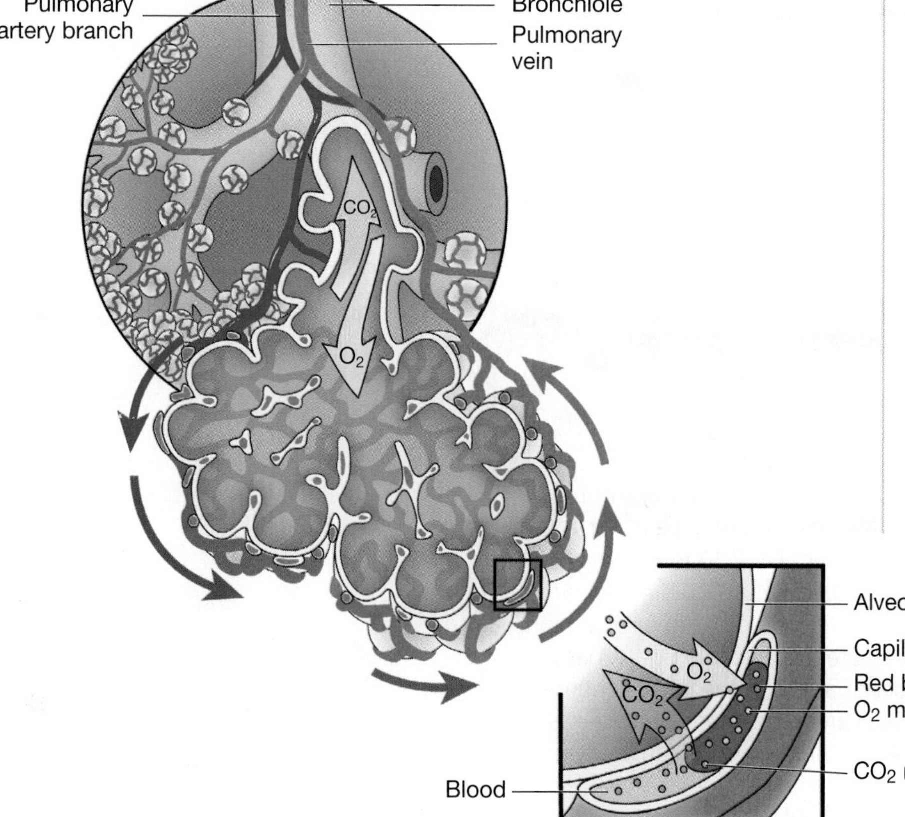

Figure 4-6 ■ Gas exchange.

Oxygen from the alveoli moves into the blood, binds to red blood cells, and is carried to the body. Carbon dioxide dissolved in the blood or carried by red blood cells moves into the alveoli and is exhaled by the lungs.

Internal respiration includes what happens to oxygen and carbon dioxide at the cellular level. Oxygen molecules leave the capillaries, enter the cells, and are used to produce energy for the cells. This process is known as **metabolism.** Carbon dioxide molecules, a byproduct of metabolism, leave the cells and enter the capillaries. These carbon dioxide molecules remain in the blood or combine with hemoglobin in the red blood cells to form carbaminohemoglobin. This **deoxygenated** blood from all the cells travels back to the heart and then to the lungs where carbon dioxide enters the alveoli and is exhaled.

internal (in-TER-nal)
intern/o- *inside*
-al *pertaining to*

metabolism (meh-TAB-oh-lizm)
metabol/o- *change, transformation*
-ism *process; disease from a specific cause*

metabolic (MET-ah-BAWL-ik)
metabol/o- *change, transformation*
-ic *pertaining to*

deoxygenated (dee-AWK-see-jen-aa-ted)
de- *reversal of; without*
ox/y- *oxygen*
gen/o- *arising from; produced by*
-ated *pertaining to a condition; composed of*

Word Alert

SOUND-ALIKE WORDS

breath (noun) the air that flows in and out of the lungs
Example: The breath of a diabetic patient can have a fruity odor to it.

breathe (verb) the action of inhaling and exhaling
Example: If you ask an asthmatic patient to breathe deeply, you might hear a wheezing sound.

mucosa (noun) a Latin word that means *mucous membrane*
Example: If a patient needs more oxygen, the oral mucosa might have a bluish coloration to it.

mucous (adjective) a descriptive word for a membrane that secretes mucus
Example: Allergies make the mucous membranes of the nose swollen and inflamed.

mucus (noun) a secretion from a mucous membrane
Example: A chronic smoker coughs often and produces a significant amount of mucus.

Across the Life Span

In the uterus, the fetus does not breathe, and its lungs are collapsed. Instead it receives oxygen from the mother's lungs via the placenta and umbilical cord. The lungs of the fetus do not function until the very first breath after birth. At that time, they must expand fully and stay expanded, as facilitated by the presence of surfactant.

The normal respiratory rate for a newborn infant is 30 to 60 breaths per minute. The normal respiratory rate for an adult is 15 to 20 breaths per minute. One inhalation and one exhalation are counted as one respiration.

As a person ages, some alveoli deteriorate. Because the body does not repair or replace alveoli, the total number of alveoli in the lungs continues to decline with age, and the remaining alveoli are less elastic. The thorax is stiff and less able to expand on inhalation. All of these changes cause decreased pulmonary function in the elderly.

Vocabulary Review

Anatomy and Physiology

Now that you have studied the anatomy and physiology of the respiratory system, take time to review those new words and descriptions. Memorize the combining forms and their definitions before going on to the next section.

Word or Phrase	Combining Form and Definition	Description
alveolus	**alveol/o-** *alveolus (air sac)*	Hollow sphere of cells in the lungs where oxygen and carbon dioxide are exchanged
apex	**apic/o-** *apex (tip)*	The rounded top of each lung
bronchus	**bronchi/o-, bronch/o-** *bronchus*	Tubular air passageway that branches off the trachea to the right or left and enters each lung. It carries inhaled and exhaled air to and from the bronchiole.
bronchiole	**bronchiol/o-** *bronchiole*	Small tubular air passageway that branches off the bronchus. It carries inhaled and exhaled air to and from the alveoli.
carbon dioxide		Exhaled gas that is a waste product of cellular metabolism
cardiopulmonary	**cardi/o-** *heart* **pulmon/o-** *lung*	Pertaining to the heart and lungs
cilia		Small hairs that flow in waves to move foreign particles away from the lungs toward the nose and the throat where they can be expelled
deoxygenated	**ox/y-** *oxygen*	Blood that contains low levels of oxygen and high levels of carbon dioxide
diaphragm	**diaphragmat/o-** *diaphragm* **phren/o-** *diaphragm; mind*	Muscular sheet that divides the thoracic cavity from the abdominal cavity. Nerve impulses from the **phrenic nerve** cause the diaphragm to contract and move inferiorly to expand the thoracic cavity during inspiration.
epiglottis	**glott/o-** *glottis (of the larynx)*	Lidlike structure that seals off the larynx, so that swallowed food goes into the esophagus
eupneic	**pne/o-** *breathing*	Pertaining to a normal rate and rhythm of breathing (eupnea)
exhalation	**hal/o-** *breathe*	Breathing out. Also known as expiration.
expiration	**spir/o-** *breathe*	Breathing out. Also known as exhalation.
hilum	**hil/o-** *hilum*	Indentation on the medial side of each lung where the bronchus, pulmonary artery, and nerves enter the lung and the pulmonary vein exits
inhalation	**hal/o-** *breathe*	Breathing in. Also known as inspiration.

Word or Phrase	Combining Form and Definition	Description
inspiration	**spir/o-** *breathe*	Breathing in. Also known as inhalation.
intercostal muscles	**cost/o-** *rib*	Muscles between the ribs that contract to pull the ribs together to forcefully expel air from the lungs
larynx	**laryng/o-** *larynx (voice box)*	Structure that contains the vocal cords and is a passageway for inhaled and exhaled air. Also known as the voice box.
lobe	**lob/o-** *lobe*	Large division of the lung, visible on the outer surface
lumen		Central opening through which air flows inside the trachea, bronchus, or bronchiole
lung	**pulmon/o-** *lung*	Organ of respiration that contains alveoli
mediastinum	**mediastin/o-** *mediastinum*	Smaller cavity within the thoracic cavity that contains the trachea and other structures not related to the respiratory system
metabolism	**metabol/o-** *change, transformation*	Process of using oxygen and glucose to produce energy for cells. Metabolism also produces byproducts like carbon dioxide and other waste products.
mucosa	**mucos/o-** *mucous membrane*	Mucous membrane that lines the respiratory tract. It warms and humidifies incoming air. It produces mucus to trap foreign particles.
nasal cavity	**nas/o-** *nose*	Hollow area inside the nose
oxygen	**ox/y-** *oxygen*	Inhaled gas that is used by each cell to produce energy in the process of metabolism
oxygenated	**ox/y-** *oxygen*	Blood that contains high levels of oxygen
oxyhemoglobin	**ox/y-** *oxygen* **hem/o-** *blood* **glob/o-** *shaped like a globe; comprehensive*	Compound that transports oxygen in the blood and is formed by the combination of oxygen with the hemoglobin of red blood cells
parenchyma	**parenchym/o-** *parenchyma (functional cells of an organ)*	Functional part of the lung (i.e., the alveoli) as opposed to the connective tissue framework
parietal pleura	**pariet/o-** *wall of a cavity*	One of the two membranes of the pleura. It lines the thoracic cavity.
pharynx	**pharyng/o-** *pharynx (throat)*	The throat. A shared passageway for both air and food.
phrenic nerve	**phren/o-** *diaphragm; mind*	Nerve that, when stimulated, causes the diaphragm to contract and initiate respiration
pleura	**pleur/o-** *pleura (lung membrane)*	Serous membrane that lines the thoracic cavity (parietal pleura) and folds back on itself (visceral pleura) to cover the surface of the lung. It secretes pleural fluid into the pleural space (space between the two layers).

Word or Phrase	Combining Form and Definition	Description
respiration	**spir/o-** *breathe* **extern/o-** *outside* **intern/o-** *inside*	The movement of air through the respiratory system and into the lungs during inhalation or inspiration and out of the lungs with exhalation or expiration. Oxygen and carbon dioxide are exchanged in the alveoli during **external** respiration. Oxygen and carbon dioxide are exchanged at the cellular level during **internal** respiration.
respiratory system	**spir/o-** *breathe*	Body system that includes the nose, nasal cavity, pharynx, larynx, trachea, bronchi, bronchioles, alveoli, and lungs. Its purpose is to bring oxygen into the body and expel carbon dioxide. Also known as the respiratory tract.
ribs	**cost/o-** *rib*	Curved bones that form the lateral parts of the bony thorax
septum	**sept/o-** *septum*	Wall of cartilage and bone that divides the nasal cavity into right and left sides
sternum	**stern/o-** *sternum (breast bone)*	Bone that forms the anterior middle part of the bony thorax
surfactant		Protein-fat compound that creates surface tension and keeps the walls of the alveolus from collapsing inward with each inhalation
thoracic cavity	**thorac/o-** *thorax (chest)* **cav/o-** *hollow space*	Hollow space within the thorax that is filled with the lungs and structures in the mediastinum
thorax	**thorac/o-** *thorax (chest)*	Bony cage of the sternum and ribs that surrounds the lungs
trachea	**trache/o-** *trachea (windpipe)*	Rigid tubular air passageway between the larynx and the bronchi. It carries inhaled and exhaled air to and from the bronchi.
tracheobronchial tree	**trache/o-** *trachea (windpipe)* **bronchi/o-** *bronchus*	Branching structures of the respiratory system that resemble an upside-down tree trunk and its branches. It includes the trachea, bronchi, and bronchioles. Also known as the bronchial tree.
turbinates		Three long bony projections (superior, middle, and inferior) in the wall of the nasal cavity. They break up and slow down inhaled air.
visceral pleura	**viscer/o-** *viscera (internal organs)*	One of the two membranes of the pleura. It covers the surface of the lung.

Labeling Exercise

A. *Match each anatomy word or phrase to its numbered structure in Figure 4-7 ■. Write that word or phrase on the blank line next to its number. Use the Answer Key at the end of the book to check your answers.*

apex of lung	bronchus	larynx	rib
base of lung	cluster of alveoli	nasal cavity	sternum
bronchioles	diaphragm	pharynx	trachea

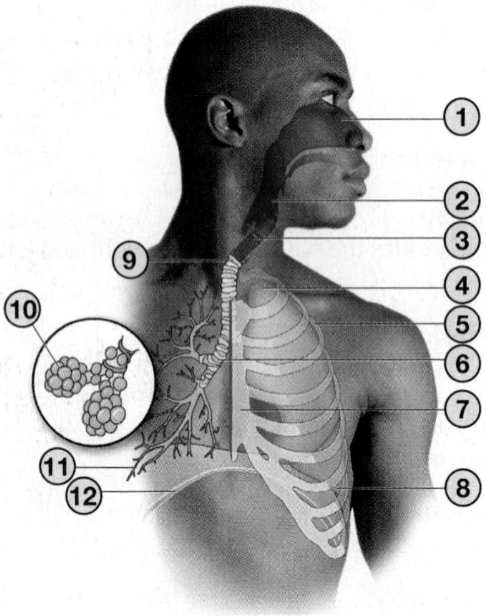

1. ____________
2. ____________
3. ____________
4. ____________
5. ____________
6. ____________
7. ____________
8. ____________
9. ____________
10. ____________
11. ____________
12. ____________

Figure 4-7 ■

B. *Match each anatomy word or phrase to its numbered structure in Figure 4-8 ■. Write that word or phrase on the blank line next to its number.*

bronchiole	carbon dioxide	oxygen
capillary	cluster of alveoli	red blood cell

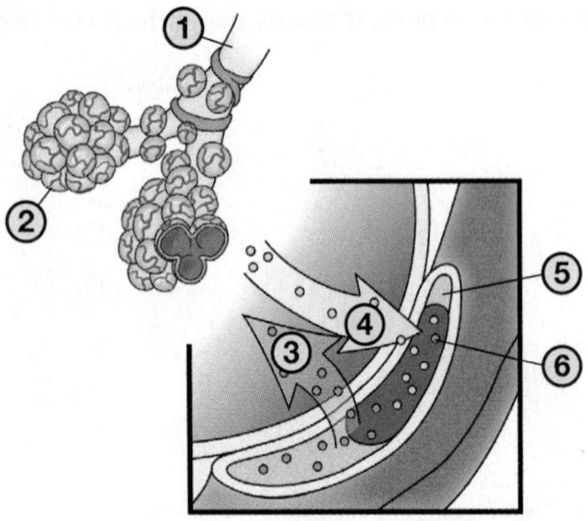

1. ____________
2. ____________
3. ____________
4. ____________
5. ____________
6. ____________

Figure 4-8 ■

Building Medical Words

Combining Forms

Here are the combining forms you have learned so far. Next to each combining form, write its meaning. Use the Answer Key at the end of the book to check your answers. The first one has been done for you.

Combining Form	Medical Meaning	Combining Form	Medical Meaning
1. alveol/o-	alveolus (air sac)	21. metabol/o-	________
2. apic/o-	________	22. muc/o-	________
3. bronchi/o-	________	23. mucos/o-	________
4. bronchiol/o-	________	24. nas/o-	________
5. bronch/o-	________	25. ox/y-	________
6. cardi/o-	________	26. parenchym/o-	________
7. cav/o-	________	27. pariet/o-	________
8. cost/o-	________	28. pharyng/o-	________
9. diaphragmat/o-	________	29. phren/o-	________
10. extern/o-	________	30. pleur/o-	________
11. gen/o-	________	31. pne/o-	________
12. glob/o-	________	32. pulmon/o-	________
13. glott/o-	________	33. sept/o-	________
14. hal/o-	________	34. ser/o-	________
15. hem/o-	________	35. spir/o-	________
16. hil/o-	________	36. stern/o-	________
17. intern/o-	________	37. thorac/o-	________
18. laryng/o-	________	38. trache/o-	________
19. lob/o-	________	39. turbin/o-	________
20. mediastin/o-	________	40. viscer/o-	________

Combining Forms and Suffixes

Read the definition hint for the medical word you are to build. Look at the combining form that is given. Write the correct suffix on the blank line. Then write the medical word. (Remember: You may need to remove the combining vowel. Always remove the hyphens and slash.) Use the Answer Key at the end of the book to check your answers. The first one has been done for you.

SUFFIX LIST

-al (pertaining to)	-ary (pertaining to)	-ole (small)
-ar (pertaining to)	-ic (pertaining to)	-ous (pertaining to)

Definition Hint	Combining Form	Suffix	Write the Medical Word
1. Pertaining to the alveolus	alveol/o-	-ar	alveolar
2. Pertaining to the nose	nas/o-	________	________
3. Pertaining to the trachea	trache/o-	________	________
4. Pertaining to the lungs	pulmon/o-	________	________

Definition Hint	Combining Form	Suffix	Write the Medical Word
5. Pertaining to a membrane that secretes a watery fluid like serum	ser/o-	________	________________
6. Pertaining to the nerve that makes the diaphragm contract	phren/o-	________	________________
7. Small bronchus	bronchi/o-	________	________________
8. Pertaining to the chest	thorac/o-	________	________________
9. Pertaining to the apex or tip	apic/o-	________	________________
10. Pertaining to a lobe of the lung	lob/o-	________	________________
11. Pertaining to the functional cells of an organ	parenchym/o-	________	________________
12. Pertaining to the ribs	cost/o-	________	________________

Combining Forms and Prefixes

Read the definition hint for the medical word you are to build. Look at the medical word or word part that is given. It already contains a combining form and a suffix. Write the correct prefix on the blank line. Then write the medical word. (Remember: You may need to remove the combining vowel. Always remove the hyphens and slash.) Use the Answer Key at the end of the book to check your answers. The first one has been done for you.

PREFIX LIST

epi- (upon, above)	ex- (out, away from)	inter- (between)
eu- (normal, good)	in- (in; without; not)	re- (again and again; backward; unable to)

Definition Hint	Prefix	Medical Word or Word Part	Write the Medical Word
1. Process of breathing in	in-	spiration	inspiration
2. Pertaining to between the ribs	________	costal	________________
3. Process of breathing again and again	________	spiration	________________
4. Pertaining to above the glottis	________	glottic	________________
5. Process of breathing out	________	halation	________________
6. Pertaining to normal breathing	________	pneic	________________

Symptoms, Signs, and Diseases

NOTE: Symptoms, signs, and diseases of the nose, nasal cavity, pharynx, and larynx are discussed in Otolaryngology (Chapter 16).

Bronchi and Bronchioles

Word or Phrase	Word Part and Definition	Description
asthma	**asthma** (AZ-mah) *Asthma* is a Greek word meaning *panting.* **bronchospasm** (BRONG-koh-spazm) **bronch/o-** *bronchus* **-spasm** *sudden, involuntary muscle contraction* **asthmatic** (az-MAT-ik) **asthm/o-** *asthma* **-atic** *pertaining to* **status asthmaticus** (STAT-us az-MAT-ih-kus) *Status* is a Latin word meaning *standing still.* A person with status asthmaticus stays in a state of continuous, severe asthma.	Sudden onset of hyperreactivity of the bronchi and bronchioles with **bronchospasm** (contraction of the smooth muscle). Inflammation and swelling severely narrow the lumens. Attacks recur intermittently and are triggered by exposure to dust, mold, cigarette smoke, inhaled chemicals, exercise, cold air, or emotional stress. Also known as reactive airway disease because the asthma is a hypersensitive reaction to a triggering agent. Symptoms include severe shortness of breath, mucus production, cough, audible wheezing, and difficulty exhaling. Patients with asthma are said to be **asthmatic. Status asthmaticus** is a prolonged, extremely severe, life-threatening asthma attack. Treatment: Inhaled bronchodilator drugs during attacks. Oxygen and epinephrine (Adrenalin) for severe attacks. **Connections** **Public Health.** Asthma is prevalent in inner-city poor children. Researchers found that exposure to cockroaches appears to be a strong asthma trigger. Extermination of live cockroaches does not eliminate the problem because cockroach droppings and carcasses remain behind the walls of apartment buildings.
bronchitis	**bronchitis** (brong-KY-tis) **bronch/o-** *bronchus* **-itis** *inflammation of*	Acute or chronic inflammation or infection of the bronchi. Inflammation due to pollution or smoking causes a constant cough, mucus production, and wheezing. Chronic bronchitis is one of the component parts of chronic obstructive pulmonary disease (COPD). Infection of the bronchi is caused by bacteria or viruses. Symptoms include coughing, mucus production, and wheezing, with a fever (if there is an infection). Treatment: Antibiotic drugs for acute bacterial bronchitis. **Did You Know?** Pack-years is a standardized way to express the amount and duration of cigarette smoking as a single number. The number of pack-years equals the number of packs smoked per day multiplied by the number of years the patient has been smoking.
bronchiectasis	**bronchiectasis** (BRONG-kee-EK-tah-sis) **bronchi/o-** *bronchus* **-ectasis** *dilation*	Chronic, permanent enlargement and loss of elasticity of the bronchi and bronchioles. Chronic inflammation destroys the smooth muscle in the walls, and the bronchi become markedly dilated. Symptoms include production of large amounts of mucus and coughing. Commonly seen in patients with cystic fibrosis. Treatment: Correct the underlying cause.

Lungs

Word or Phrase	Word Part and Definition	Description
abnormal breath sounds		Normal inspiration sounds like a soft wind rushing through a tunnel. Abnormal breath sounds include a pleural friction rub, rales, rhonchi, stridor, or wheezes.

A Closer Look

	Pleural friction rub is a creaking, grating, or rubbing sound when the two layers of the inflamed pleura rub against each other during respiration.
rales (RAWLZ)	**Rales** are irregular crackling or bubbling sounds during inspiration. Wet rales are caused by obstruction of the alveoli by fluid or infection. Dry rales are caused by chronic irritation or fibrosis.
rhonchi (RONG-kigh) *Rhonchi* is a Latin word meaning *snoring.*	**Rhonchi** are humming, whistling, or snoring sounds during inspiration or expiration. They are caused by swelling, mucus, or a foreign body that partially obstructs the bronchi.
stridor (STRY-dor)	**Stridor** is a high-pitched, harsh, crowing sound due to obstruction in the trachea or larynx.
wheezes (WHEE-zes)	**Wheezes** are high-pitched whistling or squeaking sounds during inspiration or expiration. They can often be heard without a stethoscope. They are caused by extreme narrowing of the bronchi due to bronchospasm.

Word or Phrase	Word Part and Definition	Description
adult respiratory distress syndrome (ARDS)		Precipitated by a severe infection or burns that affect the entire body. Can also be caused by direct injury to the lungs (aspiration of vomit or inhalation of chemical fumes). The alveoli are damaged because of lack of blood flow, are unable to make surfactant, and they collapse with each breath. Treatment: Oxygen. Mechanical ventilation. Treat any underlying infection.
atelectasis	**atelectasis** (AT-eh-LEK-tah-sis) **atel/o-** *incomplete* **-ectasis** *dilation* **atelectatic** (AT-eh-lek-TAT-ik)	Incomplete expansion or collapse of part or all of a lung due to mucus, tumor, trauma, or a foreign body that blocks the bronchus. The lung is said to be **atelectatic.** Also known as collapsed lung. Can develop postoperatively in patients who are breathing shallowly and have no cough reflex. Treatment: Treat the underlying condition. A chest tube may be inserted to reinflate the lung.

Word or Phrase	Word Part and Definition	Description
chronic obstructive pulmonary disease (COPD)	**chronic** (KRAW-nik) **chron/o-** *time* **-ic** *pertaining to* **obstructive** (awb-STRUK-tiv) **obstruct/o-** *blocked by a barrier* **-ive** *pertaining to* **bronchitis** (brong-KY-tis) **bronch/o-** *bronchus* **-itis** *inflammation of* **emphysema** (EM-fih-SEE-mah) **em-** *in* **phys/o-** *inflate or distend; grow* **-ema** *condition* Add words to make a correct and complete definition of *emphysema: Condition in [the lungs of excessive] inflation.* **sputum** (SPYOO-tum) *Sputum* is a Latin word meaning *to spit.*	Combination of **chronic bronchitis** and **emphysema** caused by chronic exposure to pollution or smoking. In emphysema the alveoli rupture, creating large air spaces in the lungs. Air can be inhaled but not exhaled. Symptoms include severe coughing, shortness of breath (dyspnea), **sputum** production, fatigue, and sometimes cyanosis. Due to chronic overexpansion of the lungs, the thorax becomes deformed (barrel chest). Treatment: Inhaled bronchodilator drugs and corticosteroid drugs. Oxygen therapy, if needed.
cystic fibrosis (CF)	**cystic** (SIS-tik) **cyst/o-** *bladder; fluid-filled sac; semisolid cyst* **-ic** *pertaining to* Some word parts have more than one definition. The best definition of *cystic* (in *cystic fibrosis*) is *pertaining to semisolid cysts [in the pancreas].* **fibrosis** (fy-BROH-sis) **fibr/o-** *fiber* **-osis** *condition; abnormal condition; process*	Inherited, eventually fatal disease caused by a recessive gene. Cystic fibrosis affects all the exocrine cells (those that secrete mucus, digestive enzymes, and sweat), but the respiratory system is particularly affected. Mucus is excessively viscous (thick) and blocks the alveoli and bronchioles, causing dyspnea. Constant coughing results in bronchiectasis. There are frequent bacterial infections in the lungs. The chronic lack of oxygen results in cyanosis and a unique deformity of the fingertips known as clubbing (see Figure 4-9■). Thick mucus blocks pancreatic *(continued)*

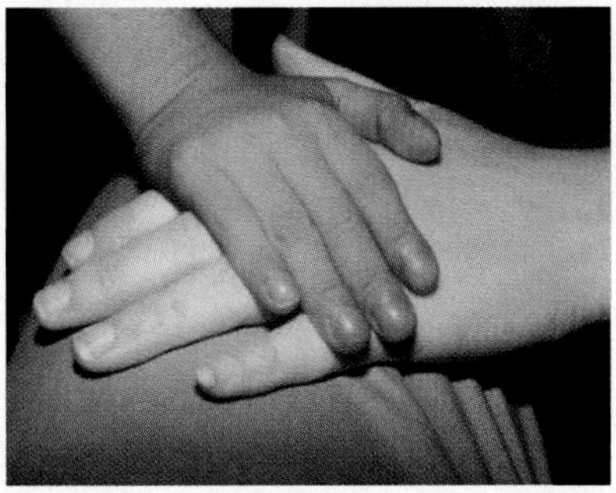

Figure 4-9 ■ Cystic fibrosis.

Cyanosis and clubbing of the fingertips are common symptoms of cystic fibrosis. Low levels of oxygen cause the blood in the arteries to be bluish rather than bright red. This is reflected in the color of the skin. The chronic lack of oxygen causes the fingertips to grow in an abnormal way.

Word or Phrase	Word Part and Definition	Description
cystic fibrosis (CF) *(continued)*		digestive enzymes and so fat is not digested properly. The patient has diarrhea and is undernourished. The pancreas develops cysts that become fibrous tissue, hence the name cystic fibrosis. The sweat glands are overactive; the patient perspires excessively, losing large amounts of salt (sodium). Life expectancy is only to young adulthood. Treatment: Daily postural drainage and chest percussion to remove mucus. Inhaled corticosteroid drugs and bronchodilator drugs, digestive enzyme supplements. High-salt diet.
influenza	**influenza** (IN-floo-EN-zah) *Influenza* is derived from an Italian word meaning *caused by the influence of the heavenly bodies.*	Acute viral infection of the upper and lower respiratory tracts. Symptoms include fever, severe muscle aches, and cough. Various strains of the virus cause flu to occur annually in the fall and winter months. Treatment: Rest, analgesic drugs, and fluids. Antibiotic drugs for a secondary bacterial infection.

Across the Life Span

Reye (RYE)

syndrome (SIN-drohm)
syn- *together*
-drome *a running*
Every medical word must contain a combining form. The suffix of *syndrome* contains the combining form *drom/o-*.

The use of aspirin to relieve the symptoms of the flu can cause **Reye's syndrome** in children. The reason for this is not known. Symptoms include very high levels of ammonia in the blood and brain, vomiting, seizures, and liver failure. These symptoms are acute and occasionally fatal. Prevention: Use of acetaminophen (Tylenol) instead of aspirin to treat symptoms of any viral infection.

Influenza plus a secondary bacterial infection can cause pneumonia and death in the elderly. Prevention: An annual flu shot is recommended for the elderly and persons with chronic disease.

Word or Phrase	Word Part and Definition	Description
empyema	**empyema** (EM-py-EE-mah) **em-** *in* **py/o-** *pus* **-ema** *condition* Add words to make a correct and complete definition of *empyema: Condition in [the lungs of] pus.* **purulent** (PYOOR-yoo-lent) **purul/o-** *pus* **-ent** *pertaining to* **pyothorax** (PY-oh-THOR-aks) **py/o-** *pus* **-thorax** *thorax (chest)*	Localized collection of **purulent** material (pus) in the thoracic cavity from an infection in the lungs. Also known as **pyothorax.** Treatment: Antibiotic drugs or surgery.

Word Alert

SOUND-ALIKE WORDS

emphysema Chronic, irreversibly damaged alveoli that become large air spaces that trap air in the lungs.
Example: Emphysema has caused this patient to have a barrel chest.

empyema Localized collection of pus in the thoracic cavity.
Example: She will be started immediately on intravenous antibiotic drugs for her empyema.

Word or Phrase	Word Part and Definition	Description
Legionnaire's disease	**Legionnaire** (lee-jen-AIR) Legionnaire's disease was named for the Legionnaires who participated in an American Legion convention where a large outbreak of the disease occurred. This is an example of an eponym: a person or thing from whom something takes its name.	Severe, sometimes fatal, bacterial infection that begins with flu-like symptoms, body aches and fever, followed by severe pneumonia with possible liver and kidney degeneration. Treatment: Antibiotic drug that is effective against this bacterium.

Did You Know?

Legionella (LEE-jeh-NEL-ah)

pneumophilia (NOO-moh-FIL-ee-ah)
- **pneum/o-** *lung; air*
- **phil/o-** *attraction to, fondness for*
- **-ia** *condition, state, thing*

Legionnaire's disease was first identified in 1976 when many people at an American Legion convention in Philadelphia became sick. They were breathing air from an air conditioning system contaminated by a bacterium that is attracted to the environment of the lungs and was subsequently named ***Legionella pneumophilia***.

Word or Phrase	Word Part and Definition	Description
lung cancer	**cancer** (KAN-ser) *Cancer* is a Latin word meaning *a crab.* Cancer begins in one location and spreads in all directions like the legs of a crab spreading out from its body. **malignant** (mah-LIG-nant) **malign/o-** *intentionally causing harm; cancer* **-ant** *pertaining to* **carcinoma** (KAR-sih-NOH-mah) **carcin/o-** *cancer* **-oma** *tumor, mass* **adenocarcinoma** (AD-eh-noh-KAR-sih-NOH-mah) **aden/o-** *gland* **carcin/o-** *cancer* **-oma** *tumor, mass*	Cancerous tumor of the lungs. More common in smokers than nonsmokers. Begins in the bronchi and causes obstruction of the airway as the tumor grows. There are several different types of lung cancer, which are named for the characteristics of the original **malignant** cell or tissue: squamous cell **carcinoma, adenocarcinoma,** large cell carcinoma, small cell carcinoma, and oat cell carcinoma. Treatment: Surgery, chemotherapy, or radiation therapy.

Word or Phrase	Word Part and Definition	Description
occupational lung diseases	**anthracosis** (AN-thrah-KOH-sis) **anthrac/o-** *coal* **-osis** *condition; abnormal condition; process* Add words to make a correct and complete definition of *anthracosis: Abnormal condition [of the lungs from inhaling] coal [dust].* **asbestosis** (AS-bes-TOH-sis) **asbest/o-** *asbestos* **-osis** *condition; abnormal condition; process* **pneumoconiosis** (NOO-moh-KOH-nee-OH-sis) **pneum/o-** *lung; air* **coni/o-** *dust* **-osis** *condition; abnormal condition; process*	Constant exposure to inhaled particles causes pulmonary fibrosis in which the alveoli lose their elasticity. **Anthracosis** (also known as coal miner's lung or black lung disease) is caused by coal dust. **Asbestosis** is caused by asbestos fibers. **Pneumoconiosis** is a general word for any occupational lung disease caused by chronically inhaling some type of dust or particle. Treatment: Inhaled bronchodilator and corticosteroid drugs.
pneumonia	**pneumonia** (noo-MOH-nee-ah) **pneumon/o-** *lung; air* **-ia** *condition, state, thing*	Inflammation or infection of some or all of the lobes of the lungs and the bronchi (see Figure 4-10■). The pneumonia is named according to its cause or its location in the lungs. Fluid from inflamed tissues, plus microorganisms and white blood cells fill the alveoli and air passages. Symptoms include difficulty breathing, cough, and sputum production. Inflammation of the pleura results in pain on inspiration. Treatment: Antibiotic drugs and oxygen therapy. Mechanical ventilation, if needed. 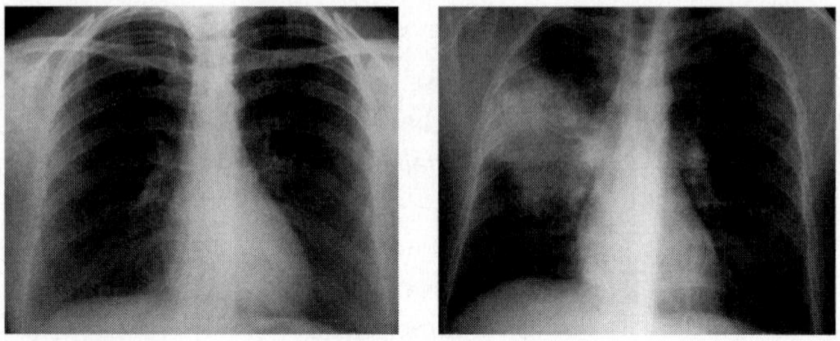 **Figure 4-10 ■ Pneumonia.** Compare the normal chest x-ray on the left with the chest x-ray on the right that shows patchy gray-white areas of pneumonia in the right upper and middle lobes.
aspiration pneumonia	**aspiration** (AS-pih-RAY-shun) **aspir/o-** *to breathe in, to suck in* **-ation** *a process; being or having*	Caused by foreign matter such as vomit that is inhaled into the lungs
bacterial pneumonia	**bacterial** (bak-TEER-ee-al) **bacteri/o-** *bacteria* **-al** *pertaining to*	Pneumonia caused by a bacterium

Word or Phrase	Word Part and Definition	Description
broncho-pneumonia	**bronchopneumonia** (BRONG-koh-noo-MOH-nee-ah) **bronch/o-** *bronchus* **pneumon/o-** *lung; air* **-ia** *condition, state, thing*	Affects the bronchi, bronchioles, and the adjacent lung tissue and alveoli
double pneumonia		Involves both lungs
lobar pneumonia	**lobar** (LOH-bar) **lob/o-** *lobe of an organ* **-ar** *pertaining to* **panlobar** (pan-LOH-bar) **pan-** *all* **lob/o-** *lobe of an organ* **-ar** *pertaining to*	Affects one part or all of a lobe of a lung. **Panlobar** pneumonia affects all the lobes of one lung.
pneumococcal pneumonia	**pneumococcal** (NOO-moh-KAW-kal) **pneum/o-** *lung; air* **cocc/o-** *spherical bacterium* **-al** *pertaining to* Add words to make a correct and complete definition of *pneumococcal: Pertaining to lungs [that are infected by a] spherical bacterium.*	Acute pneumonia caused by the bacterium *Streptococcus pneumoniae.* Prevention: Pneumococcal vaccine given to elderly patients.
***Pneumocystis carinii* pneumonia (PCP)**	***Pneumocystis carinii*** (NOO-moh-SIS-tis kah-REE-nee-eye) **opportunistic** (AWP-or-too-NIS-tik) **opportun/o-** *well-timed; taking advantage of an opportunity* **-istic** *pertaining to*	Severe form of pneumonia caused by the amoeba *Pneumocystis carinii.* Most people are infected with this microorganism in childhood. It causes a mild infection, and then lies dormant in the body within small cystlike structures. In debilitated patients, particularly those with AIDS, it emerges from the cyst and causes disease. This is known as an **opportunistic infection** because the microorganism waits for an opportunity to cause disease. Treatment: Special antibiotic drugs that are effective against amoebae. Also treat the underlying AIDS.
viral pneumonia	**viral** (VY-ral) **vir/o-** *virus* **-al** *pertaining to*	Pneumonia caused by a virus
walking pneumonia		Mild form of pneumonia caused by the bacterium *Mycoplasma pneumoniae.* The patient does not feel well but can continue daily activities.
pulmonary edema	**edema** (eh-DEE-mah) *Edema* is derived from a Greek word meaning *a swelling.*	Fluid in the alveoli because of failure of the left side of the heart to adequately pump blood. There is backup of blood in the pulmonary circulation. Symptoms include dyspnea and orthopnea. Treatment: Correct the underlying heart failure.

Word or Phrase	Word Part and Definition	Description
pulmonary embolism	**embolism** (EM-boh-lizm) **embol/o-** *embolus (occluding plug)* **-ism** *process; disease from a specific cause* **embolus** (EM-boh-lus) *Embolus* is a Greek word meaning *a plug or wedged stopper.*	Blockage of one of the pulmonary arteries by an **embolus** (blood clot or fat globule). A blood clot can develop in the legs of a patient on prolonged bedrest, or it can be a fat globule that is released from yellow marrow when a long bone is fractured. The embolus travels to the heart and into the pulmonary artery. As the pulmonary artery divides into smaller branches, the embolus becomes trapped and blocks the arterial blood flow going to that part of the lung. Symptoms include dyspnea and chest pain. A large pulmonary embolus can be fatal. Treatment: Oxygen therapy, thrombolytic drugs (to dissolve a blood clot), and anticoagulant drugs (to prevent more blood clots from forming).

Across the Life Span

sternal (STER-nal)
stern/o- *sternum (breast bone)*
-al *pertaining to*

retraction (re-TRAK-shun)
re- *again and again; backward; unable to*
tract/o- *pulling*
-ion *action; condition*

intercostal (IN-ter-KAWS-tal)
inter- *between*
cost/o- *rib*
-al *pertaining to*

Respiratory distress syndrome (RDS) develops in premature infants who lack sufficient levels of surfactant in their lungs. Signs include nasal flaring (the nostrils flare outward with each breath to draw in more air), grunting (the epiglottis closes to maintain extra pressure in the lungs to keep them from collapsing), and retractions. **Sternal retractions** bend the flexible breast bone inwards. **Intercostal retractions** pull in the soft tissue between the ribs. Also known as hyaline membrane disease (HMD). Treatment: Surfactant drug given through the endotracheal tube; oxygen therapy and ventilator support.

Word or Phrase	Word Part and Definition	Description
severe acute respiratory syndrome (SARS)		Acute viral respiratory illness that can be fatal. Symptoms include fever, dyspnea, and cough, together with a history of travel in an airplane or close contact with another SARS patient. Chest x-ray shows pneumonia or adult respiratory distress syndrome. Treatment: Oxygen therapy and ventilator support. Antibiotic drugs are not effective against viral illnesses.
tuberculosis (TB)	**tuberculosis** (too-BER-kyoo-LOH-sis) **tubercul/o-** *nodule* **-osis** *condition; abnormal condition; process* **tubercle** (TOO-ber-kl) **tuber/o-** *nodule* **-cle** *small thing* **hemoptysis** (hee-MAWP-tih-sis) **hem/o-** *blood* **-ptysis** *abnormal condition of coughing up*	Lung infection caused by the bacterium *Mycobacterium tuberculosis* and spread by airborne droplets expelled by coughing. Initially, the infection may cause few symptoms. If the patient's immune system is strong, the bacteria can remain dormant for years without causing symptoms. If the patient's immune system is depressed, the bacteria multiply, producing **tubercles** (soft nodules of necrosis) in the lungs. Symptoms include fever, cough, weight loss, night sweats, and **hemoptysis** (coughing up blood).This bacterium holds an acid stain and so it is known as an acid-fast bacillus (AFB). Its waxy, external coating resists the action of regular antibiotic drugs. Treatment: Because of a unique waxy coating around the bacterial wall of *Mycobacterium tuberculosis,* it is difficult to kill and developed a resistance to the first antitubercular drug. Now several antitubercular drugs must be used in combination for nine months to effectively treat tuberculosis.

Pleura and Thorax

Word or Phrase	Word Part and Definition	Description
hemothorax	**hemothorax** (HEE-moh-THOR-aks) **hem/o-** *blood* **-thorax** *thorax (chest)*	Presence of blood in the thoracic cavity, usually from trauma. Treatment: Thoracocentesis or insertion of a chest tube to remove blood and fluid.
pectus excavatum	**pectus excavatum** (PEK-tus EKS-kah-VAH-tum)	Congenital deformity in which the inferior tip of the sternum is positioned posteriorly, creating a hollow depression in the anterior chest wall. Treatment: Usually none.
pleural effusion	**effusion** (ee-FYOO-zhun) **effus/o-** *a pouring out* **-ion** *action; condition*	Accumulation of fluid within the pleural space due to inflammation or infection of the pleura and lungs. Treatment: Antibiotic drugs or thoracocentesis.
pleurisy	**pleurisy** (PLOOR-ih-see) **pleur/o-** *pleura (lung membrane)* **-isy** *condition of inflammation* **pleuritis** (ploo-RY-tis) **pleur/o-** *pleura (lung membrane)* **-itis** *inflammation of* **pleuritic** (ploo-RIT-ik) **pleur/o-** *pleura (lung membrane)* **-itic** *pertaining to*	Inflammation of the pleura as a result of pneumonia or other infection, trauma, or tumor. Also known as **pleuritis.** The inflamed parietal pleura and visceral pleura rub against each other, causing pain, particularly when the patient takes a deep breath. The sound heard through the stethoscope is known as a pleural friction rub. A patient with pleurisy is said to be **pleuritic.** Treatment: Treat the underlying cause.
pneumothorax	**pneumothorax** (NOO-moh-THOR-aks) **pneum/o-** *lung; air* **-thorax** *thorax (chest)*	Large volume of air that forms in the pleural space and progressively separates the two pleural membranes. This compresses or even collapses the lung. Can be caused by a penetrating injury that allows outside air to flow into the thoracic cavity. It can also occur when alveoli rupture from lung disease and release air into the thoracic cavity. Treatment: Thoracocentesis or insertion of a chest tube to remove the air.

Respiration

Word or Phrase	Word Part and Definition	Description
apnea	**apnea** (AP-nee-ah) **a-** *away from, without* **-pnea** *breathing* **obstructive** (awb-STRUK-tiv) **obstruct/o-** *blocked by a barrier* **-ive** *pertaining to* **apneic** (AP-nee-ik) **a-** *away from, without* **pne/o-** *breathing* **-ic** *pertaining to*	Brief or prolonged absence of spontaneous respirations. Causes include respiratory arrest or respiratory failure. In premature infants, the immature central nervous system fails to maintain a consistent respiratory rate, and there are occasional long pauses between periods of regular breathing. Patients with **obstructive sleep apnea** stop breathing multiple times each night because of obstruction of the airway by the soft palate or neck tissues. Apnea is followed by a gasping breath that often awakens the patient. Patients experience sleep deprivation, fatigue, and difficulty concentrating during the day. Occurs most often in middle-aged, obese men who snore excessively. Patients having an episode of apnea are said to be **apneic.** Treatment: Home apnea monitors for infants. CPAP apparatus to keep the airway open in adults.
bradypnea	**bradypnea** (brad-ip-NEE-ah) **brady-** *slow* **-pnea** *breathing*	Abnormally slow rate of breathing. May be caused by a chemical imbalance or neurological damage that affects the respiratory center of the brain. Treatment: Correct the underlying cause.

Word or Phrase	Word Part and Definition	Description
cough	**cough** (KAWF) **expectoration** (ek-SPEK-toh-RAY-shun) **ex-** *out, away from* **pector/o-** *chest* **-ation** *a process; being or having* Add words to make a correct and complete definition of *expectoration: Process [of expelling sputum] out [of the] chest.*	Protective mechanism to forcefully expel accidentally inhaled food, irritating particles (smoke, dust), or internally produced mucus. A cough may be nonproductive or productive of sputum. The process of coughing up sputum from the lungs is known as **expectoration.** Coughing up blood-tinged sputum is known as hemoptysis. Treatment: expectorant drugs for a productive cough, antitussive drugs for a nonproductive cough. Correct the underlying cause.
dyspnea	**dyspnea** (DISP-nee-ah) **dys-** *painful, difficult, abnormal* **-pnea** *breathing* **paroxysmal** (PAIR-awk-SIZ-mal) **paroxysm/o-** *sudden, sharp attack* **-al** *pertaining to* **dyspneic** (DISP-nee-ik) **dys-** *painful, difficult, abnormal* **pne/o-** *breathing* **-ic** *pertaining to*	Difficult, labored, or painful respiration due to lung disease. Also known as shortness of breath (SOB). Dyspnea on exertion (DOE) can occur after minimal activity in patients with severe COPD. **Paroxysmal nocturnal dyspnea (PND)** is shortness of breath that occurs at night (nocturnal). It is caused by fluid in the lungs because the patient is lying down. Patients are said to be **dyspneic.** Treatment: Sleeping propped up on pillows or in a chair. Oxygen therapy. Correct the underlying cause.
orthopnea	**orthopnea** (or-THAWP-nee-ah) **orth/o-** *straight* **-pnea** *breathing* Add words to make a correct and complete definition of *orthopnea: Breathing [in a] straight [up position].* **orthopneic** (or-THAWP-nee-ik) **orth/o-** *straight* **pne/o-** *breathing* **-ic** *pertaining to*	Lung disease that causes the patient to assume an upright or semi-upright position in order to breathe and sleep comfortably. Dyspnea and congestion in the lungs occur when lying down. The patient is said to be **orthopneic.** The degree of orthopnea is expressed as the number of pillows the patient needs (i.e., two-pillow orthopnea). Treatment: Oxygen therapy. Correct the underlying cause.
tachypnea	**tachypnea** (TAK-ip-NEE-ah) **tachy-** *fast* **-pnea** *breathing* **tachypneic** (TAK-ip-NEE-ik) **tachy-** *fast* **pne/o-** *breathing* **-ic** *pertaining to*	Abnormally rapid rate of breathing caused by lung disease. Patients who have tachypnea are said to be **tachypneic.** Treatment: Oxygen therapy. Correct the underlying cause.

Oxygen and Carbon Dioxide Levels

Word or Phrase	Word Part and Definition	Description
anoxia	**anoxia** (an-AWK-see-ah) **an-** *without, not* **ox/o-** *oxygen* **-ia** *condition, state, thing* **anoxic** (an-AWK-sik) **an-** *without, not* **ox/o-** *oxygen* **-ic** *pertaining to*	Complete lack of oxygen in the arterial blood and body tissues. Caused by a lack of oxygen in the inhaled air or by an obstruction that prevents oxygen from reaching the lungs. Patients are said to be **anoxic.** Treatment: Correct the underlying cause.

Across the Life Span

asphyxia (as-FIK-see-ah)
Asphyxia is a Greek word meaning *without a pulse.*

Birth **asphyxia** occurs when the fetus does not get enough oxygen through the umbilical cord and placenta before or during birth. This can be caused by a premature separation of the placenta from the uterine wall, an umbilical cord that is wrapped tightly around the neck, or an umbilical cord that is compressed by the baby's head during delivery. Asphyxia can occur at any age if a person chokes, drowns, or suffocates.

Sudden infant death syndrome (SIDS) is an acute event in which an apparently healthy infant under one year of age suddenly dies. The cause is unknown, but has been attributed to respiratory arrest from aspiration of stomach contents or asphyxiation from soft bedding blocking the flow of air. Parents are cautioned to position babies on their backs to sleep.

Word or Phrase	Word Part and Definition	Description
cyanosis	**cyanosis** (SY-ah-NOH-sis) **cyan/o-** *blue* **-osis** *condition; abnormal condition; process* **circumoral** (SER-kum-OR-al) **circum-** *around* **or/o-** *mouth* **-al** *pertaining to* **cyanotic** (SY-ah-NAWT-ik) **cyan/o-** *blue* **-tic** *pertaining to*	Bluish-gray discoloration of the skin from abnormally low levels of oxygen and abnormally high levels of carbon dioxide in the tissues. It can be seen around the mouth (**circumoral cyanosis**) or in the nailbeds (see Figure 4-9). Patients with cyanosis are said to be **cyanotic.** Treatment: Correct the underlying cause. **Connections** **Forensic Science.** When a person drowns or suffocates, there is a high level of carbon dioxide (CO_2) in the blood, and the skin shows cyanosis. When a person dies in a fire or from inhaling the fumes from car exhaust or a faulty space heater, there is a high level of carbon monoxide (CO) in the blood. Carbon monoxide binds so tightly that the hemoglobin is unable to carry any oxygen. Carbon monoxide poisoning causes a characteristic cherry red skin color.
hypercapnia	**hypercapnia** (HY-per-KAP-nee-ah) **hyper-** *above; more than normal* **capn/o-** *carbon dioxide* **-ia** *condition, state, thing*	Abnormally high level of carbon dioxide (CO_2) in the arterial blood. Treatment: Correct the underlying cause.

Word or Phrase	Word Part and Definition	Description
hypoxemia	**hypoxemia** (HY-pawk-SEE-mee-ah) **hypo-** *below; deficient* **ox/o-** *oxygen* **-emia** *condition of the blood; substance in the blood* **hypoxia** (hy-PAWK-see-ah) **hypo-** *below; deficient* **ox/o-** *oxygen* **-ia** *condition, state, thing* **hypoxic** (hy-PAWK-sik) **hypo-** *below; deficient* **ox/o-** *oxygen* **-ic** *pertaining to*	Abnormally low level of oxygen in the arterial blood. **Hypoxia** is an abnormally low level of oxygen at the cellular level. Patients with hypoxia are said to be **hypoxic.** Treatment: Correct the underlying cause.

Diagnostic Procedures

Word or Phrase	Word Part and Definition	Description
arterial blood gases (ABG)	**arterial** (ar-TEER-ee-al) **arteri/o-** *artery* **-al** *pertaining to*	Blood test to measure the partial pressure (P) of the gases oxygen (PO_2) and carbon dioxide (PCO_2) in arterial blood. The pH, how acid or alkaline the blood is, is also measured. The more carbon dioxide, the more acidic the blood and the lower the pH.
carboxyhemo-globin	**carboxyhemoglobin** (kar-BAWK-see-HEE-moh-gloh-bin) **carbox/y-** *carbon dioxide* **hem/o-** *blood* **glob/o-** *shaped like a globe; comprehensive* **-in** *a substance*	Blood test to measure the level of carbon monoxide in the blood. Carbon monoxide is a byproduct of fires or engines that burn fuel. In unventilated spaces, carbon monoxide from smoke or car exhaust builds up, combining with hemoglobin in the blood to form carboxyhemo-globin. This prevents the hemoglobin from carrying oxygen or carbon dioxide molecules. Carboxyhemoglobin blood levels above 50% are fatal.
pulmonary function tests (PFTs)	**spirometry** (spih-RAWM-eh-tree) **spir/o-** *breathe* **-metry** *process of measuring*	Diagnostic procedure to measure the capacity of the lungs and the volume of air during inhalation and exhalation. The FVC (forced vital capacity) measures the amount of air that can be forcefully exhaled from the lungs after the deepest inhalation. The FEV_1 (forced expiratory volume in one second) measures the volume of air that can be forcefully exhaled during the first second of measuring the FVC. **Spirometry,** the measurement of the FEV_1 and FVC, produces a tracing on a graph.

Word or Phrase	Word Part and Definition	Description
pulse oximetry	**oximetry** (awk-SIM-eh-tree) **ox/i-** *oxygen* **-metry** *process of measuring* **oximeter** (awk-SIM-eh-ter) **ox/i-** *oxygen* **-meter** *instrument used to measure*	Diagnostic procedure in which a pulse **oximeter**, a small, noninvasive clip device, is placed on the patient's index finger or earlobe to measure the degree of oxygen saturation of the blood (see Figure 4-11■). It emits light waves that penetrate the skin and are absorbed or reflected by saturated hemoglobin bound to oxygen versus unsaturated hemoglobin. The oximeter then calculates the oxygen saturation. The oximeter does not measure CO_2 levels. 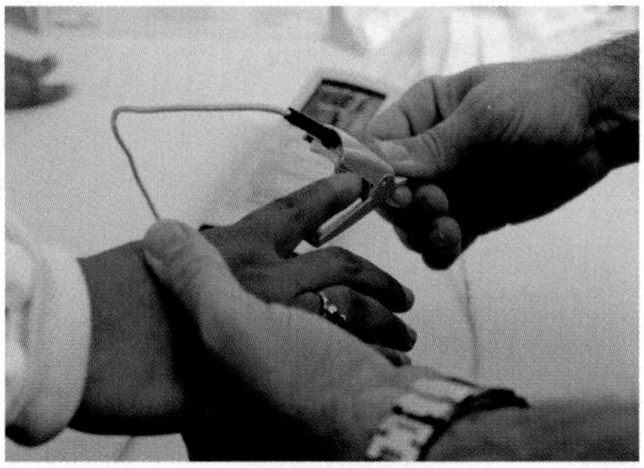 **Figure 4-11 ■ Pulse oximeter.** This device is used in ambulances and in hospitals (at the patient's bedside, and in the intensive care unit, operating room, and recovery room) to provide a quick and accurate readout of the degree of oxygen saturation of the patient's blood.
sputum culture and sensitivity (C&S)	**sensitivity** (SEN-sih-TIV-ih-tee) **sensitiv/o-** *affected by, sensitive to* **-ity** *state; condition*	Diagnostic test to identify which bacterium is causing a pulmonary infection and then determine its sensitivity to various antibiotic drugs (see Figure 4-12■). Material from a sputum specimen or needle aspiration of pleural fluid is tested. 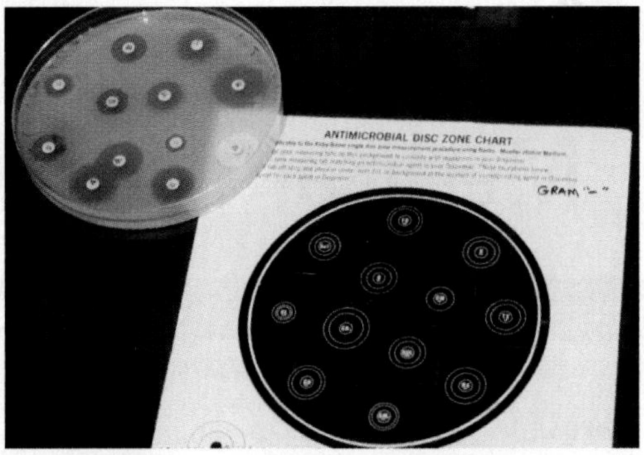 **Figure 4-12 ■ Culture and sensitivity.** Paper disks containing various antibiotics are placed in a bacterial culture. If the bacteria are sensitive to that particular antibiotic drug, there will be a zone of inhibition or no growth around that particular disk.

Word or Phrase	Word Part and Definition	Description
tuberculosis tests	**Mantoux** (man-TOO)	Screening tests used to determine if a patient has been exposed to tuberculosis recently or in the past. The tine test uses a four-pronged device (similar to the tines on a fork) that punctures the skin and introduces PPD (purified protein derivative), part of the bacterium *Mycobacterium tuberculosis.* In the **Mantoux test,** a more definitive test, an intradermal injection of PPD is given. A raised skin reaction after 48 to 72 hours indicates antibodies to the bacterium because of prior exposure. A positive Mantoux test is followed up with a chest x-ray to confirm whether or not active tuberculosis is present.
Radiology and Nuclear Medicine Procedures		
chest radiography	**radiography** (RAY-dee-AWG-rah-fee) **radi/o-** *radius (forearm bone); x-rays; radiation* **-graphy** *process of recording*	Radiologic procedure that uses x-rays to create an image of lung fields. Also known as a chest x-ray (CXR). In an AP (anteroposterior) chest x-ray, the x-rays enter the patient's body through the anterior chest and then penetrate the x-ray plate. In a PA (posteroanterior) chest x-ray, the x-rays enter through the patient's back. In a lateral chest x-ray, the x-rays enter through the patient's side. A PA and left lateral chest x-ray are commonly ordered together.
CT scan and MRI scan	**tomography** (toh-MAWG-rah-fee) **tom/o-** *a cut, slice, or layer* **-graphy** *process of recording*	Radiologic procedures that scan a narrow slice of tissue and create an image. A computer then assembles all of the "slices" into a three-dimensional image. This process is known as **tomography.** CT and MRI scans are more sensitive than radiography and are able to detect small primary tumors in the lung as well as areas of metastases.
lung scan	**ventilation** (VEN-tih-LAY-shun) **ventil/o-** *movement of air* **-ation** *a process; being or having* **perfusion** (per-FYOO-zhun) **per-** *through* **fus/o-** *pouring* **-ion** *action; condition*	Nuclear medicine procedure that uses inhaled radioactive gas to show air flow (ventilation) in the lungs. Areas of decreased uptake ("cold spots") indicate pneumonia, atelectasis, or pleural effusion. A radioactive solution is given intravenously for the perfusion part of the scan. Areas of decreased uptake indicate poor blood flow to that part of the lung. If the same area shows decreased uptake on both scans, this indicates a pulmonary embolus. Also known as a **ventilation-perfusion (V/Q) scan.**

Medical and Surgical Procedures

Medical Procedures

Word or Phrase	Word Part and Definition	Description
auscultation	**auscultation** (AWS-kul-TAY-shun) **auscult/o-** *listening* **-ation** *a process; being or having* **stethoscope** (STETH-oh-skohp) **steth/o-** *chest* **-scope** *instrument used to examine*	Medical procedure that uses a **stethoscope** to listen to breath sounds (see Figure 4-15).

Word or Phrase	Word Part and Definition	Description
cardiopulmonary resuscitation (CPR)	**cardiopulmonary** (KAR-dee-oh-PUL-moh-nair-ee) **cardi/o-** *heart* **pulmon/o-** *lung* **-ary** *pertaining to* **resuscitation** (ree-SUS-ih-TAY-shun) **resuscit/o-** *revive or raise up again* **-ation** *a process; being or having*	Medical procedure to ventilate the lungs and artificially circulate the blood if the patient has stopped breathing and the heart has stopped. Mouth-to-mouth resuscitation involves forcing air into the victim's lungs and doing chest compressions to manually pump blood through the heart.
endotracheal intubation	**endotracheal** (EN-doh-TRAY-kee-al) **endo-** *innermost, within* **trache/o-** *trachea (windpipe)* **-al** *pertaining to* **intubation** (IN-too-BAY-shun) **in-** *in; within; not* **tub/o-** *tube* **-ation** *a process; being or having* **laryngoscope** (lah-RING-goh-skohp) **laryng/o-** *larynx (voice box)* **-scope** *instrument used to examine*	Medical procedure that inserts an endotracheal tube (ETT) between the vocal cords in the larynx and into the trachea in order to establish an airway for the patient to breathe through or to manually or mechanically ventilate the patient (see Figure 4-13■). A battery-powered, lighted **laryngoscope** helps visualize the vocal cords. This procedure is performed by paramedics in the field, by physicians in the emergency department, and by anesthesiologists in the operating room. 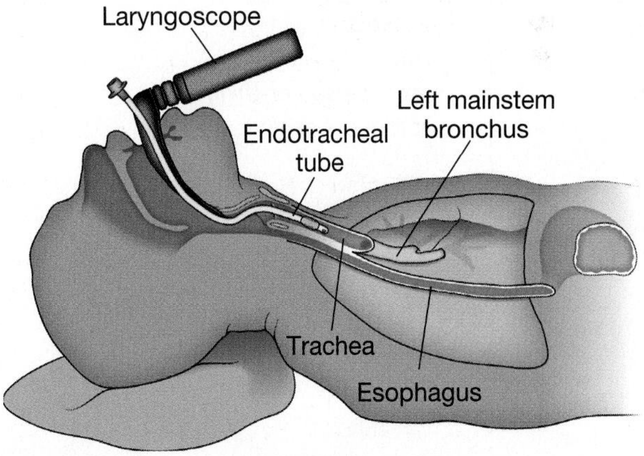 **Figure 4-13 ■ Endotracheal intubation.** A laryngoscope is used to visualize the vocal cords prior to insertion of the endotracheal tube. The endotracheal tube is positioned in the trachea, just above the bronchi. A small balloon at the tip of the tube is inflated to hold the tube in place. The external part of the tube is also taped to the patient's cheek.
Heimlich maneuver	**Heimlich** (HYM-lik) The Heimlich maneuver was developed in 1974 by Harry Heimlich, M.D. (1920–), an American thoracic surgeon. This is an example of an eponym: a person from whom something takes its name.	Medical procedure to assist a choking victim with an airway obstruction. The rescuer stands behind the victim and places a fist on the victim's abdominal wall just below the diaphragm, grasps the fist with the other hand and, with both hands, gives a sudden push inward and upward. This generates a burst of air that pushes the obstruction into the mouth where it can be expelled.

Word or Phrase	Word Part and Definition	Description
incentive spirometry	**spirometry** (spih-RAWM-eh-tree) **spir/o-** *breathe* **-metry** *process of measuring* **spirometer** (spih-RAWM-eh-ter) **spir/o-** *breathe* **-meter** *instrument used to measure*	Medical procedure to encourage patients to breathe deeply. A **spirometer** is a portable plastic device with a mouthpiece and balls that move as the patient inhales forcefully.
oxygen therapy	**cannula** (KAN-yoo-lah) *Cannula* is a Latin word meaning *a little hollow reed.* **ventilator** (VEN-tih-LAY-tor) **ventil/o-** *movement of air* **-ator** *person or thing that produces or does* **respirator** (RES-pih-RAY-tor) **re-** *again and again; backward; unable to* **spir/o-** *breathe* **-ator** *person or thing that produces or does*	Medical procedure to provide supplemental oxygen to patients with pulmonary disease. Room air is 21% oxygen. Patients with respiratory conditions may require amounts of oxygen ranging from 22% to 100%. Oxygen can be delivered to a patient via a **nasal cannula** (see Figure 4-14■) or a face mask. An infant can receive oxygen through a rigid plastic hood placed over the head or an oxygen tent. Oxygen alone is very drying, so it is always humidified (bubbled through water). Patients who require respiratory assistance as well as oxygen are placed on a **ventilator (respirator),** a mechanical device that breathes

Figure 4-14 ■ Nasal cannula.

This patient is receiving oxygen therapy through a nasal cannula, a plastic tube with two short, flexible prongs that rest just inside the patient's nostrils. A nasal cannula can provide an oxygen concentration up to 45%.

(continued)

Word	Word Part and Definition	Description
oxygen therapy *(continued)*	**Ambu** (AM-boo)	for the patient with every breath or assists with some breaths. Ventilators can provide oxygen up to 100%, as well as pressure to keep the lungs expanded. An **Ambu bag** is a hand-held device that is used to manually breathe for the patient on a temporary basis. It is attached to a face mask or to an endotracheal tube and squeezed to force air into the lungs (see Figure 4-15■). **Figure 4-15 ■ Endotracheal tube and Ambu bag.** This infant in the pediatric intensive care unit has an endotracheal tube to assist with breathing. One nurse is using a stethoscope to auscultate the infant's breath sounds. The other nurse is squeezing the Ambu bag to breathe for the infant until the endotracheal tube is reconnected to the ventilator. This infant's left chest is bandaged because a chest tube was inserted. The chest tube is visible as the yellow tubing at the right-hand bottom of the picture.
vital signs		Medical procedure during a physical examination in which the temperature, pulse, and respirations (TPR) are measured. The respirations are measured by counting the rise and fall of the thorax as one breath.
Surgical Procedures		
bronchoscopy	**bronchoscopy** (brong-KAWS-koh-pee) **bronch/o-** *bronchus* **-scopy** *process of using an instrument to examine* **bronchoscope** (BRONG-koh-skohp) **bronch/o-** *bronchus* **-scope** *instrument used to examine*	Surgical procedure that uses a flexible, lighted **bronchoscope** inserted through the mouth to examine the trachea and bronchi. Attachments on the bronchoscope can be used to remove foreign bodies, suction thick mucus, or perform a biopsy.
chest tube insertion		Surgical procedure that uses a clear plastic tube inserted between the ribs into the thoracic cavity to remove air or blood due to trauma or infection. The tube is connected to a measuring container. Used to treat pneumothorax, pyothorax, and hemothorax.

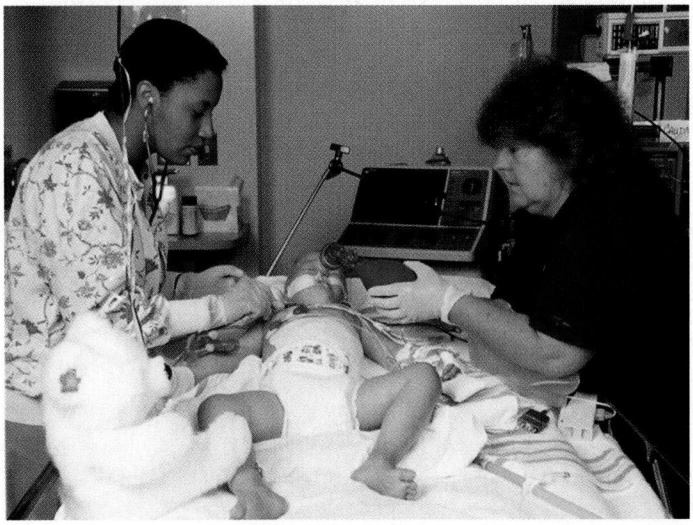

Word or Phrase	Word Part and Definition	Description
lung resection	**resection** (ree-SEK-shun) **resect/o-** *to cut out and remove* **-ion** *action; condition* **lobectomy** (loh-BEK-toh-mee) **lob/o-** *lobe of an organ* **-ectomy** *surgical excision* **pneumonectomy** (NOO-moh-NEK-toh-mee) **pneumon/o-** *lung; air* **-ectomy** *surgical excision*	Surgical procedure to remove a part or all of a lung. A wedge resection removes a small wedge-shaped piece of tissue from one lobe. A segmental resection removes a large piece or segment of one lobe. A **lobectomy** removes an entire lobe. A **pneumonectomy** removes an entire lung. Usually performed to treat lung cancer.
thoracocentesis	**thoracocentesis** (THOR-ah-koh-sen-TEE-sis) **thorac/o-** *thorax (chest)* **-centesis** *procedure to puncture*	Surgical procedure that uses a needle and syringe to remove pleural fluid from the pleural space. Used to treat pleural effusion or obtain fluid for the diagnosis of lung cancer. Also known as thoracentesis.
thoracotomy	**thoracotomy** (THOR-ah-KAWT-oh-mee) **thorac/o-** *thorax (chest)* **-tomy** *process of cutting or making an incision*	Incision into the thoracic cavity as the first step in some surgical procedures on the thoracic cavity and lungs.
tracheostomy	**tracheostomy** (TRAY-kee-AWS-toh-mee) **trache/o-** *trachea (windpipe)* **-stomy** *surgically created opening* **tracheotomy** (TRAY-kee-AWT-oh-mee) **trache/o-** *trachea (windpipe)* **-tomy** *process of cutting or making an incision*	Incision into the trachea (**tracheotomy**) and creation of a permanent opening. A plastic or metal tracheostomy tube is then inserted to keep the opening patent (see Figure 4-16■). Tracheostomies are performed to provide permanent access to the lungs in patients who need long-term respiratory support, usually with a ventilator. 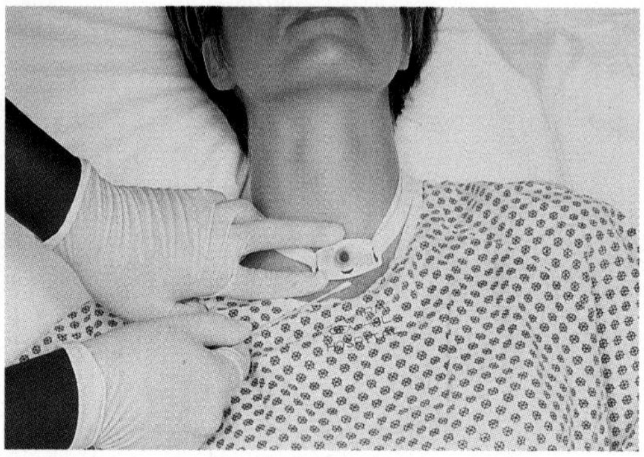 **Figure 4-16 ■ Tracheostomy tube.** This patient has a permanent tracheostomy. The tracheostomy tube has a wide flange around it with slots where cotton tape can be inserted and tied around the neck to secure the tube in the trachea.

Drug Categories

Several different categories of drugs are used to treat the symptoms, signs, and diseases of the respiratory system. The most common drugs in each category are listed.

Category	Word Part and Definition	Description	Example
antibiotic drugs	**antibiotic** (AN-tee-by-AWT-ik) (AN-tih-by-AWT-ik) **anti-** *against* **bi/o-** *life; living organisms; living tissue* **-tic** *pertaining to*	Treat bacterial respiratory infections, including acute bronchitis and pneumonia. Antibiotic drugs are not effective against viral respiratory infections.	ampicillin, amoxicillin, Cipro, Rocephin, Tequin
antitubercular drugs	**antitubercular** (AN-tee-too-BER-kyoo-lar) **anti-** *against* **tubercul/o-** *nodule; tuberculosis* **-ar** *pertaining to*	Treat tuberculosis. Several of these drugs must be used together in combination to be effective.	isoniazid (INH), Myambutol, rifampin
antitussive drugs	**antitussive** (AN-tee-TUS-iv) **anti-** *against* **tuss/o-** *cough* **-ive** *pertaining to*	Suppress the cough center in the brain. Used to treat chronic bronchitis and nonproductive coughs. Some of these drugs contain a narcotic.	dextromethorphan, Hycodan
bronchodilator drugs	**bronchodilator** (BRONG-koh-DY-lay-tor) **bronch/o-** *bronchus* **dilat/o-** *dilate, widen* **-or** *person or thing that produces or does*	Dilate constricted airways by relaxing the smooth muscles that surround the bronchioles and bronchi. Used to treat asthma, COPD, emphysema, and cystic fibrosis. Given orally or inhaled through a metered-dose inhaler (MDI) (see Figure 4-17■).	Proventil, Serevent, theophylline (Theo-Dur)
chemotherapy drugs	**chemotherapy** (KEE-moh-THAIR-ah-pee) **chem/o-** *chemical, drug* **-therapy** *treatment*	Kill rapidly dividing cancer cells in the lungs.	Adriamycin, Cytoxan, methotrexate, VePesid

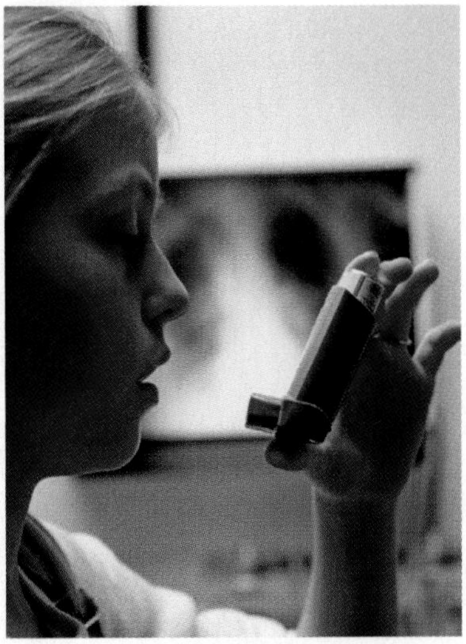

Figure 4-17 ■ Metered-dose inhaler.
A metered-dose inhaler (MDI) automatically delivers a premeasured dose of medication—a bronchodilator or corticosteroid—into the lungs as the patient inhales through the mouth. The dosage is prescribed as the number of metered sprays which are known as puffs.

Category	Word Part and Definition	Description	Example
corticosteroid drugs	**corticosteroid** (KOR-tih-koh-STAIR-oyd) **cortic/o-** *cortex (outer region)* **-steroid** *steroid* Corticosteroids produced in the cortex (outer region) of the adrenal glands have a powerful, natural anti-inflammatory effect. Synthetic corticosteroids are manufactured and used as drugs.	Block the immune system from causing inflammation in the lung. Used to treat asthma and COPD. Inhaled via metered-dose inhaler.	Azmacort, Flovent
expectorant drugs	**expectorant** (ek-SPEK-toh-rant) **ex-** *out, away from* **pector/o-** *chest* **-ant** *pertaining to*	Reduce the thickness of sputum so that it can be coughed up. Used to treat productive coughs.	guaifenesin
leukotriene receptor blockers	**leukotriene** (LOO-koh-TRY-een)	Block leukotriene which causes inflammation and edema. Used to treat asthma.	Singulair
mast cell stabilizer drugs		Stabilize mast cells in the respiratory tract and prevent them from releasing histamine that causes bronchospasm during an allergic reaction. Used to treat asthma.	cromolyn (Intal)

Abbreviations

ABG	arterial blood gases
AFB	acid-fast bacillus
A&P	auscultation and percussion
AP	anteroposterior (view on chest x-ray)
ARDS	adult respiratory distress syndrome; acute respiratory distress syndrome
bagged	manually ventilated with an Ambu bag (slang)
BS	breath sounds
C&S	culture and sensitivity
CF	cystic fibrosis
CO	carbon monoxide
CO_2	carbon dioxide
COPD	chronic obstructive pulmonary disease
CPAP	continuous positive airway pressure
CPR	cardiopulmonary resuscitation
CXR	chest x-ray
DOE	dyspnea on exertion
ETT	endotracheal tube
FEV_1	forced expiratory volume (in one second)
FiO_2	fraction (percentage) of inspired oxygen
FVC	forced vital capacity
HMD	hyaline membrane disease
LLL	left lower lobe (of the lung)
LUL	left upper lobe (of the lung)
MDI	metered-dose inhaler
O_2	oxygen
PA	posteroanterior (view on chest x-ray)
PCO_2	partial pressure of carbon dioxide (also pCO_2)
PCP	*Pneumocystis carinii* pneumonia
PFTs	pulmonary function tests
PND	paroxysmal noctural dyspnea
PO_2	partial pressure of oxygen (also pO_2)
PPD	protein purified derivative (TB test); packs per day (of cigarettes)
RA	room air (no supplemental oxygen)
RDS	respiratory distress syndrome
RLL	right lower lobe (of the lung)
RML	right middle lobe (of the lung)
RRT	registered respiratory therapist
RUL	right upper lobe (of the lung)
SARS	severe acute respiratory syndrome
SIDS	sudden infant death syndrome
SOB	shortness of breath
TB	tuberculosis
TPR	temperature, pulse, and respiration
trach	tracheostomy (slang)
URI	upper respiratory infection
V/Q	ventilation-perfusion (scan)

Word Alert

MEDICAL ABBREVIATIONS

Abbreviations are commonly used in all types of medical documents; however, they can mean different things to different people and their meaning can be misinterpreted. Always verify the meaning of an abbreviation.

A&P stands for *auscultation and percussion,* but it can also stand for *anatomy and physiology.*

BS stands for *breath sounds,* but it can also stand for *bowel sounds.*

C&S stands for *culture and sensitivity,* but it can be confused with the sound-alike word *CNS,* which stands for *central nervous system.*

PCP stands for *Pneumocystis carinii pneumonia,* but it can also stand for *primary care physician* or for the illegal drug *phencyclidine* (street name *angel dust*).

PND stands for *paroxysmal nocturnal dyspnea,* but it can also stand for *postnasal drip.*

PPD stands for *purified protein derivative* (TB test), but it can also stand for *packs [of cigarettes smoked] per day.*

RA stands for *room air,* but it can also stand for *rheumatoid arthritis* or *right atrium* (of the heart).

Career Focus

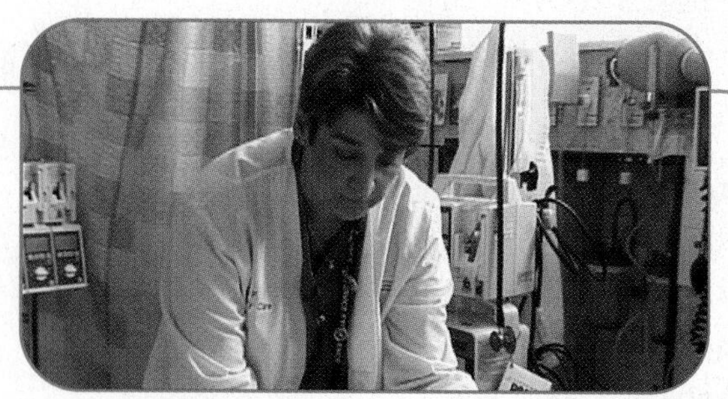

Meet Susan, a respiratory therapist in a hospital.

"I love my job. I've been doing it for 36 years. I probably could retire, but I choose not to. We treat neonates to geriatrics. We treat asthma, COPD, and pulmonary fibrosis patients and the patient's family. We also manage oxygen therapy, nebulizer therapy, medication therapy. We do pulmonary function technology and blood gases. I feel that being a respiratory therapist allows me to feel respected and appreciated, not only by the medical staff, but with patient care. You are dealing with the patient directly, as well as the physician. You feel good by the end of the day when you leave."

Respiratory therapists are allied health professionals who perform pulmonary function tests and administer respiratory therapy with various types of equipment that provide oxygen or respiratory assistance to a patient.

Pulmonologists are physicians who practice in the medical specialty of pulmonology. They diagnose and treat patients with respiratory problems. When pulmonologists perform surgery, they are known as thoracic surgeons. Physicians can take additional training and become board certified in the subspecialty of pediatric pulmonology. Cancerous tumors of the lungs are treated medically by an oncologist or surgically by a thoracic or **cardiothoracic** surgeon.

therapist (THAIR-ah-pist)
therap/o- *treatment*
-ist *one who specializes in*

pulmonologist (PUL-moh-NAWL-oh-jist)
pulmon/o- *lung*
log/o- *the study of*
-ist *one who specializes in*

cardiothoracic (KAR-dee-oh-thoh-RAS-ik)
cardi/o- *heart*
thorac/o- *thorax (chest)*
-ic *pertaining to*

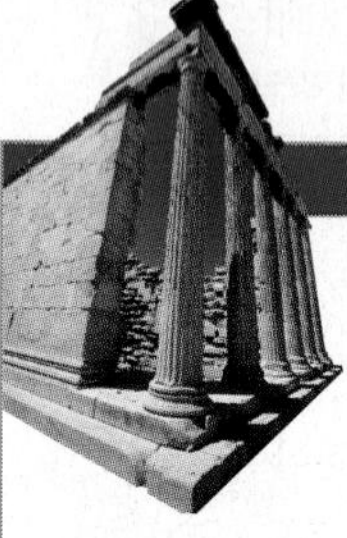

It's Greek to Me!

Did you notice that some pulmonary words have two different combining forms? Combining forms from both Greek and Latin languages remain a part of medical language today.

English Word	Greek	Latin	Examples of Medical Words
breathe, air	spir/o-	hal/o-	respiration, inspiration, inhalation, exhalation
	pne/o-		eupnea, bradypnea, tachypnea
chest	thorac/o	steth/o-	thoracic, stethoscope
	pector/o-		expectorant
lung	pneum/o-	pulmon/o-	pneumococcus, pneumoconiosis, pulmonary
	pneumon/o-		pneumonia, pneumonectomy
pus	py/o-	purul/o-	pyothorax, empyema, purulent

CHAPTER REVIEW EXERCISES

Review all the material in this chapter by completing the review exercises in this section. Use the Answer Key at the end of the book to check your answers.

Anatomy and Physiology

Matching Exercise

Match each numbered word or phrase to its description.

1. apex	____ Small passageways that end in several alveoli
2. turbinates	____ Impulse from this structure causes diaphragm to contract
3. cilia	____ Projections of bone in the nasal cavity that break up the inhaled air
4. trachea	____ Small hairs in the mucosa that move in waves
5. bronchi	____ Connecting passageways between the trachea and the bronchioles
6. bronchioles	____ Air sacs that are the functional units of the lung
7. alveoli	____ Double-layer membrane around the lungs and thoracic cavity
8. pleura	____ Muscular wall that moves on inhalation
9. diaphragm	____ Topmost part of either lung
10. thorax	____ Bony cage surrounding the lungs
11. phrenic nerve	____ Connecting passageway between the larynx and the bronchi

Circle Exercise

Circle the correct word from the choices given.

1. The top of the lung is known as the (**alveolus, apex, capillary**).
2. The (**bronchi, lungs, pleura**) have smooth muscle around them that can contract.
3. The bronchus, pulmonary artery, and pulmonary veins enter and exit the lung at the (**alveolus, base, hilum**).
4. The functional part of the lung that is made up of the alveoli is known collectively as the (**bronchioles, mediastinum, parenchyma**).
5. Swallowed food does not go into the trachea because of the (**epiglottis, pharynx, turbinates**).
6. (**Carbon dioxide, Oxygen, Surfactant**) keeps the alveoli from collapsing with each breath.
7. The (**diaphragm, phrenic nerve, thorax**) carries an impulse from the respiratory center of the brain to initiate inspiration.

True or False

Indicate whether each statement is true or false by writing T or F on the line.

1. ____ *Inhalation* is another word for *inspiration*.
2. ____ A serous membrane secretes mucus.
3. ____ The upper respiratory system includes the nose, throat, and lungs.
4. ____ Oxygen is carried in the blood in the form of oxyhemoglobin in a red blood cell.
5. ____ The pharynx is an air passageway between the nasal cavity and the bronchi.
6. ____ The alveoli are divided into lobes.
7. ____ The visceral pleura is a mucous membrane on the surface of the lung.
8. ____ A normal depth and rate of respirations is known as eupnea.
9. ____ Deoxygenated blood contains low levels of oxygen.

Sequencing Exercise

Beginning where air enters the nose, use the list of anatomical structures given here to help you sequence the structures of the respiratory tract in their correct order. The first one has been done for you

nose	trachea	larynx
bronchioles	pharynx	bronchi
nasal cavity	alveoli	hilum

1. nose ________ → 2. ________ → 3. ________ →
4. ________ → 5. ________ → 6. ________ →
7. ________ → 8. ________ → 9. ________

Medical Language Word Parts

Name that Word Part

Identify each of the word parts given here by writing in the correct letter (P, C, or S) on the line beside it. Then write the definition of the word part on the blank line. The first one has been done for you.

Prefix = P **Combining Form = C** **Suffix = S**

	Word Part	Definition		Word Part	Definition
1. -al	S	pertaining to	24. basil/o-	____	________
2. a-	____	________	25. bi/o-	____	________
3. aden/o-	____	________	26. brady-	____	________
4. alveol/o-	____	________	27. bronchi/o-	____	________
5. an-	____	________	28. bronchiol/o-	____	________
6. -ant	____	________	29. bronch/o-	____	________
7. anti-	____	________	30. capn/o-	____	________
8. anthrac/o-	____	________	31. carbox/y-	____	________
9. apic/o-	____	________	32. carcin/o-	____	________
10. -ar	____	________	33. cardi/o-	____	________
11. arteri/o-	____	________	34. cav/o-	____	________
12. -ary	____	________	35. -centesis	____	________
13. aspir/o-	____	________	36. chron/o-	____	________
14. asthm/o-	____	________	37. circum-	____	________
15. -ate	____	________	38. cocc/o-	____	________
16. -ated	____	________	39. coni/o-	____	________
17. atel/o-	____	________	40. cortic/o-	____	________
18. -atic	____	________	41. cost/o-	____	________
19. -ation	____	________	42. cyan/o-	____	________
20. -ator	____	________	43. cyst/o-	____	________
21. -atory	____	________	44. de-	____	________
22. auscult/o-	____	________	45. diaphragmat/o-	____	________
23. bacteri/o-	____	________	46. dilat/o-	____	________

		Word Part	Definition			Word Part	Definition
47.	dys-	______	______	89.	mediastin/o-	______	______
48.	-eal	______	______	90.	metabol/o-	______	______
49.	-ectasis	______	______	91.	-meter	______	______
50.	-ectomy	______	______	92.	-metry	______	______
51.	effus/o-	______	______	93.	mucos/o-	______	______
52.	em-	______	______	94.	nas/o-	______	______
53.	-ema	______	______	95.	obstruct/o-	______	______
54.	embol/o-	______	______	96.	-ole	______	______
55.	-emia	______	______	97.	-oma	______	______
56.	endo-	______	______	98.	opportun/o-	______	______
57.	epi-	______	______	99.	or/o-	______	______
58.	eu-	______	______	100.	orth/o-	______	______
59.	ex-	______	______	101.	-or	______	______
60.	extern/o-	______	______	102.	-ory	______	______
61.	fibr/o-	______	______	103.	-osis	______	______
62.	fus/o-	______	______	104.	-ous	______	______
63.	gen/o-	______	______	105.	ox/i-	______	______
64.	glob/o-	______	______	106.	ox/o-	______	______
65.	glott/o-	______	______	107.	ox/y-	______	______
66.	-graphy	______	______	108.	pan-	______	______
67.	hal/o-	______	______	109.	parenchym/o-	______	______
68.	hem/o-	______	______	110.	pariet/o-	______	______
69.	hil/o-	______	______	111.	paroxysm/o-	______	______
70.	hyper-	______	______	112.	pector/o-	______	______
71.	hypo-	______	______	113.	per-	______	______
72.	-ia	______	______	114.	pharyng/o-	______	______
73.	-ic	______	______	115.	phren/o-	______	______
74.	in-	______	______	116.	phys/o-	______	______
75.	-in	______	______	117.	pleur/o-	______	______
76.	inter-	______	______	118.	-pnea	______	______
77.	intern/o-	______	______	119.	pne/o-	______	______
78.	-ion	______	______	120.	pneum/o-	______	______
79.	-ism	______	______	121.	pneumon/o-	______	______
80.	-istic	______	______	122.	-ptysis	______	______
81.	-isy	______	______	123.	pulmon/o-	______	______
82.	-itis	______	______	124.	py/o-	______	______
83.	-ity	______	______	125.	radi/o-	______	______
84.	-ive	______	______	126.	re-	______	______
85.	laryng/o-	______	______	127.	resect/o-	______	______
86.	lob/o-	______	______	128.	resuscit/o-	______	______
87.	-logy	______	______	129.	-scope	______	______
88.	malign/o-	______	______	130.	-scopy	______	______

		Word Part	Definition
131.	sept/o-	______	______________
132.	ser/o-	______	______________
133.	-spasm	______	______________
134.	spir/o-	______	______________
135.	steth/o-	______	______________
136.	stern/o-	______	______________
137.	-steroid	______	______________
138.	-stomy	______	______________
139.	tachy-	______	______________
140.	thorac/o-	______	______________
141.	-thorax	______	______________
142.	-tic	______	______________
143.	tom/o-	______	______________
144.	-tomy	______	______________
145.	-tor	______	______________
146.	-tous	______	______________
147.	trache/o-	______	______________
148.	tract/o-	______	______________
149.	tubercul/o-	______	______________
150.	tub/o-	______	______________
151.	turbin/o-	______	______________
152.	tuss/o-	______	______________
153.	ventil/o-	______	______________
154.	vir/o-	______	______________
155.	viscer/o-	______	______________

Combining Form Exercise

Define each combining form and give one example of a pulmonology word that contains that combining form. Then define that medical word. The first one has been done for you.

Combining Form	Definition	Medical Word Example	Medical Word Definition
1. trache/o-	trachea	bronchotracheal	pertaining to bronchi and trachea
2. auscult/o-	________	______________	______________________
3. ventil/o-	________	______________	______________________
4. cyan/o-	________	______________	______________________
5. pector/o-	________	______________	______________________
6. steth/o-	________	______________	______________________

Symptoms, Signs, and Diseases

Matching Exercise

Match each numbered word or phrase to its description.

1. apnea ______ Caused by trauma, treated with a chest tube
2. asthma ______ Blood clot or fat globule in the pulmonary artery
3. hemothorax ______ Creates a pleural friction rub
4. pleurisy ______ Premature babies often have this
5. pectus excavatum ______ Congenital deformity of the sternum and chest
6. pneumoconiosis ______ Caused by allergies, exercise, or stress
7. pulmonary embolus ______ Sternal and intercostal are two types
8. retractions ______ Caused by taking aspirin during a viral illness
9. Reye's syndrome ______ Occupational lung disease

True or False

Indicate whether each statement is true or false by writing T or F on the line.

1. ____ Bronchospasm occurs during an asthma attack.
2. ____ Patients who have orthopnea use pillows to prop themselves up to sleep.
3. ____ Hemoptysis means blood in the thoracic cavity.
4. ____ Asthma is also known as reactive airway disease.
5. ____ The two components of COPD are chronic bronchitis and emphysema.
6. ____ Lobar pneumonia is caused by aspirating food while eating.
7. ____ Tuberculosis is spread by air-borne droplets from an infected person coughing.
8. ____ Purulent sputum contains pus.
9. ____ Double penumonia is twice as serious as regular pneumonia.

Fill in the Blank Exercise

Select the correct word from the word list and write it on the blank line.

carcinoma	Legionnaire's disease	tachypnea
cystic fibrosis	pulmonary edema	tuberculosis
bronchopneumonia	status asthmaticus	wheezing

1. Infection that affects the bronchi, bronchioles, and adjacent lung tissue ____________
2. Severe, sustained attack of wheezing and difficulty exhaling ____________
3. High-pitched whistling or squeaking breath sound ____________
4. Eventually fatal, inherited disease of the mucus glands ____________
5. Abnormally rapid breathing ____________
6. First identified in 1976 ____________
7. Malignant tumor of the lung ____________
8. Fluid in the lungs from heart failure ____________
9. Bacterium that causes this disease has a waxy coating ____________

Laboratory, Radiology, Surgery, and Drugs

Word-Building Exercise

Use the combining forms, prefixes, and suffixes given here to build medical words that match the definitions given. Write the word that you build on the blank line. Some word parts may be used more than once.

Word Parts

-al (pertaining to)	meter- (instrument used to measure)	thorac/o- (thorax)
anti- (against)	ox/i- (oxygen)	-tomy (process of cutting or making an incision)
bronch/o- (bronchus)	-scopy (process of using an instrument to examine)	trache/o- (trachea)
endo- (within)	spir/o- (breathe)	tuss/o- (cough)
-ive (pertaining to)		

1. Pertaining to intubation of the trachea ____________________
2. Instrument used to measure breathing ____________________
3. Procedure to visually examine the bronchi with an instrument ____________________
4. This clips on the finger and measures oxygen saturation ____________________
5. To make an incision in the chest to do lung surgery ____________________
6. Pertaining to a medicine to prevent coughing ____________________

Circle Exercise

Circle the correct word from the choices given.

1. A pneumonectomy involves surgical removal of the (**alveoli, lung, trachea**).
2. Oxygen therapy is administered by using a/an (**ABG, nasal cannula, tracheotomy**).
3. (**Carboxyhemoglobin, CXR, Pulmonary function test**) measures the amount of carbon monoxide in the blood.
4. Expectorants are used to treat (**hypoxia, productive coughs, tuberculosis**).

Abbreviations

Matching Exercise

Match each numbered abbreviation to its description.

1. SOB		____ Inhaler used to give bronchodilator drugs
2. FVC		____ Forced vital capacity
3. PFT		____ Disease that includes bronchitis and emphysema
4. PCP		____ Pneumonia that often affects AIDS patients
5. TB		____ Resuscitation
6. COPD		____ Synonym for *dyspnea*
7. CXR		____ Tuberculosis
8. MDI		____ Radiology test of the chest
9. CPR		____ Includes FVC and FEV_1

Applied Skills

Plural Noun and Adjective Spelling

Fill in the blanks with the correct word form. Be sure to check your spelling. The first one has been done for you.

Singular Noun	Plural Noun	Adjective
1. nose		nasal
2. alveolus	______	______
3. anoxia		______
4. apex	______	______
5. apnea		______
6. asthma		______
7. atelectasis		______
8. bronchiole	______	______
9. bronchus	______	______
10. cilium	______	
11. cyanosis		______
12. diaphragm		______
13. epiglottis		______
14. hilum	______	______
15. hypoxia		______
16. larynx		______
17. lobe	______	______
18. lung	______	______
19. mediastinum		______
20. mucosa		______
21. pharynx		______
22. pleura		______
23. pus		______
24. rib	______	______
25. septum		______
26. sternum		______
27. tachypnea		______
28. trachea		______

English and Medical Word Equivalents

For each English word, write its equivalent medical word. The first one has been done for you.

English Word	Medical Word
1. throat	pharynx
2. black lung disease	______
3. breast bone	______
4. chest	______
5. collapsed lung	______
6. crib death	______
7. flu	______
8. shortness of breath	______
9. throat	______
10. voice box	______
11. windpipe	______

Dictionary Challenge

On the job, you will often encounter new medical words. Practice your medical dictionary skills by looking up the phrases ***cystic fibrosis*** *and* ***status asthmaticus****. Did you find the complete definition under the first word or the second word of the phrase? Which way of word searching is more effective? Write a wordsearching rule to help you remember how to look up these phrases.*

1. cystic fibrosis
   Complete definition is under: **cystic** **fibrosis** (Circle one)
2. status asthmaticus
   Complete definition is under: **status** **asthmaticus** (Circle one)
3. Wordsearching rule: ______________________________

____

Analysis of a Medical Report

This exercise contains a report of a pulmonary admission to an acute care hospital. Read the report and answer the questions.

ADMISSION HISTORY AND PHYSICAL EXAMINATION

PATIENT NAME: OTT, GEORGE
HOSPITAL NUMBER: 208-333-7943
DATE OF ADMISSION: November 19, 20xx

HISTORY OF PRESENT ILLNESS
This 65-year-old Caucasian male was evaluated by me in the emergency department on the above date, complaining of progressive shortness of breath, coughing, fever, and fatigue.

PAST HISTORY
The patient was a coal miner for 25 years before he retired on disability with black lung at age 55. He currently smokes 2 packs of cigarettes per day and has done so for the past 22 years. Past surgical history of an appendectomy in the remote past. Bronchoscopy in the past with biopsy of suspicious lesion on chest x-ray with negative results.

PHYSICAL EXAMINATION
VITAL SIGNS: Pulse 110, respiratory rate 42 per minute, temperature 100.6, blood pressure 156/96.
GENERAL: The patient appears older than his stated age and quite tired at this time.
HEENT: Negative, except for slight cyanosis of the lips. The neck is supple and free of any masses.
CHEST: There is an increased anteroposterior diameter to the chest. There is no use of accessory muscles of respiration. There are diffuse expiratory wheezes, but no rales or rhonchi.
HEART: Normal heart sounds without murmur, gallop, or rub.
ABDOMEN: Soft and nontender.
EXTREMITIES: Normal with full range of motion noted. There was no digital clubbing noted.

LABORATORY DATA
CBC showed an elevated white blood cell count of 17,600 with 80 segs, 4 bands, and 2 lymphs. Pulse oximeter showed 70% saturation. Sputum was sent for C&S. Chest x-ray: Patchy infiltrates from the apex to the midlung on the right with some consolidative changes involving the entire right lower lobe. There is no pleural fluid noted. There is a density seen in the left lower lobe posterolaterally, which extends to the pleural surface. It is most probably focal scarring or atelectasis from old inflammation.

IMPRESSION
1. Right lower lobe pneumonia.
2. Chronic obstructive pulmonary disease, secondary to anthracosis.

Christina S. Jencks, M.D.
Christina S. Jencks, M.D.

CSJ: lcc
D: 11/19/xx
T: 11/19/xx

WORD ANALYSIS QUESTIONS

1. What is the medical abbreviation for shortness of breath? ____________________
2. The patient has dyspnea. If you wanted to use the adjective form of dyspnea, you would say, "The patient is ____________________."
3. Divide *dyspneic* into its three word parts and define each word part.

Word Part	Definition
__________	__________________________
__________	__________________________
__________	__________________________

4. Divide *bronchoscopy* into its two word parts and define each word part.

Word Part	Definition
__________	__________________________
__________	__________________________

5. Divide *cyanosis* into its two word parts and define each word part.

Word Part	Definition
__________	__________________________
__________	__________________________

6. What do these abbreviations stand for?
   a. C&S ____________________
   b. CPR ____________________
   c. COPD ____________________
   d. RLL ____________________

FACT FINDING QUESTIONS

1. What is the medical word for *black lung disease*?

   ____

2. On what part of the body did the physician look for digital clubbing?

   ____

3. What respiratory surgery did this patient have in the past?

   ____

4. What other surgery has this patient had in the past?

   ____

5. Circle all of the abnormalities that were seen on the CXR.

intercostal muscles	density in LLL
atelectasis	oximeter
consolidative change	patchy infiltrate
cyanosis	pleural fluid

CRITICAL THINKING QUESTIONS

1. Of the four medical complaints the patient had on presenting to the emergency department, which is directly related to an infection?

   ____

2. What is the descriptive name that laypersons give for the medical condition of increased anteroposterior diameter of the chest?

   ____

3. What method of examination would the physician use to hear the patient's expiratory wheezes? (Circle one)

   auscultation **percussion** **postural drainage** **pulse oximeter**

4. The patient has an elevated white blood cell count of 17,600 which indicates an infection. This is due to which of the two diagnoses listed in the IMPRESSION section?

   ____

5. Calculate the number of pack-years for this patient's history of smoking.

   ____

Pronunciation Checklist

Read each word and its pronunciation. Practice pronouncing each word. Verify your pronunciation by listening to the Pronunciation List on the CD-ROM. Check the box next to the word after you have mastered its pronunciation.

- ❑ adenocarcinoma (AD-eh-noh-KAR-sih-NOH-mah)
- ❑ alveolar (al-VEE-oh-lar)
- ❑ alveoli (al-VEE-oh-ligh)
- ❑ alveolus (al-VEE-oh-lus)
- ❑ Ambu bag (AM-boo BAG)
- ❑ anoxia (an-AWK-see-ah)
- ❑ anoxic (an-AWK-sik)
- ❑ anthracosis (AN-thrah-KOH-sis)
- ❑ antibiotic drug (AN-tee-by-AWT-ik DRUHG) (AN-tih-by-AWT-ik DRUHG)
- ❑ antitubercular drug (AN-tee-too-BER-kyoo-lar DRUHG)
- ❑ antitussive drug (AN-tee-TUS-iv DRUHG)
- ❑ apex (AA-peks)
- ❑ apical (AP-ih-kal)
- ❑ apices (AA-pih-sees)
- ❑ apnea (AP-nee-ah)
- ❑ apneic (AP-nee-ik)
- ❑ arterial blood gases (ar-TEER-ee-al BLUD GAS-ez)
- ❑ asbestosis (AS-bes-TOH-sis)
- ❑ asphyxia (as-FIK-see-ah)
- ❑ aspiration pneumonia (AS-pih-RAY-shun noo-MOH-nee-ah)
- ❑ asthma (AZ-mah)
- ❑ asthmatic (az-MAT-ik)
- ❑ atelectasis (AT-eh-LEK-tah-sis)
- ❑ atelectatic (AT-eh-lek-TAT-ik)
- ❑ auscultation (AWS-kul-TAY-shun)
- ❑ bacterial pneumonia (bak-TEER-ee-al noo-MOH-nee-ah)
- ❑ bradypnea (brad-ip-NEE-ah)
- ❑ bronchi (BRONG-kigh)
- ❑ bronchial (BRONG-kee-al)
- ❑ bronchiectasis (BRONG-kee-EK-tah-sis)
- ❑ bronchiolar (BRONG-kee-OH-lar)
- ❑ bronchiole (BRONG-kee-ohl)
- ❑ bronchitis (brong-KY-tis)
- ❑ bronchodilator drug (BRONG-koh-DY-lay-ter DRUHG)
- ❑ bronchopneumonia (BRONG-koh-noo-MOH-nee-ah)
- ❑ bronchopulmonary (BRONG-koh-PUL-moh-nair-ee)
- ❑ bronchoscope (BRONG-koh-skohp)
- ❑ bronchoscopy (brong-KAWS-koh-pee)
- ❑ bronchospasm (BRONG-koh-spazm)
- ❑ bronchus (BRONG-kus)
- ❑ cancer (KAN-ser)
- ❑ cannula (KAN-yoo-lah)
- ❑ carbon dioxide (KAR-bon dy-AWK-side)
- ❑ carboxyhemoglobin (kar-BAWK-see-HEE-moh-gloh-bin)
- ❑ carcinoma (KAR-sih-NOH-mah)
- ❑ cardiopulmonary (KAR-dee-oh-PUL-moh-nair-ee)
- ❑ cardiopulmonary resuscitation (KAR-dee-oh-PUL-moh-nair-ee ree-SUS-ih-TAY-shun)
- ❑ cardiothoracic surgeon (KAR-dee-oh-thoh-RAS-ik SER-jun)
- ❑ chemotherapy drug (KEE-moh-THAIR-ah-pee DRUHG)
- ❑ chronic obstructive pulmonary disease (KRAW-nik awb-STRUK-tiv PUL-moh-nair-ee dih-ZEEZ)
- ❑ cilia (SIL-ee-ah)
- ❑ cilium (SIL-ee-um)
- ❑ circumoral cyanosis (SER-kum-OR-al SY-ah-NOH-sis)
- ❑ concha (CON-kah)
- ❑ conchae (CON-kee)
- ❑ corticosteroid drug (KOR-tih-koh-STAIR-oyd DRUHG)
- ❑ costal (KAWS-tal)
- ❑ cough (KAWF)
- ❑ culture and sensitivity (KUL-chur and SEN-sih-TIV-ih-tee)
- ❑ cyanosis (SY-ah-NOH-sis)
- ❑ cyanotic (SY-ah-NAWT-ik)
- ❑ cystic fibrosis (SIS-tik fy-BROH-sis)
- ❑ deoxygenated (dee-AWK-see-jen-aa-ted)
- ❑ diaphragm (DY-ah-fram)
- ❑ diaphragmatic (DY-ah-frag-MAT-ik)
- ❑ dyspnea (DISP-nee-ah)
- ❑ dyspneic (DISP-nee-ik)
- ❑ effusion (ee-FYOO-zhun)
- ❑ emphysema (EM-fih-SEE-mah)
- ❑ empyema (EM-py-EE-mah)
- ❑ endotracheal intubation (EN-doh-TRAY-kee-al IN-too-BAY-shun)
- ❑ epiglottic (EP-ih-GLAWT-ik)
- ❑ epiglottis (EP-ih-GLAWT-is)
- ❑ eupnea (YOOP-nee-ah)
- ❑ eupneic (YOOP-nik)
- ❑ exhalation (EKS-hah-LAY-shun)
- ❑ expectorant (ek-SPEK-toh-rant)
- ❑ expectoration (ek-SPEK-toh-RAY-shun)
- ❑ expiration (EKS-pih-RAY-shun)
- ❑ external (eks-TER-nal)
- ❑ Heimlich maneuver (HYM-lik mah-NOO-ver)
- ❑ hemoptysis (hee-MAWP-tih-sis)
- ❑ hemothorax (HEE-moh-THOR-aks)
- ❑ hila (HY-lah)
- ❑ hilar (HY-lar)
- ❑ hilum (HY-lum)
- ❑ histamine (HIS-tah-meen)
- ❑ hypercapnia (HY-per-KAP-nee-ah)
- ❑ hypoxemia (HY-pawk-SEE-mee-ah)
- ❑ hypoxia (hy-PAWK-see-ah)
- ❑ hypoxic (hy-PAWK-sik)
- ❑ influenza (IN-floo-EN-zah)
- ❑ inhalation (IN-hah-LAY-shun)
- ❑ inspiration (IN-spih-RAY-shun)
- ❑ intercostal retraction (IN-ter-KAWS-tal ree-TRAK-shun)
- ❑ internal (in-TER-nal)
- ❑ intubation (IN-too-BAY-shun)
- ❑ laryngeal (lah-RIN-jee-al)
- ❑ laryngoscope (lah-RING-goh-skohp)
- ❑ larynx (LAIR-ingks)
- ❑ *Legionella pneumophilia* (LEE-jeh-NEL-ah NOO-moh-FIL-ee-ah)
- ❑ legionnaires' disease (lee-jen-AIRS dih-ZEEZ)
- ❑ leukotriene (LOO-koh-TRY-een)
- ❑ lobar (LOH-bar)
- ❑ lobe (LOHB)
- ❑ lobar pneumonia (LOH-bar noo-MOH-nee-ah)
- ❑ lobectomy (loh-BEK-toh-mee)
- ❑ lumen (LOO-men)
- ❑ malignant (mah-LIG-nant)
- ❑ Mantoux test (man-TOO TEST)
- ❑ mediastinal (MEE-dee-as-TY-nal)
- ❑ mediastinum (MEE-dee-as-TY-num)
- ❑ metabolic (MET-ah-BAWL-ik)
- ❑ metabolism (meh-TAB-oh-lizm)
- ❑ mucosa (myoo-KOH-sah)
- ❑ mucosal (myoo-KOH-sal)
- ❑ mucous (MYOO-kus)
- ❑ mucus (MYOO-kus)
- ❑ nasal cavity (NAY-zal KAV-ih-tee)
- ❑ obstructive apnea (awb-STRUK-tiv AP-nee-ah)
- ❑ opportunistic infection (AWP-or-too-NIS-tik in-FEK-shun)

- ❏ orthopnea (or-THAWP-nee-ah)
- ❏ orthopneic (or-THAWP-nee-ik)
- ❏ oximeter (awk-SIM-eh-ter)
- ❏ oximetry (awk-SIM-eh-tree)
- ❏ oxygen (AWK-seh-jen)
- ❏ oxygenated (AWK-see-jen-aa-ted)
- ❏ oxyhemoglobin (AWK-see-HEE-moh-GLOH-bin)
- ❏ panlobar pneumonia (pan-LOH-bar noo-MOH-nee-ah)
- ❏ parenchyma (pah-RENG-kih-mah)
- ❏ parenchymal (pah-RENG-kih-mal)
- ❏ parietal (pah-RY-eh-tal)
- ❏ paroxysmal nocturnal dyspnea (PAIR-awk-SIZ-mal nawk-TER-nal DISP-nee-ah)
- ❏ pectus excavatum (PEK-tus EKS-kah-VAH-tum)
- ❏ perfusion (per-FYOO-zhun)
- ❏ pharyngeal (fah-RIN-jee-al)
- ❏ pharynx (FAIR-ingks)
- ❏ phrenic nerve (FREN-ik NERV)
- ❏ pleura (PLOOR-ah)
- ❏ pleural (PLOOR-al)
- ❏ pleural effusion (PLOOR-al ee-FYOO-shun)
- ❏ pleurisy (PLOOR-ih-see)
- ❏ pleuritic (ploo-RIT-ik)
- ❏ pleuritis (ploo-RY-tis)
- ❏ pneumococcal pneumonia (NOO-moh-KAW-kal noo-MOH-nee-ah)
- ❏ pneumoconiosis (NOO-moh-KOH-nee-OH-sis)
- ❏ *Pneumocystis carinii* (NOO-moh-SIS-tis kah-REE-nee-eye)
- ❏ pneumonectomy (NOO-moh-NEK-toh-mee)
- ❏ pneumonia (noo-MOH-nee-ah)
- ❏ pneumothorax (NOO-moh-THOR-aks)
- ❏ pulmonary (PUL-moh-nair-ee)
- ❏ pulmonary edema (PUL-moh-nair-ee eh-DEE-mah)
- ❏ pulmonary embolism (PUL-moh-nair-ee EM-boh-lizm)
- ❏ pulmonary embolus (PUL-moh-nair-ee EM-boh-lus)
- ❏ pulmonologist (PUL-moh-NAWL-oh-jist)
- ❏ pulmonology (PUL-moh-NAWL-oh-jee)
- ❏ purulent (PYOOR-yoo-lent)
- ❏ pyothorax (PY-oh-THOR-aks)
- ❏ radiography (RAY-dee-AWG-rah-fee)
- ❏ rales (RAWLZ)
- ❏ resection (ree-SEK-shun)
- ❏ respiration (RES-pih-RAY-shun)
- ❏ respirator (RES-pih-RAY-tor)
- ❏ respiratory system (RES-pih-rah-TOR-ee SIS-tem) (reh-SPYR-ah-tor-ee)
- ❏ respiratory therapist (RES-pih-rah-TOR-ee THAIR-ah-pist)
- ❏ resuscitation (ree-SUS-ih-TAY-shun)
- ❏ retraction (re-TRAK-shun)
- ❏ Reye's syndrome (RYZ SIN-drohm)
- ❏ rhonchi (RONG-kigh)
- ❏ septal (SEP-tal)
- ❏ septum (SEP-tum)
- ❏ serous (SEER-us)
- ❏ spirometer (spih-RAWM-eh-ter)
- ❏ spirometry (spih-RAWM-eh-tree)
- ❏ sputum (SPYOO-tum)
- ❏ status asthmaticus (STAT-us az-MAT-ih-kus)
- ❏ sternal (STER-nal)
- ❏ sternal retraction (STER-nal ree-TRAK-shun)
- ❏ sternum (STER-num)
- ❏ stethoscope (STETH-oh-skohp)
- ❏ stridor (STRY-dor)
- ❏ surfactant (ser-FAK-tant)
- ❏ tachypnea (TAK-ip-NEE-ah)
- ❏ tachypneic (TAK-ip-NEE-ik)
- ❏ therapist (THAIR-ah-pist)
- ❏ thoracocentesis (THOR-ah-koh-sen-TEE-sis)
- ❏ thoracic (thoh-RAS-ik)
- ❏ thoracic cavity (thoh-RAS-ik KAV-ih-tee)
- ❏ thoracotomy (THOR-ah-KAWT-oh-mee)
- ❏ thorax (THOR-aks)
- ❏ tomography (toh-MAWG-rah-fee)
- ❏ trachea (TRAY-kee-ah)
- ❏ tracheal (TRAY-kee-al)
- ❏ tracheobronchial (TRAY-kee-oh-BRONG-kee-al)
- ❏ tracheostomy (TRAY-kee-AWS-toh-mee)
- ❏ tracheotomy (TRAY-kee-AWT-oh-mee)
- ❏ tubercle (TOO-ber-kl)
- ❏ tuberculosis (too-BER-kyoo-LOH-sis)
- ❏ turbinate (TER-bih-nayt)
- ❏ ventilation (VEN-tih-LAY-shun)
- ❏ ventilator (VEN-tih-LAY-tor)
- ❏ viral pneumonia (VY-ral noo-MOH-nee-ah)
- ❏ visceral (VIS-eh-ral)
- ❏ wheezes (WHEE-zes)

Experience Multimedia

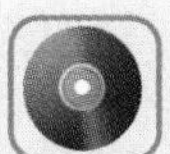

CD-ROM Learning Activities Checklist

Check off the box as you complete each learning activity.

❑ **CD-ROM Learning Activity 4.1: *ANATOMY WORD PARTS FLASHCARDS***
Use flashcards to help you memorize word parts. Make your own flashcards or print out prepared flashcards. Also see the electronic flashcard game. Time: 20 minutes.

❑ **CD-ROM Learning Activity 4.2: *MEDICINE IN ACTION***
Listen to normal and abnormal breath sounds. Time: 5 minutes.

❑ **CD-ROM Learning Activity 4.3: *DISEASE AND OTHER WORD PARTS FLASHCARDS***
A continuation of the flashcard learning activity. Time: 20 minutes.

❑ **CD-ROM Learning Activity 4.4: *MEMORY AIDS***
Use memory aids to help you memorize medical words and meanings. Time: 5 minutes.

❑ **CD-ROM Learning Activity 4.5: *MEDICAL LANGUAGE SPOKEN HERE***
Listen to actual medical reports and spell the missing medical words. Time: 20 minutes.

❑ **CD-ROM Learning Activity 4.6: *SPELLING CHALLENGE***
Listen to a pronounced medical word and then spell it. Time: 5 minutes.

❑ **CD-ROM Learning Activity 4.7: *MEDICAL LANGUAGE PRONUNCIATION***
Listen to a pronounced medical word and then practice pronouncing it. Time: 30 minutes.

❑ **CD-ROM Learning Activity 4.8: *EDUCATIONAL FUN AND GAMES***
Enjoy these fun activities while reinforcing your knowledge. Time: 15 minutes.

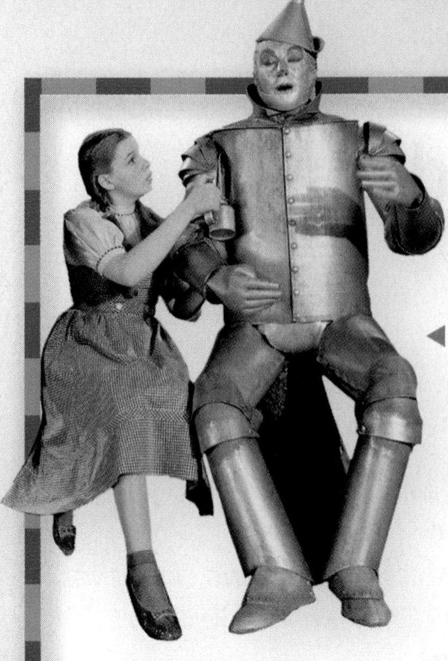

Everyone needs a heart. Just ask the Tin Man from the classic story *The Wizard of Oz.*

Dive In!

- The heart beats about 2.5 billion times and pumps about 50 million gallons of blood during an average lifetime.
- If your blood vessels were laid from end to end, they would reach around the world four times!
- Turn the page to keep your finger on the pulse of cardiology. In this chapter we'll explore the language that describes cardiovascular system structures, functions, diseases, and conditions.
- You'll be pumped up once you master the language of cardiology!

The body's pump is also the universal symbol of love. In pagan and early Christian eras it was thought to be the center of emotion.

Medicine Through HISTORY

1847

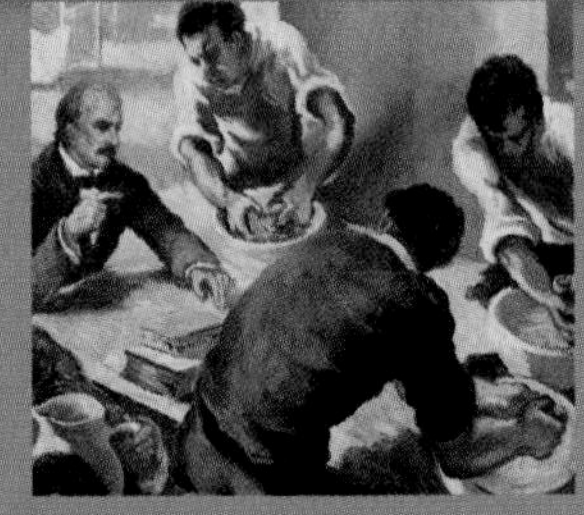

Handwashing is found to prevent the spread of disease, as discovered by Ignaz Semmelweis, a Hungarian physician

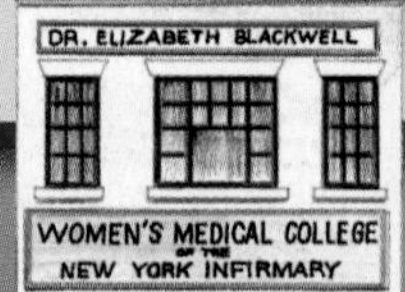

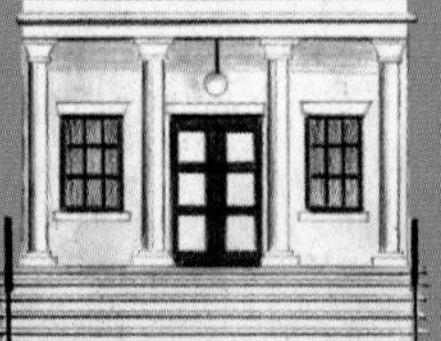

1849

Elizabeth Blackwell becomes the first woman physician

1849

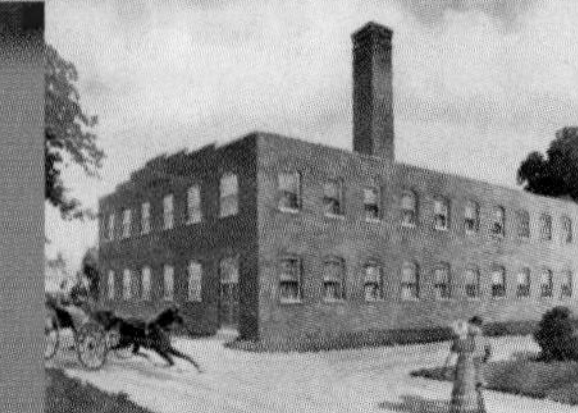

Pfizer pharmaceutical company is founded in Brooklyn, NY

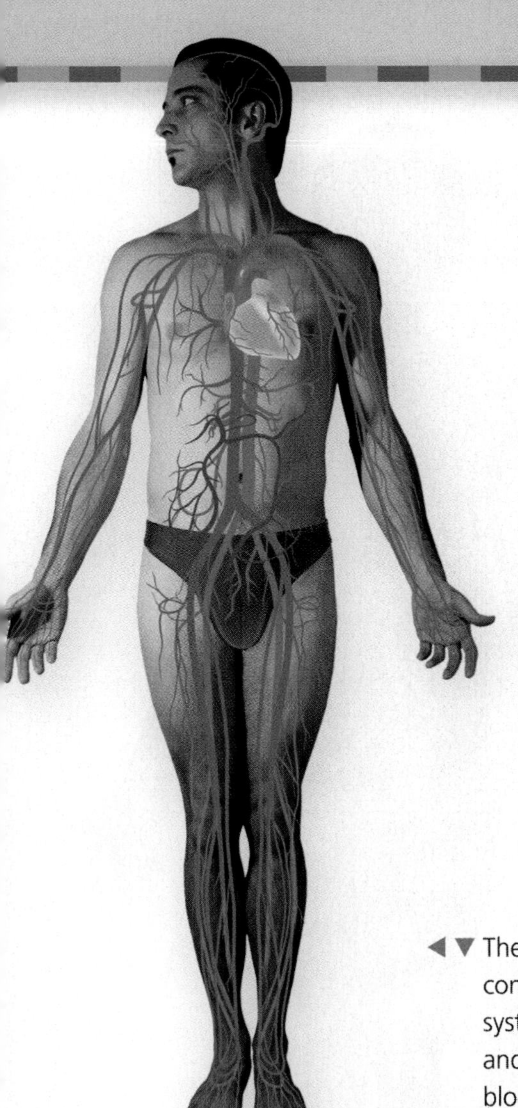

CHAPTER 5

Cardiology

Cardiovascular System

Cardiology (KAR-dee-AWL-oh-jee) is the medical specialty that studies the anatomy and physiology of the cardiovascular system and uses diagnostic tests, medical and surgical procedures, and drugs to treat cardiovascular diseases.

◀ ▼ The cardiovascular system is a continuous, circular body system—containing the heart and blood vessels—that moves blood throughout the body to transport oxygen, nutrients, and waste products.

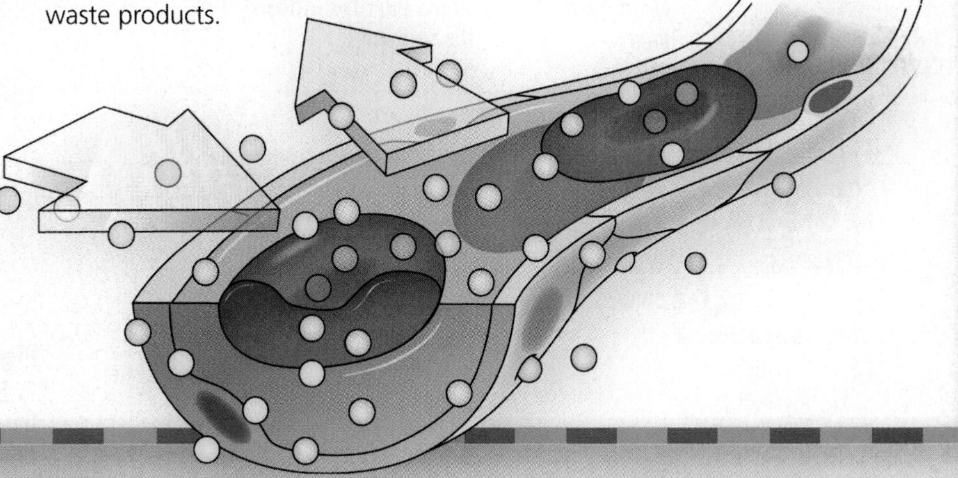

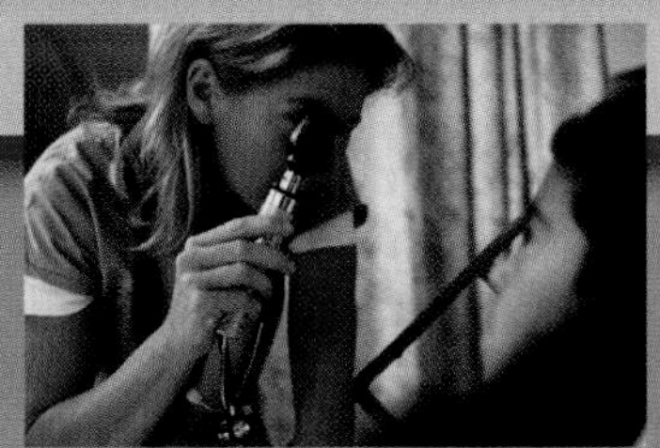

1851

The ophthalmoscope, an instrument used to view the inside of the eye, is invented by Hermann von Helmholtz, a German physiologist

1853

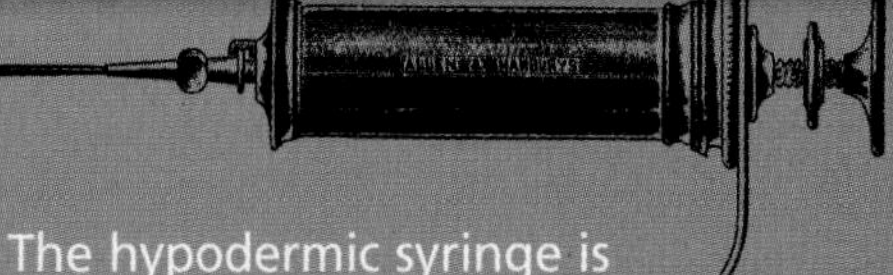

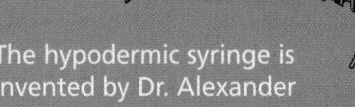

The hypodermic syringe is invented by Dr. Alexander Wood of Scotland

Measure Your Progress: Learning Objectives

After you study this chapter, you should be able to

1. Identify the anatomical structures of the cardiovascular system by correctly labeling them on anatomical illustrations.
2. Describe the process of circulation.
3. Build cardiovascular words from combining forms, prefixes, and suffixes.
4. Describe common cardiovascular diseases.
5. Describe common cardiovascular diagnostic laboratory and radiology tests.
6. Describe common cardiovascular medical and surgical procedures and drug categories.
7. Define common cardiovascular abbreviations.
8. Correctly spell and pronounce cardiovascular words.
9. Apply your skills by analyzing a cardiology report.
10. Test your knowledge of cardiology by completing review exercises at the end of the chapter and learning activities on the CD-ROM.

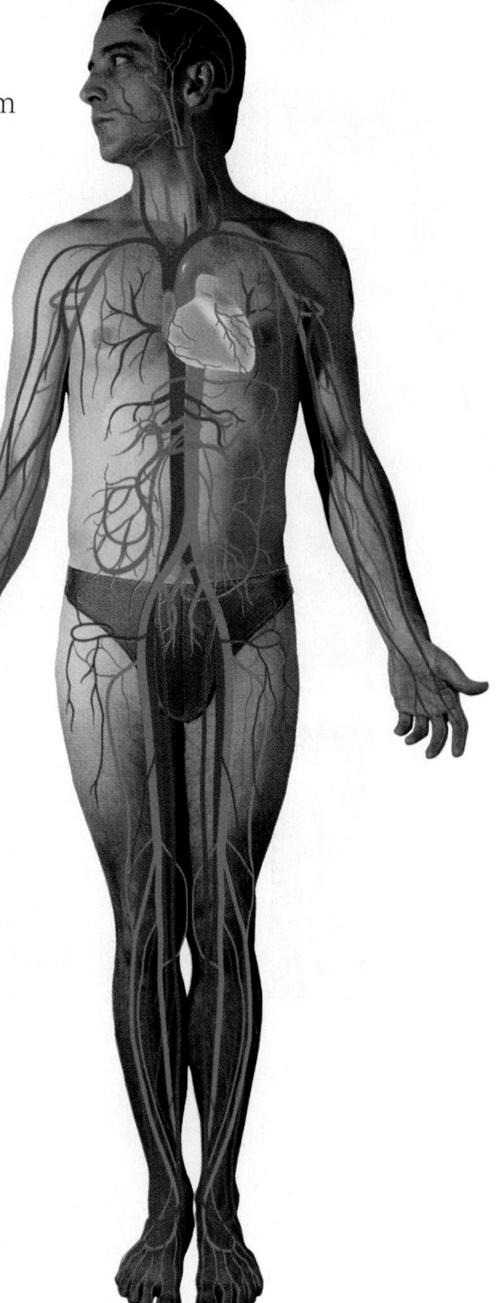

Figure 5-1 ■ The cardiovascular system.

The cardiovascular system consists of the heart and blood vessels connected in a common pathway that carries blood to and from all parts of the body.

Medical Language Key

To unlock the meaning of a medical word, first define each word part. Then put the word part definitions in order, beginning with the suffix, followed by the first word part.

	Word Part	Word Part Definition
SUFFIX	-logy	the study of
COMBINING FORM	cardi/o-	heart

Cardiology: ***The study of the heart.***

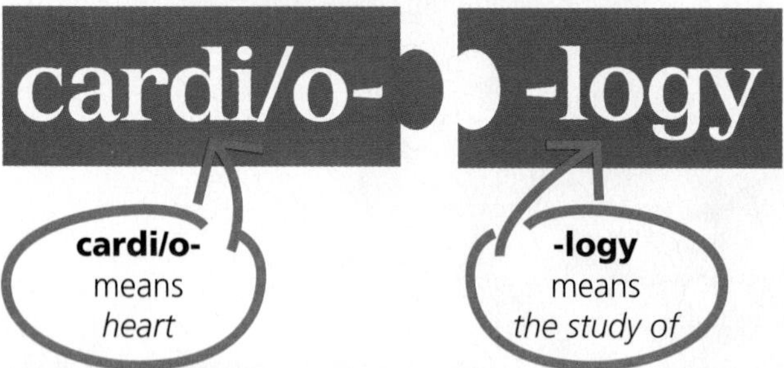

www.prenhall.com/turley

For interactive flashcards, real-life video clips, games, exercises, and audio pronunciations please explore the companion CD-ROM in the back of the book. Click on the companion website for bonus chapters, additional resources, and links to on-line learning.

Anatomy and Physiology

The **cardiovascular system** is a continuous, circular body system that includes the heart and all of the **vascular** structures or blood vessels (arteries, capillaries, veins) (see Figure 5-1■). To study the cardiovascular system, you can begin with the heart, which is located in the thoracic cavity, or you can begin with the capillaries, the tiniest blood vessels in the most distal parts of the body. Either way you will eventually reach every part of the cardiovascular system. The purpose of the cardiovascular system is to move blood throughout the body and transport oxygen, nutrients, and waste products in the blood. The blood itself is discussed in Hematology (Chapter 6).

cardiovascular (KAR-dee-oh-VAS-kyoo-lar)
cardi/o- *heart*
vascul/o- *blood vessel*
-ar *pertaining to*

system (SIS-tem)
System is derived from a Greek word meaning *combination of parts to make an organized whole.*

vascular (VAS-kyoo-lar)
vascul/o- *blood vessel*
-ar *pertaining to*

Anatomy of the Cardiovascular System

Heart

The heart is perhaps the best-known organ in the body and certainly one of the most important. It is a muscular organ that contracts at least once every second to pump blood through the body. It also has an extensive electrical system that regulates the rhythm of its contractions.

Heart Chambers Inside the heart are four hollow chambers, two on the top and two on the bottom (see Figure 5-2■). Each small upper

cardiac (KAR-dee-ak)
cardi/o- *heart*
-ac *pertaining to*
Cardiac is the adjective form for *heart*. The Latin word *cor*, which means *heart*, is sometimes used in medical reports.

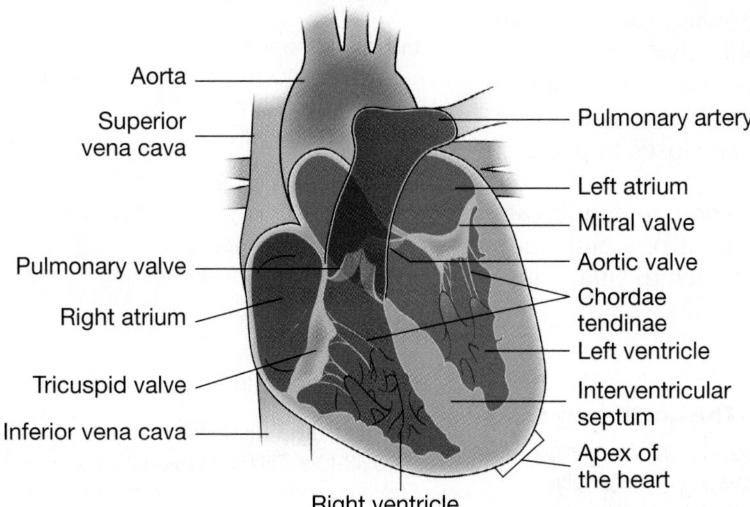

Figure 5-2 ■ The four chambers and four valves of the heart.
The heart has four chambers: the right atrium, the right ventricle, the left atrium, and the left ventricle. The heart has four valves: the tricuspid valve (between the right atrium and right ventricle), the pulmonary valve (between the right ventricle and the pulmonary artery), the mitral valve (between the left atrium and the left ventricle), and the aortic valve (between the left ventricle and the aorta).

chamber is known as an **atrium.** Each large lower chamber is known as a **ventricle.** A partitioning wall or **septum** divides the heart into right and left halves. The inferior tip of the heart is known as the **apex**.

Word Alert:

SOUND-ALIKE WORDS

The prefix "intra-" means *within*. The prefix "inter-" means *between*.

interatrial	(adjective)	Located between the right and left atria *Example: The interatrial septum is the dividing wall between the right and left atria.*
intra-atrial	(adjective)	Located within the atrium *Example: Intra-atrial blood is found within the right and left atria.*
interventricular	(adjective)	Located between the two ventricles *Example: The interventricular septum is the dividing wall between the right and left ventricles.*
intraventricular	(adjective)	Located within the ventricle *Example: Intraventricular blood is found within the right and left ventricles.*

Heart Valves **Valves** control the flow of blood through the heart. There are four valves in the heart: tricuspid valve, pulmonary valve, mitral valve, and aortic valve (see Figure 5-2).

The **tricuspid valve** is located between the right atrium and the right ventricle. This valve with its three triangular cusps (leaflets) is open as blood flows into the right ventricle and then closes to prevent blood from going back into the right atrium (see Figure 5-3■).

The **pulmonary valve** is located between the right ventricle and the pulmonary arteries that carry blood to the lungs. The pulmonary valve is open as blood flows into the pulmonary artery and then closes to prevent blood from flowing back into the right ventricle.

The **mitral valve** is located between the left atrium and the left ventricle. This valve with its two cusps is open as blood flows into the left ventricle and then closes to prevent blood from flowing back into the left atrium. This valve is also known as the **bicuspid valve.**

The **aortic valve** is located between the left ventricle and the aorta, the large artery that carries blood away from the heart. The aortic valve is open as blood flows into the aorta and then closes to prevent blood from flowing back into the left ventricle.

The tricuspid and mitral valves have many **chordae tendineae,** ropelike structures at their bases (see Figure 5-2). At one end, they attach to the valve leaflets. At the other end, they attach to small mus-

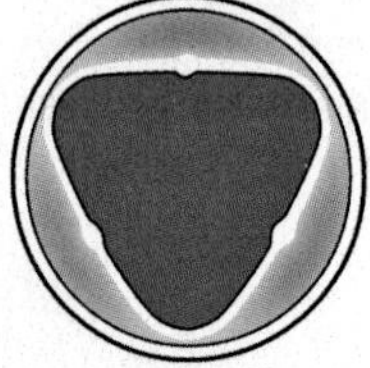

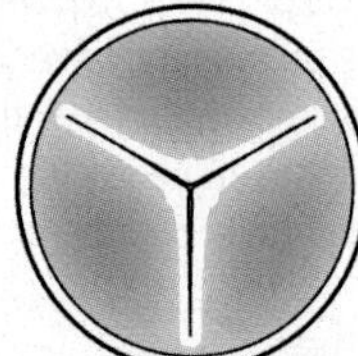

Figure 5-3 ■ The aortic valve.
With the valve leaflets open, blood flows freely through the valve. When the valve leaflets close, their edges seal tightly against one another, preventing the backflow of blood.

atrium (AA-tree-um)
atria (AA-tree-ah)
Atrium is a Latin singular neuter noun meaning *entrance hall.* Form the plural by changing *-um* to *-a.*

atrial (AA-tree-al)
atri/o- *atrium (upper heart chamber)*
-al *pertaining to*

ventricle (VEN-trih-kl)

ventricular (ven-TRIK-yoo-lar)
ventricul/o- *ventricle (lower heart chamber; chamber in the brain)*
-ar *pertaining to*

septum (SEP-tum)
Septum is derived from a Latin word meaning *a partition.*

septal (SEP-tal)
sept/o- *septum (dividing wall)*
-al *pertaining to*

apex (AA-peks)
Apex is a Latin word meaning *tip.*

apical (AP-ih-kal)
apic/o- *apex (tip)*
-al *pertaining to*

valve (VALV)

valvular (VAL-vyoo-lar)
valvul/o- *valve*
-ar *pertaining to*

tricuspid (try-KUS-pid)
tri- *three*
cusp/o- *projection, point*
-id *resembling; source or origin*

pulmonary (PUL-moh-nair-ee)
pulmon/o- *lung*
-ary *pertaining to*

mitral (MY-tral)
mitr/o- *structure like a miter (tall hat with two points)*
-al *pertaining to*

bicuspid (by-KUS-pid)
bi- *two*
cusp/o- *projection, point*
-id *resembling; source or origin*

aortic (aa-OR-tik)
aort/o- *aorta*
-ic *pertaining to*

chordae tendineae
(KOHR-dee TEN-dih-nee-ee)
Chordae tendineae is a Latin phrase meaning *cords like tendons.*

cles on the inner surface of the ventricles. When the ventricle contracts, the small muscles attached to the chordae tendineae also contract. This stabilizes the valve leaflets and keeps them firmly sealed together, so that the strong force of the ventricular blood cannot push them open.

The sounds of the valves closing are commonly known as "lubb-dupp" (a phonetic approximation of the actual sounds). The "lubb" is made as the mitral and tricuspid valves close. This first heart sound is abbreviated as S_1. The "dupp" is made as the pulmonary and aortic valves close. This second heart sound is abbreviated as S_2.

Heart Muscle The **myocardium** is the muscular layer that makes up the bulk of the heart (see Figure 5-4■ and Table 5-1). The myocardium is composed of special muscle fibers found only in the heart. These muscle fibers respond to electrical impulses generated by a node within the heart itself. This process is discussed in a later section.

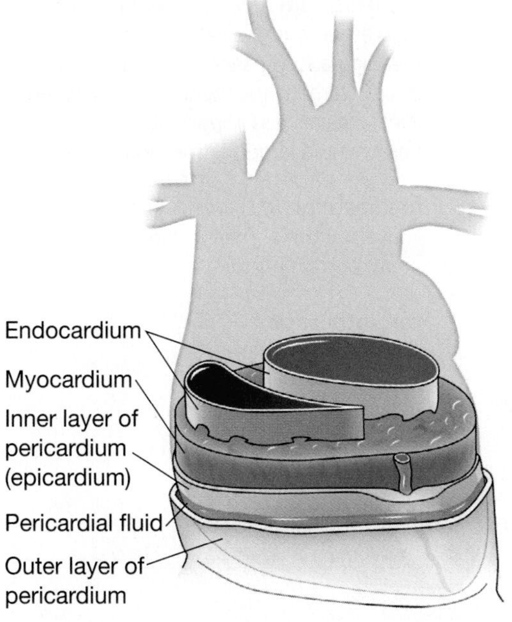

Figure 5-4 ■ Layers and membranes of the heart.

The endocardium lines the inside of the heart. The myocardium is the muscular layer of the heart. The epicardium is a membrane that covers the heart. The pericardium is a membrane that includes the epicardium and a second, more fibrous, membrane. Together these two membranes form the pericardial sac.

Table 5-1 Layers and Membranes of the Heart

endocardium	smooth membrane that lines the chambers of the heart and the heart valves. It extends into the blood vessels where it is known as endothelium.
myocardium	muscular layer of the heart
epicardium	serous membrane that covers the outer surface of the myocardium. It is the inner part of the continuous pericardium that folds back on itself to form the pericardial sac. Also known as the visceral pericardium.
parietal pericardium	part of the pericardium that forms the outer wall of the **pericardial sac.** The pericardium secretes **pericardial fluid,** a slippery, watery fluid that allows the two membranes of the pericardium to slide smoothly past one another as the heart contracts and relaxes.

myocardium (MY-oh-KAR-dee-um)
my/o- *muscle*
cardi/o- *heart*
-um *a structure*

myocardial (MY-oh-KAR-dee-al)
my/o- *muscle*
cardi/o- *heart*
-al *pertaining to*

endocardium (EN-doh-KAR-dee-um)
endo- *innermost, within*
cardi/o- *heart*
-um *a structure*

endocardial (EN-doh-KAR-dee-al)
endo- *innermost, within*
cardi/o- *heart*
-al *pertaining to*

epicardium (EP-ih-KAR-dee-um)
epi- *upon, above*
cardi/o- *heart*
-um *a structure*

epicardial (EP-ih-KAR-dee-al)
epi- *upon, above*
cardi/o- *heart*
-al *pertaining to*

pericardium (PAIR-ih-KAR-dee-um)
peri- *around*
cardi/o- *heart*
-um *a structure*

pericardial (PAIR-ih-KAR-dee-al)
peri- *around*
cardi/o- *heart*
-al *pertaining to*

The myocardium contracts in a coordinated way to pump blood. First the two atria contract, forcing blood into the two ventricles. Then the two ventricles contract, forcing blood from the right ventricle into the pulmonary artery to the lungs and blood from the left ventricle into the aorta to the entire body. The myocardium is thickest on the left side of the heart because it is the left ventricle that must work the hardest to pump blood to the entire body.

Thoracic Cavity and Mediastinum

The **thoracic cavity** contains the lungs and the **mediastinum,** a partition that surrounds an irregularly shaped central area between the lungs. The mediastinum contains the heart and parts of the "great vessels" (aorta, both venae cavae, and the pulmonary arteries and veins), as well as the thymus, trachea, and the esophagus (see Figure 5-5■). The word **cardiothoracic** reflects the relationship of the heart and the thoracic cavity.

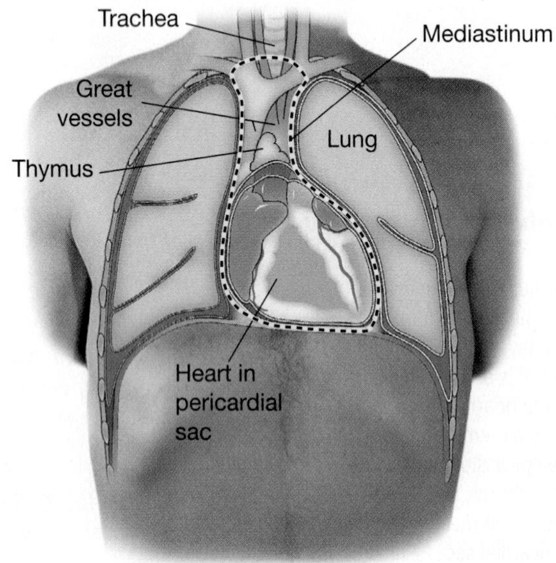

Figure 5-5 ■ The mediastinum.
The connective tissue of the mediastinum holds the heart and pericardial sac, great vessels, trachea, esophagus, and thymus in place within the thoracic cavity.

thoracic (thoh-RAS-ik)
thorac/o- *thorax (chest)*
-ic *pertaining to*

cavity (KAV-ih-tee)
cav/o- *hollow space*
-ity *state; condition*

mediastinum (MEE-dee-as-TY-num)
Mediastinum is derived from a Latin word meaning *a lower servant who performs duties.* Perhaps the mediastinum seemed like a smaller, less important area compared to the larger, active thoracic cavity.

mediastinal (MEE-dee-as-TY-nal)
mediastin/o- *mediastinum*
-al *pertaining to*

cardiothoracic
(KAR-dee-oh-thoh-RAS-ik)
cardi/o- *heart*
thorac/o- *thorax (chest)*
-ic *pertaining to*

Blood Vessels

The blood vessels are vascular channels through which blood circulates in the body. **Vasculature** refers to the network of blood vessels associated with a particular organ. All blood vessels have a central opening or **lumen** through which the blood flows. All blood vessels are lined with **endothelium,** a smooth inner layer that promotes the flow of blood. This layer is also known as the **intima.**

There are three different kinds of blood vessels in the body: arteries, capillaries, and veins. Each type of blood vessel performs a different function in the circulatory system.

vasculature (VAS-kyoo-lah-chur)
vascul/o- *blood vessel*
-ature *system composed of*

lumen (LOO-men)
Lumen is a Latin word meaning *window.*

endothelium (EN-doh-THEE-lee-um)
endo- *innermost, within*
theli/o- *tissue layer*
-um *a chemical element; a structure*

Arteries **Arteries** are located throughout the body. The smallest branches of an artery are known as **arterioles.** All arteries share some important characteristics and functions.

1. All arteries carry blood away from the heart (see Figure 5-6 ■).

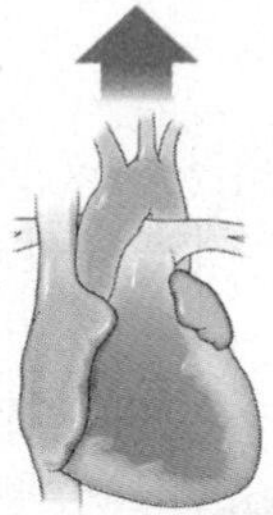

Figure 5-6 ■

2. All arteries (except the pulmonary arteries) carry bright red blood that contains high levels of oxygen (O_2). The pulmonary arteries carry dark red-purple blood with high carbon dioxide levels from the heart to the lungs.
3. Most arteries lie deep beneath the skin. Some, however, lie near the surface. Their walls bulge outward each time the heart contracts, and this can be felt as a **pulse** beneath the skin (see Figure 5-7 ■).

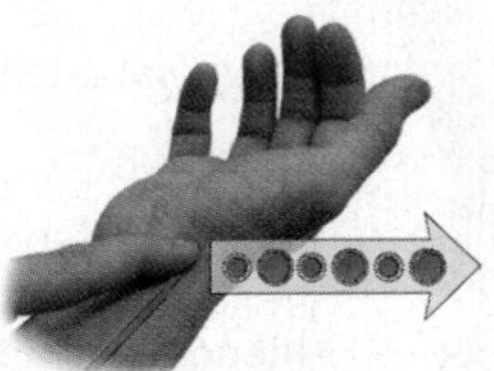

Figure 5-7 ■

4. All arteries have smooth muscle in their walls. When this smooth muscle contracts, the lumen of the artery decreases in size (**vasoconstriction**) and the blood pressure increases (see Figure 5-8 ■). When the smooth muscle relaxes, the lumen of the artery increases in size (**vasodilation**), and the blood pressure decreases. This is an important way in which the body regulates the blood pressure.

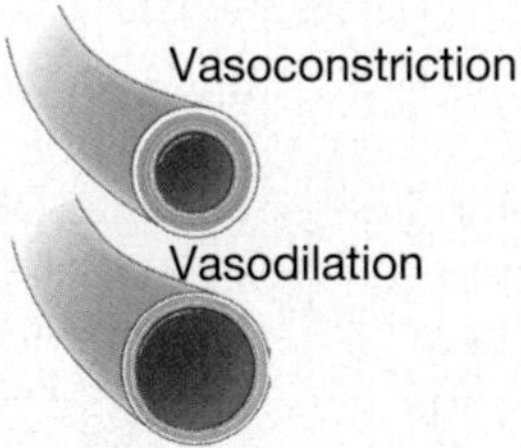

Figure 5-8 ■

endothelial (EN-doh-THEE-lee-al)
endo- *innermost, within*
theli/o- *a cellular layer*
-al *pertaining to*

intima (IN-tih-mah)
Intima is part of the Latin phrase *tunica intima,* meaning *innermost coat.*

artery (AR-ter-ee)

arterial (ar-TEER-ee-al)
arteri/o- *artery*
-al *pertaining to*

arteriole (ar-TEER-ee-ohl)
arteri/o- *artery*
-ole *small thing*

arteriolar (ar-TEER-ee-OH-lar)
arteriol/o- *arteriole*
-ar *pertaining to*

pulse (PUHLS)
Pulse is derived from a Latin word meaning *a beating motion.*

vasoconstriction (VAY-soh-con-STRIK-shun)
vas/o- *blood vessel; vas deferens*
constrict/o- *drawn together, narrowed*
-ion *action; condition*

vasodilation (VAY-soh-dy-LAY-shun)
vas/o- *blood vessel; vas deferens*
dilat/o- *dilate, widen*
-ion *action; condition*

This section describes some of the major arteries of the body (see Figure 5-9■).

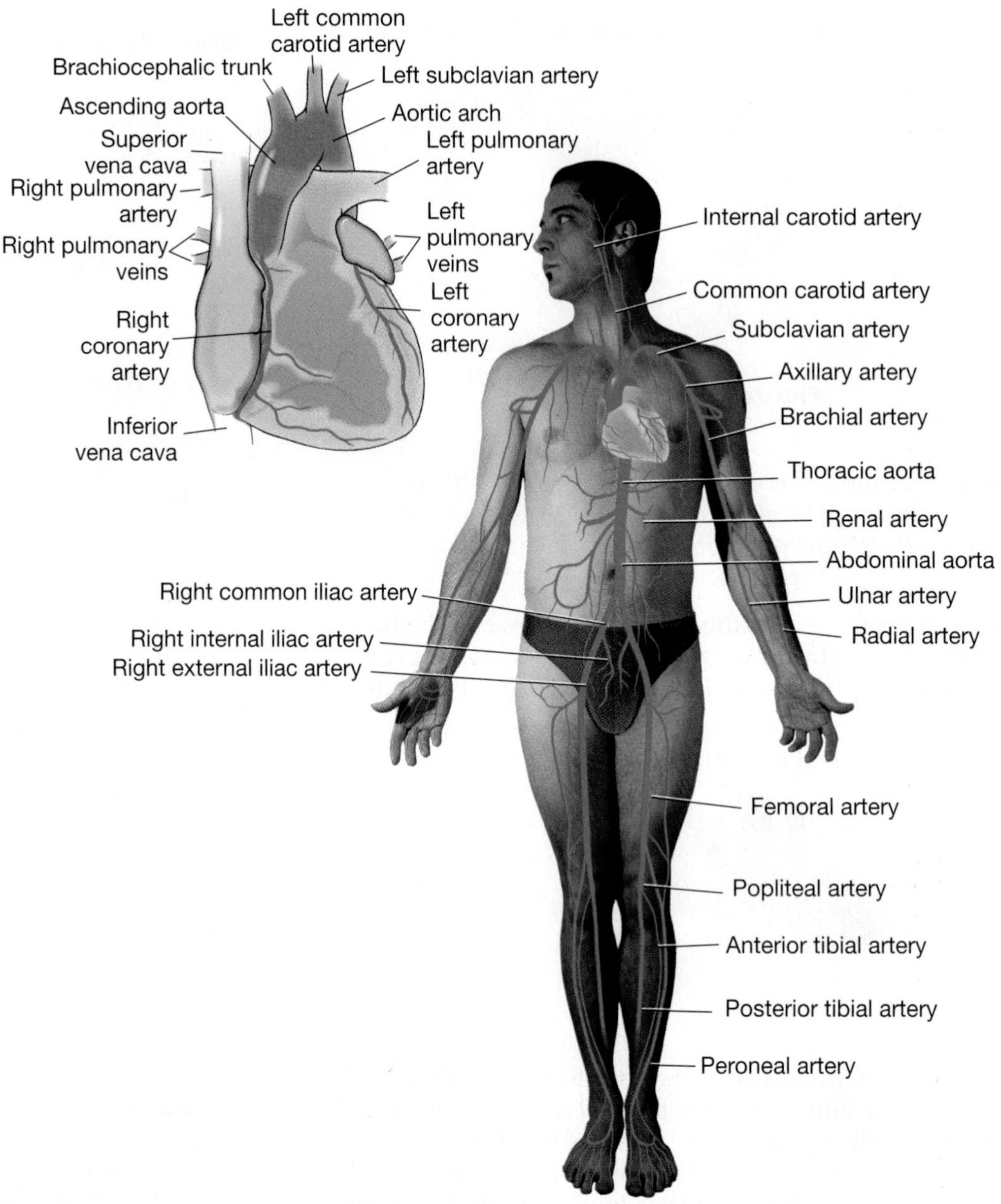

Figure 5-9 ■ The major arteries of the body.
The aorta is the largest artery of the body. It receives oxygenated blood from the heart. Arteries branch off from the aorta and carry blood to the head, arms, chest, abdomen, and legs.

Aorta The **aorta** is the largest artery in the body. It receives blood from the left ventricle of the heart. The ascending aorta proceeds superiorly from the heart. The aortic arch is the inverted, U-shaped segment of aorta superior to the heart. The thoracic aorta descends through the thoracic cavity. After it passes through the diaphragm, the thoracic aorta becomes the abdominal aorta. In the pelvic cavity, the abdominal aorta ends as it splits in two (a bifurcation) to form an inverted Y.

aorta (aa-OR-tah)
Aorta is a Latin word meaning *something that is hung up.* This may refer to the hooklike shape of the aortic arch.

aortic (aa-OR-tik)
aort/o- *aorta*
-ic *pertaining to*

Major Arteries of the Head and Chest The **coronary arteries** are the first arteries to branch off from the aorta. This is because of their importance in bringing oxygenated blood to the myocardium.

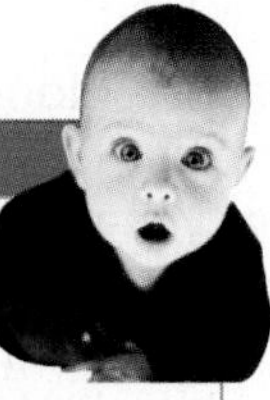

Did You Know?

Even though the chambers of the heart are filled with blood, the myocardium cannot use this blood. It must get its oxygen from the blood that flows through the coronary arteries.

Three major arteries branch off from the aortic arch: the left subclavian artery, the left common carotid artery, and the brachiocephalic trunk (that branches into the right common carotid and right subclavian arteries).

The **common carotid arteries** bring oxygenated blood from the aorta to the right and left sides of the neck, head, and brain. The common carotid artery in the neck branches into the external carotid artery to the neck, mouth, and face and the internal carotid artery to the brain.

The pulmonary arteries originate from a common pulmonary trunk coming out of the right ventricle of the heart, not the aorta. They are unlike any other artery in that they carry blood that is low in oxygen and high in carbon dioxide. They bring deoxygenated blood from the right ventricle to the right and left lungs.

Major Arteries of the Arms The **subclavian arteries** bring oxygenated blood from the aorta to the right and left shoulders and arms. Each subclavian artery goes underneath the collar bone, continues into the **axillary artery** (armpit), and then divides into the **brachial artery** (upper arm), the **radial artery** (thumb side of the lower arm), and the **ulnar artery** (little finger side of the lower arm).

Major Arteries of the Abdomen Several different arteries bring oxygenated blood from the abdominal aorta to organs in the abdominal cavity. Some arteries bring blood to more than one organ. (Example: The common hepatic artery brings blood to the liver, part of the stomach, the gallbladder, and part of the duodenum.) The **renal arteries** bring blood to the right and left kidneys. Arteries from the abdominal aorta also bring oxygenated blood to the adrenal glands, reproductive organs, and the rest of the intestines.

Major Arteries of the Hips and Legs The **common iliac arteries** begin where the abdominal aorta divides. They bring oxygenated blood to the right and left legs. Each common iliac artery divides into the external and internal iliac arteries. Each **internal iliac artery** brings blood to the pelvic organs, groin, and hip. Each **external iliac artery** continues into the **femoral artery** (upper leg) and its branches, and the **popliteal artery** (behind the knee) and its branches, and then divides into the **tibial arteries** (front and back of the lower leg), and a **peroneal artery** (lateral aspect of the lower leg).

coronary (KOR-oh-nair-ee)
coron/o- *encircling structure*
-ary *pertaining to*
Coronary is derived from a Latin word meaning *crown.* The coronary arteries sit on the surface of the heart and encircle it like a crown.

carotid (kah-ROT-id)
carot/o- *stupor, sleep*
-id *resembling; source or origin*
Ancient Greeks knew that pressing on the carotid arteries produced unconsciousness.

subclavian (sub-KLAY-vee-an)
sub- *below; underneath; less than*
clav/o- *clavicle (collar bone)*
-ian *pertaining to*

axillary (AK-sil-air-ee)
axill/o- *axilla (armpit)*
-ary *pertaining to*
Axilla is a Latin word meaning *armpit.*

brachial (BRAY-kee-al)
brachi/o- *arm*
-al *pertaining to*

radial (RAY-dee-al)
radi/o- *radius (forearm bone); x-ray; radiation*
-al *pertaining to*
Some word parts have more than one definition. The best definition of *radial* is *pertaining to the radius (forearm bone).*

ulnar (UL-nar)
uln/o- *ulna (forearm bone)*
-ar *pertaining to*

renal (REE-nal)
ren/o- *kidney*
-al *pertaining to*

iliac (IL-ee-ak)
ili/o- *ilium (hip bone)*
-ac *pertaining to*

femoral (FEM-oh-ral)
femor/o- *femur (thigh bone)*
-al *pertaining to*

popliteal (pop-LIT-ee-al) (pop-lih-TEE-al)
poplite/o- *back of the knee*
-al *pertaining to*

tibial (TIB-ee-al)
tibi/o- *tibia (shin bone)*
-al *pertaining to*

peroneal (PAIR-oh-NEE-al)
perone/o- *fibula (lower leg bone)*
-al *pertaining to*

Capillaries Arterioles divide into smaller blood vessels until they become capillaries. A **capillary** is the smallest blood vessel in the body. The lumen of a capillary is so small that blood cells must pass through in single file.

Veins Capillaries combine to form larger blood vessels known as **venules,** which then combine to form **veins.** The venae cavae are the two major veins of the body. The **superior vena cava** carries blood from the head, neck, arms and chest to the right atrium of the heart. The **inferior vena cava** carries blood from the rest of the body (except the lungs) to the right atrium. Other major veins include the **jugular veins** (carry blood from the head to the superior vena cava), the **portal vein** (carries blood from the intestines to the liver), and the **saphenous and femoral veins** (carry blood from the leg to the groin). Many veins have the same anatomical name as the arteries in that particular area of the body.

All veins share some important characteristics and functions.

1. All veins carry blood back to the heart (see Figure 5-10 ■).

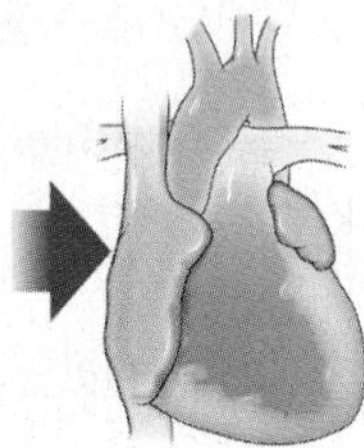

Figure 5-10 ■

2. All veins (except the pulmonary veins) carry dark red-purple blood that contains high levels of carbon dioxide (CO_2). The pulmonary veins carry bright red oxygenated blood from the lungs back to the heart.
3. Some large veins have cup-shaped valves that keep the blood flowing in one direction—toward the heart. The movement of skeletal muscles in the arms and legs compresses the veins and helps move blood toward the heart (see Figure 5-11 ■).

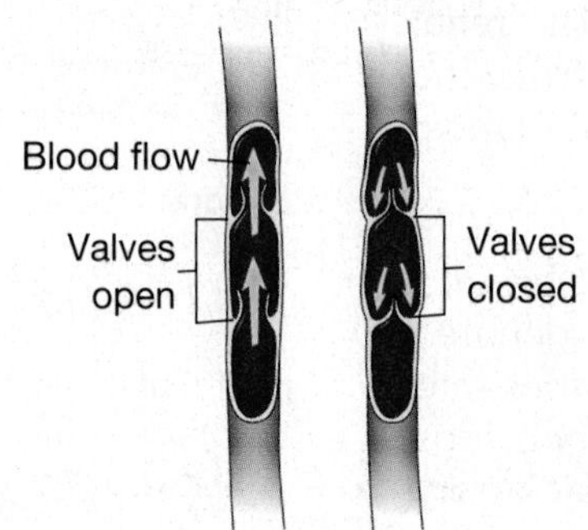

Figure 5-11 ■

4. Many veins are near the surface of the body and can easily be seen just under the skin as a bluish, sometimes bulging line.

capillary (KAP-ih-lair-ee)
capill/o- *hairlike structure*
-ary *pertaining to*
Capillary is derived from a Latin word meaning *resembling a hair.* A capillary is extremely thin, like a hair.

venule (VEN-yool)
ven/o- *vein*
-ule *small thing*

vein (VAYN)

venous (VEE-nus)
ven/o- *vein*
-ous *pertaining to*

vena cava (VEE-nah KAY-vah)
Vena is a Latin singular feminine noun meaning *vein.* Form the plural by changing *-a* to *-ae* (*venae cavae*).

jugular (JUG-yoo-lar)
jugul/o- *jugular (throat)*
-ar *pertaining to*

portal (POR-tal)
port/o- *point of entry*
-al *pertaining to*
The portal vein enters the liver through an area called the *porta hepatis* or *gate of the liver.*

saphenous (sah-FEE-nus)
saphen/o- *standing*
-ous *pertaining to*

The Circulatory System

The cardiovascular system is also known as the **circulatory system** because the heart circulates the blood through the blood vessels. The blood circulates through two different pathways (see Figure 5-12■). The **systemic circulation** includes the arteries, capillaries, and veins everywhere in the body, except in the lungs. The pulmonary circulation includes the arteries, capillaries, and veins going to, within, and coming from the lungs. The word **cardiopulmonary** reflects the close connection between the heart, circulatory system, and the lungs.

Now let's trace the route that blood takes through the systemic and pulmonary circulations as it makes one complete trip through the whole body.

circulatory (SER-kyoo-lah-TOH-ree)
circulat/o- *movement in a circular route*
-ory *having the function of*

systemic (sis-TEM-ik)
system/o- *the body as a whole*
-ic *pertaining to*

circulation (SER-kyoo-LAY-shun)
circulat/o- *movement in a circular route*
-ion *action; condition*

cardiopulmonary (KAR-dee-oh-PUL-moh-nair-ee)
cardi/o- *heart*
pulmon/o- *lung*
-ary *pertaining to*

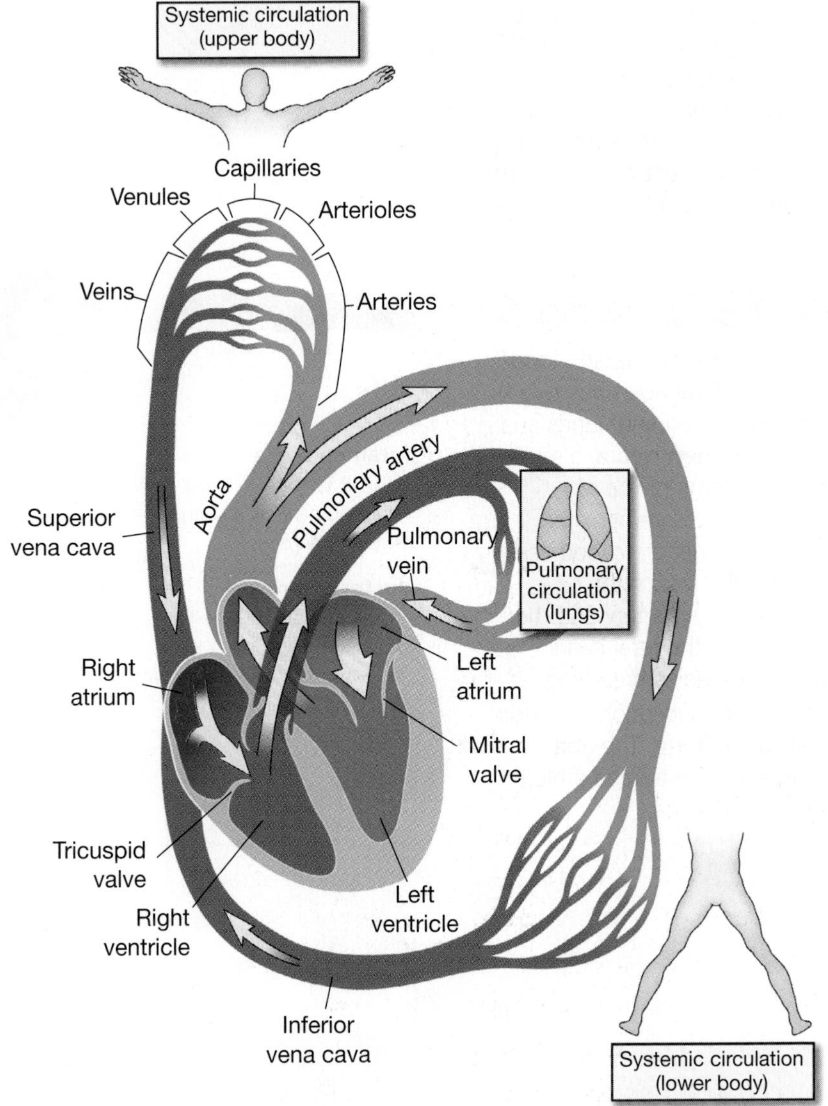

Figure 5-12 ■ Circulation of the blood.

Each time it contracts, the heart pumps blood from the right ventricle through the pulmonary circulation and from the left ventricle through the systemic circulation.

Systemic Circulation Blood coming back from the body via the systemic circulation enters the heart. This dark red-purple blood has a high level of carbon dioxide and a low level of oxygen. It travels through the right atrium, the tricuspid valve, and the right ventricle.

Pulmonary Circulation Blood then flows through the pulmonary valve and into the pulmonary arteries. The pulmonary arteries carry this blood to the lungs. In the lungs, the blood releases carbon dioxide, picks up oxygen, and becomes bright red. The pulmonary veins carry this oxygenated blood to the left atrium of the heart.

At this point, the blood returns to the systemic circulation. It travels through the left atrium, the mitral valve, the left ventricle, the aortic valve, and into the aorta. The aorta, the arteries, arterioles, and capillaries distribute this oxygenated blood to every part of the body. Oxygen moves through the capillary wall to the surrounding cells, and carbon dioxide and other cellular waste products move through the capillary wall and into the blood. This exchange takes place only in the capillaries, not in the arteries or veins. Now this dark red-purple blood has a high level of carbon dioxide and a low level of oxygen. This blood travels through venules, veins, and the superior vena cava (from the head and neck) and the inferior vena cava (from the rest of the body) back to the right atrium of the heart to complete the cycle.

Across the Life Span

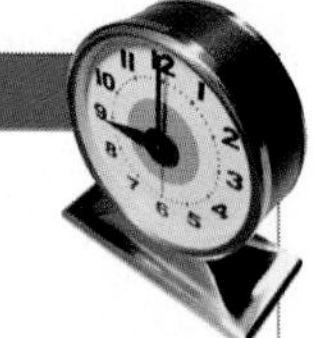

In the uterus, the right atrium of the fetal heart receives oxygenated blood from the mother via arteries in the umbilical cord. The fetal heart has two unique structures that allow it to bypass the (not yet functioning) lungs and send oxygenated blood throughout the body. The **foramen ovale,** a small, oval opening in the septum between the atria, allows some of the oxygenated blood to enter the left side of the heart where it is immediately pumped out to the body. The **ductus arteriosus,** a connecting blood vessel between the pulmonary artery and the aorta, allows the rest of the oxygenated blood to go into the right ventricle and pulmonary artery and then be diverted to the aorta. These two unique structures in the fetal heart should close automatically when the baby is born and begins breathing.

The fetal heart begins to beat just four weeks after conception. The normal heart rate for a newborn is 110 to 150 beats per minute. The normal heart rate for an adult is 70 to 80 beats per minute. A well-trained athlete can have a resting heart rate lower than 60 beats per minute.

foramen ovale
(foh-RAY-men oh-VAH-lee)
Foramen ovale is a Latin phrase meaning *an oval opening.*

ductus arteriosus
(DUK-tus ar-TEER-ee-OH-sus)
Ductus arteriosus is a Latin phrase meaning *duct that leads through a structure like an artery.*

Physiology of a Heartbeat

The heart contracts and relaxes in a regular rhythm that is coordinated by a series of nodes and nerve tissues in the **conduction system** of the heart (see Figure 5-13■). The **sinoatrial node (SA node)** or pacemaker of the heart is a small area of tissue in the posterior wall of the right atrium. The SA node initiates the electrical impulse that begins each heartbeat. The electrical impulse causes both atria to contract simultaneously. Then the electrical impulse travels through the **atrioventricular node (AV node)** to the **bundle of His** and down its left and right bundle branches in the interventricular septum. At the apex of the heart, the right and left bundles separate, and the electrical impulse spreads across the ventricles in a network of nerves (the **Purkinje fibers**), causing both ventricles to contract simultaneously.

A contraction is known as **systole,** and the resting period between contractions when the heart fills with blood is known as **diastole.**

It is important to know that many other small areas of cells in the atria and ventricles can spontaneously produce electrical impulses. These impulses are usually too weak to overpower the rhythm of the SA node. However, if the SA node fails to produce impulses or its impulses are blocked, these **ectopic** sites can take over and control the rhythm of the heart.

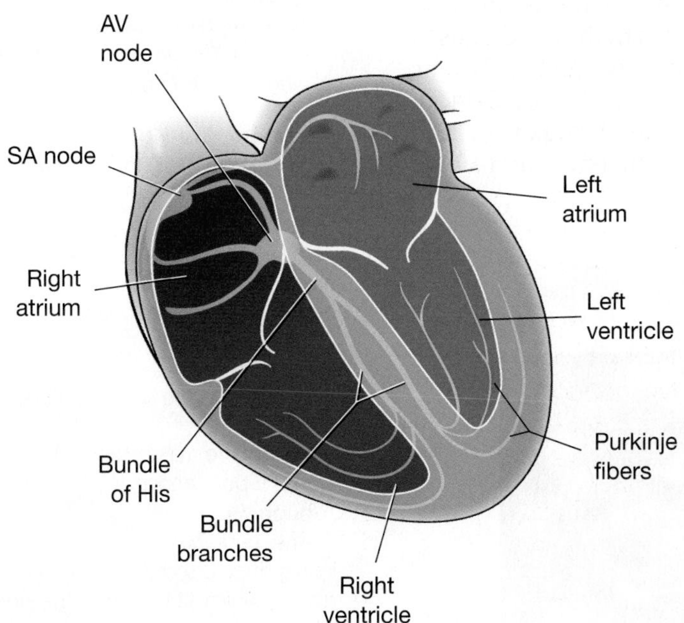

Figure 5-13 ■ The conduction system of the heart.

The SA node (pacemaker) initiates an electrical impulse that travels through the AV node, the bundle of His, the right and left bundle branches, and then to the Purkinje fibers, causing the atria and then the ventricles to contract.

conduction (con-DUK-shun)
conduct/o- *carrying, conveying*
-ion *action; condition*

sinoatrial (SY-noh-AA-tree-al)
sin/o- *hollow cavity; channel*
atri/o- *atrium (upper heart chamber)*
-al *pertaining to*
The sinoatrial node is located in a small groove that once was a sinus (hollow cavity or channel) in the fetal heart.

node (NOHD)
Node is derived from a Latin word meaning *a knob or mass of tissue.*

atrioventricular (AA-tree-oh-ven-TRIK-yoo-lar)
atri/o- *atrium (upper heart chamber)*
ventricul/o- *ventricle (lower heart chamber; chamber in the brain)*
-ar *pertaining to*

bundle of His (HISS)

Purkinje (per-KIN-jee)
Purkinje fibers were named by Johannes Purkinje (1787–1869), a Czechoslovakian anatomist. This is an example of an eponym: a person or thing from whom something takes its name.

systole (SIS-toh-lee)
Systole is a Greek word meaning *a contracting.*

systolic (sis-TAWL-ik)
systol/o- *contracting*
-ic *pertaining to*

diastole (dy-AS-toh-lee)
Diastole is a Greek word meaning *an expansion.*

diastolic (DY-ah-STAWL-ik)
diastol/o- *dilating*
-ic *pertaining to*

ectopic (ek-TOP-ik)
ectop/o- *outside of a place*
-ic *pertaining to*

On a molecular level, an elegant and intricate system allows the heart to contract tirelessly, approximately 100,000 times each day. The electrical impulse from the SA node changes the permeability of the myocardial cell membrane. This process is known as **depolarization.** Potassium **ions** (K^+) leave the cell, but sodium ions (Na^+) in the **extracellular fluid** rush into the cell, followed (more slowly) by calcium ions (Ca^{++}). This gives the **intracellular fluid** a positive charge, which triggers the release of calcium ions stored inside the cell. The calcium ions cause the myocardial cell to contract. As one myocardial cell depolarizes, it triggers the next myocardial cell to do the same. So that the contraction does not continue indefinitely, tiny molecular pumps move potassium and sodium back to where they were before. This restores the normal electrical state, and the myocardial cell returns to a resting state. This is known as **repolarization.** The myocardial cell cannot respond to another electrical impulse from the SA node until the full cycle of depolarization and repolarization is complete. This period of unresponiveness is known as the **refractory period.** A contraction and a rest period equal a cardiac cycle.

The refractory period is very, very short, and technically the heart could contract again almost instantly, but this would not allow enough time for the chambers of the heart to completely fill with blood and eventually the heart would tire. The optimum heart rate allows the heart chambers to completely fill with blood and allows the heart some time to rest between beats. This is the rate set by the SA node and it is known as **normal sinus rhythm (NSR).**

Sometimes the heart needs to beat faster than the SA node-controlled rhythm. **Epinephrine** (a neurotransmitter from the sympathetic nervous system) overrides the normal sinus rhythm and causes the heart to beat faster to support increased activity during danger (the "fight or flight" response) or during exercise (see Figure 5-14■). **Acetylcholine** (a neurotransmitter from the vagus nerve of the parasympathetic nervous system) exerts the opposite effect and slows the heart rate to a normal sinus rhythm.

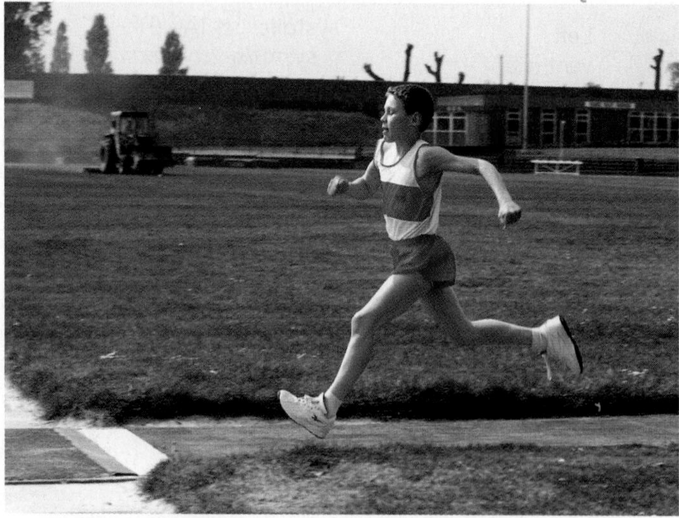

Figure 5-14 ■ Exercise increases the heart rate.

Epinephrine released during exercise increases the heart rate, constricts blood vessels to increase the blood pressure, and dilates the bronchi to increase the flow of air into the lungs.

depolarization (dee-POHL-ar-ih-ZAY-shun)
de- *reversal of, without*
polar/o- *two opposite poles*
-ization *the process of making, creating, or inserting*
Some word parts have more than one definition. The best definition of *depolarization* is *the process of making [a condition] without two oppositely charged poles*

ion (EYE-on)

extracellular (EKS-trah-SEL-yoo-lar)
extra- *outside of*
cellul/o- *cell*
-ar *pertaining to*

intracellular (IN-trah-SEL-yoo-lar)
intra- *within*
cellul/o- *cell*
-ar *pertaining to*

repolarization (ree-POHL-ar-ih-ZAY-shun)
re- *again and again; backward; unable to*
polar/o- *two opposite poles*
-ization *the process of making, creating, or inserting*

refractory (ree-FRAK-tor-ee)
re- *again and again; backward; unable to*
fract/o- *break up*
-ory *pertaining to*
Some word parts have more than one definition. The best definition of *refractory* is *pertaining to [being] unable to break up.*

sinus (SY-nus)
Sinus refers to the *sinoatrial node.*

epinephrine (EP-ih-NEF-rin)
epi- *upon, above*
nephr/o- *kidney*
-ine *pertaining to*
Epinephrine is secreted by the adrenal glands, which sit on top of the kidneys.

acetylcholine (AS-eh-til-KOH-leen)

Vocabulary Review

Anatomy and Physiology

Now that you have studied the anatomy and physiology of the cardiovascular system, take time to review those new words and descriptions. Memorize the combining forms and their definitions before going on to the next section.

Word or Phrase	Combining Form and Definition	Description
acetylcholine		Neurotransmitter for the parasympathetic nervous system. It is released by the vagus nerve and slows the heart rate.
aorta	aort/o- *aorta*	Largest artery in the body. It receives blood from the left ventricle of the heart. Parts of the aorta include the **ascending aorta,** the **aortic arch,** the **thoracic aorta,** and the **abdominal aorta.**
aortic valve	aort/o- *aorta*	Heart valve located between the left ventricle and the aorta
apex	apic/o- *apex (tip)*	Lower tip of the heart. The ventricles lie beneath the apex.
arteriole	arteriol/o- *arteriole*	Smallest branch of an artery
artery	arteri/o- *artery*	Blood vessel that carries oxygen-rich blood away from the heart. The exception is the pulmonary arteries that carry oxygen-poor blood to the lungs.
atrioventricular (AV) node	nod/o- *node (knob of tissue)*	Small knot of tissue located between the right atrium and right ventricle. The **AV node** is part of the conduction system of the heart and receives electrical impulses from the SA node.
atrium	atri/o- *atrium*	Two upper chambers of the heart
axillary artery	axill/o- *axilla (armpit)*	Major artery that carries blood to the axilla and shoulder
blood vessels	vascul/o- *blood vessel*	Channels through which the blood circulates throughout the body. These include arteries, capillaries, and veins. Also known as **vascular structures.**
brachial artery	brachi/o- *arm*	Major artery that carries blood to the upper arm
bundle of His		Section of the conduction system of the heart after the AV node. It splits into the right and left bundle branches.
bundle branches		Parallel fiber bundles of the conduction system of the heart that begin at the bundle of His and travel down the interventricular septum. At the apex of the heart, the right bundle branch turns to the right ventricle and the left bundle branch turns to the left ventricle. Then each bundle divides into the Purkinje fibers.
calcium		Ion (Ca^{++}) that causes the myocardium to contract
capillary	capill/o- *hairlike structure*	Smallest blood vessel in the body. It connects the arterioles to the venules. The exchange of oxygen and carbon dioxide takes place in the capillaries.

Word or Phrase	Combining Form and Definition	Description
cardiac cycle		One contraction of the heart and the rest period that follows
cardiopulmonary	**cardi/o-** *heart* **pulmon/o-** *lung*	Pertaining to the heart and lungs
cardiothoracic	**cardi/o-** *heart* **thorac/o-** *thorax (chest)*	Pertaining to the heart and thoracic cavity
cardiovascular system	**cardi/o-** *heart* **vascul/o-** *blood vessel*	Body system that includes the heart and the blood vessels
carotid artery	**carot/o-** *stupor, sleep*	Major artery that carries blood to the face, head, and brain. If these arteries are compressed, the lack of blood to the brain will cause a person to become unconscious.
chordae tendineae		Ropelike strands that support the tricuspid and mitral valves and keep their leaflets tightly closed when the ventricles are contracting.
circulatory system	**circulat/o-** *movement in a circular route*	Circular route that the blood takes as it moves through the body. **Circulation** is the process of moving the blood through the system.
conduction system	**conduct/o-** *carrying, conveying*	System that conveys the electrical impulse that makes the heart beat. It consists of the SA node, AV node, bundle of His, bundle branches, and Purkinje fibers.
coronary arteries	**coron/o-** *encircling structure*	Arteries that bring blood to the myocardium
depolarization	**polar/o-** *two oppositely charged poles*	Changing of the permeability of a myocardial cell to allow potassium ions to flow out of the cell, and sodium and calcium ions to flow into the cell. This is triggered by the electrical impulse of the conduction system.
diastole		Resting period between contractions. It is when the heart fills with blood.
ductus arteriosus		Temporary, small blood vessel in the fetal heart that connects the pulmonary artery to the aorta. It should close when the baby is born.
ectopic sites	**ectop/o-** *outside of a place*	Areas of tissue within the heart that can generate weak electrical impulses but are not part of the normal conduction system of the heart.
endocardium	**cardi/o-** *heart*	Innermost layer of the heart. It covers the inside of the heart chambers and valves.
endothelium	**theli/o-** *cellular layer*	Smooth innermost layer of the wall of a blood vessel. Also known as the **intima.**
epicardium	**cardi/o-** *heart*	Inner membrane of the double-layered pericardium. It covers the myocardium of the heart.
epinephrine	**nephr/o-** *kidney*	Neurotransmitter for the sympathetic nervous system. It increases the heart rate to prepare for exercise or the "flight or fight" response.
extracellular fluid	**cellul/o-** *cell*	Fluid outside a cell

Word or Phrase	Combining Form and Definition	Description
femoral artery	**femor/o-** *femur (thigh bone)*	Major artery that carries blood to the upper leg
foramen ovale		Temporary, oval-shaped opening in the interatrial septum of the fetal heart. It should close when the baby is born.
great vessels		Collective phrase for the aorta (the largest artery), the superior and inferior venae cavae (the largest veins), and the pulmonary arteries and veins
heart	**cardi/o-** *heart*	Organ that pumps blood through the body
iliac artery	**ili/o-** *ilium (hip bone)*	Major artery that carries blood to the pelvic cavity and lower extremity
intracellular fluid	**cellul/o-** *cell, cells*	Fluid inside a cell
ion		A positively or negatively charged atom
jugular vein	**jugul/o-** *jugular (throat)*	Major vein that carries blood from the head to the superior vena cava
lumen		Central opening inside a blood vessel through which the blood flows
mediastinum		Central area in the thoracic cavity that lies between the lungs and contains the heart, great vessels, thymus, trachea, and esophagus.
mitral valve	**mitr/o-** *(structure like a miter or tall hat with two points)*	Heart valve located between the left atrium and the left ventricle. Also known as the **bicuspid valve.** It has two (*bi-*) pointed **leaflets** or **cusps.**
myocardium	**my/o-** *muscle*	Muscular wall of the heart
normal sinus rhythm		A heart rate of 70 to 80 beats per minute that is the normal resting rate set by the SA node
parietal pericardium	**cardi/o-** *heart*	Part of the pericardium that forms the outer wall of the pericardial sac. This pouch is filled with pericardial fluid. The parietal pericardium is also known as the visceral pericardium.
peroneal artery	**perone/o-** *fibula*	Major artery that carries blood to the lateral aspect of the lower leg
popliteal artery	**poplit/o-** *back of the knee*	Major artery that carries blood to the back of the knee
portal vein	**port/o-** *point of entry*	Major vein that carries blood from the intestines to the liver
potassium		Ion (K^+) that plays a role in the contraction of the myocardium
pulmonary artery	**pulmon/o-** *lung*	Artery that carries blood from the heart to the lungs. The pulmonary artery is the only artery in the body that carries oxygen-poor blood.
pulmonary circulation	**pulmon/o-** *lung*	The blood, arteries, capillaries, and veins that go in and out of the lungs, but not to the rest of the body
pulmonary valve	**pulmon/o-** *lung*	Heart valve located between the right ventricle and the pulmonary artery
pulmonary vein	**pulmon/o-** *lung*	Vein that carries blood from the lungs to the heart. The pulmonary vein is the only vein in the body that carries oxygen-rich blood.

Word or Phrase	Combining Form and Definition	Description
pulse		The bulging of an artery wall from blood pumped by the heart
Purkinje fibers		Network of interlacing fibers of the conduction system of the heart. They arise from the bundle branches and spread throughout the ventricles.
radial artery	**radi/o-** *radius (forearm bone)*	Major artery that carries blood to the lower arm along the side by the thumb
refractory period	**fract/o-** *break up*	Short period of time when the myocardium is resting and unresponsive to electrical impulses
renal artery	**ren/o-** *kidney*	Major artery that carries blood to the kidney
repolarization	**polar/o-** *two opposite poles*	The opposite of depolarization. Pumps in the cell move calcium and sodium ions out of the cell. Potassium ions come back into the cell. This restores the normal electrical state of the cell and puts it in a resting state.
saphenous vein	**saphen/o-** *standing*	Major vein that carries blood from the foot and leg to the groin
septum	**sept/o-** *septum (dividing wall)*	Partitioning wall that divides the right atrium from the left atrium (**interatrial septum**) and the right ventricle from the left ventricle (**interventricular septum**)
sinoatrial node	**sin/o-** *hollow cavity; channel*	Pacemaker of the heart. Small knot of tissue located in the posterior wall of the right atrium. The **SA node** dictates the heart rate at 70 to 80 beats per minute when the body is at rest. It originates the electrical impulse for the entire conduction system of the heart.
sodium		Ion (Na^+) that plays a role in the contraction of the myocardium
subclavian artery	**clav/o-** *clavicle (collar bone)*	Major artery that carries blood to the upper extremities. It goes under the clavicle before it reaches the arm.
systemic circulation	**system/o-** *the body as a whole*	The blood, arteries, capillaries, and veins everywhere in the body except the lungs
systole		Combined contractions of the atria and the ventricles
thoracic cavity	**thorac/o-** *thorax (chest)*	Major body cavity in the chest. It contains the lungs and mediastinum (that contains the heart and great vessels).
tibial artery	**tibi/o-** *tibia (shin bone)*	Major artery that carries blood to the anterior and posterior aspects of the lower leg
tricuspid valve	**cusp/o-** *projection, point*	Heart valve located between the right atrium and right ventricle. It has three (*tri-*) pointed leaflets or cusps.
ulnar artery	**uln/o-** *ulna*	Major artery that carries blood to the lower arm along the side of the little finger
vasculature	**vascul/o-** *blood vessel*	Network of blood vessels in a particular organ
vasoconstriction	**vas/o-** *blood vessel; vas deferens* **constrict/o-** *drawn together, narrowed*	Constriction of the smooth muscle in the artery wall causes the artery to become smaller in diameter

Word or Phrase	Combining Form and Definition	Description
vasodilation	**dilat/o-** *dilate, widen*	Relaxation of the smooth muscle in the artery wall causes the artery to become larger in diameter
vein	**ven/o-** *vein*	Blood vessel that carries oxygen-poor blood as well as carbon dioxide and waste products of cellular metabolism away from the cells and back to the heart. The exception is the pulmonary vein, which carries oxygenated blood from the lungs to the heart.
vena cava		Largest vein in the body. The **superior vena cava** receives blood from the head, neck, arms, and chest and takes it to the heart. The **inferior vena cava** receives blood from the abdomen, pelvis, and legs and takes it to the heart.
venule	**ven/o-** *vein*	Smallest branch of a vein
valve	**valvul/o-** *valve*	Structure that opens and closes to control the flow of blood. The heart valves include the tricuspid valve, pulmonary valve, mitral valve, and aortic valve. There are also valves in some of the large veins that prevent backflow of blood.
ventricle	**ventricul/o-** *ventricle*	Two lower chambers of the heart

Word Alert

cardia (noun) Small region of the stomach where the esophagus enters

Example: The cardia is the first part of the stomach to receive food from the esophagus.

cardiac (adjective) Pertaining to the heart

Example: During a cardiac arrest, the heart stops beating.

cardiac sphincter (noun) Ring of muscle at the end of the esophagus that constricts

Example: If the cardiac sphincter does not close tightly, acid from the stomach goes into the esophagus and causes heartburn.

cardiac valve (noun) Structure between two chambers of the heart that opens and closes to regulate the flow of blood

Example: A stethoscope allows you to hear the sound that a cardiac valve makes as it opens and closes.

Labeling Exercise

A. *Match each anatomy word or phrase to its numbered structure in Figure 5-15■. Write that word or phrase on the blank line next to its number. Use the Answer Key at the end of the book to check your answers.*

aorta	inferior vena cava	mitral valve	right ventricle
aortic valve	interventricular septum	pulmonary artery	superior vena cava
apex	left atrium	pulmonary valve	tricuspid valve
chordae tendinae	left ventricle	right atrium	

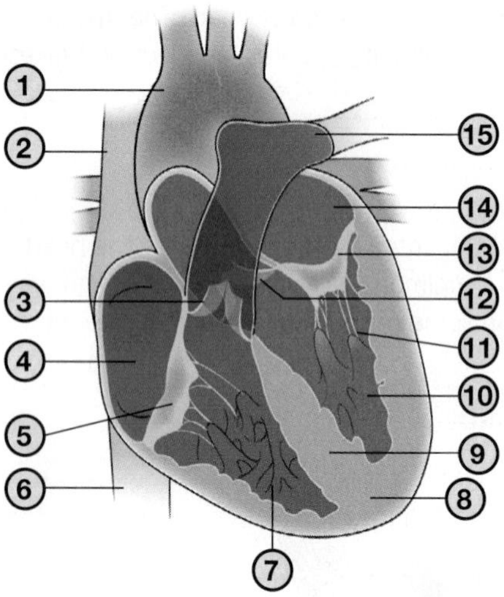

Figure 5-15 ■

1. ______________________
2. ______________________
3. ______________________
4. ______________________
5. ______________________
6. ______________________
7. ______________________
8. ______________________
9. ______________________
10. ______________________
11. ______________________
12. ______________________
13. ______________________
14. ______________________
15. ______________________

B. *Match each anatomy word or phrase to its numbered structure in Figure 5-16■. Write that word or phrase on the blank line next to its number.*

atrioventricular node	bundle of His	sinoatrial node
bundle branches	Purkinje fibers	

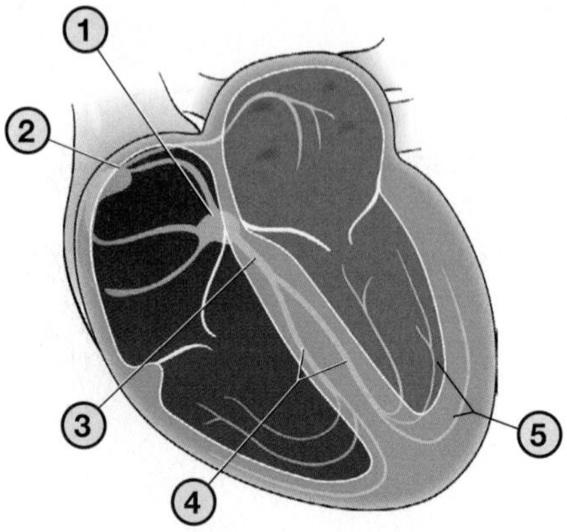

Figure 5-16 ■

1. ______________________
2. ______________________
3. ______________________
4. ______________________
5. ______________________

C. *Match each anatomy word or phrase to its numbered structure in Figure 5-17 ■. Write that word or phrase on the blank line next to its number.*

abdominal aorta	common carotid artery	internal carotid artery	radial artery
anterior tibial artery	common iliac artery	internal iliac artery	renal artery
aortic arch	coronary artery	peroneal artery	subclavian artery
ascending aorta	external iliac artery	popliteal artery	thoracic aorta
axillary artery	femoral artery	posterior tibial artery	ulnar artery
brachial artery			

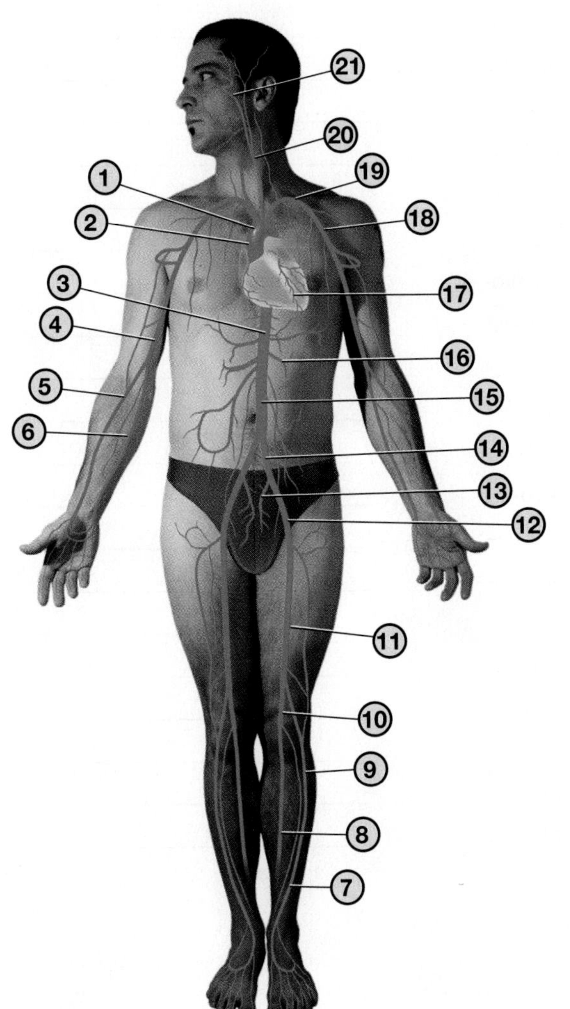

Figure 5-17 ■

1. ____________________
2. ____________________
3. ____________________
4. ____________________
5. ____________________
6. ____________________
7. ____________________
8. ____________________
9. ____________________
10. ____________________
11. ____________________
12. ____________________
13. ____________________
14. ____________________
15. ____________________
16. ____________________
17. ____________________
18. ____________________
19. ____________________
20. ____________________
21. ____________________

Building Medical Words

Combining Forms

Here are the combining forms you have learned so far. Next to each combining form, write its meaning. Use the Answer Key at the end of the book to check your answers. The first one has been done for you.

	Combining Form	Medical Meaning		Combining Form	Medical Meaning
1.	axill/o-	axilla (armpit)	24.	mitr/o-	
2.	aort/o-		25.	my/o-	
3.	apic/o-		26.	perone/o-	
4.	arteri/o-		27.	poplite/o-	
5.	arteriol/o-		28.	port/o-	
6.	atri/o-		29.	pulmon/o-	
7.	brachi/o-		30.	radi/o-	
8.	capill/o-		31.	ren/o-	
9.	cardi/o-		32.	saphen/o-	
10.	carot/o-		33.	sept/o-	
11.	cellul/o-		34.	sin/o-	
12.	circulat/o-		35.	system/o-	
13.	conduct/o-		36.	systol/o-	
14.	constrict/o-		37.	theli/o-	
15.	coron/o-		38.	thorac/o-	
16.	cusp/o-		39.	tibi/o-	
17.	diastol/o-		40.	uln/o-	
18.	dilat/o-		41.	valvul/o-	
19.	ectop/o-		42.	vascul/o-	
20.	femor/o-		43.	vas/o-	
21.	ili/o-		44.	ven/o-	
22.	jugul/o-		45.	ventricul/o-	
23.	mediastin/o-				

Combining Forms and Suffixes

Read the definition hint for the medical word you are to build. Look at the combining form that is given. Write the correct suffix on the blank line. Then write the medical word. (Remember: You may need to remove the combining vowel. Always remove the hyphens and slash.) Use the Answer Key at the end of the book to check your answers. The first one has been done for you.

SUFFIX LIST		
-ac (pertaining to)	-ary (pertaining to)	-ion (action; condition)
-al (pertaining to)	-ature (system composed of)	-ity (state; condition)
-ar (pertaining to)	-ic (pertaining to)	-ous (pertaining to)

	Definition Hint	Combining Form	Suffix	Write the Medical Word
1.	Pertaining to the thorax (chest)	thorac/o-	-ic	thoracic
2.	Pertaining to an artery	arteri/o-	______	______
3.	Pertaining to a valve	valvul/o-	______	______
4.	Action of movement in a circular route	circulat/o-	______	______
5.	Pertaining to the heart	cardi/o-	______	______
6.	Pertaining to a hairlike structure (blood vessel)	capill/o-	______	______
7.	Pertaining to a vein	ven/o-	______	______
8.	Pertaining to the body as a whole	system/o-	______	______
9.	Pertaining to the atrium	atri/o-	______	______
10.	Pertaining to the arm	brachi/o-	______	______
11.	Pertaining to the back of the knee	poplite/o-	______	______
12.	Pertaining to standing	saphen/o-	______	______
13.	Pertaining to the aorta	aort/o-	______	______
14.	System composed of blood vessels	vascul/o-	______	______
15.	Pertaining to a contracting	systol/o-	______	______
16.	Condition of a hollow space	cav/o-	______	______

Two Combining Forms and Suffixes

Read the definition hint for the medical word you are to build. Look at the suffix that is given. Write the correct combining forms on the blank lines. Then write the medical word on the next blank line. (Remember: You may need to remove the combining vowel. Always remove the hyphens and slash.) Use the Answer Key at the end of the book to check your answers. The first one has been done for you.

COMBINING FORM LIST

atri/o- (atrium)	my/o- (muscle)	vascul/o- (blood vessel)
cardi/o- (heart)	pulmon/o- (lung)	vas/o- (blood vessel; vas deferens)
constrict/o- (drawn together, narrowed)	sin/o- (hollow cavity; channel)	ventricul/o- (ventricle)
dilat/o- (dilate, widen)		

Definition Hint	Combining Form	Combining Form	Suffix	Write the Medical Word
1. Condition of dilation of blood vessels	vas/o-	dilat/o-	-ion	*vasodilation*
2. Pertaining to the heart and lungs	______	______	-ary	______
3. Pertaining to the heart and blood vessels	______	______	-ar	______
4. Pertaining to the SA node	______	______	-al	______
5. Condition of constriction of the blood vessels	______	______	-ion	______
6. Pertaining to the heart muscle	______	______	-al	______
7. Pertaining to the atrium and ventricle	______	______	-ar	______

Combining Forms and Prefixes

Read the definition hint for the medical word you are to build. Look at the medical word or word part that is given. It already contains a combining form and a suffix. Write the correct prefix on the blank line. Then write the entire medical word on the next blank line. (Remember: You may need to remove the combining vowel. Always remove the hyphens and slash.) Use the Answer Key at the end of the book to check your answers. The first one has been done for you.

PREFIX LIST

endo- (innermost, within)	extra- (outside of)	peri- (around)
epi- (upon, above)	intra- (within)	tri- (three)

Definition Hint	Prefix	Medical Word or Word Part	Write the Medical Word
1. Pertaining to outside the cell	extra-	cellular	*extracellular*
2. Pertaining to around the heart	______	cardial	______
3. Pertaining to within the ventricle	______	ventricular	______
4. Pertaining to being upon or above the heart	______	cardial	______
5. Pertaining to inside of the cell	______	cellular	______
6. Resembling three points or projections	______	cuspid	______
7. Pertaining to a cellular layer within a blood vessel	______	thelial	______

Symptoms, Signs, and Diseases

Myocardium

Word or Phrase	Word Part and Definition	Description
acute coronary syndrome		General category that includes acute ischemia of the myocardium with unstable angina pectoris. Treatment: Nitroglycerin drugs, oxygen.
angina pectoris	**angina** (AN-jih-nah) (an-JY-nah) *Angina* is a Latin word meaning *sore throat.* Its meaning changed to *chest pain that radiates to the throat and neck.* **anginal** (AN-jih-nal) (an-JY-nal) **angin/o-** *angina* **-al** *pertaining to* **pectoris** (PEK-toh-ris) *Pectoris* is a Latin word meaning *of the chest.* **ischemia** (is-KEE-mee-ah) **isch/o-** *keep back; block* **-emia** *condition of the blood; substance in the blood*	Mild-to-severe chest pain caused by **ischemia** of the myocardium. Atherosclerosis blocks the flow of oxygenated blood through the coronary arteries to the myocardium. The patient may feel a crushing, pressurelike sensation in the chest, with pain extending up into the neck or down the left arm, often accompanied by extreme sweating (diaphoresis) and a sense of doom. Angina pectoris can occur during exercise or while resting. Angina is a warning sign of an impending myocardial infarction. Treatment: Nitroglycerin drugs, oxygen. **Did You Know?** For many years, newspaper and magazine articles described the classic symptoms of angina pectoris in order to raise public awareness and encourage those with angina to promptly seek medical help. Now it is known that those symptoms occur in men, but women most often experience angina as indigestion, nausea, anxiety, extreme fatigue, or trouble sleeping.
cardiomegaly	**cardiomegaly** (KAR-dee-oh-MEG-ah-lee) **cardi/o-** *heart* **-megaly** *enlargement*	Enlargement of the heart, usually due to congestive heart failure. Treatment: Correct the underlying cause.
cardiomyopathy	**cardiomyopathy** (KAR-dee-oh-my-AWP-ah-thee) **cardi/o-** *heart* **my/o-** *muscle* **-pathy** *disease, suffering* **idiopathic** (ID-ee-oh-PATH-ik) **idi/o-** *unknown; individual* **path/o-** *disease, suffering* **-ic** *pertaining to*	Any disease condition of the heart muscle that includes heart enlargement and heart failure. In **dilated cardiomyopathy,** the left ventricle is dilated and the myocardium is so stretched that it can no longer contract to pump blood. **Idiopathic cardiomyopathy** has an unknown cause. Treatment: Correct the underlying cause, if known.
congestive heart failure (CHF)	**congestive** (con-JES-tiv) **congest/o-** *accumulation of fluid* **-ive** *pertaining to* **hypertrophy** (hy-PER-troh-fee) **hyper-** *above; more than normal* **-trophy** *process of development*	Inability of the heart to pump sufficient amounts of blood. Caused by chronic coronary artery disease or hypertension. During early CHF, the myocardium undergoes **hypertrophy** (enlargement). This temporarily improves blood flow, and the patient is said to be in **compensated** heart failure. In the later stages of CHF, the heart can no longer enlarge. Instead, the myocardium becomes dilated (dilated cardiomyopathy), flabby, and progressively loses its ability to contract, and the patient is said to be in **decompensated heart failure.** *(continued)*

Word or Phrase	Word Part and Definition	Description
congestive heart failure (CHF) *(continued)*	Every medical word must contain a combining form. The suffix of *hypertrophy* contains the combining form *troph/o-*. **hypertrophic** (HY-per-TROH-fik) **hyper-** *above; more than normal* **troph/o-** *development* **-ic** *pertaining to* **compensated** (KAWM-pen-SAY-ted) **compens/o-** *counterbalance; compensate* **-ated** *pertaining to a condition; composed of* **decompensated** (dee-KAWM-pen-SAY-ted) **de-** *reversal of, without* **compens/o-** *counterbalance; compensate* **-ated** *pertaining to a condition; composed of* **distention** (dis-TEN-shun) **distent/o-** *distended, stretched* **-ion** *action; condition* **peripheral** (peh-RIF-eh-ral) **peripher/o-** *outer aspects* **-al** *pertaining to* **edema** (eh-DEE-mah) *Edema* is derived from a Greek word meaning *a swelling*. **cor pulmonale** (KOR PUL-moh-NAL-ee)	In right-sided congestive heart failure, the right ventricle is unable to adequately pump blood. Blood backs up in the superior vena cava, causing **jugular venous distention** (dilated jugular veins in the neck). Blood also backs up in the inferior vena cava, causing hepatomegaly (enlargement of the liver), and **peripheral edema** in the legs, ankles, and feet (see Figure 5-18■). When there is lung disease and the right ventricle enlarges to pump harder, this condition is known as **cor pulmonale.** 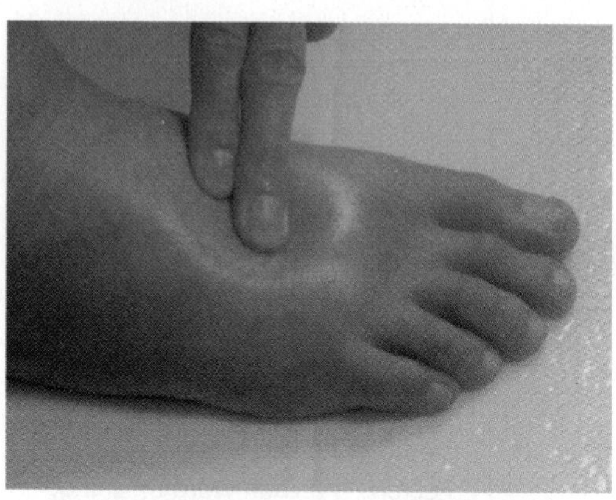 **Figure 5-18 ■ Peripheral edema.** Swollen, fluid-filled soft tissues in the legs and feet can be a sign of right-sided congestive heart failure. Pressure on the area produces a deep indentation that takes several minutes to resolve. This is known as pitting edema. In left-sided congestive heart failure, the left ventricle is unable to adequately pump blood, and blood backs up into the lungs, causing pulmonary edema, which can be seen on a chest x-ray. Other symptoms include shortness of breath, cough, and an inability to sleep while lying flat. Treatment: Diuretic drugs, digitalis, and antihypertensive drugs. Severe left-sided heart failure is life-threatening and may require a heart transplant or a left ventricular assist device (LVAD).
myocardial infarction (MI)	**myocardial** (MY-oh-KAR-dee-al) **my/o-** *muscle* **cardi/o-** *heart* **-al** *pertaining to* **infarction** (in-FARK-shun) **infarct/o-** *area of dead tissue* **-ion** *action; condition* **necrosis** (neh-KROH-sis) **necr/o-** *death* **-osis** *condition; abnormal condition; process*	Death of myocardial cells due to severe ischemia. The flow of oxygenated blood in a coronary artery is blocked by a blood clot or atherosclerosis. The patient may experience severe angina pectoris, may have mild symptoms like indigestion, or may have no symptoms at all (a silent MI). The infarcted area of myocardium has **necrosis.** If the area of necrosis is small, it will eventually be replaced by scar tissue. If the area is large, the heart muscle may be unable to contract. Treatment: Thrombolytic drugs to dissolve a clot during an MI.

Heart Valves and Layers of the Heart

Word or Phrase	Word Part and Definition	Description
endocarditis	**endocarditis** (EN-doh-kar-DY-tis) **endo-** *innermost, within* **card/i-** *heart* **-itis** *inflammation of* The combining vowel *i* of *card/i-* is deleted before it is joined to the suffix *-itis*. **subacute** (sub-ah-KYOOT) *Subacute* is a combination of the prefix *sub- (below; underneath; less than)* and the word *acute* *(severe, intense)*.	Inflammation and bacterial infection of the endocardium and the valves. This occurs in patients who already have a structural defect of the valves or heart. Bacteria from an infection elsewhere in the body travel through the blood, are trapped by the structural defect, and cause infection. Acute endocarditis causes a high fever and shock, while **subacute bacterial endocarditis (SBE)** causes fever, fatigue, and aching muscles. Treatment: Antibiotic drugs.
murmur	**murmur** (MER-mer)	Abnormal heart sound created by turbulence as blood leaks past a defective heart valve. Murmurs are described according to their volume (soft or loud), their sound, and when they occur during the cardiac cycle. Functional murmurs are mild murmurs that are not associated with disease and are not clinically significant. Treatment: Correct the defective heart valve, if needed. **Did You Know?** Heart murmurs can sound like the call of a sea gull, blowing wind, the clatter of machinery, high-pitched musical notes, or like churning, humming, or clicking.
pericarditis	**pericarditis** (PAIR-ee-kar-DY-tis) **peri-** *around* **card/i-** *heart* **-itis** *inflammation of* **tamponade** (tam-poh-NAYD) **tampon/o-** *stop up* **-ade** *action; process*	Inflammation or infection of the pericardial sac with an accumulation of pericardial fluid. When the fluid presses on the heart and prevents it from beating, this is known as **cardiac tamponade.** Treatment: Antibiotic drugs. Pericardiocentesis, if necessary.

Word or Phrase	Word Part and Definition	Description
rheumatic heart disease	**rheumatic** (roo-MAT-ik) **rheumat/o-** *watery discharge* **-ic** *pertaining to* This refers to the collection of fluid in the joints, not the heart. **vegetation** (VEJ-eh-TAY-shun) **vegetat/o-** *growth* **-ion** *action; condition* **stenosis** (steh-NOH-sis) **sten/o-** *narrowness, constriction* **-osis** *condition; abnormal condition; process*	Autoimmune response to a previous streptococcal infection, like a strep throat. It occurs most often in children and is known as rheumatic fever. The body makes antibodies to fight the bacteria, but after the infection is gone the antibodies attack the connective tissue in the body, particularly the joints and/or the heart. The joints become swollen with fluid and inflamed. The mitral and aortic valves of the heart become inflamed and damaged. **Vegetations** (irregular collections of platelets, fibrin, and bacteria) form on the valves (see Figure 5-19 ■). The valves become scarred and narrowed, a condition known as **stenosis.** Treatment: Antibiotic drug to treat the initial infection. After rheumatic heart disease has occurred, a prophylactic (preventative) antibiotic drug is given prior to any dental or surgical procedure that might release bacteria that could further damage the valves. 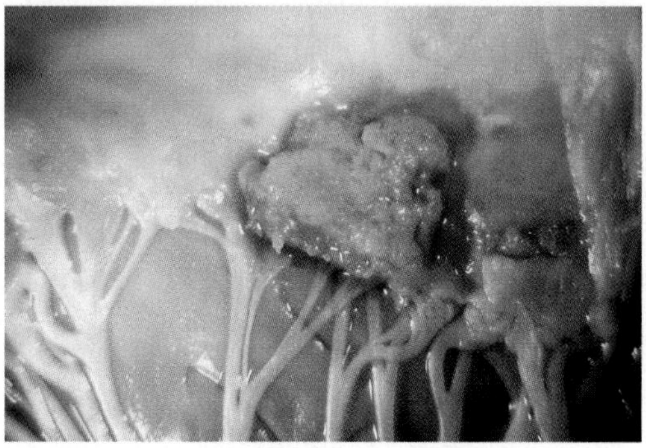 **Figure 5-19 ■ Vegetation on the mitral valve.** This close-up of the mitral valve shows an irregular brown vegetation growing on the otherwise smooth surface of the valve. The multiple ropelike structures below are the chordae tendineae of the valve.

Word or Phrase	Word Part and Definition	Description
mitral valve prolapse (MVP)	**prolapse** (PROH-laps) *Prolapse* is derived from a Greek word meaning *falling down.* **regurgitation** (ree-GER-jih-TAY-shun) **regurgitat/o-** *flow backward* **-ion** *action; condition*	Structural abnormality in which the leaflets of the mitral valve do not close tightly. This can be a congenital condition or can occur if the valve is damaged by infection. There is **regurgitation** as blood flows backwards into the left atrium with each contraction. Slight prolapse is a common condition and does not require treatment. Treatment: Surgical correction with a valvoplasty or valve replacement.

Across the Life Span

These congenital abnormalities can occur in the fetal heart as it develops:

coarctation (KOH-ark-TAY-shun)
coarct/o- *pressed together*
-ation *a process; being or having*

tetralogy (tet-RAL-oh-jee)
tetr/a- *four*
-logy *the study of*

Fallot (fah-LOW)
These congenital heart defects were first described by Ètienne-Louis Fallot (1850–1911), a French physician.

1. **Coarctation of the aorta.** The aorta is abnormally narrow.
2. **Atrial septal defect (ASD).** There is a permanent hole in the interatrial septum.
3. **Ventricular septal defect (VSD).** There is a permanent hole in the interventricular septum.
4. **Tetralogy of Fallot.** There are four defects, including a ventricular septal defect, narrowing of the pulmonary artery valve and trunk, hypertrophy of the right ventricle, and malposition of the aorta.
5. **Transposition of the great vessels.** The aorta incorrectly originates from the right ventricle, and the pulmonary artery incorrectly originates from the left ventricle.

These abnormalities occur at the time of birth during the change from fetal circulation to normal newborn circulation:

patent (PAY-tent)
pat/o- *to lie open*
-ent *pertaining to*

1. **Patent ductus arteriosus (PDA).** The ductus arteriosus fails to close.
2. **Patent foramen ovale.** The foramen ovale fails to close.

Conduction System

Word or Phrase	Word Part and Definition	Description
arrhythmia	**arrhythmia** (aa-RITH-mee-ah) **a-** *away from, without* **rrhythm/o-** *rhythm* **-ia** *condition, state, thing* **dysrrhythmia** (dis-RITH-mee-ah) **dys-** *painful, difficult, abnormal* **rrhythm/o-** *rhythm* **-ia** *condition, state, thing* Some word parts have more than one definition. The best definition of *dysrrhythmia* is *condition of an abnormal rhythm.* A dysrrhythmia is never painful.	Any type of irregularity in the rate or rhythm of the heart. Also known as **dysrrhythmia.** Arrhythmia includes bradycardia, tachycardia, heart block, flutter, and fibrillation. Treatment: Antiarrhythmic drugs, cardioversion, or pacemaker, depending on the type of arrhythmia.

Word or Phrase	Word Part and Definition	Description
bradycardia	**bradycardia** (BRAD-ee-KAR-dee-ah) **brady-** *slow* **card/i-** *heart* **-ia** *condition, state, thing* **bradycardic** (BRAD-ee-KAR-dik) **brady-** *slow* **card/i-** *heart* **ic-** *pertaining to*	Arrhythmia in which the heart beats too slowly. A patient with bradycardia is said to be **bradycardic.** Treatment: Atropine (an antiarrhythmic drug specifically for bradycardia).
cardiac arrest	**asystole** (aa-SIS-toh-lee) *Asystole* is a combination of the prefix *a-* (away from, without) and the word *systole* (contracting).	Complete absence of a heartbeat. Also known as **asystole.** Treatment: cardiopulmonary resuscitation (CPR).
flutter		Arrhythmia in which there is a very fast but regular rhythm (250 beats per minute) of the atria or ventricles. The chambers of the heart do not have time to completely fill with blood before the next contraction. Flutter can progress to fibrillation. Treatment: Antiarrhythmic drugs.
fibrillation	**fibrillation** (FIB-rih-LAY-shun) **fibrill/o-** *muscle fiber; nerve fiber* **-ation** *a process; being or having*	Arrhythmia in which there is a very fast, uncoordinated quivering of the myocardium (see Figure 5-20■). It can affect the atria or ventricles. Ventricular fibrillation, a life-threatening emergency in which the heart is unable to pump blood, it can progress to cardiac arrest. Treatment: Cardioversion. **Figure 5-20 ■ Ventricular fibrillation.** In the middle of this EKG tracing, the patient's regular heart rate changed to ventricular fibrillation. In fibrillation, the heart muscle twitches as parts of it contract independently but ineffectively.

Word or Phrase	Word Part and Definition	Description
heart block		Arrhythmia in which electrical impulses cannot travel normally from the AV node to the Purkinje fibers. In **first-degree heart block,** the electrical impulses reach the ventricles but are very delayed. In **second-degree heart block,** only some of the electrical impulses reach the ventricles. In **third-degree heart block** (complete heart block), no electrical impulses reach the ventricles. In **right or left bundle branch block,** the electrical impulses are unable to travel down the right or left bundle of His. Treatment: Antiarrhythmic drugs. Surgical insertion of a pacemaker.
palpitation	**palpitation** (PAL-pih-TAY-shun) **palpit/o-** *to throb* **-ation** *a process; being or having*	An uncomfortable sensation felt in the chest during a premature contraction of the heart. It is often described as a "thump." Treatment: None, unless it progresses to an arrhythmia.
premature contraction	**contraction** (con-TRAK-shun) **contract/o-** *pull together* **-ion** *action; condition* **extrasystole** (EKS-trah-SIS-toh-lee) *Extrasystole* is a combination of the prefix *extra-* (outside of) and the word *systole* (contracting). **bigeminy** (by-JEM-ih-nee) **bigeminal** (by-JEM-ih-nal) **bi-** *two* **gemin/o-** *twins, paired set* **-al** *pertaining to* Gemini is the constellation that has two bright, paired stars, like twins. **trigeminy** (try-JEM-ih-nee) **trigeminal** (try-JEM-ih-nal) **tri-** *three* **gemin/o-** *twins, paired set* **-al** *pertaining to*	Arrhythmia in which there are one or more extra contractions within a cardiac cycle. Also known as an **extrasystole.** There are two types of premature contractions: **premature atrial contractions (PACs)** and **premature ventricular contractions (PVCs).** A repeating pattern of one normal contraction followed by one premature contraction is known as **bigeminy.** A repeating pattern of two normal contractions followed by one premature contraction is known as **trigeminy.** Two premature contractions occurring together is known as a **couplet.** Treatment: Antiarrhythmic drugs. Surgical insertion of a pacemaker.
sick sinus syndrome		Arrhythmia in which bradycardia alternates with tachycardia. Occurs when the sinoatrial node and ecoptic sites elsewhere in the myocardium take turns being the heart's pacemaker. Treatment: Antiarrhythmic drugs. Surgical insertion of a pacemaker.
tachycardia	**tachycardia** (TAK-ih-KAR-dee-ah) **tachy-** *fast* **card/i-** *heart* **-ia** *condition, state, thing*	Arrhythmia in which there is a fast but regular rhythm (up to 200 beats/minute). A patient with tachycardia is said to be **tachycardic.** Sinus tachycardia occurs because of an abnormality in the sinoatrial (SA) node. Atrial tachycardia occurs when an ectopic group of cells somewhere in the atrium produces an electrical impulse that overrides the SA

(continued)

Word or Phrase	Word Part and Definition	Description
tachycardia *(continued)*	**tachycardic** (TAK-ih-KAR-dik) **tachy-** fast **card/i-** heart **-ic** pertaining to **supraventricular** (SOO-prah-ven-TRIK-yoo-lar) **supra-** *above* **ventricul/o-** *ventricle (lower heart chamber; chamber in the brain)* **-ar** *pertaining to* **paroxysmal** (PAIR-awk-SIZ-mal) **paroxysm/o-** *sudden, sharp attack* **-al** *pertaining to*	node rhythm. **Supraventricular tachycardia** occurs when the ectopic group of cells is located superior to the ventricles. **Paroxysmal tachycardia** is an episode of tachycardia that occurs suddenly and then goes away without treatment. Treatment: Antiarrhythmic drugs. Surgical insertion of a pacemaker.
Blood Vessels		
aneurysm	**aneurysm** (AN-yoo-rizm) *Aneurysm* is derived from a Greek word meaning *a dilation.* **dissecting** (dy-SEK-ting) **dissect/o-** *to cut apart* **-ing** *doing* **aneurysmal** (AN-yoo-RIZ-mal) **aneurysm/o-** *aneurysm (dilation)* **-al** *pertaining to*	Area of dilation and weakness in the wall of an artery (see Figure 5-21 ■). This can be congenital or where arteriosclerosis has damaged the artery. With each heartbeat, the weakened artery wall balloons outward. Aneurysms can rupture without warning. A **dissecting aneurysm** is one that enlarges by tunneling between the layers of the artery wall. Treatment: Placement of a metal clip on the neck of a small **aneurysmal** dilation to occlude the blood flow. An abdominal aortic aneurysm (AAA) may need to be replaced with a synthetic tubular graft. **Figure 5-21 ■ An aneurysm.** This arteriogram shows contrast dye outlining an artery in the brain. A bulging aneurysm can be seen at the arrow.

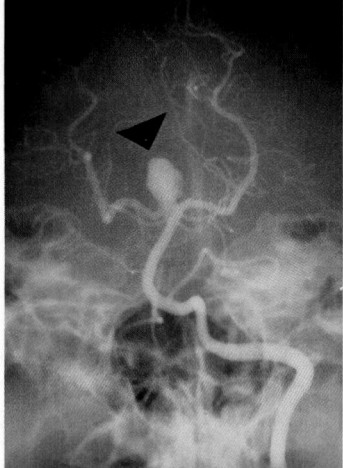

Word or Phrase	Word Part and Definition	Description
arteriosclerosis	**arteriosclerosis** (ar-TEER-ee-oh-skleh-ROH-sis) **arteri/o-** *artery* **scler/o-** *hard; sclera (white of the eye)* **-osis** *condition; abnormal condition; process* Some word parts have more than one definition. The best definition of *arteriosclerosis* is *process [in which the] artery [becomes] hard.* **atheroma** (ATH-eh-ROH-mah) **ather/o-** *soft, fatty substance* **-oma** *tumor, mass* The combining form *ather/o-* means *gruel* in Latin, a reference to its thick appearance. **atheromatous** (ATH-eh-ROH-mah-tus) **atheromat/o-** *fatty deposit or mass* **-ous** *pertaining to* **plaque** (PLAHK) *Plaque* is a French word meaning *plate.* **atherosclerosis** (ATH-eh-roh-skleh-ROH-sis) **ather/o-** *soft, fatty substance* **scler/o-** *hard; sclera (white of the eye)* **-osis** *condition; abnormal condition; process* **arteriosclerotic** (ar-TEER-ee-oh-skleh-RAW-tik) **arteri/o-** *artery* **scler/o-** *hard; sclera (white of the eye)* **-tic** *pertaining to*	Progressive degenerative changes that produce a narrowed, hardened artery. The process begins with a small tear in the endothelium that is caused by chronic hypertension. Then high-density lipoproteins (HDLs) in the blood deposit cholesterol and form an **atheroma** or **atheromatous plaque** inside the artery (see Figure 5-22 ■). These fatty plaque deposits enlarge more rapidly in patients who eat high-fat, high-sugar diets, have diabetes, or have a genetic predisposition (family history). As plaque grows on an artery wall, it makes the lumen narrower and narrower (see Figure 5-23 ■). Collagen fibers form underneath the plaque, so that the artery wall becomes hard and nonelastic. This process is known as **atherosclerosis.** Arteriosclerosis is hardening of the arteries, most commonly associated with atherosclerosis, but it can also be caused by other less common diseases. An artery with arteriosclerosis is said to be **arteriosclerotic.** Also known as arteriosclerotic cardiovascular disease (ASCVD). Arteriosclerosis of the carotid arteries to the brain can cause a stroke. Arteriosclerosis of the coronary arteries can cause angina pectoris and a myocardial infarction. Arteriosclerosis of the arteries to the kidneys can cause kidney failure. *(continued)* 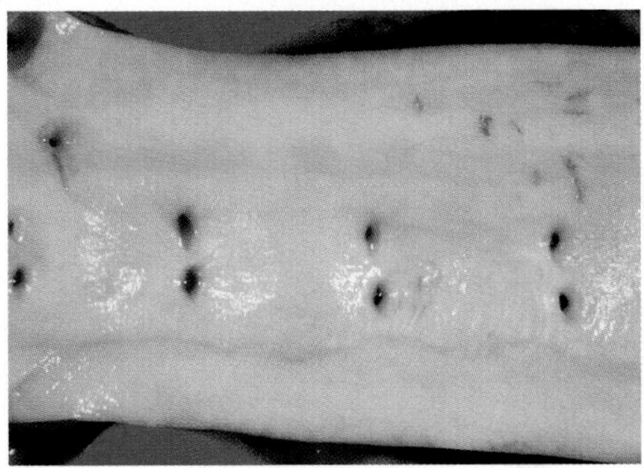 **Figure 5-22 ■ Mild atheromatous plaque.** This aorta from a cadaver shows mild, slightly raised plaque formation along the wall of the aorta. The pairs of dark areas are where right and left arteries branch off from the aorta to go to different parts of the body. The plaque has not yet occluded the lumens of these arteries.

Connections

Dietetics. The body produces its own supply of cholesterol that is used to make bile, neurotransmitters, and sex hormones. The diet contains additional cholesterol in foods derived from animal sources. An excessive amount of animal fat in the diet increases the cholesterol level in the blood. An excessive amount of sugar in the diet is converted by the body to triglycerides and results in an increased triglyceride level in the blood and increased storage as adipose tissue (fat).

Lipoproteins are carrier molecules produced in the liver. They transport lipids (fats such as cholesterol and triglycerides) in the blood. There are three types of lipoproteins. High-density lipoprotein (HDL) carries cholesterol to the liver where it is excreted in the bile, and so HDL is known as "good cholesterol." Low-density lipoprotein (LDL) carries cholesterol but deposits it on the walls of the arteries, and so it is known as "bad cholesterol." Very low-density lipoprotein (VLDL) carries triglycerides and deposits them on the walls of the arteries.

Word or Phrase	Word Part and Definition	Description
arteriosclerosis *(continued)*		Atheromatous plaque is friable and pieces can break off, travel through the blood, and block other arteries. The rough edges of the plaque can trap red blood cells and form a blood clot. Treatment: Lipid-lowering drugs. Surgery: Angioplasty or stent to press down the plaque or endarterectomy to remove the plaque. 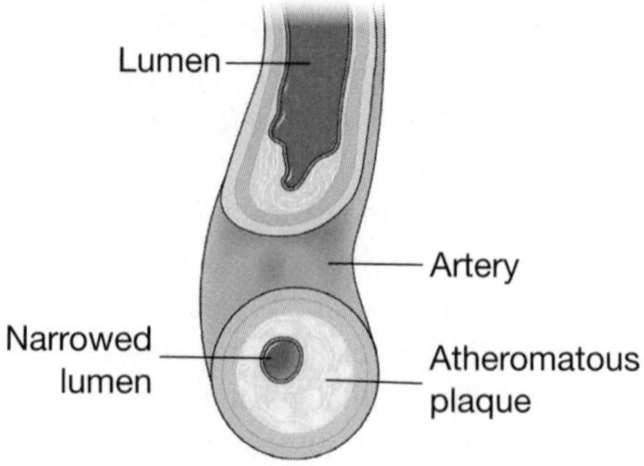 **Figure 5-23 ■ Severe atherosclerotic plaque in an artery.** The lumen of the artery is now so small that little blood can flow through.
bruit	**bruit** (BROO-ee)	A harsh rushing sound made by blood passing through an artery narrowed and roughened by atherosclerosis. The bruit can be heard when a stethoscope is placed over the artery.
coronary artery disease (CAD)		Arteriosclerosis of the coronary arteries. They are filled with atheromatous plaque, and their narrowed lumens cannot carry enough oxygenated blood to the myocardium. This results in angina pectoris. Severe arteriosclerosis (or a blood clot that forms on an atherosclerotic plaque) can completely block the lumen of a coronary artery. This causes a myocardial infarction. Treatment: Lipid-lowering drugs. Surgery: Percutaneous transluminal coronary angioplasty (PTCA) or coronary artery bypass grafting (CABG). **Connections** **Public Health.** There are many factors that contribute to the development of coronary artery disease. These are known as cardiac risk factors. They include demographic factors (heredity, gender, age), medical factors (hypertension, hypercholesterolemia, diabetes, obesity), and lifestyle factors (smoking, lack of exercise, poor diet, stress, alcoholism).
hypertension (HTN)	**hypertension** (HY-per-TEN-shun) **hyper-** *above; more than normal* **tens/o-** *pressure, tension* **-ion** *action; condition*	Elevated blood pressure. Normal blood pressure readings in an adult are less than 120/80 mm Hg. Those between 120/80 mm Hg and 140/90 mm Hg are categorized as **prehypertension.** Blood pressures above 140/90 mm Hg are categorized as hypertension, and the patient is said to be **hypertensive.** Several blood pressure readings, not just one, are needed to make a diagnosis. Essential hypertension, the most common *(continued)*

Word or Phrase	Word Part and Definition	Description
hypertension *(continued)*	**prehypertension** (pree-HY-per-TEN-shun) **pre-** *before, in front of* **hyper-** *above; more than normal* **tens/o-** *pressure, tension* **-ion** *action; condition* **hypertensive** (HY-per-TEN-siv) **hyper-** *above; more than normal* **tens/o-** *pressure, tension* **-ive** *pertaining to*	type of hypertension, is one in which the exact cause is not known. Secondary hypertension has a known cause, like kidney disease. Treatment: Lifestyle changes (decreased salt intake, increased exercise, weight loss) followed by antihypertensive drugs. **Did You Know?** Some people have increased blood pressure readings just because they are nervous from being in a doctor's office. This is known as white-coat hypertension. This is not a true hypertension because as soon as they leave the doctor's office, their blood pressure returns to normal.
hypotension	**hypotension** (HY-poh-TEN-shun) **hypo-** *below; deficient* **tens/o-** *pressure, tension* **-ion** *action; condition* **hypotensive** (HY-poh-TEN-siv) **hypo-** *below; deficient* **tens/o-** *pressure, tension* **-ive** *pertaining to* **orthostatic** (OR-thoh-STAT-ik) **orth/o-** *straight* **stat/o-** *standing still; staying in one place* **-ic** *pertaining to* *Orthostatic* refers to standing up straight.	Blood pressure lower than 90/60 mm Hg, usually because of a loss of blood volume. A patient with hypotension is said to be **hypotensive. Orthostatic hypotension** is the sudden, temporary, but self-correcting decrease in systolic blood pressure that occurs when the patient changes from a lying to a standing position and experiences lightheadedness. Treatment: Correct the underlying cause.
peripheral artery disease (PAD)	**peripheral** (peh-RIF-eh-ral) **peripher/o-** *outer aspects* **-al** *pertaining to* **perfusion** (per-FYOO-zhun) **per-** *through, throughout* **fus/o-** *pouring* **-ion** *action; condition* **claudication** (KLAW-dih-KAY-shun) **claudicat/o-** *limping pain* **-ion** *action; condition* **necrotic** (neh-KRAWT-ik) **necr/o-** *death* **-tic** *pertaining to*	Arteriosclerosis of the arteries of the legs. Blood flow (**perfusion**) to the extremities is poor, and there is ischemia of the tissues. While walking, the patient experiences pain in the calf (intermittent **claudication**). In severe PAD, the feet and toes remain cool and cyanotic and may become **necrotic** as the tissues die. Treatment: Lipid-lowering drugs. Surgery: Angioplasty.
peripheral vascular disease (PVD)	**peripheral** (peh-RIF-eh-ral) **peripher/o-** *outer aspects* **-al** *pertaining to*	Any disease of the arteries of the extremities. It includes peripheral artery disease as well as Raynaud's disease.

Word or Phrase	Word Part and Definition	Description
phlebitis	**phlebitis** (fleh-BY-tis) **phleb/o-** *vein* **-itis** *inflammation of* **thrombophletibis** (THRAWM-boh-fleh-BY-tis) **thromb/o-** *thrombus (blood clot)* **phleb/o-** *vein* **-itis** means *inflammation of*	Inflammation of a vein, usually accompanied by infection. The area around the vein is painful, and the skin may show a red streak that follows the course of the vein. A severe inflammation can partially occlude the vein and slow the flow of blood. **Thrombophlebitis** is phlebitis with the formation of a thrombus (blood clot). Treatment: Analgesic drugs for pain, anti-inflammatory drugs for inflammation. Antibiotic drugs, if needed. Thrombolytic drugs to dissolve a clot.
Raynaud's disease	**Raynaud** (ray-NO) Raynaud's disease was named by Maurice Raynaud (1834–1881), a French physician.This is an example of an eponym: a person from whom something takes its name.	Sudden, severe vasoconstriction and spasm of the arterioles in the fingers and toes, often triggered by cold or emotional upset. They become white or cyanotic and numb for minutes or hours until the attack passes. Can lead to necrosis. Treatment: Vasodilator drugs.
varicose veins	**varicose** (VAR-ih-kohs) **varic/o-** *varix; varicose vein* **-ose** *full of*	Damaged or incompetent valves in a vein that let blood flow backward and collect in the preceding section of vein. Eventually the vein becomes engorged with blood, twisting and bulging under the surface of the skin (see Figures 5-24■). Varicose veins can be caused by phlebitis, injury, long periods of sitting with the legs crossed, or occupations that require constant standing. Also, during pregnancy, pressure from the enlarging uterus restricts the flow of blood in the lower extremities and causes the leg veins to dilate. There is a family tendency to develop varicose veins. Symptoms include pain and aching; the legs feel heavy and leaden. Treatment: Destruction of the vein by injecting a sclerosing solution or foam to harden and occlude it. Laser or radiowaves to destroy the vein. **Figure 5-24 ■ Severe varicose veins in the leg.** Superficial varicose veins are unsightly and easily injured because they protrude. Patients often have varicose veins treated to achieve an improved cosmetic appearance, but treatment also helps decrease the chance of injury and thrombophlebitis. **Connections** **Gastroenterology (Chapter 3).** Varicose veins of the esophagus and stomach are known as esophageal and gastric varices. Varicose veins of the rectum are known as hemorrhoids.

Word or Phrase	Word Part and Definition	Description
hyperlipidemia	**hyperlipidemia** (HY-per-LIP-ih-DEE-mee-ah) **hyper-** *above; more than normal* **lipid/o-** *lipid (fat)* **-emia** *condition of the blood; substance in the blood* **hypercholesterolemia** (HY-per-koh-LES-ter-awl-EE-mee-ah) **hyper-** *above; more than normal* **cholesterol/o-** *cholesterol* **-emia** *condition of the blood; substance in the blood* **hypertriglyceridemia** (HY-per-try-GLIS-er-ih-DEE-mee-ah) **hyper-** *above; more than normal* **triglycerid/o-** *triglyceride* **-emia** *condition of the blood; substance in the blood*	Elevated levels of lipids (fats) in the blood. Lipids include cholesterol and triglycerides. **Hypercholesterolemia** is an elevated level of cholesterol in the blood. **Hypertriglyceridemia** is an elevated level of triglycerides in the blood. Normal levels are below 200 mg/dL for cholesterol and below 150 mg/dL for triglycerides. Treatment: Lipid-lowering drugs.

Diagnostic Procedures

Blood Tests

Word or Phrase	Word Part and Definition	Description
cardiac enzymes	**enzyme** (EN-zime) The suffix *-ase* indicates an enzyme. **creatine phosphokinase** (KREE-ah-teen FAWS-foh-KY-nays) **lactate dehydrogenase** (LAK-tayt dee-HY-droh-jen-ase)	Blood test to measure the levels of enzymes that are released into the blood when myocardial cells die. **Creatine kinase (CK)** is found in skeletal muscle cells, but a specific form of it (CK-MB) is found exclusively in myocardial cells. The CK-MB level begins to rise 2–6 hours after a myocardial infarction. Also known as **creatine phosphokinase (CPK). Lactate dehydrogenase (LDH)** is found in many different cells, including the heart. The LDH level begins to rise 12 hours after a myocardial infarction. An elevated LDH can support the CK-MB results but cannot be the sole basis of diagnosing a myocardial infarction. Cardiac enzymes are measured every few hours for several days.
C-reactive protein (CRP)		Blood test to measure the level of inflammation in the body. Inflammation from sites other than the cardiovascular system (like inflammation of the gums or chronic urinary tract infections) can produce inflammation of the walls of the blood vessels. This can lead to blood clot formation and a myocardial infarction.

Word or Phrase	Word Part and Definition	Description
lipid profile	**lipid** (LIP-id) **lip/o-** *lipid (fat)* **-id** *resembling*	Blood test that provides a comprehensive picture of the levels of cholesterol and triglycerides and their lipoprotein carriers in the blood: HDL, LDL, and VLDL.
troponin	**troponin** (troh-POH-nin)	Blood test to measure the level of two proteins that are released into the blood when myocardial cells die. Troponin I and troponin T are only found in the myocardium. The troponin levels begin to rise 4–6 hours after a myocardial infarction. More importantly, they remain elevated for up to 10 days, so they can be used to diagnose a myocardial infarction many days after it occurred. Troponin levels are done in conjunction with CK-MB and LDH levels.
Diagnostic Heart Procedures		
cardiac catheterization	**catheterization** (KATH-eh-ter-ih-ZAY-shun) **catheter/o-** *catheter* **-ization** *process of making, creating, or inserting* *Catheter* is derived from a Greek word meaning *to send down.*	Diagnostic procedure performed to evaluate the right or left side of the heart. For a right heart catheterization, a catheter is inserted into the femoral or brachial vein and threaded to the right atrium. The catheter is used to record right heart pressures. Then a radiopaque contrast dye is injected through the catheter to outline the chambers of the heart. A right heart catheterization is used to diagnose congenital heart defects. For a left heart catheterization, a catheter is inserted into the femoral or brachial artery and threaded to the left atrium. Then radiopaque contrast dye is injected to outline the coronary arteries and show narrow or blocked areas. If blockages of the coronary arteries are present, an angioplasty may be performed at that time.
electrocardiography (ECG, EKG)	**electrocardiography** (ee-LEK-troh-KAR-dee-AWG-rah-fee) **electr/o-** *electricity* **cardi/o-** *heart* **-graphy** *process of recording* **electrocardiogram** (ee-LEK-troh-KAR-dee-oh-gram) **electr/o-** *electricity* **cardi/o-** *heart* **-gram** *a record or picture*	Diagnostic procedure that records the electrical activity of the heart during contractions and rest (see Figure 5-25■). Electrodes (metal pieces in adhesive patches) are placed on the limbs (both arms and one leg) to record the electrical impulses of the heart to the EKG machine. These are the three limb leads (leads I through III). Electrodes placed on the chest are known as the precordial leads (V_1 through V_6). A 12-lead EKG records 12 different leads that show the electrical activity between different combinations of electrodes to give an electrical picture of the heart from 12 different angles. Samples of each of these 12 tracings are mounted on a backing. A longer sample of just the lead II tracing is known as a rhythm strip.

(continued)

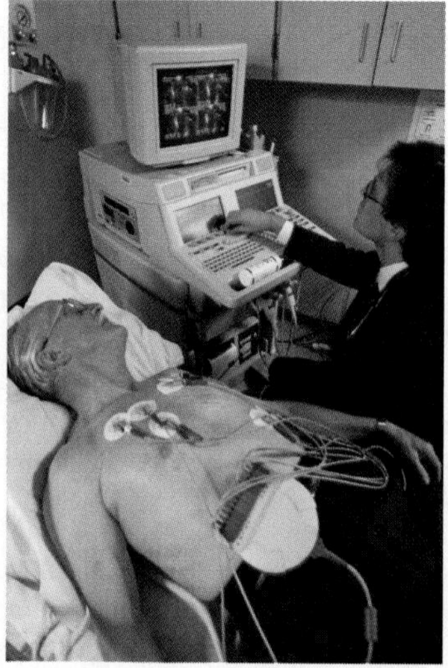

Figure 5-25 ■ Electrocardiography.

Electrode patches attached to wire leads are placed on the body to pick up the electrical impulses of the heart from many different angles. Interpretation of an EKG involves determining the heart rate, the heart rhythm, and identifying abnormalities in the shape of the electrical pattern.

Word or Phrase	Word Part and Definition	Description
electrocardiography *(continued)*		**A Closer Look** The electrical image generated by the contraction and relaxation of the heart has a characteristic pattern (see Figure 5-26 ■). The P wave corresponds to depolarization of the SA node and both atria. The QRS complex corresponds to depolarization of the septum and both ventricles. The T wave corresponds to repolarization of the ventricles. The repolarization of the atria is hidden by the QRS complex. **Figure 5-26 ■ An EKG tracing.** Each heart contraction has a characteristic P wave, QRS complex, and T wave. **Did You Know?** The *K* in the abbreviation *EKG* comes from the Greek word *kardia* (heart).

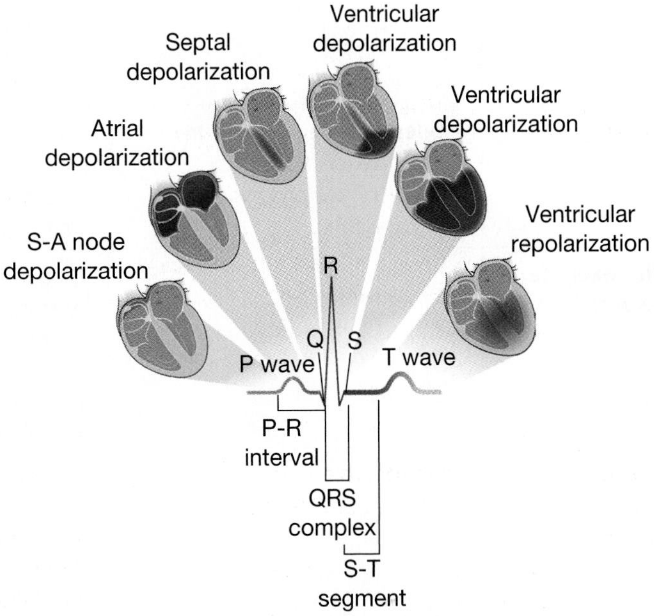

Word or Phrase	Word Part and Definition	Description
electrophysiologic study (EPS)	**electrophysiologic** (ee-LEK-troh-FIZ-ee-oh-LAW-jik) **electr/o-** *electricity* **physi/o-** *physical function* **log/o-** *the study of* **-ic** *pertaining to*	Diagnostic procedure to map the heart's conduction system in patients with arrhythmias. While an EKG is performed, catheters are inserted into the femoral vein and the subclavian vein. X-rays are used to guide the catheters to the heart. The catheters send out electrical impulses to stimulate the heart and try to induce an arrhythmia to pinpoint where the arrhythmias are originating from in the heart.
Holter monitor		Diagnostic procedure during which the patient's heart rate and rhythm are continuously monitored as an outpatient for 24 hours. The patient wears electrodes attached to a small, portable EKG monitor (carried in a vest or placed in a pocket). The patient also keeps a diary of activities, meals, and symptoms. This procedure is used to document infrequently occurring arrhythmias and to link them to activities or symptoms such as chest pain.
telemetry	**telemetry** (teh-LEM-eh-tree) **tele/o-** *distance* **-metry** *the process of measuring*	Diagnostic procedure to monitor a patient's heart rate and rhythm in the hospital. The patient wears electrodes that continuously transmit the EKG tracing to a central monitoring station, usually in the coronary care unit or intensive care unit.
cardiac exercise stress test	**pharmacologic** (FAR-mah-koh-LAWJ-ik) **pharmac/o-** *medicine, drug* **log/o-** *study of* **-ic** *pertaining to*	Diagnostic procedure performed to evaluate the heart's response to exercise in patients with chest pain, palpitations, or arrhythmias. The patient walks on a motorized treadmill (**treadmill exercise stress test**) or rides a stationary bicycle while an EKG is performed. The speed of the treadmill and the steepness of its incline (or the resistance of the bicycle) are gradually increased while the patient's heart rate, blood pressure, and EKG are monitored. The procedure is stopped if the patient complains of angina, palpitations, shortness of breath, or tiredness, or if the EKG pattern becomes abnormal. The patient's resting heart rate and maximum heart rate are compared to standards for other people of the same age and sex. Any abnormalities in the EKG pattern are analyzed. A **pharmacologic stress test** is performed in patients who cannot exercise vigorously. A vasodilator drug like adenosine or dipyridamole (Persantine) is given to cause normal coronary arteries to dilate. Occluded arteries cannot dilate, and this stresses the heart in a way that is similar to exercise and provokes angina.

Radiology and Nuclear Medicine Procedures

Word or Phrase	Word Part and Definition	Description
angiography	**angiography** (AN-jee-AWG-rah-fee) **angi/o-** *blood vessel; lymph vessel* **-graphy** *process of recording* **arteriography** (ar-TEER-ee-AWG-rah-fee) **arteri/o-** *artery* **-graphy** *process of recording* **venography** (vee-NAWG-rah-fee) **ven/o-** *vein* **-graphy** *process of recording* **angiogram** (AN-jee-oh-gram) **angi/o-** *blood vessel; lymph vessel* **-gram** *a record or picture* **arteriogram** (ar-TEER-ee-oh-gram) **arteri/o-** *artery* **-gram** *a record or picture* **venogram** (VEE-noh-gram) **ven/o-** *vein* **-gram** *a record or picture*	Radiologic procedure in which radiopaque contrast dye is injected into a blood vessel to fill and outline it. In **arteriography,** it is injected into an artery and shows blockage, narrowed areas, or aneurysms (see Figure 5-21). In **venography,** it is injected into a vein and shows weakened valves and dilated walls. The x-ray image is known as an **angiogram,** or specifically as an **arteriogram** or **venogram.** In coronary angiography, a catheter is inserted into the femoral artery and threaded to the aorta. The radiopaque contrast dye outlines the coronary arteries and shows narrowing, stenosis, or blockage. The x-ray is known as a coronary angiogram. In rotational angiography, multiple x-rays are taken as the x-ray arm moves around the patient. This technique is particularly helpful in documenting tortuous blood vessels in three dimensions. Digital subtraction angiography (DSA) combines two x-ray images. The first is taken without radiopaque contrast dye. The second image is taken after radiopaque contrast dye has been injected to outline the blood vessel. A computer then compares the images and digitally "subtracts" or removes the soft tissues, bones, and muscles, leaving just the image of the arteries.
aortography	**aortography** (AA-or-TAWG-rah-fee) **aort/o-** *aorta* **-graphy** *process of recording* **aortogram** (aa-OR-toh-gram) **aort/o-** *aorta* **-gram** *a record or picture*	Radiologic procedure in which an radiopaque contrast dye is used to outline the aorta to look for stenosis or an aortic aneurysm. The x-ray image is known as an **aortogram.**

Word or Phrase	Word Part and Definition	Description
myocardial perfusion scan	**perfusion** (per-FYOO-zhun) **per-** *through* **fus/o-** *pouring* **-ion** *action; condition* **thallium** (THAL-ee-um)	Nuclear medicine procedure that combines a cardiac exercise stress test with intravenous injections of a radioactive tracer. In a **thallium stress test,** thallium-201 is used as the radioactive tracer or thallium-201 and technetium-99m can be used. Technetium-99m is joined to a synthetic molecule (sestamibi). The combination of technetium-99m with sestamibi is known as Cardiolite, so this test is also known as a Cardiolite stress test. The radioactive tracers collect in those parts of the myocardium that have the best perfusion (blood flow). A gamma camera records gamma rays emitted by the radioactive tracers and creates a two-dimensional image of the heart. Areas of decreased uptake ("cold spots") on the image indicate poor perfusion from a blocked coronary artery. The artery must be about 70% blocked before any abnormality is evident on the image. Areas of no uptake indicate dead tissue from a previous myocardial infarction.
multiple-gated acquisition (MUGA) scan	**radionuclide** (RAY-dee-oh-NOO-klide) **radi/o-** *radius (forearm bone); x-rays; radiation* **nucle/o-** *nucleus (of an atom)* **-ide** *chemically modified* A radionuclide is a substance whose nucleus has been chemically modified to make it radioactive. **ventriculography** (ven-TRIK-yoo-LAWG-rah-fee) **ventricul/o-** *ventricle* **-graphy** *process of recording*	Nuclear medicine procedure that uses the radioactive tracer technetium-99m. First pyrophosphate is injected intravenously to prepare the patient's red blood cells to bind with technetium-99m. Then technetium-99m is injected. A gamma camera records gamma rays emitted by a radioactive tracer that is bound to red blood cells. The camera is coordinated (gated) with the patient's EKG so that images of the heart chambers are taken at various times during the cardiac cycle. A MUGA scan also calculates the ejection fraction (how much blood the ventricle can eject with one contraction). The ejection fraction is the most accurate indicator of overall heart function. This procedure is also known as a **radionuclide ventriculography (RNV)** or **gated blood pool scan.**
single-photon emission computed tomography (SPECT) scan	**tomography** (toh-MAWG-rah-fee) **tom/o-** *a cut, slice, or layer* **-graphy** *process of recording* A photon is another name for a gamma ray.	During a myocardial perfusion scan or a MUGA scan, the gamma camera is normally kept in a stationary position above the patient's chest. However, if the gamma camera is moved in a circle around the patient, then this becomes a SPECT scan. The computer creates many individual images or "slices" (tomography) and compiles them into a three-dimensional image of the heart.

Word or Phrase	Word Part and Definition	Description
echocardiography	**echocardiography** (EK-oh-KAR-dee-AWG-rah-fee) **ech/o-** *echo (sound wave)* **cardi/o-** *heart* **-graphy** *process of recording* **echocardiogram** (EK-oh-KAR-dee-oh-gram) **ech/o-** *echo (sound wave)* **cardi/o-** *heart* **-gram** *a record or picture*	Radiologic procedure that uses a transducer to produce ultrahigh-frequency sound waves (ultrasound) that are bounced off the heart to create an image. **Two-dimensional echocardiography** (2-D echo) creates a real-time picture of the heart and its chambers and valves as it contracts and relaxes. The image is known as an **echocardiogram** (see Figure 5-27 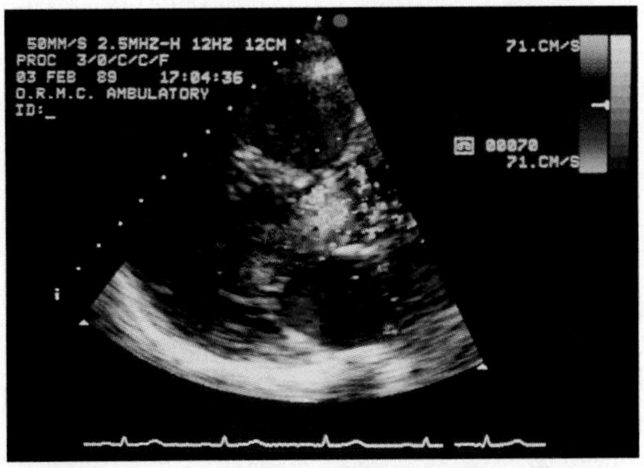 ■). **Figure 5-27 ■ An echocardiogram.** This photo was taken as a two-dimensional echocardiography produced real-time, moving images of the heart on the display screen. An echocardiogram uses sound waves to create images.
	transesophageal (TRANS-ee-SAWF-ah-JEE-al) **trans-** *across, through* **esophag/o-** *esophagus* **-eal** *pertaining to* **ultrasonography** (UL-trah-soh-NAWG-rah-fee) **ultra-** *beyond; higher* **son/o-** *sound* **-graphy** *process of recording* **duplex** (DOO-pleks) **Doppler** (DAWP-ler)	A **transesophageal echocardiogram (TEE)** may be ordered when a standard echocardiogram produces a poor quality image. For a TEE, the patient swallows an endoscopic tube that contains a tiny sound-emitting transducer. This is positioned in the esophagus directly behind the heart. **Color flow duplex ultrasonography** combines a two-dimensional ultrasound image with another image generated by Doppler ultrasonography that color-codes images according to their velocity and direction. The image shows turbulence and variation in velocity by different degrees of brightness. This test is the "gold standard" for evaluating tortuous varicose veins. **Doppler ultrasonography** images the flow of blood in the arteries. The reflected sound waves vary depending on how fast the blood is traveling in an artery or vein. The image can also show blockages or clots in the vessel. Doppler technology is also used in automatic blood pressure machines, in hand-held devices that give the heart rate if placed on the skin over an artery, and in fetal monitors that, when placed on the mother's abdomen, give the heart rate of the fetus.

Medical and Surgical Procedures

Medical Procedures

Word or Phrase	Word Part and Definition	Description
auscultation	**auscultation** (AWS-kul-TAY-shun) **auscult/o-** *listening* **-ation** *a process; being or having* **stethoscope** (STETH-oh-skohp) **steth/o-** *chest* **-scope** *instrument used to examine*	Medical procedure that uses a **stethoscope** to listen to the heart sounds and detect murmurs and other abnormal sounds.
cardioversion	**cardioversion** (KAR-dee-oh-VER-zhun) **cardi/o-** *heart* **vers/o-** *to turn; to travel* **-ion** *action; condition* **defibrillator** (dee-FIB-rih-lay-ter) **de-** *reversal of, without* **fibrill/o-** *muscle fiber, nerve fiber* **-ator** *person or thing that does or produces*	Medical procedure to treat a life-threatening arrhythmia (ventricular fibrillation) and restore the heart to normal sinus rhythm. A **defibrillator** is the device used for the procedure (see Figure 5-28■). Two large, handheld paddles are placed on either side of the patient's chest while the defibrillator generates an electrical shock to override the arrhythmia or to stimulate a nonbeating heart after a cardiac arrest. An automatic implantable cardioverter/defibrillator (AICD) is a small device that is implanted in a patient who is at high risk for developing a serious arrhythmia. The AICD is implanted under the skin of the chest. It has leads (wires) that go to the heart, sense its rhythm, and deliver an electrical shock, if needed. An automatic external defibrillator (AED) is a portable computerized device kept on emergency response vehicles and in public places like airports. It analyzes the patient's heart rhythm and delivers an electrical shock to stimulate a heart in cardiac arrest. An AED is designed to be used by nonmedical persons. 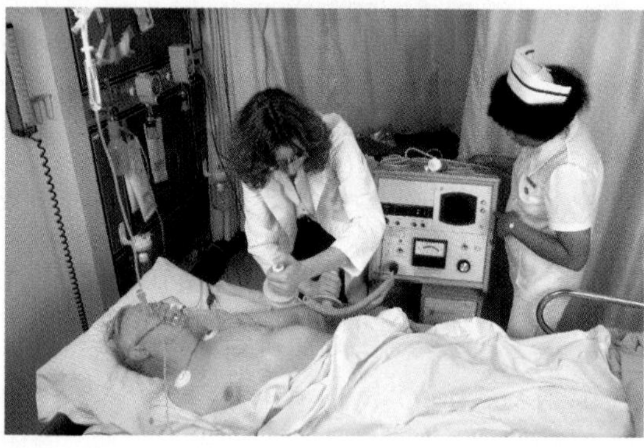 **Figure 5-28 ■ Cardioversion.** This physician is about to apply defibrillator paddles to the patient's chest to convert a life-threatening arrhythmia. Emergency departments, operating rooms, and intensive care units are all equipped with defibrillators that can be brought to the patient's bedside.

Word or Phrase	Word Part and Definition	Description
radiofrequency catheter ablation	**ablation** (ah-BLAY-shun) **ablat/o-** *take away; destroy* **-ion** *action; condition* **occlusion** (oh-KLOO-zhun) **occlus/o-** *close against* **-ion** *action; condition*	Medical procedure to destroy ectopic areas in the heart that are emitting electrical impulses and producing arrhythmias. A catheter is inserted into the heart. Electromagnetic energy produced by a generator produces enough heat at the site to kill the cells causing the arrhythmia. **Radiofrequency catheter occlusion** uses heat to collapse and seal large varicose veins.
sclerotherapy	**sclerotherapy** (SKLER-oh-THAIR-ah-pee) **scler/o-** *hard; sclera (white of the eye)* **-therapy** *treatment*	Medical procedure in which a sclerosing drug (liquid or foam) is injected into a varicose vein. The drug causes irritation and inflammation that later hardens as fibrosis that occludes the vein.
vital signs		Medical procedure during a physical examination to measure the temperature, pulse, and respirations (TPR) as well as the blood pressure. The heart rate is measured by counting the pulse. The pulse can be felt in several different parts of the body (see Figure 5-29 ■). Pulse points include the carotid pulse in the neck, apical pulse on the anterior chest, axillary pulse in the armpit, brachial pulse at the inner elbow, radial pulse at the wrist, femoral pulse in the inguinal area (groin), popliteal pulse at the back of the knee, the posterior tibial pulse at the back of the lower leg, and the dorsalis pedis pulse on the dorsum of the foot. The **radial pulse** in the wrist is the most commonly used site. In an emergency, the carotid pulse can be felt (see Figure 5-30 ■), particularly if the patient is in shock and little blood is flowing to the

(continued)

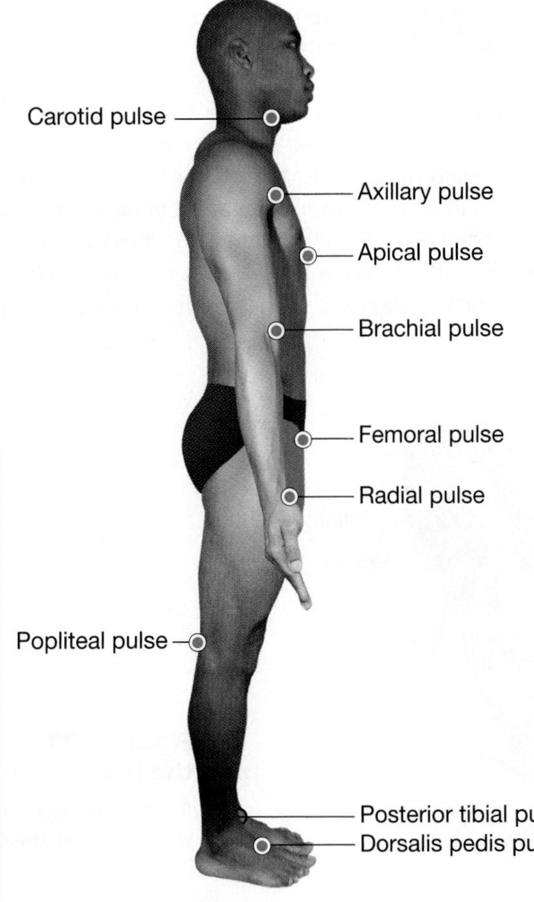

Figure 5-29 ■ Pulse points.

A pulse point is where a pulse can be felt on the surface of the body when the heart contracts and sends blood through the artery. Pulse points are felt to determine the heart rate.

Word or Phrase	Word Part and Definition	Description
vital signs *(continued)*		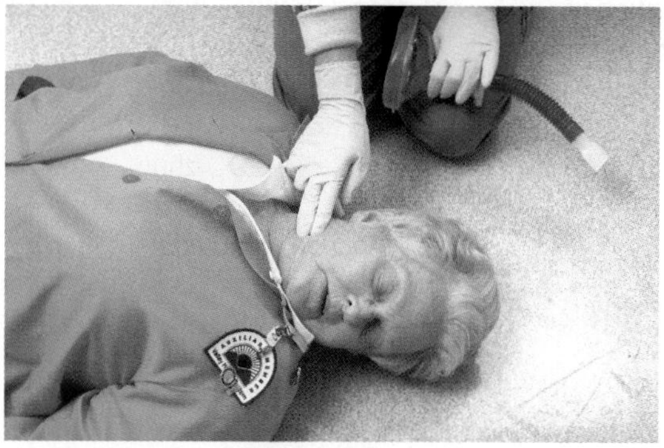 **Figure 5-30 ■ The carotid pulse.** The pulse of the carotid artery can be easily felt in the neck. Emergency medical technicians use this site to quickly assess a patient's heartbeat. extremities. The **apical pulse** (at the apex of the heart) can be heard with a stethoscope and is also used to evaluate the heart sounds. The presence of peripheral vascular disease can be determined by comparing the strength of the pulse in the right leg to the same pulse on the left.
	sphygmomanometer (SFIG-moh-mah-NAWM-eh-ter) **sphygm/o-** *pulse* **man/o-** *thin* **-meter** *instrument used to measure* Add words to make a correct and complete definition of *sphygmomanometer: instrument used to measure [the pressure of the] pulse [by using a] thin [inflatable cuff].*	The blood pressure is measured with a **sphygmomanometer** and a stethoscope. The sphygmomanometer consists of a thin, inflatable cuff that wraps around the arm (or leg), a hand bulb that is pumped to increase the pressure in the cuff, a regulating valve that is opened to release the pressure from the cuff, and a calibrated gauge that is used to read the pressure (see Figure 5-31 ■). Blood pressure cuffs come in several different sizes to accommodate very thin to very large arms. There are even blood pressure cuffs for newborn and premature infants. The correct size blood pressure cuff must be used or the blood pressure reading will be either too high or too low. The stethoscope is placed at the inner elbow over the brachial pulse. As pressure increases in the cuff, it cuts off the flow of blood. The cuff pressure is decreased. When the cuff pressure is lower than the pressure in the artery, the blood spurts through and creates the first sound. This is the **systolic pressure,**

(continued)

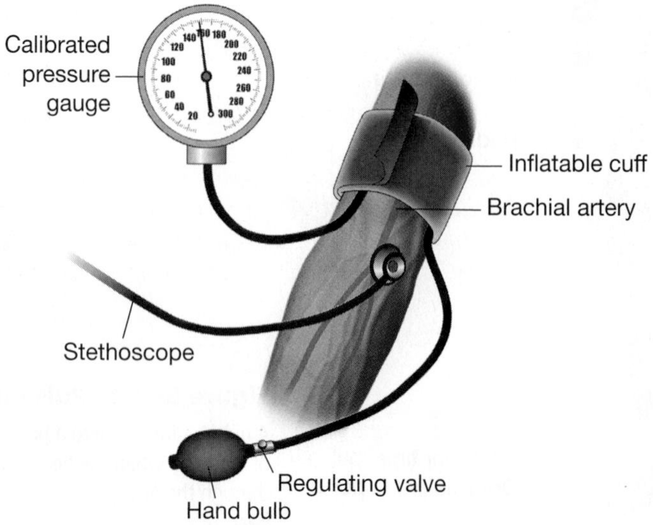

Figure 5-31 ■ Measuring the blood pressure.
A sphygmomanometer and a stethoscope are used to measure the blood pressure.

Word or Phrase	Word Part and Definition	Description
vital signs *(continued)*		the top number in a blood pressure reading. When cuff pressure reaches the resting pressure in the artery, this is the **diastolic pressure.** A blood pressure measurement is recorded as two numbers: the systolic pressure over the diastolic pressure. Blood pressure is measured in millimeters of mercury (mm Hg).
Surgical Procedures		
aneurysmectomy	**aneurysmectomy** (AN-yoo-riz-MEK-toh-mee) **aneurysm/o-** *aneurysm (dilatation)* **-ectomy** *surgical excision*	Surgical procedure to remove an aneurysm and repair the defect in the artery wall. If a dissecting aneurysm involves a large segment of artery, a flexible, tubular synthetic graft is used to replace that segment.
cardiopulmonary bypass	**cardiopulmonary** (KAR-dee-oh-PUL-moh-nair-ee) **cardi/o-** *heart* **pulmon/o-** *lung* **-ary** *pertaining to*	Technique used during open-heart surgery in which the patient's blood is rerouted through a cannula in the femoral vein to a heart-lung machine. There, the blood is oxygenated, carbon dioxide and waste products are removed, and the blood is pumped back into the body via a cannula in the femoral artery. Cardiopulmonary bypass takes over the functions of the heart and lungs during the surgery.
carotid endarterectomy	**endarterectomy** (END-ar-ter-EK-toh-mee) **endo-** *innermost, within* **arter/o-** *artery* **-ectomy** *surgical excision*	Surgical procedure to remove plaque from an occluded carotid artery. Used to treat carotid stenosis due to atherosclerosis.
coronary artery bypass graft (CABG)	**anastomosis** (ah-NAS-toh-MOH-sis) **anastom/o-** *unite two tubular structures* **-osis** *condition; abnormal condition; process*	Surgical procedure to bypass an occluded coronary artery and restore blood flow to the myocardium. A blood vessel (either the saphenous vein from the leg or the internal mammary artery from the chest) is used as the bypass graft. If the saphenous vein is used, it must be placed in a reversed position so that its valves will not obstruct the flow of blood. The suturing of one blood vessel to another is known as an **anastomosis.** Oxygenated blood flows through the graft, past the blockage, and back into the coronary artery. The abbreviation CABG is pronounced "cabbage."
heart transplantation	**transplantation** (TRANS-plan-TAY-shun) **transplant/o-** *move something to another place* **-ation** *a process; being or having* **donor** (DOH-nor) *Donor* is derived from a Latin word meaning *one who gives.*	Surgical procedure to remove a severely damaged heart from a patient with end-stage heart failure and insert a new heart from a **donor** (a patient who has recently died). The patient is matched by blood type and tissue type to the donor. Heart transplant patients must take immunosuppressant drugs for the rest of their lives to keep their bodies from rejecting the foreign tissue of their new heart. Some patients receive an artificial heart made of plastic, metal, and other synthetic materials. While awaiting a donor heart, the patient may have a left ventricular assist device (LVAD) temporarily implanted. This battery- or pneumatic-powered pump is placed in the abdomen and connected via tubes to the left ventricle and the aorta. In some patients, it becomes a permanent solution.

Word or Phrase	Word Part and Definition	Description
pacemaker insertion		Surgical procedure in which an automated device is implanted to control the heart rate and rhythm (see Figure 5-32■). Pacemakers use two or three wires (or leads) positioned on the heart to coordinate the heartbeat with an electrical impulse. 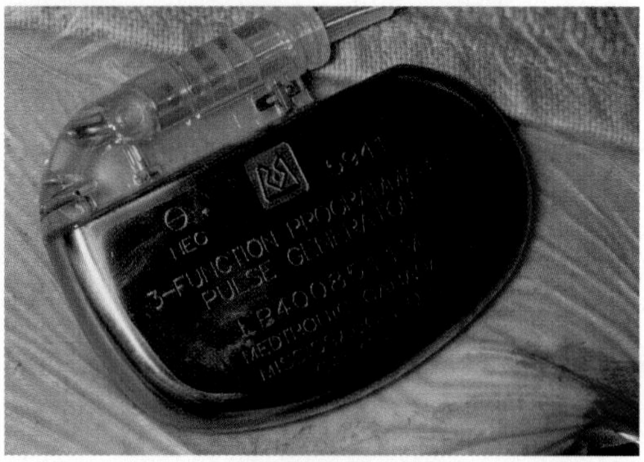 **Figure 5-32 ■ A pacemaker.** This Medtronic pacemaker is placed under the skin of the anterior chest, and its wires are positioned on the heart.
percutaneous transluminal coronary angioplasty (PTCA)	**percutaneous** (PER-kyoo-TAY-nee-us) **per-** *through* **cutane/o-** *skin* **-ous** *pertaining to* **transluminal** (trans-LOO-mih-nal) **trans-** *across, through* **lumin/o-** *lumen (opening)* **-al** *pertaining to* **angioplasty** (AN-jee-oh-PLAS-tee) **angi/o-** *blood vessel; lymph vessel* **-plasty** *process of reshaping by surgery*	Surgical procedure to reconstruct an artery that is narrowed because of atheriosclerosis. A catheter is inserted into the femoral artery and threaded to the site of the stenosis. In a **balloon angioplasty,** a balloon within the catheter is inflated, compressing the atheromatous plaque and widening the lumen of the artery. The catheter and balloon are then removed (see Figure 5-33■). 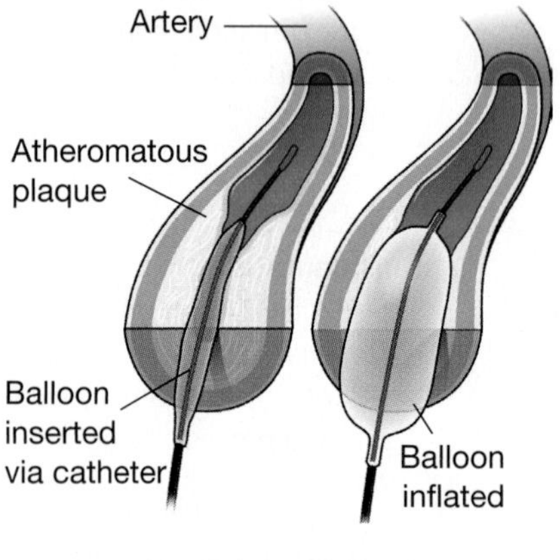 Artery Atheromatous plaque Balloon inserted via catheter Balloon inflated **Figure 5-33 ■ Balloon angioplasty.** The inflated balloon compresses atheromatous plaque in the artery, opening the lumen, and reestablishing blood flow.

Word or Phrase	Word Part and Definition	Description
percutaneous transluminal coronary angioplasty (PTCA) *(continued)*		Alternatively, an intravascular stainless steel mesh **stent** can be inserted on the catheter (see Figure 5-34■). The catheter is removed, but the expanded stent remains in the artery. 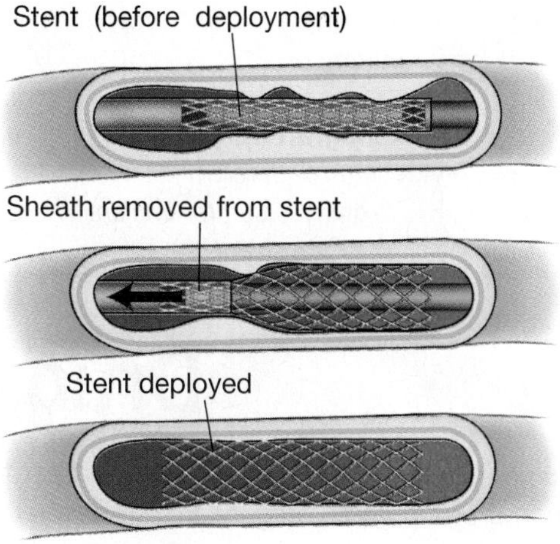 **Figure 5-34 ■ A stent.** A stent is expanded inside the artery to compress the atheromatous plaque and increase the blood flow. It provides continuing support to keep the lumen of the artery open.
pericardiocentesis	**pericardiocentesis** (PAIR-ih-KAR-dee-oh-sen-TEE-sis) **peri-** *around* **cardi/o-** *heart* **-centesis** *procedure to puncture*	Surgical procedure that uses a needle to puncture the pericardium and withdraw inflammatory fluid accumulated in the pericardial sac. Used to treat pericarditis and cardiac tamponade.
valvoplasty	**valvoplasty** (VAL-voh-plas-tee) **valv/o-** *valve* **-plasty** *process of reshaping by surgery* **valvulotome** (VAL-vyoo-loh-tohm) **valvul/o-** *valve* **-tome** *instrument used to cut; an area with distinct edges* **valvuloplasty** (VAL-vyoo-loh-PLAS-tee) **valvul/o-** *valve* **-plasty** *process of reshaping by surgery*	Surgical procedure to reconstruct a heart valve to correct stenosis or prolapse. A **valvulotome** is used to cut the valve. This procedure is also known as a **valvuloplasty.**

Word or Phrase	Word Part and Definition	Description
valve replacement	**prosthetic** (praws-THET-ik) **prosthet/o-** *artificial part* **-ic** *pertaining to* *Prosthesis* is a Greek word meaning *an addition to; a putting on.* **xenograft** (ZEN-oh-graft) **xen/o-** *foreign* **-graft** *tissue for implant or transplant*	Surgical procedure to replace a severely damaged or prolapsed heart valve. There are several types of **prosthetic** (replacement) heart valves that can be used. If the replacement valve comes from an animal, it is known as a **xenograft.**

Drug Categories

Several different categories of drugs are used to treat the symptoms, signs, and diseases of the cardiovascular system. The most common drugs in each category are listed.

Category	Word Part and Definition	Description	Example
ACE (angiotensin-converting enzyme) inhibitor drugs	**angiotensin** (AN-jee-oh-TEN-sin) **angi/o-** *blood vessel; lymphatic vessel* **tens/o-** *pressure, tension* **-in** *a substance*	Treat congestive heart failure and hypertension. Also increase the survival rate after myocardial infarction. ACE inhibitor drugs produce vasodilation and decrease the blood pressure by blocking an enzyme that converts angiotensin I to angiotensin II (a vasoconstrictor).	Capoten, Prinivil, Vasotec, Zestril
antiarrhythmic drugs	**antiarrhythmic** (AN-tee-aa-RITH-mik) **anti-** *against* **a-** *away from, without* **rrhythm/o-** *rhythm* **-ic** pertaining to	Treat arrhythmias.	atropine (only for bradycardia). Xylocaine (only for ventricular arrhythmia). See beta blockers and calcium channel blockers.
antibiotic drugs	**antibiotic** (AN-tee-by-AWT-ik) (AN-tih-by-AWT-ik) **anti-** *against* **bi/o-** *life, living organisms; living tissue* **-tic** *pertaining to*	Treat bacterial endocarditis. Antibiotic drugs are not effective against viral infections.	penicillin, Rocephin
antihypertensive drugs	**antihypertensive** (AN-tee-HY-per-TEN-siv) **anti-** *against* **hyper-** *above; more than normal* **tens/o-** *pressure, tension* **-ive** *pertaining to*	Treat hypertension.	See ACE inhibitors, beta-blockers, calcium channel blockers, and diuretic drugs.
aspirin		Prevents heart attacks. Prevents blood clots from forming by keeping platelets from sticking together.	Bayer aspirin, St. Joseph aspirin

Category	Word Part and Definition	Description	Example
beta-blocker drugs		Treat angina pectoris and hypertension. Beta blockers decrease the heart rate and dilate the arteries by blocking beta receptors in cells in the heart and arteries.	Corgard, Inderal, Lopressor
calcium channel blocker drugs		Treat angina pectoris, congestive heart failure, and hypertension. Calcium channel blockers block the movement of calcium ions into myocardial cells and smooth muscle cells of the artery walls, causing the heart rate and blood pressure to decrease.	Adalat, Calan, Procardia
digitalis drugs	**digitalis** (DIJ-ih-TAL-is)	Treat congestive heart failure. Digitalis decreases the heart rate and strengthens the heart's contraction.	digoxin (Lanoxin)

Did You Know?

Digitalis drugs are derived from *Digitalis* (foxglove plant). Its flowers were thought to resemble fingerlike projections or digits.

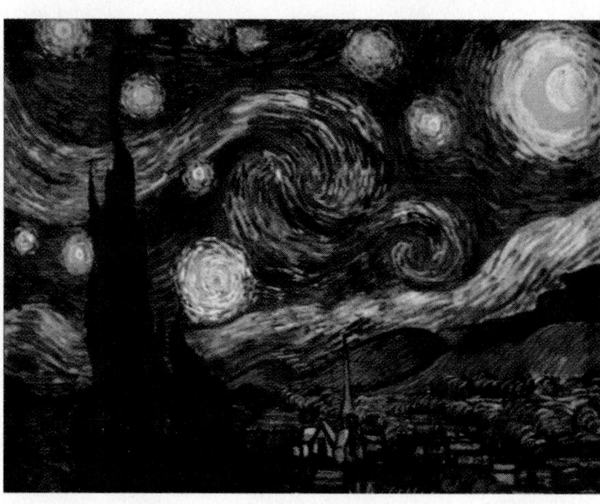

Figure 5-35 ■ The Starry Night

Vincent van Gogh's "The Starry Night" (1889) is believed by some physicians to show evidence of digitalis toxicity in the way the Dutch painter depicted the yellow-green halos around the stars. Van Gogh (1853–1890) suffered from mania and epilepsy and may have been given digitalis for lack of a more specific drug therapy available at that time. Digitalis can easily reach toxic levels in the blood. Symptoms of toxicity include nausea and vomiting, decreased heart rate, and sometimes visual halos. Van Gogh may simply have painted what he actually saw because of digitalis toxicity.

Category	Word Part and Definition	Description	Example
diuretic drugs	**diuretic** (DY-yoo-RET-ik) **dia-** *complete; completely through* **ur/o-** *urine; urinary system* **-etic** *pertaining to* The *a* is dropped from the prefix *dia-* when the word parts are combined to form *diuretic.*	Block sodium from being absorbed from the tubule back into the blood. As the sodium is excreted in the urine, it brings water and potassium with it because of osmotic pressure. This process is known as diuresis. This decreases the volume of blood and is useful in the treatment of hypertension, congestive heart failure, and nephrotic syndrome.	Aldactone, Esidrix, Hygroton, Lasix, Zaroxolyn
drugs for cardiac arrest		Treat a nonbeating heart by stimulating it to contract.	epinephrine (Adrenalin)
drugs for hyperlipidemia		Treat hypercholesterolemia and hypertriglyceridemia.	Lipitor, Vytorin, Zocor (for hypercholesterolemia); Lopid (for hypertriglyceridemia); Crestor (for hyperlipidemia)
nitrate drugs	nitrate (NY-trayt)	Treat angina pectoris. Nitrates dilate arteries and increase blood flow to the myocardium.	nitroglycerin (Nitro-Bid, Transderm-Nitro)
thrombolytic drugs	thrombolytic (THRAWM-boh-LIT-ik) **thromb/o-** *thrombus (blood clot)* **ly/o-** *to separate or dissolve* **-tic** *pertaining to*	Treat a blood clot that is blocking blood flow through an artery. Thrombolytic drugs lyse (break apart) a clot.	Activase

Did You Know?

In the mid-1890s, physicians observed that the pain of angina pectoris seemed to be relieved in those patients who worked in dynamite factories where nitroglycerin was an ingredient in the manufacturing process. This led to the practice of prescribing nitroglycerin for angina.

Abbreviations

AAA	abdominal aortic aneurysm
ACE	angiotensin-converting enzyme (inhibitor)
ACS	acute coronary syndrome
AED	automatic external defibrillator
A fib	atrial fibrillation
AI	aortic insufficiency
AICD	automatic implantable cardioverter-defibrillator
AMI	acute myocardial infarction
AS	aortic stenosis
ASCVD	arteriosclerotic cardiovascular disease
ASD	atrial septal defect
ASHD	arteriosclerotic heart disease
AV	atrioventricular
BP	blood pressure
BPM, bpm	beats per minute
CABG	coronary artery bypass graft
CAD	coronary artery disease
cath	(cardiac) catheterization
CCU	coronary care unit
CHF	congestive heart failure
CK-MB	creatine kinase-M band
CPK-MB	creatine phosphokinase-M band
CPR	cardiopulmonary resuscitation
CRP	C-reactive protein
CV	cardiovascular
DSA	digital subtraction angiography
ECG	electrocardiography
echo	echocardiogram
EKG	electrocardiography
HDL	high-density lipoprotein
HTN	hypertension
JVD	jugular venous distention
LA	left atrium
LBBB	left bundle branch block
LDH	lactic dehydrogenase
LDL	low-density lipoprotein
LV	left ventricle
LVAD	left ventricular assist device
LVH	left ventricular hypertrophy
MI	myocardial infarction
mm Hg	millimeters of mercury
MR	mitral regurgitation
MUGA	multiple-gated acquisition (scan)

MVP	mitral valve prolapse
NSR	normal sinus rhythm
P	pulse
PAC	premature atrial contraction
PAD	peripheral artery disease
PDA	patent ductus arteriosus
PMI	point of maximum impulse
PTCA	percutaneous transluminal coronary angioplasty
PVC	premature ventricular contraction
PVD	peripheral vascular disease
RA	right atrium
RBBB	right bundle branch block
RFA	radiofrequency catheter ablation
RNV	radionuclide ventriculography
RV	right ventricle
S_1	first heart sound
S_2	second heart sound
S_3	third heart sound
S_4	fourth heart sound
SA	sinoatrial
SBE	subacute bacterial endocarditis
SPECT	single photon emission computerized tomography
SVT	supraventricular tachycardia
TEE	transesophageal echocardiogram
TPR	temperature, pulse, and respiration
V fib	ventricular fibrillation
VLDL	very low-density lipoprotein
VSD	ventricular septal defect
V tach	ventricular tachycardia

Word Alert

ABBREVIATIONS

Abbreviations are commonly used in all types of medical documentation; however, they can mean different things to different people and their meaning can be misinterpreted. Always verify the meaning of an abbreviation.

RA stands for *right atrium,* but it can also stand for *rheumatoid arthritis* or *room air.*

S1 stands for *first heart sound,* but it can also stand for *first sacral vertebra.*

Do not confuse the abbreviation *CPR* (cardiopulmonary resuscitation) with *CRP* (C-reactive protein).

Career Focus

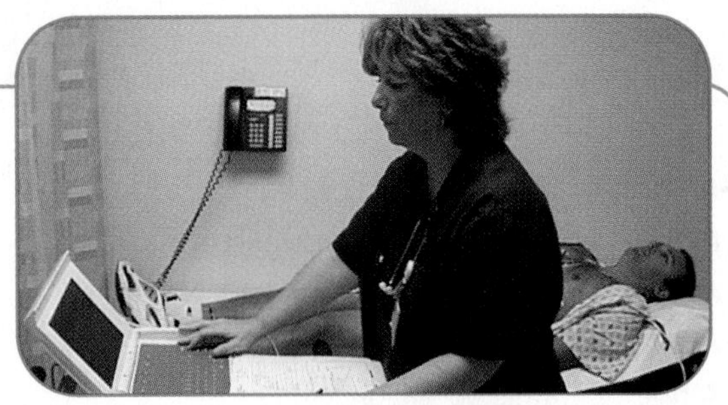

Meet Laurie, a cardiac stress test technologist in a hospital.

"Cardiology is a very important department. I use medical terminology during all aspects of my job. My daughter was born with a heart defect. Wanting to know more information about what was happening to her, I started to take a class here, a class there, and then just wound up in a certificate program. The most rewarding part of my job is if I can get a patient through the test and at the end of the test they say, 'You made that so much easier for me.' "

Cardiac stress test technologists are allied health professionals who perform ECGs, Holter monitor tests, and cardiac stress tests in a hospital setting or a cardiologist's office.

Cardiologists are physicians who practice in the medical specialty of cardiology. They diagnose and treat patients with diseases of the heart and circulatory system. When cardiologists perform surgery, they are known as heart surgeons, cardiothoracic surgeons, or cardiovascular surgeons. Physicians can take additional training and become board certified in the subspecialty of pediatric cardiology. Cancerous tumors of the heart or blood vessels are treated medically by an oncologist or surgically by a cardiothoracic or cardiovascular surgeon.

technologist (tek-NAWL-oh-jist)
techn/o- *technical skill*
log/o- *the study of*
-ist *one who specializes in*

cardiologist (KAR-dee-AWL-oh-jist)
cardi/o- *heart*
log/o- *the study of*
-ist *one who specializes in*

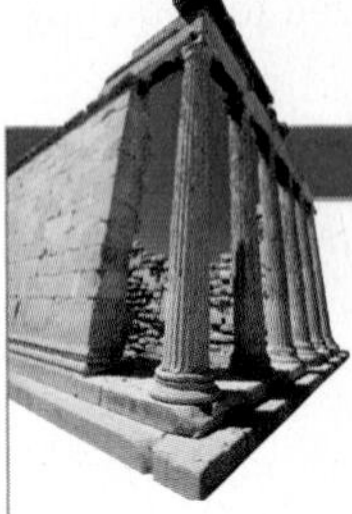

It's Greek to Me!

Did you notice that some cardiovascular words have two different combining forms? Combining forms from both Greek and Latin languages remain a part of medical language today.

English Word	Greek	Latin	Example of Medical Word
blood vessel	angi/o-	vas/o- vascul/o-	angiography, angiogram, vasoconstriction, vasodilator vascular, vasculature
heart	cardi/o-	cor	cardiac, cardiology, cardiopulmonary, cardiothoracic, cor pulmonale
vein	phleb/o-	ven/o-	phlebitis, thrombophlebitis, venous, venography, venogram

CHAPTER REVIEW EXERCISES

Review all the material in this chapter by completing the review exercises in this section. Use the Answer Key at the end of the book to check your answers.

Anatomy and Physiology

Matching Exercise

Match each numbered word or phrase to its description.

1. mediastinum	_____ Another name for the mitral valve
2. pericardium	_____ Network of blood vessels related to a particular organ
3. myocardium	_____ Dividing wall between the atria and ventricles
4. ventricle	_____ Double-layered membrane around the heart
5. tricuspid valve	_____ Bottom chamber of the heart
6. septum	_____ Area between the lungs that contains the heart
7. aortic valve	_____ Valve between the right atrium and right ventricle
8. vasculature	_____ Heart muscle
9. bicuspid valve	_____ Valve that blood flows through as it leaves the left ventricle
10. chordae tendineae	_____ Ropelike strands that strengthen the tricuspid and mitral valves

True or False

Indicate whether each statement is true or false by writing T or F on the line.

1. ____ The aorta is the largest vein in the body.
2. ____ The sympathetic nervous system releases epinephrine, which increases the heart rate and blood pressure.
3. ____ The blood flows from the inferior vena cava to the right atrium to the right ventricle to the pulmonary vein and to the lungs.
4. ____ The refractory period is the time during which the ventricles contract.
5. ____ Little veins are known as capillaries.
6. ____ The interventricular septum is within the ventricle.
7. ____ The endocardium is a serous membrane that lies on the surface of the heart.
8. ____ All arteries carry blood away from the heart.
9. ____ The subclavian artery carries blood to the leg.
10. ____ The peroneal artery carries blood to the lateral aspect of the lower leg.
11. ____ The blood in veins is a dark blue-purple color because it is carrying high levels of carbon dioxide.
12. ____ The systemic circulation carries blood to the whole body with the exception of the lungs.
13. ____ Intracellular fluids are within the cell.
14. ____ Vasodilation is the opposite of vasoconstriction.

Circle Exercise

Circle the correct word from the choices given.

1. The great vessels include the superior and inferior vena cavae and the (**aorta, artery, mediastinum**).
2. The vascular structures of the body include all of the following EXCEPT (**arteries, capillaries, valves, veins**).
3. Listening to a patient's heart sounds with a stethoscope is known as (**auscultation, diastole, repolarization**).
4. This is a unique structure found only in the fetal heart: (**apex, foramen ovale, vasculature**).
5. This vein brings blood from the head to the superior vena cava: (**jugular, portal, saphenous**).
6. The (**AV node, Purkinje fiber, SA node**) is the pacemaker of the heart.

Medical Language Word Parts

Name That Word Part

Identify each of the word parts given here by writing in the correct letter (P, C, or S) on the line beside it. Then write the definition of the word part on the blank line. The first one has been done for you.

Prefix = P **Combining Form = C** **Suffix = S**

		Word Part	Definition			Word Part	Definition
1.	-al	S	pertaining to	35.	cholesterol/o-		
2.	a-			36.	circulat/o-		
3.	ablat/o-			37.	claudicat/o-		
4.	-ac			38.	clav/o-		
5.	anastom/o-			39.	coarct/o-		
6.	aneurysm/o-			40.	compens/o-		
7.	angi/o-			41.	conduct/o-		
8.	anti-			42.	congest/o-		
9.	aort/o-			43.	constrict/o-		
10.	apic/o-			44.	contract/o-		
11.	-ar			45.	coron/o-		
12.	arteri/o-			46.	cusp/o-		
13.	arteriol/o-			47.	cutane/o-		
14.	arter/o-			48.	de-		
15.	-ary			49.	diastol/o-		
16.	-ated			50.	dilat/o-		
17.	ather/o-			51.	distent/o-		
18.	atheromat/o-			52.	dys-		
19.	-ation			53.	-eal		
20.	atri/o-			54.	ech/o-		
21.	-ature			55.	-ectomy		
22.	auscult/o-			56.	ectop/o-		
23.	axill/o-			57.	electr/o-		
24.	bi-			58.	-emia		
25.	bi/o-			59.	emiss/o-		
26.	brachi/o-			60.	endo-		
27.	brady-			61.	-ent		
28.	capill/o-			62.	epi-		
29.	card/i-			63.	esophag/o-		
30.	cardi/o-			64.	extra-		
31.	carot/o-			65.	femor/o-		
32.	cav/o-			66.	fibrill/o-		
33.	cellul/o-			67.	fract/o-		
34.	-centesis			68.	fus/o-		

		Word Part	Definition			Word Part	Definition
69.	gemin/o-	______	______________	110.	-ose	______	______________
70.	-gram	______	______________	111.	-osis	______	______________
71.	-graphy	______	______________	112.	-ous	______	______________
72.	hyper-	______	______________	113.	nephr/o-	______	______________
73.	hypo-	______	______________	114.	palpit/o-	______	______________
74.	-ia	______	______________	115.	-pathy	______	______________
75.	-ian	______	______________	116.	pat/o-	______	______________
76.	-ic	______	______________	117.	per-	______	______________
77.	-id	______	______________	118.	peri-	______	______________
78.	-ide	______	______________	119.	peripher/o-	______	______________
79.	ili/o-	______	______________	120.	perone/o-	______	______________
80.	-in	______	______________	121.	pharmac/o-	______	______________
81.	-ine	______	______________	122.	phleb/o-	______	______________
82.	infarct/o-	______	______________	123.	physi/o-	______	______________
83.	inter-	______	______________	124.	-plasty	______	______________
84.	intra-	______	______________	125.	polar/o-	______	______________
85.	-ion	______	______________	126.	poplite/o-	______	______________
86.	isch/o-	______	______________	127.	port/o-	______	______________
87.	-itis	______	______________	128.	pre-	______	______________
88.	-ity	______	______________	129.	prosthet/o-	______	______________
89.	-ive	______	______________	130.	pulmon/o-	______	______________
90.	-ization	______	______________	131.	radi/o-	______	______________
91.	jugul/o-	______	______________	132.	re-	______	______________
92.	lipid/o-	______	______________	133.	regurgitat/o-	______	______________
93.	lip/o-	______	______________	134.	ren/o-	______	______________
94.	log/o-	______	______________	135.	rheumat/o-	______	______________
95.	-logy	______	______________	136.	rotat/o-	______	______________
96.	lumin/o-	______	______________	137.	rrhythm/o-	______	______________
97.	ly/o-	______	______________	138.	saphen/o-	______	______________
98.	man/o-	______	______________	139.	scler/o-	______	______________
99.	-megaly	______	______________	140.	-scope	______	______________
100.	-meter	______	______________	141.	sept/o-	______	______________
101.	-metry	______	______________	142.	sin/o-	______	______________
102.	mitr/o-	______	______________	143.	son/o-	______	______________
103.	my/o-	______	______________	144.	sphygm/o-	______	______________
104.	necr/o-	______	______________	145.	stat/o-	______	______________
105.	nucle/o-	______	______________	146.	sten/o-	______	______________
106.	-ole	______	______________	147.	steth/o-	______	______________
107.	-oma	______	______________	148.	sub-	______	______________
108.	orth/o-	______	______________	149.	supra-	______	______________
109.	-ory	______	______________	150.	system/o-	______	______________

	Word Part	Definition
151. systol/o-	______	______________
152. tachy-	______	______________
153. tele/o-	______	______________
154. tens/o-	______	______________
155. tetr/a-	______	______________
156. theli/o-	______	______________
157. -therapy	______	______________
158. tibi/o-	______	______________
159. thorac/o-	______	______________
160. thromb/o-	______	______________
161. -tic	______	______________
162. -tome	______	______________
163. tom/o-	______	______________
164. trans-	______	______________
165. transplant/o-	______	______________
166. tri-	______	______________
167. triglycerid/o-	______	______________
168. -trophy	______	______________
169. -ule	______	______________
170. uln/o-	______	______________
171. ultra-	______	______________
172. -um	______	______________
173. valv/o-	______	______________
174. valvul/o-	______	______________
175. varic/o-	______	______________
176. vascul/o-	______	______________
177. vas/o-	______	______________
178. vegetat/o-	______	______________
179. ven/o-	______	______________
180. ventricul/o-	______	______________
181. vers/o-	______	______________

Word-Building Exercise

Use the combining forms, prefixes, and suffixes given here to build medical words that match the definitions given. Write the word that you build on the blank line. Some word parts may be used more than once. The first one has been done for you.

Word Parts

-al (pertaining to)	cardi/o- (heart)	peri- (around)	-um (a structure)
aort/o- (aorta)	-ic (pertaining to)	pulmon/o- (lung)	vascul/o- (blood vessel)
-ary (pertaining to)	inter- (between)	sin/o- (hollow cavity; channel)	ven/o- (vein)
atri/o- (atrium)	my/o- (muscle)	system/o- (the body as a whole)	ventricul/o- (ventricle)
-ature (system composed of)	-ous (pertaining to)	-ule (small thing)	

1. Pertaining to a vein (You think *ven/o-* + *-ous*). You write venous
2. Pertaining to around the heart ____________________
3. System composed of blood vessels ____________________
4. Heart muscle ____________________
5. Pertaining to the heart and the lungs ____________________
6. The node that originates the heartbeat ____________________
7. Pertaining to the body as a whole ____________________
8. Small vein ____________________
9. Pertaining to the aorta ____________________
10. Pertaining to between the ventricles ____________________

Symptoms, Signs, and Diseases

Matching Exercise

Match each numbered word or phrase to its description.

1.	arrhythmia	_____ Normal contraction followed by a premature contraction
2.	cardiac arrest	_____ Fatty deposit
3.	extrasystole	_____ Dysrrhythmia
4.	bigeminy	_____ Any kind of premature contraction
5.	cardiomegaly	_____ Chest sensation during premature contraction
6.	thrombus	_____ Cell death
7.	palpitation	_____ Asystole
8.	coarctation	_____ Blood clot
9.	necrosis	_____ Enlarged heart
10.	atheroma	_____ Abnormal narrowing
11.	tetralogy of Fallot	_____ Congenital heart defect

Circle Exercise

Circle the correct word from the choices given.

1. (**Asystole, Bradycardia, Fibrillation**) is an abnormally slow heart rate.
2. Narrowing of an artery is known as (**arteriosclerosis, endocarditis, stenosis**).
3. A weakness in the wall of an artery is known as a/an (**aneurysm, varicose vein, ecchymosis**).
4. (**Patent foramen ovale, Heart block, Aneurysm**) is a congenital heart defect.

True or False

Indicate whether each statement is true or false by writing T or F on the line.

1. ____ Angina pectoris is chest pain that means the myocardial cells have died.
2. ____ Prolapse of a valve is when the cusps hang down and do not close completely.
3. ____ Raynaud's disease is severe vasocontriction of the extremities triggered by cold or emotional stress.
4. ____ Hyperlipidemia can mean either hypercholesterolemia or hypertriglyceridemia.
5. ____ Regurgitation is an infection of the heart caused by bacteria.
6. ____ To check for arteriosclerosis in the arteries of the legs, you would feel the pulse in the radial artery.
7. ____ Auscultation is using a stethoscope to listen to the heart sounds.
8. ____ S_1 and S_2 are abnormal heart sounds.
9. ____ In patients with right-sided congestive heart failure, the neck may show signs of pitting edema.
10. ____ A sphygmomanometer measures the blood pressure in millimeters of mercury (mm Hg).

Laboratory, Radiology, Surgery, and Drugs

Laboratory Test Exercise

Review this form for ordering laboratory tests (see Figure 5-37■). Find each of the following tests related to cardiology and put a checkmark in the box next to it.

cardio CRP	digoxin	lipid panel
cardio CRP w/ lipid profile	HDL cholesterol	triglycerides
cholesterol		

PANELS AND PROFILES			TESTS		
968T		Lipid Panel	19687W		Bilirubin (Direct)
315F		Electrolyte Panel	265F		HBsAg
10256F		Hepatic Function Panel	51870R		HB Core Antibody
10165F		Basic Metabolic Panel	1012F		Cardio CRP
10231A		Comprehensive Metabolic Panel	23242E		GGT
10306F		Hepatitis Panel, Acute	28852E		Protein, Total
182Aaa		Obstetric Panel	141A		CBC Hemogram
18T		Chem-Screen Panel (Basic)	21105R		hCG, Qualitative, Serum
554T		Chem-Screen Panel (Basic with HDL)	10321A		ANA
7971A		Chem-Screen Panel (Basic with HDL, TIBC)	80185		Cardio CRP with Lipid Profile
TESTS			26F		PT with INR
56713E		Lead, Blood	232Aaa		UA, Dipstick
2782A		Antibody Screen	42A		CBC with Diff
3556F		Iron, TIBC	20867W		HDL Cholesterol
20933E		Cholesterol	31732E		PTT
3084111E		Uric Acid	34F		UA, Dipstick and Microscopic
53348W		Rubella Antibody	20396R		CEA
27771E		Phosphate	45443E		Hematocrit
2111600E		Creatinine	28571E		PSA, Total
29868W		Testosterone, Total	66902E		WBC count
9704F		Creatinine Clearance	20750E		Chloride
19752E		Bilirubin (Total)	7187W		Hemoglobin
30536Rrr		T3, Total	4259T		HIV-1 Antibody
687T		Protein Electrophoresis	45484R		Hemoglobin A1c
3563444R		Digoxin	67868R		Alk Phosphatase
15214R		Glucose, 2-Hour Postprandial	24984R		Iron
30502E		T3, Uptake	28512E		Sodium
7773E		Platelet Count	17426R		ALT
39685R		Dilantin (phenytoin)	MICROBIOLOGY		
30494R		Triglycerides	112680E		Group A Beta Strep Culture, Throat
26013E		Magnesium	5827W		Group B Beta Strep Culture, Genitals
15586R		Glucose, Fasting	49932E		Chlamydia, Endocervix/Urethra
30237W		T4, Free	6007W		Culture, Blood
28233E		Potassium	2692E		Culture, Genitals
19208W		AST	2649T		Culture, HSV
30163E		TSH	612A		Culture, Sputum
22764R		Ferritin	6262E		Culture, Throat
20008W		Calcium	6304R		Culture, Urine
54726F		Occult Blood, Stool	50286R		Gonococcus, Endocervix/Urethra
51839W		HAV Antibody, Total	6643E		Gram Stain
430A		Blood Group and Rh Type	STOOL PATHOGENS		
28399W		Progesterone	10045F		Culture, Stool
30262E		T4, Total	4475F		Culture, Campylobacter
20289W		Carbon Dioxide	10018T		Culture, Salmonella
1156F		RPR	86140A		E. coli Toxins
30940E		Urea Nitrogen	1099T		Ova and Parasites
17417W		Albumin	VENIPUNCTURE		
28423E		Prolactin	63180		Venipuncture

Figure 5-37 ■

Word-Building Exercise

Use the combining forms, prefixes, and suffixes here to build medical words that match the definitions given. Write the word that you build on the blank line. Some word parts may be used more than once. The first one has been done for you.

aneurysm/o- (aneurysm)	-gram (a record or picture)	-therapy (treatment)
angi/o- (blood vessel; lymphatic vessel)	-graphy (process of recording)	-tome (instrument used to cut)
cardi/o- (heart)	phleb/o- (vein)	-tomy (process of cutting or making an incision)
-ectomy (surgical excision)	scler/o- (hard; white of the eye)	ultra- (beyond; higher)
electr/o- (electricity)	son/o- (sound)	valvul/o- (valve)

1. Therapy used to harden a varicose vein (You think *scler/o-* + *-therapy*) You write sclerotherapy
2. Radiology test that outlines the blood vessel by using contrast material ____________
3. A written record of the electrical activity of the heart ____________
4. Test that uses ultra high-frequency sound waves to outline the heart ____________
5. Surgery to remove an aneurysm ____________
6. Instrument used to cut diseased valves ____________

True or False

Indicate whether each statement is true or false by writing T or F on the line.

1. ____ Antiarrhythmic drugs are used to treat hypertension.
2. ____ Thrombolytic drugs break apart blood clots.
3. ____ An artificial valve is also known as a prosthesis.
4. ____ A stent is inserted during a MUGA scan.
5. ____ Sclerotherapy is used to treat arteriosclerosis (hardening of the arteries).

Abbreviations

Matching Exercise

Match each abbreviation to its description.

1. LVAD ____ "Good cholesterol," a high-density lipoprotein
2. AAA ____ High blood pressure
3. SBE ____ Bacterial infection inside the heart
4. CRP ____ The heart rate set by the SA node
5. mm Hg ____ Test to detect inflammation in the heart
6. HTN ____ A hole in the septum between the ventricles
7. NSR ____ Can be dissecting-type of aneurysm
8. TPR ____ Vital signs
9. TEE ____ Measurement of blood pressure
10. VSD ____ Heart test that goes into the esophagus
11. HDL ____ May be used instead of heart transplantation

Applied Skills

Plural Noun and Adjective Spelling

Fill in the blanks with the correct word form. Be sure to check your spelling. The first one has been done for you.

Singular Noun	Plural Noun	Adjective	Singular Noun	Plural Noun	Adjective
1. endothelium		*endothelial*	7. valve	____	____
2. pericardium		____	8. aorta		____
3. atrium	____	____	9. vein	____	____
4. ventricle	____	____	10. heart		____
5. septum		____	11. valve	____	____
6. myocardium		____			

Analysis of a Medical Report

This exercise contains a hospital Admission History and Physical Examination report. Read the report and answer the questions. Use the Answer Key at the end of the book to check your answers.

ADMISSION HISTORY AND PHYSICAL EXAMINATION

PATIENT NAME: COVINGTON, Victoria

HOSPITAL NUMBER: 62-700245

DATE OF ADMISSION: January 21, 20xx

HISTORY OF PRESENT ILLNESS

The patient is a 76-year-old white female who was transferred emergently from home via ambulance to this emergency department. Apparently, the patient had just finished eating breakfast when her family noticed that she was standing in the middle of the hallway with her walker, seemingly dazed. She was assisted to her bed, but rest did not improve her mental status. The family stated that she continued to be confused, incoherent, and unable to answer simple questions. At that point, the family called 911.

PAST MEDICAL HISTORY

The past medical history was obtained from the patient's daughter-in-law. The patient has a history of CHF, which has been slowly worsening over about the past 8 years. She also has a history of hypertension. The patient has been diagnosed with type 2 diabetes mellitus. The daughter-in-law remembers that the patient's last fasting blood sugar in the doctor's office last month was over 250. She is usually noncompliant with her diet, eating foods that are high in fat and calories. The patient does not take a pill or insulin for her diabetes. In the past week, the patient has had no appetite, has eaten little, but reportedly gained 2 pounds anyway. The daughter-in-law does not know the names of all of the patient's medications, except for Lasix. The patient smokes 1 pack of cigarettes per day and has done so for the past 40+ years. The patient has no known allergies.

PHYSICAL EXAMINATION

The patient is an obese female, lying in bed. She is stuporous, opening her eyes to commands but she is unable to answer questions. Heart: Regular rate and rhythm. The PMI is displaced to the left. The neck veins are slightly distended. The breath sounds reveal rales in both bases bilaterally. The abdomen is soft with hypoactive bowel sounds. Physical examination of the lower extremities shows pitting edema in both feet with 2+ pretibial edema in the legs.

COURSE IN THE EMERGENCY DEPARTMENT

The patient was placed on a cardiac monitor and given a stat dose of intravenous Lasix. Labs were sent for CBC with WBC differential, electrolytes, CK-MB, troponin, and glucose. An arterial blood gas was drawn. Portable chest x-ray in the emergency department showed cardiomegaly with an LVH configuration. There was significant pulmonary vascular congestion. While awaiting the results of the blood chemistries, the patient suddenly went into cardiac arrest. CPR was initiated. She responded to aggressive drug intervention and defibrillation, and we were able to establish a normal sinus rhythm. The patient was then transferred to the intensive care unit in critical condition, intubated, and on the ventilator.

Alfred P. Molina, M.D.

Alfred P. Molina, M.D.

APM:mtt
D: 01/21/xx
T: 01/21/xx

WORD ANALYSIS QUESTIONS

1. What is the medical abbreviation for hypertension? ____________________

2. The patient has hypertension. If you wanted to use the adjective form of *hypertension,* you would say, "The patient is ____________________."

3. What do these abbreviations stand for?

   a. CHF ____________________

   b. CK-MB ____________________

   c. CPR ____________________

   d. LVH ____________________

   e. PMI ____________________

4. Divide *defibrillation* into its three word parts and define each word part.

Word Part	Definition
____________	____________________
____________	____________________
____________	____________________

5. Divide *vascular* into its two word parts and define each word part.

Word Part	Definition
____________	____________________
____________	____________________

6. Divide *cardiomegaly* into its two word parts and define each word part.

Word Part	Definition
____________	____________________
____________	____________________

7. Dictionary Skills

   These medical words were not covered in this chapter, but you need to know their meanings in order to understand this medical report. Look up these words in a medical or English dictionary amd write their definitions.

Word	Definition
incoherent	____________________
stuporous	____________________
emergently	____________________

FACT FINDING QUESTIONS

1. What is the range of beats per minute for normal sinus rhythm in an adult? ____________________
2. Name 3 cardiac risk factors that this patient has.
   a. ________________________________
   b. ________________________________
   c. ________________________________
3. Defibrillation was used to treat what condition? (Circle one)
   cardiomegaly **hypertension** **cardiac arrest** **diabetes mellitus**
4. The PMI was displaced to the left. What diagnostic test was done in the emergency room that confirmed this finding from the physical examination? (Circle one)
   troponin **portable chest x-ray** **blood glucose** **intubation**

CRITICAL THINKING QUESTIONS

1. The pitting edema and the pretibial edema in the patient's extremities reflected congestion and backup of blood due to failure of which side of the heart?
   ____
2. The pulmonary vascular congestion seen on chest x-ray reflected failure of which side of the heart?
   ____
3. Lasix is a diuretic drug that removes fluid from the body by excreting it in the urine. For which of the patient's medical conditions was this drug prescribed? (Circle one)
   congestive heart failure **lack of appetite** **obesity**
4. If the patient ate little food in the past week, why did she gain two pounds?
   ____

Pronunciation Checklist

Read each word and its pronunciation. Practice pronouncing each word. Verify your pronunciation by listening to the Pronunciation List on the CD-ROM. Check the box next to the word after you have mastered its pronunciation.

- ❑ acetylcholine (AS-eh-til-KOH-leen)
- ❑ anastomosis (ah-NAS-toh-MOH-sis)
- ❑ aneurysm (AN-yoo-rizm)
- ❑ aneurysmal (AN-yoo-RIZ-mal)
- ❑ aneurysmectomy (AN-yoo-riz-MEK-toh-mee)
- ❑ angina (AN-jih-nah) (an-JY-nah)
- ❑ anginal (AN-jih-nal) (an-JY-nal)
- ❑ angina pectoris (AN-jih-nah PEK-toh-ris)
- ❑ angiogram (AN-jee-oh-gram)
- ❑ angiography (AN-jee-AWG-rah-fee)
- ❑ angioplasty (AN-jee-oh-PLAS-tee)
- ❑ angiotensin (AN-jee-oh-TEN-sin)
- ❑ antiarrhythmic drug (AN-tee-aa-RITH-mik DRUHG)
- ❑ antibiotic drug (AN-tee-by-AWT-ik DRUHG) (AN-tih-by-AWT-ik)
- ❑ antihypertensive drug (AN-tee-HY-per-TEN-siv DRUHG)
- ❑ aorta (aa-OR-tah)
- ❑ aortic valve (aa-OR-tik VALV)
- ❑ aortogram (aa-OR-toh-gram)
- ❑ aortography (AA-or-TAWG-rah-fee)
- ❑ apex (AA-peks)
- ❑ apical (AP-ih-kal)
- ❑ arrhythmia (aa-RITH-mee-ah)
- ❑ arterial (ar-TEER-ee-al)
- ❑ arteriogram (ar-TEER-ee-oh-gram)
- ❑ arteriography (ar-TEER-ee-AWG-rah-fee)
- ❑ arteriolar (ar-TEER-ee-OH-lar)
- ❑ arteriole (ar-TEER-ee-ohl)
- ❑ arteriosclerosis (ar-TEER-ee-oh-skleh-ROH-sis)
- ❑ arteriosclerotic (ar-TEER-ee-oh-skleh-RAW-tik)
- ❑ artery (AR-ter-ee)
- ❑ asystole (aa-SIS-toh-lee)
- ❑ atheroma (ATH-eh-ROH-mah)
- ❑ atheromatous (ATH-eh-ROH-mah-tus)
- ❑ atherosclerosis (ATH-eh-roh-skleh-ROH-sis)
- ❑ atria (AA-tree-ah)
- ❑ atrial (AA-tree-al)
- ❑ atrioventricular (AA-tree-oh-ven-TRIK-yoo-lar)
- ❑ atrium (AA-tree-um)
- ❑ auscultation (AWS-kul-TAY-shun)
- ❑ axillary artery (AK-sil-air-ee AR-ter-ee)
- ❑ bicuspid valve (by-KUS-pid VALV)
- ❑ bigeminal rhythm (by-JEM-ih-nal RITH-um)
- ❑ bigeminy (by-JEM-ih-nee)
- ❑ brachial artery (BRAY-kee-al AR-ter-ee)
- ❑ bradycardia (BRAD-ee-KAR-ee-ah)
- ❑ bradycardic (BRAD-ee-KAR-dik)
- ❑ bruit (BROO-ee)
- ❑ bundle of His (BUN-dl of HISS)
- ❑ capillary (KAP-ih-lair-ee)
- ❑ cardiac (KAR-dee-ak)
- ❑ cardiac catheterization (KAR-dee-ak KATH-eh-ter-ih-ZAY-shun)
- ❑ cardiac enzymes (KAR-dee-ak EN-zimez)
- ❑ cardiologist (KAR-dee-AWL-oh-jist)
- ❑ cardiology (KAR-dee-AWL-oh-jee)
- ❑ cardiomegaly (KAR-dee-oh-MEG-ah-lee)
- ❑ cardiomyopathy (KAR-dee-oh-my-AWP-ah-thee)
- ❑ cardiopulmonary (KAR-dee-oh-PUL-moh-nair-ee)
- ❑ cardiopulmonary resuscitation (KAR-dee-oh-PUL-moh-nair-ee ree-SUS-ih-TAY-shun)
- ❑ cardiothoracic (KAR-dee-oh-thoh-RAS-ik)
- ❑ cardiovascular system (KAR-dee-oh-VAS-kyoo-lar SIS-tem)
- ❑ cardioversion (KAR-dee-oh-VER-zhun)
- ❑ carotid artery (kah-ROT-id AR-ter-ee)
- ❑ cavity (KAV-ih-tee)
- ❑ chordae tendineae (KOHR-dee TEN-dih-nee-ee)
- ❑ circulation (SER-kyoo-LAY-shun)
- ❑ circulatory (SER-kyoo-lah-TOH-ree)
- ❑ claudication (KLAW-dih-KAY-shun)
- ❑ coarctation (KOH-ark-TAY-shun)
- ❑ compensated heart failure (KAWM-pen-SAY-ted HART FAYL-yer)
- ❑ conduction (con-DUK-shun)
- ❑ congestive (con-JES-tiv)
- ❑ contraction (con-TRAK-shun)
- ❑ cor pulmonale (KOR PUL-moh-NAL-ee)
- ❑ coronary artery (KOR-oh-nair-ee AR-ter-ee)
- ❑ creatine phosphokinase (KREE-ah-teen FAWS-foh-KY-nays)
- ❑ decompensated heart failure (dee-KAWM-pen-SAY-ted HART FAYL-yer)
- ❑ defibrillator (dee-FIB-rih-lay-ter)
- ❑ depolarization (dee-POHL-ar-ih-ZAY-shun)
- ❑ diastole (dy-AS-toh-lee)
- ❑ diastolic (DY-ah-STAWL-ik)
- ❑ digitalis (DIJ-ih-TAL-is)
- ❑ dissecting aneurysm (dy-SEK-ting AN-yoo-rizm)
- ❑ distention (dis-TEN-shun)
- ❑ Doppler ultrasonography (DAWP-ler UL-trah-soh-NAWG-rah-fee)
- ❑ dorsalis pedis (dohr-SAH-lis PEE-dis)
- ❑ ductus arteriosus (DUK-tus ar-TEER-ee-OH-sus)
- ❑ duplex ultrasonography (DOO-pleks UL-trah-soh-NAWG-rah-fee)
- ❑ dysrrhythmia (dis-RITH-mee-ah)
- ❑ echocardiogram (EK-oh-KAR-dee-oh-gram)
- ❑ echocardiography (EK-oh-KAR-dee-AWG-rah-fee)
- ❑ ectopic (ek-TOP-ik)
- ❑ edema (eh-DEE-mah)
- ❑ electrocardiogram (ee-LEK-troh-KAR-dee-oh-gram)
- ❑ electrocardiographic technician (ee-LEK-troh-KAR-dee-oh-GRAF-ik tek-NISH-un)
- ❑ electrocardiography (ee-LEK-troh-KAR-dee-AWG-rah-fee)
- ❑ electrophysiologic (ee-LEK-troh-FIZ-ee-oh-LAW-jik)
- ❑ endarterectomy (END-ar-ter-EK-toh-mee)
- ❑ endocardial (EN-doh-KAR-dee-al)
- ❑ endocarditis (EN-doh-kar-DY-tis)
- ❑ endocardium (EN-doh-KAR-dee-um)
- ❑ endothelial (EN-doh-THEE-lee-al)
- ❑ endothelium (EN-doh-THEE-lee-um)
- ❑ epicardial (EP-ih-KAR-dee-al)
- ❑ epicardium (EP-ih-KAR-dee-um)
- ❑ epinephrine (EP-ih-NEF-rin)
- ❑ extracellular (EKS-trah-SEL-yoo-lar)
- ❑ extrasystole (EKS-trah-SIS-toh-lee)

- ❑ femoral artery (FEM-oh-ral AR-ter-ee)
- ❑ fibrillation (FIB-rih-LAY-shun)
- ❑ foramen ovale (foh-RAY-men oh-VAH-lee)
- ❑ heart donor (HART DOH-nor)
- ❑ heart transplantation (HART TRANS-plan-TAY-shun)
- ❑ hypercholesterolemia (HY-per-koh-LES-ter-awl-EE-mee-ah)
- ❑ hyperlipidemia (HY-per-LIP-ih-DEE-mee-ah)
- ❑ hypertension (HY-per-TEN-shun)
- ❑ hypertensive (HY-per-TEN-siv)
- ❑ hypertriglyceridemia (HY-per-try-GLIS-er-ih-DEE-mee-ah)
- ❑ hypertrophic (HY-per-TROH-fik)
- ❑ hypertrophy (hy-PER-troh-fee)
- ❑ hypotension (HY-poh-TEN-shun)
- ❑ hypotensive (HY-poh-TEN-siv)
- ❑ idiopathic (ID-ee-oh-PATH-ik)
- ❑ iliac artery (IL-ee-ak AR-ter-ee)
- ❑ infarction (in-FARK-shun)
- ❑ interatrial septum (IN-ter-AA-tree-al SEP-tum)
- ❑ interventricular septum (IN-ter-ven-TRIK-yoo-lar SEP-tum)
- ❑ intima (IN-tih-mah)
- ❑ intra-atrial (IN-trah-AA-tree-al)
- ❑ intracellular (IN-trah-SEL-yoo-lar)
- ❑ intraventricular (IN-trah-ven-TRIK-yoo-lar)
- ❑ ion (EYE-on)
- ❑ ischemia (is-KEE-mee-ah)
- ❑ jugular vein (JUG-yoo-lar VAYN)
- ❑ lactate dehydrogenase (LAK-tayt dee-HY-droh-jeh-nays)
- ❑ lipid (LIP-id)
- ❑ lipoprotein (LIP-oh-PROH-teen)
- ❑ lumen (LOO-men)
- ❑ mediastinal (MEE-dee-as-TY-nal)
- ❑ mediastinum (MEE-dee-as-TY-num)
- ❑ mitral valve (MY-tral VALV)
- ❑ mitral regurgitation (MY-tral ree-GER-jih-TAY-shun)
- ❑ murmur (MER-mer)
- ❑ myocardial (MY-oh-KAR-dee-al)
- ❑ myocardial infarction (MY-oh-KAR-dee-al in-FARK-shun)
- ❑ myocardial perfusion scan (MY-oh-KAR-dee-al per-FYOO-zhun SKAN)
- ❑ myocardium (MY-oh-KAR-dee-um)
- ❑ necrosis (neh-KROH-sis)
- ❑ necrotic (neh-KRAWT-ik)
- ❑ nitrate drug (NY-trayt DRUHG)
- ❑ nitrates (NY-trayts)
- ❑ node (NOHD)
- ❑ occlusion (oh-KLOO-zhun)
- ❑ orthostatic hypotension (OR-thoh-STAT-ik HY-poh-TEN-shun)
- ❑ palpitation (PAL-pih-TAY-shun)
- ❑ paroxysmal tachycardia (PAR-awk-SIZ-mal TAK-ih-KAR-dee-ah)
- ❑ patent (PAY-tent)
- ❑ percutaneous transluminal angioplasty (PER-kyoo-TAY-nee-us trans-LOO-mih-nal AN-jee-oh-PLAS-tee)
- ❑ perfusion (per-FYOO-shun)
- ❑ pericardial sac (PAIR-ih-KAR-dee-al SAK)
- ❑ pericardiocentesis (PAIR-ih-KAR-dee-oh-sen-TEE-sis)
- ❑ pericarditis (PAIR-ee-kar-DY-tis)
- ❑ pericardium (PAIR-ih-KAR-dee-um)
- ❑ peripheral (peh-RIF-eh-ral)
- ❑ peroneal artery (PAIR-oh-NEE-al AR-ter-ee)
- ❑ phlebitis (fleh-BY-tis)
- ❑ plaque (PLAHK)
- ❑ popliteal artery (pop-LIT-ee-al AR-ter-ee) (pop-lih-TEE-al)
- ❑ portal vein (POR-tal VAYN)
- ❑ prehypertension (pree-HY-per-TEN-shun)
- ❑ prosthetic valve (praws-THET-ik VALV)
- ❑ pulmonary artery (PUL-moh-nair-ee AR-ter-ee)
- ❑ pulmonary valve (PUL-moh-nair-ee VALV)
- ❑ pulmonary vein (PUL-moh-nair-ee VAYN)
- ❑ pulse (PUHLS)
- ❑ Purkinje fiber (per-KIN-jee FY-ber)
- ❑ radial artery (RAY-dee-al AR-ter-ee)
- ❑ radiofrequency catheter ablation (RAY-dee-oh-FREE-kwen-see KATH-eh-ter ah-BLAY-shun)
- ❑ radionuclide ventriculography (RAY-dee-oh-NOO-klide ven-TRIK-yoo-LAWG-rah-fee
- ❑ Raynaud's disease (ray-NOZ dih-ZEEZ)
- ❑ refractory (ree-FRAK-tor-ee)
- ❑ renal artery (REE-nal AR-ter-ee)
- ❑ repolarization (ree-POH-lar-ih-ZAY-shun)
- ❑ rheumatic heart disease (roo-MAT-ik HART dih-ZEEZ)
- ❑ saphenous vein (sah-FEE-nus VAYN)
- ❑ sclerotherapy (SKLAIR-oh-THAIR-ah-pee)
- ❑ septal (SEP-tal)
- ❑ septum (SEP-tum)
- ❑ sinoatrial node (SY-noh-AA-tree-al NOHD)
- ❑ sinus rhythm (SY-nus RITH-um)
- ❑ sphygmomanometer (SFIG-moh-mah-NAWM-eh-ter)
- ❑ stenosis (steh-NOH-sis)
- ❑ stethoscope (STETH-oh-skohp)
- ❑ subacute (sub-ah-KYOOT)
- ❑ subclavian artery (sub-KLAY-vee-an AR-ter-ee)
- ❑ supraventricular tachycardia (SOO-prah-ven-TRIK-yoo-lar TAK-ih-KAR-dee-ah)
- ❑ systemic (sis-TEM-ik)
- ❑ systole (SIS-toh-lee)
- ❑ systolic (sis-TAWL-ik)
- ❑ tachycardia (TAK-ih-KAR-dee-ah)
- ❑ tachycardic (TAK-ih-KAR-dik)
- ❑ tamponade (tam-poh-NAYD)
- ❑ telemetry (teh-LEM-eh-tree)
- ❑ tetralogy of Fallot (tet-RAL-oh-jee of feh-LOW)
- ❑ thallium stress test (THAL-ee-um STRES TEST)
- ❑ thoracic cavity (thoh-RAS-ik KAV-ih-tee)
- ❑ thrombolytic drug (THRAWM-boh-LIT-ik DRUHG)
- ❑ thrombophlebitis (THRAWM-boh-fleh-BY-tis)
- ❑ tibial artery (TIB-ee-al AR-ter-ee)
- ❑ tomography (toh-MAWG-rah-fee)
- ❑ transesophageal echocardiogram (TRANS-ee-SAWF-ah-JEE-al EK-oh-KAR-dee-oh-gram)
- ❑ tricuspid valve (try-KUS-pid VALV)
- ❑ trigeminal rhythm (try-JEM-ih-nal RITH-um)
- ❑ trigeminy (try-JEM-ih-nee)
- ❑ troponin (troh-POH-nin)
- ❑ ulnar artery (UL-nar AR-ter-ee)
- ❑ ultrasonography (UL-trah-soh-NAWG-rah-fee)
- ❑ valve (VALV)

- ❑ valve prolapse (VALV PROH-laps)
- ❑ valvoplasty (VAL-voh-plas-tee)
- ❑ valvular (VAL-vyoo-lar)
- ❑ valvuloplasty (VAL-vyoo-loh-PLAS-tee)
- ❑ valvulotome (VAL-vyoo-loh-tohm)
- ❑ varicose vein (VAR-ih-kohs VAYN)
- ❑ vascular (VAS-kyoo-lar)
- ❑ vasculature (VAS-kyoo-lah-chur)
- ❑ vasoconstriction (VAY-soh-con-STRIK-shun)
- ❑ vasodilation (VAY-soh-dy-LAY-shun)
- ❑ vegetation (VEJ-eh-TAY-shun)
- ❑ vein (VAYN)
- ❑ vena cava (VEE-nah KAY-vah)
- ❑ venogram (VEE-noh-gram)
- ❑ venography (vee-NAWG-rah-fee)
- ❑ venous (VEE-nus)
- ❑ ventricle (VEN-trih-kl)
- ❑ ventricular (ven-TRIK-yoo-lar)
- ❑ ventriculography (ven-TRIK-yoo-LAWG-rah-fee)
- ❑ venule (VEN-yool)
- ❑ xenograft (ZEN-oh-graft)

Experience Multimedia

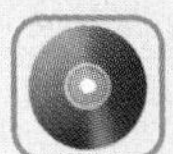

CD-ROM Learning Activities Checklist

Check off the box as you complete each learning activity.

- ❑ **CD-ROM Learning Activity 5.1: *ANATOMY WORD PARTS FLASHCARDS***
  Use flashcards to help you memorize word parts. Make your own flashcards or print out prepared flashcards. Also see the electronic flashcard game. Time: 20 minutes.
- ❑ **CD-ROM Learning Activity 5.2: *MEDICINE IN ACTION***
  Listen to normal and abnormal heart sounds. Time: 5 minutes.
- ❑ **CD-ROM Learning Activity 5.3: *DISEASE AND OTHER WORD PARTS FLASHCARDS***
  A continuation of the flashcard learning activity. Time: 20 minutes.
- ❑ **CD-ROM Learning Activity 5.4: *MEMORY AIDS***
  Use memory aids to help you memorize medical words and meanings. Time: 5 minutes.
- ❑ **CD-ROM Learning Activity 5.5: *MEDICAL LANGUAGE SPOKEN HERE***
  Listen to actual medical reports and spell the missing medical words. Time: 20 minutes.
- ❑ **CD-ROM Learning Activity 5.6: *SPELLING CHALLENGE***
  Listen to a pronounced medical word and then spell it. Time: 5 minutes.
- ❑ **CD-ROM Learning Activity 5.7: *MEDICAL LANGUAGE PRONUNCIATION***
  Listen to a pronounced medical word and then practice pronouncing it. Time: 30 minutes.
- ❑ **CD-ROM Learning Activity 5.8: *EDUCATIONAL FUN AND GAMES***
  Enjoy these fun activities while reinforcing your knowledge. Time: 15 minutes.

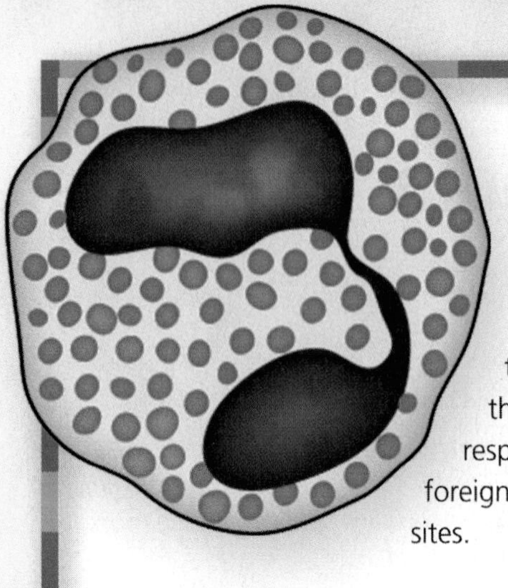

◀ An eosinophil is a type of white blood cell that, as part of the immune response, destroys foreign cells and parasites.

Dive In!

- Human blood circles the body in about 20 seconds, traveling thousands of miles per day.
- 15 million blood cells are produced and destroyed in the human body every second.
- To score an A or B (or AB or O), keep reading. In this chapter we'll explore the language that describes blood and lymphatic system structures, functions, diseases, and conditions.
- Your knowledge will be flowing once you master the language of hematology and immunology!

▶ Blood contains proteins that female mosquitoes need to lay their eggs. That's why only the females bite.

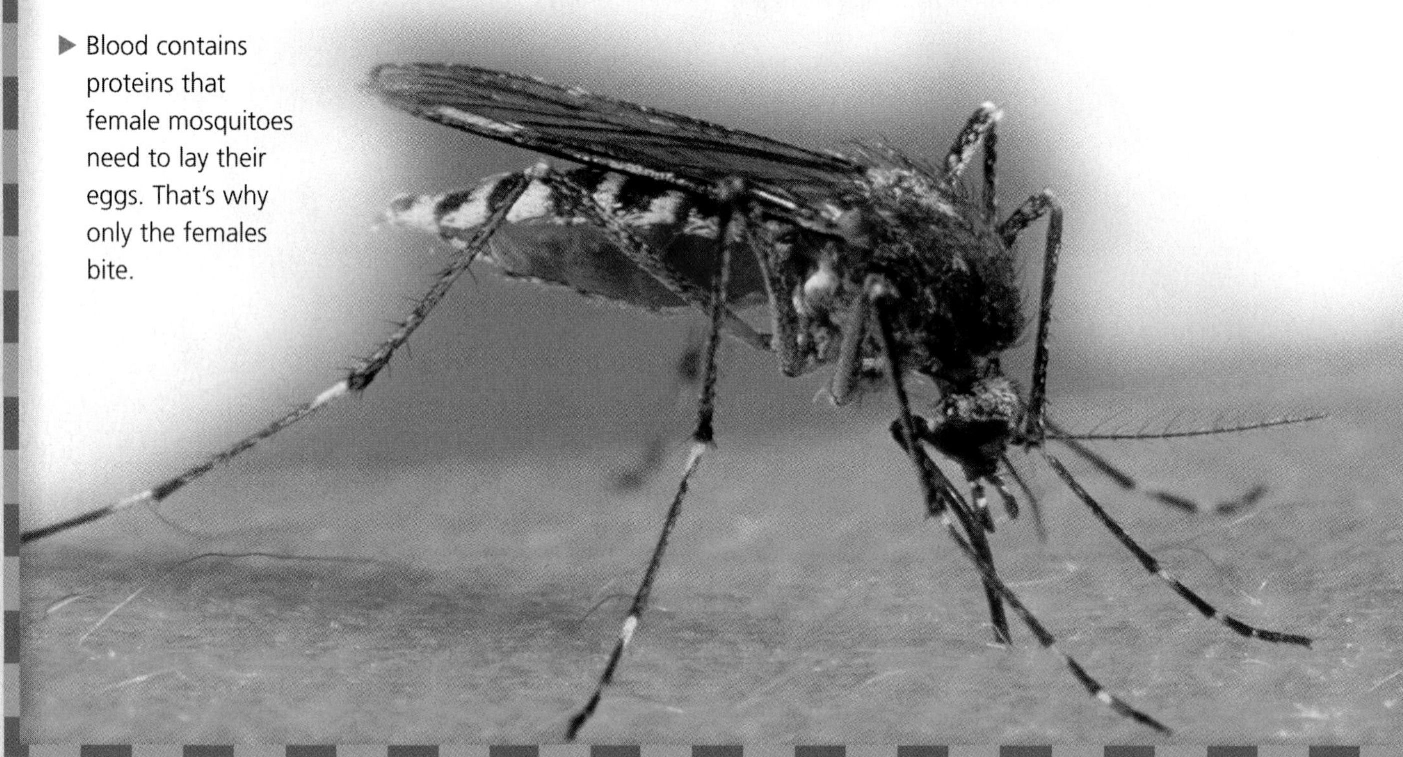

Medicine Through HISTORY

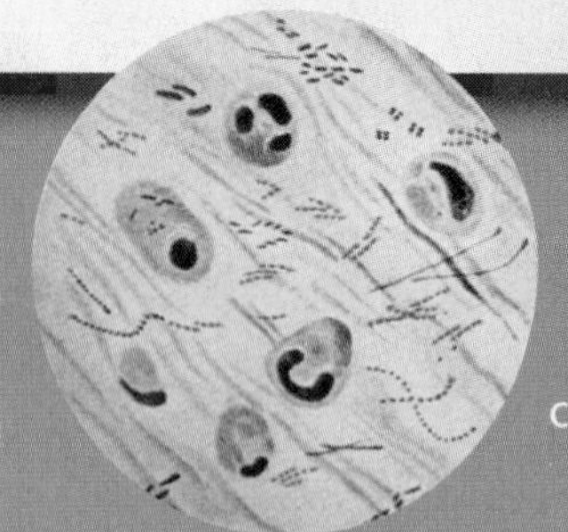

1859

Louis Pasteur suggests that microscopic organisms cause disease

1862

Dutch physician Hermann Snellen invents the Snellen chart for testing distance vision

1864

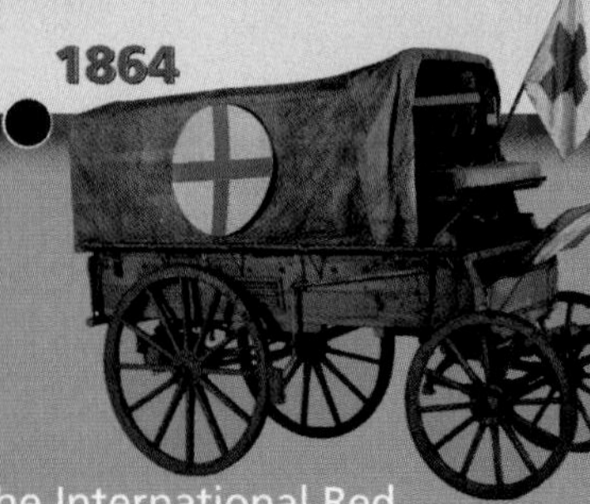

The International Red Cross is founded

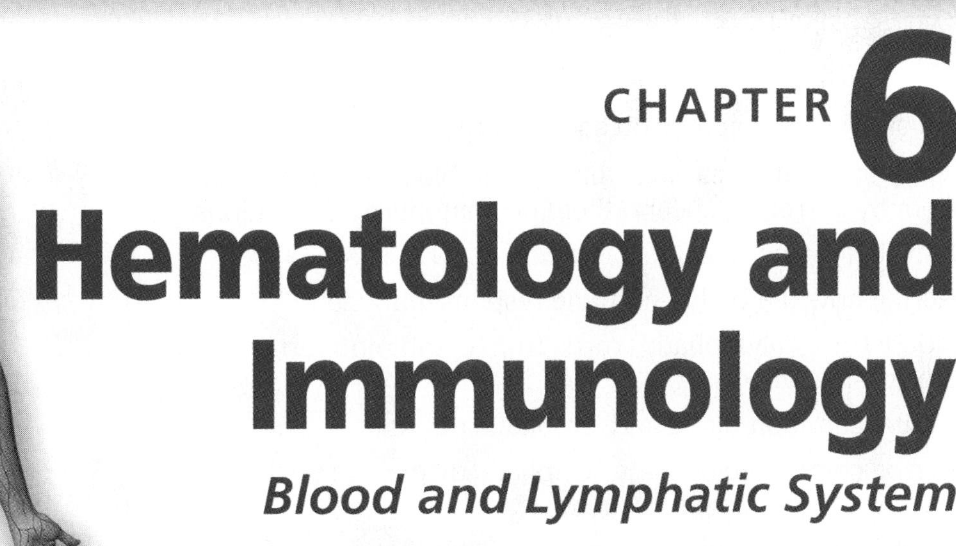

CHAPTER 6 Hematology and Immunology

Blood and Lymphatic System

Hematology (HEE-mah-TAWL-oh-jee) is the medical specialty that studies the anatomy and physiology of the blood and uses diagnostic tests, medical and surgical procedures, and drugs to treat blood diseases. Immunology (IM-yoo-NAWL-oh-jee) is the medical specialty that studies the immune response and uses diagnostic tests, medical and surgical procedures, and drugs to treat immune response diseases.

◀ The lymphatic system is a pathway of vessels and nodes that defend the body via the immune response.

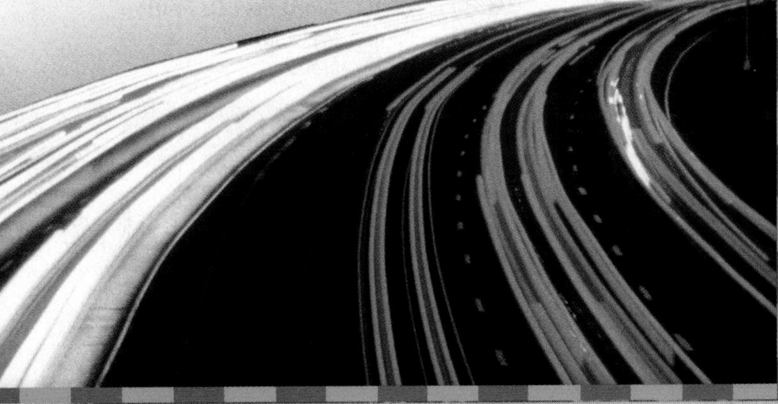

▶ Blood is an essential transport system, largely composed of red and white blood cells.

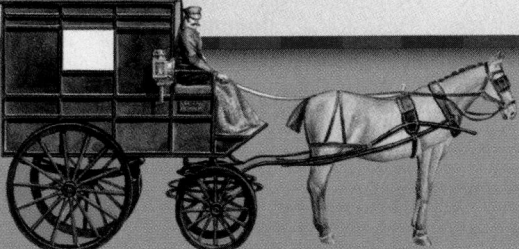

1865

Johann Gregor Mendel formulates the laws for genetics while crossbreeding pea plants

1869

The first ambulance service was established at Bellevue Hospital in New York by Dr. Edward Dalton

Measure Your Progress: Learning Objectives

After you study this chapter, you should be able to

1. Identify the anatomical structures of the blood and lymphatic system by correctly labeling them on anatomical illustrations.
2. Describe how the blood forms a clot.
3. Describe how the body's immune response functions.
4. Build blood and lymphatic words from combining forms, prefixes, and suffixes.
5. Describe common blood and lymphatic diseases.
6. Describe common blood and lymphatic diagnostic laboratory and radiology tests.
7. Describe common blood and lymphatic medical and surgical procedures and drug categories.
8. Define common blood and lymphatic abbreviations.
9. Correctly spell and pronounce blood and lymphatic words.
10. Apply your skills by analyzing a hematology and immunology report.
11. Test your knowledge of hematology and immunology by completing review exercises at the end of the chapter and learning activities on the CD-ROM.

Medical Language Key

To unlock the meaning of a medical word, first define each word part. Then put the word part definitions in order, beginning with the suffix, followed by the first word part.

	Word Part	Word Part Definition
SUFFIX	-logy	*the study of*
COMBINING FORM	hemat/o-	*blood*

Hematology: ***The study of the blood.***

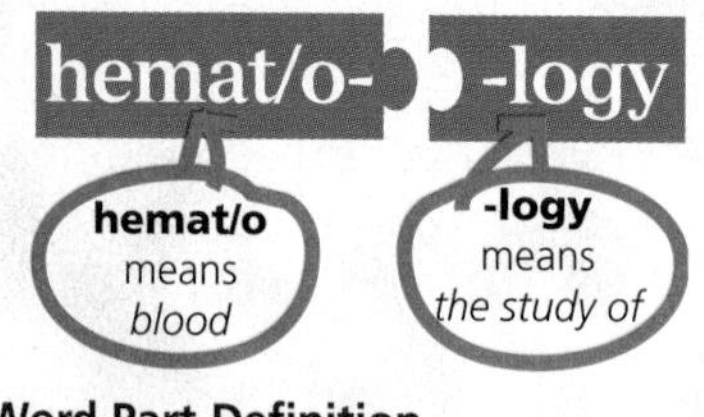

	Word Part	Word Part Definition
SUFFIX	-logy	*the study of*
COMBINING FORM	immun/o-	*immune response*

Immunology: ***The study of the immune response.***

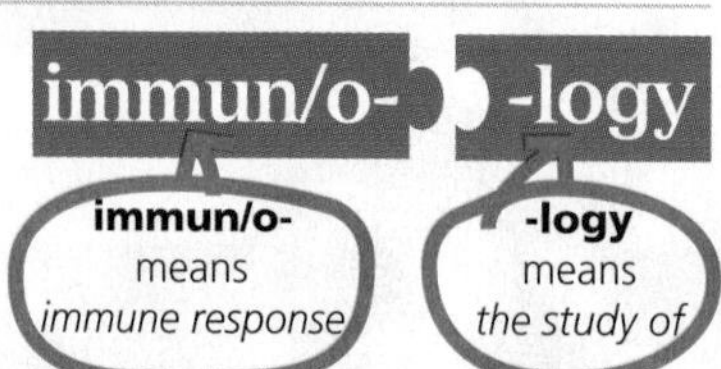

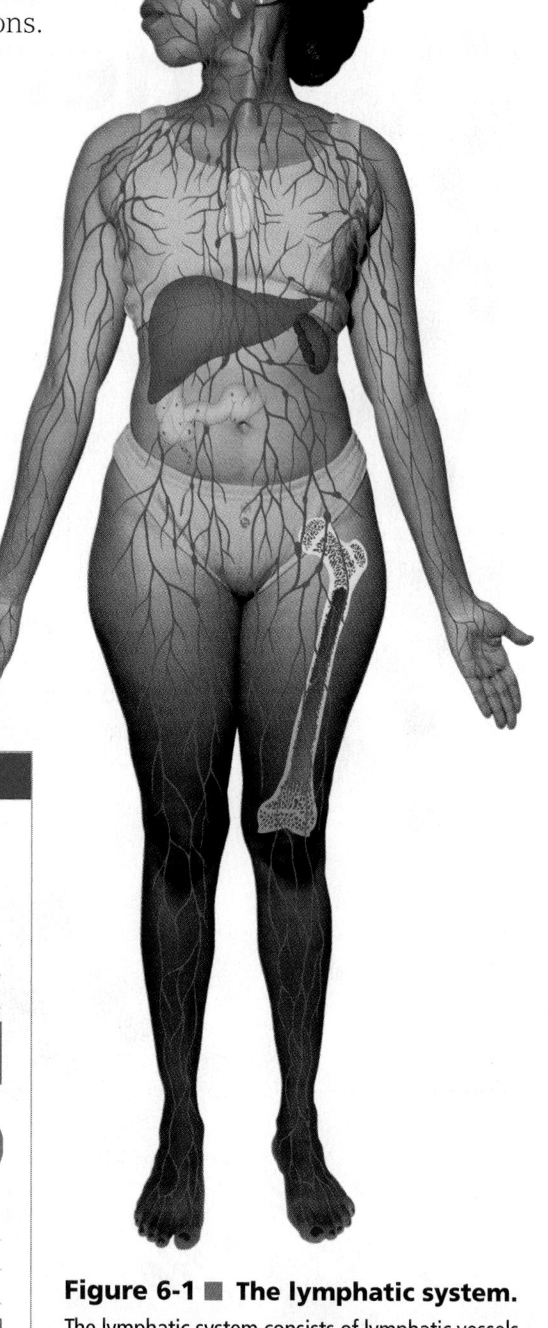

Figure 6-1 ■ The lymphatic system.

The lymphatic system consists of lymphatic vessels, lymph nodes, lymph fluid, lymphoid tissues, and lymphoid organs. The lymphatic system shares common elements with the blood: lymphocytes and macrophages (white blood cells).

www.prenhall.com/turley

For interactive flashcards, real-life video clips, games, exercises, and audio pronunciations please explore the companion CD-ROM in the back of the book. Click on the companion website for bonus chapters, additional resources, and links to on-line learning.

Anatomy and Physiology

Blood is classified as a type of connective tissue because it comes in contact with all the organs and tissues of the body. Blood contains fluid, cells, and a variety of other substances (proteins, clotting factors, and so forth). The purpose of the blood is to transport oxygen, carbon dioxide, nutrients, and the waste products of metabolism. The blood also carries within itself the means to stop its own flow at the site of an injury.

The lymphatic system (see Figure 6-1■) consists of the lymphatic vessels, lymph nodes, lymph fluid, lymphoid tissues, and lymphoid organs. The lymphatic system forms a pathway of lymphatic vessels and nodes throughout the body that is separate from that of the cardiovascular system that contains the blood. The purpose of the lymphatic system is to defend the body against microorganisms and cancerous cells via the immune response.

Anatomy of the Blood

Plasma

The fluid portion of blood, **plasma,** is a clear, straw-colored liquid that makes up about 55% of the total volume of blood (see Figure 6-2■). The plasma itself is about 90% water. The amount of plasma in the blood is dependent upon how much water is taken into the body and how much is excreted from the body. Decreased intake of water or an increased loss of water (for example, from diarrhea, increased urination, or excessive sweating) will decrease the percentage of plasma in the blood. Blood cells are suspended in the plasma. When clotting factors in the plasma are activated to form a blood clot, the fluid portion of plasma that remains is known as **serum.**

plasma (PLAZ-mah)

serum (SEER-um)
Serum is a Latin word meaning *whey.* When milk curdles, it separates into the curds and whey (the liquid).

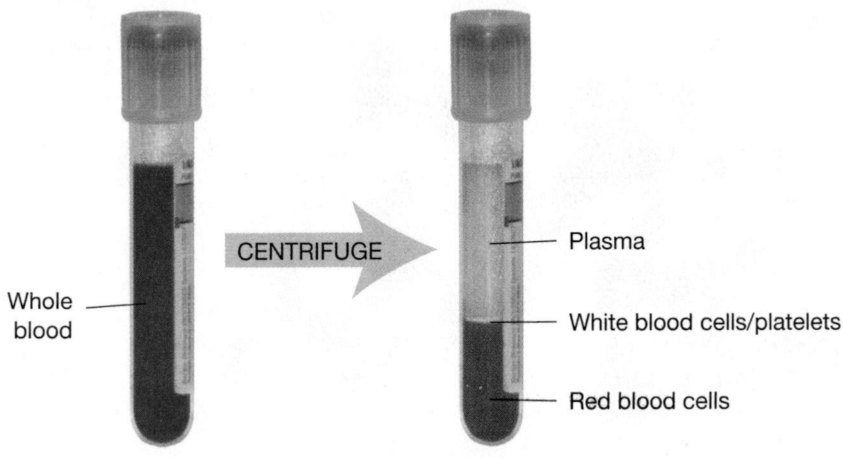

Figure 6-2 ■ Plasma.
Blood is composed of plasma and several different kinds of blood cells. When a specimen of whole blood is placed in a centrifuge and spun quickly, the heavier parts (blood cells) are pulled to the bottom, and the clear, straw-colored plasma remains on the top.

Erythrocytes

Erythrocytes are the most numerous type of blood cell. An **erythrocyte** or **red blood cell (RBC)** is a round, somewhat flattened, red disk. Its depressed center, where the cell is not as thick, is paler in color (see Figure 6-3■). Erythrocytes are unique among the other blood cells because they have no cell nucleus when they are mature.

erythrocyte (eh-RITH-roh-site)
erythr/o- *red*
-cyte *cell*

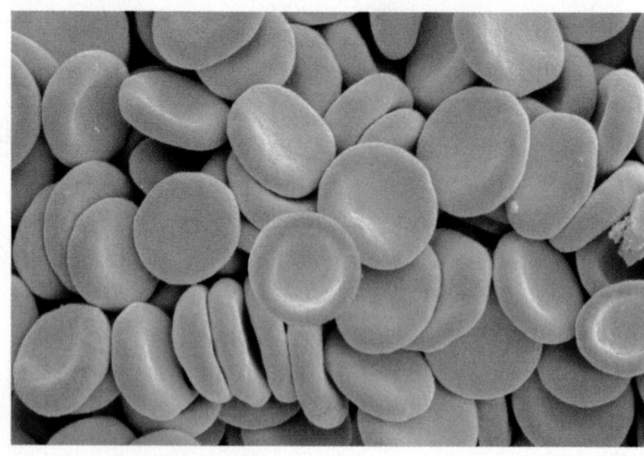

Figure 6-3 ■ Erythrocytes.
Notice the characteristic deep red color of erythrocytes (red blood cells) and their unique "donut" shape. Each erythrocyte has a depressed center and no cell nucleus.

All erythrocytes contain **hemoglobin,** a red, iron-containing molecule. It is the hemoglobin molecules in the erythrocyte that carry oxygen from the lungs to every cell in the body. Hemoglobin carries oxygen molecules as **oxyhemoglobin.** Hemoglobin also carries carbon dioxide from every cell back to the lungs. Hemoglobin carries carbon dioxide as carbaminohemoglobin.

hemoglobin (HEE-moh-GLOH-bin)
(HEE-moh-GLOH-bin)
hem/o- *blood*
glob/o- *shaped like a globe; comprehensive*
-in *a substance*

oxyhemoglobin
(AWK-see-HEE-moh-GLOH-bin)
ox/y- *oxygen*
hem/o- *blood*
glob/o- *shaped like a globe; comprehensive*
-in *a substance*

A Closer Look

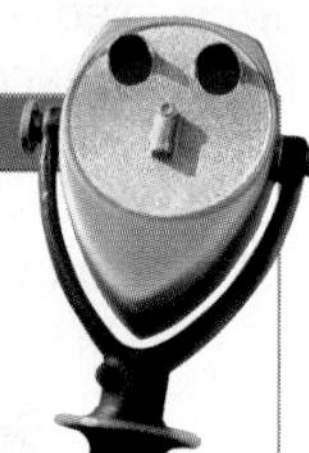

Hemoglobin is composed of **globins:** four chains of proteins (two alpha and two beta) that twist to form a globe-shaped molecule. Each chain contains a **heme** molecule. Each heme molecule contains an atom of iron that gives hemogloblin its red color.

globin (GLOH-bin)
glob/o- *shaped like a globe; comprehensive*
-in *a substance*

heme (HEEM)
Heme is derived from a Greek word meaning *blood.*

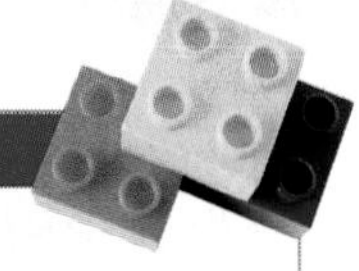

Connections

Forensic Science. When a person drowns or suffocates, there is a high level of carbon dioxide (CO_2) in the blood. This causes the skin to have a deep bluish-purple color known as cyanosis. When a person dies in a fire or from inhaling the fumes from car exhaust or a faulty space heater, there is a high level of carbon monoxide (CO) in the blood. Unlike oxygen and carbon dioxide, **carbon monoxide** binds so tightly and irreversibly that the hemoglobin is unable to carry any other molecule. Carbon monoxide poisoning causes a characteristic cherry red skin color.

carbon monoxide
(KAR-bon mawn-AWK-side)
Carbon monoxide is a descriptin of the chemical content of the molecule; it contains one carbon atom and one oxygen atom. *Mon/o-* is a combining form meaning *one, single.*

Hematopoiesis, the process by which all blood cells are formed, occurs in the red marrow of long or flat bones (such as the sternum, ribs, hip bones, bones of the spinal column, and the long bones of the legs). Every blood cell begins as a very immature cell known as a stem cell. For an erythrocyte the stem cell matures and its nucleus decreases in size, as it becomes an **erythroblast** and then a **normoblast.** When it is released into the blood, it has no nucleus but is still in a slightly immature form known as a **reticulocyte.** Within a day, the reticulocyte becomes a mature erythrocyte. The body produces several million erythrocytes every second. Any time the body experiences a significant blood loss, the kidneys secrete **erythropoietin,** a hormone that dramatically increases the speed at which erythrocytes are produced and become mature.

Because it does not have a nucleus, an erythrocyte is unable to divide or repair itself. It lasts only 120 days before it begins to deteriorate. Specialized cells (macrophages) in the spleen engulf old erythrocytes, breaking down their hemoglobin molecules into globins and heme. The globins are further broken down into amino acids that are used by the body to build other cells. Iron stripped from the heme molecule is stored in the liver and spleen and is used to build more erythrocytes when the diet does not contain enough iron. The remainder of the heme molecule is converted to bilirubin. Bilirubin plays an important role as an antioxidant, protecting body cells from damage by free radicals.

hematopoiesis (HEE-mah-toh-poy-EE-sis)
hemat/o- *blood*
-poiesis *condition of formation*

erythroblast (eh-RITH-roh-blast)
erythr/o- *red*
-blast *immature cell*

normoblast (NOR-moh-blast)
norm/o- *normal, usual*
-blast *immature cell*

reticulocyte (reh-TIK-yoo-loh-site)
reticul/o- *small network*
-cyte *cell*
A reticulocyte has a network of ribosomes in its cytoplasm.

erythropoietin (eh-RITH-roh-POY-eh-tin)
erythr/o- *red*
-poietin *a substance that forms*
Add words to make a correct definition of *erythropoietin: a substance that forms red [blood cells].*

Connections

Gastroenterology (Chapter 3). Bilirubin is also used by the liver to make bile. Bilirubin is a yellow pigment that gives bile its characteristic yellow-green appearance. The combining form *rub/o-* (red) indicates that bilirubin comes from the breakdown of red blood cells, not that it is a red pigment.

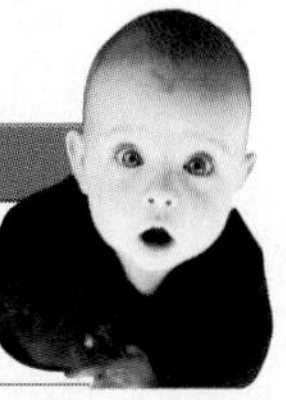

Did You Know?

Erythrocytes and leukocytes are also known as red corpuscles and white corpuscles. *Corpuscle* is a Latin word meaning *a little body.*

Leukocytes

Leukocytes or **white blood cells (WBCs)** are unique in that they include five different cells, each of which performs a different function in the body's immune response. The five leukocytes include neutrophils, eosinophils, basophils, lymphocytes, and monocytes (see Table 6-1).

Each type of leukocyte can be identified by the presence or absence of granules in its cytoplasm and by the shape of its nucleus. These differences can be seen when blood cells are stained and examined under a microscope. A leukocyte with large granules in its cytoplasm and a segmented nucleus is categorized as a granulocyte. **Granulocytes** include neutrophils, eosinophils, and basophils. A leukocyte with nearly invisible granules in its cytoplasm and a round or kidney bean–shaped nucleus is categorized as an agranulocyte. **Agranulocytes** includes lymphocytes and monocytes.

leukocyte (LOO-koh-site)
leuk/o- *white*
-cyte *cell*

granulocyte (GRAN-yoo-loh-SITE)
granul/o- *granule*
-cyte *cell*

agranulocyte (aa-GRAN-yoo-loh-SITE)
a- *away from, without*
granul/o- *granule*
-cyte *cell*

Neutrophils

Neutrophils are the most common leukocyte, comprising 40 to 60% of the leukocytes in the blood. Neutrophils are categorized as granulocytes. The large granules in their cytoplasm are "neutral" in that they do not readily stain with either a red, acidic dye (eosin) or with a blue, alkaline dye (hematoxylin) (see Figure 6-4 ■). Neutrophils derive their name from their neutral reaction to these dyes. Because the nucleus is in segments or lobes, the cell is known as a segmented neutrophil, segmenter, seg, or a **polymorphonucleated leukocyte (PMN)** or poly.

neutrophil (NOO-troh-fil)
neutr/o- *not taking part*
-phil *attraction to, fondness for*

polymorphonucleated (PAWL-ee-MOR-foh-NOO-klee-aa-ted)
poly- *many, much*
morph/o- *shape*
nucle/o- *nucleus*
-ated *pertaining to a condition; composed of*

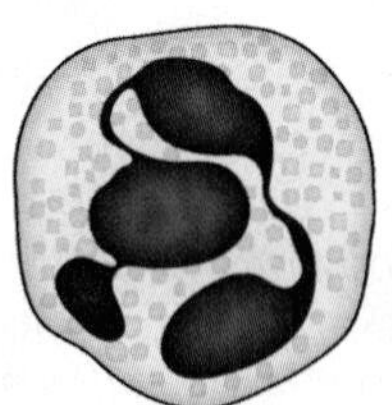

Figure 6-4 ■ Neutrophil.
A neutrophil has cytoplasm that contains granules that do not readily stain with either a red or blue dye. It has a nucleus with three or more lobes.

Neutrophils develop in the red marrow from stem cells that become **myeloblasts,** then **myelocytes,** and then bands. A band is an immature neutrophil that has a nucleus shaped like a curved band. Bands are also known as stabs (the German word for *band*). There are always a few bands present in the blood, but, during severe bacterial infections, the number of bands rises as the need for more neutrophils increases.

Mature neutrophils are part of the immune response because they function as phagocytes. **Phagocytes** are cells that engulf microorganisms and destroy them with enzymes. This process is known as **phagocytosis.** Neutrophils specifically act as phagocytes for bacteria. Neutrophils only live a few days or even just a few hours if they are actively destroying bacteria. One neutrophil can destroy about 10 bacteria before it dies.

myeloblast (MY-eh-loh-blast)
myel/o- *bone marrow; spinal cord; myelin*
-blast *immature cell*
Some word parts have more than one definition. The best definition of *myeloblast* is *an immature cell [that develops in the] bone marrow.*

myelocyte (MY-eh-loh-site)
myel/o- *bone marrow; spinal cord; myelin*
-cyte *cell*

phagocyte (FAG-oh-site)
phag/o- *eating, swallowing*
-cyte *cell*

phagocytosis (FAG-oh-sy-TOH-sis)
phag/o- *eating, swallowing*
cyt/o- *cell*
-osis *condition; abnormal condition; process*

Eosinophils **Eosinophils** are one of the least common leukocytes, comprising just 1 to 4% of the leukocytes in the blood. Eosinophils are categorized as granulocytes. The granules in their cytoplasm are large and stain bright pink to red with the red, acidic dye eosin (see Figure 6-5 ■). Eosinophils derive their name from their reaction to this dye. The nucleus of an eosinophil has two lobes. Eosinophils are also known as eos.

eosinophil (EE-oh-SIN-oh-fil)
eosin/o- *eosin (acidic red dye)*
-phil *attraction to, fondness for*

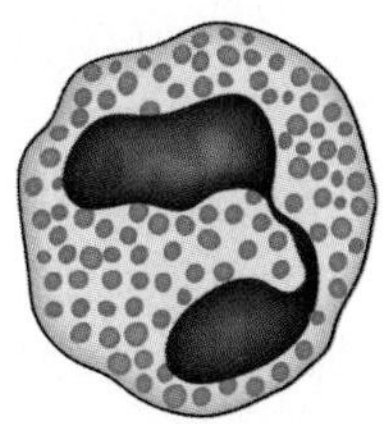

Figure 6-5 ■ Eosinophil.
An eosinophil has cytoplasm that contains granules that stain bright pink to red. It has a nucleus with two lobes.

Eosinophils develop in the red marrow from stem cells that become myeloblasts, then myelocytes, and then mature eosinophils. As part of the immune response, eosinophils are phagocytes that engulf and destroy foreign cells (pollen, animal dander, and so forth). Eosinophils also release chemicals that kill parasites that invade the body.

Basophils **Basophils** are the least common leukocyte, comprising just 0.5 to 1% of the leukocytes in the blood. Basophils are categorized as granulocytes. The granules in their cytoplasm are very large and stain dark blue to purple with the blue, alkaline dye hematoxylin (see Figure 6-6 ■). This alkaline dye has a high pH, which makes it a base (as opposed to an acid). Basophils derive their name from their reaction to this dye. The nucleus of a basophil has more than one lobe. Basophils are also known as basos.

basophil (BAY-soh-fil)
bas/o- *basic (alkaline)*
-phil *attraction to, fondness for*

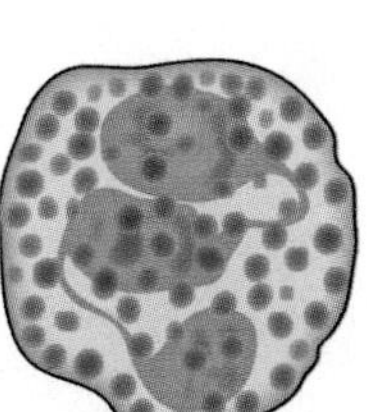

Figure 6-6 ■ Basophil.
A basophil has cytoplasm that contains granules that stain dark blue to purple. It has a nucleus with more than one lobe.

Basophils develop in the red marrow from stem cells that become myeloblasts, then myelocytes, and then mature basophils. As part of the immune response, basophils release histamine at the site of tissue damage. As part of the blood clotting process, basophils release heparin, an anticoagulant that limits the size of blood clots that form at the site of tissue damage.

Lymphocytes **Lymphocytes** are the second most common leukocyte, comprising 20 to 40% of the leukocytes in the blood. Lymphocytes are categorized as agranulocytes because the granules in their cytoplasm are nearly invisible. The cytoplasm is often no more than a thin edge around the nucleus (see Figure 6-7 ■). Lymphocytes are the smallest leukocytes. Some lymphocytes live for just a few days, while others live for many years. Lymphocytes are also known as lymphs.

lymphocyte (LIM-foh-site)
lymph/o- *lymph; lymphatic system*
-cyte *cell*

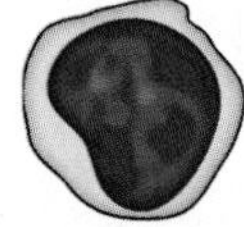

Figure 6-7 ■ Lymphocyte.
A lymphocyte has little cytoplasm with nearly invisible granules and a round nucleus.

Lymphocytes begin their development in the red marrow from stem cells that then become **lymphoblasts.** Lymphoblasts that remain in the red marrow become B lymphocytes (B cells) or NK (natural killer) cells. Other lymphoblasts migrate to the thymus, where the presence of thymosins (hormones) causes them to become T lymphocytes (T cells). Mature lymphocytes of all types are present in the blood, lymph nodes, and lymphoid tissues. The function of these cells is discussed in the section on the immune response.

lymphoblast (LIM-foh-blast)
lymph/o- *lymph; lymphatic system*
-blast *immature cell*

Monocytes **Monocytes** are one of the least common leukocytes, comprising just 2 to 4% of the leukocytes in the blood. Monocytes are categorized as agranulocytes because the granules in their cytoplasm are nearly invisible. A monocyte has a large amount of cytoplasm, and its nucleus is shaped like a kidney bean (see Figure 6-8 ■). Monocytes are the largest leukocytes. Monocytes are also known as monos.

monocyte (MAWN-oh-site)
mon/o- *one, single*
-cyte *cell*
Add words to make a correct and complete definition of *monocyte: Cell [that has a] single [lobe in its nucleus].*

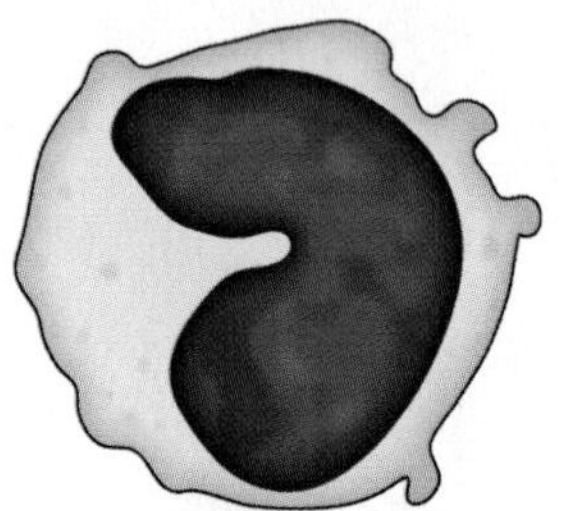

Figure 6-8 ■ Monocyte.
A monocyte has cytoplasm with nearly invisible granules and a kidney bean-shaped nucleus.

Monocytes develop in the red marrow from stem cells that become **monoblasts** and then mature monocytes. As part of the immune response, monocytes are phagocytes that engulf and destroy microorganisms, cancerous cells, dead leukocytes, and cellular debris. Because they are able to engulf large numbers of cells and cellular debris, monocytes are also known as **macrophages.** Monocytes are found in the blood and in the lymph nodes of the lymphatic system.

monoblast (MAWN-oh-blast)
mon/o- *one, single*
-blast *immature cell*

macrophage (MAK-roh-fayj)
macr/o- *large*
-phage *thing that eats*

Table 6-1 Leukocyte Types and Characteristics

Leukocyte Type	Nucleus	Cytoplasm	Category
neutrophil segmented neutrophil seg, segmenter polymorphonuclear leukocyte (PMN), poly	3 or more lobes	large granules that do not stain either red or blue	granulocyte
eosinophil eo	2 lobes	large granules that stain bright pink to red	granulocyte
basophil baso	more than 1 lobe	large granules that stain dark blue to purple	granulocyte
lymphocyte lymph	round	nearly invisible granules	agranulocyte
monocyte mono	kidney bean shaped	nearly invisible granules	agranulocyte

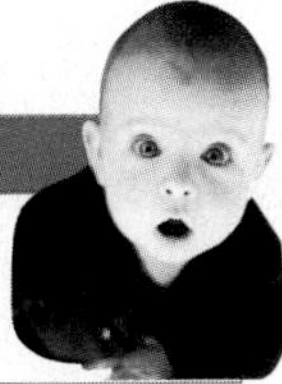

Did You Know?

Of the 5 to 6 quarts of blood in the body, leukocytes make up 1½ fluid ounces and thrombocytes make up only 1 teaspoonful.

Thrombocytes

A **thrombocyte** or **platelet** is different from other blood cells because it is only a cell fragment. Thrombocytes are active in the blood clotting process. Within seconds of an injury, they form clumps that help to block the flow of blood. Thrombocytes also contain some clotting factors that they release to begin the formation of a blood clot.

An individual thrombocyte begins in the red marrow as a stem cell that then becomes a **megakaryoblast.** Then it matures into a **megakaryocyte,** a very large cell with a great deal of cytoplasm and a large nucleus with several lobes. The cytoplasm of the megakaryocyte constantly breaks away at the edges to form the cell fragments (thrombocytes) that are released into the blood. When all of the cytoplasm is gone, the nucleus of the megakaryocyte is broken down and its amino acids are recycled to build other cells.

thrombocyte (THRAWM-boh-site)
thromb/o- *thrombus (blood clot)*
-cyte *cell*

platelet (PLAYT-let)
Platelet is a combination of the English word *plate* and the suffix *-let* (little).

megakaryoblast (MEG-ah-KAIR-ee-oh-blast)
meg/a- *large*
kary/o- *nucleus*
-blast *immature cell*

megakaryocyte (MEG-ah-KAIR-ee-oh-site)
meg/a- *large*
kary/o- *nucleus*
-cyte *cell*

Substances in the Blood

The blood contains many substances that are dissolved in the plasma besides blood cells. These include water, amino acids, cholesterol, triglycerides, electrolytes, glucose, minerals, and vitamins from digested foods absorbed into the blood from the intestines. Albumin, clotting factors, complement proteins, conjugated bilirubin, lipoproteins (carry fats through the blood) and other substances produced by the liver are present as well as unconjugated bilirubin produced by the spleen. Hormones from various endocrine glands are also present. Finally, creatinine and urea, the waste products of cellular metabolism, are present in the blood.

Did You Know?

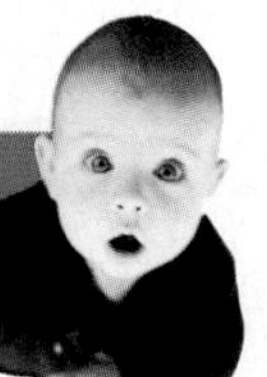

Blood tastes salty because the electrolytes sodium and chloride in the plasma are the same ingredients that make up table salt.

A Closer Look

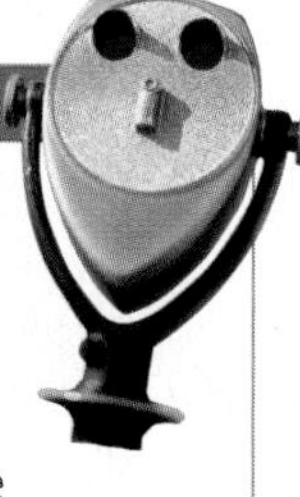

Plasma proteins like **albumin** are in the blood. Their molecules are too large to pass through the wall of the blood vessel. They exert an osmotic pressure that keeps water in the blood from moving out into the surrounding tissues.

Electrolytes are chemical elements that carry a positive or negative electrical charge. Electrolytes in the plasma include sodium (Na^+), potassium (K^+), chloride (Cl^-), calcium (Ca^{++}), and bicarbonate (HCO_3^-). Sodium plays an important role in maintaining the volume and pressure of the blood. Sodium, potassium, and calcium are important in the contraction of the heart and skeletal muscles. Calcium is also important in the formation of bone and for blood clotting. Bicarbonate acts as a buffer to maintain the correct blood pH.

albumin (al-BYOO-min)

electrolyte (ee-LEK-troh-lite)
electr/o- *electricity*
-lyte *dissolved substance*
An electrolyte is so named because it will conduct electricity when it is in a solution.

Word Alert

SOUND-ALIKE WORDS

albumen (noun) the white of an egg
Example: Albumen in egg whites is a good source of dietary protein.

albumin (noun) protein molecule in the blood
Example: Albumin is the most abundant of all the plasma proteins.

Blood Type

Each person's erythrocytes have a unique combination of inherited genetic material that determines the blood type. The most important blood types or blood groups are the ABO and Rh groups, although there are 22 other minor groups. Each blood group is represented by **antigens,** proteins on the surface of the cell membrane of the erythrocyte.

antigen (AN-tih-jen)
anti- *against*
-gen *that which produces*
In this word, the prefix *anti-* is actually a shortened form of the word *antibody.*

The **ABO blood group** contains A, B, AB, and O antigens (see Table 6-2). A person with type A blood has A antigens on their erythrocytes and so forth. A person with type O blood has neither A nor B antigens on their erythrocytes. In addition, each person's plasma contains antibodies against blood types other than its own.

Table 6-2 ABO Blood Group

Blood Type	Antigen on RBC	Antigen in Plasma
A	A antigen	anti-B antibodies
B	B antigen	anti-A antibodies
AB	A and B antigens	none
O	none	anti-A and anti-B antibodies

Did You Know?

The Austrian pathologist Dr. Karl Landsteiner discovered the first two antigens on an erythrocyte in 1900. He named them A and B and categorized blood into four blood types: A, B, AB, and O. He won a Nobel prize for this in 1930. Lansteiner and other scientists discovered the Rh blood group in the blood of a rhesus monkey in 1940.

The **Rh blood group** has 47 different antigens. As a group, they are known as the **Rh factor.** When these antigens are present on erythrocytes, the blood type is Rh positive. When these antigens are not present, the blood type is Rh negative.

The ABO and the Rh blood group systems are always considered together, so that type A blood is either A positive or A negative, and so forth.

Blood type O negative is known as the universal donor because it can be given to patients with any other blood type without causing a transfusion reaction (see Figure 6-9■).

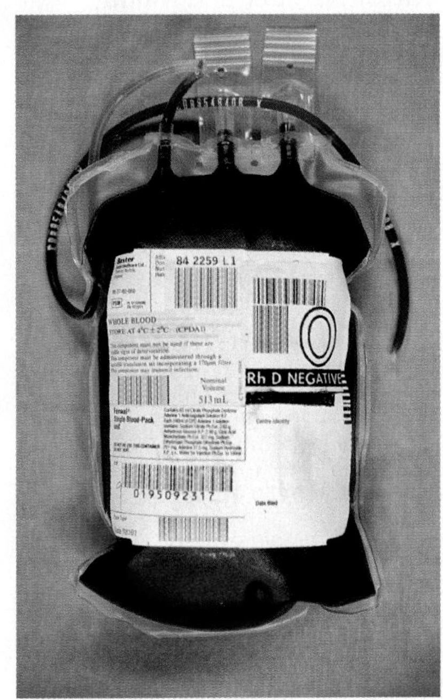

Figure 6-9 ■ A unit of blood.
This donated unit of blood is blood type O negative, the universal donor. A donated unit of blood contains 500 cc of blood (one half of a liter). This is nearly the same as 1 pint. There are approximately 10 to 12 pints of blood in the body.

Physiology of Blood Clotting

When the body is injured, the injured blood vessel constricts to decrease the amount of blood flow. Thrombocytes stick to the damaged area of the blood vessel wall and form clumps to block the blood flow. This process is known as **platelet aggregation.** Then clotting factors in the plasma are activated and begin to produce strands of **fibrin** that trap erythrocytes and form a **thrombus** or blood clot. This process is known as **coagulation,** and the cessation of bleeding is known as **hemostasis.** The final size of a blood clot is limited by the action of heparin, a natural anticoagulant released from basophils.

All of the clotting factors must be present and at normal levels for the blood to clot. There are 12 clotting factors, numbered as Roman numerals I through XIII (there is no factor VI) (see Table 6-3). Although the clotting factors are listed in numeral order, they are not activated in this order.

aggregation (AG-reh-GAY-shun)
aggreg/o- *crowding together*
-ation *a process; being or having*

fibrin (FY-brin)
fibr/o- *fiber*
-in *a substance*

thrombus (THRAWM-bus)
thrombi (THRAWM-by)
Thrombus is a Latin singular masculine noun meaning *a clot.* Form the plural by changing *-us* to *-i.*

coagulation (koh-AG-yoo-LAY-shun)
coagul/o- *clotting*
-ation *a process; being or having*

hemostasis (HEE-moh-STAY-sis)
hem/o- *blood*
-stasis *condition of standing still or staying in one place*

Connections

Dietetics. The liver needs vitamin K in order to produce clotting factors. Vitamin K is present in green leafy vegetables, grains, and liver. Vitamin K is also manufactured by bacteria in the small intestine.

Table 6-3 Blood Clotting Factor

Factor Number and Name		Source	Word Part and Definition
I	**fibrinogen**	liver	**fibrinogen** (fy-BRIN-oh-jen) **fibrin/o-** *fibrin* **-gen** *that which produces*
II	**prothrombin**	liver	**prothrombin** (pro-THRAWM-bin) **pro-** *before* **thromb/o-** *thrombus (blood clot)* **-in** *a substance* Prothrombin is the clotting factor activated just before the thrombus is formed.
III	tissue factor (thromboplastin)	injured tissue	
IV	calcium	platelets	
V	prothrombin accelerator	liver	
VII	prothrombin conversion accelerator	liver	
VIII	antihemophilic factor	platelets	
IX	plasma thromboplastin factor	liver	
X	Stuart-Power factor	liver	
XI	plasma **thromboplastin** antecedent	liver	**thromboplastin** (THRAWM-boh-PLAS-tin) **thromb/o-** *thrombus (blood clot)* **plast/o-** *being formed or shaped* **-in** *a substance*
XII	Hageman factor	liver	
XIII	fibrin-stabilizing factor	liver and platelets	

Although the blood and lymphatic system move through the body in physically separate paths, they are interdependent in several important ways.

1. The blood and lymphatic system share lymphocytes and macrophages. These cells are present in the blood and in lymph nodes and other lymphatic tissues, where they function as part of the immune response.
2. The thymus. Some immature leukocytes are released into the blood and travel to the thymus. There they develop into a specific type of leukocyte (lymphocyte) that fights viruses. This leukocyte is present in the blood and in the lymphatic system.
3. The spleen. The spleen serves as a storage area for reserve supplies of blood. The spleen also breaks down and recycles old erythrocytes (red blood cells). Another part of the spleen is composed of lymphatic tissue that contains lymphocytes.

Anatomy of the Lymphatic System

Lymphatic Vessels, Lymph Nodes, and Lymph

Lymphatic vessels are similar in structure to blood vessels, but with several important differences. Lymphatic vessels begin as tiny lymphatic capillaries in the tissues. Tissue fluid enters a lymphatic capillary and becomes **lymph,** the fluid that circulates through the lymphatic system. Lymphatic capillaries have large openings in their walls that allow microorganisms and cancerous cells to enter. Lymphatic capillaries become larger lymphatic vessels that bring lymph to the lymph nodes. One-way valves keep lymph flowing toward the larger lymphatic vessels. **Lymph nodes** are small, encapsulated structures that are round, oval, or bean shaped. They range in size from the head of a pin to about 1 inch. The lymph node filters the lymph, and lymphocytes and macrophages in the lymph node destroy any microorganisms or cancerous cells that are present.

Lymph nodes are closely grouped together in chains in areas where there is a high risk of invasion by microorganisms or cancerous cells (see Figure 6-10■). All lymphatic vessels end at ducts in the thoracic cavity. The right lymphatic duct receives lymph from the right side of the head, right arm, right chest, and back. The thoracic duct receives lymph from the rest of the body. Both lymphatic ducts then empty into large veins in the neck.

lymphatic (lim-FAT-ik)
lymph/o- *lymph; lymphatic system*
-atic *pertaining to*

lymph (LIMF)
Lymph is derived from a Latin word meaning *clear spring water.*

node (NOHD)
Node is derived from a Latin word meaning *a knob or mass of tissue.*

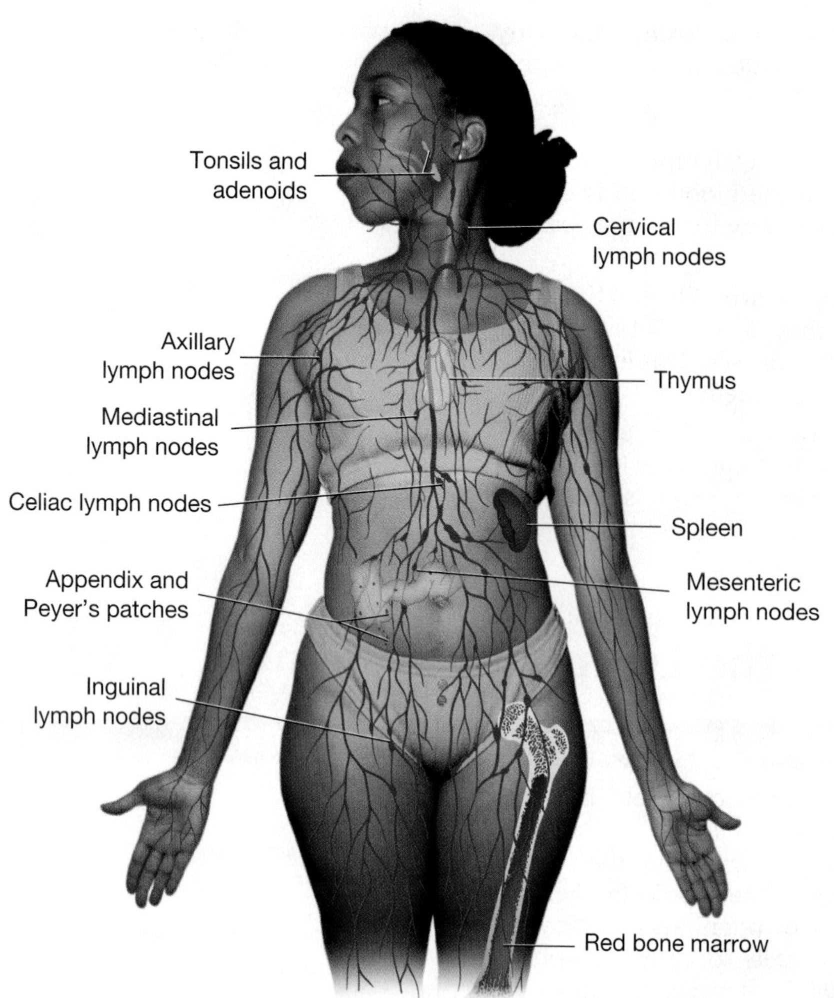

Figure 6-10 ■ The lymphatic system. Lymphatic capillaries in all parts of the body carry lymph to the lymph nodes. The lymph nodes are arranged in chains in areas of the body where invading microorganisms or cancerous cells are likely to be found. The lymphatic system also consists of the tonsils and adenoids in the posterior oral cavity, the thymus, the spleen, and Peyer's patches and the appendix in the intestines. The immune response of the lymphatic system also utilizes lymphocytes and monocytes formed in the red bone marrow.

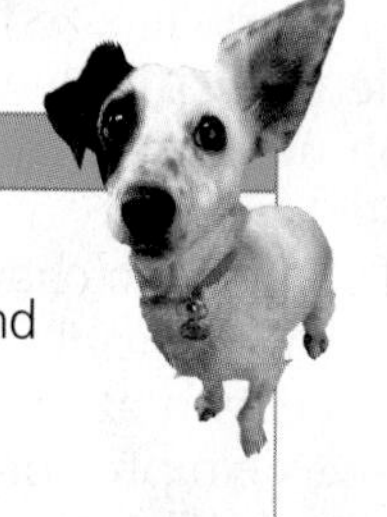

Word Alert

SOUND-ALIKE WORDS

lymph	(noun)	Fluid that flows through lymphatic vessels and lymph nodes
lymphs	(noun)	Another name for *lymphocytes*

Lymphoid Tissues and Organs

Lymphoid tissues include the tonsils and adenoids in the posterior oral cavity, discussed in Otolaryngology (Chapter 16), and the appendix and Peyer's patches in the small intestine, discussed in Gastroenterology (Chapter 3) (see Figure 6-10). Lymphoid tissues contain lymphocytes that are active in the immune response.

The **thymus,** a lymphoid organ with a pink color and a grainy consistency, is located in the mediastinum, posterior to the sternum. During childhood and adolescence, the thymus gland is large, but becomes much smaller during adulthood. The thymus functions as part of the lymphatic system and the endocrine system. As part of the lymphatic system, the thymus receives lymphoblasts that migrate from the red marrow. As part of the endocrine system, the thymus secretes

lymphoid (LIM-foyd)
lymph/o- *lymph; lymphatic system*
-oid *resembling*

thymus (THY-mus)

thymic (THY-mik)
thym/o- *thymus; rage*
-ic *pertaining to*
Some word parts have more than one definition. The best definition of *thymic* is *pertaining to the thymus.*

several hormones, collectively known as **thymosins,** which cause lymphoblasts to become mature T cell lymphocytes.

The **spleen,** a rounded lymphoid organ, is located on the left side of the abdominal cavity, behind the stomach. The spleen is the largest organ of the lymphatic system. It is surrounded by the firm **splenic capsule,** but has a soft, pulpy interior. The spleen functions as part of the lymphatic system and the blood and cardiovascular system. The white pulp of the spleen contains lymphoid tissue with mature B and T lymphocytes. As part of the blood and cardiovascular system, the spleen filters the blood, removing old erythrocytes and breaking down the hemoglobin into globins and heme. Iron from the heme molecule is stored in the spleen. The spleen also acts as a storage area for whole blood. During times of danger or injury, the release of epinephrine by the sympathetic nervous system causes the spleen to contract and release the stored blood into the circulatory system. Because of its location and soft consistency, the spleen can rupture from sports trauma or accidents.

thymosin (thy-MOH-sin)
Thymosin is a combination of the Greek word *thymos* (thymus) and the suffix *-in* (a substance).

spleen (SPLEEN)

splenic (SPLEH-nik)
splen/o- *spleen*
-ic *pertaining to*

Physiology of the Immune Response

The **immune response** involves a coordinated effort between the blood and the lymphatic system to destroy invading microorganisms and cancerous cells that arise internally.

immune (ih-MYOON)
Immune is derived from a Latin word meaning *protected from.*

Connections

Dermatology (Chapter 7). The skin is the body's first line of defense. Intact skin acts as a protective barrier that repels microorganisms. Openings in the skin (like the nose, ears, throat, urethra, rectum, and vagina are high-risk areas where microorganisms can enter the body.

The immune response begins with the detection of an invading microorganism. Microorganisms such as bacteria, viruses, and protozoa, as well as plant cells like fungi or yeast that cause disease are known as **pathogens.** The immune response also detects and destroys cancerous cells that arise within the body.

Once a pathogen is detected in the blood or lymphatic system, the body attacks it in several different ways.

pathogen (PATH-oh-jen)
path/o- *disease, suffering*
-gen *that which produces*

1. **Cytokines** are chemicals released by injured body tissues. They summon leukocytes to the area.
2. **Neutrophils.** Neutrophils engulf and destroy bacteria coated with complement proteins or antibodies.
3. **Eosinophils.** Eosinophils release chemicals that destroy parasitic worms and their eggs. They engulf and destroy foreign cells (pollen, animal dander, and so forth).
4. **Basophils.** Basophils release histamine in response to the presence of microorganisms. **Histamine** dilates blood vessels and increases blood flow, which brings more leukocytes to the area. Histamine also changes the permeability of the blood vessel walls, allowing large protein molecules and water to leak out into the tissues. This causes edema and swelling. Redness and edema are both signs of

cytokine (SY-toh-kyne)
cyt/o- *cell*
-kine *movement*

histamine (HIS-tah-meen)

inflammation or infection associated with the presence of microorganisms.

5. **Monocytes.** Monocytes engulf and destroy all types of pathogens that have been coated with complement proteins or antibodies. They also eat dead leukocytes and cellular debris. Because they eat so much, they are also known as macrophages. A macrophage takes fragments of the pathogen it has eaten and presents them to a B cell (lymphocyte). This stimulates the B cell to become a plasma cell and make antibodies against that specific pathogen. Macrophages also produce special immune response chemicals: interferon, interleukin, and tumor necrosis factor.
   a. **Interferon** is released by macrophages that have engulfed a virus. Interferon stimulates cells to produce an antiviral substance that keeps a virus from entering a cell and reproducing. This keeps viral infections from spreading through the body. Interferon also stimulates NK cells to attack viruses.
   b. **Interleukin** stimulates B cell and T cell lymphocytes and activates NK cells. It also produces the fever associated with inflammation and infection. An increased body temperature stimulates leukocyte activity. Interferon is also produced by the lymphocytes themselves.
   c. **Tumor necrosis factor (TNF)** destroys **endotoxins** produced by certain bacteria. It also destroys cancer cells.
6. **Lymphocytes**
   a. **NK (natural killer) cells** are special lymphocytes that recognize a pathogen by the **antigens** on its cell wall and release chemicals to destroy it. NK cells can recognize a pathogen before it is coated with antibodies or complement proteins.
   b. **B cells** (lymphocytes that mature in the red marrow) are inactive until a macrophage presents them with fragments from a pathogen. Then the B cell changes into a plasma cell and produces antibodies (immunoglobulins) against that pathogen. B cells also activate helper T cells.
   c. **T cells** (lymphocytes that mature in the thymus) have four different subsets.
      - **Helper T cells** stimulate the production of cytotoxic T cells. Helper T cells also produce memory T cells. Helper T cells are known as **CD4 cells** because of a special protein marker on their cell membranes.
      - **Memory T cells** are created when a helper T cell is exposed to a pathogen. Memory T cells are inactive until the next time that pathogen enters the body. Then memory cells remember the pathogen and become cytotoxic T cells.
      - **Cytotoxic T cells** engulf and destroy all types of pathogens as well as body cells infected with viruses.
      - **Suppressor T cells** limit the extent and duration of the immune response by inhibiting B cells and cytotoxic T cells. Suppressor T cells are also known as CD8 cells because of a special protein marker on their cell membranes.
7. **Antibodies.** If NK cells do not immediately destroy a pathogen, it must be marked so that it can be recognized and destroyed by other leukocytes. This marking process involves coating the pathogen with antibodies, also known as **immunoglobulins.**

interferon (IN-ter-FEER-on)
Interferon is a combination of the English word *interfere* and the suffix *-on* (substance; structure).

interleukin (IN-ter-LOO-kin)
inter- *between*
leuk/o- *white*
-in *a substance*

endotoxin (EN-doh-TAWK-sin)
endo- *innermost, within*
tox/o- *poison*
-in *substance; structure*

antigen (AN-tih-jen)
Antigen is a combination of the word *antibody* (with *body* deleted) and the suffix *-gen* (that which produces).

cytotoxic (SY-toh-TAWK-sik)
cyt/o- *cell*
tox/o- *poison*
-ic *pertaining to*

suppressor (soo-PRES-or)
suppress/o- *press down*
-or *person or thing that produces or does*

antibody (AN-tih-bawd-ee)
anti- *against*
-body *a structure or thing*

immunoglobulin (IM-yoo-noh-GLAWB-yoo-lin)
immun/o- *immune response*
globul/o- *shaped like a globe*
-in *a substance*

8. **Complement proteins.** Complement is a group of 9 proteins (C1 through C9) that activate each other. When antibodies attach to a pathogen or a virus-infected cell, complement attaches to the antibodies and drill holes in the pathogen's cell wall.

complement (KAWM-pleh-ment)
Complement is so named because its proteins complement the work of antibodies. The English word *complement* means *to provide something that was lacking in order to complete the whole.*

A Closer Look

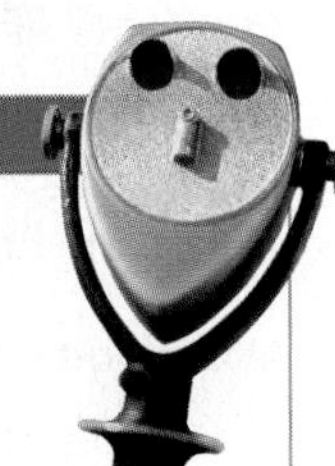

There are five classes of antibodies or immunoglobulins: IgA, IgD, IgE, IgG, and IgM.

Class	Function
IgA	Present in body secretions (tears; saliva; mucus in the nose, lungs, and intestines). IgA is present in colostrum, the first milk produced by the breastfeeding mother. This maternal IgA provides **passive immunity** until 18 months of age when the infant begins to make its own antibodies.
IgD	Present in B cells. It activates a B cell to become a plasma cell.
IgE	Present in basophils. It causes them to release heparin and histamine during inflammatory and allergic reactions.
IgG	Produced by plasma cells. This forms the basis of **active immunity,** the body's response and defense against pathogens it has seen before. IgG is also the most abundant of all the immunoglobulins. IgG is the smallest immunoglobulin. It is able to pass from the mother's blood through the placenta and provide **passive immunity** to the fetus for all the diseases the mother ever had.
IgM	Produced by plasma cells the first time they encounter a pathogen. IgM also reacts to incompatible blood types during a blood transfusion. IgM is the largest immunoglobulin.

immunity (ih-MYOO-nih-tee)
immun/o- *immune response*
-ity *state; condition*

Across the Life Span

Childhood immunizations against polio, diphtheria, pertussis, and tetanus and adult immunizations against the flu or pneumococcal pneumonia use a vaccine made of dead or weakened pathogens or inactivated endotoxins. The vaccination causes the body to produce antibodies and gives active immunity without exposure to the actual disease.

Word Alert

SOUND-ALIKE WORDS

globin (noun) Breakdown product of the hemoglobin molecule
Example: The spleen breaks down old erythrocytes to form heme and globin molecules.

globulin (noun) Protein molecule that makes up immunoglobulins
Example: Globulin is used by a plasma cell to build antibodies.

Vocabulary Review

Anatomy and Physiology

Now that you have studied the anatomy and physiology of the blood and lymphatic system, take time to review those new words and descriptions. Memorize the combining forms and their definitions before going on to the next section.

Word or Phrase	Combining Form and Definition	Description
ABO blood group		Category that includes blood types A, B, AB, and O. Blood types are hereditary. Each blood type has antigens on its erythrocytes and antibodies in the plasma against other blood types.
active immunity	**immun/o-** *immune response*	The body's continuing immune response and defense against pathogens it has seen before
aggregation	**aggreg/o-** *crowding together*	Process of platelets sticking to a damaged area in the blood vessel wall and forming clumps
agranulocyte	**granul/o-** *granule*	Category of leukocytes with nearly invisible granules in the cytoplasm. Includes lymphocytes and monocytes.
albumin		Most abundant plasma protein
antibody		Produced by a B cell that becomes a plasma cell. Also known as an immunoglobulin.
antigen		A protein marker on the cell membrane of an erythrocyte that indicates the blood type. Also, a protein marker on the cell wall of pathogens (bacteria, viruses, and so forth) and cancerous cells that the body recognizes as foreign.
B cell		Type of lymphocyte that matures in the red marrow. B cells are activated by macrophages and become plasma cells that make antibodies. B cells also activate helper T cells.
band		Immature neutrophil in the blood. It has a nucleus shaped like a curved band. Also known as a stab.
basophil	**bas/o-** *basic (alkaline)*	Least numerous of the leukocytes. It is classified as a granulocyte because granules in its cytoplasm stain dark blue to purple with basic dye. It releases histamine and heparin at the site of tissue damage. Basophils are also known as basos.
blood	**hem/o-** *blood* **hemat/o-** *blood*	Type of connective tissue that contains plasma and blood cells. The blood transports oxygen, carbon dioxide, nutrients, and waste products of metabolism.
clotting factors		A series of 12 protein factors that are released either from platelets or injured tissue or are produced by the liver. They activate each other in a series of steps that eventually forms fibrin strands that trap erythrocytes and form a blood clot.
coagulation	**coagul/o-** *clotting*	The formation of a blood clot by platelets and the clotting factors
complement proteins		Group of 9 proteins in the plasma that are activated by the presence of bacteria, viruses, or parasites. They coat the pathogen and kill it by making holes in it. Complement proteins also cause basophils to release histamine in areas where the tissue has been injured.

Word or Phrase	Combining Form and Definition	Description
cytokines	cyt/o- *cell*	Protein molecules released by damaged tissues. Cytokines call leukocytes to that area.
electrolytes	electr/o- *electricity*	Chemical elements that carry a positive or negative electrical charge: sodium (Na^+), potassium (K^+), chloride (Cl^-), calcium (Ca^{++}), and bicarbonate (HCO_3^-). They are carried in the plasma.
endotoxin	tox/o- *poison*	Toxic substance produced by some bacteria. It acts as a poison in the body and can cause decreased blood pressure.
eosinophil	eosin/o- *eosin (red acidic dye)*	Type of leukocyte. It is classified as a granulocyte because granules in its cytoplasm stain bright pink to red with eosin dye. The nucleus has two lobes. It is a phagocyte that eats foreign cells like pollen and animal dander and also parasites. Eosinophils are also known as eos.
erythroblast	erythr/o- *red*	Immature erythrocyte that develops from a stem cell in the red marrow
erythrocyte	erythr/o- *red*	A red blood cell. Erythrocytes contain hemoglobin and carry oxygen and carbon dioxide to and from the lungs and cells of the body.
erythropoietin	erythr/o- *red*	Hormone produced by the kidneys that stimulates the production of erythrocytes
fibrin	fibr/o- *fiber*	Fiber strands formed by the activation of clotting factors. Fibrin traps erythrocytes to form a blood clot.
fibrinogen	fibrin/o- *fibrin*	Blood clotting factor
globins	glob/o- *shaped like a globe; comprehensive*	Chains of protein molecules in hemoglobin
granulocyte	granul/o- *granule*	Category of leukocytes with large granules in the cytoplasm. Includes neutrophils, eosinophils, and basophils.
hematopoiesis	hemat/o- *blood*	Process by which blood cells are formed in the red marrow
heme		Molecule in hemoglobin that contains iron and gives erythrocytes their red color
hemoglobin	hem/o- *blood* glob/o- *shaped like a globe; comprehensive*	Substance in an erythrocyte that binds to oxygen and carbon dioxide. Made of a heme molecule and globin chains
hemostasis	hem/o- *blood*	The cessation of bleeding after the formation of a blood clot.
histamine		Released by basophils. It dilates blood vessels and increases blood flow to damaged tissue. It also allows protein molecules to leak out of blood vessels into the tissue, which produces redness and swelling.
IgA		Immunglobulin A. Antibody present in body secretions (tears, saliva, mucus, and breast milk). It gives passive immunity to a breastfeeding infant.
IgD		Immunoglobulin D. Antibody present on the surface of B cells. It stimulates the B cell to become a plasma cell.

… or Phrase	Combining Form and Definition	Description
		Immunoglobulin E. Antibody present on the surface of basophils. It causes them to release histamine and heparin during inflammatory and allergic reactions.
IgG		Immunoglobulin G. Antibody that is produced by plasma cells the second time a specific pathogen enters the body; IgG forms the basis for active immunity. Smallest of all the immunoglobulins. Most abundant of all the immunoglobulins. During pregnancy, it crosses the placenta to the fetus and provides passive immunity.
IgM		Immunoglobulin M. Antibody that is produced by plasma cells during the initial exposure to a pathogen. IgM also reacts to incompatible blood types during a blood transfusion. Largest of the immunglobulins.
immune response	**immun/o-** *immune response*	Coordinated effort between the blood and lymphatic system to identify and destroy invading microorganisms or cancerous cells produced within the body
immunoglobulins	**immun/o-** *immune response* **globul/o-** *shaped like a globe*	Antibodies. There are five classes of immunoglobulins: IgA, IgD, IgE, IgG, and IgM.
interferon		Substance released by macrophages that have engulfed a virus. It stimulates normal body cells to produce an antiviral substance that prevents the virus from entering them to reproduce itself.
interleukin		Substance released by macrophages that stimulates B cell and T cell lymphocytes and activates NK cells. It also produces fever.
leukocyte	**leuk/o-** *white*	A white blood cell. There are five different types of mature leukocytes: neutrophils, eosinophils, basophils, lymphocytes, and monocytes.
lymph		Fluid that flows through the lymphatic system
lymphatic system	**lymph/o-** *lymph; lymphatic system*	Body system that includes a network of lymphatic vessels, circulating lymph fluid, lymph nodes, the lymphoid organs (thymus, spleen), and lymphoid tissues (tonsils and adenoids, appendix, and Peyer's patches). Also includes the blood cells lymphocytes and macrophages.
lymphatic vessels	**lymph/o-** *lymph; lymphatic system*	Vessels that begin as capillaries carrying lymph, continue through lymph nodes, and empty into the right lymphatic duct or the thoracic duct
lymph nodes		Small, encapsulated pieces of lymphoid tissue located along the lymphatic vessels. Lymph nodes filter and destroy invading microorganisms and cancerous cells present in the lymph.
lymphoblast	**lymph/o-** *lymph; lymphatic system*	Immature cell that comes from a stem cell in the red marrow and develops into a lymphocyte
lymphocyte	**lymph/o-** *lymph; lymphatic system*	Second most abundant leukocyte, but the smallest in size. It is classified as an agranulocyte, and the cytoplasm is only a thin ring that edges the round nucleus. Lymphocytes in the red marrow become NK cells or B lymphocytes that produce antibodies. Lymphocytes in the thymus become T lymphocytes. Lymphocytes are also known as lymphs
macrophage	**macr/o-** *large*	Another name for a monocyte because it is able to engulf large numbers of cells and cellular debris

Word or Phrase	Combining Form and Definition	Description
megakaryoblast	kary/o- *nucleus*	Immature cell that comes from a stem cell in the red marrow and develops into a megakaryocyte
megakaryocyte	kary/o- *nucleus*	Very large cell whose cytoplasm breaks away at the edges to form individual thrombocytes
monoblast	mon/o- *one, single*	Immature cell that comes from a stem cell in the red marrow and develops into a monocyte
monocyte	mon/o- *one, single*	Largest of the leukocytes. It is classified as an agranulocyte. The nucleus is shaped like a kidney bean. Monocytes are also known as *monos.* Because it is the largest of the phagocytes, it is also called a *macrophage.*
myeloblast	myel/o- *bone marrow; spinal cord; myelin*	Immature cell that comes from a stem cell in the red marrow and develops into a myelocyte
myelocyte	myel/o- *bone marrow; spinal cord; myelin*	Immature cell that comes from a myeloblast in the red marrow and develops into either a neutrophil, eosinophil, or basophil
natural killer (NK) cell		Type of lymphocyte that matures in the red marrow and, without the help of antibodies or complement, recognizes and destroys pathogens
neutrophil	neutr/o- *not taking part* morph/o- *shape*	Most numerous type of leukocyte. It is classified as a granulocyte, but granules in its cytoplasm do not readily stain red or blue. The nucleus has several segmented lobes. It is a phagocyte that eats bacteria and cellular debris. Neutrophils are also known as segmented neutrophils, segmenters, segs, polymorphonucleated leukocytes, polys, or PMNs.
normoblast	norm/o- *normal, usual*	Immature erythrocyte that develops from an erythroblast in the red marrow
oxyhemoglobin	ox/y- *oxygen*	Compound formed when hemoglobin binds to an oxygen molecule
passive immunity		Immune response and defense against pathogens that is conveyed by the mother's antibodies to the fetus via the placenta or to the breast-feeding baby. These maternal antibodies provide protection from all the diseases the mother has had.
pathogen	path/o- *disease, suffering*	Microorganism that causes a disease. Pathogens include bacteria, viruses, protozoa, and other microorganisms, as well as plant cells like fungi or yeast.
phagocyte	phag/o- *eating, swallowing*	Category of leukocytes that engulfs foreign cells and cellular debris and destroy them with digestive enzymes. Phagocytes include neutrophils, eosinophils, and monocytes.
phagocytosis	phag/o- *eating, swallowing* cyt/o- *cell*	The process by which a phagocyte destroys a foreign cell or cellular debris
plasma		Clear, straw-colored fluid portion of the blood that carries blood cells and contains dissolved substances like proteins, glucose, minerals, electrolytes, clotting factors, complement proteins, hormones, bilirubin, urea, and creatinine.

Word or Phrase	Combining Form and Definition	Description
plasma proteins		Protein molecules in the blood. The most important one is albumin.
prothrombin	thromb/o- *thrombus (blood clot)*	Blood clotting factor that is activated just before the thrombus is formed
reticulocyte	reticul/o- *small network*	Immature erythrocyte that is released into the blood. It has no nucleus, but contains a network of ribosomes in its cytoplasm.
Rh blood group		Category of blood type. When the Rh factor is present, the blood is Rh positive. Without the Rh factor, the blood is Rh negative.
serum		Fluid portion of the plasma that remains after the clotting factors are activated to form a blood clot
spleen	splen/o- *spleen*	Lymphoid organ located in the abdominal cavity behind the stomach. The spleen destroys old erythrocytes, breaking their hemoglobin into heme and globins. It also acts as a storage area for whole blood. Its white pulp is lymphoid tissue that contains B and T lymphocytes.
stem cell		Extremely immature cell in the red marrow that is the precursor to all types of blood cells
T cell		Type of lymphocyte that matures in the thymus. There are four subsets of T cells: helper T cells (CD4 cells), memory T cells, cytotoxic T cells, and suppressor T cells (CD8 cells).
thrombocyte	thromb/o- *thrombus (blood clot)*	Cell fragment that does not have a nucleus. It is active in the blood clotting process. Thrombocytes are also known as platelets.
thromboplastin	plast/o- *being formed or shaped*	Blood clotting factor. Also known as tissue factor because it is released when an object penetrates the tissue.
thrombus	thromb/o- *thrombus (blood clot)*	A blood clot
thymus	thym/o- *thymus; rage*	Lymphoid organ in the thoracic cavity. As an endocrine gland, it releases hormones known as thymosins. The thymosins cause lymphoblasts in the thymus to mature into T lymphocytes.
tumor necrosis factor (TNF)		Substance released by macrophages. It destroys endotoxins produced by certain bacteria. It also destroys cancerous cells.

Labeling Exercise

A. Match each anatomy word or phrase to its numbered structure in Figure 6-11■. Write that word or phrase on the blank line next to its number. Use the Answer Key at the end of the book to check your answers.

basophil	lymphocyte	neutrophil
eosinophil	monocyte	

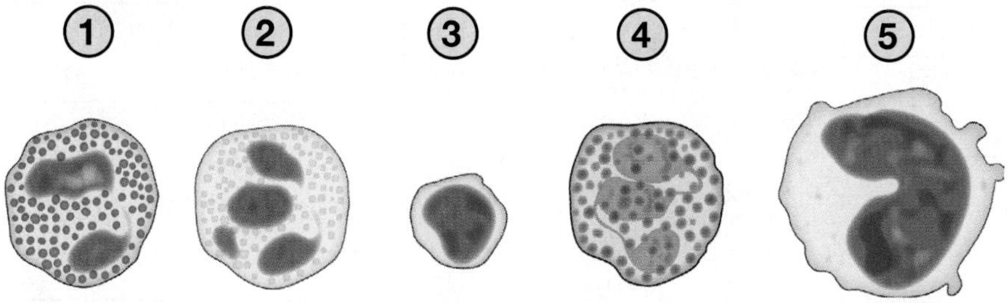

1. ______________
2. ______________
3. ______________
4. ______________
5. ______________

Figure 6-11 ■

B. Match each anatomy word or phrase to its numbered structure in Figure 6-12■. Write that word or phrase on the blank line next to the number.

appendix and Peyer's patches	cervical lymph nodes	inguinal lymph nodes	thymus
axillary lymph nodes	mediastinal lymph nodes	red bone marrow	tonsils and adenoids
celiac lymph nodes	mesenteric lymph nodes	spleen	

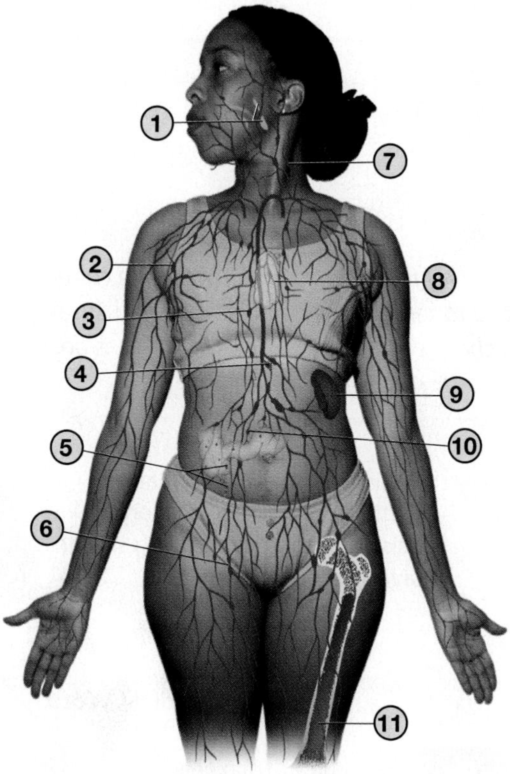

1. ______________
2. ______________
3. ______________
4. ______________
5. ______________
6. ______________
7. ______________
8. ______________
9. ______________
10. ______________
11. ______________

Figure 6-12 ■

Building Medical Words

Combining Forms

Here are the combining forms you have learned so far. Next to each combining form, write its meaning. Use the Answer Key at the end of the book to check your answers. The first one has been done for you.

Combining Form	Medical Meaning	Combining Form	Medical Meaning
1. aggreg/o-	crowding together	20. meg/a-	______
2. bas/o-	______	21. mon/o-	______
3. coagul/o-	______	22. morph/o-	______
4. cyt/o-	______	23. myel/o-	______
5. electr/o-	______	24. neutr/o-	______
6. eosin/o-	______	25. norm/o-	______
7. erythr/o-	______	26. nucle/o-	______
8. fibrin/o-	______	27. ox/y-	______
9. fibr/o-	______	28. path/o-	______
10. glob/o-	______	29. phag/o-	______
11. globul/o-	______	30. plast/o-	______
12. granul/o-	______	31. reticul/o-	______
13. hemat/o-	______	32. rub/o-	______
14. hem/o-	______	33. splen/o-	______
15. immun/o-	______	34. suppress/o-	______
16. kary/o-	______	35. thromb/o-	______
17. leuk/o-	______	36. thym/o-	______
18. lymph/o-	______	37. tox/o-	______
19. macr/o-	______		

Combining Forms and Suffixes

Read the definition hint for the medical word you are to build. Look at the combining form that is given. Write the correct suffix on the blank line. Then write the medical word. (Remember: You may need to remove the combining vowel. Always remove the hyphens and slash.) Use the Answer Key at the end of the book to check your answers. The first one has been done for you.

SUFFIX LIST

-ation (a process; being or having)
-blast (immature cell)
-cyte (cell)
-gen (that which produces)
-ic (pertaining to)
-ity (state; condition)
-logy (the study of)
-lyte (dissolved substance)
-oid (resembling)
-phil (attraction to, fondness for)
-poiesis (condition of formation)
-poietin (a substance that forms)
-stasis (condition of standing still or staying in one place)

Definition Hint	Combining Form	Suffix	Write the Medical Word
1. Condition of formation of blood	hemat/o-	-poiesis	hematopoiesis
2. White blood cell	leuk/o-	______	______
3. Process of clotting	coagul/o	______	______

Definition Hint	Combining Form	Suffix	Write the Medical Word
4. Pertaining to the spleen	splen/o-	________	________________
5. Cell that eats	phag/o-	________	________________
6. Resembling the lymph or lymphatic system	lymph/o-	________	________________
7. The study of the blood	hemat/o-	________	________________
8. Substance that forms red blood cells	erythr/o-	________	________________
9. Cell that has an attraction to a red acidic dye	eosin/o-	________	________________
10. That which produces disease and suffering	path/o-	________	________________
11. Condition where the blood stops flowing (after injury to an area)	hem/o-	________	________________
12. Cell that helps form a blood clot	thromb/o-	________	________________
13. That which produces fibrin strands	fibrin/o-	________	________________
14. Very immature white blood cell	myel/o-	________	________________
15. Substance that conducts electricity when dissolved in water	electr/o-	________	________________
16. State of readiness of immune system	immun/o-	________	________________

Combining Forms and Prefixes

Read the definition hint for the medical word you are to build. Look at the medical word or word part that is given. It already contains a combining form and a suffix. Write the correct prefix on the blank line. Then write the medical word. (Remember: You may need to remove the combining vowel. Always remove the hyphens and slash.) Use the Answer Key at the end of the book to check your answers. The first one has been done for you.

PREFIX LIST			
a- (away from, without)	endo- (innermost, within)	poly- (many, much)	pro- (before)

Definition Hint	Prefix	Medical Word or Word Part	Write the Medical Word
1. Substance produced by some bacteria that is poisonous to body cells	endo-	toxin	endotoxin
2. Cell without granules in its cytoplasm	________	granulocyte	________________
3. Many-shaped nucleus	________	morphonucleated	________________
4. Substance that comes before thrombin	________	thrombin	________________

Symptoms, Signs, and Diseases

Blood

Word or Phrase	Word Part and Definition	Description
blood dyscrasia	**dyscrasia** (dis-KRAY-zee-ah) **dys-** *painful, difficult, abnormal* **-crasia** *a mixing* *Dyscrasia* is derived from a Greek word meaning *disease caused by an abnormal mixing* of the four "humors": blood, black bile, yellow bile, and phlegm (mucus).	Any disease condition involving blood cells. Treatment: Correct the underlying cause.
hemorrhage	**hemorrhage** (HEM-oh-rij) **hem/o-** *blood* **-rrhage** *excessive flow or discharge*	Loss of a large amount of blood, externally or internally. Injury to an artery causes a forceful spurting of a large amount of bright red blood. Treatment: Tourniquet, pressure, or suturing to stop the bleeding.
pancytopenia	**pancytopenia** (PAN-sy-toh-PEE-nee-ah) **pan-** *all* **cyt/o-** *cell* **-penia** *condition of deficiency*	Decreased numbers of all types of blood cells due to failure of the bone marrow to produce stem cells. Treatment: Correct the underlying cause.
septicemia	**septicemia** (SEP-tih-SEE-mee-ah) **septic/o-** *infection* **-emia** *condition of the blood; substance in the blood* *Sepsis* is a Greek word meaning *putrefaction or decay.*	Severe bacterial infection of the tissues that spreads to the blood. Both the bacteria and their toxins cause severe systemic symptoms. Also known as sepsis or blood poisoning. Treatment: Antibiotic drugs.

Erythrocytes

Word or Phrase	Word Part and Definition	Description
abnormal red blood cell morphology	**morphology** (mor-FAWL-oh-jee) **morph/o-** *shape* **-logy** *the study of*	Disease category that includes erythrocytes that have an abnormality of size or shape. These are associated with anemia and deficiency diseases. Treatment: Correct underlying cause.
anisocytosis	**anisocytosis** (an-EYE-soh-sy-TOH-sis) **anis/o-** *unequal* **cyt/o-** *cell* **-osis** *condition; abnormal condition; process* **macrocyte** (MAK-roh-site) **macr/o-** *large* **-cyte** *cell* **microcyte** (MY-kroh-site) **micr/o-** *small* **-cyte** *cell*	Erythrocytes that are either too large or too small. A **macrocyte** is an abnormally large erythrocyte seen in folic acid anemia (folic acid deficiency) and pernicious anemia (vitamin B_{12} deficiency). A **microcyte** is an abnormally small erythrocyte seen in iron deficiency anemia.

Word or Phrase	Word Part and Definition	Description
poikilocytosis	**poikilocytosis** (POY-kih-loh-sy-TOH-sis) **poikil/o-** *irregular* **cyt/o-** *cell* **-osis** *condition; abnormal condition; process*	Erythrocytes that vary in shape. A sickle cell is a crescent-shaped erythrocyte seen in sickle cell anemia. Erythrocytes can also be shaped like spheres (spherocytes), ovals, teardrops, or have spike-like projections on their surface. Treatment: None, as these are genetic defects of the erythrocyte.
anemia	**anemia** (ah-NEE-mee-ah) **an-** *without, not* **-emia** *condition of the blood; substance in the blood* Add words to make a correct and complete definition of *anemia: Condition of the blood [of] not [enough red blood cells].* Every medical word must contain a combining form. The suffix of *anemia* contains a combining form based on the Greek word *haima* (blood). **anemic** (ah-NEE-mik) **an-** *without, not* **-emic** *pertaining to a condition of the blood or a substance in the blood*	The number of erythrocytes in the blood is decreased. This can be due to any of the following reasons: 1. Too few erythrocytes are produced because of insufficient amounts of amino acids, folic acid, iron, vitamin B_6, or vitamin B_{12}. 2. Too few erythrocytes are produced because disease, cancer, radiation, or chemotherapy drugs have damaged or destroyed the red marrow. 3. Many erythrocytes have been destroyed because of lysis or increased cell fragility. 4. Many erythocytes have been lost because of hemorrhage, excessive menstruation, or chronic blood loss. Anemias can be classified by their cause or by the size, shape, and appearance of their erythrocytes. A patient with anemia is said to be **anemic.** Treatment: Correct the underlying cause.
aplastic anemia	**aplastic** (aa-PLAS-tik) **a-** *away from, without* **plast/o-** *being formed or shaped* **-ic** *pertaining to* **normocytic** (NOR-moh-SIT-ik) **norm/o-** *normal, usual* **cyt/o-** *cell* **-ic** *pertaining to* **normochromic** (NOR-moh-KROH-mik) **norm/o-** *normal, usual* **chrom/o-** *color* **-ic** *pertaining to*	Failure of the bone marrow to produce erythrocytes because it has been damaged by disease, cancer, radiation, or chemotherapy drugs. The total number of erythrocytes is decreased, even though individual erythrocytes are **normocytic** (normal in size) and **normochromic** (normal in color). Treatment: Blood transfusion, erythropoietin drug to stimulation erythrocyte production, or bone marrow transplantation.

Word or Phrase	Word Part and Definition	Description
iron deficiency anemia	**microcytic** (MY-kroh-SIT-ik) **micr/o-** *small* **cyt/o-** *cell* **-ic** *pertaining to* **hypochromic** (HY-poh-KROH-mik) **hypo-** *below; deficient* **chrom/o-** *color* **-ic** *pertaining to*	Caused by a deficiency of iron in the diet. Also caused by increased loss of iron due to menstruation, hemorrhage, or chronic blood loss. The erythrocytes are **microcytic** (small in size) and **hypochromic** (pale in color) (see Figure 6-13a ■ and b ■). Infant formulas include supplemental iron to prevent iron deficiency anemia. Treatment: Dietary iron supplements, correction of cause of blood loss.

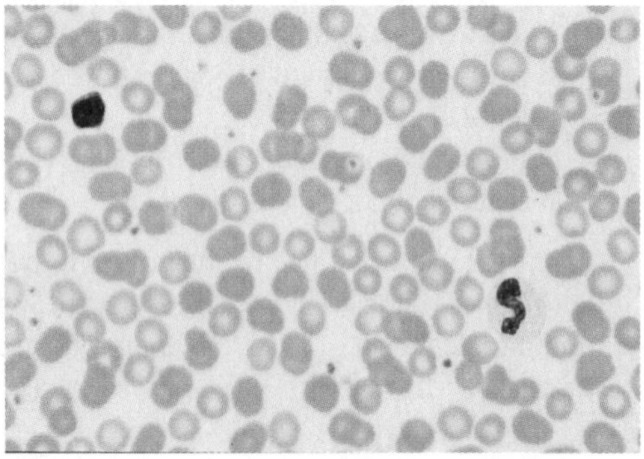

Figure 6-13a ■ Normal erythrocytes.
This blood smear shows erythrocytes that are normal in size and color.

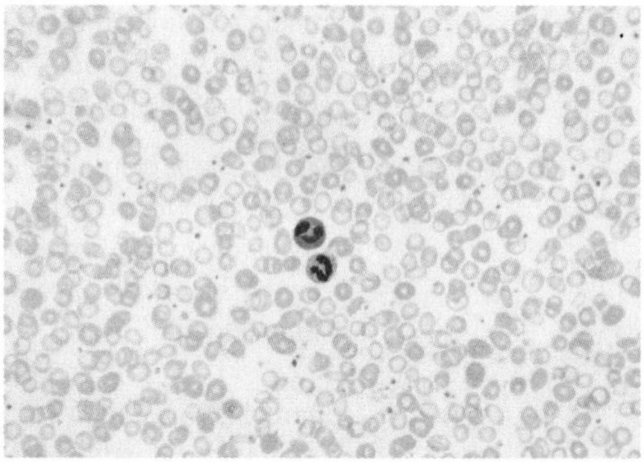

Figure 6-13b ■ Microcytic, hypochromic erythrocytes.
This blood smear shows small, pale erythrocytes that are characteristic of iron deficiency anemia.

Word or Phrase	Word Part and Definition	Description
folic acid deficiency anemia	**megaloblast** (MEG-ah-loh-blast) **megal/o-** *large* **-blast** *immature cell*	Caused by a deficiency of folic acid in the diet. Commonly seen in patients who are malnourished (the elderly, poor, alcoholics), those who have malabsorption diseases, and pregnant women. The erythrocytes are abnormally large and very immature (**megaloblasts**). Treatment: Balanced diet, folic acid supplements.
pernicious anemia	**pernicious** (per-NISH-us) *Pernicious* is derived from a Latin word meaning *destructive.*	Caused by a lack of vitamin B_{12} in the diet (from animal foods) or a lack of intrinsic factor in the stomach. Can be seen in vegetarians. Untreated, it can cause permanent damage to the nerves. The erythrocytes are abnormally large and very immature (megaloblasts). Treatment: Intramuscular or nasal spray vitamin B_{12}.

Across the Life Span

As a person ages, the stomach produces less secretions, including hydrochloric acid and intrinsic factor. Both of these must be present for vitamin B_{12} in food to be absorbed into the blood. A decreased level of vitamin B_{12} in the body causes pernicious anemia.

Word or Phrase	Word Part and Definition	Description
sickle cell anemia	Sickle cells are shaped like a sickle, a handheld tool with a curved blade that is used to cut tall grass or wheat.	Inherited genetic abnormality of an amino acid in hemoglobin. If there is one abnormal amino acid, the patient has sickle cell trait and is a carrier for sickle cell disease but does not have the disease. If there are two abnormal amino acids, the patient has sickle cell disease. Low oxygen levels in the blood cause the erythrocyte to become distorted into a crescent or sickle shape (see Figure 6-14■). Sickle cells do not move easily through the capillaries, blocking the flow of blood, causing small clots and pain, particularly in the joints and abdomen. Sickle cells are fragile (because they frequently change shape), and they have a shortened life span, which results in anemia. Treatment: Pain medication, avoidance of situations that lower blood oxygen levels. Hydroxyurea (a drug that stimulates the production of fetal hemoglobin that does not sickle). **Figure 6-14 ■ Sickle cell.** The abnormal crescent shape and sharp edges of this sickled erythrocyte are very different from the smooth, rounded contour of a normal erythrocyte. Repeated sickling causes these fragile erythrocytes to have a shortened life span, resulting in anemia.
polycythemia vera	**polycythemia vera** (PAWL-ee-sy-THEE-mee-ah VER-ah) **poly-** *many, much* **cyt/o-** *cell* **hem/o-** *blood* **-ia** *condition, state, thing* **viscosity** (vis-KAWS-ih-tee) **viscos/o-** *thickness* **-ity** *state; condition*	Increased number of erythrocytes due to uncontrolled production by the red marrow. The cause is unknown. The **viscosity** of the blood increases and the total blood volume is increased. Initial symptoms include dizziness, headache, fatigue, and splenomegaly. Patients are prone to develop blood clots and high blood pressure. Treatment: Periodic phlebotomy to remove blood and keep the hematocrit at a normal level.
thalassemia	**thalassemia** (THAL-ah-SEE-mee-ah) *Thalassemia* is derived from a Greek word meaning *sea* because the disease was first identified in persons living in countries around the Mediterranean Sea.	Inherited genetic abnormality that affects the synthesis of globin chains in the hemoglobin molecule. The erythrocytes are small (microcytic), pale (hypochromic), and of variable size (anisocytosis). Target cells (erythrocytes with a central dark spot) are seen. Symptoms include anemia, weakness, and splenomegaly. Thalassemia major is the severe form of the disease; thalassemia minor produces fewer symptoms and signs. Treatment: Blood transfusions.

Word or Phrase	Word Part and Definition	Description
transfusion reaction	**transfusion** (trans-FYOO-shun) **trans-** *across, through* **fus/o-** *pouring* **-ion** *action; condition* **hemolysis** (hee-MAWL-ih-sis) **hem/o-** *blood* **-lysis** *process of breaking down or dissolving* **hemolytic** (HEE-moh-LIT-ik) **hem/o-** *blood* **ly/o-** *break down, separate, dissolve* **-tic** *pertaining to*	Reaction that occurs when a patient receives a blood transfusion with an incompatible blood type. Antibodies in the patient's serum attack antigens on the erythrocytes of the donor blood causing **hemolysis** of the donor erythrocytes. This is known as a **hemolytic reaction.** Fever, chills, and hypotension occur almost immediately. The patient has flank pain because hemolyzed erythrocytes clog the filtering membrane of the kidneys and cause kidney failure. Transfusion reactions can be fatal. Treatment: Stop the transfusion immediately and treat the patient's symptoms and signs.
Leukocytes		
acquired immunodeficiency syndrome (AIDS)	**immunodeficiency** (IM-yoo-noh-deh-FISH-en-see) **immun/o-** *immune response* **defici/o-** *lacking, inadequate* **-ency** *condition of being* **immunocompromised** (IM-yoo-noh-COM-proh-myzd) **immun/o-** *immune response* **compromis/o-** *exposed to danger* **-ed** *pertaining to*	Severe infection caused by the human immunodeficiency virus (HIV). AIDS is primarily a sexually transmitted disease, but is also transmitted by shared needles in drug abusers, accidental needle sticks, exposure to contaminated blood, blood transfusions, and via breast milk from an infected mother to a nursing baby. Initially, AIDS causes fevers, night sweats, weight loss, enlarged lymph nodes, and diarrhea. It takes about three months for the body to develop enough antibodies against HIV to give a positive serology test. A patient with HIV antibodies is said to be HIV positive. Like all viruses, HIV cannot reproduce itself. It must enter a body cell and use the cell's DNA to replicate itself. The body cell is destroyed as the new viruses are released. HIV uses helper T cells (CD4 lymphocytes) to reproduce. As large numbers of helper T cells are destroyed, the action of suppressor T cells (CD8 lymphocytes) is unopposed. This suppresses the normal immune response and leaves the patient **immunocompromised** and defenseless against infection and cancer. A diagnosis of AIDS is made when the CD4 cell count is below

Word or Phrase	Word Part and Definition	Description
acquired immunodeficiency syndrome (AIDS) *(continued)*	**opportunistic** (AWP-or-too-NIS-tik) **opportun/o-** *well timed, taking advantage of an opportunity* **-ist** *one who specializes in* **-ic** *pertaining to*	200 (normal is 500–1500 cells/mm^3) and there is an **opportunistic infection** such as *Pneumocystis carinii* pneumonia, oral or esophageal candidiasis (see Figure 6-15■), cytomegalovirus retinitis, or unusual cancers (like Kaposi's sarcoma). AIDS wasting syndrome is characterized by weight loss and loss of muscle mass and strength. Treatment: Antiretroviral drugs. There is no cure for AIDS. **Figure 6-15 ■ Oral candidiasis.** This 25-year-old man with AIDS has oral candidiasis, an opportunistic infection caused by the yeast *Candida albicans.*
leukemia	**leukemia** (loo-KEE-mee-ah) **leuk/o-** *white* **-emia** *condition of the blood; substance in the blood* The word *leukemia* was coined by Rudolph Virchow (1821–1902), a German physician. **cancer** (KAN-ser) *Cancer* is a Latin word meaning *a crab.* Cancer begins in one location and spreads in all directions like the legs of a crab spreading out from its body. **myelogenous** (MY-eh-LAWJ-eh-nus) **myel/o-** *bone marrow; spinal cord; myelin* **gen/o-** *arising from; produced by* **-ous** *pertaining to* **lymphocytic** (LIM-foh-SIT-ik) **lymph/o-** *lymph; lymphatic system* **cyt/o-** *cell* **-ic** *pertaining to*	**Cancer** of the leukocytes. The excessive numbers of leukocytes crowd out other cells in the bone marrow. Patients have anemia (from too few erythrocytes), easy bruising and hemorrhages (from too few thrombocytes), fever, and susceptibility to infection (from too many immature leukocytes). Leukemia is named according to the type of leukocyte that is most prevalent and whether the onset of symptoms is acute or chronic. Leukemia can be caused by exposure to radiation or toxic chemicals and drugs. Patients with chronic myelogenous leukemia have an abnormal chromosome known as the Philadelphia chromosome. Most cases of leukemia occur in persons over age 60. The most common leukemia in children is acute lymphocytic leukemia. acute **myelogenous** leukemia (AML): too many myeloblasts and myelocytes chronic myelogeous leukemia (CML): too many myeloblasts,myelocytes, and mature neutrophils, eosinophils, and basophils acute **lymphocytic** leukemia (ALL): too many lymphoblasts chronic lymphocytic leukemia (CLL): too many mature lymphocytes *(continued)*

Word or Phrase	Word Part and Definition	Description
leukemia *(continued)*		Diagnosis is made by examination of the blood (see Figure 6-16■) and bone marrow aspiration.Treatment: Chemotherapy, radiation therapy, bone marrow or stem cell transplantation. **Figure 6-16 ■ Acute lymphocytic leukemia.** This blood smear was taken from a patient with acute lymphocytic leukemia. There is a tremendous increase in the number of lymphoblasts with some mature lymphocytes present in the blood.
mononucleosis	**mononucleosis** (MAWN-oh-noo-klee-OH-sis) **mon/o-** *one, single* **nucle/o-** *nucleus* **-osis** *condition; abnormal condition; process*	Infectious disease caused by the Epstein-Barr virus (EBV). Symptoms include lymphadenopathy, fever, and fatigue. Often called "the kissing disease" because it commonly affects young adults and is transmitted through contact with saliva that contains the virus. Treatment: Rest. (There is no antiviral drug that is effective against mononucleosis. Antibiotic drugs are not effective against any viral illness.)
multiple myeloma	**myeloma** (MY-eh-LOH-mah) **myel/o-** *bone marrow; spinal cord; myelin* **-oma** *tumor, mass* **hypercalcemia** (HY-per-kal-SEE-mee-ah) **hyper-** *above; more than normal* **calc/o-** *calcium* **-emia** *condition of the blood; substance in the blood*	Cancer of the plasma cells that produce antibodies. Symptoms include weakness, anemia, and increased susceptibility to infections. Multiple tumors in the bone destroy the red marrow and cause pain, fractures, and **hypercalcemia** (as calcium is released from destroyed bone). The abnormal plasma cells produce Bence Jones protein, an abnormal immunoglobulin that can be detected in the urine. Treatment: Radiation therapy and chemotherapy.

Thrombocytes

Word or Phrase	Word Part and Definition	Description
coagulopathy	**coagulopathy** (koh-AG-yoo-LAWP-ah-thee) **coagul/o-** *clotting* **-pathy** *disease, suffering*	Any disease that affects the ability of the blood to clot normally. Treatment: Correct the underlying cause.
deep venous thrombosis (DVT)	**thrombus** (THRAWM-bus) **thrombosis** (thrawm-BOH-sis) **thromb/o-** *thrombus (blood clot)* **-osis** *condition; abnormal condition; process* **stasis** (STAY-sis) *Stasis* is a Greek word meaning *a standing still.* **embolus** (EM-boh-lus) *Embolus* is a Greek word meaning *an occluding plug.* **embolism** (EM-boh-liz-em) **embol/o-** *embolus (occluding plug)* **-ism** *process; disease from a specific cause*	A **thrombus** (blood clot) in one of the deep veins of the lower leg, often after surgery or in patients on bedrest. Lack of exercise causes the blood to pool in the veins (**venous stasis**) and form a clot. Sometimes a thrombus becomes an **embolus** that travels through the circulatory system until it becomes trapped and blocks the blood flow in a small artery of the brain, heart, or lungs. This obstruction is known as an **embolism.** Treatment: Anticoagulant drugs to prevent clot formation; thrombolytic drugs to break up a thrombus.
disseminated intravascular coagulation (DIC)	**disseminated** (dih-SEM-ih-NAYT-ed) **dissemin/o-** *widely scattered throughout the body* **-ated** *pertaining to a condition; composed of* **intravascular** (IN-trah-VAS-kyoo-lar) **intra-** *within* **vascul/o-** *blood vessel* **-ar** *pertaining to* **coagulation** (koh-AG-yoo-LAY-shun) **coagul/o-** *clotting* **-ation** *a process; being or having*	Severe disorder of clotting in which multiple small thrombi are formed throughout the body. These blood clots use up platelets and fibrinogen from the plasma to the extent that there is spontaneous bleeding from the nose, mouth, IV sites, and incisions. DIC can be triggered by severe injuries, burns, cancer, or systemic infections. Treatment: Intravenous fibrinogen and platelets.

Word or Phrase	Word Part and Definition	Description
hemophilia	**hemophilia** (HEE-moh-FIL-ee-ah) **hem/o-** *blood* **phil/o-** *attraction to, fondness for* **-ia** *condition, state, thing* **hemophiliac** (HEE-moh-FIL-ee-ak) **hem/o-** *blood* **phil/o-** *attraction to, fondness for* **-iac** *pertaining to*	Inherited genetic abnormality of a gene on the X chromosome. This causes a lack or a deficiency of a specific clotting factor. When injured, hemophiliac patients continue to bleed for long periods of time. Minor injuries produce large hematomas under the skin and bleeding inside body cavities, joints, and organs. The abnormal gene is carried by a female on the X chromosome, but she does not have the disease. If a male inherits the abnormal gene, it causes hemophilia. A patient who has hemophilia is known as a **hemophiliac.** Hemophilia A is due to a lack of clotting factor VIII and is the most common type of hemophilia. Hemophilia B is caused by a lack of factor IX. Hemophilia C is caused by a lack of factor XI. Treatment: Intravenous administration of the specific clotting factor that is lacking.
thrombocytopenia	**thrombocytopenia** (THRAWM-boh-SY-toh-PEE-nee-ah) **thromb/o-** *thrombus (blood clot)* **cyt/o-** *cell* **-penia** *condition of deficiency* **petechiae** (peh-TEE-kee-ee) **ecchymosis** (EK-ih-MOH-seez) **idiopathic** (ID-ee-oh-PATH-ik) **idi/o-** *unknown; individual* **path/o-** *disease, suffering* **-ic** *pertaining to* **purpura** (PER-peh-rah) *Purpura* is derived from a Greek word meaning *purple.* Purpura includes both petechiae and ecchymoses.	Deficiency in the number of thrombocytes due to exposure to radiation or chemicals or drugs that damage stem cells in the bone marrow. It also occurs when leukemia cells take over the red marrow and crowd out the stem cells that produce thrombocytes. Also, some patients have antibodies that destroy their own thrombocytes. This causes small, pinpoint hemorrhages (**petechiae**) and larger hemorrhages (**ecchymoses**) or bruises on the skin. **Idiopathic thrombocytopenia purpura** has no identifiable cause. Treatment: Correct the underlying cause.

Lymphatic System

Word or Phrase	Word Part and Definition	Description
graft-versus-host disease (GVHD)		Immune reaction originating from the donor tissue or organ (graft) against the patient (host). This can occur after bone marrow transplantation or any type of organ transplantation. This may cause a rash and fever, or it can be severe enough to cause death. Treatment: Oral corticosteroid drugs.
lymphadenopathy	**lymphadenopathy** (lim-FAD-eh-NAWP-eh-thee) **lymph/o-** *lymph; lymphatic system* **aden/o-** *gland* **-pathy** *disease, suffering* *Lymph glands* is an alternate term for *lymph nodes,* although nodes are not really glands.	Enlarged lymph nodes. Lymph nodes in the neck, axillae and groin can be easily felt if they are enlarged. A sore throat will cause the lymph nodes in the neck to enlarge (see Figure 6-17■). A severe infection or cancer will cause the lymph nodes in that area to become enlarged. Treatment: Correct the underlying cause. **Figure 6-17 ■ Lymphadenopathy.** The physician is palpating the cervical lymph nodes of this patient. The cervical lymph nodes trap and destroy pathogens or cancerous cells from infection or cancer in the nose, mouth, or throat, but large numbers can overwhelm the lymph nodes and cause them to become enlarged.
lymphedema	**lymphedema** (LIM-fah-DEE-mah) **lymph/o-** *lymph; lymphatic system* **-edema** *swelling*	Generalized swelling of an arm or a leg that occurs after surgery when a chain of lymph nodes has been removed. Tissue fluid in that area cannot drain into the lymphatic vessels at the normal rate, and this causes edema. Treatment: Elevation of the body part.
lymphoma	**lymphoma** (lim-FOH-mah) **lymph/o-** *lymph; lymphatic system* **-oma** *tumor, mass*	Cancerous tumor of lymphocytes in the lymph nodes or lymphoid tissue. A lymphoma that originates in a lymph node should not be confused with metastasis to a lymph node from a primary site of cancer located elsewhere in the body. Treatment: Radiation therapy, chemotherapy.
Hodgkin's lymphoma	**Hodgkin** (HAWJ-kin) Named by Thomas Hodgkin (1798–1866), a British physician. This is an example of an eponym: a person or thing from whom something takes its name.	Most common type of lymphoma. It occurs most often in young adults and is discovered on physical examination as a painless, enlarged cervical lymph node in the neck. There is fever, weakness, weight loss, and splenomegaly. A biopsy of the lymph node shows abnormal lymphocytes known as Reed-Sternberg cells. Also known as **Hodgkin's disease.**
non-Hodgkin's lymphoma		A group of more than 20 different types of lymphomas that occur in older adults and do not show Reed-Sternberg cells.

Word or Phrase	Word Part and Definition	Description
splenomegaly	**splenomegaly** (SPLEH-noh-MEG-ah-lee) **splen/o-** *spleen* **-megaly** *enlargement*	Enlargement of the spleen, felt on palpation of the abdomen. Can be caused by mononucleosis, Hodgkin's disease, hemolytic anemia, polycythemia vera, or leukemia. Treatment: Correct the underlying cause.
thymoma	**thymoma** (thy-MOH-mah) **thym/o-** *thymus; rage* **-oma** *tumor, mass*	Usually benign tumor of the thymus. May cause cough and chest pain. Often seen in patients who already have an autoimmune disorder such as myasthenia gravis. Treatment: Thymectomy.
	Autoimmune Disorders	
autoimmune diseases	**autoimmune** (AW-toh-ih-MYOON) **auto-** *self* **-immune** *immune response* Every medical word must contain a combining form. The suffix of *autoimmune* contains the combining form *immun/o-*.	Diseases in which the body makes antibodies against its own tissues. Specific tissues are attacked, causing pain and loss of function. The following autoimmune diseases are further described in other chapters: **Autoimmune Disease** — **Area Affected** diabetes mellitus, type 1 — pancreas Graves' disease — thyroid Hashimoto's thyroiditis — thyroid inflammatory bowel disease — intestines multiple sclerosis — nerves myasthenia gravis — muscles psoriasis — skin rheumatoid arthritis — joints scleroderma — skin and blood vessels systemic lupus erythematosus — connective tissue, skin, kidneys, lungs

Diagnostic Procedures

Blood Cell Tests

Word or Phrase	Word Part and Definition	Description
blood type	**agglutination** (ah-GLOO-tih-NAY-shun) **agglutin/o-** *clumping, sticking* **-ation** *a process; being or having* *Agglutination* is derived from a Latin word meaning *glue*.	Blood test that determines the blood type (A, B, AB, or O) and Rh factor (positive or negative) of the patient's blood. **Type and crossmatch** is done when a patient needs to receive a blood transfusion. The donor's blood was typed when it was stored in the blood bank. The patient's (recipient's) blood is then typed. The patient's plasma is mixed with the donor's red blood cells (crossmatching). If the donor's red blood cells clump together (**agglutination**), the blood types are not compatible.

Word or Phrase	Word Part and Definition	Description
complete blood count (CBC) with differential	**differential** (DIF-er-EN-shal) **different/o-** *being distinct, different* **-ial** *pertaining to*	Group of blood tests that are performed automatically by machine to determine the number, type, and characteristics of various cells in the blood (see Table 6-4). **A Closer Look** A severe bacterial infection will increase the number of bands in the differential count. This is known as a **shift to the left.** It refers back to when the differential count was done manually. There was a column on the tally sheet for each type of leukocyte. While counting the leukocytes under the microscope, the laboratory technician put tally marks in the appropriate columns. The column to the far left was for bands. When there were more tally marks in that column than usual, the differential count was said to show a shift to the left.

Table 6-4 Complete Blood Count (CBC) with Differential

Test Name	Description	Word Part and Definition
erythrocytes (red blood cells, RBCs)	Number (millions) per cubic millimeter (m/cmm)	
hematocrit (HCT)	Percentage of RBCs	**hematocrit** (hee-MAT-oh-krit) **hemat/o-** *blood* **-crit** *separation of*
hemoglobin (Hgb)	Amount (grams) per deciliter (g/dL)	
red blood cell **indices** **mean** cell volume (MCV) mean cell hemoglobin (MCH) mean cell hemoglobin concentration (MCHC)	 Average volume of one RBC Average weight of hemoglobin in one RBC Average concentration of hemoglobin in one RBC	**index** (IN-deks) **indices** (IN-dih-seez) *Index* is a Latin singular noun meaning *something that points out.* Form the plural by changing *-ex* to *-ices.* **mean** (MEEN) *Mean* is an English word meaning *the arithmetic average.*
leukocytes (white blood cells, WBCs)	Number (thousands) per cubic millimeter (**k**/cmm)	The *k* in k/cmm stands for *kilo-*, a prefix meaning *one thousand.*
WBC differential neutrophils lymphocytes monocytes eosinophils basophils	Percentage of each type of WBC per 100 WBCs	
thrombocytes (platelets)	Number (thousands) per cubic millimeter (k/cmm)	

Word or Phrase	Word Part and Definition	Description
peripheral blood smear	**peripheral** (peh-RIF-eh-ral) **peripher/o-** *outer aspects* **-al** *pertaining to* *Peripheral* refers to circulating blood taken from an extremity (usually from the arm) as opposed to blood contained in the heart, spleen, or bone marrow.	Blood test done manually to examine the characteristics of erythrocytes and leukocytes under the microscope. A drop of blood is spread as a thin smear on a glass slide and then hematoxylin and eosin dyes are used to stain the blood cells. A blood smear is used to investigate abnormal blood cells discovered on the automated CBC, or a blood smear can be ordered by the physician when there is reason to suspect blood cell abnormalities.
Coagulation Tests		
activated clotting time (ACT)		Blood test to monitor the effectiveness of the anticoagulant drug heparin when it is given in high dosages. A prolonged (rather than normal) activated clotting time would be expected.
partial thromboplastin time (PTT)		Blood test to monitor the effectiveness of the anticoagulant drug heparin when it is given in regular dosages. A prolonged (rather than normal) PTT would be expected. An activated partial thromboplastin time (aPTT) test uses a chemical activator to get faster PTT test results.
prothrombin time (PT)		Blood test to evaluate the effectiveness of the anticoagulant drug Coumadin. A prolonged (rather than normal) PT would be expected. The **international normalized ratio (INR)** reports the PT value in a standardized way, regardless of what laboratory performed the PT test.
Other Blood Tests		
blood chemistries		Blood test used to determine the levels of various chemicals in the blood (see Figure 6-18■). These include electrolytes, albumin, total protein, ALT, AST, BUN and creatinine, bilirubin, glucose, LDH, total cholesterol, uric acid, and alkaline phosphatase. A Chem-20 includes 20 individual chemistry tests performed at the same time. Also called a metabolic panel. **Figure 6-18 ■ Blood chemistry analyzer.** This clinical laboratory scientist is reviewing the results of a blood chemistry analysis. Multiple tests can be performed together automatically on this computerized equipment.

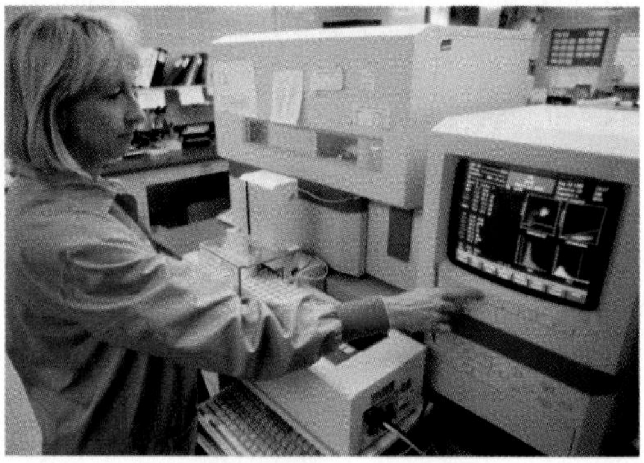

Word or Phrase	Word Part and Definition	Description
ferritin	**ferritin** (FAIR-ih-tin) **ferrit/o-** *iron* **-in** *a substance*	Blood chemistry test that indirectly measures the amount of iron (ferritin) stored in the body by measuring the small amount that is always present in the blood. Used to diagnose iron deficiency anemia.
total iron binding capacity (TIBC)	**transferrin** (trans-FAIR-in) **trans-** *across, through* **ferr/o-** *iron* **-in** *a substance*	Blood chemistry test that measures the level of **transferrin,** a protein that carries iron in the blood. Used to diagnose iron deficiency anemia.
	Serum Tests	
electrophoresis	**electrophoresis** (ee-LEK-troh-foh-REE-sis) **electr/o-** *electricity* **phor/o-** *to bear, to carry* **-esis** *condition* Add words to make a correct and complete definition of *electrophoresis: condition [of a test that uses] electricity to carry [immunoglobulins].*	Immunoglobulin electrophoresis determines the amounts of immunoglobulins IgA, IgD, IgE, IgG, and IgM in the blood. A sample of serum is placed in a gel. An electric current causes the immunoglobulins to become charged and move toward a positive or negative electrode. Each immunoglobulin travels a different distance and direction through the gel, depending on its size and charge, and appears as a spike in a different area on the graph paper. The size of the spike corresponds to how much immunoglobulin is present.
human immunodeficiency virus (HIV) tests		Serology tests that detect antibodies against HIV in the serum. HIV serology tests are reported as either HIV negative or HIV positive.
ELISA		This HIV test can also be positive if the patient has antibodies against lupus erythematosis, Lyme disease, or syphilis. ELISA stands for enzyme-linked immunosorbent assay.
Western blot		Serum test for antibodies against HIV. Used to confirm the findings of a positive ELISA and make a diagnosis of HIV infection.
viral load test		Measures tiny amounts of HIV RNA that are present in the serum during the six weeks before antibodies against HIV can be detected. Uses the RT-PCR or bDNA test. Also used to monitor the progression of the disease and response to antiretroviral drugs.
p24 antigen test		Detects p24, a protein in HIV. The results are reported as a titer. This test is also used to screen donated blood for the presence of HIV.
CD4 count		Measures the number of CD4 cells (helper T cells). Used to monitor the progression of the disease and response to antiretroviral drugs. The CD4:CD8 ratio is also monitored.
MonoSpot test	**heterophil** (HET-er-oh-fil) **heter/o-** *other* **-phil** *attraction to, fondness for*	Rapid test that uses the patient's serum mixed with horse erythrocytes. If the patient has infectious mononucleosis, **heterophil antibodies** in the patient's serum will cause the horse's erythrocytes to clump. Also called heterophil antibody test.
	Saliva Test	
OraSure		Doctor's office or clinic quick screening test that detects antibodies to HIV in the saliva.

Urine Tests

Word or Phrase	Word Part and Definition	Description
Bence Jones protein	Bence Jones protein was named by Henry Bence Jones (1814–1873), an English physician.	Urine test used to monitor the course of multiple myeloma. The cancerous plasma cells produce this abnormal immunoglobulin that can be detected in the urine.
Schilling test		Urine test used to diagnose pernicious anemia. It measures the amount of radioactive vitamin B_{12} excreted in the urine. The patient swallows a capsule that contains intrinsic factor and vitamin B_{12} labeled with a radioactive tracer. The patient swallows a second capsule that contains vitamin B_{12} labeled with a different radioactive tracer but no intrinsic factor. If the patient has pernicious anemia, only the capsule that contained vitamin B_{12} and intrinsic factor will be absorbed into the blood and then excreted in the urine.

Radiologic Procedures

Word or Phrase	Word Part and Definition	Description
lymphangiography	**lymphangiography** (lim-FAN-jee-AWG-rah-fee) **lymph/o-** *lymph; lymphatic system* **angi/o-** *blood vessel; lymph vessel* **-graphy** *process of recording* **lymphangiogram** (lim-FAN-jee-oh-gram) **lymph/o-** *lymph; lymphatic system* **angi/o-** *blood vessel; lymph vessel* **-gram** *a record or picture*	Radiologic procedure in which a radiopaque contrast dye is injected into a lymphatic vessel. X-rays are taken as the dye travels through the lymphatic vessels and lymph nodes. Used to demonstrate enlarged lymph nodes, lymphomas, and areas of blocked lymphatic drainage. The x-ray image is known as a **lymphangiogram.**
color flow duplex ultrasonography	**ultrasonography** (UL-trah-soh-NAWG-rah-fee) **ultra-** *beyond, higher* **son/o-** *sound* **-graphy** *process of recording*	Radiologic procedure that combines a two-dimensional ultrasound image with Doppler **ultrasonography** that color codes images of the blood according to their velocity and direction. It shows turbulence and variation in velocity by variations in brightness. This test is the "gold standard" for evaluating tortuous varicose veins and diagnosing deep venous thrombosis.

Medical and Surgical Procedures

Medical Procedures

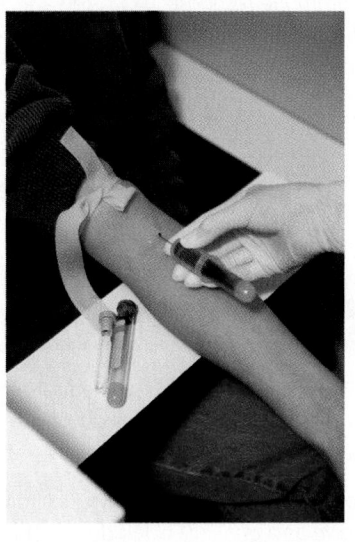

Word or Phrase	Word Part and Definition	Description
bone marrow aspiration	**aspiration** (AS-pih-RAY-shun) **aspir/o-** *to breathe in, to suck in* **-ation** *a process; being or having*	Procedure to remove red bone marrow from the posterior iliac crest of the hip bone. This is done in patients with leukemia, lymphoma, and anemia to examine the different stages of development (stem cell to mature cell) of the blood cells. It is also done to harvest bone marrow from a healthy donor to give to a patient who needs a bone marrow transplantation.
phlebotomy	**phlebotomy** (fleh-BAWT-oh-mee) **phleb/o-** *vein* **-tomy** *process of cutting or making an incision* **venipuncture** (VEE-nih-PUNK-chur) **ven/i-** *vein* **punct/o-** *hole, perforation* **-ure** *system, result of*	Medical procedure for drawing a sample of venous blood into a vacuum tube. The vacuum tubes have different colored rubber stoppers that indicate what additive or anticoagulant is in the tube; this determines what blood test can be performed on the blood in that tube (see Figure 6-19■). Also known as **venipuncture.** 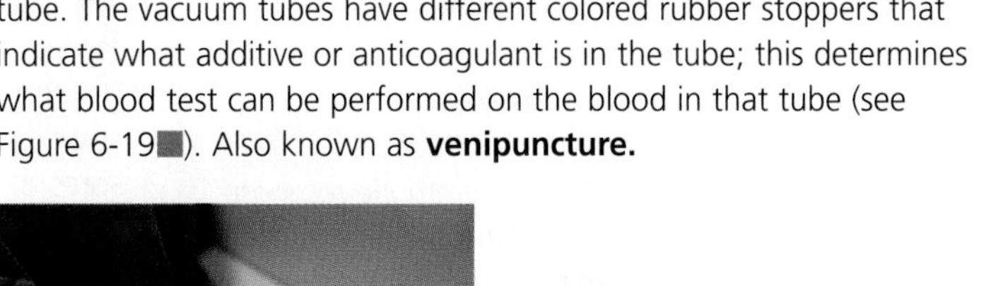 **Figure 6-19 ■ Phlebotomy.** This patient is having blood drawn. The lavender-top tube is used for a complete blood count. The red-top tube is used for blood chemistry tests. The technician placed a tourniquet around the patient's upper arm to distend the veins in the lower arm. The patient's arm is supported to keep the elbow straight so that the needle goes into the lumen of the vein, not through it. A vacuum tube is placed into the plastic holder and the vacuum draws blood into the tube. The tubes of blood are sent to the laboratory for testing.

Word or Phrase	Word Part and Definition	Description
vaccination	**vaccination** (VAK-sih-NAY-shun) **vaccin/o-** *giving a vaccine* **-ation** *a process; being or having* **vaccine** (vak-SEEN) *Vaccine* is derived from a Latin word meaning *pertaining to a cow* **attenuated** (ah-TEN-yoo-aa-ted) **attenu/o-** *weakened* **-ated** *pertaining to a condition; composed of* **immunization** (IM-yoo-nih-ZAY-shun **immun/o-** *immune response* **-ization** *the process of making, creating, or inserting*	Medical procedure that injects a vaccine into the body. The **vaccine** consists of killed or **attenuated** bacterial or viral cells or cell fragments. The body produces antibodies and memory B lymphocytes specific to that pathogen. If the vaccinated patient encounters that pathogen again, the patient will have mild or no symptoms of the disease. Vaccinations are routinely used to prevent diseases that could be fatal or cause serious disability if contracted (polio, diphtheria, tetanus, and so forth). Immunoglobins (antibodies) against some diseases (rabies or tetanus) can be given to provide passive immunity if the person has just been exposed. Also known as **immunization.** **A Closer Look** The principles of vaccination were established in 1796 by Edward Jenner, an English physician. He noticed that milkmaids did not get the serious disease smallpox because they first contracted cowpox, a viral disease of cows. Jenner took fluid from the skin sores of a milkmaid with cowpox. He made cuts in the skin of a young boy and introduced the fluid, and the boy later developed cowpox. Later, Jenner gave the boy the smallpox virus, and the boy did not develop smallpox. This medical practice was successful, but it horrified people. Cartoonists drew pictures of patients with cow parts coming out of their bodies. However, several years later, most doctors were using Jenner's technique to protect their patients from smallpox.
Blood Donation and Tranfusion Procedures		
apheresis	**apheresis** (AF-ah-REE-sis) *Apheresis* is a Greek word meaning *removal.*	Medical procedure that separates out one specific type of blood cell. The rest of the blood is returned to the donor. The collected cells are then given as a transfusion to a patient.
blood donation	**donation** (doh-NAY-shun) **donat/o-** *give as a gift* **-ion** *action; condition*	Medical procedure in which a unit of whole blood is collected from a donor. The unit is labeled as to blood type and stored in a blood bank. A unit of whole blood can be given as a transfusion, or the unit can be divided into its component parts (erythrocytes, platelets, plasma), and just that part can be given as a transfusion to meet the needs of a specific patient. **Connections** **Public Health.** All donated blood must be tested for syphilis, hepatitis, and HIV. The Food and Drug Administration (FDA) is responsible for the safety of blood and blood products used in the United States. The FDA has banned people from donating blood if they lived in or visited Europe for a certain length of time because of the possibility of contamination with the microorganism that causes mad cow disease.

Word or Phrase	Word Part and Definition	Description
blood transfusion	**transfusion** (trans-FYOO-shun) **trans-** *across, through* **fus/o-** *pouring* **-ion** *action; condition*	Whole blood, blood cellular products, or plasma can be given by intravenous transfusion. Transfusions of whole blood provide a complete correction of blood loss. Packed red blood cells (PRBCs) are a concentrated preparation of RBCs in a small amount of plasma. Transfusion with PRBCs avoids fluid overload in patients with congestive heart failure or in premature infants. Platelets are given to patients with thrombocytopenia or leukemia and to cancer patients whose bone marrow is depressed after radiation therapy or chemotherapy. Plasma is given to hemophiliac patients who need clotting factors.

A Closer Look

autologous (aw-TAWL-oh-gus)
auto- *self*
log/o- *relation*
-ous *pertaining to*
Here *log/o-* means *relation* rather than its usual meaning of *the study of.*

Patients scheduled to have certain types of surgery may be asked to donate a unit of their own blood in advance so they can receive it during surgery. This is known as an **autologous blood transfusion.** Also, blood in the operative field can be suctioned, collected, filtered, and returned to the patient during the surgery. At the conclusion of every surgery, the surgeon estimates the amount of blood loss and records this in the patient's operative report.

Word or Phrase	Word Part and Definition	Description
bone marrow transplantation (BMT)	**transplantation** (TRANS-plan-TAY-shun) **transplant/o-** *to move something to another place* **-ation** *a process; being or having*	Medical procedure used to treat patients with leukemia and lymphoma. Red marrow is harvested by aspirating it from the hip bone of a matched donor. The patient is treated with high-dose chemotherapy drugs or radiation to destroy all cancerous cells (this also destroys all the cells in the red marrow). The donor marrow is then filtered and given to the patient intravenously. The donated bone marrow cells travel through the blood to the bones where they implant. After two to four weeks, the patient's marrow begins to produce normal blood cells.

A Closer Look

allogeneic (AL-oh-jeh-NEE-ik)
all/o- *other; strange*
gene/o- *gene*
-ic *pertaining to*
Add words to make a correct definition of *allogeneic: pertaining to [someone] other [than the patient and that person's] genes.*

Unlike blood transfusions where donor blood and patient blood are crossmatched for compatibility of the ABO and Rh blood groups systems, bone marrow donors and recipient patients are matched for a different set of proteins called human leukocyte-associated (HLA) antigens. In **autologous transplants,** patients provide their own bone marrow or stem cells (which are treated to destroy any cancerous cells). In **allogeneic transplants,** patients receive bone marrow or stem cells donated by another person.

Word or Phrase	Word Part and Definition	Description
plasmapheresis	**plasmapheresis** (PLAZ-mah-feh-REE-sis) **plasm/o-** *plasma; formed substance* **apher/o-** *withdrawal* **-esis** *condition*	Medical procedure in which plasma is separated from the blood cells. A donor gives a unit of blood, which is rapidly spun in a centrifuge. Centrifugal force pulls the blood cells to the bottom of the bag. The plasma portion at the top is siphoned off and pooled with plasma from other donors to make fresh frozen plasma, albumin, or clotting factors. The blood cells are given back to the donor.
stem cell transplantation		Medical treatment for leukemia and lymphoma. Stem cells from the patient or matched donor are collected by apheresis. Matched stem cells from umbilical cord blood can also be used. The stem cells are given intravenously. They migrate to the red marrow and begin producing normal blood cells.

Surgical Procedures

Word or Phrase	Word Part and Definition	Description
lymph node biopsy	**biopsy** (BY-awp-see) **bi/o-** *life; living organisms; living tissue* **-opsy** *process of viewing* **excisional** (ek-SIZH-un-al) **excis/o-** *to cut out* **-ion** *action; condition* **-al** *pertaining to*	Surgical process that uses a fine needle to aspirate material from a lymph node. The lymph node may also be completely removed by doing an **excisional biopsy.**
lymph node dissection	**dissection** (dy-SEK-shun) **dissect/o-** *to cut apart* **-ion** *action; condition*	Surgical removal of several or all of the lymph nodes in a lymph node chain during extensive surgery for cancer.
splenectomy	**splenectomy** (spleh-NEK-toh-mee) **splen/o-** *spleen* **-ectomy** *surgical excision*	Surgical removal of the spleen when it has ruptured due to trauma. **Word Alert** **spleen** (noun) organ of the lymphatic system **splenectomy** (noun) surgical removal of the spleen **splenic** (adjective) pertaining to the spleen **splenomegaly** (noun) enlargement of the spleen
thymectomy	**thymectomy** (thy-MEK-toh-mee) **thym/o-** *thymus; rage* **-ectomy** *surgical excision*	Surgical removal of the thymus because of a benign or cancerous tumor. Thymectomy is also performed on patients with myasthenia gravis. After a thymectomy, the level of antibodies against acetylcholine receptors falls, and patients with myasthenia gravis can be treated with fewer immunosuppressant drugs. The reason for the improvement is not known.

Drug Categories

Several different categories of drugs are used to treat the symptoms, signs, and diseases of the blood and lymphatic system. The most common drugs in each category are listed.

Category	Word Part and Definition	Description	Examples
anticoagulant drugs	**anticoagulant** (AN-tee-koh-AG-yoo-lant) (AN-tih-koh-AG-yoo-lant) **anti-** *against* **coagul/o-** *clotting* **-ant** *pertaining to*	Prevent blood clot from forming by inhibiting the clotting factors or by inhibiting the production of vitamin K, which is needed to form the clotting factors.	Coumadin (oral), heparin (subcutaneous or intravenous)
chemotherapy drugs	**chemotherapy** (KEE-moh-THAIR-ah-pee) **chem/o-** *chemical, drug* **-therapy** *treatment*	Kill rapidly dividing cancer cells in the blood or lymphatic system.	Cytoxan, Myleran, VePesid

Category	Word Part and Definition	Description	Examples
colony-stimulating factor (CSF) drugs		In the body, colony-stimulating factor stimulates stem cells to mature into leukocytes. G-CSF stimulates the production of granulocytes; GM-CSF stimulates the production of granulocytes and macrophages.	Leukine (GM-CSF), Neupogen (G-CSF)
corticosteroid drugs	**corticosteroid** (KOR-tih-koh-STAIR-oyd) **cortic/o-** *cortex (outer region)* **-steroid** *steroid*	Anti-inflammatory drugs given to suppress the immune response and decrease inflammation. Also given to organ transplant patients to prevent rejection of the donor organ.	Decadron, prednisone, Solu-Medrol
erythropoietin	**erythropoietin** (eh-RITH-roh-POY-eh-tin) **erythr/o-** *red* **-poietin** *a substance that forms*	In the body, erythropoietin from the kidneys stimulates the red marrow to make erythrocytes. As a drug, erythropoietin has the same effect.	Epogen, Procrit
immuno-suppressant drugs	**immunosuppressant** (IM-yoo-noh-soo-PRES-ant) **immun/o-** *immune response* **suppress/o-** *press down* **-ant** *pertaining to*	Given to suppress the immune response. Prevents rejection of transplanted organ.	CellCept, Neoral, Prograf, Sandimmune
platelet aggregation inhibitor drugs	**inhibitor** (in-HIB-ih-tor) **inhibit/o-** *block; hold back* **-or** *person or thing that produces or does*	Prevent platelets from aggregating (clumping together), the first step in forming a blood clot.	Aggrastat, aspirin, Plavix, ReoPro, Ticlid
protease inhibitor drugs	**protease** (PROH-tee-ace) **prote/o-** *protein* **-ase** *enzyme*	Inhibit protease, an enzyme the virus needs to reproduce itself	Crixivan, Fortovase, Invirase
reverse transcriptase inhibitor drugs	**transcriptase** (trans-KRIP-tays)	Inhibit reverse transcriptase, an enzyme the virus needs to reproduce itself.	Epivir, Hivid, Retrovir, Sustiva, Viramune
thrombolytic enzyme drugs	**thrombolytic** (THRAWM-boh-LIT-ik) **thromb/o-** *thrombus (blood clot)* **ly/o-** *break down, separate, dissolve* **-tic** *pertaining to*	Dissolve blood clots that have already formed by breaking the fibrin strands.	Streptase The suffix *-ase* indicates that the drug is an enzyme.
tissue plasminogen activator (TPA) drugs	**plasminogen** (plaz-MIN-oh-jen)	Dissolve blood clots that have already formed by converting plasminogen to an enzyme that breaks the fibrin strands.	Activase, Retavase
vitamin B_{12} drugs		Used to treat pernicious anemia. Given by intramuscular injection or by nasal spray.	hydroxycobalamin, Nascobal

A Closer Look

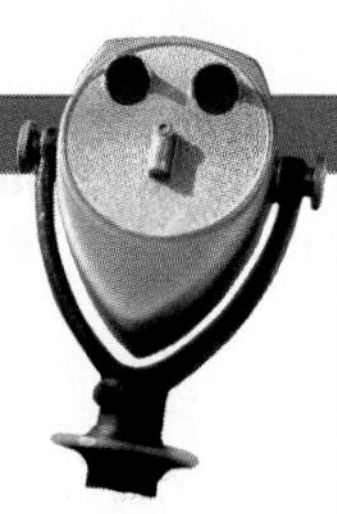

Some antiretroviral drugs exert their action on reverse transcriptase. *Retro-* refers to reverse transcriptase, an enzyme associated with the process of making viral RNA. Viral reverse transcriptase tells the DNA in a human cell to make more viral RNA and more viruses. This is backwards (retro-) from the normal process in which human DNA tells its own RNA what to produce.

antiretroviral
(AN-tee-REH-troh-VY-ral)
(AN-tih-REH-troh-VY-ral)
anti- *against*
retro- *behind, backward*
vir/o- *virus*
-al *pertaining to*

Abbreviations

A	a blood type in the ABO blood group
AB	a blood type in the ABO blood group
AIDS	acquired immunodeficiency syndrome
ALL	acute lymphocytic leukemia
AML	acute myelogenous leukemia
B	a blood type in the ABO blood group
basos	basophils
BMT	bone marrow transplantation
CBC	complete blood count
CLL	chronic lymphocytic leukemia
CML	chronic myelogenous leukemia
cmm	cubic millimeter
DIC	disseminated intravascular coagulation
diff	differential count of WBCs (slang)
EBV	Epstein-Barr virus
ELISA	enzyme-linked immunosorbent assay
eos	eosinophils
G-CSF	granulocyte colony-stimulating factor
GM-CSF	granulocyte-macrophage colony-stimulating factor
GVHD	graft-versus-host disease
HCT	hematocrit
Hgb	hemoglobin
H&H	hemoglobin and hematocrit
HIV	human immunodeficiency virus
HLA	human leukocyte antigen
IgA	immunoglobulin A
IgD	immunoglobulin D
IgE	immunoglobulin E
IgG	immunoglobulin G
IgM	immunoglobulin M
lymphs	lymphocytes
MCH	mean cell hemoglobin
MCHC	mean cell hemoglobin concentration
MCV	mean cell volume
mm^3	cubic millimeter
mono	mononucleosis (slang)
monos	monocytes
O	a blood type in the ABO blood group
PMN	polymorphonucleated leukocytes
polys	polymorphonucleated leukocytes
PRBCs	packed red blood cells
pro time	prothrombin time (slang)
PT	prothrombin time
PTT	partial thromboplastin time
RBC	red blood cell
segs	segmented neutrophils
TNF	tumor necrosis factor
TPA	tissue plasminogen activator (drug)
WBC	white blood cell

Word Alert

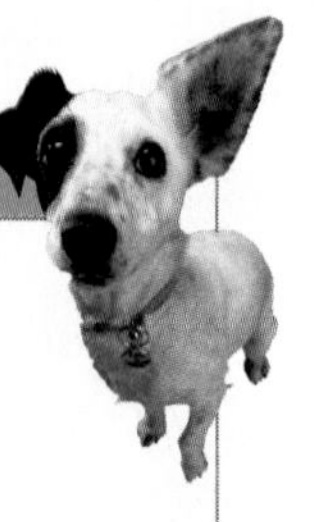

MEDICAL ABBREVIATIONS

Abbreviations are commonly used in all types of medical documents; however, they can mean different things to different people and their meaning can be misinterpreted. Always verify the meaning of an abbreviation.

Monos is a brief form that stands for *monocytes,* but the slang *mono* stands for *mononucleosis.*

PT stands for *prothrombin time,* but it can also stand for *physical therapy* or *physical therapist.*

Career Focus

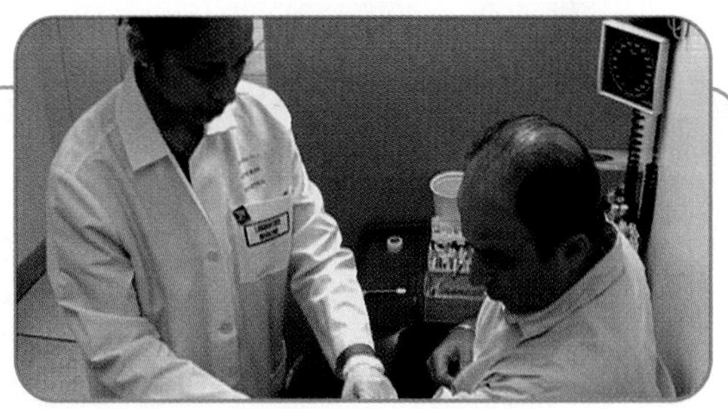

Meet Adriana, a phlebotomist in a hospital.

"A phlebotomist's job description is to draw blood, the collection of blood. On a daily basis, I draw about 30 to 50 patients. Every time it's someone different, so every time it's a different challenge. That's why I love it."

Phlebotomists are allied health professionals who use venipuncture techniques to draw blood. They follow procedures for storing and transporting blood specimens for diagnostic testing in the laboratory.

Hematologists are physicians who practice in the medical specialty of hematology. They diagnose and treat patients with diseases of the blood. Malignancies of the blood and lymphatic system are treated medically by an oncologist or surgically by a general surgeon.

Immunologists are physicians or they are scientists who have a Ph.D. in cellular biology or pharmacology. They practice in the medical specialty of immunology. Clinical immunologists diagnose and treat patients who have autoimmune diseases, immunodeficiency diseases, cancer, or who are undergoing transplantation (organ, bone marrow, or stem cell).

phlebotomist (fleh-BAWT-oh-mist)
phleb/o- *vein*
tom/o- *a cut, slice, or layer*
-ist *one who specializes in*

hematologist (HEE-mah-TAWL-oh-jist)
hemat/o- *blood*
log/o- *the study of*
-ist *one who specializes in*

immunologist (IM-yoo-NAWL-oh-jist)
immun/o- *immune response*
log/o- *the study of*
-ist *one who specializes in*

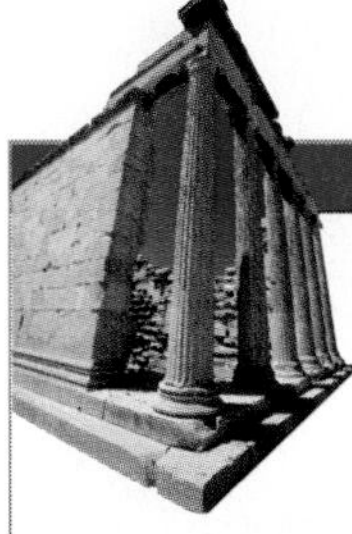

It's Greek to Me!

Did you notice that some blood and lymphatic system words have two different combining forms? Combining forms from both Greek and Latin languages remain a part of medical language today.

English Word	Greek	Latin	Examples of Medical Words
cell	cyt/o-	cellul/o-	pancytopenia, cellular
form, shape	morph/o-	plast/o-	polymorphonucleated, aplastic
nucleus	kary/o-	nucle/o-	megakaryocyte, polymorphonucleated
red	eosin/o-	rub/o-	eosinophil, bilirubin
	erythr/o-		erythrocyte
vein	phleb/o-	ven/o-	phlebotomy, venous

Chapter Review Exercises

Review all the material in this chapter by completing the review exercises in this section. Use the Answer Key at the end of the book to check your answers.

Anatomy and Physiology

Matching Exercise

Match each numbered word or phrase to its description.

1. albumin	____	Secreted by the kidneys to increase RBCs
2. B cell	____	The most immature cell in the red marrow
3. bilirubin	____	Cell fragment
4. eosinophil	____	Maternal antibodies cross placenta to fetus
5. erythrocyte	____	Cessation of bleeding
6. erythropoietin	____	Has granules that stain red with eosin
7. hematopoiesis	____	Process of engulfing foreign cells
8. hemoglobin	____	Carries oxygen and carbon dioxide
9. hemostasis	____	Red blood cell
10. macrophage	____	Clear yellow liquid part of blood
11. lymphocyte	____	Type of agranulocyte
12. passive immunity	____	Process by which blood cells are formed
13. phagocytosis	____	Antioxidant that protects from damage by free radicals
14. plasma	____	Most abundant plasma protein
15. stem cell	____	Monocytes in lymph nodes that eat pathogens
16. thrombocyte	____	Lymphocyte that develops in the red marrow

True or False

Indicate whether each statement is true or false by writing T or F on the line.

1. ____ The fluid portion of blood without the clotting factors is known as serum.
2. ____ Carbon monoxide poisoning causes the skin to become cherry red.
3. ____ IgG is the smallest immunoglobulin.
4. ____ Blood type AB negative is known as the universal donor.
5. ____ The three different categories of blood cells are erythrocytes, lymphocytes, and platelets.
6. ____ Bands are also known as segs.
7. ____ The formation of a blood clot is known as coagulation.
8. ____ Megakaryoblasts are large cells whose cytoplasm breaks off to form platelets.
9. ____ Endotoxins are poisons produced by some bacteria.
10. ____ Plasma cells produce the plasma portion of blood.

Circle Exercise

Circle the correct word from the choices given.

1. (**Blood, Serum, Thymus**) is a connective tissue that travels to every part of the body.
2. (**Hemoglobin, Platelets, Red blood cells**) are cells that have no nucleus.
3. Strong elastic bands that trap erythrocytes to form a clot are known as (**antigens, fibrin, lymph nodes**).
4. Microorganisms that cause disease are known as (**antibodies, antigens, pathogens**).
5. Chemicals with a positive or negative charge are known as (**clotting factors, electrolytes, plasma proteins**).
6. (**IgA, IgD, IgM**) is the immunoglobulin present in tears, saliva, and breast milk.
7. Iron is carried in the (**globin, globulin, heme**) part of the erythrocyte.
8. The process of platelets clumping together at the site of an injury is known as (**aggregation, coagulation, hemostasis**).

Multiple Choice

Select the choice that best completes the statement.

1. Red blood cells are known by the name ________________.
   a. monocytes
   b. lymphocytes
   c. basophils
   d. erythrocytes
   e. none of the above

2. Immature forms of erythrocytes include all of the following EXCEPT ________________.
   a. reticulocytes
   b. myelocytes
   c. erythroblasts
   d. normoblasts
   e. stem cells

3. All of the following are breakdown products of hemoglobin EXCEPT ________________.
   a. globin chains
   b. iron
   c. heme
   d. monocytes
   e. bilirubin

4. ________________ is a cytokine produced by macrophages that produces fever and stimulates the production of helper T cells.
   a. Thymosin
   b. Endotoxin
   c. Interleukin
   d. Infection
   e. Antigen

Fill in the Blank

Answer each of these questions by filling in the correct answers in the blanks provided.

1. Name the four blood types in the ABO blood group system.

   ________________ ________________ ________________ ________________

2. Granulocytes is a category that includes which three types of white blood cells?

   ________________ ________________ ________________

3. Give three names for a neutrophil.

   ________________ ________________ ________________

4. Name the two lymphoid organs of the lymphatic system.

   ________________ ________________

Matching Exercise

Match each numbered word or phrase to its description.

1.	adenoids	_____	Limit the extent and duration of the immune response
2.	CD4 cell	_____	Released from basophils and mast cells
3.	cytokines	_____	Protein molecule messengers that communicate between cells
4.	histamine	_____	Makes antibodies
5.	Peyer's patches	_____	Destroys pathogens not coated by antibodies or complement proteins
6.	plasma cell	_____	Hormones produced by the thymus
7.	skin	_____	Filters blood and removes old erythrocytes
8.	spleen	_____	Lymphatic tissue in the nasopharynx
9.	suppressor T cells	_____	Body's first line of defense
10.	NK cell	_____	Lymphatic tissue areas in the small intestines
11.	thymosins	_____	Helper T cell

Medical Language Word Parts

Name that Word Part

Identify each of the word parts given here by writing the correct letter (P, C, or S) on the line beside it. Then write the definition of the word part on the blank line. The first one has been done for you.

Prefix = P **Combining Form = C** **Suffix = S**

		Word Part	Definition			Word Part	Definition
1.	a-	P	away from, without	21.	bas/o-	_____	_____
2.	aden/o-	_____	_____	22.	bi/o-	_____	_____
3.	agglutin/o-	_____	_____	23.	-blast	_____	_____
4.	aggreg/o-	_____	_____	24.	-body	_____	_____
5.	-al	_____	_____	25.	calc/o-	_____	_____
6.	an-	_____	_____	26.	chrom/o-	_____	_____
7.	angi/o-	_____	_____	27.	coagul/o-	_____	_____
8.	anis/o-	_____	_____	28.	compromis/o-	_____	_____
9.	-ant	_____	_____	29.	cortic/o-	_____	_____
10.	anti-	_____	_____	30.	-crasia	_____	_____
11.	apher/o-	_____	_____	31.	-cyte	_____	_____
12.	-ar	_____	_____	32.	cyt/o-	_____	_____
13.	-ase	_____	_____	33.	defici/o-	_____	_____
14.	aspir/o-	_____	_____	34.	different/o-	_____	_____
15.	-ate	_____	_____	35.	dissect/o-	_____	_____
16.	-ated	_____	_____	36.	dissemin/o-	_____	_____
17.	-atic	_____	_____	37.	dys-	_____	_____
18.	-ation	_____	_____	38.	-ectomy	_____	_____
19.	attenu/o-	_____	_____	39.	-ed	_____	_____
20.	auto-	_____	_____	40.	-edema	_____	_____

		Word Part	Definition
41.	electr/o-	______	______
42.	embol/o-	______	______
43.	-emia	______	______
44.	-ency	______	______
45.	endo-	______	______
46.	eosin/o-	______	______
47.	erythr/o-	______	______
48.	-esis	______	______
49.	excis/o-	______	______
50.	ferrit/o-	______	______
51.	ferr/o-	______	______
52.	fibrin/o-	______	______
53.	fibr/o-	______	______
54.	fus/o-	______	______
55.	-gen	______	______
56.	gen/o-	______	______
57.	glob/o-	______	______
58.	globul/o-	______	______
59.	-gram	______	______
60.	granul/o-	______	______
61.	-graphy	______	______
62.	hemat/o-	______	______
63.	hem/o-	______	______
64.	heter/o-	______	______
65.	hyper-	______	______
66.	hypo-	______	______
67.	-ia	______	______
68.	-iac	______	______
69.	-ial	______	______
70.	-ic	______	______
71.	idi/o-	______	______
72.	-immune	______	______
73.	immun/o-	______	______
74.	-in	______	______
75.	inhibit/o-	______	______
76.	inter-	______	______
77.	intra-	______	______
78.	-ion	______	______
79.	-ism	______	______
80.	-ist	______	______
81.	-ity	______	______
82.	-ization	______	______

		Word Part	Definition
83.	kary/o-	______	______
84.	-kine	______	______
85.	leuk/o-	______	______
86.	log/o-	______	______
87.	-logy	______	______
88.	lymph/o-	______	______
89.	ly/o-	______	______
90.	-lysis	______	______
91.	-lyte	______	______
92.	macr/o-	______	______
93.	meg/a-	______	______
94.	megal/o-	______	______
95.	-megaly	______	______
96.	micr/o-	______	______
97.	mon/o-	______	______
98.	morph/o-	______	______
99.	myel/o-	______	______
100.	neutr/o-	______	______
101.	norm/o-	______	______
102.	nucle/o-	______	______
103.	-oid	______	______
104.	-oma	______	______
105.	opportun/o-	______	______
106.	-opsy	______	______
107.	-or	______	______
108.	-osis	______	______
109.	-ous	______	______
110.	ox/y-	______	______
111.	pan-	______	______
112.	path/o-	______	______
113.	-pathy	______	______
114.	-penia	______	______
115.	peripher/o-	______	______
116.	-phage	______	______
117.	phag/o-	______	______
118.	-phil	______	______
119.	phil/o-	______	______
120.	phleb/o-	______	______
121.	phor/o-	______	______
122.	plasm/o-	______	______
123.	plast/o-	______	______
124.	-poiesis	______	______

		Word Part	Definition
125.	-poietin	_____	_______________
126.	poikil/o-	_____	_______________
127.	poly-	_____	_______________
128.	pro-	_____	_______________
129.	prote/o-	_____	_______________
130.	punct/o-	_____	_______________
131.	reticul/o-	_____	_______________
132.	-rrhage	_____	_______________
133.	rub/o-	_____	_______________
134.	septic/o-	_____	_______________
135.	son/o-	_____	_______________
136.	splen/o-	_____	_______________
137.	-stasis	_____	_______________
138.	-steroid	_____	_______________
139.	suppress/o-	_____	_______________
140.	-therapy	_____	_______________
141.	thromb/o-	_____	_______________
142.	thym/o-	_____	_______________
143.	-tic	_____	_______________
144.	-tomy	_____	_______________
145.	tox/o-	_____	_______________
146.	trans-	_____	_______________
147.	transplant/o-	_____	_______________
148.	ultra-	_____	_______________
149.	-ure	_____	_______________
150.	vaccin/o-	_____	_______________
151.	vascul/o-	_____	_______________
152.	ven/i-	_____	_______________
153.	viscos/o-	_____	_______________

Symptoms, Signs, and Diseases

Matching Exercise

Match each numbered word or phrase to its definition.

1. acute lymphocytic	____ Abnormal immunoglobulin seen in multiple myeloma
2. AIDS	____ Caused by exposure to chemicals or radiation
3. anisocytosis	____ Cancerous tumor of a lymph node
4. aplastic anemia	____ Seen in Hodgkin's lymphoma
5. Bence Jones protein	____ Enlargement of the spleen
6. dyscrasia	____ Causes hemolysis of erythrocytes
7. hemophilia	____ Transmitted on the X chromosome of females
8. lymphoma	____ Any disease condition of the blood
9. megaloblasts	____ Caused by genetic abnormality of hemoglobin
10. polycythemia vera	____ Severe bacterial infection in the blood
11. Reed-Sternberg cells	____ Sexually transmitted viral disease
12. septicemia	____ Most common leukemia in childhood
13. sickle cell anemia	____ Erythrocytes vary in size from very small to very large
14. splenomegaly	____ Abnormally large, very immature erythrocytes seen in some anemias
15. transfusion reaction	____ Blood becomes thick with erythrocytes

True or False

Indicate whether each statement is true or false by writing T or F on the line.

1. ____ Pancytopenia is a condition of decreased numbers of platelets in the blood.
2. ____ In iron deficiency anemia, the erythrocytes are microcytic and hypochromic.
3. ____ Opportunistic infections cause diseases in people if they already have hemophilia.
4. ____ *Coagulopathy* is a general word for any disease that affects the ability of the blood to clot.
5. ____ In sickle cell anemia, once an erthrocyte become sickled (bent), it stays that way for the rest of the life span of the cell.
6. ____ All patients with HIV also have AIDS.
7. ____ AIDS is a sexually transmitted disease that is also known as the kissing disease.
8. ____ The most common type of hemophilia is lacking blood clotting factor I.
9. ____ Petechiae are pinpoint hemorrhages in the skin.
10. ____ A thymoma is a usually benign tumor of the thymus.

Multiple Choice

Circle the choice that best answers the question or completes the statement.

1. Which of the following is an autoimmune disease?
   a. hemorrhage c. rheumatoid arthritis
   b. hemophilia d. leukemia

2. Which of the following is an inherited genetic disease?
   a. hemophilia c. HIV
   b. thymoma d. iron deficiency anemia

3. Poikilocytosis includes all of these abnormally shaped cells EXCEPT ____________.
   a. sphereocyte c. target cell
   b. blast d. sickle cell

4. Pernicious anemia is most commonly seen in ____________.
   a. children c. women
   b. patients with cancer d. the elderly

5. Which of the following diseases is caused by the Epstein-Barr virus (EBV)?
   a. leukemia c. mononucleosis
   b. anemia d. thalassemia

Word-Building Exercise

Use the combining forms, prefixes, and suffixes given here to build medical words that match the definitions given. Write the word that you build on the blank line. Some word parts may be used more than once. The first one has been done for you.

Word Parts List

-ation (a process; being or having)	hem/o- (blood)	-oma (tumor, mass)
chrom/o- (color)	hypo- (below; deficient)	pan- (all)
coagul/o- (clotting)	-ia (condition, state, thing)	-penia (condition of deficiency)
-cyte (cell)	-ic (pertaining to)	phil/o- (attraction to, fondness for)
cyt/o- (cell)	leuk/o- (white)	-rrhage (excessive flow or discharge)
-emia (condition of the blood; substance in the blood)	lymph/o- (lymph; lymphatic system)	thromb/o- (thrombus, blood clot)
erythr/o- (red)	-lysis (process of breaking down or dissolving)	

Definition	Word Parts	Write the Medical Word
1. Red blood cell	erythro- + -cyte	erythrocyte
2. Excessive loss of a large amount of blood	______ + ______	______
3. Pertaining to decreased color (in RBCs)	______ + ______ + ______	______
4. Blood cancer with increased leukocytes	______ + ______	______
5. Process of breaking down blood cells during a transfusion reaction	______ + ______	______
6. Condition of deficiency of all types of blood cells	______ + ______ + ______	______
7. Inherited problem with blood clotting	______ + ______ + ______	______
8. Process of blood clotting	______ + ______	______
9. White blood cell	______ + ______	______
10. Condition of deficiency of platelets	______ + ______ + ______	______
11. Cancerous tumor of lymph node	______ + ______	______

Laboratory, Radiology, Surgery, and Drugs

Circle Exercise

Circle the correct word from the choices given.

1. The physician would order a (**ferritin level, lymphangiogram, type and crossmatch**) to see if the patient had iron deficiency anemia.
2. A bone marrow aspiration is done by taking red marrow from the (**blood, iliac crest, spleen**).
3. The red blood cell indices include (**HCT, MCV, WBC**).
4. The (**DNA, HCT, INR**) is given in a standardized international measurement along with the PT.
5. This test uses gel and an electric current to separate proteins: (**electrophoresis, prothrombin time, Schilling test**).
6. The (**CBC, CD4 count, heterophil antibodies test**) measures the number of helper T lymphocytes.
7. (**Anticoagulant, Antiretroviral, Antithrombolytic**) drugs are used to break apart an already formed blood clot.

Matching Exercise

Match each numbered word or phrase to its description.

1. blood smear	_____	Counts the number of different types of leukocytes
2. blood type	_____	Manual test to look for abnormal blood cells
3. bone marrow aspiration	_____	Used to diagnose mononucleosis
4. differential	_____	Also known as harvesting
5. hematocrit	_____	Uses attenuated or killed bacteria
6. lymphangiogram	_____	Uses dye to outline the lymphatic system
7. MonoSpot test	_____	Used to diagnose pernicious anemia
8. Schilling test	_____	Percentage of erythrocytes in a sample of blood
9. shift to the left	_____	ABO and Rh systems
10. vaccine	_____	Presence of immature neutrophils indicates a severe bacterial infection on blood smear

Abbreviations

Match each numbered abbreviation to its description.

1. ABO	_____	Hemoglobin and hematocrit tests
2. CBC	_____	Another name for a neutrophil
3. DIC	_____	A type of leukemia
4. EBV	_____	Causes AIDS
5. H&H	_____	Must be matched for blood transfusions
6. HIV	_____	Concentrated erythrocytes for transfusion
7. HLA	_____	Disease with both clotting and hemorrhage at the same time
8. PMN	_____	Common test on blood
9. PRBCs	_____	Must be matched for bone marrow and organ transplantation
10. PT	_____	Causes mononucleosis
11. CML	_____	Test that measures coagulation time of blood

Applied Skills

Analysis of a Laboratory Report

This exercise contains a laboratory report. Read the report and answer the questions. Use the Answer Key at the end of the book to check your answers.

ACCESSION NUMBER: 309-019
LOCATION: Central Lab
DATE DRAWN: 11/19/xx
DATE RECEIVED: 11/19/xx
TIME RECEIVED: 0900

PATIENT NAME: THOMAS, Irene
PATIENT ID NUMBER: 365-14-3972
DATE OF BIRTH: 07/29/xx
SEX: Female

Procedure	Result	Normal Range	Technician
Complete Blood Count (CBC)			
RBC	4.70 m/cmm	4.2–5.7 m/cmm	JRT
HEMOGLOBIN	14.7 g/dL	12.6–16.6 g/dL	JRT
HEMATOCRIT	42.9%	38.0–50.0%	JRT
MCV	91.2 fL	80–100 fL	JRT
MCH	31.3 pg	28.0–33.0 pg	JRT
MCHC	34.3 g/dL	32–36 g/dL	JRT
WBC	7.7 k/cmm	4.3–10.5 k/cmm	JRT
PLATELETS	142 k/cmm	150–450 k/cmm	JRT

FACT FINDING QUESTIONS

1. What is the name of the group of tests done on this patient? ____________________
2. What unit of measurement is used to report RBCs? ____________________
3. Write out this unit of measurement in words. ____________________
4. What individual test result was not within the normal range of values? ____________________
5. What does the *k* stand for in the unit of measurement k/cmm? ____________________

Analysis of a Medical Report

This exercise contains an Emergency Department Report. Read the report and answer the questions.

EMERGENCY DEPARTMENT REPORT

PATIENT NAME: JONES, JEROME

HOSPITAL NUMBER: 635-64-46223

DATE: November 19, 20xx

HISTORY OF PRESENT ILLNESS

This 42-year-old black male presented to the emergency room today with complaints of dysphagia, extreme weakness, fevers, diarrhea, and weight loss.

PAST MEDICAL HISTORY

He has a prior history of intravenous heroin usage for many years and was diagnosed with HIV about 6 years ago. At that time, he was HIV positive on serology testing, but was asymptomatic with a CD4 count of 500. He was subsequently lost to follow-up until recently. In the last few months, his health has deteriorated rapidly, but he refused to seek medical attention. Last month, however, he was admitted to this hospital through the emergency department in respiratory distress with a CD4 count of 100 and was diagnosed with *Pneumocystis carinii* pneumonia and AIDS. He was given a 14-day course of intravenous pentamidine. He was discharged on a triple-drug regimen of Retrovir, Epivir, and Sustiva. He was also given a prescription for aerosolized pentamidine to prevent future episodes of PCP. He has been noncompliant with his drug therapy, stating that he does not take his AIDS drugs on a regular basis.

PHYSICAL EXAMINATION

GENERAL: Physical examination today showed a black male appearing much older than his stated age. Temperature 101.2, pulse 100, respirations 26, blood pressure 110/76. Height: 5 feet 11 inches. Weight 128 pounds. HEENT exam: Normocephalic, atraumatic. Eyes: Sclerae and conjunctivae pale and nonicteric. Brisk pupillary response. Extraocular movements intact. Dilated funduscopic examination revealed no retinal abnormalities indicative of cytomegalovirus retinitis. Mouth: White plaque coating on the tongue. When the plaque is scraped away with a tongue depressor, the tongue underneath is beefy red and bleeds slightly. Examination with a laryngeal mirror reveals plaques on the tonsils and in the oropharynx. Neck: The neck is supple with cervical lymphadenopathy.
HEART: Regular rate and rhythm with no murmurs, gallops, or rubs.
CHEST: Clear.
ABDOMEN: Soft, nontender, with normal bowel sounds.
EXTREMITIES: Wasting of the extremities. Extreme weakness with muscle strength 2/5 bilaterally. Deep tendon reflexes intact bilaterally. The skin is negative.

DIAGNOSES

1. Oral candidiasis.
2. Wasting syndrome, secondary to acquired immunodeficiency syndrome (AIDS).
3. Acquired immunodeficiency syndrome (AIDS).
4. Past history of *Pneumocystis carinii* pneumonia.

PLAN

Blood work was sent for CBC and differential, CD4 total count, and CD4:CD8 ratio. The patient was restarted on his antiretroviral 3-drug regimen of Retrovir 300 mg b.i.d., Epivir 150 mg b.i.d., and Sustiva 600 mg q.d. h.s. He was given nystatin oral suspension 5 cc q.i.d., swish and swallow, to treat his oral infection with *Candida albicans*. He will be begun on Megace oral suspension, 20 mg/0.5 cc, to stimulate his appetite and help him gain weight.

Joseph K. McAdams, M.D.

Joseph K. McAdams, M.D.

JKM:ltt
D: 11/19/xx
T: 11/19/xx

FACT FINDING QUESTIONS

1. Six years ago, the patient was "asymptomatic," which means that ____________________.
   a. he did not have an HIV infection
   b. he did not have any symptoms of an HIV infection
   c. he was healthy

2. What two opportunistic infections have complicated this patient's AIDS?

   ____

   ____

3. What do these abbreviations stand for?

   AIDS ____

   PCP ____

4. What was the patient's CD4 count six years ago? ____________________

   What was the patient's CD4 count when he was diagnosed with AIDS? ____________________

5. What three drugs were prescribed for the patient's AIDS?

   ____

   ____

   ____

6. What category of drugs do these three drugs belong to? ____________________

7. What laboratory test was ordered to show the current number of helper T lymphocytes? ____________________

CRITICAL THINKING QUESTIONS

1. What is the probable source of the patient's HIV infection? ____________________

2. Which of these symptoms is related to the patient's oral candidiasis?
   a. extreme weakness
   b. fevers
   c. dysphagia
   d. diarrhea

3. When the patient was admitted to the hospital last month with *Pneumocystis carinii* pneumonia, why was his diagnosis changed from HIV positive to AIDS? ____________________

4. The patient is diagnosed with wasting syndrome due to AIDS. What three pieces of information support this diagnosis?
   a. Hint: Look for a phrase at the beginning of the History of Present Illness.

      ____

   b. Hint: Look for a measurement in the "General" section of the Physical Examination.

      ____

   c. Hint: Look for a phrase in the "Extremities" section of the Physical Examination.

      ____

5. Serology is laboratory testing that detects the ____________________.
   a. symptoms of HIV.
   b. presence of HIV in the saliva.
   c. presence of antibodies to HIV.

6. In what part of the body did the physician find enlarged lymph nodes? ____________________

Pronunciation Checklist

Read each word and its pronunciation. Practice pronouncing each word. Verify your pronunciation by listening to the Pronunciation List on the CD-ROM. Check the box next to each word after you master its pronunication.

- ❑ agglutination (ah-GLOO-tih-NAY-shun)
- ❑ aggregation (AG-reh-GAY-shun)
- ❑ agranulocyte (aa-GRAN-yoo-loh-site)
- ❑ albumin (al-BYOO-min)
- ❑ allogeneic (AL-oh-jeh-NEE-ik)
- ❑ anemia (ah-NEE-mee-ah)
- ❑ anemic (ah-NEE-mik)
- ❑ anisocytosis (an-EYE-soh-sy-TOH-sis)
- ❑ antibody (AN-tee-BAWD-ee) (AN-tih-BAWD-ee)
- ❑ anticoagulant drug (AN-tee-koh-AG-yoo-lant DRUHG) (AN-tih-koh-AG-yoo-lant DRUHG)
- ❑ antigen (AN-tih-jen)
- ❑ apheresis (AF-ah-REE-sis)
- ❑ aplastic (aa-PLAS-tik)
- ❑ attenuated vaccine (ah-TEN-yoo-aa-ted vak-SEEN)
- ❑ autoimmune (AW-toh-ih-MYOON)
- ❑ basophil (BAY-soh-fil)
- ❑ biopsy (BY-awp-see)
- ❑ blood donation (BLUD doh-NAY-shun)
- ❑ bone marrow aspiration (BOHN MAIR-oh AS-pih-RAY-shun)
- ❑ bone marrow transplantation (BOHN MAIR-oh TRANS-plan-TAY-shun)
- ❑ cancer (KAN-ser)
- ❑ chemotherapy drug (KEE-moh-THAIR-ah-pee DRUHG)
- ❑ coagulation (koh-AG-yoo-LAY-shun)
- ❑ coagulopathy (koh-AG-yoo-LAWP-ah-thee)
- ❑ complement protein (COM-pleh-ment PRO-teen)
- ❑ corticosteroid drug (KOR-tih-koh-STAIR-oyd DRUHG)
- ❑ cytokine (SY-toh-kine)
- ❑ cytotoxic (SY-toh-TAWK-sik)
- ❑ differential (DIF-er-EN-shal)
- ❑ disseminated intravascular coagulation (dih-SEM-ih-NAYT-ed IN-trah-VAS-kyoo-lar koh-AG-yoo-LAY-shun)
- ❑ dyscrasia (dis-KRAY-zee-ah)
- ❑ ecchymoses (EK-ih-MOH-seez)
- ❑ electrolyte (ee-LEK-troh-lite)
- ❑ electrophoresis (ee-LEK-troh-foh-REE-sis)
- ❑ embolism (EM-boh-liz-em)
- ❑ embolus (EM-boh-lus)
- ❑ endotoxin (EN-doh-TAWK-sin)
- ❑ eosinophil (EE-oh-SIN-oh-fil)
- ❑ erythroblast (eh-RITH-roh-blast)
- ❑ erythrocyte (eh-RITH-roh-site)
- ❑ erythropoietin (eh-RITH-roh-POY-eh-tin)
- ❑ excisional biopsy (ek-SIH-zhun-al BY-awp-see)
- ❑ ferritin (FAIR-ih-tin)
- ❑ fibrin (FY-brin)
- ❑ fibrinogen (fy-BRIN-oh-jen)
- ❑ globin (GLOH-bin)
- ❑ granulocyte (GRAN-yoo-loh-site)
- ❑ hematocrit (hee-MAT-oh-krit)
- ❑ hematologist (HEE-mah-TAWL-oh-jist)
- ❑ hematology (HEE-mah-TAWL-oh-jee)
- ❑ hematopoiesis (HEE-mah-toh-poy-EE-sis)
- ❑ heme (HEEM)
- ❑ hemoglobin (HEE-moh-GLOH-bin) (hee-moh-GLOH-bin)
- ❑ hemolysis (hee-MAWL-ih-sis)
- ❑ hemolytic anemia (HEE-moh-LIT-ik ah-NEE-mee-ah)
- ❑ hemophilia (HEE-moh-FIL-ee-ah)
- ❑ hemophiliac (HEE-moh-FIL-ee-ak)
- ❑ hemorrhage (HEM-oh-rij)
- ❑ hemostasis (HEE-moh-STAY-sis)
- ❑ heterophil antibody (HET-er-oh-fil AN-tee-BAWD-ee)
- ❑ Hodgkin disease (HAWJ-kin dih-ZEEZ)
- ❑ hypochromic (HY-poh-KROH-mik)
- ❑ idiopathic (ID-ee-oh-PATH-ik)
- ❑ immune (ih-MYOON)
- ❑ immunity (ih-MYOO-nih-tee)
- ❑ immunocompromised (IM-yoo-noh-COM-proh-myzd)
- ❑ immunodeficiency (IM-yoo-noh-deh-FISH-en-see)
- ❑ immunoglobulin (IM-yoo-noh-GLAWB-yoo-lin)
- ❑ immunologist (IM-yoo-NAWL-oh-jist)
- ❑ immunology (IM-yoo-NAWL-oh-jee)
- ❑ immunosuppressant drug (IM-yoo-noh-soo-PRES-ant DRUHG)
- ❑ immunization (IM-yoo-nih-ZAY-shun)
- ❑ index (IN-deks)
- ❑ indices (IN-dih-seez)
- ❑ inhibitor (in-HIB-ih-tor)
- ❑ interferon (IN-ter-FEER-on)
- ❑ interleukin (IN-ter-LOO-kin)
- ❑ intravascular (IN-trah-VAS-kyoo-lar)
- ❑ leukemia (loo-KEE-mee-ah)
- ❑ leukocyte (LOO-koh-site)
- ❑ lymph (LIMF)
- ❑ lymph node (LIMF NOHD)
- ❑ lymph node dissection (LIMF NOHD dy-SEK-shun)
- ❑ lymphadenopathy (lim-FAD-eh-NAWP-eh-thee)
- ❑ lymphangiogram (lim-FAN-jee-oh-gram)
- ❑ lymphangiography (lim-FAN-jee-AWG-rah-fee)
- ❑ lymphatic system (lim-FAT-ik SIS-tem)
- ❑ lymphedema (LIM-fah-DEE-mah)
- ❑ lymphoblast (LIM-foh-blast)
- ❑ lymphocyte (LIM-foh-site)
- ❑ lymphocytic leukemia (LIM-foh-SIT-ik loo-KEE-mee-ah)
- ❑ lymphoid (LIM-foyd)
- ❑ lymphoma (lim-FOH-mah)
- ❑ macrocyte (MAK-roh-site)
- ❑ macrophage (MAK-roh-fayj)
- ❑ megakaryoblast (MEG-ah-KAIR-ee-oh-blast)
- ❑ megakaryocyte (MEG-ah-KAIR-ee-oh-site)
- ❑ megaloblast (MEG-ah-loh-blast)
- ❑ microcyte (MY-kroh-site)
- ❑ microcytic (MY-kroh-SIT-ik)
- ❑ monoblast (MAWN-oh-blast)
- ❑ monocyte (MAWN-oh-site)
- ❑ mononucleosis (MAWN-oh-noo-klee-OH-sis)
- ❑ morphology (mor-FAWL-oh-jee)
- ❑ myeloblast (MY-eh-loh-blast)
- ❑ myelocyte (MY-eh-loh-site)
- ❑ myelogenous leukemia (MY-eh-LAWJ-eh-nus loo-KEE-mee-ah)
- ❑ myeloma (MY-eh-LOH-mah)
- ❑ neutrophil (NOO-troh-fil)
- ❑ normoblast (NOR-moh-blast)
- ❑ normochromic (NOR-moh-KROH-mik)
- ❑ normocytic (NOR-moh-SIT-ik)
- ❑ opportunistic infection (AWP-or-too-NIS-tik in-FEK-shun)
- ❑ oxyhemoglobin (AWK-see-HEE-moh-GLOH-bin)
- ❑ pancytopenia (PAN-sy-toh-PEE-nee-ah)
- ❑ pathogen (PATH-oh-jen)

- ❑ peripheral (peh-RIF-eh-ral)
- ❑ pernicious (per-NISH-us)
- ❑ petechiae (peh-TEE-kee-ee)
- ❑ phagocyte (FAG-oh-site)
- ❑ phagocytosis (FAG-oh-sy-TOH-sis)
- ❑ phlebotomist (fleh-BAWT-oh-mist)
- ❑ phlebotomy (fleh-BAWT-oh-mee)
- ❑ plasma (PLAZ-mah)
- ❑ plasmapheresis (PLAZ-mah-feh-REE-sis)
- ❑ plasminogen (plaz-MIN-oh-jen)
- ❑ platelet (PLAYT-let)
- ❑ poikilocytosis (POY-kih-loh-sy-TOH-sis)
- ❑ polycythemia vera (PAWL-ee-sy-THEE-mee-ah VER-ah)
- ❑ polymorphonucleated leukocyte (PAWL-ee-MOR-foh-NOO-klee-aa-ted LOO-koh-site)
- ❑ protease inhibitor drug (PROH-tee-ace in-HIB-ih-tor DRUHG)
- ❑ prothrombin (proh-THRAWM-bin)
- ❑ purpura (PER-peh-rah)
- ❑ reticulocyte (reh-TIK-yoo-loh-site)
- ❑ reverse transcriptase inhibitor drug (ree-VERS trans-KRIP-tays in-HIB-ih-tor DRUHG)
- ❑ septic (SEP-tic)
- ❑ septicemia (SEP-tih-SEE-mee-ah)
- ❑ serum (SEER-um)
- ❑ spleen (SPLEEN)
- ❑ splenectomy (spleh-NEK-toh-mee)
- ❑ splenic (SPLEH-nik)
- ❑ splenomegaly (SPLEH-noh-MEG-ah-lee)
- ❑ suppressor (soo-PRES-or)
- ❑ thalassemia (THAL-ah-SEE-mee-ah)
- ❑ thrombocyte (THRAWM-boh-site)
- ❑ thrombocytopenia (THRAWM-boh-SY-toh-PEE-nee-ah)
- ❑ thrombolytic drug (THRAWM-boh-LIT-ik DRUHG)
- ❑ thromboplastin (THRAWM-boh-PLAS-tin)
- ❑ thrombosis (thrawm-BOH-sis)
- ❑ thrombus (THRAWM-bus)
- ❑ thymectomy (thy-MEK-toh-mee)
- ❑ thymic (THY-mik)
- ❑ thymoma (thy-MOH-mah)
- ❑ thymosin (thy-MOH-sin)
- ❑ thymus (THY-mus)
- ❑ transferrin (trans-FAIR-in)
- ❑ transfusion (trans-FYOO-shun)
- ❑ ultrasonography (UL-trah-soh-NAWG-rah-fee)
- ❑ vaccination (VAK-sih-NAY-shun)
- ❑ vaccine (vak-SEEN)
- ❑ venipuncture (VEE-nih-PUNK-chur)
- ❑ viscosity (vis-KAWS-ih-tee)

Experience Multimedia

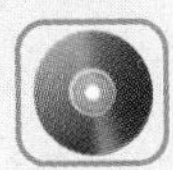

CD-ROM Learning Activities Checklist

Check off the box as you complete each learning activity.

❑ ***CD-ROM Learning Activity 6.1: ANATOMY WORD PARTS FLASHCARDS***
Use flashcards to help you memorize word parts. Make your own flashcards or print out prepared flashcards. Also see the electronic flashcard game. Time: 20 minutes.

❑ ***CD-ROM Learning Activity 6.2: MEDICINE IN ACTION***
Watch a video clip about sickle cell anemia. Time: 5 minutes

❑ ***CD-ROM Learning Activity 6.3: DISEASE AND OTHER WORD PARTS FLASHCARDS***
A continuation of the flashcard learning activity. Time: 20 minutes.

❑ ***CD-ROM Learning Activity 6.4: MEMORY AIDS***
Use memory aids to help you memorize medical words and meanings. Time: 5 minutes.

❑ ***CD-ROM Learning Activity 6.5: MEDICAL LANGUAGE SPOKEN HERE***
Listen to actual medical reports and spell the missing medical words. Time: 20 minutes.

❑ ***CD-ROM Learning Activity 6.6: SPELLING CHALLENGE***
Listen to a pronounced medical word and then spell it. Time: 5 minutes.

❑ ***CD-ROM Learning Activity 6.7: MEDICAL LANGUAGE PRONUNCIATION***
Listen to a pronounced medical word and then practice pronouncing it. Time: 30 minutes.

❑ ***CD-ROM Learning Activity 6.8: EDUCATIONAL FUN AND GAMES***
Enjoy these fun activities while reinforcing your knowledge. Time: 15 minutes.

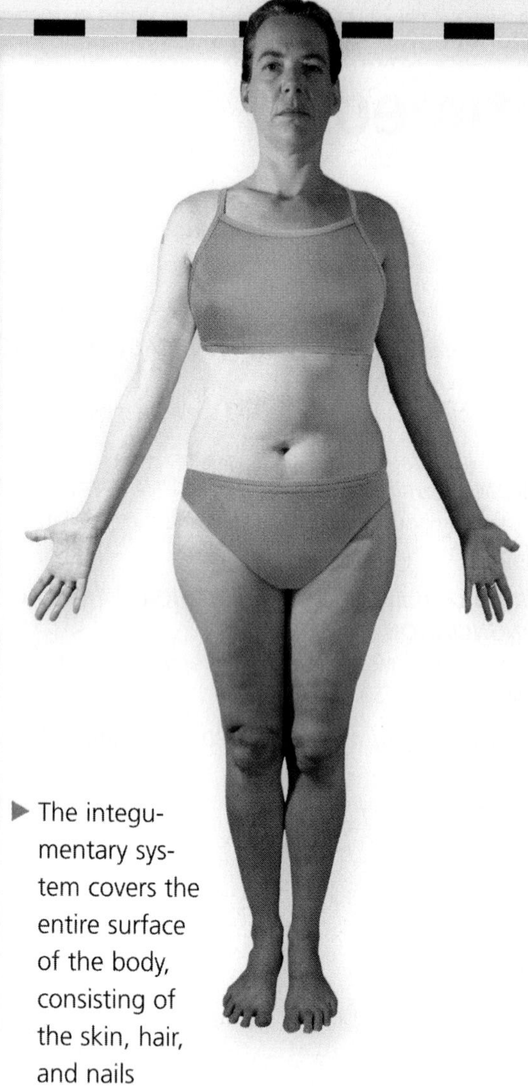

▶ The integumentary system covers the entire surface of the body, consisting of the skin, hair, and nails

Dive In!

- There are more living organisms on the skin of a single human being than there are human beings on the surface of the earth.
- The thumbnail grows the slowest; the middle nail grows the fastest.
- Ready to explore deeper layers of knowledge? In this chapter we'll explore the language that describes integumentary system structures, functions, diseases, and conditions.
- You'll move beyond scratching the surface once you master the language of dermatology!

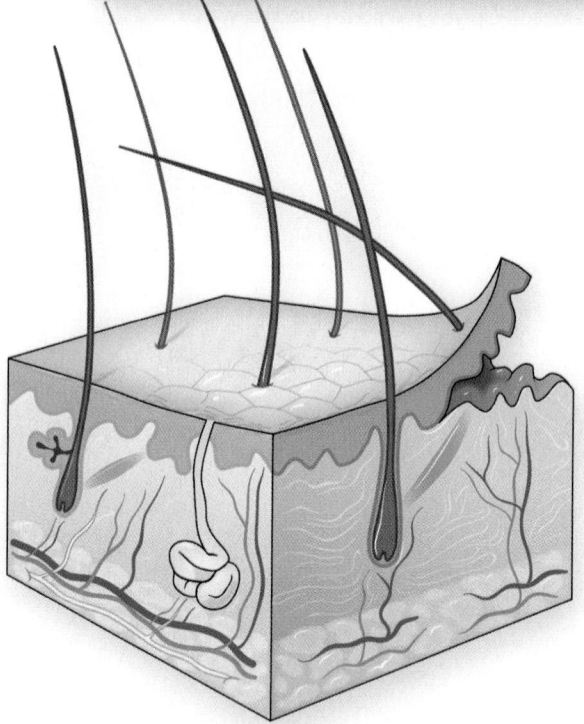

▶ There are many components within the epidermis and the dermis, which collectively comprise the skin.

Medicine Through HISTORY

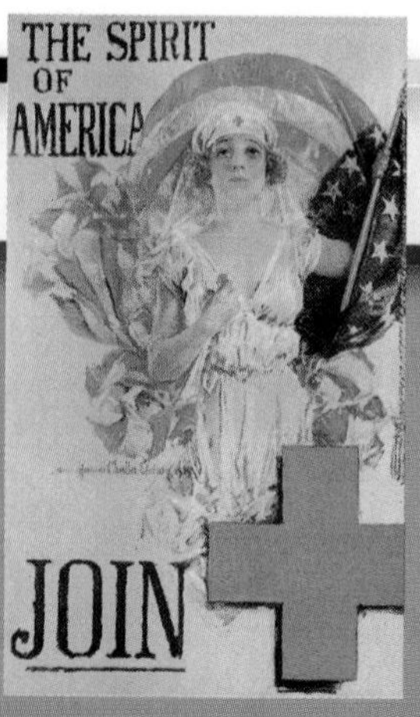

1881

The American Red Cross is founded

1885

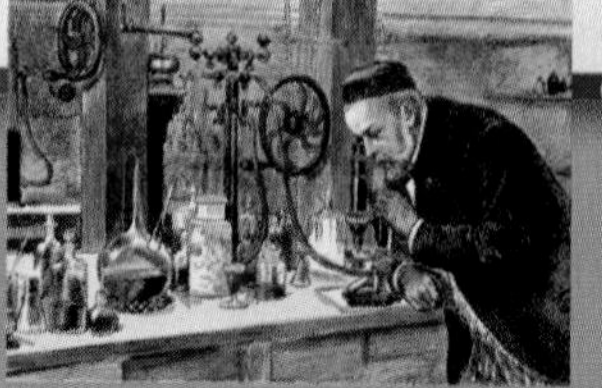

Louis Pasteur develops a vaccine for rabies

1838

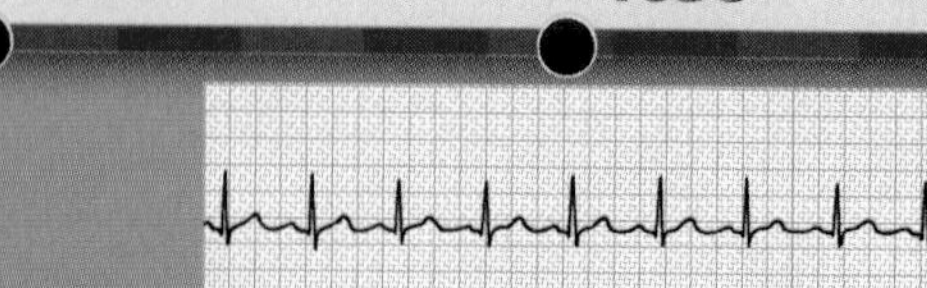

British physiologist Augustus Waller performs the first electrocardiography (ECG)

CHAPTER 7

Dermatology

Integumentary System

Dermatology (DER-mah-TAWL-oh-jee) is the medical specialty that studies the anatomy and physiology of the integumentary system and uses diagnostic tests, medical and surgical procedures, and drugs to treat integumentary diseases.

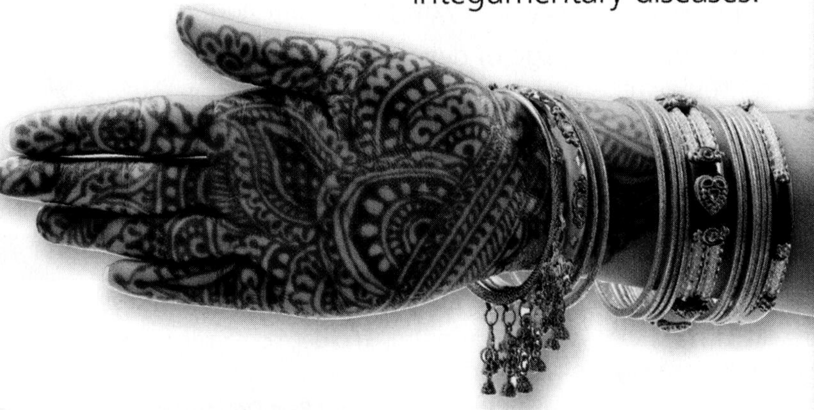

◀ ▲ Hair and skin often hold cultural distinctions, thus resulting in so many different styles and rituals around the world.

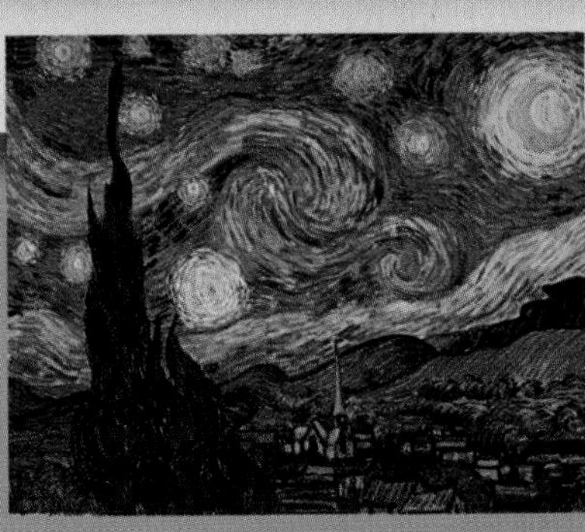

1889

"The Starry Night" is painted by Vincent van Gogh. The artist may have been suffering from digitalis overdose, the toxic effects of which are known to include visual halos around lights

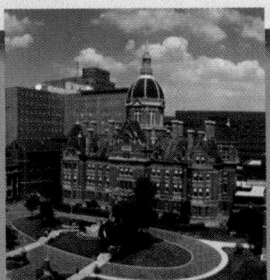

1893

The first medical school in America opens at Johns Hopkins University in Maryland

Measure Your Progress: Learning Objectives

After you study this chapter, you should be able to

1. Identify the anatomical structures of the integumentary system by correctly labeling them on anatomical illustrations.
2. Describe the process of an allergic reaction.
3. Build integumentary words from combining forms, prefixes, and suffixes.
4. Describe common integumentary diseases.
5. Describe common integumentary diagnostic laboratory tests.
6. Describe common integumentary medical and surgical procedures and drug categories.
7. Define common integumentary abbreviations.
8. Correctly spell and pronounce integumentary words.
9. Apply your skills by analyzing a dermatology report.
10. Test your knowledge of dermatology by completing review exercises at the end of the chapter and learning activities on the CD-ROM.

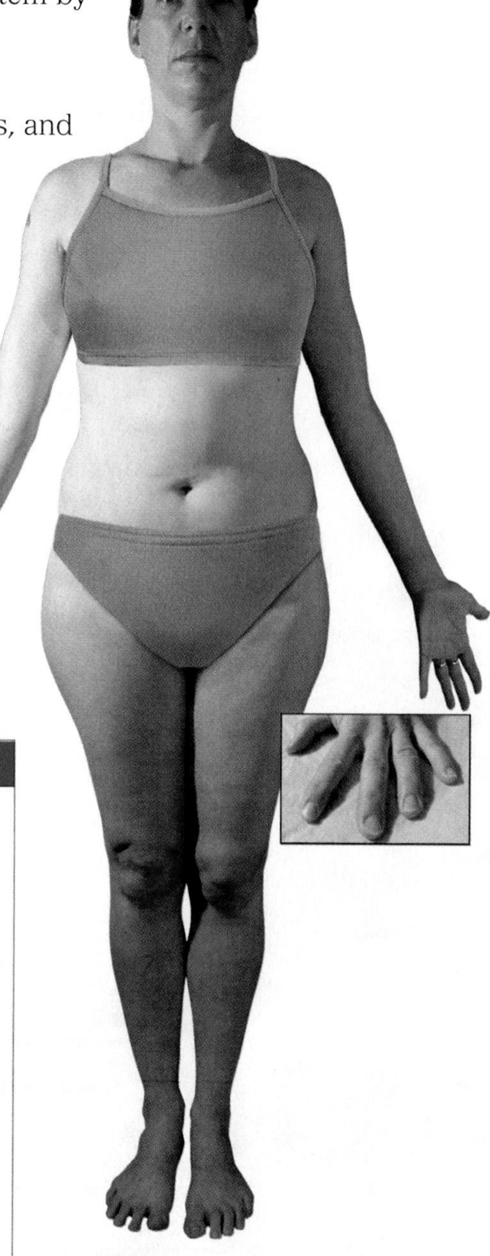

Figure 7-1 ■ The integumentary system.

The integumentary system covers the entire surface of the body and consists of the skin, hair, and the nails.

Medical Language Key

To unlock the meaning of a medical word, first define each word part. Then put the word part definitions in order, beginning with the suffix, followed by the first word part.

	Word Part	Word Part Definition
SUFFIX	-logy	*the study of*
COMBINING FORM	dermat/o-	*skin*

Dermatology: The study of the skin.

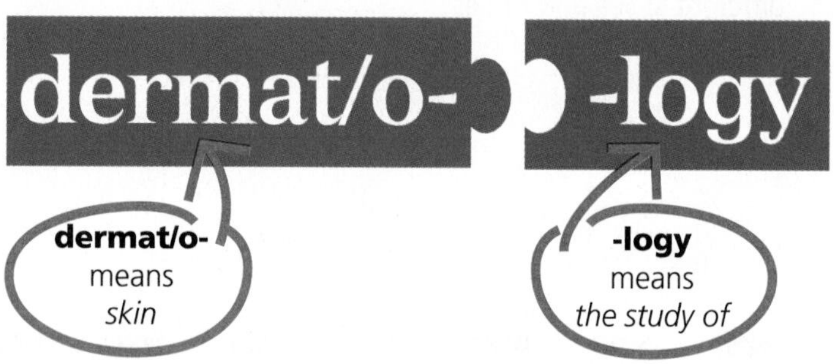

www.prenhall.com/turley

For interactive flashcards, real-life video clips, games, exercises, and audio pronunciations please explore the companion CD-ROM in the back of the book. Click on the companion website for bonus chapters, additional resources, and links to on-line learning.

Anatomy and Physiology

The **integumentary system** (see Figure 7-1■) is an extremely large, flat, flexible body system that covers the entire surface of the body. It consists of the skin, hair, and nails. The purpose of the integumentary system is to protect the body; it is the body's first line of defense against invading microorganisms. The sense of touch is also part of the integumentary system.

integumentary (in-TEG-yoo-MEN-tair-ee)
integument/o- *skin*
-ary *pertaining to*
Integumentary is derived from a Latin word meaning *a covering.*

system (SIS-tem)
System is derived from a Greek word meaning *combination of parts to make an organized whole.*

Anatomy of the Integumentary System

Skin

The skin or **integument** is categorized as **epithelium** or **epithelial tissue.** The epithelium covers the external surface of the body (in the form of the skin), but also includes the mucous membranes that line the walls of internal cavities that connect to the outside of the body. The skin itself consists of two different layers: the epidermis and the dermis.

Epidermis The **epidermis** is the thin, outermost layer of the skin (see Figure 7-2■). The most superficial part of the epidermis contains cells that have no nuclei and are filled with **keratin,** a hard, fibrous protein. These cells form a protective layer, but they are dead cells so they are constantly being shed or sloughed off. This process is known as

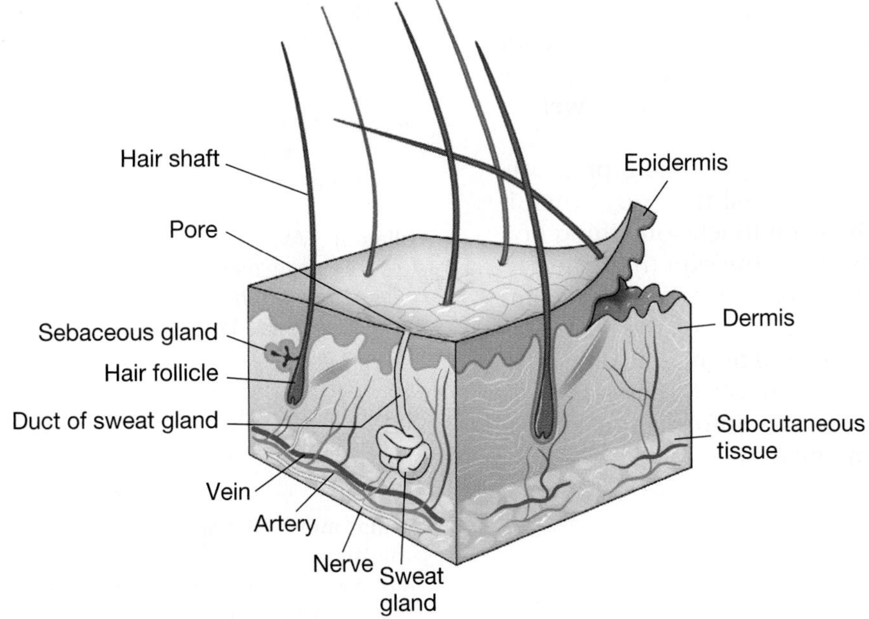

Figure 7-2 ■ Epidermis and dermis.

The skin is composed of the epidermis and the dermis. The epidermis has dead protective cells on its surface and living, actively dividing cells at its base. The dermis contains hair follicles, sebaceous glands, and sweat glands. The subcutaneous tissue is a type of connective tissue that lies beneath the dermis.

integument (in-TEG-yoo-ment)
integu/o- *to cover*
-ment *action; state*

cutaneous (kyoo-TAY-nee-us)
cutane/o- *skin*
-ous *pertaining to*
Both *cutaneous* and *integumentary* are adjective forms for skin. *Cutaneous* is derived from a Latin word meaning *skin.*

epithelium (EP-ih-THEE-lee-um)
epi- *upon, above*
theli/o- *cellular layer*
-um *a structure*

epithelial (EP-ih-THEE-lee-al)
epi- *upon, above*
theli/o- *cellular layer*
-al *pertaining to*

epidermis (EP-ih-DER-mis)

epidermal (EP-ih-DER-mal)
epi- *upon, above*
derm/o- *skin*
-al *pertaining to*

keratin (KAIR-ah-tin)
kerat/o- *hard, fibrous protein*
-in *a substance*

exfoliation. In contrast, the deepest part (**basal layer**) of the epidermis is composed of living cells that are constantly dividing and working their way to the surface. The epidermis does not contain any blood vessels. It receives nutrients and oxygen from the blood vessels in the dermis.

The epidermis also contains **melanocytes,** pigment cells that produce **melanin,** a dark brown or black pigment. Melanin in the epidermis absorbs ultraviolet light from the sun to protect the DNA in skin cells from undergoing genetic mutations. Some sunlight is beneficial, however, because the sun's ultraviolet rays convert cholesterol in the epidermis to a compound that is then made into vitamin D. The amount of vitamin D produced depends on the time of day and the season of the year. Usually about 20 to 45 minutes of exposure to sunlight per week produces sufficient amounts of vitamin D. Vitamin D is stored in fat cells in the subcutaneous tissue. It helps the body absorb and use calcium and phosphorus in foods.

exfoliation (eks-FOH-lee-AA-shun)
ex- *out, away from*
foli/o- *leaf*
-ation *a process; being or having*
Add words to make a correct and complete definition of *exfoliation: A process [of skin cells moving] away from [the body like a] leaf [falling off a tree].*

basal (BAY-sal)
bas/o- *base of a structure*
-al *pertaining to*

melanocyte (meh-LAN-oh-site) (MEL-ah-noh-site)
melan/o- *black*
-cyte *cell*
Add words to make a correct and complete definition of *melanocyte: A cell [in the skin that produces a dark brown or] black [pigment].*

melanin (MEL-ah-nin)
melan/o- *black*
-in *a substance*

Did You Know?

All races have the same number of melanocytes in the skin. The differences in skin color occur because of differing levels of melanin production. Dark-skinned people produce more melanin than fair-skinned people. Albinos have a normal number of melanocytes in their skin, but the cells do not produce any melanin. Exposure to the sun's ultraviolet rays increases the rate of melanin production in all people and causes a suntan. During prolonged sun exposure, the melanin is unable to absorb all the ultraviolet light, and the result is a sunburn.

Dermis The **dermis** is a thicker layer beneath the epidermis (see Figure 7-2). It is both firm and elastic because it is composed of **collagen** fibers (firm, white protein) and **elastin** fibers (elastic, yellow protein). The dermis contains arteries, veins, and nerves, as well as hair follicles, sebaceous glands, and sweat glands.

The nerves in the dermis are stimulated by light touch, pressure, vibration, pain, and temperature. These nerves tell the body when it has come in contact with something. When you touch something hot, the sensation is carried as a nerve impulse from the skin to the nerves of the spinal cord. The spinal cord immediately sends a motor command to a muscle for you to move your hand away from the heat. This takes place without any conscious input from the brain. It is only after your hand has already moved that your brain thinks "That was hot!" Each nerve of the spinal cord receives sensory information from a specific area of the skin known as a **dermatome** (see Figure 7-3 ■).

dermis (DER-mis)
Dermis is derived from a Greek word meaning *skin.*

dermal (DER-mal)
derm/o- *skin*
-al *pertaining to*

collagen (KAWL-lah-jen)
coll/a- *fibers that hold together*
-gen *that which produces*
Collagen is derived from a Greek word meaning *glue.*

elastin (ee-LAS-tin)
elast/o- *flexing, stretching*
-in *a substance*

dermatome (DER-mah-tohm)
derm/a- *skin*
-tome *instrument used to cut; an area with distinct edges*

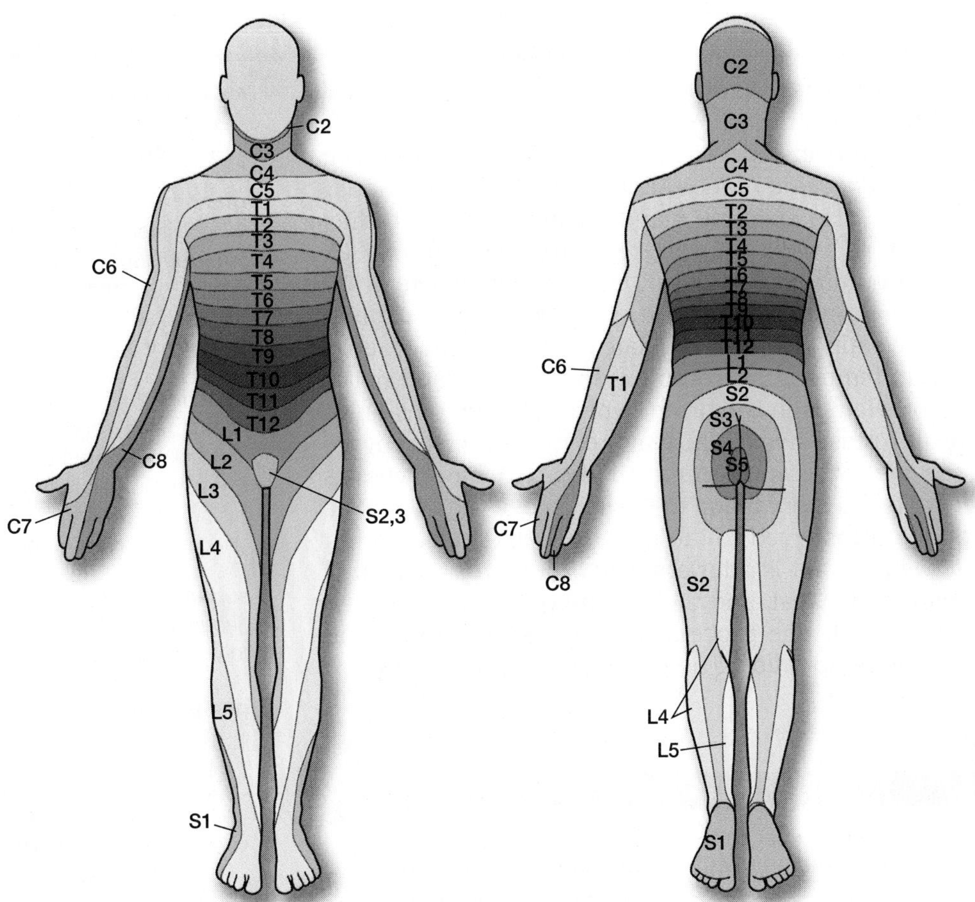

Figure 7-3 ■ Dermatomes of the body.

A dermatome is a specific area of the skin that sends sensory information through a single spinal nerve to the spinal cord. Each dermatome is named according to the level at which its spinal nerve leaves the spinal cord. *C* stands for the cervical spinal nerves that leave the spinal cord at the level of the neck, *T* stands for the thoracic spinal nerves that leave the spinal cord at the level of the thorax, *L* stands for the lumbar spinal nerves that leave the spinal cord at the level of the lower back, and *S* stands for the sacral spinal nerves that leave the spinal cord at the level of the sacrum (last bone in the spinal column). The skin of the face sends sensory information through the cranial nerves to the brain.

Subcutaneous Tissue

The **subcutaneous tissue** is a loose, connective tissue directly beneath the dermis of the skin (see Figure 7-2). It is composed of **adipose tissue** or fat that is made up of **lipocytes** (fat-storing cells). These cells contain stored fat (triglycerides) as an energy reserve. The amount of fat in adipose tissue usually far exceeds any energy needs the body might have! The subcutaneous tissue also provides a layer of insulation to conserve internal body heat. The subcutaneous tissue can be thin or as thick as several inches in areas like the abdomen, depending on a person's metabolism, dietary intake of sugars and fats, and how much fat is stored in the lipocytes. The subcutaneous layer also acts as a cushion to protect the bones and internal organs.

subcutaneous (SUB-kyoo-TAY-nee-us)
sub- *below; underneath; less than*
cutane/o- *skin*
-ous *pertaining to*

adipose (AD-ih-pohs)
adip/o- *fat*
-ose *full of*

lipocyte (LIP-oh-site)
lip/o- *lipid (fat)*
-cyte *cell*

Sebaceous and Sweat Glands

The **sebaceous glands** are a type of **exocrine gland** located in the dermis. They secrete **sebum** through a duct into a hair follicle (see Figure 7-2). Sebum consists of oil that coats and protects the hair shaft to keep it from becoming brittle. Sebaceous glands are also known as oil glands.

The sweat glands are also exocrine glands. The sweat gland duct opens onto the surface of the skin through a pore (see Figure 7-2). Sweat contains water, sodium, and small amounts of body waste products like urea, ammonia, and creatinine. It is the sodium that gives sweat its salty taste. Sweating helps to regulate the body temperature. When the body is hot, temperature receptors in the skin send nerve impulses to the hypothalamus in the brain, which then sends signals to the sweat glands to release sweat. The water content of sweat evaporating from the surface of the skin cools the body. Also, blood vessels in the dermis dilate to bring more blood to the surface of the body. The heat from the blood is transferred to the epidermis and radiated out from the body. Although sweat is odorless, bacteria on the surface of the skin digest sebum and sweat, and their waste products cause the odor associated with sweat. The process of sweating and the sweat itself are both known as **perspiration.** The sweat glands are also known as the **sudoriferous glands.**

Connections

Forensic Science. Oil from the sebaceous glands leaves a fingerprint when a person touches something. Each person's fingerprints are a unique combination of whorls, loops, or arches that can be matched to fingerprints on file in a database. Cells from a hair follicle can be analyzed for DNA. Hair can be tested for evidence of toxins or poisons. White horizontal bands on the fingernails indicate arsenic poisoning. If a body is buried in moist dirt, the adipose tissue decomposes and forms a characteristic waxy substance known as **adipocere.**

sebaceous (seh-BAY-shus)
sebace/o- *sebum (oil)*
-ous *pertaining to*

gland (GLAND)
Gland is derived from a Latin word meaning *acorn.* Some glands are the size of acorns, but others are much smaller, even microscopic. All glands produce and secrete specific substances.

exocrine (EK-soh-krin) (EK-soh-krine)
exo- *away from, external, outward*
-crine *a thing that secretes*
Every medical word must contain a combining form. The suffix of *exocrine* contains the combining form *crin/o-.*

sebum (SEE-bum)
Sebum is a Latin word meaning *suet or tallow* (animal fat).

perspiration (PER-spih-RAY-shun)
per- *through, throughout*
spir/o- *breathe*
-ation *a process; being or having*

sudoriferous (SOO-doh-RIF-er-us)
sudor/i- *sweat*
fer/o- *to bear*
-ous *pertaining to*
Sudor is a Latin word meaning *sweat.*

adipocere (AD-ih-poh-SEER)
adip/o- *fat*
-cere *waxy substance*

Hair

Hair covers most of the body, although its consistency and color vary from one part of the body to the other and from one person to the next. Additional facial, axillary, and pubic hairs appear during puberty.

Each hair forms in a hair **follicle** in the dermis (see Figure 7-2). Melanocytes give color to the hair. Hair cells are filled with keratin, which makes the hair shaft strong. Usually, the hair lies flat on the surface of the skin, but when the skin is cold, tiny erector muscles at the base of the hair follicle contract and cause the hair to stand up (**piloerection**). The contracted muscle forms a goose bump. The contraction produces heat, and the erect hair traps some of this heat near the skin.

Did You Know?

The scalp contains about 100,000 hairs. Dark hair contains melanin, but blond hair and red hair contain a variant of melanin that contains more sulfur, so the hair appears more yellow or orange. As we age, melanocytes in the dermis die, so the hair contains no melanin and appears gray or white.

follicle (FAWL-ih-kl)

follicular (foh-LIK-yoo-lar)
follicul/o- *follicle (small sac)*
-ar *pertaining to*

piloerection (PY-loh-ee-REK-shun)
pil/o- *hair*
erect/o- *to stand up*
-ion *action; condition*

Nails

The nails cover and protect the distal ends of the fingers and toes because these areas are easily traumatized. Each nail consists of several parts (see Figure 7-4 ■). The outer layer—the tough, opaque **nail plate**—is composed of dead cells that contain hard keratin. The nail plate rests on the **nail bed,** a layer of living tissue that contains nerves and blood vessels. The blood vessels in the nail bed give the nail plate its color: pink normally or bluish-purple if there is decreased blood flow (because of cold temperatures or if there is not enough oxygen in the blood). The nail bed is also known as the quick. The **cuticle** is an edge of dead cells, arising from the skin along the proximal end of the nail. The cuticle is adherent to the nail plate to prevent microorganisms from gaining access to the nail root. The **lunula,** the whitish half-moon under the proximal nail plate, is the tip of the nail root. The **nail root,** which is located beneath the skin of the finger, produces the keratin-containing cells that form the nail plate. These cells are white at first (in the lunula), but gradually become opaque as the nail plate grows. Trauma to or infection in the nail root results in a malformed nail plate.

ungual (UNG-gwal)
ungu/o- *nail*
-al *pertaining to*
Ungual is the adjective form for *nail.*

cuticle (KYOO-tih-kl)
cut/i- *skin*
-cle *small thing*

lunula (LOO-nyoo-lah)
lun/o- *moon*
-ula *small thing*
Lunula is a Latin word meaning *little moon.*

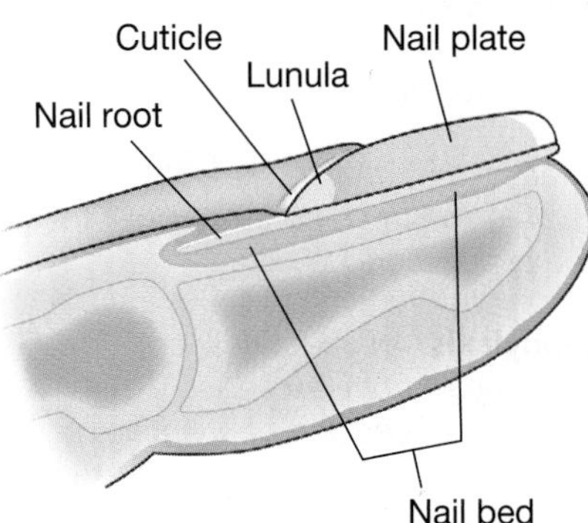

Figure 7-4 ■ Nail.
The nail is composed of both living and dead cells. The nail root constantly produces keratin-containing cells that form the lunula. As the nail plate grows, these cells die and harden to form a protective covering for the distal end of the finger.

A Closer Look

The skin is the body's first line of defense against disease and injury. The dead cells of the outer epidermis present a dry and slightly acidic environment that discourages the growth of microorganisms. The constant shedding of epidermal cells prevents microorganisms from multiplying and invading the dermis. Sweat and sebum contain antibodies and enzymes that kill bacteria. Normal skin flora (bacteria that are able to thrive under these conditions) do not cause disease. They also inhibit the growth of disease-causing microorganisms by competing with them for space and nutrients.

Physiology of an Allergic Reaction

Allergic reactions anywhere in the body almost always manifest themselves in the skin and mucous membranes. An **allergy** or **allergic reaction** is a **hypersensitivity** response to certain types of antigens known as allergens. **Allergens** include cells from plant and animal sources (foods, pollens, molds, animal dander), as well as dust, chemicals, and drugs. The basis of all allergic reactions is the release of histamine from basophils in the blood and mast cells in the connective tissue.

A **local reaction** occurs when an allergen touches the skin or mucous membranes of a hypersensitive individual. Histamine causes redness, swelling (edema), irritation, and itching in that specific area. Examples: Chemicals in deodorant applied to the skin or pollen in the air that enters the nose.

A **systemic reaction** occurs when allergens are inhaled by, ingested by, or injected into a hypersensitive person, causing symptoms in several body systems. Histamine constricts the bronchi, dilates the blood vessels throughout the body, and causes hives in various places on the skin. Examples: Inhaled pollens, molds, or dust trigger asthma attacks; ingested foods or drugs cause hives on the skin. **Anaphylaxis** is a severe systemic allergic reaction that can be life threatening. Symptoms include bronchoconstriction with respiratory distress, hypotension, and shock. Eating peanuts, being stung by a bee, taking a drug they are already allergic to, or being exposed to latex gloves are all common causes of anaphylaxis in hypersensitive individuals. It is also known as **anaphylactic shock.**

allergy (AL-er-jee)
all/o- *other; strange*
-ergy *activity; process of working*

allergic (ah-LER-jik)
all/o- *other; strange*
erg/o- *activity; work*
-ic *pertaining to*

hypersensitivity (HY-per-SEN-sih-TIV-ih-tee)
hyper- *above, more than normal*
sensitiv/o- *affected by, sensitive to*
-ity *state; condition*

allergen (AL-er-jen)
all/o- *other; strange*
erg/o- *activity; work*
-gen *that which produces*
Note: The duplicated letter *g* is deleted before forming the word.

local (LOH-kal)
loc/o- *in one place*
-al *pertaining to*

systemic (sis-TEM-ik)
system/o- *the body as a whole*
-ic *pertaining to*

anaphylaxis (AN-ah-fih-LAK-sis)
ana- *apart from; excessive*
-phylaxis *condition of guarding or protecting*

anaphylactic (AN-ah-fih-LAK-tik)
ana- *apart from; excessive*
phylact/o- *guarding or protecting*
-ic *pertaining to*

Across the Life Span

The skin of an infant is smooth and very flexible (see Figure 7-5■). It has few wrinkles because of the large amount of elastin in the dermis and a thick layer of fat in the subcutaneous tissue. This fat layer conserves body heat and protects the internal organs as the infant learns to walk. In the elderly, the amount of elastin in the skin decreases, and the skin develops sags and wrinkles. The fat in the subcutaneous layer thins, making the skin appear translucent and revealing large arteries and veins especially in the hands. Up to 40% of the melanocytes stop functioning with age, but other melanocytes overproduce, causing variable areas of pigmentation.

In persons who smoke, the nicotine in cigarettes decreases oxygen levels in the skin and destroys the collagen fibers. This causes deep wrinkles and gives a leathery quality to the skin, even in middle age.

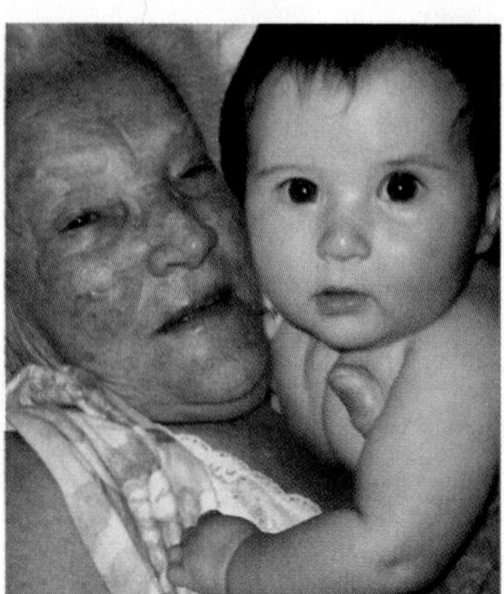

Figure 7-5 ■ Aging skin.
As a person ages, the skin loses subcutaneous fat, the amount of elastin decreases, and the melanocytes underproduce or overproduce melanin.

Vocabulary Review

Anatomy and Physiology

Now that you have studied the anatomy and physiology of the integumentary system, take time to review those new words and descriptions. Memorize the combining forms and their definitions before going on to the next section.

Word or Phrase	Combining Form and Definition	Description
adipose tissue	adip/o- *fat*	Fatty tissue in the subcutaneous layer. It contains lipocytes.
allergen	all/o- *other; strange*	Cells from plants or animals (foods, pollens, molds, animal dander), as well as dust, chemicals, and drugs that cause an allergic response in a hypersensitive person.
allergic reaction	all/o- *other; strange*	Response to an allergen in a hypersensitive person. An allergic reaction is based on the release of histamine. Also known as an **allergy.**
anaphylaxis	phylact/o- *guarding or protecting*	Severe systemic allergic reaction characterized by bronchoconstriction, hypotension, and shock. Also known as **anaphylactic shock.**
collagen	coll/a- *fibers that hold together*	Firm, white protein connective tissue fibers throughout the dermis
cutaneous	cutane/o- *skin*	Pertaining to the skin
cuticle	cut/i- *skin*	Layer of dead skin that arises from the epidermis around the proximal end of the nail. It keeps microorganisms from entering the nail root.
dermatome	derm/a- *skin*	Area of the skin that sends sensory information to one spinal nerve
dermis	derm/o- *skin*	Layer of skin under the epidermis. It is composed of collagen and elastin fibers. It contains arteries, veins, nerves, sebaceous glands, sweat glands, and hair follicles.
elastin	elast/o- *flexing, stretching*	Elastic, yellow protein fibers in the dermis
epidermis	derm/o- *skin* bas/o- *base of a structure*	Thin, outermost layer of skin. The most superficial part of the epidermis consists of dead cells filled with keratin. The deepest part (**basal layer**) contains constantly dividing cells and melanocytes.
epithelium	theli/o- *cellular layer*	Category that includes the skin and all of its structures that cover the external surface of the body, but also includes the mucous membranes that line the walls of internal cavities that connect to the outside of the body. Also known as **epithelial tissue.**
exfoliation	foli/o- *leaf*	Normal process of constant shedding of dead skin cells from the most superficial part of the epidermis
exocrine gland	crin/o- *thing that secretes*	Type of gland that secretes substances through a duct. Example: Sebaceous (oil) and sudoriferous (sweat) glands of the skin.
follicle	follicul/o- *follicle (small sac)*	Site where a hair is formed. The follicle is located in the dermis.
hypersensitivity	sensitiv/o- *affected by, sensitive to*	Individually unique response to an allergen that provokes an allergic response in some people

Word or Phrase	Combining Form and Definition	Description
integument	**integu/o-** *to cover*	The skin, hair, and nails
integumentary system	**integument/o-** *skin*	Body system that covers the entire surface of the body and consists of the skin, hair, and nails
keratin	**kerat/o-** *hard, fibrous protein*	Hard protein found in the cells of the outermost part of the epidermis and in the nails
lipocyte	**lip/o-** *lipid (fat)*	Cell in the subcutaneous layer that stores fat
local reaction	**loc/o-** *in one place*	Allergic reaction that takes place on a certain area of the skin that was exposed to an allergen
lunula	**lun/o-** *moon*	Whitish half-moon visible under the proximal portion of the nail plate. It is the visible tip of the nail root.
melanocyte	**melan/o-** *black*	Pigment-containing cell in the epidermis that produces **melanin,** a dark brown or black pigment that gives color to the skin and hair.
nail bed		Layer of living tissue beneath the nail plate. It contains blood vessels and nerves. Also known as the quick.
nail plate	**ungu/o-** *nail*	Hard, flat, protective covering over the distal end of each finger and toe. It is composed of dead cells that contain keratin. Also known as the nail.
nail root		Produces cells that form the lunula and nail plate
perspiration	**spir/o-** *breathe*	Process of sweating and the sweat itself. Sweat is produced by sudoriferous glands. It contains sodium and waste products. As its water content evaporates from the skin, it cools the body.
piloerection	**pil/o-** *hair* **erect/o-** *to stand up*	Process in which erector muscles contract (to form a goose bump) and the body hair becomes erect when the skin is cold. This generates heat that is trapped as a layer of warm air near the surface of the skin.
sebaceous gland	**sebace/o-** *sebum (oil)*	An exocrine gland of the skin that secretes **sebum** through a duct. Sebaceous glands are located in the dermis. The duct joins with a hair, and sebum coats the hair shaft as it moves toward the surface of the skin. Also known as an oil gland.
skin	**cutane/o-** *skin* **integument/o-** *skin*	Tissue covering of the body that consists of two layers (epidermis and dermis). Skin is categorized as an epithelial tissue. The skin is one part of the integumentary system.
subcutaneous tissue	**cutane/o-** *skin*	Loose, connective tissue directly beneath the dermis. It is composed of adipose tissue.
sudoriferous gland	**sudor/i-** *sweat* **fer/o-** *to bear*	An exocrine gland of the skin that secretes sweat through a duct. These glands are located in the dermis. The duct opens at a pore on the surface of the skin. Also known as sweat glands.
systemic reaction	**system/o-** *the body as a whole*	Allergic reaction that takes place throughout the body in a hypersensitive person after contact with an allergen that was ingested, inhaled, or injected

Labeling Exercise

A. *Match each anatomy word or phrase to its numbered structure in Figure 7-6■. Write that word or phrase on the blank line next to its number. Use the Answer Key at the end of the book to check your answers.*

artery	epidermis	nerve	subcutaneous tissue
dermis	hair follicle	pore	sweat gland
duct of sweat gland	hair shaft	sebaceous gland	vein

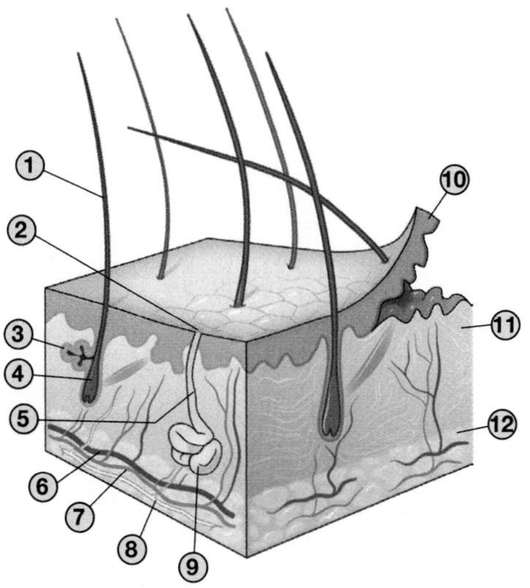

1. ____________
2. ____________
3. ____________
4. ____________
5. ____________
6. ____________
7. ____________
8. ____________
9. ____________
10. ____________
11. ____________
12. ____________

Figure 7-6 ■

B. *Match each anatomy word or phrase to its numbered structure in Figure 7-7■. Write that word or phrase on the blank line next to its number.*

cuticle	lunula	nail bed	nail plate	nail root

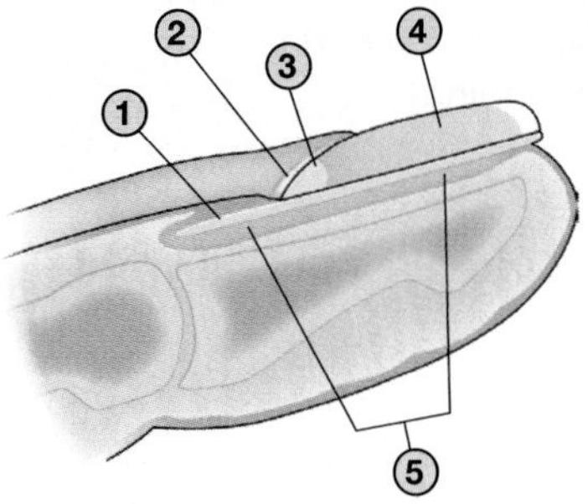

1. ____________
2. ____________
3. ____________
4. ____________
5. ____________

Figure 7-7 ■

Building Medical Words

Combining Forms

Here are the combining forms you have learned so far. Next to each combining form, write its meaning. Use the Answer Key at the end of the book to check your answers. The first one has been done for you.

Combining Form	Medical Meaning	Combining Form	Medical Meaning
1. follicul/o-	follicle (small sac)	14. kerat/o-	
2. adip/o-		15. lip/o-	
3. all/o-		16. loc/o-	
4. coll/a-		17. lun/o-	
5. cutane/o-		18. melan/o-	
6. cut/i-		19. pil/o-	
7. derm/a-		20. phylact/o-	
8. dermat/o-		21. sebace/o-	
9. derm/o-		22. sudor/i-	
10. elast/o-		23. system/o-	
11. erect/o-		24. theli/o-	
12. integu/o-		25. ungu/o-	
13. integument/o-			

Combining Forms and Suffixes

Read the definition hint for the medical word you are to build. Look at the combining form that is given. Write the correct suffix on the blank line. Then write the medical word. (Remember: You may need to remove the combining vowel. Always remove the hyphens and slash.) Use the Answer Key at the end of the book to check your answers. The first one has been done for you.

SUFFIX LIST

-al (pertaining to)	-cyte (cell)	-ment (action; state)	-tome (instrument used to cut; an area with distinct edges)
-ary (pertaining to)	-gen (that which produces)	-ose (full of)	-ula (small thing)
-cle (small thing)	-in (a substance)	-ous (pertaining to)	

Definition Hint	Combining Form	Suffix	Write the Medical Word
1. Substance that flexes, stretches	elast/o-	-in	elastin
2. Pertaining to the nail	ungu/o-		
3. A skin area with distinct edges	derm/a-		
4. Substance made of hard, fibrous protein	kerat/o-		
5. Pertaining to the skin	derm/o-		
6. That which produces fibers that hold together	coll/a-		

Definition Hint	Combining Form	Suffix	Write the Medical Word
7. Full of fat (type of tissue)	adip/o-	________	________________
8. Cell that makes dark brown and black pigment	melan/o-	________	________________
9. Pertaining to the skin	cutane/o-	________	________________
10. Pertaining to sebum (oil)	sebace/o-	________	________________
11. Small edge of skin	cut/i-	________	________________
12. Fat cell	lip/o-	________	________________
13. Pertaining to the skin	integument/o-	________	________________
14. Little moon	lun/o-	________	________________
15. A state of having a covering	integu/o-	________	________________

Combining Forms and Prefixes

Read the definition hint for the medical word you are to build. Look at the medical word or word part that is given. It already contains a combining form and a suffix. Write the correct prefix on the blank line. Then write the entire medical word. (Remember: You may need to remove the combining vowel. Always remove the hyphens and slash.) Use the Answer Key at the end of the book to check your answers. The first one has been done for you.

PREFIX LIST

epi- (upon, above)	exo- (away from, external, outward)	sub- (below; underneath; less than)
ex- (out, away from)	per- (through, throughout)	

Definition Hint	Prefix	Medical Word or Word Part	Write the New Medical Word
1. Process of something falling away like a leaf	ex-	foliation	*exfoliation*
2. Pertaining to above the dermis	________	dermal	________________
3. Pertaining to underneath the skin	________	cutaneous	________________
4. Pertaining to a cellular layer that is upon the body	________	thelial	________________
5. Process of breathing through the skin	________	spiration	________________
6. A gland that secretes to the external surface of the body	________	-crine	________________

Symptoms, Signs, and Diseases

General

Word or Phrase	Word Part and Definition	Description
dermatitis	**dermatitis** (DER-mah-TY-tis) **dermat/o-** *skin* **-itis** *inflammation of*	Any disease condition involving inflammation of the skin. Treatment: Correct the underlying cause.
edema	**edema** (eh-DEE-mah) *Edema* is derived from a Greek word meaning *a swelling.*	Excessive amounts of fluid move from the blood into the dermis or subcutaneous tissue and cause swelling. Localized areas of edema occur with inflammation, allergic reactions, and infections. Large areas of edema occur with cardiovascular or urinary system diseases. Treatment: Correct the underlying cause.
hemorrhage	**hemorrhage** (HEM-oh-rij) **hem/o-** *blood* **-rrhage** *excessive flow or discharge* **extravasation** (eks-TRAV-ah-SAY-shun) **extra-** *outside of* **vas/o-** *blood vessel; vas deferens* **-ation** *a process; being or having* **petechia** (peh-TEE-kee-ah) **petechiae** (peh-TEE-kee-ee) *Petechia* is a Latin singular feminine noun. Form the plural by changing *-a* to *-ae*. **petechial** (peh-TEE-kee-al) **petechi/o-** *petechia* **-al** *pertaining to* **contusion** (con-TOO-zhun) **contus/o-** *bruising* **-ion** *action; condition* **ecchymosis** (EK-ih-MOH-sis) **ecchymoses** (EK-ih-MOH-seez) *Ecchymosis* is a Greek singular noun. Form the plural by changing *-is* to *-es*. **ecchymotic** (EK-ih-MAWT-ik) **ecchym/o-** *blood in the tissues* **-osis** *condition; abnormal condition; process* **hematoma** (HEE-mah-TOH-ma) **hemat/o-** *blood* **-oma** *tumor, mass*	Trauma to the skin releases a small or large amount of blood. **Extravasation** is the process by which that blood flows into the surrounding tissues. **Petechiae** are pinpoint hemorrhages in the skin from ruptured capillaries. A **contusion** is an area of any size of hemorrhage under the skin. An **ecchymosis** is a 3 cm in diameter or larger area of hemorrhage under the skin. Both are classified as bruises. A **hematoma** is an elevated, localized collection of blood under the skin. Treatment: None.

Word or Phrase	Word Part and Definition	Description
lesion	**lesion** (LEE-shun) *Lesion* is derived from a Latin word meaning *to injure*.	Any area of visible damage on the skin, whether it is from disease or injury (see Figure 7-8■). Treatment: Correct the underlying cause.

LESION	DESCRIPTION	COLOR	CONTENTS	EXAMPLE
Cyst	Elevated circular mound	Skin color or erythema	Semisolid or partly fluid filled	Acne sebaceous cyst
Fissure	Small, cracklike crevice	Erythema	None; some fluid exudate	Dry, chapped skin
Macule	Flat circle	Pigmented; brown or black	None	Freckle, age spot
Papule	Elevated	Skin color or erythema	Solid	Acne pimple
Pustule	Elevated	White top	Pus	Acne whitehead
Scale	Flat to slightly elevated thin flake	White	None	Dandruff, psoriasis
Vesicle	Elevated with pointed top	Erythema; transparent top	Clear fluid	Herpes, chickenpox, shingles
Wheal	Elevated with broad, flat top	Erythema; pale top	Clear fluid	Insect bites, urticaria

Figure 7-8 ■ Types of skin lesions.

cyst (SIST)
Cyst is derived from a Greek word meaning *bladder or fluid-filled sac.*

fissure (FISH-ur)
fiss/o- *splitting*
-ure *system; result of*

macule (MAK-yool)
Macule is derived from a Latin word meaning *a spot.*

papule (PAP-yool)
Papule is derived from a Latin word meaning *pimple.*

pustule (PUS-chool)
Pustule is derived from a Latin word meaning *little pimple containing pus.*

vesicle (VES-ih-kl)
vesic/o- *bladder; fluid-filled sac*
-cle *small thing*

vesicular (veh-SIK-yoo-lar)
vesicul/o- *bladder; fluid-filled sac*
-ar *pertaining to*

wheal (HWEEL)

Word or Phrase	Word Part and Definition	Description
neoplasm	**neoplasm** (NEE-oh-plazm) **ne/o-** *new* **-plasm** *growth; formed substance* **benign** (bee-NINE) *Benign* is derived from a Latin word meaning *kind, not cancerous.* **malignant** (mah-LIG-nant) **malign/o-** *intentionally causing harm; cancer* **-ant** *pertaining to*	Any **benign** or **malignant** new growth that occurs on or in the skin. Treatment: Excision for large benign neoplasms. Excision and chemotherapy or radiation therapy for malignant neoplasms.
pruritus	**pruritus** (proo-RY-tus) *Pruritus* is derived from a Latin word meaning *to itch.* **pruritic** (proo-RIT-ik) **prurit/o-** *itching* **-ic** *pertaining to*	Itching. Pruritus is associated with many skin diseases. It is also present during an allergic reaction because of the release of histamine. A patient with pruritus is said to be **pruritic.** Treatment: Topical or oral antihistamine drugs or corticosteroid drugs.
rash		Any type of skin lesion that is pink to red, flat or raised, pruritic or nonpruritic. Certain systemic diseases (chickenpox, measles) have distinctive characteristic rashes. Treatment: Topical or oral antihistamine drugs or corticosteroid drugs.
wound		Any area of visible damage to the skin that is caused by physical means (rubbing, trauma, and so forth). Treatment: Apply a protective covering and topical antibiotic drug to prevent infection.
xeroderma	**xeroderma** (ZEER-oh-DER-mah) **xer/o-** *dry* **-derma** *skin* **turgor** (TER-gor) *Turgor* is derived from a Latin word meaning *fullness.*	Excessive dryness of the skin that can result in a fissure. Can be caused by aging, cold weather with low humidity, vitamin A deficiency, or dehydration. The level of hydration of the body can be determined by assessing the **skin turgor.** A fold of skin gently pinched between the thumb and fingertips should flatten out immediately when released. Dehydration causes the skin to remain elevated (tenting of the skin) or flatten out very slowly. Treatment: Correct the underlying cause.
	Changes in Skin Color	
albinism	**albinism** (AL-by-niz-em) **albin/o-** *white* **-ism** *process; disease from a specific cause* **albino** (al-BY-noh)	White-to-light pink skin coloration. Genetic mutation associated with melanocytes that do not produce melanin. There is a lack of pigment in the skin, hair, and iris of the eyes. The patient is said to be an **albino.** Treatment: None.

Word or Phrase	Word Part and Definition	Description
cyanosis	**cyanosis** (SY-ah-NOH-sis) **cyan/o-** *blue* **-osis** *condition; abnormal condition; process* **cyanotic** (SY-ah-NAWT-ik) **cyan/o-** *blue* **-tic** *pertaining to*	Bluish-purple discoloration of the skin and nails due to decreased oxygen levels in the blood. Caused by cardiac or respiratory disease. The patient is said to be **cyanotic.** In healthy persons, areas of skin exposed to the cold also exhibit cyanosis. Treatment: Correct the underlying cause.
erythema	**erythema** (AIR-eh-THEE-mah) *Erythema* is a Greek word meaning *flushed skin.* **erythematous** (AIR-eh-THEM-eh-tus) **erythemat/o-** *redness* **-ous** *pertaining to*	Reddish discoloration of the skin. It can be confined to one area of local inflammation or infection, or it can affect large areas of the skin surface as in sunburn. The area is said to be **erythematous.** Treatment: Correct the underlying cause.
jaundice	**jaundice** (JAWN-dis) *Jaundice* is derived from a French word meaning *yellow.* **icterus** (IK-ter-us) **icteric** (ik-TAIR-ik) **icter/o-** *jaundice* **-ic** *pertaining to*	Yellowish discoloration of the skin and whites of the eyes. It is associated with liver disease. The liver cannot process bilirubin, and high levels of unconjugated bilirubin in the blood move into the tissues and color the skin yellow. Also known as **icterus.**The patient is said to be jaundiced or **icteric.**
necrosis	**necrosis** (neh-KROH-sis) **necr/o-** *death* **-osis** *condition; abnormal condition; process* **necrotic** (neh-KRAWT-ik) **necr/o-** *death* **-tic** *pertaining to* **gangrene** (GANG-green) **gangrenous** (GANG-greh-nus) **gangren/o-** *gangrene* **-ous** *pertaining to*	Gray-to-black discoloration of the skin in areas where the tissue has died (see Figure 7-9 ■). **Necrotic** tissue can occur in a burn, decubitus ulcer, wound, or any tissue with a poor blood supply. Necrosis of the tissue with subsequent bacterial invasion and decay is known as **gangrene,** and the area is said to be **gangrenous.** Treatment: Correct the underlying cause. 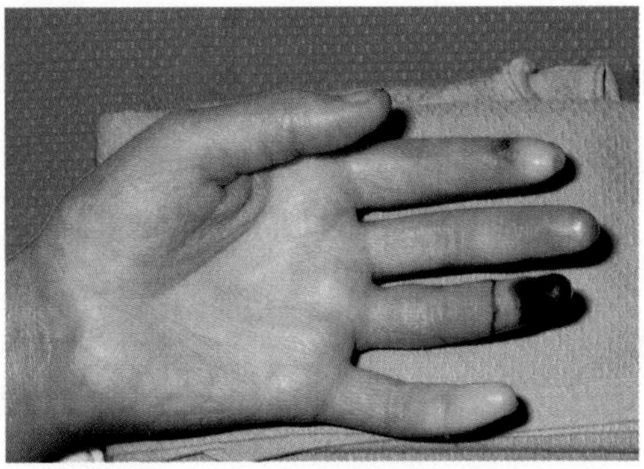 **Figure 7-9 ■ Necrosis and pallor.** This patient's ring finger has necrosis and gangrene following severe frostbite. The ring finger has been marked to show the location where an amputation will be performed. The tips of the index and little fingers show pallor, indicating poor blood flow.

Word or Phrase	Word Parts and Definition	Description
pallor	**pallor** (PAL-or) *Pallor* is a Latin word meaning *paleness.*	Unnatural paleness due to a lack of blood supply to the tissue (see Figure 7-9). Treatment: Correct the underlying cause.
vitiligo	**vitiligo** (VIT-ih-LY-goh) *Vitiligo* is derived from a Latin word meaning *defect or blemish.* **depigmentation** (dee-PIG-men-TAY-shun) **de-** *reversal of, without* **pigment/o-** *pigment* **-ation** *a process; being or having*	White, depigmented patches interspersed with normally pigmented skin. An autoimmune response slowly destroys melanocytes in ever-enlarging patches of skin. The rate of **depigmentation** is variable (see Figure 7-10 ■). Treatment: None. **Figure 7-10 ■ Vitiligo.** This patient has variable areas of depigmentation on both hands due to vitiligo, a progressive autoimmune disease.

Connections

chloasma (kloh-AZ-mah)

linea nigra (LIN-ee-ah NY-grah)
Linea nigra is a Latin phrase meaning *black line.*

striae (STRY-ee)

Obstetrics (Chapter 13). Melanocyte-stimulating hormone (from the anterior pituitary gland in the brain) can become active during pregnancy and cause dark, hyperpigmented areas on the face. This condition is known as **chloasma** or the mask of pregnancy. This hormone can also causes a dark hyperpigmented line on the skin of the abdomen from the umbilicus to the pubis. This is known as the **linea nigra.**

Stretch marks (**striae**) in the skin of the abdomen and buttocks are the result of small tears in the dermis as the skin stretches to accommodate the pregnant uterus. These are irregular, reddened lines that later become lighter and shiny as they heal and become scar tissue.

Skin Injuries

Word or Phrase	Word Parts and Definition	Description
abrasion	**abrasion** (ah-BRAY-zhun) **abras/o-** *scrape off* **-ion** *action; condition*	Sliding injury that mechanically removes the epidermal layer of the skin to reveal the dermis beneath. Also known as a brush burn. Treatment: Apply a protective covering.
blister	**blister** (BLIS-ter)	Repetitive rubbing injury that mechanically separates the epidermis from the dermis and releases tissue fluid. A blister is a fluid-filled sac with a thin, transparent covering of epidermis. Blisters often form on the heel from poorly fitting shoes or on the hand where a tool rubs. Treatment: Apply a protective covering.

Word or Phrase	Word Part and Definition	Description
burns		Heat (fire, hot objects, steam, boiling water), electrical current (lightning, electrical outlets or cords), chemicals, or radiation or x-rays (sunshine or prescribed radiation therapy) can injure superficial or deep tissues. Treatment: Topical anti-infective drugs. Second-degree burns over a large area and all third-degree burn require debridement and skin grafting.
first-degree burn		Involves only the epidermis. Causes erythema, pain, and swelling, but not blisters.
second-degree burn	**bulla** (BUL-ah) **bullae** (BUL-ee) *Bulla* is a Latin singular feminine noun meaning *bubble*. Form the plural by changing *-a* to *-ae*.	Involves the epidermis and the upper layer of the dermis. Causes erythema, pain, and swelling. There are small blisters or larger **bullae,** formed as the epidermis detaches from the dermis and the space between them fills with tissue fluid (see Figure 7-11■). Also known as a partial-thickness burn. 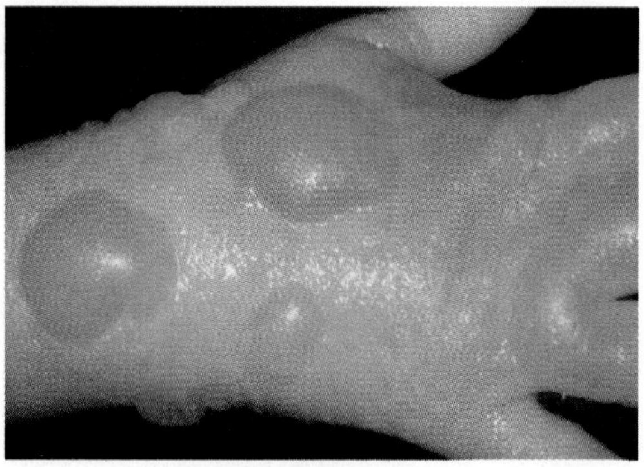 **Figure 7-11 ■ Second-degree burn of the hand.** The burn caused the epidermis to separate from the dermis. Tissue fluid caused the epidermis to swell into large, fluid-filled bullae.
third-degree burn	**anesthesia** (AN-es-THEE-zee-ah) an- *without, not* esthes/o- *sensation, feeling* -ia *condition, state, thing* **eschar** (ES-kar) *Eschar* is derived from a Greek word meaning *a burn scab.*	Involves the epidermis and entire dermis. The subcutaneous tissue and even the muscle layer may be involved. The area is black where the skin is charred. If the nerves in the dermis were destroyed, there is local **anesthesia** (no sensation of pain). Also known as a full-thickness burn. An **eschar** is a thick, crusty scar of necrotic tissue that forms on a third-degree burn. Because an eschar traps fluid released by the burned tissue, delays healing, and can become the site of infection, it is removed.
callus	**callus** (KAL-us)	Repetitive rubbing injury that causes the epidermis to gradually thicken into a wide, elevated pad. A **corn** is a callus with a hard central area with a pointed tip that causes pain and inflammation of deeper skin tissues. Treatment: Removal.

Word or Phrase	Word Part and Definition	Description
cicatrix	**cicatrix** (SIK-ah-triks) *Cicatrix* is a Latin word meaning *scar.* **keloid** (KEE-loyd) **kel/o-** *tumor* **-oid** *resembling*	Fibrous tissue composed of collagen that replaces injured skin tissue as the injury heals. Also known as a scar. A **keloid** is a very firm, abnormally large scar that is bigger than the original injury. It is due to an overproduction of collagen fibers (see Figure 7-12 ■). Unlike a scar, a keloid does not fade or decrease in size over time. Treatment: Removal, although keloids often grow back if they are removed. 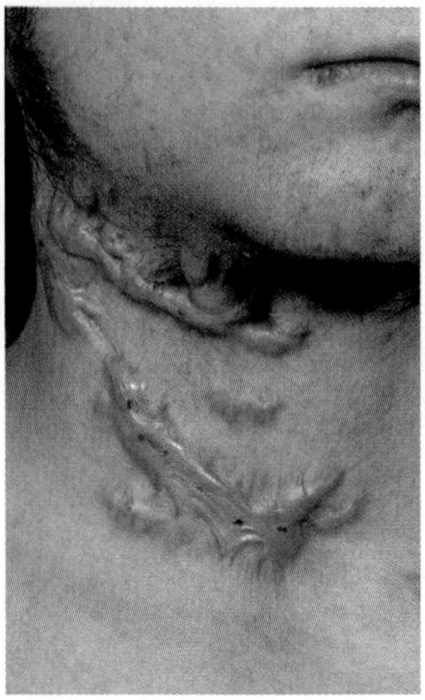 **Figure 7-12 ■ Keloid.** A keloid is a scar that continues to grow until it is larger than the original injury. Depending on its location, a keloid can be cosmetically unacceptable.
decubitus ulcer	**decubitus** (dee-KYOO-bih-tus) *Decubitus* is derived from a Latin word meaning *lying down.* **ulcer** (UL-ser) *Ulcer* is derived from a Latin word meaning *a sore.* 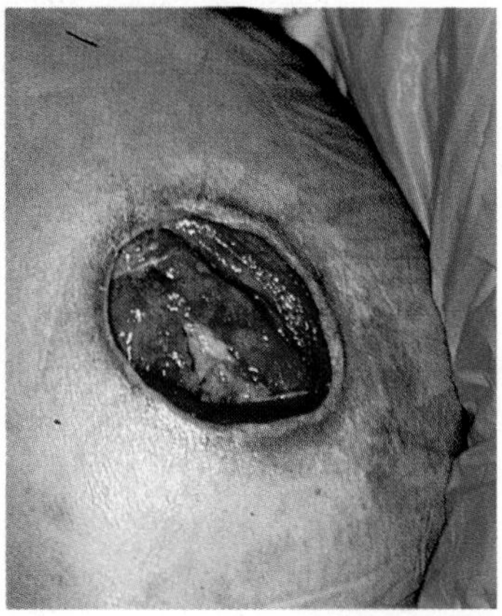 **Figure 7-13 ■ Decubitus ulcer.** This stage III decubitus ulcer involves the loss of the epidermis and dermis, exposing the subcutaneous tissue.	Pressure injury from constantly lying in one position that prevents blood flow to the tissues. The epidermis and then dermis break down and slough off, resulting in a shallow or deep wound (see Figure 7-13 ■). Decubitus ulcers occur at pressure points overlying bony prominences such as the hip or sacrum. Also known as pressure sores or bed sores. Treatment: Frequent repositioning, increased protein intake to rebuild tissue, and debridement of any necrotic tissue to promote healing. **Across the Life Span** Decreased fat in the subcutaneous tissue, poor nutrition, long-standing circulatory problems, and confinement to a bed or wheelchair predispose elderly patients to developing decubitus ulcers. Frequent repositioning of the patient and keeping the skin free of urine and stool help prevent decubitus ulcers. The level of protein in the blood (serum albumin) indicates whether the patient is able to build healthy tissue and heal an existing decubitus ulcer. A low serum albumin is treated nutritionally by offering the patient high-protein snacks.

Word or Phrase	Word Part and Definition	Description
excoriation	**excoriation** (eks-KOH-ree-AA-shun) **excori/o-** *to take out skin* **-ation** *a process; being or having*	Superficial injury with a sharp object such as a fingernail or thorn that creates a linear scratch in the skin. Treatment: Apply a protective covering.
laceration	**laceration** (LAS-er-AA-shun) **lacer/o-** *a tearing* **-ation** *a process; being or having*	Deep, penetrating wound with cleanly cut or torn, ragged skin edges (see Figure 7-14■). Treatment: Suturing. 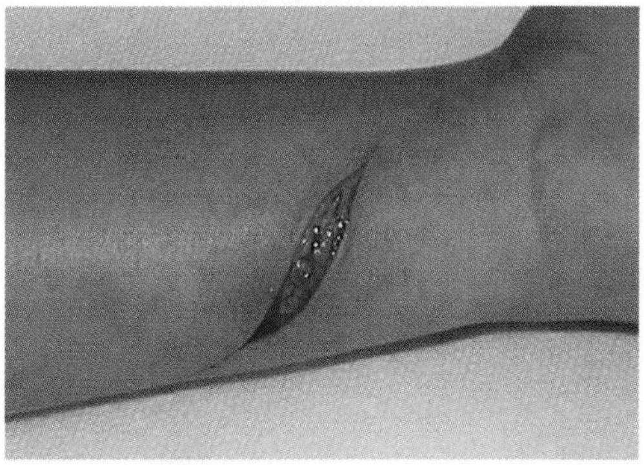 **Figure 7-14 ■ Laceration.** This deep laceration of the forearm was caused by a piece of glass that penetrated to adipose tissue in the subcutaneous layer.
Skin Infections		
abscess	**abscess** (AB-ses) **furuncle** (FYOO-rung-kl) *Furuncle* is derived from a Latin word meaning *petty thief.* **carbuncle** (KAR-bung-kl) *Carbuncle* is derived from a Latin word meaning *a live coal.*	Localized, pus-containing pocket caused by a bacterial infection. The infection is usually caused by *Staphylococcus aureus,* a common bacterium on the skin. A **furuncle** is a localized abscess around a hair follicle that causes the skin to be elevated, painful, and red. Also known as a boil. A **carbuncle** is composed of large furuncles with connecting channels through the subcutaneous tissue or to the skin surface. Treatment: Incision and drainage, oral antibiotic drugs.
cellulitis	**cellulitis** (SEL-yoo-LY-tis) **cellul/o-** *cell* **-itis** *inflammation of* Add words to make a correct and complete definition of *cellulitis: Inflammation of [many] cells [and tissue layers].*	Spreading inflammation and infection of the connective tissues of the skin and muscle. It develops from a superficial cut, scratch, insect bite, blister, or splinter that becomes infected. The infecting bacteria produce enzymes that allow the infection to spread between the tissue layers. Signs of cellulitis include erythema (often as a red streak), warmth, and tenderness. Treatment: Oral antibiotic drugs.

Word or Phrase	Word Part and Definition	Description
herpes	**herpes** (HER-peez) **herpes simplex** (HER-peez SIM-pleks) **herpes whitlow** (HER-peez WHIT-loh) **herpes varicella-zoster** (HER-peez VAIR-ih-SEL-lah ZAWS-ter) **shingles** (SHING-glz) *Shingles* is derived from a Latin word for *girdle,* as the lesions follow the dermatome as it wraps around the body.	Skin infection caused by the herpes virus. There are clustered vesicles, erythema, edema, and pain. The vesicles rupture, releasing clear fluid that forms crusts. Treatment: Topical or oral antiviral drugs. **Herpes simplex virus (HSV) type 1** occurs on the lips. These lesions tend to recur during illness and stress. Also known as cold sores or fever blisters. **Herpes simplex virus (HSV) type 2** is a sexually transmitted disease that causes vesicles in the genital area. These lesions tend to recur during illness and stress. Also known as genital herpes. **Herpes whitlow** is a herpes simplex infection at the base of the fingernail caused by contact with herpes simplex type 1 of the mouth or type 2 of the genitals. The virus enters through a small tear in the cuticle. **Herpes varicella-zoster** causes the skin rash of chickenpox during childhood. The virus then remains dormant in the body until it is activated in later life by illness or emotional stress. Then it forms painful vesicles and crusts along some dermatomes. Also known as **shingles** (see Figure 7-15 ■). **Figure 7-15 ■ Shingles.** The vesicles and crusts of shingles. The lesions occur along the dermatomes of individual spinal nerves.
tinea	**tinea** (TIN-ee-ah) *Tinea* is a Latin word meaning *worm.* **capitis** (KAP-ih-tis) *Capitis* is a Latin word meaning *of the head.* **corporis** (KOR-por-is) *Corporis* is a Latin word meaning *of the body.* **cruris** (KROOR-is) *Cruris* is a Latin word meaning *of the leg.*	Skin infection caused by a microscopic fungi that feeds on epidermal cells. It multiplies quickly in the warm, moist environment of body creases and areas enclosed by clothing or shoes. Tinea is characterized by severe itching and burning with red, scaly lesions. Tinea is named according to where it occurs on the body. **Tinea capitis** occurs on the scalp and causes hair loss. **Tinea corporis** occurs on any part of the body. The round lesions led to the erroneous conclusion that the disease was caused by a worm, and so it was originally named ringworm. **Tinea cruris** occurs in the groin and perineum and is known as jock itch. **Tinea pedis** occurs on the feet and toes and is known as athlete's foot (see Figure 7-16 ■).

Word or Phrase	Word Part and Definition	Description
tinea *(continued)*	**pedis** (PEE-dis) *Pedis* is a Latin word meaning *of the foot.*	**Figure 7-16 ■ Tinea pedis.** This fungal infection, also known as athlete's foot, causes severe itching and burning. The erythematous, scaly lesions eventually become soft and white and begin to peel due to moisture between the toes.
verruca	**verruca** (veh-ROO-kah) **verrucae** (veh-ROO-kee) *Verruca* is a Latin singular feminine noun meaning *a wart.* Form the plural by changing *-a* to *-ae.*	Irregular, rough skin lesion caused by human papillomavirus transmitted by contact. Commonly found on the hand and fingers or the sole of the foot (plantar wart). Also known as a wart.
Skin Infestations		
pediculosis	**pediculosis** (peh-DIK-yoo-LOH-sis) **pedicul/o-** *lice* **-osis** *condition; abnormal condition; process*	Infestation of lice and their eggs in the scalp, hair, eyelashes, or pubic hair. Lice are easily transmitted from one person to another by means of combs or hats. Treatment: Shampoo and skin lotion to kill lice.
scabies	**scabies** (SKAY-beez) *Scabies* is derived from a Latin word meaning *to scratch.*	Infestation of parasitic mites that tunnel under the skin and produce vesicles. These lesions are pruritic. Treatment: Shampoo and skin lotion to kill mites.

Allergic Skin Conditions

Word or Phrase	Word Part and Definition	Description
contact dermatitis	**dermatitis** (DER-mah-TY-tis) **dermat/o-** *skin* **-itis** *inflammation of*	Topical reaction to physical contact with a substance that is an allergen or an irritant. Examples: Chemicals (deodorant, soaps, detergents, makeup, urine), metals, fabrics (Spandex bathing suit or girdle), plants (poison ivy), or animals (see Figure 7-17 ■). The skin becomes inflamed and pruritic. Small vesicles may also appear. Treatment: Topical or oral antihistamine or corticosteroid drugs. **Figure 7-17 ■ Severe contact dermatitis.** This was caused by the application of a new deodorant whose chemical ingredients caused irritation.
urticaria	**urticaria** (ER-tih-KAIR-ee-ah) *Urticaria* is derived from *Urtica*, a genus of stinging plants commonly known as nettle.	Condition of edema and wheals that appear suddenly and may also disappear rapidly. Scratching tends to cause the areas to enlarge. Urticaria is caused by an allergic reaction to food, plants, animals, insect bites, or drugs. Urticaria is also known as hives. A large wheal is known as a welt. Treatment: Topical or oral antihistamine or corticosteroid drugs.

Benign Skin Markings and Neoplasms

Word or Phrase	Word Part and Definition	Description
actinic keratoses	**actinic** (ak-TIN-ik) **actin/o-** *rays of the sun* **-ic** *pertaining to* **keratosis** (KAIR-ah-TOH-sis) **keratoses** (KAIR-ah-TOH-seez) **kerat/o-** *hard, fibrous protein* **-osis** *condition; abnormal condition; process* **solar** (SOH-lar) *Solar* is derived from a Latin word meaning *sun*.	Raised, irregular, rough areas of skin that are dry and feel like sandpaper. These develop in middle-aged persons in areas chronically exposed to the sun. They can become squamous cell carcinoma. Also known as **solar keratoses.** Treatment: Avoid more sun exposure.

Word or Phrase	Word Part and Definition	Description
dysplastic nevus	**dysplastic** (dis-PLAS-tik) dys- *painful, difficult, abnormal* plast/o- *growth, formation* -ic *pertaining to* **nevus** (NEE-vus) *Nevus* is a Latin word meaning *mole.*	A mole (nevus) with irregular edges and variations in color. It can develop into malignant melanoma. Treatment: None; observe for changes.
freckle	**freckle** (FREK-l) **benign** (bee-NINE) *Benign* is derived from a Latin word meaning *kind, not cancerous.*	**Benign,** pigmented, flat macule that develops after sun exposure. Freckles contain groups of melanocytes. Freckles fade over time without continued sun exposure.
hemangioma	**hemangioma** (hee-MAN-jee-OH-mah) hem/o- *blood* angi/o- *blood vessel; lymph vessel* -oma *tumor, mass*	Congenital growth composed of a mass of superficial and dilated blood vessels (see Figure 7-18 ■). Treatment: Most hemangiomas disappear without treatment by age 3. **Figure 7-18 ■ Hemangioma.** The bright red color comes from the large number of dilated blood vessels. Most hemangiomas disappear without treatment by age 3.
lipoma	**lipoma** (ly-POH-mah) lip/o- *lipid (fat)* -oma *tumor, mass*	Benign growth composed of adipose tissue from the subcutaneous layer. It causes a soft, rounded, nontender elevation of the skin. Treatment: Excision, if desired.
nevus	**nevus** (NEE-vus) *Nevus* is a Latin word meaning *mole or birthmark.*	Benign skin lesion that is present at birth and comes in a variety of colors and shapes. **Moles** are darkly pigmented nevi that can be flat or round and elevated and often contain hairs. **Port-wine stains** are slightly elevated, red-to-purple vascular nevi with distinct, but irregularly shaped margins. They can involve large areas of skin on the face and neck. Their shape and color resemble a puddle of spilled wine. They are also known as birthmarks. Treatment: Excision of a mole if clothing irritates it. Laser treatment to remove port-wine stains.
papilloma	**papilloma** (PAP-ih-LOH-mah) papill/o- *elevated structure* -oma *tumor, mass*	Small, soft, flesh-colored growth of epidermis and dermis that protrudes outwardly. It comes in a variety of shapes: irregular mounds, globes, flaps, or polyps with round tops on slender stalks. It occurs on the eyelid, neck, or trunk of the body. Also known as a skin tag. Treatment: Removal by cryotherapy, electrocautery, or surgical excision, if desired.

Word or Phrase	Word Part and Definition	Description
premalignant skin lesions	**premalignant** (PREE-mah-LIG-nant) **pre-** *before; in front of* **malign/o-** *intentionally causing harm; cancer* **-ant** *pertaining to*	Abnormal but not yet clearly cancerous lesions. Over time and with continued exposure to sunlight or irritation, these lesions can become cancerous. Treatment: None; observe for changes.
senile lentigo	**senile** (SEE-nile) **sen/o-** *old age* **-ile** *pertaining to* **lentigo** (len-TY-goh) *Lentigo* is derived from a Latin word meaning *a lentil (a small, flat, round, brownish dried seed).*	Light-to-dark brown macules with irregular edges. They occur most often on the hands and face, areas that are chronically exposed to the sun. Also called age spots or liver spots.
syndactyly	**syndactyly** (sin-DAK-tih-lee) **syn-** *together* **-dactyly** *condition of fingers or toes* Every medical word must contain a combining form. The suffix of *syndactyly* contains the combining form *dactyl/o.* **polydactyly** (PAWL-ee-DAK-tih-lee) **poly-** *many, much* **-dactyly** *condition of fingers or toes*	Congenital abnormality in which the skin and soft tissues are joined between the fingers or toes (see Figure 7-19■). In some cases the fingernails or toenails are also fused. **Polydactyly** is a congenital abnormality in which there are extra fingers or toes. Treatment: Surgical correction, if desired. **Figure 7-19 ■ Syndactyly.** The skin and soft tissues of the second and third toes are fused together in this patient with syndactyly.
xanthoma	**xanthoma** (zan-THOH-mah) **xanth/o-** *yellow* **-oma** *tumor, mass* **xanthelasma** (ZAN-theh-LAZ-mah) **xanth/o-** *yellow* **-elasma** *platelike structure*	Benign growth that occurs as a yellow nodule or plaque on the hands, elbows, knees, or feet. It is most often seen in patients who have high levels of lipids in the blood or diabetes mellitus. A xanthoma that occurs on the eyelid is known as a **xanthelasma.** Treatment: Excision, if desired.

Malignant Neoplasms of the Skin

Word or Phrase	Word Part and Definition	Description
cancer of the skin	**cancer** (KAN-ser) *Cancer* is a Latin word meaning *a crab.* Cancer reaches into other tissues like the legs of a crab reach out from its center. **malignancy** (mah-LIG-nan-see) **malign/o-** *intentionally causing harm; cancer* **-ancy** *state of*	**Malignancy** that occurs in areas of the skin that are chronically exposed to ultraviolet light radiation from the sun. Skin cancer is more common in the elderly (life time of sun exposure) and in fair-skinned persons (less melanin to absorb radiation). Treatment: Excision, chemotherapy drugs, photodynamic therapy.
basal cell carcinoma	**carcinoma** (KAR-sih-NOH-mah) **carcin/o-** *cancer* **-oma** *tumor, mass*	Arises from the basal layer of the epidermis. It is the most common type of skin cancer. It most often appears as a raised, pearly bump. A slow-growing cancer that does not metastasize to other parts of the body.
malignant melanoma	**malignant** (mah-LIG-nant) **malign/o-** *intentionally causing harm; cancer* **-ant** *pertaining to* **melanoma** (MEL-ah-NOH-mah) **melan/o-** *black* **-oma** *tumor, mass*	Arises from melanocytes in the epidermis (see Figure 7-20 ■). A malignant melanoma grows quickly and metastasizes to other parts of the body. Malignant melanomas have these four characteristics: A Asymmetry. Each side of the lesion has a different shape. B Border or edge is irregular and ragged. C Color varies from black to brown to red within the same lesion. D Diameter is variable and is growing.

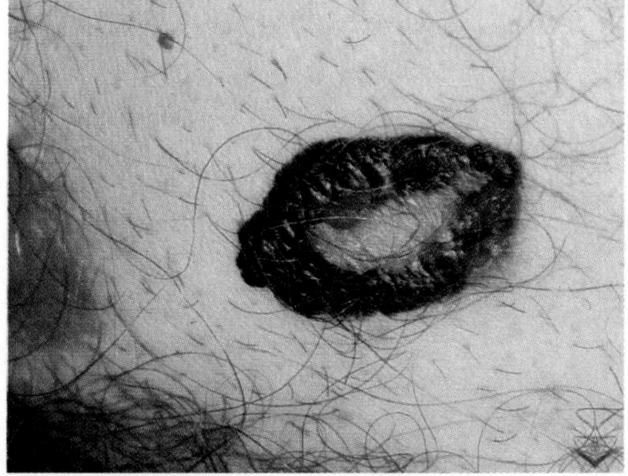

Figure 7-20 ■ Malignant melanoma.

This lesion reveals three of the four typical characteristics of malignant melanoma: asymmetry; ragged, irregular edges; and varying shades of color. The fourth characteristic—an increase in size—would be noted over time.

Connections

Public Health. Depletion of the earth's ozone layer has lead to an increased number of cases of malignant melanoma. The use of sunscreen and avoiding prolonged sun exposure, particularly during midday, helps to decrease this risk. A self-examination of the skin should be done regularly. Irregular or changing skin lesions should be examined by a dermatologist.

Word or Phrase	Word Part and Definition	Description
squamous cell carcinoma	**squamous** (SKWAY-mus) **squam/o-** *scalelike cell* **-ous** *pertaining to*	Arises from the flat squamous cells of the outer part of the epidermis. It often begins as an actinic keratosis. It most often appears as a red bump or ulcer. It is the second most common type of skin cancer, but it grows slowly.

Word or Phrase	Word Part and Definition	Description
Kaposi's sarcoma	**Kaposi** (kah-POH-see) Named by Moritz Kaposi (1837–1902), a Hungarian dermatologist. This is an example of an eponym: a person from whom something takes its name. **sarcoma** (sar-KOH-mah) **sarc/o-** *connective tissue* **-oma** *tumor, mass*	Arises from connective tissue or lymph nodes. Tumors on the skin are elevated, irregular, and dark reddish-blue. This was once a relatively rare malignancy, but is now commonly seen in AIDS patients. Treatment: Excision of single lesions, radiation therapy for multiple lesions.
Autoimmune Diseases with Skin Symptoms		
psoriasis	**psoriasis** (soh-RY-ah-sis) **psor/o-** *itching* **-iasis** *state of; process of* **psoriatic** (SOH-ree-AT-ik) **psor/o-** *itching* **-iatic** *pertaining to a state or process*	Autoimmune disorder characterized by the production of excessive amounts of epidermal cells. Skin lesions are itchy and show erythema covered with silvery scales and plaques, particularly on the scalp, elbows, hands, and knees (see Figure 7-21■). Illness and stress tend to cause flare-ups, and psoriasis has a hereditary component. Treatment: Topical coal tar, vitamin D, and corticosteroid drugs; oral vitamin A and oral corticosteroid drugs. Light therapy with a psoralen drug and ultraviolet light A (PUVA). **Figure 7-21 ■ Psoriasis.** Psoriasis produces characteristic elevated, erythematous lesions that are topped by silvery scales and plaques.
systemic lupus erythematosus (SLE)	**systemic** (sis-TEM-ik) **system/o-** *the body as a whole* **-ic** *pertaining to* **lupus erythematosus** (LOO-pus AIR-ih-THEM-ah-TOH-sus) *Lupus* is a Latin word meaning *wolf.* The erythematous rash on the face was thought to resemble a wolf bite.	Autoimmune disorder characterized by deterioration of collagen in the skin and connective tissues. There is a rash, joint pain, sensitivity to sunlight, and fatigue. Often there is a characteristic butterfly-shaped, erythematous rash that covers the nose and cheeks. Treatment: Oral corticosteroid drugs.

Word or Phrase	Word Part and Definition	Description
scleroderma	**scleroderma** (SKLER-oh-DER-mah) **scler/o-** *hard; sclera (white of the eye)* **-derma** *skin*	Autoimmune disorder that causes the skin and internal organs to become progressively hardened due to deposits of collagen. Treatment: Oral corticosteroid drugs.
Diseases of the Sebaceous Glands		
acne vulgaris	**acne vulgaris** (AK-nee vul-GAIR-is) *Acne* is derived from a Latin word meaning *a pointed thing.* *Vulgaris* is derived from a Latin word meaning *common or ordinary.* **comedo** (KOM-eh-doh) (koh-MEE-doh)	During puberty, the sebaceous glands produce large amounts of sebum, particularly on the forehead, nose, chin, shoulders, and back. Excess sebum builds up around the hair shaft, hardens, and blocks the follicle. The blocked secretions elevate the skin and form a reddish papule. In other hair follicles, the oily sebum traps dirt and enlarges the pore. The sebum turns black as its oil is oxidized from exposure to the air. This forms a **comedo** (blackhead). As bacteria feed on the sebum, they release irritating substances that produce inflammation. Large numbers of bacteria produce infection, forming pustules (whiteheads) (see Figure 7-22■). In severe cystic acne, the papules enlarge to form deep, pus-filled cysts. Treatment: Topical cleansing drugs, topical or oral antibiotic drugs to kill skin bacteria. Oral vitamin A–type drugs for severe cystic acne. 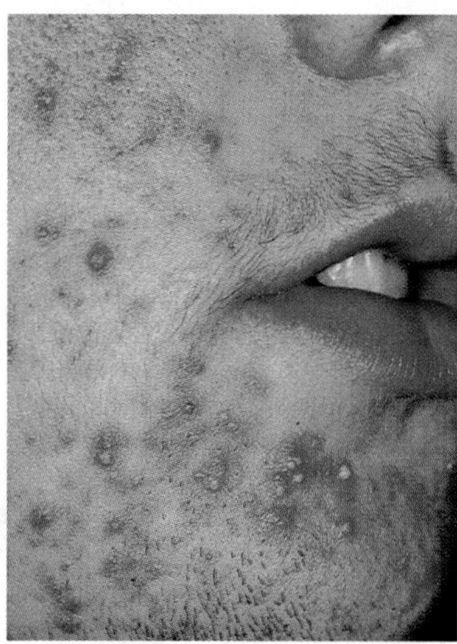 **Figure 7-22 ■ Acne vulgaris.** This adolescent boy has severe acne vulgaris with papules, comedos, and pustules. Increased secretion of the sebaceous glands during puberty triggers the onset of acne vulgaris.

Word or Phrase	Word Parts and Definition	Description
acne rosacea	**acne rosacea** (AK-nee roh-ZAY-shee-ah) *Rosacea* is derived from a Latin word meaning *rose colored.* **rhinophyma** (RY-noh-FY-mah) **rhin/o-** *nose* **-phyma** *tumor, growth*	Chronic skin condition of the face in middle-aged patients. The sebaceous glands secrete excessive amounts of sebum, causing papules and pustules. Acne rosacea is also characterized by constant blotchy erythema, dilated superficial blood vessels, and edema that are made worse by heat, stress, and sunlight (see Figure 7-23 ■). Also known as rosacea. Men can develop an erythematous, irregular enlargement of the nose known as **rhinophyma**. Treatment: Topical antibacterial drugs. Laser surgery to destroy small, superficial blood vessels.

Figure 7-23 ■ Acne rosacea.
This patient's face shows the blotchy erythema and dilated superficial blood vessels of acne rosacea. There is no evidence of pustules or swelling at this time.

Table 7-1 Comparison of Acne Vulgaris and Acne Rosacea

	Site	Comedos	Pustules and Papules	Dilated Blood Vessels	Age
Acne vulgaris	face, shoulders, chest, back	yes	yes	no	adolescence
Acne rosacea	face only	no	yes	yes	middle age

Word or Phrase	Word Part and Definition	Description
seborrhea	**seborrhea** (SEB-oh-REE-ah) **seb/o-** *sebum (oil)* **-rrhea** *flow, discharge* **seborrheic** (SEB-oh-REE-ik) **seb/o-** *sebum (oil)* **rrhe/o-** *flow, discharge* **-ic** *pertaining to* **dermatitis** (DER-mah-TY-tis) **dermat/o-** *skin* **-itis** *inflammation of* **eczema** (EK-zeh-mah)	Overproduction of sebum, particularly on the face and scalp, that occurs at a time other than puberty. In **seborrheic dermatitis,** oily areas are interspersed with patches of dry, scaly skin and dandruff. There can also be erythema and crusty, yellow exudates. In adults, seborrheic dermatitis often appears after illness or stress. It can be caused by environmental or food allergies. Called cradle cap in infants and **eczema** in infants and adults. Treatment: Topical corticosteroid drugs, medicated shampoos.
Diseases of the Sweat Glands		
anhidrosis	**anhidrosis** (AN-hy-DROH-sis) **an-** *without, not* **hidr/o-** *sweat* **-osis** *condition; abnormal condition; process*	Congenital absence of the sweat glands and inability to tolerate heat. Treatment: Avoid overheating.
diaphoresis	**diaphoresis** (DY-ah-foh-REE-sis) **diaphore/o-** *sweating* **-sis** *condition* **diaphoretic** (DY-ah-foh-RET-ik) **diaphore/o-** *sweating* **-tic** *pertaining to*	Profuse sweating. Although a high fever, emotional stress, strenuous exercise, or the hot flashes of menopause can cause profuse sweating, these are *not* referred to as diaphoresis. Diaphoresis is caused by an underlying condition such as myocardial infarction, hyperthyroidism, hypoglycemia, or withdrawal from narcotic drugs. The patient is said to be **diaphoretic.** Treatment: Correct the underlying cause.
Diseases of the Hair		
alopecia	**alopecia** (AL-oh-PEE-shee-ah) *Alopecia* is derived from a Greek word meaning *hair falling out.* This first referred to mange, a skin disease of dogs and foxes that causes hair loss. *Alopex* is the Greek word for *fox.*	Acute or chronic loss of scalp hair. Acute alopecia can be caused by chemotherapy drugs that attack rapidly dividing cancer cells, but also affect rapidly dividing hair cells. Skin diseases of the scalp can also cause acute hair loss. Chronic hair loss usually begins in early middle age in men. The influence of testosterone (male hormone), heredity, and decreased blood flow to the hair follicles cause the thickness of the hair shaft to diminish. In men, hair on the top of the scalp gradually thins and may eventually disappear, leaving a fringe of hair at the back of the head. This is known as male pattern baldness. Alopecia occurs in women during menopause when the level of androgen (produced in minute amounts by the adrenal cortex) exceeds that of estrogen produced by the ovaries. Treatment: Topical drugs that cause vasodilation of the scalp or oral drugs that block the effect of testosterone.
folliculitis	**folliculitis** (foh-LIK-yoo-LY-tis) **follicul/o-** *follicle (small sac)* **-itis** *inflammation of*	Inflammation or infection of the hair follicle. It occurs after shaving, plucking, or removing hair with hot wax. Treatment: Topical corticosteroid or antibiotic drugs.

Word or Phrase	Word Part and Definition	Description
hirsutism	**hirsutism** (HER-soo-tizm) **hirsut/o-** *hairy* **-ism** *process; disease from a specific cause*	The presence of excessive, dark hair on the forearms and over the upper lip of a woman. It is due to hypersecretion of testosterone because of a tumor in the adrenal cortex. Treatment: Correct the underlying cause.
pilonidal sinus	**pilonidal** (PY-loh-NY-dal) **pil/o-** *hair* **nid/o-** *nest; focus* **-al** *pertaining to* **sinus** (SY-nus) *Sinus* is a Latin word meaning *cavity or channel.* **fistula** (FIS-tyoo-lah) *Fistula* is a Latin word meaning *a tube.*	Abnormal passageway (**fistula**) that begins as an enlarged, abnormal hair follicle that contains a hair that is never shed. The follicle is visible as a pit or dimple on the skin in the sacral area of the back. Irritation causes the hair follicle to become infected, eventually creating a sinus into the subcutaneous tissue, with erythema, tenderness, and purulent discharge. Treatment: Incision and drainage of the sinus.
schizotrichia	**schizotrichia** (SKIZ-oh-TRIK-ee-ah) **schiz/o-** *split* **trich/o-** *hair* **-ia** *condition, state, thing*	Split ends on hairs
Diseases of the Nails		
onychomycosis	**onychomycosis** (ON-ih-koh-my-KOH-sis) **onych/o-** *nail* **myc/o-** *fungus* **-osis** *condition; abnormal condition; process*	Fungal infection of the fingernails or toenails. A fungus infects the nail root and deforms the nail as it grows. The nail is discolored, misshapen, thickened, and raised up from the nail bed (see Figure 7-24■). Treatment: Topical or oral antifungal drugs. 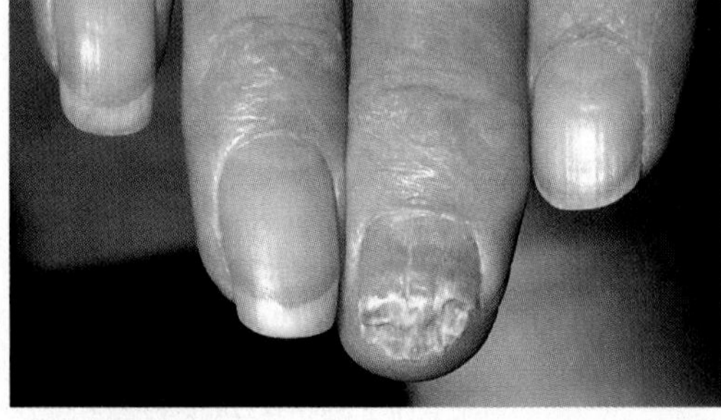 **Figure 7-24 ■ Onychomycosis.** This fungal infection can involve one or all of the nails of the hands or feet.

Word or Phrase	Word Part and Definition	Description
paronychia	**paronychia** (PAR-oh-NIK-ee-ah) par- *beside* onych/o- *nail* -ia *condition, state, thing*	Inflammation and infection of the skin along the cuticle. There is tenderness, erythema, and swelling, and an abscess with pus. Treatment: Oral antibiotic drugs.
clubbing		Abnormally curved fingernails and stunted growth of the finger associated with a chronic lack of oxygen in patients with cystic fibrosis.

Diagnostic Procedures

Word or Phrase	Word Part and Definition	Description
allergy skin testing	**intradermal** (IN-trah-DER-mal) intra- *within* derm/o- *skin* -al *pertaining to*	Solutions of various antigens (animal dander, foods, plants, pollen, and so forth) are given by **intradermal** injections in the forearm. If the patient is allergic to a particular antigen, a wheal will form at the site of that injection (see Figure 7-25■). Alternatively, the antigen is scratched into the skin, and the procedure is known as a **scratch test.** **Figure 7-25 ■ Allergy skin testing.** This patient's forearm shows a number of wheals where the body's immune response was triggered by the injected antigen. The size of the wheal corresponds to the degree of allergy to that antigen. No wheal formation means that the patient is not allergic to that antigen.
culture and sensitivity (C&S)	**sensitivity** (SEN-sih-TIV-ih-tee) sensitiv/o- *affected by, sensitive to* -ity *state; condition* **exudate** (EKS-yoo-dayt) exud/o- *oozing fluid* -ate *composed of; pertaining to*	A specimen of the **exudate** from an ulcer, wound, burn, or laceration or the pus from an infection is cultured in a Petri dish to diagnose a bacterial infection. Microorganisms present in the exudate grow into colonies. The specific disease-causing pathogen is identified and then tested to determine its sensitivity to various antibiotic drugs.

Word or Phrase	Word Part and Definition	Description
RAST		Blood test that measures the amount of IgE produced each time the blood is mixed with a specific allergen. It shows which of many allergens the patient is allergic to and how severe the allergy is. RAST stands for radioallergosorbent test.
skin scraping		A skin scraping is done with the edge of a scalpel to obtain material from skin lesions, examine it under the microscope, and make a diagnosis of ringworm.
Tzanck test	**Tzanck** (TSAHNGK) This test was developed by Arnault Tzanck (1886–1954), a Russian dermatologist. This is an example of an eponym: a person from whom something takes its name.	A skin scraping is done to obtain fluid from a vesicle. A smear of the fluid is placed on a slide, stained, and examined under a microscope. Herpes virus infections and shingles show characteristic giant cells with viruses in them.
Wood's lamp or light	Invented by Robert Wood (1868–1955), an American physicist.	Ultraviolet light used to highlight areas of skin abnormality. In a darkened room, ultraviolet light makes vitiligo appear bright white and tinea capitus (ringworm) appear blue-green because the fungus fluoresces.

Medical and Surgical Procedures

Medical Procedures

Word or Phrase	Word Part and Definition	Description
Botox injections	**Botox** (BOH-tawks)	Medical procedure in which the drug Botox is injected into the muscles that cause deep skin wrinkles on the face. The drug inhibits the release of acetylcholine and keeps these muscles from contracting. This treatment is only effective for several months. **Did You Know?** Botox is actually a neurotoxin from the bacteria *Clostridium botulinum* type A that causes food poisoning (botulism).
collagen injections		Medical procedure in which a solution of the protein collagen is injected into wrinkles or acne scars. This plumps the skin and decreases the depth of the wrinkle or scar. Collagen is from cow or human sources.
cryosurgery	**cryosurgery** (KRY-oh-SER-jer-ee) **cry/o-** *cold* **surg/o-** *operative procedure* **-ery** *process of*	Medical procedure in which liquid nitrogen is sprayed or painted onto a wart, mole, or other benign lesion, or onto a small malignant lesion. The liquid nitrogen freezes and destroys the tissue.

Word or Phrase	Word Part and Definition	Description
curettage	**curettage** (kyoo-rah-TAWZH) *Curettage* is a French word meaning *a scraping.* **curet** (kyoo-RET) *Curet* is a French word meaning *a scraper.*	Medical procedure that involves using a **curet** to scrape off the superficial part of a skin lesion. A curet is a metal instrument that ends in a small, circular or oval ring with a sharp edge. Curettage is often combined with electrodesiccation for complete removal of a lesion.
debridement	**debridement** (deh-BREED-maw) *Debridement* is a French word meaning *to unbridle.*	Medical or surgical procedure in which necrotic tissue is debrided (removed) from a burn, wound, or ulcer. Debridement is done to remove dead tissue that can become the source of infection, assess the extent or depth of a wound, and create a clean, raw surface that is ready to heal or receive a skin graft. Mechanical debridement consists of putting on a wet dressing, letting it dry, and then removing the dressing, pulling off necrotic tissue with it. Topical enzyme drugs debride necrotic tissue by chemically dissolving it. Surgical debridement is done under anesthesia using a scalpel, scissors, or curet.
electrosurgery	**electrosurgery** (ee-LEK-troh-SER-jer-ee) **electr/o-** *electricity* **surg/o-** *operative procedure* **-ery** *process of* **electrodesiccation** (ee-LEK-troh-DES-ih-KAY-shun) **electr/o-** *electricity* **desicc/o-** *to dry up* **-ation** *a process; being or having* **fulguration** (FUL-gyoo-RAY-shun) **fulgur/o-** *spark of electricity* **-ation** *a process; being or having* **electrosection** (ee-LEK-troh-SEK-shun) **electr/o-** *electricity* **sect/o-** *to cut* **-ion** *action; condition*	Medical procedure that involves the use of electrical current to remove a nevus, wart, skin tag, or small malignant lesion. The electrical current passes through an electrode and causes the intracellular contents to evaporate. In **electrodesiccation,** the electrode is touched to or inserted into the skin or lesion. In **fulguration,** the electrode is held away from the skin and transmits a spark to the skin surface. **Electrosection** uses a wire loop electrode to cut tissue.
incision and drainage (I&D)	**incision** (in-SIZH-un) **incis/o-** *to cut into* **-ion** *action; condition*	Medical procedure to treat a cyst or abscess. A scalpel is used to make an incision, and the fluid or pus inside is expressed manually or allowed to drain out.
laser surgery	**laser** (LAY-zer) *Laser* is an acronym, a word made from the first letters of the phrase ***l**ight **a**mplification by **s**timulated **e**mission of **r**adiation.*	Medical procedure that uses pulses of laser light to remove birthmarks, tattoos, superficial blood vessels of acne rosacea, and unwanted hair. A tunable laser has a specific wavelength of light that only reacts with certain colors (the dark red of a birthmark, the black pigment of a tattoo and so forth) to break up that color and the structure that contains it. Surrounding tissue is unharmed.

Word or Phrase	Word Part and Definition	Description
skin examination		Medical procedure to examine all of the patient's skin or just one skin lesion, rash, or tumor. The dermatologist uses a lens to magnify the area (see Figure 7-26■). 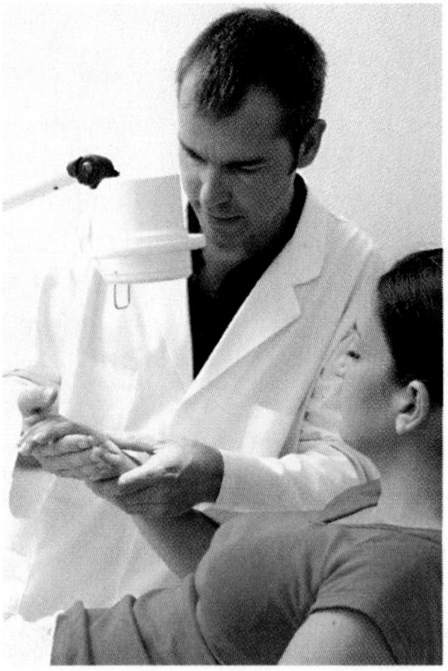 **Figure 7-26 ■ Skin examination.** This dermatologist is using a magnifying lens and strong light to examine a lesion on this patient's skin. The area may need to be biopsied to obtain a diagnosis.
skin resurfacing		Removal of superficial and deep acne scars, fine or deep wrinkles, or tattoos, and correction of large pores and skin tone irregularities by means of topical chemicals, abrasion, or laser treatments.
chemical peel		Uses a chemical to remove the epidermis. Alphahydroxy acid (glycolic acid) provides the mildest chemical peel. Stronger chemical peels using trichloroacetic acid and phenol are usually done in surgery.
dermabrasion	**dermabrasion** (DER-mah-BRAY-zhun) **derm/o-** *skin* **abras/o-** *scrape off* **-ion** *action; condition*	Uses a rapidly spinning wire brush or diamond surface to mechanically abrade (scrape away) the epidermis.
laser skin resurfacing		Uses a computer-controlled laser to vaporize the epidermis and some of the dermis. This promotes the regrowth of smooth skin. Also known as a laser peel.
microderm-abrasion	**microdermabrasion** (MY-kroh-DER-mah-BRAY-shun) **micr/o-** *small* **derm/o-** *skin* **abras/o-** *scrape off* **-ion** *action; condition*	Uses aluminum oxide crystals to abrade and remove the epidermis to produce smoother skin

Word or Phrase	Word Part and Definition	Description
suturing	**suture** (SOO-chur) *Suture* is derived from a Latin word meaning *a seam.*	Medical procedure that uses sutures to bring the edges of the skin together after a laceration or other injury (see Figure 7-27■). **Figure 7-27 ■ Sutures.** After topical and local anesthetic drugs were administered, this laceration in the forearm was sewn closed with two layers of sutures, the first to approximate the deeper layers and the second to approximate the skin edges. After a week, the skin sutures were cut and removed. The deeper sutures were made of a material that is absorbed by the body and does not need to be removed.

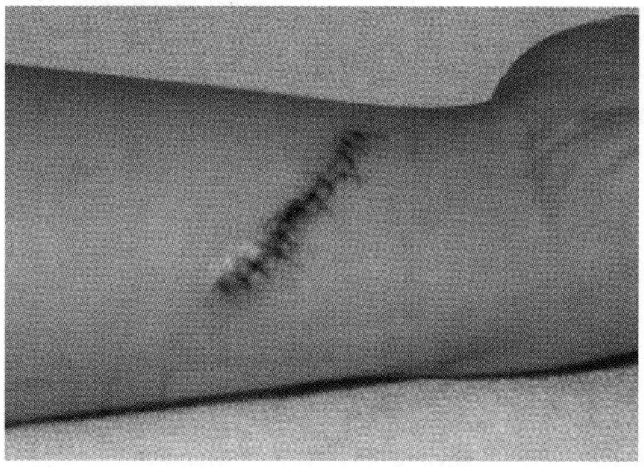

Surgical Procedures

Word or Phrase	Word Part and Definition	Description
biopsy (Bx)	**biopsy** (BY-awp-see) **bi/o-** *life; living organisms; living tissue* **-opsy** *process of viewing*	Surgical procedure to remove all or part of a skin lesion for the purpose of diagnosis. The biopsy specimen is sent to the pathology department for examination and diagnosis.
excisional biopsy	**excisional** (ek-SIZH-un-al) **excis/o-** *to cut out* **-ion** *action; condition* **-al** *pertaining to*	Uses a scalpel to remove an entire large lesion
incisional biopsy	**incisional** (in-SIZH-un-al) **incis/o-** *to cut into* **-ion** *action; condition* **-al** *pertaining to*	Uses a scalpel to make an incision into part of a large lesion to remove a wedge of it
needle aspiration	**aspiration** (AS-pih-RAY-shun) **aspir/o-** *to breathe in; to suck in* **-ation** *a process; being or having*	Uses a needle to aspirate the fluid contents in a cyst
punch biopsy		Uses a small, circular metal cutter to remove a plug-shaped core of skin that includes the epidermis, dermis, and subcutaneous tissue
shave biopsy		Uses a scalpel or razor blade to remove a superficial lesion of the epidermis and/or dermis

Word or Phrase	Word Part and Definition	Description
dermatoplasty	**dermatoplasty** (DER-mah-toh-PLAS-tee) **dermat/o-** *skin* **-plasty** *process of reshaping by surgery*	Surgical procedure for any type of plastic surgery of the skin, such as skin grafting, removal of keloids, release of skin contractures, and so forth.
liposuction	**liposuction** (LIP-oh-SUK-shun) **lip/o-** *lipid (fat)* **suct/o-** *to suck* **-ion** *action; condition* **lipectomy** (ly-PEK-toh-mee) **lip/o-** *lipid (fat)* **-ectomy** *surgical excision*	Surgical procedure to remove excessive adipose tissue deposits, usually from the abdomen, hips, legs, or buttocks. A suction cannula removes the fat through small incisions. Ultrasonic-assisted liposuction uses ultrasonic waves to break up the fat before it is removed. Also known as **suction-assisted lipectomy.**
Moh's surgery	**Moh's** (MOHZ) The technique was developed in 1936 by Dr. Frederic Mohs, and it is still the preferred method of surgery for some skin cancers.	Surgical procedure to remove skin cancer, particularly tumors with irregular shapes and depths. An operating microscope is used during the surgery to examine each layer of excised tissue. If the tissue shows cancerous cells, more tissue is removed until no trace of cancer remains.
rhytidectomy	**rhytidectomy** (RIT-ih-DEK-toh-mee) **rhytid/o-** *wrinkle* **-ectomy** *surgical excision* **blepharoplasty** (BLEF-ah-roh-PLAS-tee) **blephar/o-** *eyelid* **-plasty** *process of reshaping by surgery*	Surgical procedure to remove wrinkles and tighten loose, aging skin on the face and neck. Also known as a face-lift. A **blepharoplasty,** removal of fat and drooping skin from around the eyelids, may be performed at the same time.
skin grafting	**dermatome** (DER-mah-tohm) **derm/a-** *skin* **-tome** *instrument used to cut; an area with distinct edges*	Surgical procedure that uses human, animal, or artificial skin to provide a temporary covering or permanent layer of skin over a burn or wound. A **dermatome** is used to remove (harvest) a thin layer of skin to be used as a graft. A split-thickness skin graft contains the epidermis and part of the dermis. A full-thickness skin graft contains the epidermis and all of the dermis. Tiny holes can be cut in the skin graft to stretch it like mesh and cover a larger area. These holes allow fluid from damaged tissue to flow out and provide spaces into which the new skin can grow.
autograft	**autograft** (AW-toh-graft) **auto-** *self* **-graft** *tissue for implant or transplant* *Autograft* is a shortened form of *autologous graft.*	Uses a skin graft taken from another part of the patient's body
allograft	**allograft** (AL-oh-graft) **all/o-** *other; strange* **-graft** *tissue for implant or transplant*	Uses a skin graft taken from a cadaver. It is frozen and stored in a skin bank until needed. This is a temporary skin graft to protect the patient against infection and fluid loss.

Word or Phrase	Word Part and Definition	Description
xenograft	**xenograft** (ZEN-oh-graft) **xen/o-** *foreign* **-graft** *tissue for implant or transplant*	Uses a skin graft (dermis only) taken from an animal (pig). This is a temporary skin graft to protect the patient against infection and fluid loss.
synthetic skin grafts		Uses a skin graft made from collagen fibers arranged in a lattice pattern. The patient's body does not reject synthetic skin, and healing skin grows into it as the graft gradually disintegrates.

Word Alert

HOMONYMS

dermatome (noun) a specific area of the skin that sends sensory information through a spinal nerve.

Example: The patient had shingles on the chest and back along the T6 dermatome.

dermatome (noun) a surgical instrument used to make a shallow, continuous cut to form a skin graft.

Example: After the donor site was prepped and draped, a dermatome was used to obtain a split-thickness skin graft.

Did You Know?

The skin of frogs and lizards were used as skin grafts in the 1600s.

Drug Categories

Several different categories of drugs are used to treat the symptoms, signs, and diseases of the integumentary system. The most common drugs in each category are listed. Drugs used to treat the skin can be administered topically on the skin for a local effect or orally and intravenously for a systemic effect.

Category	Word Part and Definition	Description	Example
antibiotic drugs	**antibiotic** (AN-tee-by-AWT-ik) (AN-tih-by-AWT-ik) **anti-** *against* **bi/o-** *life; living organisms; living tissue* **-tic** *pertaining to*	Treat bacterial infections of the skin or acne vulgaris. Can be administered topically or orally.	bacitracin, neomycin, tetracycline (oral)
antifungal drugs	**antifungal** (AN-tee-FUN-gal) (AN-tih-FUN-gal) **anti-** *against* **fung/o-** *fungus* **-al** *pertaining to*	Treat ringworm (tinea). Administered topically. Treat fungal infection of the nails. Administered orally.	Desenex, Lamisil, Lotrimin, Tinactin Grifulvin, Nizoral
antipruritic drugs	**antipruritic** (AN-tee-proo-RIT-ik) (AN-tih-proo-RIT-ik) **anti-** *against* **prurit/o-** *itching* **-ic** *pertaining to*	Decrease itching. Administered topically or orally.	Benadryl, Caladryl
antiviral drugs	**antiviral** (AN-tee-VY-ral) (AN-tih-VY-ral) **anti-** *against* **vir/o-** *virus* **-al** *pertaining to*	Treat herpes simplex viral infections. Administered topically or orally.	Famvir, Valtrex, Zovirax
chemotherapy drugs	**chemotherapy** (KEE-moh-THAIR-ah-pee) **chem/o-** *chemical, drug* **-therapy** *treatment*	Kill rapidly dividing cancer cells in skin. Used to treat malignant melanoma and Kaposi's sarcoma. Other skin cancers are treated with radiation therapy.	Alkeran, Taxol, Taxotere, Velban
coal tar drugs		Treat psoriasis. They cause the epidermal cells to multiply more slowly and decrease itching. Coal tar is a by-product of the processing of bituminous coal. It contains over 10,000 different chemicals.	Neutrogena T/Gel, Zetar
corticosteroid drugs	**corticosteroid** (KOR-tih-koh-STAIR-oyd) **cortic/o-** *cortex (outer region)* **-steroid** *steroid* Corticosteroids are produced in the cortex (outer region) of the adrenal glands. They have a powerful, natural anti-inflammatory effect. Synthetic corticosteroids are manufactured and used as drugs.	Treat skin inflammation from contact dermatitis, psoriasis, and eczema. Administered topically or orally.	Cyclocort, Cutivate, hydrocortisone, Topicort, prednisone (oral)
drugs for infestations		Treat scabies (mites) and pediculosis (lice).	Lindane, Ovide

Category	Word Part and Definition	Description	Example
photodynamic therapy (PDT)	**photodynamic** (FOH-toh-dy-NAM-ik) **phot/o-** *light* **dynam/o-** *power; movement* **-ic** *pertaining to*	Treats cancer of the skin with laser light and a photosensitizing drug. Unofficially used to treat psoriasis.	Photofrin
psoralen drugs	**psoralen** (SOR-ah-len) *Psoralen* is derived from *Psoralea corylifolia,* an herb known to cause sensitivity to light when eaten.	Treat psoriasis. Psoralen sensitizes the skin to ultraviolet light therapy which then damages cellular DNA and decreases the rate of cell division. This combination is known as PUVA (psoralen drug and ultraviolet A light)	Oxsoralen, Uvadex
vitamin A–type drugs		Treat acne vulgaris or severe cystic acne. They cause the epidermal cells to multiply rapidly. This rapid turnover keeps the pores from becoming clogged.	Accutane, Retin-A

Connections

topical (TOP-ih-kal)
topic/o- *a specific area*
-al *pertaining to*

transdermal (trans-DER-mal)
trans- *across, through*
derm/o- *skin*
-al *pertaining to*

intradermal (IN-trah-DER-mal)
intra- *within*
derm/o *skin*
-al *pertaining to*

hypodermic (HY-poh-DER-mik)
hypo- *below; deficient*
derm/o- *skin*
-ic *pertaining to*

Pharmacology. Topical drugs like creams, lotions, and ointments are absorbed into the skin for a local drug effect. Topical drug patches release small amounts of a drug over time that are absorbed through the skin and exert a systemic effect. This is known as the **transdermal** route. The **intradermal** route uses a needle inserted just beneath the epidermis. This is used for the Mantoux tuberculosis test and allergy testing. Other types of drug injections are classified as **hypodermic** injections because the needle goes beneath the dermis, either into the subcutaneous tissue (subcu, subQ, SQ) or into the muscle (intramuscular, IM).

Abbreviations

Bx	biopsy
Ca	cancer (slang)
C&S	culture and sensitivity
Derm	dermatology (slang)
HSV	herpes simplex virus
I&D	incision and drainage
PDT	photodynamic therapy
PUVA	psoralen drug and ultraviolet A light (therapy)
SLE	systemic lupus erythematosus
SQ, subcu, subQ	subcutaneous

Career Focus

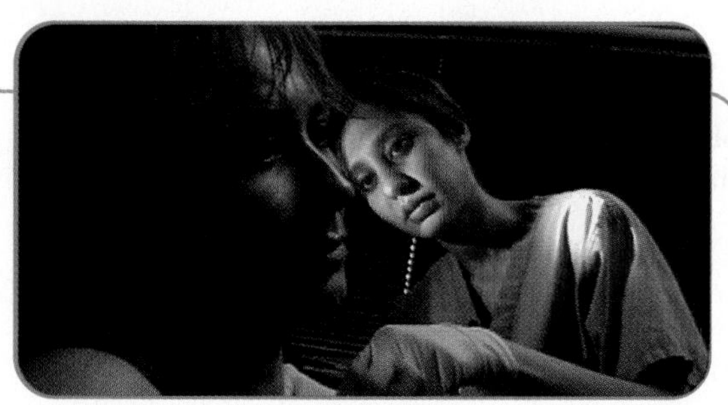

Meet Toral, a physician's assistant in a cosmetic surgeon's office.

"Growing up, I always knew I would be in medicine. At first, I entertained the idea of becoming a nurse. Then I entertained the idea of becoming a physician. Being a physician's assistant allows me to see my own patients, treat and diagnose, write my own prescriptions, care for patients, and advise them. I also assist in laser procedures and all surgical procedures. Our everyday language is medical terminology—from talking to the physician, talking to your co-workers, to charting in the charts. With so many patients being internet-savvy, they come in talking in medical terminology!"

Physician's assistants are healthcare professionals who are licensed to perform basic medical care while under the supervision of a physician. They perform physical examinations, prescribe drugs, and perform minor surgery. They can assist the physician during more extensive surgery. They work in physicians' offices, clinics, and in hospitals.

Dermatologists are physicians who practice in the medical specialty of dermatology. They diagnose and treat patients with diseases of the skin. Physicians can take additional training and become board certified in the subspecialty of pediatric dermatology. Malignancies of the skin are treated medically by an oncologist or surgically by a dermatologist, a general surgeon, or plastic surgeon.

Plastic surgeons are physicians who perform plastic and reconstructive surgery to reshape the body. They remove lesions and scars and perform liposuction and other procedures that reshape the skin and subcutaneous tissue.

dermatologist (DER-mah-TAWL-oh-jist)
dermat/o- *skin*
log/o- *the study of*
-ist *one who specializes in*

plastic (PLAS-tik)
plast/o- *growth, formation*
-ic *pertaining to*

surgeon (SER-jun)
surg/o- *operative procedure*
-eon *one who performs*
Surgeon is derived from a Latin word (*chirurgus*) meaning *hand work.*

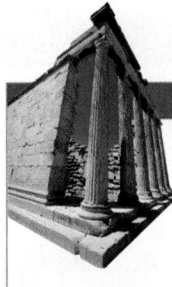

It's Greek to Me!

Did you notice that some integumentary words have two different combining forms? Combining forms from both Greek and Latin languages remain a part of medical language today.

English Word	Greek	Latin	Examples of Medical Words
fat	lip/o-	adip/o-	lipocyte, adipose tissue, adipocere
hair	trich/o-	hirsut/o-, pil/o-	schizotrichia, hirsutism, pilonidal cyst, piloerection
nail	onych/o-	ungu/o-	onychomycosis, ungual
skin	derm/a-, derm/o- dermat/o-	cutane/o-, cut/i- integument/o-	dermatome, dermal, subcutaneous, cuticle dermatologist, integumentary
sweat	diaphor/o-	hidr/o-, sudor/i-	diaphoresis, anhidrosis, sudoriferous gland

Chapter Review Exercises

Review all the material in this chapter by completing the review exercises in this section. Use the Answer Key at the end of the book to check your answers.

Anatomy and Physiology

Matching Exercise

Match each numbered word or phrase to its description.

1. basal layer	____ Consists of the epidermis, dermis, nails, and hair
2. dermis	____ Outermost layer of skin
3. epidermis	____ Another name for sweat glands
4. lipocytes	____ Half moon that contains keratin cells
5. lunula	____ Cells that make up adipose tissue
6. integument	____ Produces brown or black pigment
7. melanocyte	____ Deepest part of the epidermis
8. sudoriferous glands	____ Contains sebaceous glands and sweat glands
9. allergen	____ Substance that causes an allergic reaction

Circle Exercise

Circle the correct word from the choices given.

1. The (**nail bed, nail plate, nail root**) is also known as the quick.
2. (**Collagen, Keratin, Melanin**) is a hard, fibrous protein found in the most superficial cells of the epidermis.
3. Piloerection involves movement of a (**dermatome, hair, lipocyte**).
4. (**Anaphylaxis, Exfoliation, Perspiration**) is the normal shedding of skin cells.
5. All of the following are changes that occur in the skin during pregnancy EXCEPT (**dermatome, linea nigra, striae**).
6. *Ungual* is the adjective form for (**hair, nail, skin**).

True or False

Indicate whether each statement is true or false by writing T or F on the line.

1. ____ The integumentary system consists of the skin, hair, and nails.
2. ____ The epithelium is the outermost layer of the skin.
3. ____ Sebaceous glands are exocrine glands.
4. ____ Melanin is produced by melanocytes in the subcutaneous tissue.
5. ____ Sunlight on the skin helps manufacture vitamin D.
6. ____ Anaphylaxis is a severe, systemic allergic reaction.

Medical Language Word Parts

Name that Word Part

Identify each of the word parts given here by writing in the correct letter (P, C, or S) on the line beside it. Then write the definition of the word part on the blank line. The first one has been done for you.

Prefix = P **Combining Form = C** **Suffix = S**

		Word Part	Definition			Word Part	Definition
1.	abras/o-	C	scrape off	35.	cyan/o-		
2.	actin/o-			36.	-cyte		
3.	adip/o-			37.	-dactyly		
4.	-al			38.	de-		
5.	albin/o-			39.	-derma		
6.	all/o-			40.	derm/a-		
7.	an-			41.	dermat/o-		
8.	ana-			42.	derm/o-		
9.	-ancy			43.	desicc/o-		
10.	angi/o-			44.	diaphore/o-		
11.	-ant			45.	dynam/o-		
12.	anti-			46.	dys-		
13.	-ar			47.	ecchym/o-		
14.	-ary			48.	-ectomy		
15.	aspir/o-			49.	-elasma		
16.	-ate			50.	elast/o-		
17.	-ation			51.	electr/o-		
18.	auto-			52.	-eon		
19.	bas/o-			53.	epi-		
20.	bi/o-			54.	erect/o-		
21.	blephar/o-			55.	erg/o-		
22.	carcin/o-			56.	-ergy		
23.	cellul/o-			57.	-ery		
24.	-cere			58.	erythemat/o-		
25.	chem/o-			59.	esthes/o-		
26.	-cle			60.	ex-		
27.	coll/a-			61.	excis/o-		
28.	contus/o-			62.	excori/o-		
29.	cortic/o-			63.	exo-		
30.	-crine			64.	extra-		
31.	crin/o-			65.	exud/o-		
32.	cry/o-			66.	fer/o-		
33.	cutane/o-			67.	follicul/o-		
34.	cut/i-			68.	foli/o-		

		Word Part	Definition
69.	fulgur/o-	______	______________
70.	fung/o-	______	______________
71.	gangren/o-	______	______________
72.	-gen	______	______________
73.	-graft	______	______________
74.	hemat/o-	______	______________
75.	hem/o-	______	______________
76.	hidr/o-	______	______________
77.	hirsut/o-	______	______________
78.	hyper-	______	______________
79.	hypo-	______	______________
80.	-ia	______	______________
81.	-iasis	______	______________
82.	-iatic	______	______________
83.	-ic	______	______________
84.	icter/o-	______	______________
85.	-ile	______	______________
86.	-in	______	______________
87.	incis/o-	______	______________
88.	integument/o-	______	______________
89.	integu/o-	______	______________
90.	intra-	______	______________
91.	-ion	______	______________
92.	-ism	______	______________
93.	-ist	______	______________
94.	-itis	______	______________
95.	-ity	______	______________
96.	kel/o-	______	______________
97.	kerat/o-	______	______________
98.	lacer/o-	______	______________
99.	lip/o-	______	______________
100.	loc/o-	______	______________
101.	log/o-	______	______________
102.	-logy	______	______________
103.	lun/o-	______	______________
104.	malign/o-	______	______________
105.	melan/o-	______	______________
106.	-ment	______	______________
107.	micr/o-	______	______________
108.	myc/o-	______	______________
109.	necr/o-	______	______________

		Word Part	Definition
110.	ne/o-	______	______________
111.	nid/o-	______	______________
112.	-oid	______	______________
113.	-oma	______	______________
114.	onych/o-	______	______________
115.	-opsy	______	______________
116.	-ose	______	______________
117.	-osis	______	______________
118.	-ous	______	______________
119.	papill/o-	______	______________
120.	par-	______	______________
121.	pedicul/o-	______	______________
122.	per-	______	______________
123.	petechi/o-	______	______________
124.	phot/o-	______	______________
125.	phylact/o-	______	______________
126.	-phylaxis	______	______________
127.	-phyma	______	______________
128.	pigment/o-	______	______________
129.	pil/o-	______	______________
130.	-plasm	______	______________
131.	plas/o-	______	______________
132.	plast/o-	______	______________
133.	-plasty	______	______________
134.	poly-	______	______________
135.	pre-	______	______________
136.	prurit/o-	______	______________
137.	psor/o-	______	______________
138.	rhin/o-	______	______________
139.	rhytid/o-	______	______________
140.	-rrhage	______	______________
141.	-rrhea	______	______________
142.	rrhe/o-	______	______________
143.	sarc/o-	______	______________
144.	schiz/o-	______	______________
145.	scler/o-	______	______________
146.	sebace/o-	______	______________
147.	seb/o-	______	______________
148.	sect/o-	______	______________
149.	sen/o-	______	______________
150.	sensitiv/o-	______	______________

		Word Part	Definition
151.	-sis	______	________________
152.	spir/o-	______	________________
153.	squam/o-	______	________________
154.	-steroid	______	________________
155.	sub-	______	________________
156.	suct/o-	______	________________
157.	sudor/i-	______	________________
158.	surg/o-	______	________________
159.	syn-	______	________________
160.	system/o-	______	________________
161.	theli/o-	______	________________
162.	-therapy	______	________________
163.	-tic	______	________________
164.	-tome	______	________________
165.	topic/o-	______	________________
166.	trans-	______	________________
167.	trich/o-	______	________________
168.	-ula	______	________________
169.	-um	______	________________
170.	ungu/o-	______	________________
171.	vas/o-	______	________________
172.	vesic/o-	______	________________
173.	vesicul/o-	______	________________
174.	vir/o-	______	________________
175.	xanth/o-	______	________________
176.	xen/o-	______	________________
177.	xer/o-	______	________________

Symptoms, Signs, and Diseases

Circle Exercise

Circle the name of the skin lesion shown in each of these illustrations.

1. This skin lesion is a (**cyst, fissure, papule, wheal**).

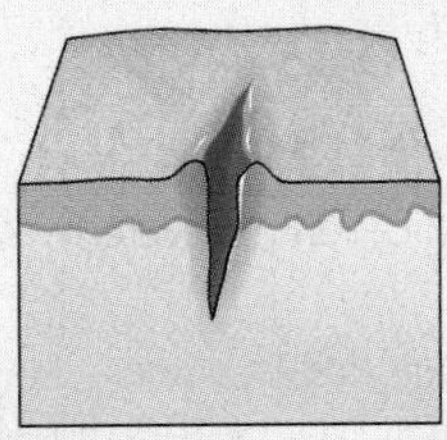

2. This skin lesion is a (**cyst, laceration, macule, vesicle**).

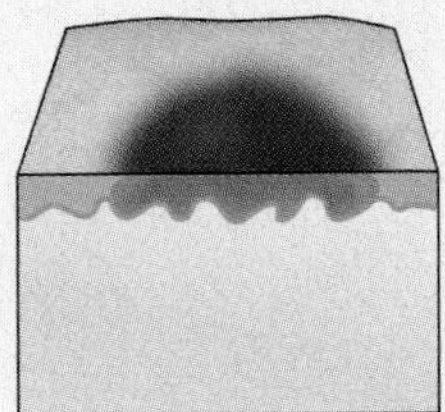

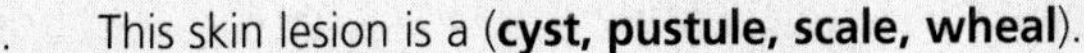

3. This skin lesion is a (**cyst, pustule, scale, wheal**).

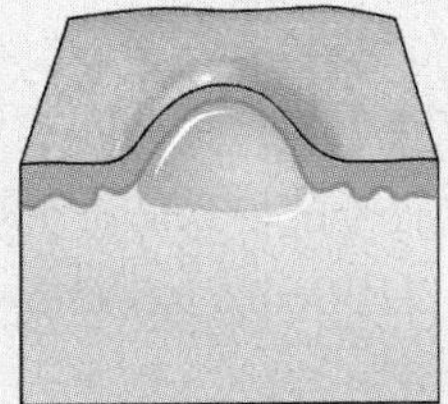

English and Medical Word Equivalents

For each English word or phrase, write the medical word that is its equivalent.

English Word	Medical Word	English Word	Medical Word
1. brush burn	____________	8. cradle cap	____________
2. boil	____________	9. port-wine stain	____________
3. ringworm	____________	10. age spots or liver spots	____________
4. wart	____________	11. skin tag	____________
5. infestation with lice	____________	12. baldness	____________
6. infestation with mites	____________	13. bed sore	____________
7. hives	____________		

Divide and Conquer

Separate these dermatology words into their component parts (prefix, combining form, and suffix). Note: Some words do not contain all three word parts.

Medical Word	Prefix	Combining Form	Suffix
1. abrasion	________	____________	________
2. anesthesia	________	____________	________
3. anhidrosis	________	____________	________
4. cyanosis	________	____________	________
5. dermatitis	________	____________	________
6. dysplastic	________	____________	________
7. lipoma	________	____________	________
8. neoplasm	________	____________	________
9. paronychia	________	____________	________
10. pruritic	________	____________	________

True or False

Indicate whether each statement is true or false by writing T or F on the line.

1. ____ A neoplasm is always a malignant growth of the skin.
2. ____ Bluish discoloration of the skin from a lack of oxygen is known as a bruise.
3. ____ An abnormally enlarged scar is known as a keloid.
4. ____ Actinic keratoses are rough, raised areas due to chronic sun exposure.
5. ____ Rhinophyma is a complication of severe acne vulgaris of the nose.
6. ____ Hirsutism is a lack of hair due to aging.
7. ____ Psoriasis is treated with coal tar drugs and PUVA.

Matching Exercise

Match each numbered word or phrase to its description.

1. abscess	_____	Inflammation of the skin
2. bullae	_____	Yellow discoloration (icterus)
3. callus	_____	Localized collection of pus
4. decubitus ulcer	_____	Often seen in AIDS patients
5. dermatitis	_____	Autoimmune disease with depigmentation patches
6. diaphoresis	_____	Thickened, firm pad on the epidermis
7. dysplastic nevus	_____	Fungal infection of the nails
8. hematoma	_____	Present in second-degree burns
9. jaundice	_____	Frequent repositioning avoids development of these
10. Kaposi's sarcoma	_____	Profuse sweating
11. onychomycosis	_____	Collection of blood under the skin
12. vitiligo	_____	Can develop into malignant melanoma

Circle Exercise

Circle the correct word from the choices given.

1. A macule is a (**crevice, elevated, flat**) lesion.
2. An acne whitehead is also called a (**cyst, pustule, wheal**).
3. (**Excoriation, Exfoliation, Laceration**) is a superficial linear scratch on the skin.
4. The thick, black crust over a third-degree burn is known as a/an (**cicatrix, eschar, keloid**).
5. Tinea corporis occurs on the skin of the (**feet, groin, trunk**).
6. A nevus includes all of the following EXCEPT (**birthmark, cellulitis, mole**).
7. A yellow plaque on the skin is known as a/an (**jaundice, xanthoma, scleroderma**).
8. Tinea pedis is a fungal infection of the skin also known as (**onychomycosis, ringworm, verruca**).

Matching Exercise

Match each numbered word or phrase to its description.

1. chickenpox	_____	Occurs at the base of the fingernail
2. cold sores	_____	Herpes simplex type 2
3. pediculosis	_____	Infestation of parasitic mites
4. furuncle	_____	First occurrence of herpes varicella-zoster
5. herpes whitlow	_____	Second occurrence of herpes varicella-zoster
6. genital herpes	_____	Herpes simplex type 1
7. shingles	_____	Caused by human papillomavirus
8. scabies	_____	Infestation of lice
9. verruca	_____	Caused by *Staphylococcus aureus*

Word-Building Exercise

Use the combining forms, prefixes, and suffixes given here to build medical words that match the definitions given. Write the word you build on the blank line. Some word parts may be used more than once.

an- (without, not)	-ia (condition, state, thing)	onych/o- (nail)	-rrhea (flow, discharge)
-derma (skin)	melan/o- (black)	-osis (condition; abnormal condition; process)	seb/o- (sebum, oil)
hemat/o- (blood)	myc/o- (fungus)	par- (beside)	xer/o- (dry)
hidr/o- (sweat)	-oma (tumor, mass)		

1. Infection of the skin along the cuticle ______________________
2. Congenital absence of sweat glands ______________________
3. Mass of blood under the skin ______________________
4. Excessively dry skin ______________________
5. Fungal infection of the nails ______________________
6. Overproduction of sebum other than at puberty ______________________
7. Cancer arising from melanocytes ______________________

Laboratory, Radiology, Surgery, and Drugs

Matching Exercise

Match each numbered word or phrase to its description.

1. allergy skin testing	____	Instrument used to make a skin graft
2. culture and sensitivity	____	Uses ultrasonic waves to break up and suction fat
3. debridement	____	Done in a Petri dish
4. dermatome	____	Remove necrotic tissue
5. liposuction	____	Uses allergens for testing
6. Tzanck test	____	Skin graft taken from an animal
7. xenograft	____	Examines scrapings of fluid from a vesicle

Circle Exercise

Circle the correct word from the choices given.

1. Electrosurgery includes all of the following EXCEPT (**debridement, fulguration, electrodesiccation**).
2. (**Cryosurgery, Curettage, Incision**) uses a curet to scrape off a skin lesion.
3. Allergy skin testing uses (**hypodermic, intradermal, transdermal**) injections.
4. Surgical procedure to remove wrinkles from the face is a (**blepharoplasty, Botox injection, rhytidectomy**).
5. A/an (**dermatoplasty, excisional biopsy, incisional biopsy**) removes just a piece of a large skin lesion.
6. All of the following are skin resurfacing techniques EXCEPT (**chemical peel, dermabrasion, incision and drainage**).
7. All of the following drugs are used to treat psoriasis EXCEPT (**antifungal drugs, coal tar drugs, psoralen**).

Abbreviations

Matching Exercise

Match each numbered abbreviation to its definition.

1.	Bx	____	Used to treat an abscess
2.	C&S	____	Autoimmune disease
3.	HSV	____	Can be excisional and incisional
4.	I&D	____	Causes genital herpes, cold sores, and shingles
5.	PUVA	____	Used to treat psoriasis
6.	SLE	____	Tissue beneath the dermis
7.	SubQ	____	Test to identify pathogen and a drug to treat it

Applied Skills

Plural Noun and Adjective Spelling

Fill in the blanks with the correct word form. Be sure to check your spelling. The first one has been done for you.

Singular Noun	Plural Noun	Adjective
1. follicle	follicles	follicular
2. skin		________ ________
3. epidermis		________
4. dermis		________
5. nail	________	________
6. epithelium		________
7. vesicle	________	________
8. pruritus		________
9. cyanosis		________

Singular Noun	Plural Noun	Adjective
10. erythema		________
11. icterus		________
12. necrosis		________
13. gangrene		________
14. verruca	________	
15. malignancy	________	________
16. keratosis	________	
17. psoriasis		________
18. seborrhea		________
19. diaphoresis		________

Dictionary Challenge

On the job, you will often encounter new medical words. Practice your medical dictionary skills by looking up the medical words in bold and writing their definitions on the blank lines.

OFFICE CHART NOTE

This 11-year-old young lady was brought in by her mother. The mother states that the patient continually bites her fingernails despite all attempts to discourage her. Her fingernails are always bitten to the quick, and the skin around them is frequently bloody. The patient does not deny this, but states she is unable to stop. When her mother stepped out of the examining room, the patient became tearful as she related pressure at school and an impending divorce between her parents.

On examination, the fingernails show evidence of chronic biting, right hand greater than left. The patient is right handed. Examination of the feet also shows evidence of nail biting. There is erythema and swelling of the tissue along the medial nail groove of her right great toe where the nail was bitten away and is growing back but is ingrown. The skin on the lower arms bilaterally shows aggressive scratching of small, isolated insect bites. The scalp shows some small, patchy areas where there is an absence of hair. The patient admits to some hair-pulling.

DIAGNOSES

1. **Onychophagia.**
2. **Onychocryptosis.**
3. **Trichotillomania**

Plan: The medial side of the nail on the right great toe was trimmed with clippers. The patient's mother was given a prescription for a 7-day course of oral antibiotics. The patient's mother was also given a referral for the patient to see a child psychologist for counseling.

1. onychophagia ______________________________
2. onychocryptosis ______________________________
3. trichotillomania ______________________________

Analysis of a Medical Report

This exercise contains an office chart note. Read the report and answer the questions.

CHART NOTE

PATIENT NAME: GUNDERSON, DENISE

PATIENT NUMBER: 191-46-3985

DATE: November 19, 20xx

S: Severe pruritus since early this morning. This began about 20 minutes after the patient took her last scheduled dose of Zithromax. She has been on Zithromax for a severe skin flare-up of erythema nodosum following a strep throat. For this, she had initial swelling and edema in her right foot. This then involved her right leg, then areas on her chest, then her left knee and, to a lesser extent her left foot. These areas were extremely painful to touch, erythematous, and her right knee developed a large, painful nodule under the skin. Other smaller nodules were scattered throughout her body. Her right foot was so painful and edematous that it was nearly impossible for her to walk. This continued for a few weeks. At one point, the dorsum of her right foot developed some cellulitis, at which time she was placed on the Zithromax. As noted, she had just taken her last scheduled dose of Zithromax. She describes suddenly having a very itchy scalp. When she scratched her scalp, she could feel multiple raised areas. About 20 minutes later, there were about twice as many raised areas on her scalp and now she could see wheals on her cheeks. She also found them on her trunk. When the hives on her face began to coalesce into large welts, she became concerned about not being able to breathe and took 2 antihistamine pills (Benadryl). One hour later, she had to take 2 more Benadryl. After that, the welts, hives, and itching began to subside. Although she was feeling better, she decided to come to the office today to be examined.

O: Integumentary system: There are a few, small, scattered hives still visible on her trunk and arms. The welts and wheals on her scalp and face have completely disappeared. The cellulitis of her right foot has cleared up and the smaller nodules from the erythema nodosum have disappeared. The largest nodule over her right knee is slowly resolving.

A:

1. Severe urticaria, secondary to an allergic drug reaction to Zithromax.
2. Right foot cellulitis, resolved.
3. Resolving erythema nodosum status post streptococcal infection (strep throat).

P: A note has been made in the patient's medical record that she is allergic to Zithromax. The acute phase of this allergic reaction is past. The patient has been instructed to never take that antibiotic or any of the other macrolide antibiotics in that class of drugs. Follow-up p.r.n. for her resolving erythema nodosum.

Bonnie R. Grant, M.D.

Bonnie R. Grant, M.D.

BRG: lcc
D: 11/19/xx
T: 11/19/xx

WORD ANALYSIS QUESTIONS

1. Divide *cellulitis* into word parts and define each word part.

Word Part	**Definition**
________________	____
________________	____

2. The patient has erythema on her legs. If you wanted to use the adjective form of *erythema,* you would say, "She has ________________ areas on her legs."

FACT FINDING QUESTIONS

1. What is the medical word for *itching*? ________________
2. Circle the word that means reddened: (**edematous, erythematous, flare-up**)
3. What three symptoms of urticaria did this patient have?

   ____

   ____

   ____

4. What skin condition did the patient develop after having a strep throat? ________________
5. Which are larger—welts or wheals? ________________
6. In the "Objective" section of this chart note, which body system is examinend? ________________
7. The patient's urticaria was due to (**cellulitis, drug reaction, strep throat**).

CRITICAL THINKING SKILLS

1. Zithromax is a member of what category of drugs? ________________
2. Which two of the patient's diagnoses were caused by bacterial infections?

   ____

   ____

Pronunciation Checklist

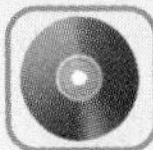

Read each word and its pronunciation. Practice pronouncing each word. Verify your pronunciation by listening to the Pronunciation List on the CD-ROM. Check the box next to the word after you master its pronunciation.

- ❑ abrasion (ah-BRAY-zhun)
- ❑ abscess (AB-ses)
- ❑ acne rosacea (AK-nee roh-ZAY-shee-ah)
- ❑ acne vulgaris (AK-nee vul-GAIR-is)
- ❑ actinic keratosis (ak-TIN-ik KAIR-ah-TOH-sis)
- ❑ adipocere (AD-ih-poh-SEER)
- ❑ adipose (AD-ih-pohs)
- ❑ albinism (AL-by-niz-em)
- ❑ albino (al-BY-noh)
- ❑ allergen (AL-er-jen)
- ❑ allergic (ah-LER-jik)
- ❑ allergy (AL-er-jee)
- ❑ allograft (AL-oh-graft)
- ❑ alopecia (AL-oh-PEE-shee-ah)
- ❑ anaphylactic shock (AN-ah-fih-LAK-tik SHAWK)
- ❑ anaphylaxis (AN-ah-fih-LAK-sis)
- ❑ anesthesia (AN-es-THEE-zee-ah)
- ❑ anhidrosis (AN-hy-DROH-sis)
- ❑ antibiotic drug (AN-tee-by-AWT-ik DRUHG) (AN-tih-by-AWT-ik)
- ❑ antifungal drug (AN-tee-FUN-gal DRUHG) (AN-tih-FUN-gal)
- ❑ antipruritic drug (AN-tee-proo-RIT-ik DRUHG) (AN-tih-proo-RIT-ik)
- ❑ antiviral drug (AN-tee-VY-ral DRUHG) (AN-tih-VY-ral)
- ❑ aspiration (AS-pih-RAY-shun)
- ❑ autograft (AW-toh-graft)
- ❑ basal layer (BAY-sal LAY-er)
- ❑ benign (bee-NINE)
- ❑ biopsy (BY-awp-see)
- ❑ blepharoplasty (BLEF-ah-roh-PLAS-tee)
- ❑ blister (BLIS-ter)
- ❑ Botox (BOH-tawks)
- ❑ bulla (BUL-ah)
- ❑ bullae (BUL-ee)
- ❑ callus (KAL-us)
- ❑ cancer (KAN-ser)
- ❑ carbuncle (KAR-bung-kl)
- ❑ carcinoma (KAR-sih-NOH-mah)
- ❑ cellulitis (SEL-yoo-LY-tis)
- ❑ cicatrix (SIK-ah-triks)
- ❑ chloasma (kloh-AZ-mah)
- ❑ collagen (KAWL-lah-jen)
- ❑ comedo (KOH-me-doh)
- ❑ contusion (con-TOO-zhun)
- ❑ corticosteroid drug (KOR-tih-koh-STAIR-oyd DRUHG)
- ❑ cryosurgery (KRY-oh-SER-jer-ee)
- ❑ curettage (kyoo-rah-TAWZH)
- ❑ curet (kyoo-RET)
- ❑ cutaneous (kyoo-TAY-nee-us)
- ❑ cuticle (KYOO-tih-kl)
- ❑ cyanosis (SY-ah-NOH-sis)
- ❑ cyanotic (SY-ah-NAWT-ik)
- ❑ cyst (SIST)
- ❑ debridement (deh-BREED-maw)
- ❑ decubitus ulcer (dee-KYOO-bih-tus UL-ser)
- ❑ depigmentation (dee-PIG-men-TAY-shun)
- ❑ dermabrasion (DER-mah-BRAY-zhun)
- ❑ dermal (DER-mal)
- ❑ dermatitis (DER-mah-TY-tis)
- ❑ dermatologist (DER-mah-TAWL-oh-jist)
- ❑ dermatology (DER-mah-TAWL-oh-jee)
- ❑ dermatome (DER-mah-tohm)
- ❑ dermatoplasty (DER-mah-toh-PLAS-tee)
- ❑ dermis (DER-mis)
- ❑ diaphoresis (DY-ah-foh-REE-sis)
- ❑ diaphoretic (DY-ah-foh-RET-ik)
- ❑ dysplastic nevus (dis-PLAS-tik NEE-vus)
- ❑ ecchymosis (EK-ih-MOH-sis)
- ❑ eczema (EK-zeh-mah)
- ❑ edema (eh-DEE-mah)
- ❑ elastin (ee-LAS-tin)
- ❑ electrodesiccation (ee-LEK-troh-DES-ih-KAY-shun)
- ❑ electrosection (ee-LEK-troh-SEK-shun)
- ❑ electrosurgery (ee-LEK-troh-SER-jer-ee)
- ❑ epidermal (EP-ih-DER-mal)
- ❑ epidermis (EP-ih-DER-mis)
- ❑ epithelial (EP-ih-THEE-lee-al)
- ❑ epithelium (EP-ih-THEE-lee-um)
- ❑ erythema (AIR-eh-THEE-mah)
- ❑ erythematous (AIR-eh-THEM-ah-tus)
- ❑ eschar (ES-kar)
- ❑ excisional (ek-SIZH-un-al)
- ❑ excoriation (eks-KOH-ree-AA-shun)
- ❑ exfoliation (eks-FOH-lee-AA-shun)
- ❑ exocrine gland (EK-soh-krin GLAND) (EK-soh-krine)
- ❑ exudate (EKS-yoo-dayt)
- ❑ fissure (FISH-ur)
- ❑ fistula (FIS-tyoo-lah)
- ❑ follicle (FAWL-ih-kl)
- ❑ follicular (foh-LIK-yoo-lar)
- ❑ folliculitis (foh-LIK-yoo-LY-tis)
- ❑ fulguration (FUL-gyoo-RAY-shun)
- ❑ furuncle (FYOO-rung-kl)
- ❑ gangrene (GANG-green)
- ❑ gangrenous (GANG-greh-nus)
- ❑ gland (GLAND)
- ❑ hemangioma (hee-MAN-jee-OH-mah)
- ❑ hematoma (HEE-mah-TOH-mah)
- ❑ herpes simplex (HER-peez SIM-pleks)
- ❑ herpes varicella-zoster (HER-peez VAIR-ih-SEL-ah ZAWS-ter)
- ❑ herpes whitlow (HER-peez WHIT-loh)
- ❑ hirsutism (HER-soo-tizm)
- ❑ hypersensitivity (HY-per-SEN-sih-TIV-ih-tee)
- ❑ hypodermic (HY-poh-DER-mik)
- ❑ icterus (IK-tair-us)
- ❑ icteric (ik-TAIR-ik)
- ❑ incision (in-SIZH-un)
- ❑ incisional (in-SIZH-un-al)
- ❑ integumentary (in-TEG-yoo-MEN-tair-ee)
- ❑ intradermal (IN-trah-DER-mal)
- ❑ jaundice (JAWN-dis)
- ❑ Kaposi's sarcoma (kah-POH-seez sar-KOH-mah)
- ❑ keloid (KEE-loyd)
- ❑ keratin (KAIR-ah-tin)
- ❑ keratoses (KAIR-ah-TOH-seez)
- ❑ keratosis (KAIR-ah-TOH-sis)
- ❑ laceration (LAS-er-AA-shun)
- ❑ laser (LAY-zer)
- ❑ lesion (LEE-shun)
- ❑ linea nigra (LIN-ee-ah NY-grah)
- ❑ lipocyte (LIP-oh-site)
- ❑ lipectomy (ly-PEK-toh-mee)
- ❑ lipoma (ly-POH-mah)
- ❑ liposuction (LIP-oh-SUK-shun)
- ❑ local (LOH-kal)
- ❑ lunula (LOO-nyoo-lah)
- ❑ lupus erythematosus (LOO-pus AIR-ih-them-ah-TOH-sus)
- ❑ macule (MAK-yool)
- ❑ malignancy (mah-LIG-nan-see)
- ❑ malignant (mah-LIG-nant)
- ❑ melanin (MEL-ah-nin)
- ❑ melanocyte (meh-LAN-oh-site) (MEL-ah-noh-site)

- ❑ melanoma (MEL-ah-NOH-mah)
- ❑ microdermabrasion (MY-kroh-DER-mah-BRAY-shun)
- ❑ necrosis (neh-KROH-sis)
- ❑ necrotic (neh-KRAWT-ik)
- ❑ neoplasm (NEE-oh-plazm)
- ❑ nevus (NEE-vus)
- ❑ onychomycosis (ON-ih-koh-my-KOH-sis)
- ❑ pallor (PAL-or)
- ❑ papilloma (PAP-ih-LOH-mah)
- ❑ papule (PAP-yool)
- ❑ paronychia (PAR-oh-NIK-ee-ah)
- ❑ pediculosis (peh-DIK-yoo-LOH-sis)
- ❑ perspiration (PER-spih-RAY-shun)
- ❑ petechiae (peh-TEE-kee-ee)
- ❑ piloerection (PY-loh-ee-REK-shun)
- ❑ pilonidal sinus (PY-loh-NY-dal SY-nus)
- ❑ plastic surgeon (PLAS-tik SER-jun)
- ❑ polydactyly (PAWL-ee-DAK-tih-lee)
- ❑ premalignant (PREE-mah-LIG-nant)
- ❑ pruritic (proo-RIT-ik)
- ❑ pruritus (proo-RY-tus)
- ❑ psoralens (SOR-ah-lens)
- ❑ psoriasis (soh-RY-ah-sis)
- ❑ psoriatic (SOH-ree-AT-ik)
- ❑ pustule (PUS-chool)
- ❑ rhinophyma (RY-noh-FY-mah)
- ❑ rhytidectomy (RIT-ih-DEK-toh-mee)
- ❑ scabies (SKAY-beez)
- ❑ scleroderma (SKLER-oh-DER-mah)
- ❑ sebaceous (seh-BAY-shus)
- ❑ seborrhea (SEB-oh-REE-ah)
- ❑ seborrheic (SEB-oh-REE-ik)
- ❑ sebum (SEE-bum)
- ❑ senile lentigo (SEE-nile len-TY-goh)
- ❑ sensitivity (SEN-sih-TIV-ih-tee)
- ❑ shingles (SHING-glz)
- ❑ squamous (SKWAY-mus)
- ❑ solar (SOH-lar)
- ❑ striae (STRY-ee)
- ❑ subcutaneous (SUB-kyoo-TAY-nee-us)
- ❑ sudoriferous (SOO-doh-RIF-er-us)
- ❑ syndactyly (sin-DAK-tih-lee)
- ❑ systemic (sis-TEM-ik)
- ❑ tinea capitis (TIN-ee-ah KAP-ih-tis)
- ❑ tinea corporis (TIN-ee-ah KOR-por-is)
- ❑ tinea cruris (TIN-ee-ah KROOR-is)
- ❑ tinea pedis (TIN-ee-ah PEE-dis)
- ❑ topical drug (TOP-ih-kal DRUHG)
- ❑ transdermal drug (trans-DER-mal DRUHG)
- ❑ turgor (TER-gor)
- ❑ Tzanck (TSAHNGK)
- ❑ ulcer (UL-ser)
- ❑ ungual (UNG-gwal)
- ❑ urticaria (ER-tih-KAIR-ee-ah)
- ❑ verruca (veh-ROO-kah)
- ❑ verrucae (veh-ROO-kee)
- ❑ vesicle (VES-ih-kl)
- ❑ vesicular (veh-SIK-yoo-lar)
- ❑ vitiligo (VIT-ih-LY-goh)
- ❑ wheal (HWEEL)
- ❑ xanthelasma (ZAN-theh-LAZ-mah)
- ❑ xanthoma (zan-THOH-mah)
- ❑ xenograft (ZEN-oh-graft)
- ❑ xeroderma (ZEER-oh-DER-mah)

Experience Multimedia

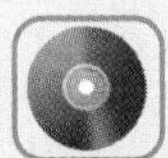

CD-ROM Learning Activities Checklist

Check off the box as you complete each learning activity.

❏ **CD-ROM Learning Activity 7.1: *ANATOMY WORD PARTS FLASHCARDS***
Use flashcards to help you memorize word parts. Make your own flashcards or print out prepared flashcards. Also see the electronic flashcard game. Time: 20 minutes.

❏ **CD-ROM Learning Activity 7.2: *MEDICINE IN ACTION***
Watch a video clip about skin cancer. Time: 5 minutes.

❏ **CD-ROM Learning Activity 7.3: *DISEASE AND OTHER WORD PARTS FLASHCARDS***
A continuation of the flashcard learning activity. Time: 20 minutes.

❏ **CD-ROM Learning Activity 7.4: *MEMORY AIDS***
Use memory aids to help you memorize medical words and meanings. Time: 5 minutes.

❏ **CD-ROM Learning Activity 7.5: *MEDICAL LANGUAGE SPOKEN HERE***
Listen to actual medical reports and spell the missing medical words. Time: 20 minutes.

❏ **CD-ROM Learning Activity 7.6: *SPELLING CHALLENGE***
Listen to a pronounced medical word and then spell it. Time: 5 minutes.

❏ **CD-ROM Learning Activity 7.7: *MEDICAL LANGUAGE PRONUNCIATION***
Listen to a pronounced medical word and then practice pronouncing it. Time: 30 minutes.

❏ **CD-ROM Learning Activity 7.8: *EDUCATIONAL FUN AND GAMES***
Enjoy these fun activities while reinforcing your knowledge. Time: 15 minutes.

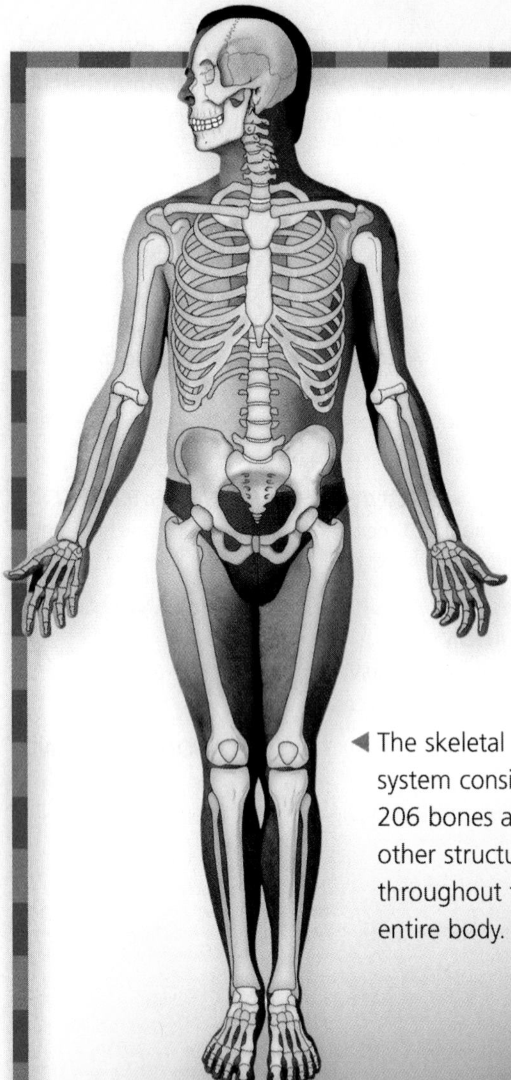

Dive In!

- Babies are born with about 100 more bones than adults.
- Humans and giraffes have the same number of bones in their necks.
- Do you want to discover some more hard facts? In this chapter, we'll explore the language that describes skeletal system structures, functions, diseases, and conditions.
- You'll have structure and support once you master the language of the skeletal system!

◀ The skeletal system consists of 206 bones and other structures throughout the entire body.

▼ Like the frame of a house, the skeleton provides structural support.

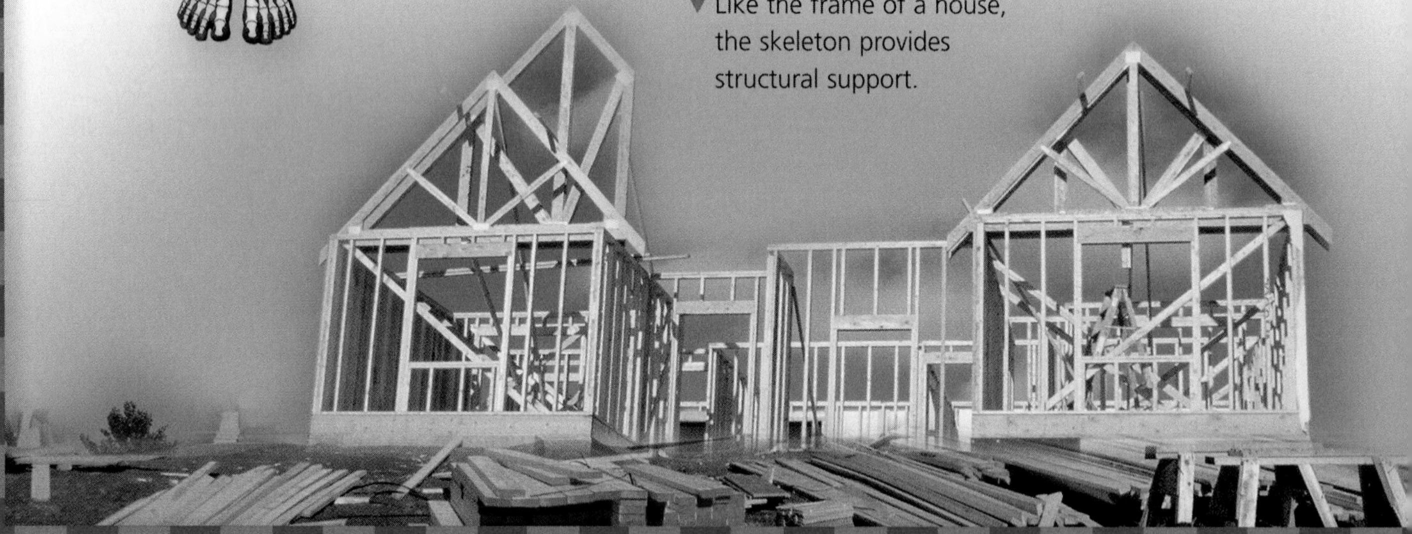

Medicine Through HISTORY

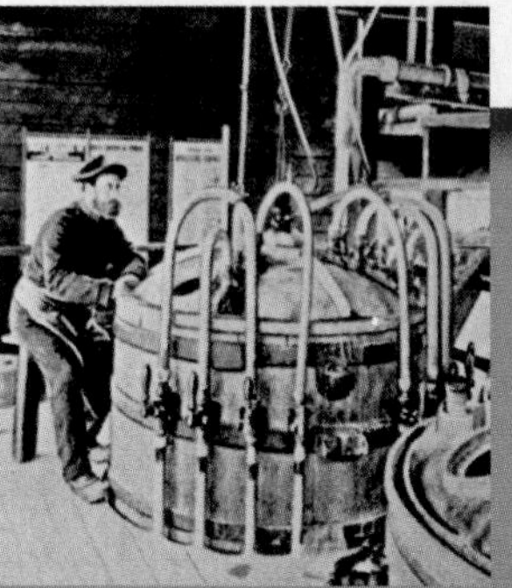

1895

Nitroglycerin is first prescribed to treat angina when workers in a dynamite factory experience relief of their chest pain. Nitroglycerin is an ingredient in dynamite

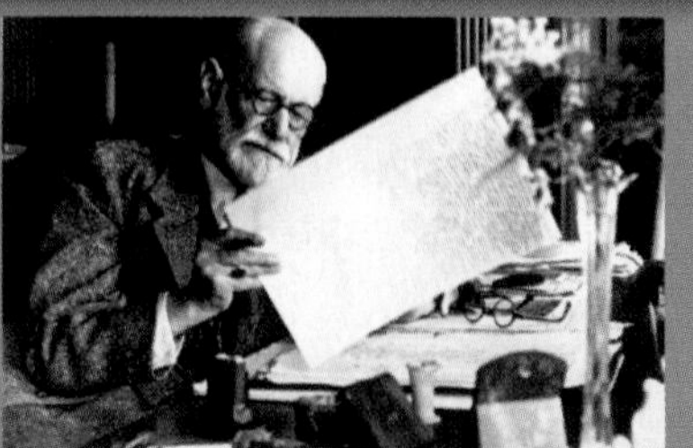

1896

Freud first uses the term psychoanalysis

CHAPTER 8

Orthopedics

Skeletal System

Orthopedics (OR-thoh-PEE-diks) is the medical specialty that studies the anatomy and physiology of the skeletal and muscular systems and uses diagnostic tests, medical and surgical procedures, and drugs to treat skeletal and muscular diseases. In this chapter, you will study orthopedics from the perspective of the skeletal system. In Chapter 9, you will study the muscular system.

▶ Bones come in a variety of shapes and sizes, and are composed of exterior and interior structures.

▶ Breaking news…injuries do occur, but so does the healing process.

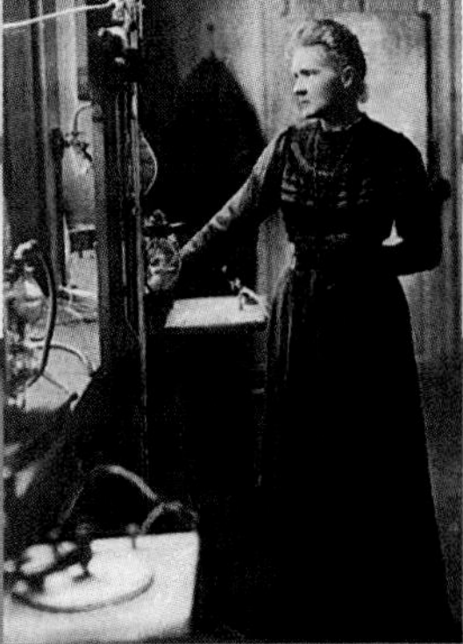

1898

Marie Curie discovers radioactivity as she works with radium

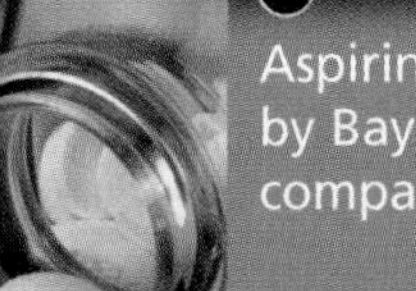

1899

Aspirin is introduced by Bayer, a German company

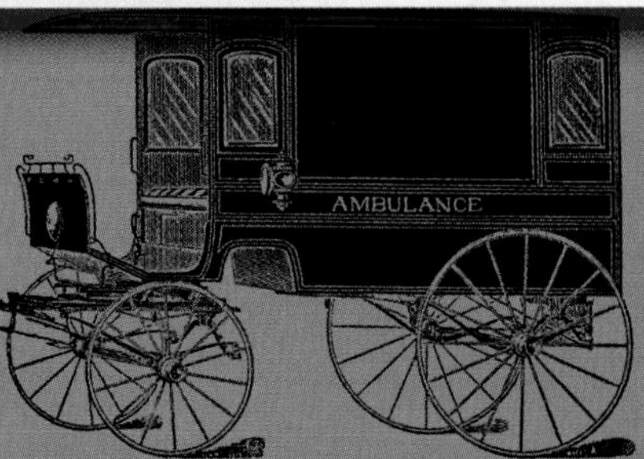

1899

First motorized ambulance company begins in Ohio

Measure Your Progress: Learning Objectives

After you study this chapter, you should be able to

1. Identify the anatomical structures of the skeletal system by correctly labeling them on anatomical illustrations.
2. Describe the process of growth.
3. Build skeletal words from combining forms, prefixes, and suffixes.
4. Describe common skeletal diseases.
5. Describe common skeletal diagnostic laboratory and radiology tests.
6. Describe common skeletal medical and surgical procedures and drug categories.
7. Define common skeletal abbreviations.
8. Correctly spell and pronounce skeletal words.
9. Apply your skills by analyzing an orthopedic (skeletal) report.
10. Test your knowledge of orthopedics (skeletal) by completing review exercises at the end of the chapter and learning activities on the CD-ROM.

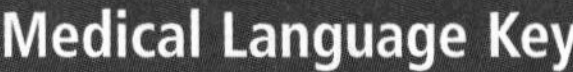

Medical Language Key

To unlock the meaning of a medical word, first define each word part. Then put the word part definitions in order, beginning with the suffix, followed by the first word part, then the other word parts in order.

	Word Part	Word Part Definition
SUFFIX	-ics	*knowledge, practice*
COMBINING FORM	orth/o-	*straight*
COMBINING FORM	ped/o-	*child*

Orthopedics: ***The knowledge and practice of producing straightness in a child or an adult.***

Orthopedics can also be spelled *orthopaedics.* Many hospitals retain this spelling in the title *Department of Orthopaedics,* although others do not. The *ae* spelling is derived from Greek.

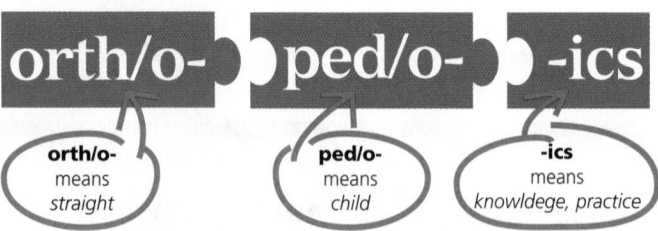

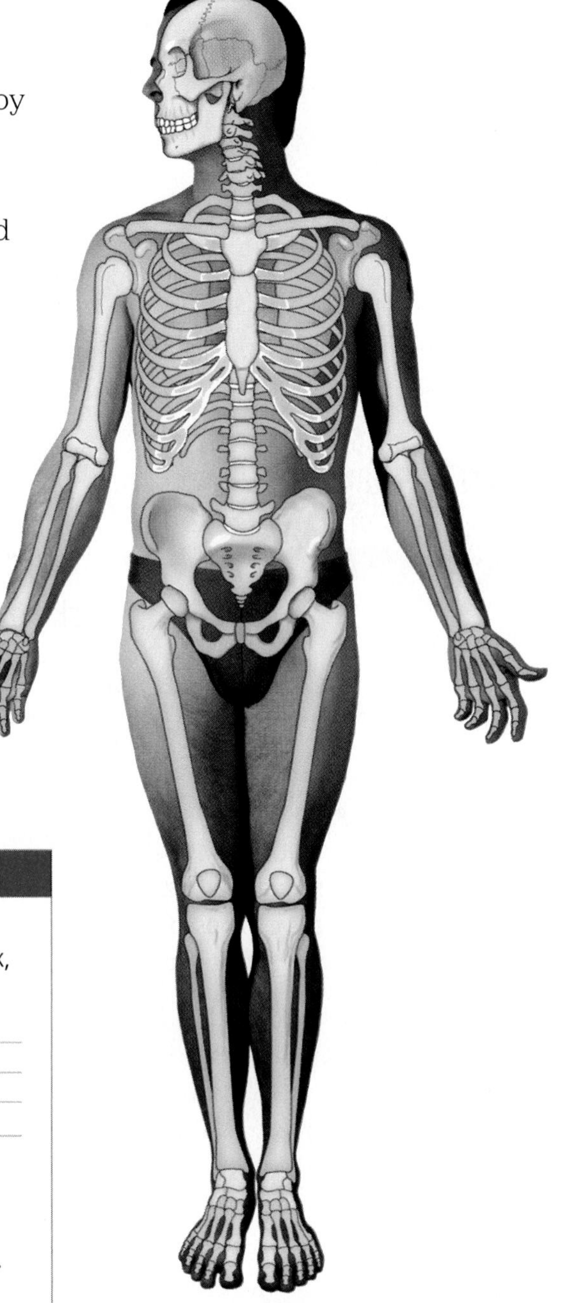

orth/o- means straight
ped/o- means child
-ics means knowldege, practice

Figure 8-1 ■ The skeletal system.

The skeletal system is a widespread, connected system that consists of 206 bones and other structures. It stretches throughout the body from the top of the head to the tips of the fingers and toes.

www.prenhall.com/turley

For interactive flashcards, real-life video clips, games, exercises, and audio pronunciations please explore the companion CD-ROM in the back of the book. Click on the companion website for bonus chapters, additional resources, and links to on-line learning.

Anatomy and Physiology

The **skeletal system** is the **bony** framework on which the body is built. The **skeleton** is composed of 206 bones as well as cartilage and ligaments (see Figure 8-1 ■). The functions of the skeletal system are to provide structural support for the body, work with the muscles in the process of movement, and protect the body's vital organs. The skeletal system is also known as the **skeletomuscular system** and **musculoskeletal system**. The bones and muscles are in close proximity to each other and dependent on each other to maintain body position and initiate movement.

skeleton (SKEL-eh-ton)

skeletal (SKEL-eh-tal)
skelet/o- *skeleton*
-al *pertaining to*
Skeleton is derived from a Greek word meaning *dried up.*

system (SIS-tem)
System is derived from a Greek word meaning *combination of parts to make an organized whole.*

bony (BOH-nee)
Osseous and *osteal* are other adjective forms for *bone.*

skeletomuscular (SKEL-eh-toh-MUS-kyoo-lar)
skelet/o- *skeleton*
muscul/o- *muscle*
-ar *pertaining to*

musculoskeletal (MUS-kyoo-loh-SKEL-eh-tal)
muscul/o- *muscle*
skelet/o- *skeleton*
-al *pertaining to*

Anatomy of the Skeletal System

Axial and Appendicular Skeleton

The skeleton can be divided into two areas of bones: the axial skeleton and the appendicular skeleton. The **axial skeleton** forms the central bony structure of the body around which other parts move. It consists of the bones of the head, chest, and spine. The **appendicular skeleton** consists of the bones of the shoulders, arms, hips, and legs.

axial (AK-see-al)
axi/o- *axis*
-al *pertaining to*
An axis is a central structure around which something rotates.

appendicular (AP-en-DIK-yoo-lar)
appendicul/o- *limb; small attached part*
-ar *pertaining to*

Bones of the Head

The **skull** is the bony structure of the head. It includes both the cranium and facial bones. The **cranium** is the domelike bone at the top of the head. Within the cranium is the **cranial** cavity, a hollow area that contains the brain. The **facial bones** are the bony structures that support the tissues of the face including the nose, cheeks, and lips. The facial bones also protect the eyes and internal structures of the nose, mouth, and upper throat.

Cranium

The cranium is composed of eight bones (see Figures 8-2 ■ and 8-3 ■). The line where one cranial bone meets another is known as a **suture.** The **frontal bone** forms the forehead and top of the cranium and ends at the **coronal suture.** Within the frontal bone, just above either eyebrow, are the two hollow frontal sinuses, discussed in Otolaryngology (Chapter 16). The **parietal bones** begin at the coronal suture and form the right and left sides of the top and back of the cranium. These two bones join at the midline **sagittal suture** that runs from front to back. The **occipital bone** forms the posterior and base of

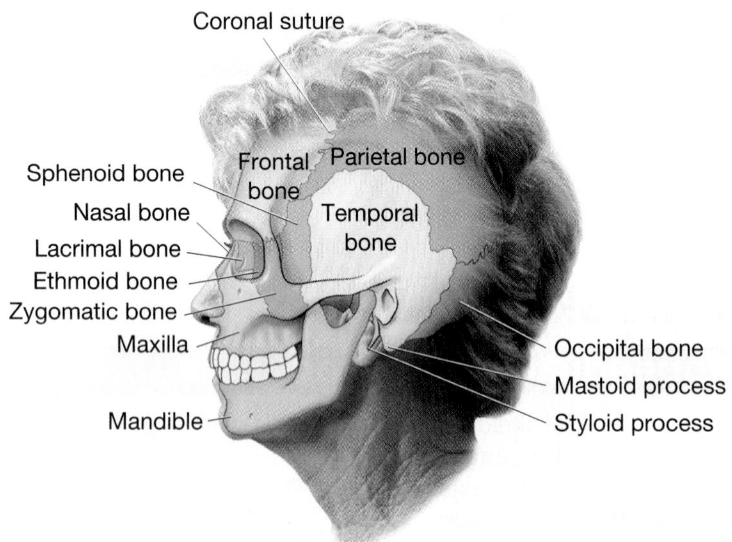

Figure 8-2 ■ Side view of the cranium and facial bones.
The frontal bone, parietal bone, occipital bone, temporal bone, sphenoid bone, and ethmoid bone form the left side of the cranium. The frontal bone joins the parietal bone at the coronal suture. From the side, these facial bones are visible: nasal bone, lacrimal bone, zygomatic bone, maxillary bone, and mandible.

skull (SKUHL)
Skull is an Old English word meaning *a bowl.*

cranium (KRAY-nee-um)
Cranium is derived from a Greek word meaning *skull.* The Latin word for skull—*calvaria*—is not used often in medicine.

cranial (KRAY-nee-al)
crani/o- *cranium (skull)*
-al *pertaining to*

facial (FAY-shal)
faci/o- *face*
-al *pertaining to*

suture (SOO-chur)
Suture is derived from a Latin word meaning *a seam.*

frontal (FRUN-tal)
front/o- *front*
-al *pertaining to*

coronal (kor-OH-nal)
coron/o- *encircling structure*
-al *pertaining to*
Coronal is derived from a Latin word meaning *crown.*

parietal (pah-RY-eh-tal)
pariet/o- *wall of a cavity*
-al *pertaining to*

sagittal (SAJ-ih-tal)
sagitt/o- *going from front to back*
-al *pertaining to*
Sagittal is derived from a Latin word meaning *an arrow,* implying the path of an arrow that goes through the body from front to back.

occiptal (awk-SIP-ih-tal)
occipit/o- *occiput (back of the head)*
-al *pertaining to*

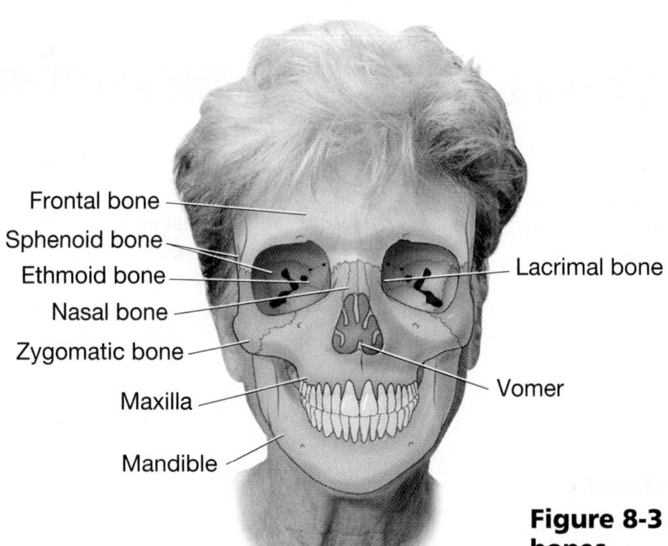

Figure 8-3 ■ Front view of the cranium and facial bones.

The facial bones connect to each other and to the bones of the cranium.

the cranium. It contains the **foramen magnum**, a large, round opening through which the spinal cord passes to join the brain. The **temporal bones** form the lower sides of the cranium. Each temporal bone contains an opening for the ear canal and a bony cavity within that houses the bones of the middle ear, discussed in Otolaryngology (Chapter 16). The **mastoid process** is a bony projection from the inferior temporal bone just behind the ear. The most inferior part of each temporal bone ends in the sharp **styloid process**, a point of attachment for ligaments that go to the hyoid bone in the throat. The **sphenoid bone** forms the central base of the cranium; it is a large, irregularly shaped bone that also travels superiorly and laterally. It forms the posterior walls of the eye sockets. The sphenoid bone behind the nose contains the hollow sphenoid sinuses, discussed in Otolaryngology (Chapter 16). The sphenoid bone also contains a bony cup that holds the pituitary gland, discussed in Endocrinology (Chapter 14). The sphenoid bone has bony projections that attach to muscles that move the soft palate and lower jaw. The **ethmoid bone** forms the anterior base of the cranium. It is a long, narrow bone that is oriented from front to back. It forms the bony nasal septum that divides the nasal cavity into right and left sides. It also forms the medial wall of each eye socket. It contains many tiny hollow areas that make up the ethmoid sinuses, discussed in Otolaryngology (Chapter 16).

foramen magnum
(foh-RAY-min MAG-num)
Foramen is a Latin word meaning *an opening. Magnum* is a Latin word meaning *large.* The foramen magnum is the largest foramen in the body. Small foramina in other parts of the body allow blood vessels to pass through the bones.

temporal (TEM-poh-ral)
tempor/o- *temple (side of the head)*
-al *pertaining to*

mastoid (MAS-toyd)
mast/o- *breast; mastoid process*
-oid *resembling*
The rounded, downward-pointing bone was thought to resemble a breast.

process (PRAWS-es)
Process is derived from a Latin word meaning *a prominence or projection.*

styloid (STY-loyd)
styl/o- *stake*
-oid *resembling*

sphenoid (SFEE-noyd)

sphen/o- *wedge shape*
-oid *resembling*

ethmoid (ETH-moyd)
ethm/o- *sieve*
-oid *resembling*
The ethmoid bone is very porous with many small, hollow spaces that resemble a sieve.

Across the Life Span

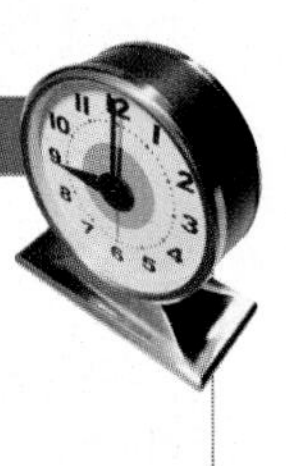

Neonatology. When the fetus is in the uterus, the bones of the cranium have large spaces between them called **fontanels** or soft spots (see Figure 8-4 ■). The fontanels allow the bones to move as the fetus passes through the birth canal, and they remain open to allow the brain to grow during childhood. The bony edges finally fuse together to become immobile in early adulthood.

fontanel (FAWN-tah-NEL)
Fontanel, also spelled *fontanelle,* is a Latin word meaning *fountain or spring,* referring to the pulse that could be felt in the fontanel and was thought to be the fountain or spring of life.

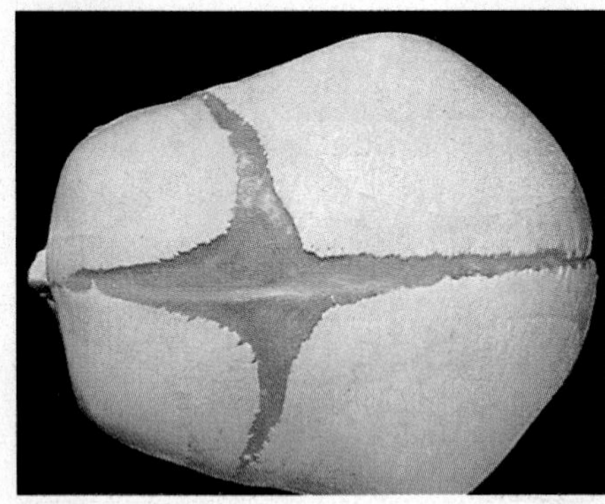

Figure 8-4 ■ Fontanel.
This fetal cranium shows the large anterior fontanel where the frontal bone has not yet joined the parietal bones. There is also a smaller, posterior fontanel at the back of the cranium. The translucent yellow membrane in the fontanel is the dura mater, a tough fibrous membrane that covers the brain.

Facial Bones

There are 14 bones in the face (see Figures 8-2 and 8-3). The **nasal bones** form the bridge of the nose and the inner roof of the nasal cavity. The **inferior nasal turbinates,** discussed in Otolaryngology (Chapter 16), are thin, bony projections that jut out from each side of the nasal cavity. The **vomer** is a narrow wall of bone that forms the inferior part of the nasal septum and continues posteriorly to the cranium where it joins the sphenoid bone. The **lacrimal bones** are very small, flat bones within the eye sockets, near the lacrimal (tear) glands. Each **zygoma** or **zygomatic bone** forms a cheek bone and the lateral edge of the eye socket. The **maxilla** covers the area above the mouth and is known as the upper jaw. It forms the inferior edge of each eye socket and the anterior hard palate. It supports the tissues of the nose and upper lip. It contains the roots of the upper teeth and the hollow maxillary sinuses, discussed in Otolaryngology (Chapter 16). The **palatine bones** are small, flat bones that form the posterior hard palate. The **mandible** is a large, irregularly shaped bone, known as the lower jaw. It is the only moveable bone in the skull. The roots of the lower teeth are in the mandible. Each side of the mandible travels superiorly, ending in two bony tips. The anterior bony tip slides under the zygoma, while the posterior bony tip forms a moveable joint with the temporal bone just in front of the ear.

nasal (NAY-zal)
nas/o- *nose*
-al *pertaining to*

turbinate (TUR-bih-nayt)
turbin/o- *scroll-like structure; turbinate*
-ate *composed of; pertaining to*
Turbinate is derived from a Latin word meaning *something that spins like a top.* The turbinate bones roll around within themselves, like a turban or like a scroll.

vomer (VOH-mer)
Vomer is derived from a Latin word meaning *plowshare,* the cutting part of a plow. The vomer bone is shaped somewhat like the blade on a plow.

lacrimal (LAK-rih-mal)
lacrim/o- *tears*
-al *pertaining to*

zygoma (zy-GOH-mah)
Zygoma is a Greek word meaning *a bar.* Form the plural by changing *-ma* to *-mata.*

zygomatic (ZY-goh-MAT-ik)
zygomat/o- *zygoma (cheek bone)*
-ic *pertaining to*

maxilla (mak-SIL-ah)
The upper jaw bone consists of a right maxilla and a left maxilla that are fused in the midline, but the plural form *maxillae* is seldom used.

Other Bones of the Head There are also three tiny bones in each ear: the malleus, incus, and stapes. Collectively, these are known as the **ossicles** or the **ossicular chain** because they are arranged in a row. They are active in the process of hearing, discussed in Otolaryngology (Chapter 16).

There is also one small bone in the anterior neck below the mandible: the **hyoid bone.** It is a flat, U-shaped bone that does not touch any other bones, but functions as a bony bridge that anchors the muscles of the tongue and larynx.

maxillary (MAK-sih-lair-ee)
maxill/o- *maxilla (upper jaw)*
-ary *pertaining to*

palatine (PAL-ah-tyne)
palat/o- *palate*
-ine *pertaining to*

mandible (MAN-dih-bl)

mandibular (man-DIB-yoo-lar)
mandibul/o- *mandible (lower jaw)*
-ar *pertaining to*

ossicle (AWS-ih-kl)
Ossicle is derived from a Latin word meaning *little bone.*

ossicular (aw-SIK-yoo-lar)
ossicul/o- *ossicle (little bone)*
-ar *pertaining to*

hyoid (HY-oyd)
hy/o- *U-shaped structure*
-oid *resembling*

Bones of the Chest

The chest contains the **thorax,** a bony cage that is also known as the rib cage. Within the thorax is the **thoracic** cavity, a hollow area that contains the heart, lungs, and other structures. The bones of the thorax include the sternum and 24 ribs (12 pairs) (see Figure 8-5■). The **sternum,** also known as the breast bone, is in the center of the anterior thorax. The **manubrium** is the triangular, most superior part of the sternum, while the **xiphoid process** is the small tip at its inferior end.

There are 12 pairs of ribs (see Figure 8-5). Beginning at the top of the sternum, rib pairs 1 through 7 are attached to the spinal column

thorax (THOH-raks)
Thorax is a Greek word meaning *breastplate.*

thoracic (thoh-RAS-ik)
thorac/o- *thorax (chest)*
-ic *pertaining to*

sternum (STER-num)

sternal (STER-nal)
stern/o- *sternum (breast bone)*
-al *pertaining to*

manubrium (mah-NOO-bree-um)
Manubrium is a Latin word meaning *handle.* The manubrium is like the handle of the sternum with the xiphoid at the other end being its pointed tip.

xiphoid (ZY-foyd)
xiph/o- *sword*
-oid *resembling*

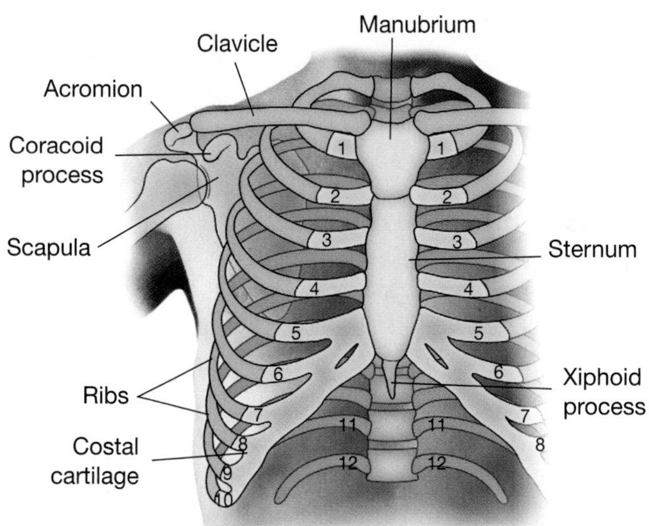

Figure 8-5 ■ Bones of the chest and shoulder.
The sternum and ribs form the thorax, a bony cage that protects the heart and lungs. The clavicle and scapula are part of the bones of the shoulder.

posteriorly and to the sternum anteriorly by **costal cartilage.** These ribs are known as true ribs. Cartilage is a smooth, firm, but flexible connective tissue. The area where the cartilage meets the rib is known as the **costochondral joint.** Rib pairs 8 through 10 are attached to the spinal column, but are only indirectly attached to the sternum by long lengths of costal cartilage. These ribs are known as false ribs. Rib pairs 11 and 12 are attached to the spinal column but not to the sternum. These ribs are known as floating ribs.

costal (KAWS-tal)
cost/o- *rib*
-al *pertaining to*
Costal is the adjective form for *rib.*

cartilage (KAR-tih-lij)

cartilaginous (KAR-tih-LAJ-ih-nus)
cartilagin/o- *cartilage*
-ous- *pertaining to*

costochondral (KAWS-toh-CON-dral)
cost/o- *rib*
chondr/o- *cartilage*
-al *pertaining to*

Bones of the Neck and Back

The **spine** or backbone is a vertical column of bones that is also known as the **spinal column** or **vertebral column** (see Figure 8-6 ■). It is composed of 24 individual vertebrae, plus the sacrum and coccyx. The spinal column supports the weight of the head, neck, and chest and protects the spinal cord.

spine (SPYN)

spinal (SPY-nal)
spin/o- *spine; backbone*
-al *pertaining to*

vertebra (VER-teh-brah)
vertebrae (VER-teh-bree)
Vertebra is a Latin singular feminine noun. Form the plural by changing *-a* to *-ae.*

vertebral (VER-teh-bral)
vertebr/o- *vertebra*
-al *pertaining to*

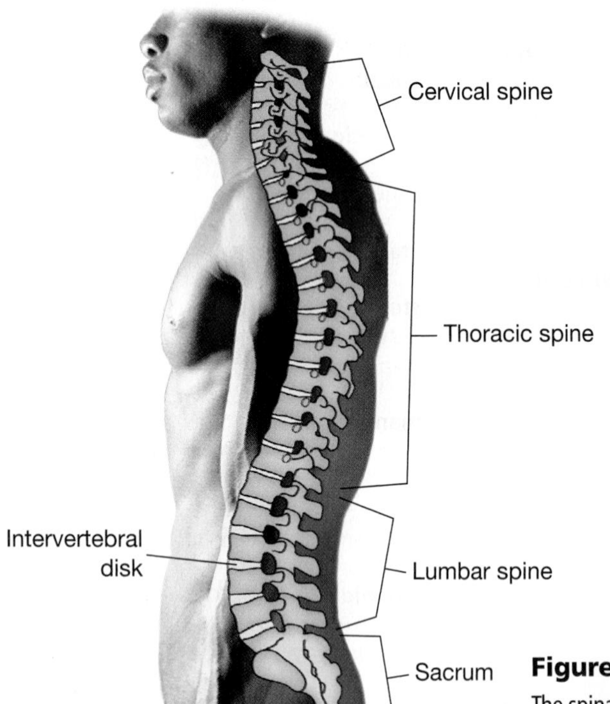

Figure 8-6 ■ Bones of the spinal column.
The spinal column consists of five regions: cervical vertebrae, thoracic vertebrae, lumbar vertebrae, sacrum, and coccyx. Notice how the vertebrae become progressively larger and sturdier as they bear more and more of the weight of the body.

The spinal column is divided into five different regions: the cervical vertebrae, the thoracic vertebrae, the lumbar vertebrae, the sacrum, and the coccyx. The **cervical vertebrae** (C1–C7) are located in the neck. The first cervical vertebra (C1) is directly below the occipital bone of the cranium and is known as the **atlas.** Its appearance is different from the other cervical vertebrae; it must conform to the occipital bone and form a joint that allows the head to nod up and down. The second cervical vertebra (C2) is known as the **axis.** It fits into the atlas to form a joint that allows the head to move from side to side. The **thoracic vertebrae** (T1–T12) are located in the chest. Each thoracic vertebra joins with one of the 12 pairs of ribs of the thoracic cage. The **lumbar vertebrae** (L1–L5) are located in the lower back. The lumbar vertebrae are larger than the cervical or thoracic vertebrae because they bear the weight of the entire head, neck, and trunk of the body. The **sacrum** is a group of five fused vertebrae that are not individually numbered, except for the first sacral vertebra (S1). The sacrum joins with the hip bones to form the most posterior part of the pelvis. The **coccyx** (tail bone) is a group of several small, fused vertebrae that are not individually numbered.

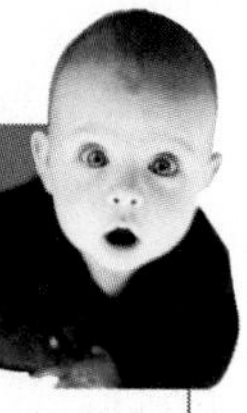

Did You Know?

Atlas was the name given to the mythological Greek god who was forced to hold the world on his shoulders. A person's head was imagined as a round globe and therefore the first vertebra was suitably named the *atlas*.

cervical (SER-vih-kal)
cervic/o- *neck; cervix*
-al *pertaining to*

atlas (AT-las)

axis (AK-sis)

thoracic (thoh-RAS-ik)
thorac/o- *thorax (chest)*
-ic *pertaining to*

lumbar (LUM-bar)
lumb/o- *lower back; area between the ribs and pelvis*
-ar *pertaining to*

sacrum (SAY-krum)
Sacrum is part of the Latin phrase *os sacrum* meaning *sacred bone.*

sacral (SAY-kral)
sacr/o- *sacrum*
-al *pertaining to*

coccyx (KAWK-siks)
Coccyx is derived from a Greek word meaning *cuckoo* because it resembles the beak of a cuckoo bird.

coccygeal (kawk-SIJ-ee-al)
coccyg/o- *coccyx (tail bone)*
-eal *pertaining to*

The vertebrae in each of these regions differ slightly in appearance but most share these common features (see Figure 8-7 ■): a vertebral body (circular, flat center), a **spinous process** (a long, bony projection that juts out along the midline of the back), two **transverse processes** (smaller bony projections on each side), and the **vertebral foramen** (the hole through which the spinal cord passes). The spinous and transverse processes are points of attachment for the spinal muscles. Between the vertebrae (beginning with C2 and ending with S1) are the **intervertebral disks,** circular disks with two flat surfaces. The outer wall of each disk is made of tough fibrocartilage. The inside of each disk is filled with a gelatinous substance known as the **nucleus pulposis.** The disk acts as a cushion to absorb impact during body movement.

spinous (SPY-nus)
spin/o- *spine; backbone*
-ous *pertaining to*

process (PRAWS-es)

transverse (trans-VERS)
trans- *across, through*
-verse *to travel; to turn*

foramen (foh-RAY-min)

intervertebral (IN-ter-VER-teh-bral)
inter- *between*
vertebr/o- *vertebra*
-al *pertaining to*

disk (DISK)
Some dictionaries prefer the spelling *disc.*

nucleus pulposis
(NOO-klee-us pul-POH-sis)
The nucleus is the central part of a structure. *Pulposis* refers to the pulpy consistency of the contents within the intervertebral disk.

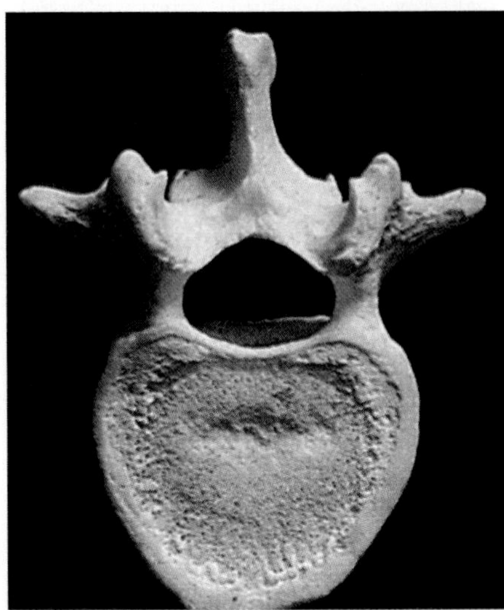

Figure 8-7 ■ Lumbar vertebra.

This vertebra shows the wide, flat surface that is characteristic of lumbar vertebrae. The lumbar vertebrae support the weight of the entire upper body.

Did You Know?

Andreas Vesalius (1514–1564) was born in Belgium and was educated in the great medical universities of France and Italy. He assembled his first human skeleton while in medical school by robbing the gallows after a public hanging. His masterpiece, *De Humani Corporis Fabrica* (*The Structure of the Human Body*), was published in 1543. His woodcuts showed dissected bodies in natural poses with scenery in the background. Prior to his work, there were almost no illustrations in medical textbooks. His beautiful, highly detailed, and anatomically correct illustrations educated a new generation of physicians (see Figure 8-8 ■).

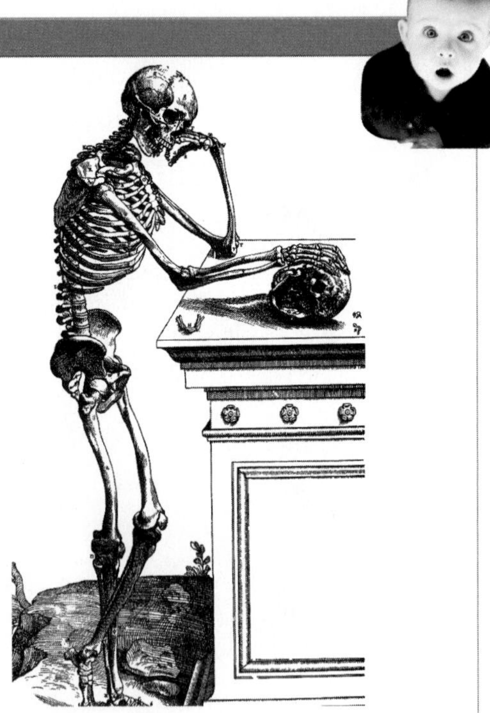

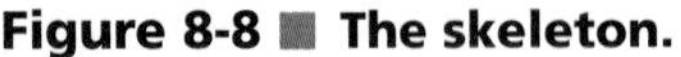

Figure 8-8 ■ The skeleton.

An anatomical illustration of the skeleton by Andreas Vesalius.

Bones of the Shoulder

The shoulder bones are also known as the shoulder girdle because they go around the shoulder on all sides. The shoulder bones include two clavicles and two scapulae (see Figures 8-5 and 8-9 ■). The **clavicle** or collar bone is a thin, rodlike bone on each side of the anterior neck. Its medial end connects to the manubrium of the sternum; its lateral end connects to the scapula. The **scapula** or shoulder blade is a triangular-shaped bone on either side of the vertebral column in the upper back. It has a long, bladelike spine along its upper half. This spine ends in a flat projection known as the **acromion** that connects to the clavicle. The **coracoid process,** a small projection that resembles a bent finger, is a point of attachment for several muscles of the arm and chest. The **glenoid fossa,** a shallow depression, is where the head of the humerus joins the scapula to make the shoulder joint.

clavicle (KLAV-ih-kl)

clavicular (klah-VIK-yoo-lar)
clavicul/o- *clavicle (collar bone)*
-ar *pertaining to*

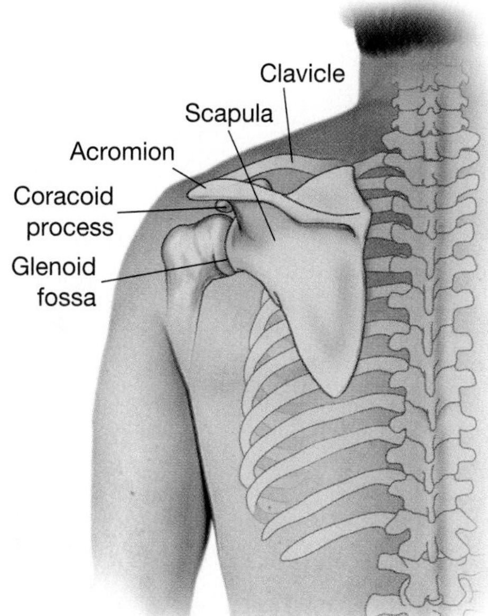

Figure 8-9 ■ Bones of the shoulder.

This posterior view shows the scapula joining the upper arm bone at the glenoid fossa. The acromion is connected to the clavicle. The scapula itself is not connected to the ribs or spinal column. This allows the scapula to move freely in several directions as the shoulder moves.

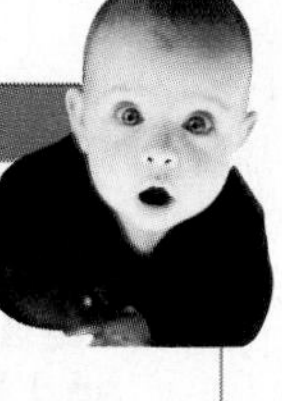

Did You Know?

During birth, it is not unusual for the clavicle to break as the baby goes through the birth canal. The fracture does not need to be treated as it heals by itself within a matter of days because of the high rate of bone growth in babies.

scapula (SKAP-yoo-lah)
scapulae (SKAP-yoo-lee)
Scapula is a Latin singular feminine noun meaning *shoulder blade*. Form the plural by changing *-a* to *-ae.*

scapular (SKAP-yoo-lar)
scapul/o- *scapula (shoulder blade)*
-ar *pertaining to*

acromion (ah-KROH-mee-on)
Acromion is derived from a Greek word meaning *tip of the shoulder.*

coracoid (KOR-ah-koyd)
Coracoid means *resembling a crow's beak.*

glenoid (GLEH-noyd)
glen/o- *socket of a joint*
-oid *resembling*

fossa (FAW-sah)
Fossa is a Latin word meaning *trench or ditch,* but in anatomy a fossa is a shallow depression in a bone.

Bones of the Arm

Upper and Lower Arm The arm, the upper **extremity** of the body, consists of the upper arm and lower arm or forearm. The arm contains the bones of the humerus, radius, and ulna (see Figure 8-10■). The **humerus** is the long bone in the upper arm. At its proximal end (the end closest to the shoulder), the head of the humerus fits into the glenoid fossa of the scapula to form the shoulder joint. At its distal end, the humerus joins with both the radius and the ulna to form the elbow joint.

Did You Know?

The "funny bone" is not a bone at all. The ulnar nerve travels across a rounded, bony projection (epicondyle) on the medial side of the distal humerus. When you accidentally bump this area, you hit the ulnar nerve and send a shock wave (that is in no way "funny") through your entire upper extremity.

The **radius** is one of the two bones in the forearm. It lies on the thumb side of the forearm. At its distal end, it connects to the bones of the wrist. The **ulna** lies on the little finger side of the forearm. At its proximal end is the **olecranon**, a large, square projection that forms the point of the elbow. At its distal end, the ulna connects to the bones of the wrist.

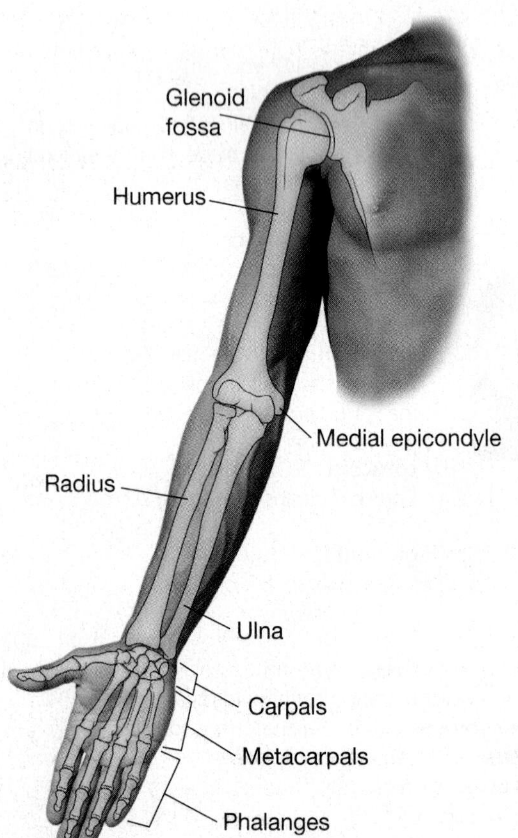

Figure 8-10 ■ Bones of the arm, wrist, hand, and fingers.

The humerus of the upper arm joins with both the radius and the ulna, the bones of the forearm. These two bones rotate around each other, which allows the hand to be turned palm up or palm down. The carpal bones in the wrist are connected to the metacarpal bones in the hand. The fingers contain three phalanageal bones; the thumb only contains two.

extremity (eks-TREM-ih-tee)
Extremity is derived from an Old English word meaning *the state of being the end part.*

humerus (HYOO-mer-us)
humeri (HYOO-mer-eye)
Humerus is a Latin singular masculine noun. Form the plural by changing *-us* to *-i.*

humeral (HYOO-mer-al)
humer/o- *humerus (upper arm bone)*
-al *pertaining to*

radius (RAY-dee-us)
radii (RAY-dee-eye)
Radius is a Latin singular masculine noun meaning *a rod.* Form the plural by changing *-us* to *-i.*

radial (RAY-dee-al)
radi/o- *radius (forearm bone); x-rays; radiation*
-al *pertaining to*
Some word parts have more than one definition. The best definition of *radial* is *pertaining to the radius (forearm bone).*

ulna (UL-nah)
ulnae (UL-nee)
Ulna is a Latin singular feminine noun meaning *elbow and arm.* Form the plural by changing *-a* to *-ae.*

ulnar (UL-nar)
uln/o- *ulna (forearm bone)*
-al *pertaining to*

olecranon (oh-LEK-rah-non)
Olecranon is a Greek word meaning *point of the elbow.*

Word Alert

SOUND-ALIKE WORDS

humerus (noun) the bone of the upper arm
Example: The patient sustained a fracture of the humerus.

humorous (adjective) descriptive English word meaning *funny*
Example: It is not very humorous when you fracture a bone.

humeral (adjective) descriptive word for the bone of the upper arm
Example: The x-ray showed a humeral fracture.

humoral (adjective) descriptive word for immunity (resistance) to infection that comes from antibodies in the blood
Example: Humoral immunity from infection occurs when B cell lymphocytes attack pathogens.

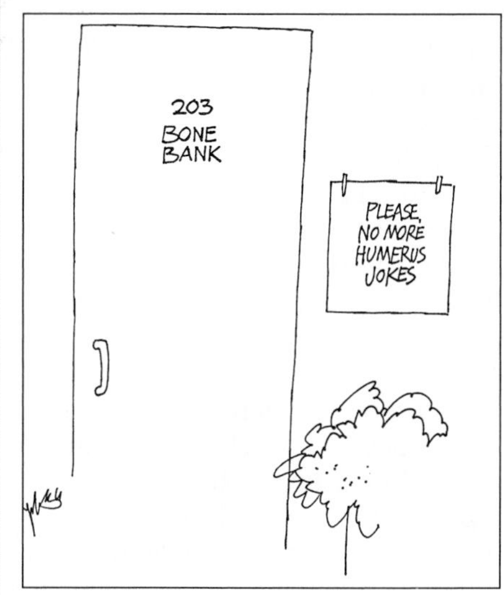

Wrist, Hand, and Fingers Each wrist contains eight small, individual **carpal bones** arranged in two rows (see Figure 8-10). One row connects to the radius and ulna. The other row connects to the bones of the hand. Each hand contains five individual **metacarpal bones,** one corresponding to each of the five fingers. Each finger or **digit** contains three individual **phalangeal bones** or **phalanges** (except the thumb, which contains two), arranged end to end. The distal **phalanx** is the final bone at the very tip of each finger. The fingers are also known as **rays.** The metacarpophalangeal (MCP) joint is between a metacarpal bone and a phalanx. The distal interphalangeal (DIP) joint is between the last two phalanges in a finger or toe.

carpal (KAR-pal)
carp/o- *wrist*
-al *pertaining to*
Carpus is a Latin word meaning *wrist.*

metacarpal (MET-ah-KAR-pal)
meta- *after; subsequent to; transition; change*
carp/o- *wrist*
-al *pertaining to*
Some word parts have more than one definition. The best definition of *metacarpal* is *pertaining to [bones that are] after or subsequent to the wrist.*

digit (DIJ-it)
Digit is derived from a Latin word meaning *a finger or toe.*

phalanx (FAY-langks)
phalanges (fah-LAN-jeez)
Phalanx is a Greek singular noun meaning *a line of soldiers.* The fingers and toes can be imagined to be soldiers in a row. Form the plural by changing *-x* to *-ges.*

phalangeal (fah-LAN-jee-al)
phalang/o- *phalanx (finger or toe)*
-eal *pertaining to*

ray (RAY)
The rays or digits extend outward from the hand like the rays of the sun.

Bones of the Hip

The bones of the hip are also known as the pelvic girdle because they go around the pelvic cavity on all sides. The **pelvis** includes the hip bones as well as the sacrum and coccyx of the spinal column. The hip bones include an ilium, ischium, and pubis on each side of the spinal column (see Figure 8-11 ■). The **ilium**, the most superior of the hip bones, has a broad, flaring rim known as the **iliac crest.** Anteriorly, a smaller bony projection is known as the anterior-superior **iliac spine.** Posteriorly, each ilium joins one side of the sacrum. The ilium travels inferiorly to form part of the **acetabulum** (the deep socket of the hip joint) and medially to join the pubis. The **ischium** is the most inferior of the hip bones. Each ischium is one of the "seat bones" that you sit on. It consists of a thick, curved bone that surrounds the **obturator foramen.** The obturator foramen is covered by a fibrous membrane and is a point of attachment for some muscles of the hip. The **pubis** or **pubic bone** is the most anterior of the hip bones. It is a small, bridgelike bone. Its two halves meet in the anterior midline, where they form the **pubic symphysis**, a nearly immobile joint that contains a cartilage pad between the bone ends. The pubis also forms part of the acetabulum.

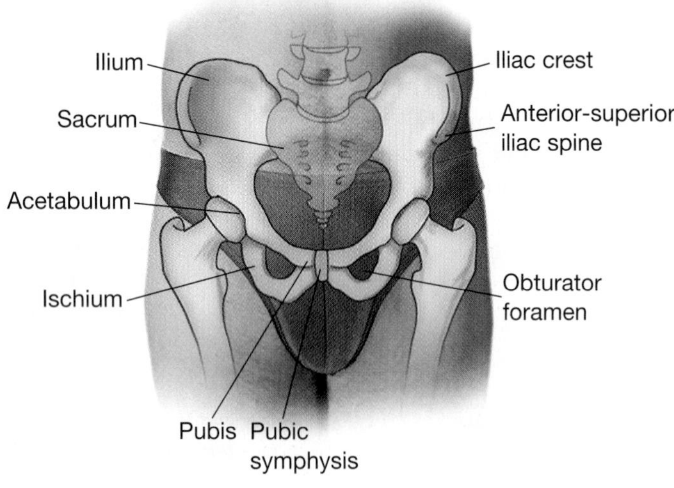

Figure 8-11 ■ Bones of the hip.

The ilium, ischium, and pubis on each side of the hip flow into each other without visible sutures or joints. However, the main part of each bone can be identified according to landmarks.

Word Alert

SOUND-ALIKE WORDS

ilium (noun) the superior flaring part of the hip bone of the pelvis
Example: During the car accident, she sustained a pelvic fracture that involved the ilium.

ileum (noun) the third part of the small intestine
Example: Inflammation of the ileum may also involve other parts of the small bowel.

ileus (noun) abnormal absence of contractions in the small intestine
Example: A postoperative ileus can occur after extensive abdominal surgery.

---

pelvis (PEL-vis)
Pelvis is a Latin word meaning *basin.* The bones of the pelvis have a flaring superior edge and a small, round, inferior outlet that resemble the shape of a basin.

pelvic (PEL-vik)
pelv/o- *pelvis (hip bone; renal pelvis)*
-ic *pertaining to*

ilium (IL-ee-um)
Ilium is a Latin word meaning *groin.* There are two ilia, but the plural form is seldom used.

iliac (IL-ee-ak)
ili/o- *ilium (hip bone)*
-ac *pertaining to*

spine (SPYN)
Spine is derived from a Latin word meaning *a thorn.* A spine is a thin projection from the surface of a bone. *Spine* can also mean *the spinal column.*

acetabulum (AS-eh-TAB-yoo-lum)
Acetabulum is a Latin word meaning *vinegar cup,* a small, shallow cup containing vinegar that the Romans served with meals.

acetabular (AS-eh-TAB-yoo-lar)
acetabul/o- *acetabulum (hip socket)*
-ar *pertaining to*

ischium (IS-kee-um)
Ischium is a Latin word meaning *hip.* There are two ischia, but the plural form is seldom used.

ischial (IS-kee-al)
ischi/o- *ischium (hip bone)*
-al *pertaining to*

obturator (AWB-too-RAY-tor)
Obturator is a Latin word meaning *to occlude.*

foramen (foh-RAY-min)
Foramen is a Latin word meaning *an opening.*

pubis (PYOO-bis)
There are two of these bones, but there is no plural form for *pubis* because it is part of the phrase *os pubis. Os* means *bone.*

pubic (PYOO-bik)
pub/o- *pubis (hip bone)*
-ic *pertaining to*

symphysis (SIM-fih-sis)
sym- *together, with*
-physis *state of growing*

Bones of the Leg

Upper and Lower Leg The leg, the lower extremity of the body, consists of the upper leg or thigh and the lower leg. The leg contains the bones of the femur, tibia, and fibula (see Figure 8-12 ■). The **femur** or thigh bone is the long bone in the upper leg. At its proximal end (the end closest to the hip bones), the head of the femur fits into the acetabulum to form the hip joint. The two bony prominences at the proximal end are the greater and lesser **trochanters.** At its distal end, the femur joins the tibia to form the knee joint.

The **tibia** or shin bone is the large bone on the medial side of the lower leg. At its distal end, it has a bony process known as the **medial malleolus.** The **fibula** is the very thin bone on the lateral side of the lower leg. Its proximal end connects to the tibia, not to the femur. It is not a weight-bearing bone in the leg. Its distal end has a small, pointed bony prominence known as the **lateral malleolus.** The adjective **peroneal** applies to the fibula bone and to the muscles and nerves in

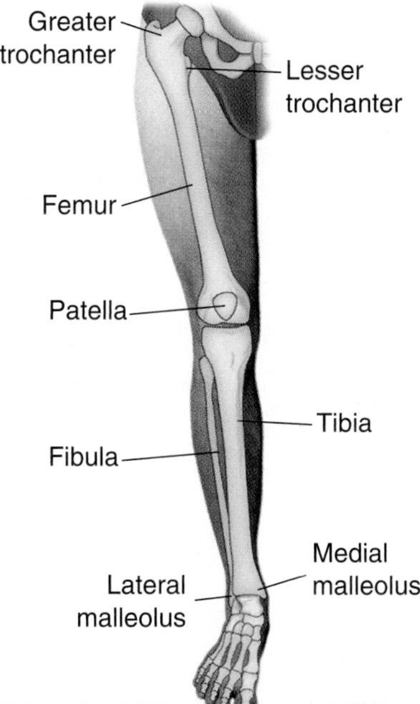

Figure 8-12 ■ Bones of the leg.
The femur of the upper leg joins the tibia of the lower leg to support the weight of the body. The fibula, the smaller of the two bones in the lower leg, is located on the side of the little toe. The patella is a small, round bone that protects the anterior aspect of the knee joint.

Did You Know?

Babies are born without kneecaps. These bones develop between the ages of 2 and 6 years old.

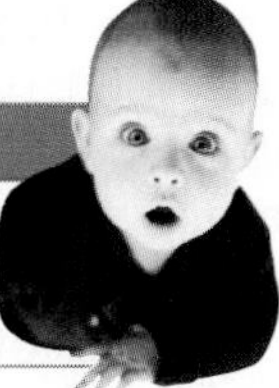

femur (FEE-mur)
femora (FEM-oh-rah)
Femur is a Latin word meaning *thigh bone.* The plural form is femora.

femoral (FEM-oh-ral)
femor/o- *femur (thigh bone)*
-al *pertaining to*

trochanter (troh-KAN-ter)
Trochanter is a Greek word meaning *a runner.*

trochanteric (troh-kan-TAIR-ik)
trochanter/o- *trochanter*
-ic *pertaining to*

tibia (TIB-ee-ah)
tibiae (TIB-ee-ee)
Tibia is a Latin singular feminine noun meaning *shin bone.* Form the plural by changing *-a* to *-ae.*

tibial (TIB-ee-al)
tibi/o- *tibia (shin bone)*
-al *pertaining to*

medial (MEE-dee-al)
medi/o- *middle*
-al *pertaining to*

malleolus (mah-LEE-oh-lus)
malleoli (mah-LEE-oh-ligh)
Malleolus is a Latin singular masculine noun. Form the plural by changing *-us* to *-i.*

malleolar (mah-LEE-oh-lar)
malleol/o- *malleolus*
-ar *pertaining to*

fibula (FIB-yoo-lah)
fibulae (FIB-yoo-lee)
Fibula is a Latin singular feminine noun meaning *a clasp or buckle.* The lateral malleolus of the fibula sticks out like a sharp buckle on the side of a shoe. Form the plural by changing *-a* to *-ae.*

fibular (FIB-yoo-lar)
fibul/o- *fibula (lower leg bone)*
-ar *pertaining to*

lateral (LAT-er-al)
later/o- *side*
-al *pertaining to*

peroneal (PAIR-oh-NEE-al)
perone/o- *fibula (lower leg bone)*
-al *pertaining to*
Peroneal is derived from a Greek word meaning *fibula.*

that area. The **patella** or kneecap is a thick, rounded bone anterior to the knee joint. It is most prominent in thin people when the knee is partially bent. The **popliteal space** is a diamond-shaped area at the back of the knee that is bordered by muscles and contains blood vessels and nerves.

Ankle, Foot, and Toes Each ankle contains seven individual **tarsal bones** (see Figure 8-13■). The talus is the first tarsal bone, and the largest is the **calcaneus** or heel bone. The midfoot contains five individual **metatarsal bones**, one corresponding to each of the five toes. The instep or arch of the foot is composed of both tarsal bones and metatarsal bones. Each toe or digit contains three individual phalangeal bones or phalanges (except the great toe, which contains two). The distal phalanx is at the very tip of the toe. The toes are also known as rays. The great toe, which is on the medial side of the foot, is known as the **hallux**. The little toe is on the lateral side of the foot.

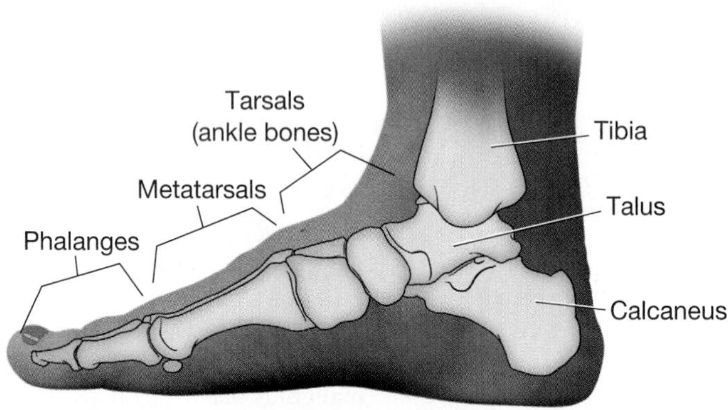

Figure 8-13 ■ Bones of the ankle and foot.

The tarsal bones in the ankle are connected to the metatarsal bones in the midfoot. The toes each contain three phalanageal bones; the great toe or hallux only contains two. In all, each foot contains 26 bones and 150 ligaments to hold the bones together.

patella (pah-TEL-ah)
patellae (pah-TEL-ee)
Patella is a Latin singular feminine noun meaning *small plate.* Form the plural by changing *-a* to *-ae.*

patellar (pah-TEL-ar)
patell/o- *patella (kneecap)*
-ar *pertaining to*

popliteal (pop-LIT-ee-al) (pop-lih-TEE-al)
poplite/o- *back of the knee*
-al *pertaining to*

tarsal (TAR-sal)
tars/o- *ankle*
-al *pertaining to*
Tarsus is a Latin word meaning *ankle.*

calcaneus (kal-KAY-nee-us)
Calcaneus is the Latin word for *heel bone.*

calcaneal (kal-KAY-nee-al)
calcane/o- *calcaneus (heel bone)*
-al *pertaining to*

metatarsal (MET-ah-TAR-sal)
meta- *after; subsequent to; transition; change*
tars/o- *ankle*
-al *pertaining to*

hallux (HAL-uks)
Hallux is a Latin word meaning *great toe.*

Joints, Cartilage, and Ligaments

A **joint** or **articulation** is an area where two bones come together. There are three types of joints. A suture joint between two cranial bones is immovable and contains no cartilage. The pubic symphysis and the joints between the vertebrae are slightly moveable joints that contain fibrocartilage pads or disks. A synovial joint, such as the elbow joint, is fully moveable and has other distinguishing characteristics.

joint (JOYNT)
Joint is derived from a Latin word meaning *junction or union.*

articulation (ar-TIK-yoo-LAY-shun)
articul/o- *joint*
-ation *a process; being or having*

Synovial joints (see Figure 8-14■) join bones whose ends are covered with **articular cartilage**. A **meniscus** is a special crescent-shaped cartilage pad found in some synovial joints, such as the knee. **Ligaments,** strong fibrous bands of connective tissue, hold the two bone ends together in a synovial joint. The entire joint is encased in a **joint capsule** that is composed of a fibrous outer layer and an inner synovial membrane. The **synovial membrane** lines the surfaces of the joint and produces **synovial fluid,** a clear, thick fluid that lubricates the joint.

There are two kinds of synovial joints: hinge-type joints (such as the elbow and knee) that only allow motion in two directions and ball-and-socket joints (such as the shoulder and hip) that allow motion in many directions.

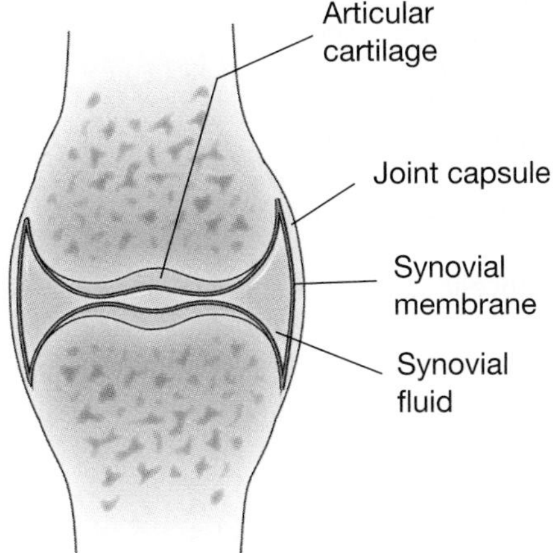

Figure 8-14 ■ Synovial joint.
Synovial joints are fully moveable joints that have a joint capsule and a synovial membrane that makes synovial fluid. Hinge-type synovial joints (like the elbow and knee) allow motion in two directions. Ball-and-socket synovial joints (like the shoulder and hip) allow motion in many directions.

synovial (sih-NOH-vee-al)
synovi/o- *synovium (membrane)*
-al *pertaining to*

articular (ar-TIK-yoo-lar)
articul/o- *joint*
-ar *pertaining to*

meniscus (meh-NIS-kus)
menisci (meh-NIS-kigh)
Meniscus is a Latin singular masculine noun meaning *a crescent.* Form the plural by changing *-us* to *-i.*

meniscal (meh-NIS-kal)
menisc/o- *meniscus (crescent-shaped cartilage)*
-al *pertaining to*

ligament (LIG-ah-ment)
Ligament is derived from a Latin word meaning *a band.*

ligamentous (LIG-ah-MEN-tus)
ligament/o- *ligament*
-ous *pertaining to*

capsule (KAP-sool)
Capsule is derived from a Latin word meaning *little box.*

capsular (KAP-soo-lar)
capsul/o- *capsule (enveloping structure)*
-ar *pertaining to*

The Structure of Bone

Bone is a type of connective tissue known as **osseous tissue.** The outside surface of a bone is covered by **periosteum,** a thick, fibrous membrane (see Figure 8-15■). A long bone such as the humerus or femur has a characteristic straight shaft or **diaphysis** and two widened ends or **epiphyses.** It is at the **epiphysial plates** that bone growth takes place.

Inside a long bone are two visibly different areas. Along the diaphysis is a layer of dense compact **cortical bone.** Beneath this is the **medullary cavity,** which is filled with yellow bone marrow that contains fatty tissue. The epiphyses contain a different type of bone known as **cancellous bone** or spongy bone. It is less dense than compact bone, and the spaces in it are filled with red bone marrow.

osseous (AW-see-us)
osse/o- *bone*
-ous *pertaining to*

periosteum (PAIR-ee-AWS-tee-um)

periosteal (PAIR-ee-AWS-tee-al)
peri- *around*
oste/o- *bone*
-al *pertaining to*

diaphysis (dy-AF-ih-sis)
diaphyses (dy-AF-ih-seez)
Diaphysis is a Greek singular noun. Form the plural by changing *-is* to *-es.*

diaphysial (DY-ah-FIZ-ee-al)
diaphys/o- *shaft of a bone*
-ial *pertaining to*
Some dictionaries prefer the spelling *diaphyseal.*

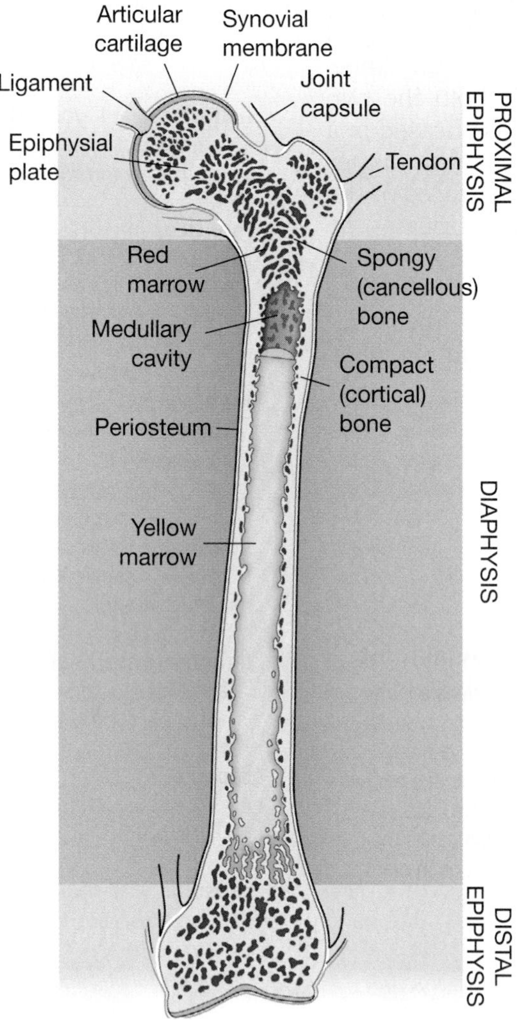

Figure 8-15 ■ Structure of a bone.

The external structure of a long bone includes the diaphysis (shaft) and epiphyses (ends). The internal structure has areas of compact bone for weight bearing, a medullary cavity that contains yellow marrow, and the bone ends of cancellous bone filled with red marrow that produces blood cells.

Connections

Hematology and Immunology (Chapter 6). Red bone marrow produces very immature stem cells that differentiate into immature red blood cells, white blood cells, and platelets that mature and then enter the blood.

epiphysis (eh-PIF-ih-sis)
epiphyses (eh-PIF-ih-seez)
Epiphysis is a Greek singular noun. Form the plural by changing *-is* to *-es*.

epiphysial (EP-ih-FIZ-ee-al)
epiphys/o- *growth area on the end of a bone*
-ial *pertaining to*
Some dictionaries prefer the spelling *epiphyseal*.

cortical (KOR-tih-kal)
cortic/o- *cortex (outer region)*
-al *pertaining to*

medullary (MED-yoo-LAIR-ee)
medull/o- *medulla (inner region)*
-ary *pertaining to*

cavity (KAV-ih-tee)
cav/o- *hollow space*
-ity *state; condition*

cancellous (kan-SEL-us)
cancell/o- *lattice structure*
-ous *pertaining to*

Physiology of Bone Growth

In a fetus, the bones are made of cartilage. During childhood, this cartilaginous tissue is gradually replaced by bony tissue in a process known as **ossification**. In addition, new bone is formed along the epiphysial growth plates at the ends of long bones as the body grows taller (see Figure 8-16■).

ossification (AWS-ih-fih-KAY-shun)
ossificat/o- *changing into bone*
-ion *action; condition*

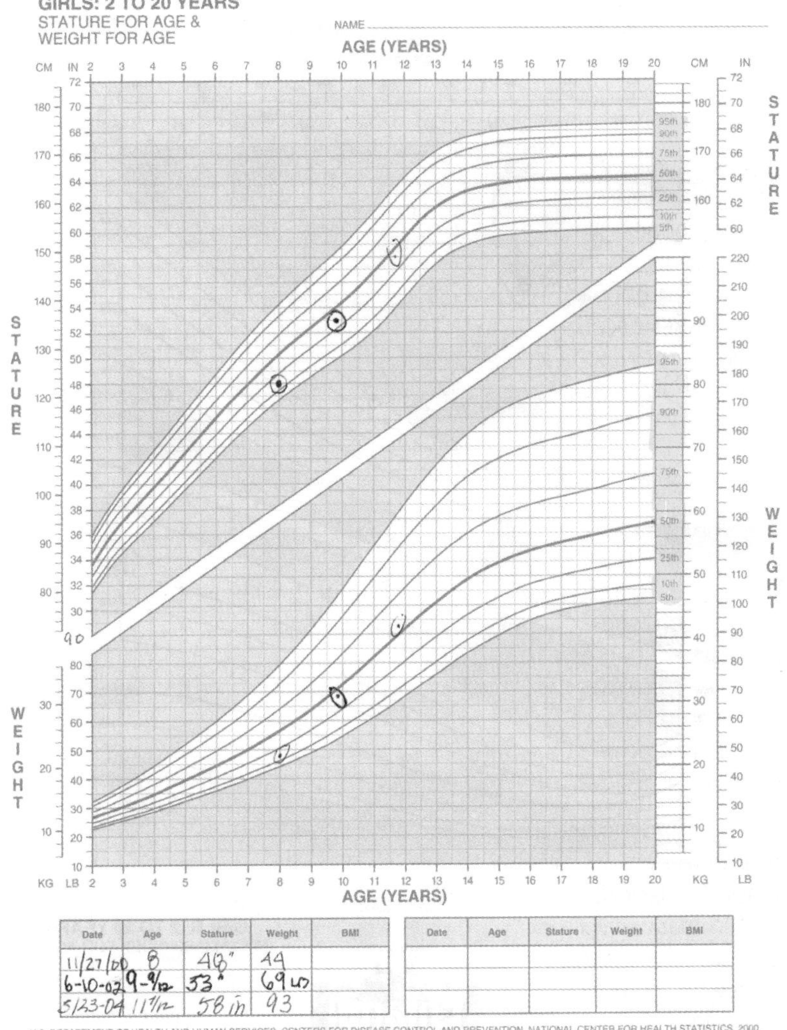

Figure 8-16 ■ Pediatric growth chart.

This chart tracks height and weight for girls ages 2 to 20 years and assigns percentiles. On the initial visit to her pediatrician, this 8-year-old child had a diagnosis of malnutrition and was in about the 15th percentile (measured on the yellow vertical bars on the right) for both height (stature) and weight. After three years of good nutrition, her most recent visit at age 11 years, 7 months, shows that she is now in about the 40th percentile for height and about the 55th percentile for weight.

Although mature bone is a hard substance, it is also a living tissue that undergoes change. About 10% of the entire skeleton is broken down and rebuilt each year. This process occurs in areas that are damaged or subjected to mechanical stress. Two types of **osteocytes** or bone cells are constantly at work on mature bone. **Osteoclasts** break down areas of old or damaged bone, while **osteoblasts** deposit new bone tissue in those areas. Almost all of the calcium in the body is stored in the bones, but this mineral is also extremely important to the proper functioning of skeletal muscles and heart to help them contract regularly and forcefully. As osteoclasts break down old or damaged bone, calcium in the bone is continuously released and made available to the rest of the body.

osteocyte (AWS-tee-oh-site)
oste/o- *bone*
-cyte *cell*

osteoclast (AWS-tee-oh-klast)
oste/o- *bone*
-clast *cell that breaks down substances*

osteoblast (AWS-tee-oh-blast)
oste/o- *bone*
-blast *immature cell*
Osteoblasts begin as immature cells, but then later become mature cells that produce either bone, cartilage, or collagen fibers.

Across the Life Span

From infancy through puberty, new bone formation exceeds bone breakdown. During adulthood, the daily formation of new bone equals the daily rate of bone breakdown. In old age, the rate of bone breakdown exceeds that of new bone formation, and the bones become fragile and prone to fracture. At all stages of life, formation of new bone is dependent on having enough calcium and phosphorus in the diet.

Connections

Endocrinology (Chapter 14). Calcium levels in the blood are controlled by parathyroid hormone secreted by the parathyroid glands. Parathyroid hormone raises calcium levels in the blood by stimulating osteoclasts to break down more bone. Calcitonin from the thyroid gland has the opposite effect, and so these two hormones constantly work to balance the blood calcium level. Estradiol and other hormones stimulate bone formation. Growth hormone from the pituitary gland influences the rate of bone growth.

Space Medicine. Astronauts who live in a weightless environment for prolonged periods of time are in danger of losing bone mass. The lack of weight-bearing stress on the bones decreases new bone formation while bone breakdown continues at its normal rate. All astronauts have regular exercise programs with resistance exercises that exert force on the bones. Patients confined to bed face this same problem of bone loss.

Vocabulary Review

Anatomy and Physiology

Now that you have studied the anatomy and physiology of the skeletal system, take time to review those new words and descriptions. Memorize the combining forms and their definitions before going on to the next section.

Word or Phrase	Combining Form and Definition	Description
acetabulum	acetabul/o- *acetabulum*	Cup-shaped socket in the hip bone that is formed by the ilium and the pubic bone. It is where the head of the femur fits to form the hip joint.
acromion		Flat, bony projection of the scapula where it connects to the clavicle
appendicular skeleton	appendicul/o- *limb; small attached part*	The bones of the shoulders, arms, hips, and legs
articular cartilage	articul/o- *joint*	Cartilage that covers the bone ends in a synovial joint
articulation	articul/o- *joint*	A joint where two bones come together and join or articulate
axial skeleton	axi/o- *axis*	The bones of the head, chest, and spine
bones	osse/o- *bone* oste/o- *bone*	The 206 individual pieces of the skeleton
calcaneus	calcane/o- *calcaneus (heel bone)*	Largest of the ankle bones. Also known as the heel bone.
cancellous bone	cancell/o- *lattice structure*	Spongy bone found in the epiphyses of long bones. Its spaces are filled with red bone marrow that makes blood cells.
carpal bones	carp/o- *wrist*	The eight small bones of the wrist joint
cervical vertebrae	cervic/o- *neck; cervix*	Vertebrae C1 through C7 in the cervical spine. C1 is also known as the **atlas;** C2 is known as the **axis.**
clavicle	clavic/o- *clavicle (collar bone)*	Horizontal bone in each shoulder that joins with the manubrium of the sternum and the acromion of the scapula. Also known as the **collar bone.**
coccyx	coccyg/o- *coccyx (tail bone)*	Group of several small, fused vertebrae below the sacrum. Also known as the **tail bone.**
coracoid process		Small projection on the scapula where muscles of the arm and chest attach. It resembles a bent finger.
coronal suture	coron/o- *encircling structure*	Suture between the frontal bone and the parietal bones of the cranium
costal cartilage	cost/o- *rib* chondr/o- *cartilage*	Smooth, firm, but flexible segments of connective tissue that join the ribs to the sternum. The area where the costal cartilage meets the rib is known as the **costochondral joint.**
cranium	crani/o- *cranium*	Bony structure of the head that contains the **cranial** cavity and the brain

Word or Phrase	Combining Form and Definition	Description
diaphysis	**diaphys/o-** *shaft of a bone*	The straight shaft of a long bone
epiphysis	**epiphys/o-** *growth area on the end of a bone*	The widened ends of a long bone. Each end contains the **epiphysial plate** where bone growth takes place.
ethmoid bone	**ethm/o-** *sieve*	Bone that forms the anterior base of the cranium, the bony nasal septum, and the medial walls of the eye sockets. It contains the many tiny hollow areas of the ethmoid sinuses.
extremity		An arm or a leg. Also known as a **limb.**
facial bones	**faci/o-** *face*	Bones that support and protect the external and internal structures of the face.
femur	**femor/o-** *femur (thigh bone)* **trochanter/o-** trochanter	Long bone of the upper leg. Also known as the **thigh bone.** The two bony prominences on the proximal end are the greater and lesser **trochanters.**
fibula	**fibul/o-** *fibula (lower leg bone)*	Smaller of the two bones in the lower leg. Located on the little toe side of the lower leg.
fontanel		Soft spot on the baby's head where the cranial sutures are still open. Also spelled fontanelle.
foramen		A hole in a bone: **foramen magnum** in the cranium, **vertebral foramen** in a vertebra, and **obturator foramen** in each ischium
frontal bone	**front/o-** *front*	Bone that forms the forehead and front of the cranium and contains the frontal sinuses
glenoid fossa	**glen/o-** *socket of a joint*	Shallow depression in the scapula where the head of the humerus articulates to form the shoulder joint
hallux		The great toe
humerus	**humer/o-** *humerus (upper arm bone)*	Long bone of the upper arm
hyoid bone	**hy/o-** *U-shaped structure*	A U-shaped bone that anchors the muscles of the tongue and larynx
ilium	**ili/o-** *ilium (hip bone)*	Most superior hip bone. Bony landmarks include the **iliac crest** and the anterior-superior **iliac spine.** Posteriorly, each ilium joins one side of the sacrum.
intervertebral disk	**vertebr/o-** *vertebra*	Circular disk between two vertebrae. It consists of an outer wall of fibrocartilage and an inner gelatinous substance, the **nucleus pulposis**, that acts as a cushion. Also spelled *disc.*
ischium	**ischi/o-** *ischium (hip bone)*	Most inferior hip bone. It contains the obturator foramen.
joint		Area where two bones come together. There are three types of joints: suture, symphysis, and synovial.
lacrimal bones	**lacrim/o-** *tears*	Facial bones within the eye socket near the lacrimal glands that produce tears
ligament	**ligament/o-** *ligament*	Fibrous bands that hold two bone ends together in a synovial joint

Word or Phrase	Combining Form and Definition	Description
lumbar vertebrae	lumb/o- *lower back; area between the ribs and pelvis*	Vertebrae L1 through L5 in the lumbar part of the spine in the lower back
malleolus	malleol/o- *malleolus*	Bony projections of the distal tibia (medial malleolus) and fibula (lateral malleolus). Often mistakenly called the ankle bones.
mandible	mandibul/o- *mandible (lower jaw)*	Facial bone that forms the lower jaw and contains the roots of the lower teeth. It is the only moveable bone in the skull and forms a moveable joint with the temporal bone just in front of the ear.
manubrium		Triangular, most superior part of the sternum
maxillary bones	maxill/o- *maxilla (upper jaw)*	Facial bones that form the immoveable upper jaw, the inferior edges of the eye sockets, and the anterior part of the hard palate. They support the nose and lips and contain the roots of the upper teeth and the hollow maxillary sinuses. Each side is known as a **maxilla.**
medullary cavity	medull/o- *medulla (inner region)* cav/o- *hollow space*	Long cavity in the center of a long bone. It contains yellow bone marrow (fatty tissue).
meniscus	menisc/o- *meniscus (crescent-shaped cartilage)*	Crescent-shaped cartilage pad found in some synovial joints like the knee
metacarpal bones	carp/o- *wrist*	The five long bones of the hand, one corresponding to each finger, that lie distal to the wrist bones
metatarsal bones	tars/o- *ankle*	The five long bones of the midfoot, one corresponding to each toe, that lie distal to the ankle bones
nasal bones	nas/o- *nose*	Facial bones that form the bridge of the nose and the inner roof of the nasal cavity
obturator foramen		Large opening in the ischium that is covered by a fibrous membrane and is a point of attachment for some muscles of the hip
occipital bone	occipit/o- *occipit (back of the head)*	Bone that forms the back of the cranium and the posterior base of the cranium
olecranon		Large, square, bony projection on the proximal ulna that forms the point of the elbow
osseous tissue	osse/o- *bone*	Bone, which is a type of connective tissue
ossicles	ossicul/o- *ossicle (little bone)*	Three tiny bones in the middle ear that function in the process of hearing. Also known as the **ossicular chain**
ossification	ossificat/o- *changing into bone*	Process by which cartilaginous tissue is changed into bone from infancy through puberty
osteoblast	oste/o- *bone*	Osteocyte that forms new bone or rebuilds bone
osteoclast	oste/o- *bone*	Osteocyte that breaks down old or damaged areas of bone
osteocyte	oste/o- *bone*	Bone cell. There are two types of osteocytes: osteoclasts and osteoblasts.

Word or Phrase	Combining Form and Definition	Description
palatine bones	**palat/o-** *palate*	Facial bones that form the posterior part of the hard palate
parietal bones	**pariet/o-** *wall of a cavity*	Bones that form the right and left sides of the top and back of the cranium
patella	**patell/o-** *patella (kneecap)*	Thick, round bone anterior to the knee joint. Also known as the **kneecap.**
pelvis	**pelv/o-** *pelvis (hip bone; renal pelvis)*	The hip bones as well as the sacrum and coccyx of the spinal column
periosteum	**oste/o-** *bone*	Thick, fibrous membrane that covers the outside surface of a bone
peroneal	**perone/o-** *fibula (lower leg bone)*	Adjective meaning *the fibula*. It applies to the fibula bone as well as muscles and nerves in that area.
phalanx	**phalang/o-** *phalanx (finger or toe)*	One of the individual bones of a finger or toe. Also known as a **digit** or a **ray.**
popliteal space	**poplite/o-** *back of the knee*	Area at the back of the knee that is bordered by muscles and contains blood vessels and nerves
pubis	**pub/o-** *pubis*	Most anterior hip bone. Bony landmark includes the **pubic symphysis,** a nearly immobile joint between the two **pubic bones.**
radius	**radi/o-** *radius (forearm bone); x-rays; radiation*	Forearm bone located along the thumb side of the lower arm
rib	**cost/o-** *rib*	The twelve pairs of bones that form the sides of the thorax. There are true ribs, false ribs, and floating ribs.
sacrum	**sacr/o-** *sacrum*	Group of five fused vertebrae below the lumbar vertebrae
sagittal suture	**sagitt/o-** *going from front to back*	Midline suture between the two parietal bones on the right and left sides of the cranium
scapula	**scapul/o-** *scapula (shoulder blade)*	Triangular-shaped bone on each side of the upper back. Also known as the **shoulder blade.** It has three distinct landmarks: the acromion, coracoid process and glenoid fossa.
skeletal system	**skelet/o-** *skeleton*	Body system that consists of all the bones, ligaments, and joints in the body
skeletomuscular system	**skelet/o-** *skeleton* **muscul/o-** *muscle*	The combined systems of the bones and muscles. The bones provide support for the muscles, and the muscles enable the bones to move. Also known as the **musculoskeletal system.**
skeleton	**skelet/o-** *skeleton*	The bony framework of the body that consists of all the bones
skull		Bony structure of the head that consists of the cranium and facial bones
sphenoid bone	**sphen/o-** *wedge shape*	Bone that forms the central base of the cranium and the posterior walls of the eye sockets. It contains the sphenoid sinuses. A bony cup in the sphenoid bone holds the pituitary gland.

Word or Phrase	Combining Form and Definition	Description
spine	**spin/o-** *spine, backbone*	Bony vertical column of vertebrae. Also known as the **spinal column, vertebral column,** or backbone. It is divided into five regions: cervical vertebrae, thoracic vertebrae, lumbar vertebrae, sacrum, and coccyx. *Spine* also refers to a bony projection, such as the spinous process on a vertebra.
sternum	**stern/o-** *sternum (breast bone)*	Vertical bone of the anterior thorax to which the clavicle and ribs are attached. Also known as the breast bone.
suture		Immoveable joint between two bones of the cranium
tarsal bones	**tars/o-** *ankle*	The seven bones in the ankle joint. The first is the tarsus; the largest is the calcaneus.
synovial joint	**synovi/o-** *synovium (membrane)* **capsul/o-** *capsule (enveloping structure)*	Fully moveable joints. There are two types: hinge-type and ball-and-socket joints. Ligaments hold the bone ends together. The entire joint is enclosed in a **joint capsule.** The inner surface of the joint capsule is lined by a **synovial membrane** that produces **synovial fluid** to lubricate the joint.
temporal bones	**tempor/o-** *temple (side of the head)* **mast/o-** *breast; mastoid process* **styl/o-** *stake*	Bones that form the right and left sides of the cranium. They contain the openings for the ear canals and house the small bones of the middle ear. Bony landmarks include the **mastoid process** behind the ear and the pointed **styloid process,** a site of attachment for ligaments to the hyoid bone.
thoracic vertebrae	**thorac/o-** *thorax (chest)*	Vertebrae T1 through T12 in the thoracic part of the spine in the chest.
thorax	**thorac/o-** *thorax (chest)*	Bony cage of the chest that contains the thoracic cavity with the heart, lungs, and other structures. Also known as the **rib cage.**
tibia	**tibi/o-** *tibia (shin bone)*	Larger of the two bones of the lower leg. Located on the great toe side of the lower leg. Also known as the **shin bone.**
turbinates	**turbin/o-** *scroll-like structure; turbinate*	Facial bones that are bony projections within the nasal cavity. The bones are formed like a scroll.
ulna	**uln/o-** *ulna (forearm bone)*	Forearm bone located along the little finger side of the lower arm
vertebra	**vertebr/o-** *vertebra*	Bony structure of the spine. Most vertebrae have a vertebral body (flat, central area), spinous process (bony projection along the midback), two transverse processes (bony projections to the side), and a foramen (hole where the spinal cord passes through).
vomer		Facial bone that forms the bottom of the nasal septum and continues to the base of the cranium to join the sphenoid bone
xiphoid process	**xiph/o-** *sword*	Inferior pointed tip of the sternum
zygomatic bones	**zygomat/o-** *zygoma (cheek bone)*	Facial bones that form the lateral edges of the eye sockets and the cheek bones. Each zygomatic bone is known as a **zygoma.**

Labeling Exercise

A. *Match each anatomy word or phrase to its numbered structure in Figure 8-17■. Write that word or phrase on the blank line next to its number. Use the Answer Key at the end of the book to check your answers.*

coronal suture	lacrimal bone	nasal bone	sphenoid bone
ethmoid bone	mandible	occipital bone	temporal bone
frontal bone	maxillary bone	parietal bone	zygomatic bone

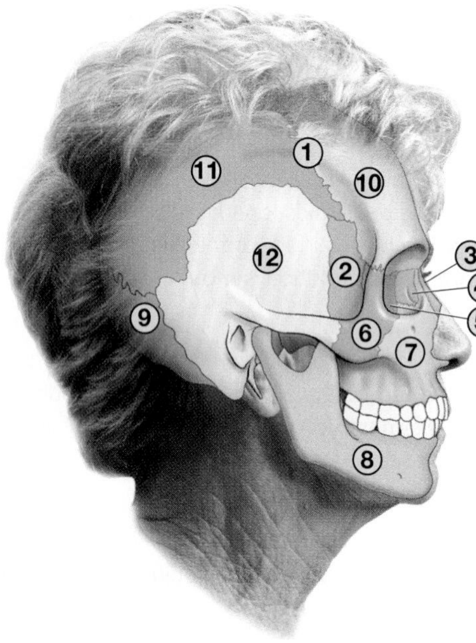

1. ______________
2. ______________
3. ______________
4. ______________
5. ______________
6. ______________
7. ______________
8. ______________
9. ______________
10. ______________
11. ______________
12. ______________

Figure 8-17 ■

B. *Match each anatomy word or phase to its numbered structure in Figure 8-18■. Write that word or phrase on the blank line next to its number.*

carpal bones	humerus	metacarpal bones	radius
glenoid fossa	medial epicondyle	phalanges	ulna

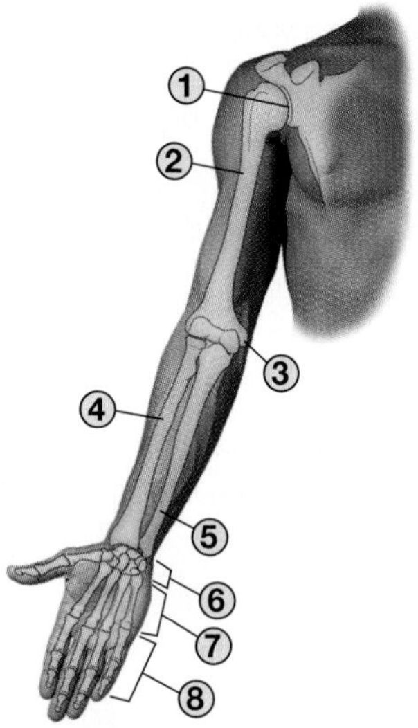

1. ______________
2. ______________
3. ______________
4. ______________
5. ______________
6. ______________
7. ______________
8. ______________

Figure 8-18 ■

C. *Match each anatomy word or phase to its numbered structure in Figures 8-19 ■ and 8-20 ■. Write that word or phrase on the blank line next to its number. Note: Some words or phrases may appear in both illustrations.*

calcaneus	fibula	medial malleolus	patella	tarsal bones
femur	lateral malleolus	metatarsal bones	phalanges	tibia

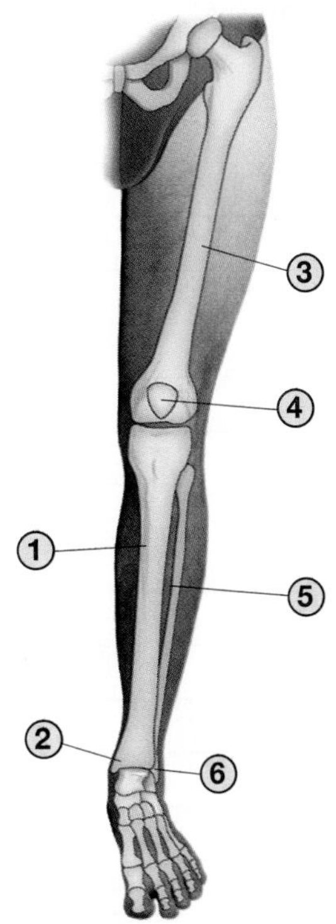

Figure 8-19 ■

1. ______________________
2. ______________________
3. ______________________
4. ______________________
5. ______________________
6. ______________________

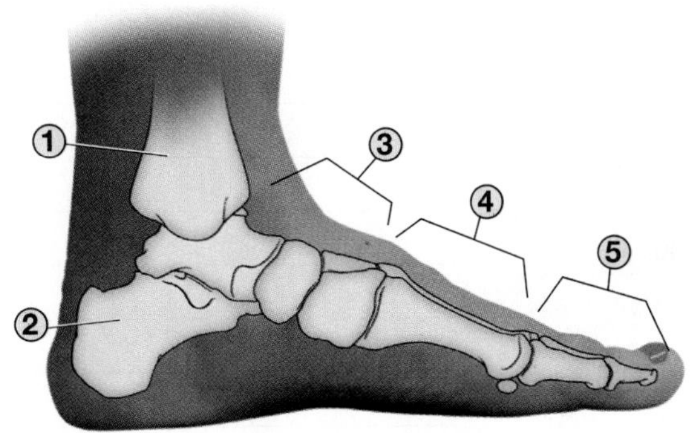

Figure 8-20 ■

1. ______________________
2. ______________________
3. ______________________
4. ______________________
5. ______________________

Building Medical Words

Combining Forms

Here are the skeletal combining forms you have learned so far. Next to each combining form, write its meaning. Use the Answer Key at the end of the book to check your answers. The first one has been done for you.

	Combining Form	Medical Meaning		Combining Form	Medical Meaning
1.	muscul/o-	muscle	35.	malleol/o-	
2.	acetabul/o-		36.	mandibul/o-	
3.	appendicul/o-		37.	mast/o-	
4.	articul/o-		38.	maxill/o-	
5.	axi/o-		39.	medi/o-	
6.	calcane/o-		40.	medull/o-	
7.	cancell/o-		41.	menisc/o-	
8.	capsul/o-		42.	nas/o-	
9.	carp/o-		43.	occipit/o-	
10.	cartilagin/o-		44.	orth/o-	
11.	cav/o-		45.	osse/o-	
12.	cervic/o-		46.	ossicul/o-	
13.	chondr/o-		47.	ossificat/o-	
14.	clavicul/o-		48.	oste/o-	
15.	coccyg/o-		49.	palat/o-	
16.	cortic/o-		50.	pariet/o-	
17.	cost/o-		51.	patell/o-	
18.	crani/o-		52.	ped/o-	
19.	diaphys/o-		53.	pelv/o-	
20.	epiphys/o-		54.	perone/o-	
21.	ethm/o-		55.	phalang/o-	
22.	faci/o-		56.	poplite/o-	
23.	femor/o-		57.	pub/o-	
24.	fibul/o-		58.	radi/o-	
25.	front/o-		59.	sacr/o-	
26.	glen/o-		60.	scapul/o-	
27.	humer/o-		61.	skelet/o-	
28.	hy/o-		62.	sphen/o-	
29.	ili/o-		63.	spin/o-	
30.	ischi/o-		64.	stern/o-	
31.	lacrim/o-		65.	styl/o-	
32.	later/o-		66.	synovi/o-	
33.	ligament/o-		67.	tars/o-	
34.	lumb/o-		68.	tempor/o-	

	Combining Form	Medical Meaning		Combining Form	Medical Meaning
69.	thorac/o-	______	73.	uln/o-	______
70.	tibi/o-	______	74.	vertebr/o-	______
71.	trochanter/o-	______	75.	xiph/o-	______
72.	turbin/o-	______	76.	zygomat/o-	______

Combining Forms and Suffixes

Read the definition hint for the medical word you are to build. Look at the combining form that is given. Write the correct suffix on the blank line. Then write the medical word. (Remember: You may need to remove the combining vowel. Always remove the hyphens and slash.) Use the Answer Key at the end of the book to check your answers. The first one has been done for you.

SUFFIX LIST

-al (pertaining to)	-clast (cell that breaks down substances)	-cyte (cell)	-ic (pertaining to)
-ar (pertaining to)		-eal (pertaining to)	-ous (pertaining to)

	Definition Hint	Combining Form	Suffix	Write the Medical Word
1.	Pertaining to the cranium	crani/o-	-al	cranial
2.	Pertaining to the thorax	thorac/o-	______	______
3.	Pertaining to the ribs	cost/o-	______	______
4.	Pertaining to the mandible	mandibul/o-	______	______
5.	Pertaining to the bones of the ankle joint	tars/o-	______	______
6.	A bone cell	oste/o-	______	______
7.	Pertaining to a ligament	ligament/o-	______	______
8.	Pertaining to the pelvis	pelv/o-	______	______
9.	Pertaining to a finger or toe	phalang/o-	______	______
10.	Pertaining to bone	osse/o-	______	______
11.	Pertaining to the heel bone	calcane/o-	______	______
12.	Breaks down old bone	oste/o-	______	______
13.	Pertaining to the vertebra	vertebr/o-	______	______
14.	Pertaining to the lower back	lumb/o-	______	______

Symptoms, Signs, and Diseases

Diseases of the Bones and Cartilage

Word or Phrase	Word Part and Definition	Description
avascular necrosis	**avascular** (aa-VAS-kyoo-lar) **a-** *away from, without* **vascul/o-** *blood vessel* **-ar** *pertaining to* **necrosis** (neh-KROH-sis) **necr/o-** *death* **-osis** *condition; abnormal condition; process*	Death of cells in the epiphysis of a long bone, often the femur. Caused by an injury, fracture, or dislocation that damages nearby blood vessels or by a blood clot that interrupts the blood supply to the bone. Treatment: Surgery (osteotomy) to remove the dead bone, then a bone graft. For large areas of avascular necrosis, a joint replacement is done.
bone tumor	**osteoma** (AWS-tee-OH-mah) **oste/o-** *bone* **-oma** *tumor, mass* **osteosarcoma** (AWS-tee-oh-sar-KOH-mah) **oste/o-** *bone* **sarc/o-** *connective tissue* **-oma** *tumor, mass* **osteogenic** (AWS-tee-oh-JEN-ik) **oste/o-** *bone* **gen/o-** *arising from; produced by* **-ic** *pertaining to* **sarcoma** (sar-KOH-mah) **sarc/o-** *connective tissue* **-oma** *tumor, mass* **Ewing** (YOO-ing) Named by James Ewing (1866–1943), an American pathologist. This is an example of an *eponym:* a person from whom something takes its name.	**Osteoma** is a benign tumor of the bone. **Osteosarcoma** is a malignant bone tumor in which osteoblasts, the cells that form new bone, multiply uncontrollably. Also known as **osteogenic sarcoma. Ewing's sarcoma** is a malignant tumor of the bone that occurs mainly in young men. Treatment: Surgical excision of the tumor or amputation of the limb followed by radiation therapy or chemotherapy.
chondroma	**chondroma** (con-DROH-mah) **chondr/o-** *cartilage* **-oma** *tumor, mass*	A benign tumor of the cartilage. Treatment: Excision, if large.
chondromalacia patellae	**chondromalacia** (CON-droh-mah-LAY-shee-ah) **chondr/o-** *cartilage* **malac/o-** *softening* **-ia** *condition, state, thing* **patellae** (pah-TEL-ee)	Abnormal softening of the patella because of thinning and uneven wear. The thigh muscle pulls the patella in a crooked path that wears away the underside of the bone. Treatment: Strengthening of the thigh muscle to straighten its contraction.

Word or Phrase	Word Part and Definition	Description
fracture	**fracture** (FRAK-chur) **fract/o-** *break up* **-ure** *system; result of* **pathologic** (PATH-oh-LAWJ-ik) **path/o-** *disease, suffering* **log/o-** *the study of* **-ic** *pertaining to* **malalignment** (MAL-ah-LINE-ment) **mal-** *bad, inadequate* **align/o-** *arranged in a straight line* **-ment** *action; state*	Broken bone due to an accident, injury, or disease process. Fractures are classified according to the way in which the bone breaks and whether or not the skin is pierced with a bony fragment (see Table 8-1 and Figure 8-21 ■). A fracture that is caused by a disease process such as osteoporosis, bone cancer, or metatases to the bone is known as a **pathologic fracture**. Fractures that are allowed to heal without treatment often show evidence of **malalignment** of the fracture fragments. Treatment: Closed reduction and manipulation to align the fracture pieces, application of a cast. Surgery: Open reduction and internal fixation using wires, pins, screws, or plates. **Figure 8-21 ■ Bone fracture.** This x-ray shows an oblique fracture of the fibula of the lower leg.

Table 8-1 Fracture Names and Descriptions

Fracture Name	Description	Illustration	Word Part and Definition
closed fracture	Any type of fracture in which the bone does not break through the overlying skin		
open fracture	Any type of fracture in which the bone breaks through the overlying skin. Also known as a **compound fracture.**		
nondisplaced fracture **displaced fracture**	Broken bone ends remain in their normal anatomical alignment Broken bone ends are pulled out of their normal anatomical alignment	Nondisplaced fracture Displaced fracture	**nondisplaced** (non-dis-PLAYSD) The prefix *non-* means *not.* The prefix *dis-* means *away from.* **displaced** (dis-PLAYSD)

(continued)

Table 8-1 Fracture Names and Descriptions (*continued*)

Fracture Name	Description	Illustration	Word Part and Definition
Colles' fracture	Distal radius is broken by falling onto an outstretched hand	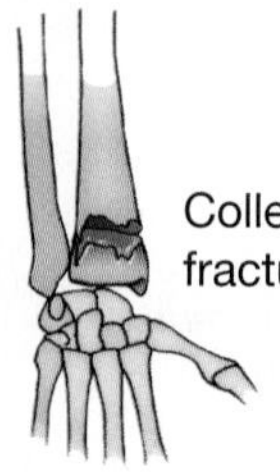	**Colles' fracture** (KOH-leez)
comminuted fracture	Bone is crushed into several pieces	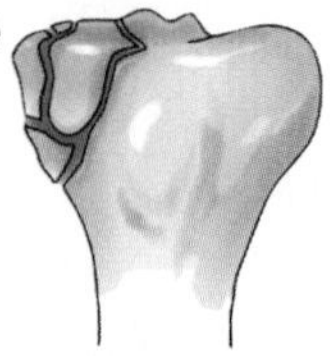	**comminuted** (COM-ih-nyoo-ted) **comminut/o-** *break into minute pieces* **-ed** *pertaining to*
compression fracture	Vertebrae are compressed together after falling onto the buttocks or a vertebra collapses in on itself because of disease	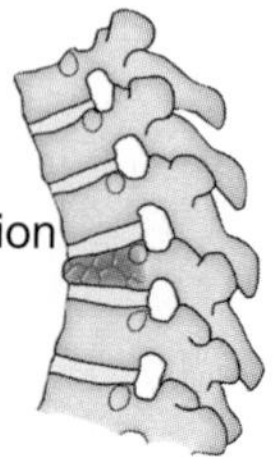	**compression** (com-PRESH-un) **compress/o-** *press together* **-ion** *action; condition*
depressed fracture	Cranium is fractured inward towards the brain	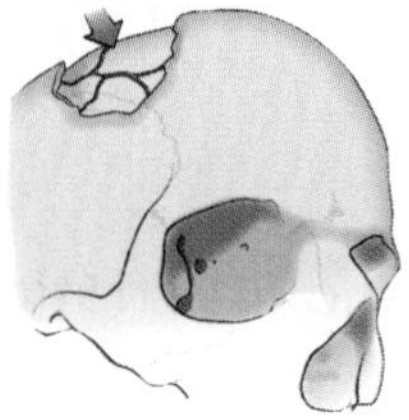	**depressed** (dee-PRESD) **depress/o-** *press down* **-ed** *pertaining to*
greenstick fracture	Bone is broken on only one side. Occurs most often in children as part of the bone is still composed of flexible cartilage.	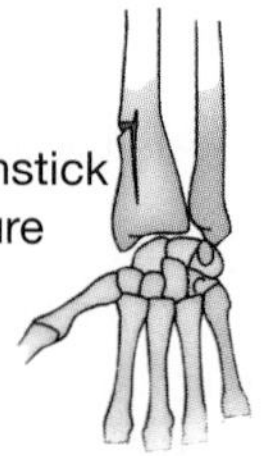	*Greenstick* refers to new branches on a tree that bend rather than break.

Table 8-1 Fracture Names and Descriptions (*continued*)

Fracture Name	Description	Illustration	Word Part and Definition
hairline fracture	Very thin break line with the bone pieces still together. May be difficult to detect on an x-ray.	Hairline fracture	
oblique fracture	Bone is broken on an oblique angle	Oblique fracture	**oblique** (awb-LEEK) *Oblique* is derived from a Latin word meaning *slanting.*
spiral fracture	Bone is broken in a spiral because of a twisting force	Spiral fracture	**spiral** (SPY-ral) **spir/o-** *a coil* **-al** *pertaining to*
transverse fracture	Bone is broken in a transverse plane perpendicular to its long axis	Transverse fracture	**transverse** (trans-VERS) **trans-** *across, through* **-verse** *to travel; to turn*

Word or Phrase	Word Part and Definition	Description
osteomalacia	**osteomalacia** (AWS-tee-oh-mah-LAY-shee-ah) oste/o- *bone* malac/o- *softening* -ia *condition, state, thing*	Abnormal softening of the bones due to a deficiency of vitamin D or inadequate exposure to the sun. In children, this causes rickets with bone pain, fractures, and muscle weakness. Treatment: Vitamin D supplements, sun exposure.
osteomyelitis	**osteomyelitis** (AWS-tee-oh-my-LIE-tis) oste/o- *bone* myel/o- *bone marrow; spinal cord; myelin* -itis *inflammation of* Some word parts have more than one definition. The best definition of *osteomyelitis* is *inflammation of the bone and bone marrow.*	Infection in the bone and the bone marrow. Bacteria enter the bone following an open fracture, crush injury, or surgical procedure. Treatment: Antibiotic drugs.
osteoporosis	**osteoporosis** (AWS-tee-oh-poh-ROH-sis) oste/o- *bone* por/o- *small openings; pores* -osis *condition; abnormal condition; process* **osteoporotic** (AWS-tee-oh-poh-RAWT-ik) oste/o- *bone* por/o- *small openings; pores* -tic *pertaining to* **demineralization** (dee-MIN-er-al-ih-ZAY-shun) de- *reversal of; without* mineral/o- *mineral; electrolyte* -ization *process of making, creating, or inserting*	Abnormal thinning of the bone structure. When bone breakdown exceeds new bone formation, the minerals calcium and phosphorus are lost, and the bone becomes porous with many small areas of **demineralization** (see Figure 8-22 ■). This can result in a compression fracture as a vertebra collapses in on itself. The spinal column decreases in length, the patient becomes shorter, and an abnormal curvature (dowager's hump) forms in the upper back and shoulders. Osteoporosis can also cause spontaneous fractures of the hip or femur. Osteoporosis occurs in postmenopausal women and elderly men. Estradiol stimulates bone formation, and loss of estradiol begins the development of osteoporosis. A lack of dietary calcium and a lack of exercise contribute to the process. Treatment: Drugs that decrease the rate of bone resorption or drugs that activate estradiol receptors, as well as calcium supplements. 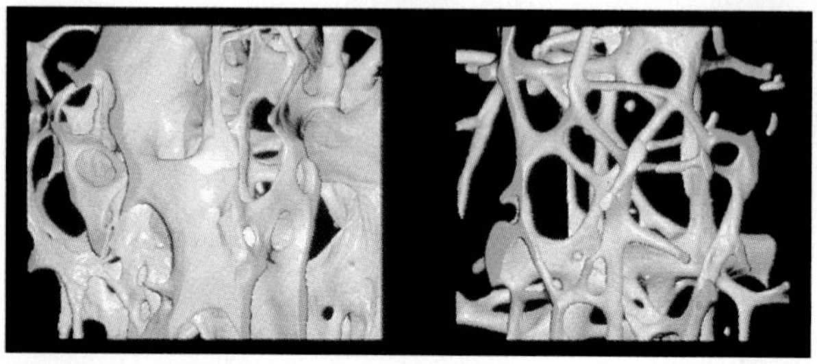 **Figure 8-22 ■ Normal bone versus osteoporotic bone.** The bone on the left shows normal mineralization and density. The bone on the right shows demineralization, large holes, and loss of density. This bone would be extremely prone to fracture.

Diseases of the Vertebrae

Word or Phrase	Word Part and Definition	Description
ankylosing spondylitis	**ankylosing** (ANG-kih-LOH-sing) ankyl/o- *fused together, stiff* -osing *a condition of doing* **spondylitis** (SPAWN-dih-LY-tis) spondyl/o- *vertebra* -itis *inflammation of* **inflammation** (IN-flah-MAY-shun) inflammat/o- *redness and warmth* -ion *action; condition*	Chronic **inflammation** of the vertebrae that leads to fibrosis, restriction of movement of the vertebrae, and stiffening of the spine. Treatment: Nonsteroidal anti-inflammatory drugs.
kyphosis	**kyphosis** (ky-FOH-sis) kyph/o- *bent; humpbacked* -osis *condition; abnormal condition; process* **kyphotic** (ky-FAWT-ik) kyph/o- *bent; humpbacked* -tic *pertaining to* **kyphoscoliosis** (KY-foh-SKOH-lee-OH-sis) kyph/o- *bent; humpbacked* scoli/o- *curved, crooked* -osis *condition; abnormal condition; process*	Abnormal, excessive, posterior curvature of the thoracic spine. Also known as **humpback** or **hunchback.** The back is said to have a **kyphotic** curvature. **Kyphoscoliosis** is a complex abnormal curvature with components of both kyphosis and scoliosis. Treatment: Back brace or surgery to fuse and straighten the spine.
lordosis	**lordosis** (lor-DOH-sis) lord/o- *swayback* -osis *condition; abnormal condition; process* **lordotic** (lor-DAWT-ik) lord/o- *swayback* -tic *pertaining to*	Abnormal, excessive, anterior curvature of the lumbar spine. Also known as **swayback.** The back is said to have a **lordotic** curvature. Treatment: Back brace or surgery to fuse and straighten the spine.

Word or Phrase	Word Part and Definition	Description
scoliosis	**scoliosis** (SKOH-lee-OH-sis) **scoli/o-** *curved, crooked* **-osis** *condition; abnormal condition; process* **scoliotic** (SKOH-lee-AWT-ik) **scoli/o-** *curved, crooked* **-tic** *pertaining to* **dextroscoliosis** (DEKS-troh-SKOH-lee-OH-sis) **dextr/o-** *right* **scoli/o-** *curved, crooked* **-osis** *condition; abnormal condition; process* **levoscoliosis** (LEE-voh-SKOH-lee-OH-sis) **lev/o-** *left* **scoli/o-** *curved, crooked* **-osis** *condition; abnormal condition; process*	Abnormal, excessive, C-shaped or S-shaped lateral curvature of the spine (see Figure 8-23 ■). The back is said to have a **scoliotic** curvature. A **dextroscoliosis** curves to the patient's right, while a **levoscoliosis** curves to the patient's left. Scoliosis can be congenital but most often the cause is unknown. It develops during childhood and may continue to progress during adolescence. It impairs movement, posture, and breathing. X-rays are used to determine the number of degrees in the curvature. Treatment: Back brace or surgery to fuse and straighten the spine. **Figure 8-23 ■ Scoliosis.** This patient with moderate scoliosis of the spine to the right shows the characteristic tilt to the shoulders and hips and a difference in arm lengths. **Connections** **Public Health.** Scoliosis screening is routinely done by a school nurse for all elementary school children. The child's back is observed while standing and then while bending over. Some cases of scoliosis become more apparent with bending over as one side of the back becomes noticeably higher and one scapula sticks out.
spondylolisthesis	**spondylolisthesis** (SPAWN-dih-LOH-lis-THEE-sis) **spondyl/o-** *vertebra* **-olisthesis** *abnormal condition and process of slipping*	Degenerative condition of the spine in which one vertebra moves anteriorly over another vertebra and slips out of proper alignment due to degeneration of the intervertebral disk. It can occur because of a sports injury or compression fracture of the vertebra from osteoporosis. Treatment: Back brace or surgery to relieve a pinched spinal nerve.

Diseases of the Joints and Ligaments

Word or Phrase	Word Part and Definition	Description
arthralgia	**arthralgia** (ar-THRAL-jee-ah) arthr/o- *joint* alg/o- *pain* -ia *condition, state, thing*	Pain in the joint from injury, inflammation, or infection from various causes. Treatment: Correct the underlying cause.
arthropathy	**arthropathy** (ar-THRAWP-ah-thee) arthr/o- *joint* -pathy *disease, suffering*	Disease of a joint from any cause. Treatment: Correct the underlying cause.
dislocation	**dislocation** (DIS-loh-KAY-shun) dis- *away from* locat/o- *a place* -ion *action; condition* **congenital** (con-JEN-ih-tal) congenit/o- *present at birth* -al *pertaining to*	Displacement of the end of a bone from its normal position within a joint. Usually caused by injury or trauma. **Congenital dislocation of the hip (CDH)** is present at birth because the acetabulum is poorly formed or the ligaments are loose. Treatment: Manipulate and return the bone to its normal position. Congenital dislocation of the hip is treated with a splint or with surgery to revise the acetabulum or ligaments.
gout	**gout** (GOWT) *Gout* is derived from a Latin word meaning *drop.* It was believed that gout was a harmful influence that went drop by drop into the joints. **tophus** (TOH-fus) **tophi** (TOH-fye) *Tophus* is a Latin singular masculine noun meaning *mineral deposit found in water.* Form the plural by changing *-us* to *-i.* **gouty** (GOW-tee) **arthritis** (ar-THRY-tis) arthr/o- *joint* -itis *inflammation of*	Metabolic disorder that occurs most often in men. There are excessive levels of uric acid in the blood. Acute attacks cause sudden, severe pain as uric acid moves from the blood into the soft tissues and forms masses of crystals with soft tissue swellings known as **tophi.** Historically, patients with gout have been pictured with throbbing big toes, although tophi can also form in the hands. Tophi in the joints is known as **gouty arthritis.** Treatment: Avoid foods that increase uric acid levels. Drugs that decrease uric acid levels.
hemarthrosis	**hemarthrosis** (HEE-mar-THROH-sis) hem/o- *blood* arthr/o- *joint* -osis *condition; abnormal condition; process*	Blood in the joint cavity from blunt trauma or a penetrating wound. It also occurs spontaneously in hemophiliac patients. Treatment: Temporary immobilization of the joint, aspiration of blood, corticosteroid drugs. Surgery: Arthroscopy.
Lyme disease	**Lyme** (LIME) Lyme disease was named in 1977 when arthritis was observed in a group of children who lived in Lyme, Connecticut.	Arthritis caused by a bacterium in the bite of an infected deer tick. There is an erythematous rash that expands outward for several weeks (bull's-eye rash) but is not itchy and joint pain, fever, chills, and fatigue. If untreated, Lyme disease can cause severe fatigue and affect the nervous system (numbness, severe headache) and the heart. Treatment: Antibiotic drugs.

Word or Phrase	Word Part and Definition	Description
osteoarthritis	**osteoarthritis** (AWS-tee-oh-ar-THRY-tis) oste/o- *bone* arthr/o- *joint* -itis *inflammation of* **crepitus** (KREP-ih-tus) *Crepitus* is a Latin word meaning a *rattle.* **osteophyte** (AWS-tee-oh-fite) oste/o- *bone* -phyte *growth* **degenerative** (dee-JEN-er-ah-tiv) de- *reversal of; without* gener/o- *production; creation* -ative *pertaining to*	Chronic inflammatory disease of the joints, particularly the large weight-bearing joints of the knees and hips, and joints that move repeatedly like the shoulders, neck, and hands. Osteoarthritis usually begins in middle age, but can develop sooner in a joint that has been overused or subject to trauma. Early symptoms include joint pain and stiffness. The inflammation is caused by constant wear and tear and is accelerated when the patient is overweight. The normally smooth cartilage becomes roughened and then wears away in spots (see Figure 8-24 ■). The bone ends rub against each other, causing additional inflammation and a grinding sound known as **crepitus.** New bone growth around the edges of the inflammation sometimes develops into a sharp bone spur or **osteophyte** that causes pain. Also known as **degenerative joint disease (DJD).** **Figure 8-24 ■ Osteoarthritis.** This patient's knee shows loss of the articular cartilage and narrowing of the joint space between the bone ends that is characteristic of degenerative joint disease.
rheumatoid arthritis	**rheumatoid** (ROO-mah-toyd) rheumat/o- *watery discharge* -oid *resembling* There is a collection of fluid in the joints. **arthritis** (ar-THRY-tis) arthr/o- *joint* -itis *inflammation of*	Acute and chronic inflammatory disease of connective tissues, particularly of the joints. This is an autoimmune disease in which the patient's own antibodies attack cartilage and connective tissues. Patients are usually young to middle-aged females. There is redness and swelling of the joints, most often of the hands and feet. The joint cartilage is slowly destroyed by inflammation. The symptoms flare and subside over time with progressive deformity of the joints (see Figure 8-25 ■). Treatment: Corticosteroid drugs. Surgery: Joint replacement surgery. 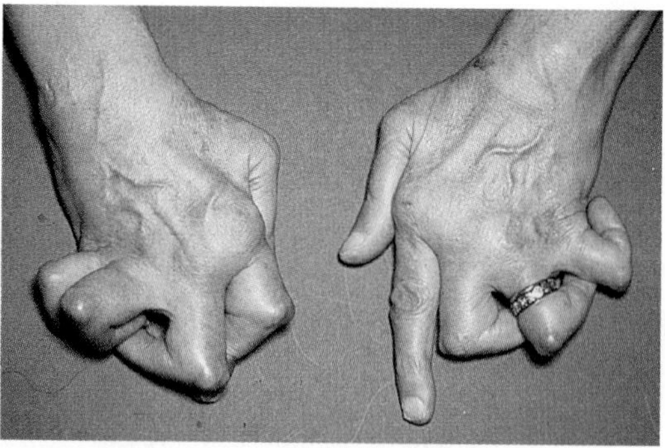 **Figure 8-25 ■ Rheumatoid arthritis.** This patient shows the severe joint deformities of the hand that are characteristic of rheumatoid arthritis.

Word or Phrase	Word Part and Definition	Description
sprain	**sprain** (SPRAYN)	Overstretching or tearing of a ligament. Treatment: Rest or surgery to repair the ligament.
torn meniscus	**meniscus** (meh-NIS-kus)	Tear of the cartilage pad of the knee because of an injury. Treatment: Arthroscopy and repair.
Diseases of the Bony Thorax		
pectus excavatum	**pectus excavatum** (PEK-tus EKS-kah-VAH-tum) *Pectus* is a Latin word meaning *sternum (breast bone). Excavatum* is derived from a Latin word meaning *to make a hole or cavity.*	Congenital deformity of the bony thorax in which the sternum, particularly the xiphoid process, is bent inward, creating a hollow depression in the anterior chest. Treatment: Surgery, if severe.
Diseases of the Bones of the Legs and Feet		
genu varum	**genu varum** (JEE-noo VAR-um) *Genu* is a Latin word meaning *knee. Varum* is derived from a Latin word meaning *bent toward the midline.*	Congenital deformity in which, beginning at the knees, the lower legs are bent toward the midline. Also known as **bowleg.** Treatment: Surgical correction, if severe.
genu valgum	**genu valgum** (JEE-noo VAL-gum) *Valgum* is derived from a Latin word meaning *bent away from the midline.*	Congenital deformity in which, beginning at the knees, the lower legs are bent outward. Also known as **knock-knee.** Treatment: Surgical correction, if severe.
hallux valgus	**hallux valgus** (HAL-uks VAL-gus) *Hallux* is a Latin word meaning *great toe. Valgus* is a Latin word meaning *bent away from the midline.* **bunion** (BUN-yun) *Bunion* is derived from a Greek word meaning *turnip* (referring to its hard consistency).	Deformity in which the great toe is angled laterally toward the other toes (see Figure 8-26■). Often a **bunion** develops at the base of the great toe with swelling and inflammation. This is a common deformity seen in women who wear pointy-toed shoes. Treatment: Wear wide-toed shoes. Bunionectomy. 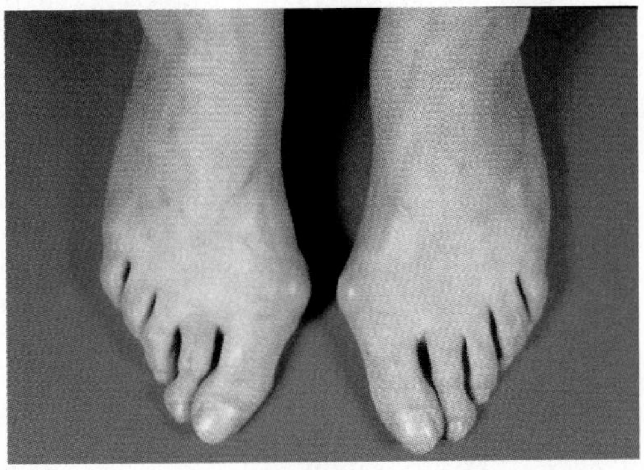 **Figure 8-26 ■ Bilateral hallus valgus.** Notice the reddened, enlarged bunions on the medial side of each foot at the bases of the great toes.

Word or Phrase	Word Part and Definition	Description
talipes equinovarus	**talipes equinovarus** (TAY-lih-peez ee-KWY-noh-VAR-us) *Talipes* is derived from two Latin words meaning *ankle* and *foot*. *Equin/o-* means *horse*. In a horse, the hooves are the equivalent of toenails. *Varus* is a Latin word meaning *bent toward the midline*.	Congenital deformity of one or both feet in which the foot is pulled downwards and laterally to the side. The heel never rests on the ground. This is the most common type of clubfoot. Clubfoot also occurs with many other abnormal positions of the foot (see Figure 8-27 ■). Treatment: Casts applied to progressively straighten the foot. Surgical correction for severe cases.

Figure 8-27 ■ Bilateral clubfeet.
This infant was born with bilateral clubfeet. Although all newborns' feet are rotated medially due to the confining environment of the uterus, the feet can be moved into an anatomically correct position. In talipes equinovarus, the feet cannot be positioned correctly and do not correct themselves over time.

Diagnostic Procedures

Laboratory Tests

Word or Phrase	Word Part and Definition	Description
rheumatoid factor		Blood test that is positive in patients with rheumatoid arthritis.
uric acid	**uric acid** (YOO-rik AS-id)	Blood test that has elevated levels in patients with gout and gouty arthritis.

Radiology and Nuclear Medicine Procedures

Word or Phrase	Word Part and Definition	Description
arthrography	**arthrography** (ar-THRAWG-rah-fee) **arthr/o-** *joint* **-graphy** *process of recording* **arthrogram** (AR-throh-gram) **arthr/o-** *joint* **-gram** *a record or picture*	Radiologic procedure that uses a radiopaque contrast dye that is injected into a joint. It coats and outlines the bone ends and joint capsule. An x-ray or CT scan is then taken. MRI arthrography uses a strong magnetic field to align protons in the atoms of the patient's body. The protons emit signals to form a series of thin, successive slices of the joint. A contrast dye can also be injected into the joint. The x-ray, CT, or MRI image is known as an **arthrogram.**

Word or Phrase	Word Part and Definition	Description
bone density tests	**DEXA scan** (DEK-sah) *DEXA* stands for *dual-energy x-ray absorptiometry. Dual energy* refers to the use of the two different x-ray beams. **tomography** (toh-MAWG-rah-fee) **tom/o-** *a cut, slice, or layer* **-graphy** *process of recording* **densitometry** (DEN-sih-TAWM-eh-tree) **densit/o-** *density* **-metry** *process of measuring*	Radiologic procedure that measures the bone mineral density (BMD) to determine if demineralization from osteoporosis has occurred. The heel or wrist bone can be tested, but the hip and spine bones give more accurate results. There are two types of bone density tests: **DEXA (or DXA) scan** and **quantitative computerized tomography (QCT).** These tests are both known as **bone densitometry.** A DEXA scan uses two x-ray beams with different energy levels to create a two-dimensional image. This scan can detect as little as a 1% loss of bone. Quantitative computerized tomography uses an x-ray beam and a CT scanner to create a three-dimensional image. QCT is able to take separate measurements for cancellous and cortical bone. Cancellous bone is the first to be affected by osteoporosis and the first to respond to therapy. **Did You Know?** Standard x-ray procedures are not used to measure bone density, because you must lose at least 30% of your bone mass before the loss can be detected.
bone scintigraphy	**scintigraphy** (sin-TIG-rah-fee) **scint/i-** *point of light* **-graphy** *process of recording* **scintigram** (SIN-tih-gram) **scint/i-** *point of light* **-gram** *a record or picture*	Nuclear medicine procedure in which phosphate compounds (DPD or MDP) are tagged with the radioactive tracer technetium-99m. They are injected intravenously and taken up into the bone. A gamma scintillation camera detects gamma rays from the radioactive tracer. Areas of increased uptake ("hot spots") indicate increased bone metabolism due to arthritis, fracture, osteomyelitis, cancerous tumors of the bone, or areas of bony metastasis. The nuclear image is known as a **scintigram.**
x-ray	**x-ray** (EKS-ray)	Radiologic procedure that uses x-rays to diagnose bony abnormalities of any part of the body. X-rays are the primary means for diagnosing fractures, dislocations, bone tumors, and so forth.

Medical and Surgical Procedures

Medical Procedures

Word or Phrase	Word Part and Definition	Description
cast	**cast** (KAST)	Medical procedure in which a cast of plaster or fiberglass is applied around a fractured bone and adjacent areas to immobilize the fracture in a fixed position to facilitate healing (see Figure 8-28 ■ and 8-29 ■). For fractures of the leg, the physician may order the patient to be non-weight bearing (putting no weight on the affected leg), toe touch (partial weight bearing), or full weight bearing (with a walking cast). Patients with leg casts are instructed in the use of crutches for ambulation.

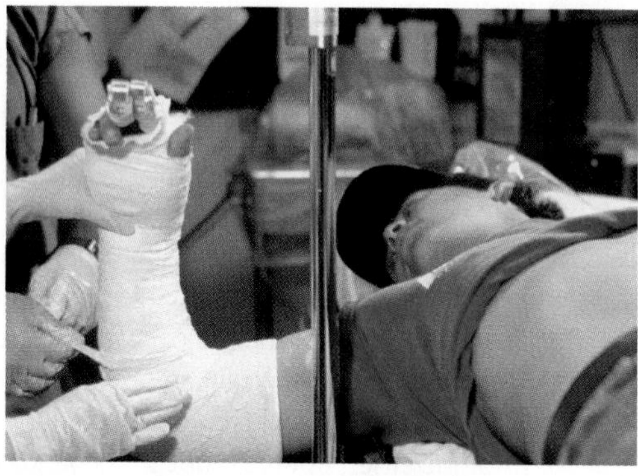

Figure 8-28 ■ Application of a cast.
This patient sustained several fractures during a dirt-bike accident. His two fractured fingers were placed in an aluminum buddy splint to immobilize them, while his fractured wrist (Colles' fracture) was placed in a long-arm cast.

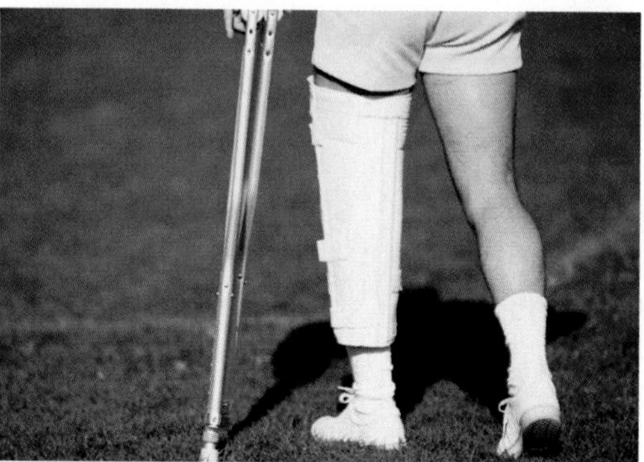

Figure 8-29 ■ Cast and crutches.
A leg cylinder cast is used to treat fractures of the knee or immobilize the knee after extensive surgery.

Word or Phrase	Word Part and Definition	Description
closed reduction	**reduction** (ree-DUK-shun) **reduct/o-** *to bring back; decrease* **-ion** *action; condition*	Medical procedure in which manual manipulation of a displaced fracture is performed so that the bone ends go back into normal alignment without the need for surgery.
cortisone injection	**cortisone** (KOR-tih-zohn) **intra-articular** (IN-trah-ar-TIK-yoo-lar) **intra-** *within* **articul/o-** *joint* **-ar** *pertaining to* **injection** (in-JEK-shun) **inject/o-** *insert or put in* **-ion** *action; condition*	Medical procedure in which the drug cortisone is given by **intra-articular injection** into one particular joint with degenerative joint disease to decrease inflammation and pain.

Word or Phrase	Word Part and Definition	Description
extracorporeal shock wave therapy (ESWT)	**extracorporeal** (EKS-trah-kor-POH-ree-al) **extra-** *outside of* **corpor/o-** *body* **-eal** *pertaining to*	Medical procedure in which sound waves originating outside the body (extracorporeal) are used to break up bony spurs and treat other minor but painful skeletal problems of the foot.
goniometry	**goniometry** (GOH-nee-AWM-eh-tree) **goni/o-** *angle* **-metry** *process of measuring* **goniometer** (GOH-nee-AWM-eh-ter) **goni/o-** *angle* **-meter** *instrument used to measure*	Medical procedure in which a protractor-like device (**goniometer**) is used to measure the angle and degrees of range of movement (ROM) of a joint.
orthosis	**orthosis** (or-THOH-sis) **orth/o-** *straight* **-osis** *condition; abnormal condition; process*	Orthopedic device like a brace, splint, or collar that is used to immobilize or correct an orthopedic problem. These are often custom made to fit the patient's specific measurements.
physical therapy	**physical** (FIZ-ih-kal) **physic/o-** *body* **-al** *pertaining to* **therapy** (THAIR-ah-pee) The combining form *therap/o-* means *treatment.*	Medical procedure that uses active or passive exercises to improve a patient's range of motion, joint mobility, and balance while walking.
prosthesis	**prosthesis** (praws-THEE-sis) *Prosthesis* is a Greek word meaning *an adding on.* **prosthetic** (praws-THET-ik) **prosthet/o-** *artificial part* **-ic** *pertaining to*	Orthopedic device like an artificial leg that is used by a patient who has had an amputation of a limb (see Figure 8-30 ■). Also known as a **prosthetic device.** **Figure 8-30 ■ Leg prosthesis.** This prosthetist is using computer-aided design to create an artificial leg for a patient. It is built according to the patient's height and weight (to match the unamputated leg) and according to where the leg was amputated.

Word or Phrase	Word Part and Definition	Description
traction	**traction** (TRAK-shun) **tract/o-** *pulling* **-ion** *action; condition*	Medical procedure that uses weights to pull the bone ends of a fracture into correct alignment. Skin traction uses elastic wraps, straps, halters, or skin adhesives connected to a pulley and weights. Skeletal traction uses pins, wires, or tongs inserted into the bone during surgery. Halo traction uses pins inserted into the cranium and attached to a circular metal frame that forms a halo around the patient's head. Bars connect the halo to a rigid vest that immobilizes the chest and back while exerting upward traction on the head to straighten a fracture of the spine.

Surgical Procedures

Word or Phrase	Word Part and Definition	Description
amputation	**amputation** (AM-pyoo-TAY-shun) **amputat/o-** *to cut off* **-ion** *action; condition* **amputee** (AM-pyoo-tee) **amput/o-** *to cut off* **-ee** *person who is the object of an action*	Surgical procedure to remove all or part of an extremity because of trauma or circulatory disease. A muscle flap is wrapped over the end of the bone to provide a cushion and support an artificial limb (prosthesis). A below-the-knee amputation (BKA) is performed at the level of the tibia and fibula. An above-the-knee amputation (AKA) is performed at the level of the femur. A patient who has had an amputation is known as an **amputee.**
arthrocentesis	**arthrocentesis** (AR-throh-sen-TEE-sis) **arthr/o-** *joint* **-centesis** *procedure to puncture*	Surgical procedure to remove an accumulation of fluid in a joint by using a needle or trocar inserted into the joint space.
arthrodesis	**arthrodesis** (AR-throh-DEE-sis) **arthr/o-** *joint* **-desis** *procedure to fuse together*	Surgical procedure to fuse the bones in a degenerated, unstable joint.
arthroscopy	**arthroscopy** (ar-THRAWS-koh-pee) **arthr/o-** *joint* **-scopy** *process of using an instrument to examine* **arthroscope** (AR-throh-skohp) **arthr/o-** *joint* **-scope** *instrument used to examine* **arthroscopic** (AR-throh-SKAW-pik) **arthr/o-** *joint* **scop/o-** *examine with an instrument* **-ic** *pertaining to*	Surgical procedure that uses an **arthroscope** inserted into the joint to visualize the inside of the joint and its structures (see Figure 8-31■). Various instruments can be inserted through the arthroscope to scrape or cut damaged cartilage and smooth sharp bone edges. **Figure 8-31 ■ Arthroscopic surgery.** The skin around the elbow was scrubbed with the orange antiseptic solution Betadine prior to surgery. The arthroscope has been inserted into the elbow joint through a surgically created portal (opening in the skin). Other portals are used to insert instruments or remove fluid. A fiberoptic light and a magnifying lens on the arthroscope give a clear picture of the inside of the joint, and this is also seen enlarged on a TV monitor in the operating room.

Word or Phrase	Word Part and Definition	Description
bone graft	**graft** (GRAFT) **autograft** (AW-toh-graft) **auto-** *self* **-graft** *tissue for implant or transplant* **allograft** (AL-oh-graft) **all/o-** *other; strange* **-graft** *tissue for implant or transplant*	Surgical procedure that uses whole bone or bone chips to repair fractures with extensive bone loss or defects due to bone cancer. Bone taken from the patient's own body is known as an **autograft.** Frozen or freeze-dried bone taken from a cadaver is known as an **allograft.**
cartilage transplantation	**transplantation** (TRANS-plan-TAY-shun) **transplant/o-** *move something to another place* **-ation** *a process; being or having*	Surgical procedure that is an alternative to a total knee replacement. Used to treat middle-aged adults (as opposed to elderly) with degenerative joint disease of the knee who have an active lifestyle. **Did You Know?** Active people walk 1 to 3 million steps each year! The average person walks 4 miles each day. Wear and tear on the knee joints can result in the need for a cartilage transplant or a total knee replacement.
bunionectomy	**bunionectomy** (BUN-yun-EK-toh-mee) **bunion/o-** *bunion* **-ectomy** *surgical excision*	Surgical procedure to remove the prominent part of a metatarsal bone that is causing the bunion.
external fixation	**external** (eks-TER-nal) **extern/o-** *outside* **-al** *pertaining to* **fixation** (fik-SAY-shun) **fixat/o-** *to make stable or still* **-ion** *action; condition*	Surgical procedure used to treat a complicated fracture. An external fixator orthopedic device has metal pins that are inserted in the bone on either side of the fracture and connected to a metal frame. This immobilizes the fracture. To lengthen a congenitally short leg, the device has screws that are turned each day to pull the bone and lengthen it.

Word or Phrase	Word Part and Definition	Description
joint replacement surgery	**arthroplasty** (AR-throh-PLAS-tee) **arthr/o-** *joint* **-plasty** *process of reshaping by surgery*	Surgical procedure to replace a joint that has been destroyed by inflammation. A prosthesis is inserted in its place (see Figure 8-32 ■). A prosthesis is a metal or plastic device that takes the place of part of the bones in a joint. This surgery is done on hips (**total hip replacement [THR]**), knees, shoulders, and even on the small joints of the fingers. For a total hip replacement, the head of the femur is sawn off. The stem (long metal projection) of the prosthesis is hammered into the femur to achieve a tight fit. The head (ball) of the prosthesis is selected to match the size of the patient's acetabulum. The cup of the prosthesis is used to replace the acetabulum, and the ball is inserted into the cup. Also known as an **arthroplasty.**

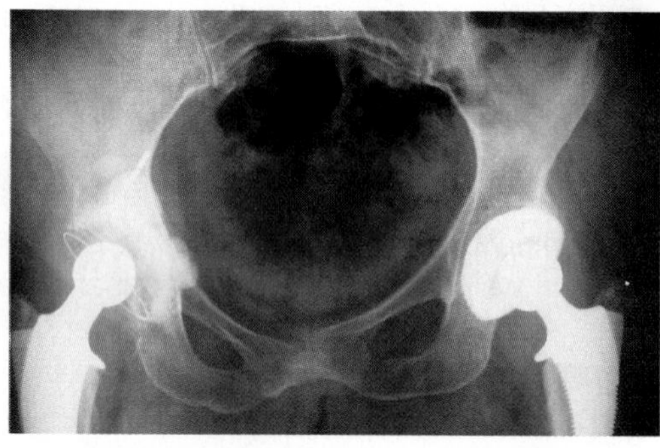

Figure 8-32 ■ Hip prostheses.

This patient has had total hip replacement surgery at two different times and received a different style of hip prosthesis each time. The metal of a prosthesis makes it stand out clearly on an x-ray.

Word or Phrase	Word Part and Definition	Description
open reduction and internal fixation (ORIF)	**reduction** (ree-DUK-shun) **reduct/o-** *to bring back;* decrease **-ion** *action; condition*	Surgical procedure to treat a complicated fracture. An incision is made at the fracture site, the fracture is reduced (realigned), and an internal fixation procedure is done using screws, nails, or plates to hold the fracture fragments in correct anatomical alignment (see Figure 8-33 ■).

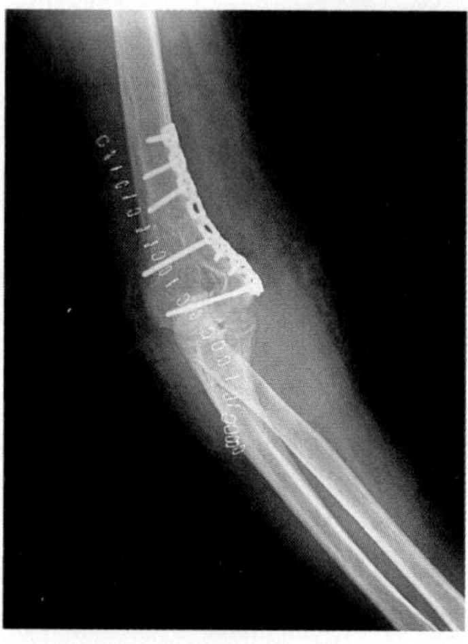

Figure 8-33 ■ Orthopedic plate and screws.

This fracture of the humerus was surgically repaired with an open reduction and internal fixation using a metal plate and screws to stabilize the bone fragments.

Did You Know?

osteotome (AWS-tee-oh-tohm)
oste/o- *bone*
-tome *instrument used to cut; an area with distinct edges*

rongeur (rawn-ZHER)
Rongeur is a French word meaning *to gnaw.*

Orthopedic surgery is not unlike carpentry. The surgical instruments commonly used are hammers, nails, screws, metal plates, chisels, mallets, gouges, and saws. An **osteotome** is used to cut bone. A **rongeur** is a forceps that is used to remove small bone fragments.

Drug Categories

Several different categories of drugs are used to treat the symptoms, signs, and diseases of the skeletal system. The most common drugs in each category are listed.

Category	Word Part and Definition	Description	Example
analgesic drugs	**analgesic** (AN-al-JEE-zik) **an-** *without, not* **alges/o-** *sensation of pain* **-ic** *pertaining to*	Over-the-counter drug aspirin and nonaspirin drugs used to suppress inflammation and decrease pain. Used to treat minor injuries, sprains, and osteoarthritis.	Bayer aspirin, Ecotrin, Tylenol
chemotherapy drugs	**chemotherapy** (KEE-moh-THAIR-ah-pee) **chem/o-** *chemical, drug* **-therapy** *treatment*	Kill rapidly dividing cancer cells in the bones.	Adriamycin, VePesid
corticosteroid drugs	**corticosteroid** (KOR-tih-koh-STAIR-oyd) **cortic/o-** *cortex (outer region)* **-steroid-** *steroid* **intra-articular** (IN-trah-ar-TIK-yoo-lar) **intra-** *within* **articul/o-** *joint* **-ar** *pertaining to*	Suppress inflammation. Given orally to treat osteoarthritis and rheumatoid arthritis. Also given by **intra-articular** injection into the joint.	hydrocortisone, prednisone Depo-Medrol (injection)
nonsteroidal anti-inflammatory drugs (NSAIDs)	**nonsteroidal** (non-stair-OY-dal) **non-** *not* **steroid/o** *steroid* **-al** *pertaining to* **anti-inflammatory** (AN-tee-in-FLAM-ah-TOR-ee) **anti-** *against* **inflammat/o-** *redness and warmth* **-ory** *having the function of* Nonsteroidal anti-inflammatory drugs are not steroids (corticosteroids) but they do resemble them in their drug action.	Suppress inflammation and decrease pain. Used to treat osteoarthritis and orthopedic injuries.	ibuprofen, Motrin, Orudis KT, Relafen, Voltaren
gold compound drugs		Inhibit the body's own immune response that attacks the joints and connective tissue in patients with rheumatoid arthritis. These drugs actually contain gold.	Ridaura, Solganal
bone resorption inhibitor drugs	**resorption** (ree-SORP-shun) **re-** *again and again; backward; unable to* **sorb/o-** *to suck up* **-tion** *a process; being or having* The *b* in *sorb/o-* (absorb) is changed to a *p*.	Inhibit bone from being broken down. Used to treat osteoporosis.	Didronel, Fosamax, Miacalcin

Abbreviations

AKA	above-the-knee amputation
AP	anteroposterior
ASIS	anterior-superior iliac spine
BKA	below-the-knee amputation
BMD	bone mineral density
C1–C7	cervical vertebrae
Ca	calcium
CDH	congenital dislocation of the hip
DEXA, DXA	dual-energy x-ray absorptiometry
DIP	distal interphalangeal (joint)
DJD	degenerative joint disease
ESWT	extracorporeal shock wave therapy
fib	fibula (slang)
Fx	fracture
L1–L5	lumbar vertebrae
LLE	left lower extremity
LUE	left upper extremity
MCP	metacarpophalangeal (joint)
NSAID	nonsteroidal anti-inflammatory drug
OA	osteoarthritis
ortho	orthopedics (slang)
P	phosphorus
PIP	proximal interphalangeal (joint)
PT	physical therapy/therapist
QCT	quantitative computerized tomography
RA	rheumatoid arthritis
RLE	right lower extremity
ROM	range of motion
RUE	right upper extremity
S1	first sacral vertebra
T1–T12	thoracic vertebrae
THR	total hip replacement
tib	tibia (slang)

Word Alert

ABBREVIATIONS

Abbreviations are commonly used in all types of medical documentation; however, they can mean different things to different people and their meaning can be misinterpreted. Always verify the meaning of an abbreviation.

AKA stands for *above-the-knee amputation,* but it can also stand for the English phrase *also known as.*

Ca stands for *calcium,* but it can also stand for *cancer.*

OA stands for *osteoarthritis,* but it can also stand for *Overeaters Anonymous.*

P stands for *phosphorus,* but it can also stand for *para* (the number of births a woman has had).

RA stands for *rheumatoid arthritis,* but it can also stand for *right atrium* (of the heart) or *room air.*

Career Focus

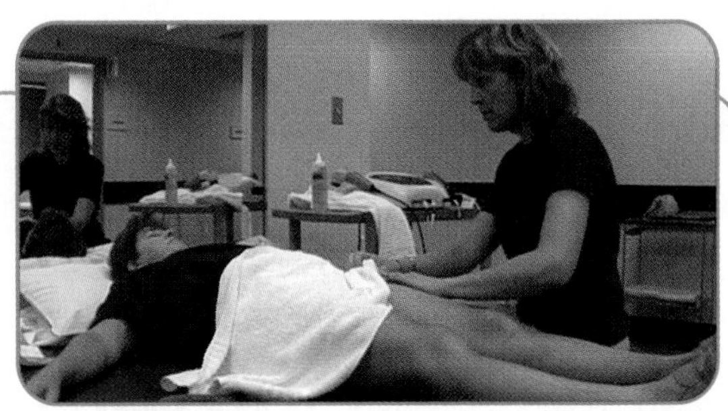

Meet Sara, a physical therapist in an outpatient physical therapy department.

"I always knew I wanted to work in health care. My mom was a nurse. I became aware of other careers in health care, and physical therapy was one of them. It sounded interesting to me, and I enjoyed anatomy. We use a lot of medical terminology on the job. Our documentation here is all narrative and it's all handwritten. That's the way we communicate to physicians and other healthcare providers."

Physical therapists are allied health professionals who develop treatment and rehabilitation plans based on a physician's order. They use strengthening exercises and assistive devices (crutches, canes, wheelchairs, and so forth) to improve patients' balance and mobility. They work in hospitals, clinics, and rehabilitation centers.

Orthopedists (or orthopaedists) are physicians who practice in the medical specialty of orthopedics. They diagnose and treat patients with skeletal and muscular problems. Orthopedists are physicians who have an M.D. (doctor of medicine) degree and have graduated from a school of medicine. When orthopedists perform surgery, they are known as orthopedic surgeons. **Rheumatologists** are physicians who specialize in treating inflammatory and degenerative diseases of the joints. Physicians can take additional training and become board certified in the subspecialty of pediatric orthopedics. Malignancies of the skeletomuscular system are treated medically by an oncologist or surgically by an orthopedic surgeon.

physical (FIZ-ih-kal)
physic/o- *body*
-al *pertaining to*

therapist (THER-ah-pist)
therap/o- *treatment*
-ist *one who specializes in*

orthopedist (OR-thoh-PEE-dist)
orth/o- *straight*
ped/o- *child*
-ist *one who specializes in*

rheumatologist (ROO-mah-TAWL-oh-jist)
rheumat/o- *watery discharge*
log/o- *the study of*
-ist *one who specializes in*

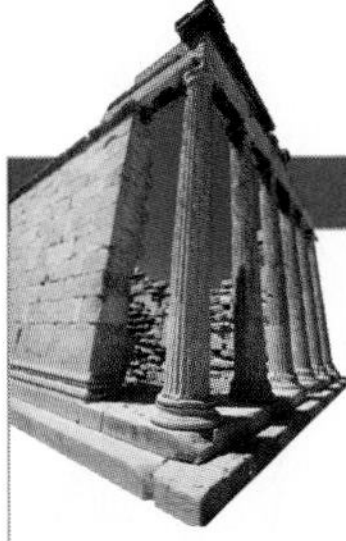

It's Greek To Me!

Did you notice that some skeletal words have two different combining forms? Combining forms from both Greek and Latin languages remain a part of medical language today.

English Word	Greek	Latin	Examples of Medical Words
bone	oste/o-	osse/o-	osteoarthritis, osseous
bent, crooked, stiff	ankyl/o-	scoli/o-	ankylosing, scoliosis
cartilage	chondr/o-	cartilag/o-	costochondral, cartilaginous
fibula	perone/o-	fibul/o-	peroneal, fibular
finger or toe	dactyl/o-	phalang/o-	polydactyly, syndactyly, phalangeal
joint	arthr/o-	articul/o-	arthroscopy, articulation
vertebra	spondyl/o-	vertebr/o-	spondylolisthesis, vertebral

CHAPTER REVIEW EXERCISES

Review all the material in this chapter by completing the review exercises in this section. Use the Answer Key at the end of the book to check your answers.

Anatomy and Physiology

Matching Exercise

Match each numbered word or phrase to its description.

1.	acetabulum	_____ Cell that breaks down bone
2.	calcaneus	_____ Cranial suture that names the plane that divides the body into anterior and posterior parts
3.	carpal bones	_____ Cranial bone that forms the back of the head
4.	coronal	_____ Facial bone that moves up and down when you chew
5.	diaphysis	_____ Pointed tip at the end of the sternum
6.	foramen	_____ Opening where the spinal cord goes through
7.	humerus	_____ Contains the glenoid fossa area of the shoulder joint
8.	ligaments	_____ Fibrous bands that connect bone to bone
9.	mandible	_____ Bone of the upper arm
10.	medial malleolus	_____ Lower arm bone that is on the same side as the thumb
11.	occipital	_____ The bones of the wrist
12.	osteoclast	_____ Another name for a finger
13.	radius	_____ Part of the hip bone where the head of the femur rests
14.	ray	_____ Bony projection on the distal tibial bone
15.	scapula	_____ The biggest of the ankle bones
16.	symphysis	_____ Slightly moveable joint that joins the two pubic bones
17.	vertebral foramen	_____ Shaft of a long bone
18.	xiphoid process	_____ Opening in a bone

Circle Exercise

Circle the correct word from the choices given.

1. The bone of the upper arm is the (**acetabulum, fibula, humerus**).
2. Replacing cartilage with hard bone is the process of (**articulation, ossification, resorption**).
3. The hip bone that has a large crest on it is the (**ilium, intervertebral disk, ischium**).
4. Mature bone cells are known as (**osteoblasts, osteoclasts, osteocytes**).
5. The tarsal bones are in the (**ankle, hand, midfoot**).
6. If you hit your "funny bone," you would have hit the nerve that runs across the (**glenoid fossa, lateral malleolus, medial epicondyle**).
7. The olecranon is located in the (**ankle, elbow, hip**).
8. (**Parietal, Peroneal, Popliteal**) means *behind the knee.*
9. The (**clavicle, coccyx, coracoid process**) is another name for the collar bone.

True or False

Indicate whether each statement is true or false by writing T or F on the line.

1. ____ The adjective form for *fibula* is *peroneal.*
2. ____ The parietal and temporal bones are in the cranium.
3. ____ The olecranon is a large, square bony projection off the ulna.
4. ____ The humorous is the name of the upper arm bone.
5. ____ The adjective form for *rib* is *costal.*
6. ____ The fibula is in the lower leg on the side of the little toe.
7. ____ The patella is a small bone that protects the knee joint.

Medical Language Word Parts

Name that Word Part

Identify each of the word parts given here by writing in the correct letter (P, C, or S) on the line beside it. Then write the definition of the word part on the blank line. The first one has been done for you.

Prefix = P **Combining Form = C** **Suffix = S**

		Word Part	Definition
1.	-al	S	pertaining to
2.	a-	____	____
3.	-ac	____	____
4.	acetabul/o-	____	____
5.	acromi/o-	____	____
6.	alg/o-	____	____
7.	alges/o-	____	____
8.	align/o-	____	____
9.	all/o-	____	____
10.	amputat/o-	____	____
11.	amput/o-	____	____
12.	an-	____	____
13.	ankyl/o-	____	____
14.	anti-	____	____
15.	appendicul/o-	____	____
16.	-ar	____	____
17.	arthr/o-	____	____
18.	articul/o-	____	____
19.	-ary	____	____
20.	-ate	____	____
21.	-ation	____	____
22.	-ative	____	____
23.	auto-	____	____
24.	axi/o-	____	____
25.	-blast	____	____

		Word Part	Definition
26.	bunion/o-	____	____
27.	calcane/o-	____	____
28.	cancell/o-	____	____
29.	capsul/o-	____	____
30.	carp/o-	____	____
31.	cartilagin/o-	____	____
32.	cav/o-	____	____
33.	-centesis	____	____
34.	cervic/o-	____	____
35.	chem/o-	____	____
36.	chondr/o-	____	____
37.	-clast	____	____
38.	clavicul/o-	____	____
39.	coccyg/o-	____	____
40.	comminut/o-	____	____
41.	compress/o-	____	____
42.	congenit/o-	____	____
43.	coron/o-	____	____
44.	corpor/o-	____	____
45.	cortic/o-	____	____
46.	cost/o-	____	____
47.	crani/o-	____	____
48.	-cyte	____	____
49.	de-	____	____
50.	densit/o-	____	____

		Word Part	Definition
51.	depress/o-		
52.	-desis		
53.	dextr/o-		
54.	diaphys/o-		
55.	dis-		
56.	disk/o-		
57.	-eal		
58.	-ectomy		
59.	-ed		
60.	-ee		
61.	epiphys/o-		
62.	ethm/o-		
63.	extern/o-		
64.	extra-		
65.	faci/o-		
66.	femor/o-		
67.	fibul/o-		
68.	fixat/o-		
69.	fract/o-		
70.	front/o-		
71.	gener/o-		
72.	gen/o-		
73.	glen/o-		
74.	goni/o-		
75.	-graft		
76.	-gram		
77.	-graphy		
78.	hem/o-		
79.	humer/o-		
80.	hy/o-		
81.	-ia		
82.	-ial		
83.	-ic		
84.	-ics		
85.	ili/o-		
86.	-ine		
87.	inflammat/o-		
88.	inject/o-		
89.	inter-		
90.	intra-		
91.	-ion		
92.	ischi/o-		
93.	-ist		
94.	-itis		
95.	-ity		
96.	-ization		
97.	kyph/o-		
98.	lacrim/o-		
99.	later/o-		
100.	lev/o-		
101.	ligament/o-		
102.	locat/o-		
103.	log/o-		
104.	lord/o-		
105.	lumb/o-		
106.	mal-		
107.	malac/o-		
108.	malleol/o-		
109.	mandibul/o-		
110.	maxill/o-		
111.	medi/o-		
112.	medull/o-		
113.	menisc/o-		
114.	-ment		
115.	meta-		
116.	-meter		
117.	-metry		
118.	mineral/o-		
119.	muscul/o-		
120.	myel/o-		
121.	nas/o-		
122.	necr/o-		
123.	non-		
124.	occipit/o-		
125.	-oid		
126.	olisthe/o-		
127.	-olisthesis		
128.	-oma		
129.	orth/o-		
130.	-ory		
131.	-osis		
132.	osse/o-		

		Word Part	Definition
133.	ossicul/o-	______	______________
134.	ossificat/o-	______	______________
135.	oste/o-	______	______________
136.	-ous	______	______________
137.	palat/o-	______	______________
138.	pariet/o-	______	______________
139.	patell/o-	______	______________
140.	path/o-	______	______________
141.	-pathy	______	______________
142.	ped/o-	______	______________
143.	pelv/o-	______	______________
144.	peri-	______	______________
145.	perone/o-	______	______________
146.	phalang/o-	______	______________
147.	physic/o-	______	______________
148.	-physis	______	______________
149.	-phyte	______	______________
150.	-plasty	______	______________
151.	poplite/o-	______	______________
152.	por/o-	______	______________
153.	prosthet/o-	______	______________
154.	pub/o-	______	______________
155.	radi/o-	______	______________
156.	re-	______	______________
157.	reduct/o-	______	______________
158.	rheumat/o-	______	______________
159.	sacr/o-	______	______________
160.	sagitt/o-	______	______________
161.	sarc/o-	______	______________
162.	scapul/o-	______	______________
163.	scint/i-	______	______________
164.	scoli/o-	______	______________
165.	-scope	______	______________
166.	scop/o-	______	______________
167.	-scopy	______	______________
168.	skelet/o-	______	______________
169.	sorb/o-	______	______________
170.	sphen/o-	______	______________
171.	spin/o-	______	______________
172.	spir/o-	______	______________
173.	spondyl/o-	______	______________
174.	stern/o-	______	______________
175.	-steroid	______	______________
176.	steroid/o-	______	______________
177.	sym-	______	______________
178.	synov/o-	______	______________
179.	tars/o-	______	______________
180.	tempor/o-	______	______________
181.	therap/o-	______	______________
182.	-therapy	______	______________
183.	thorac/o-	______	______________
184.	tibi/o-	______	______________
185.	-tic	______	______________
186.	-tion	______	______________
187.	-tome	______	______________
188.	tom/o-	______	______________
189.	tract/o-	______	______________
190.	trans-	______	______________
191.	transplant/o-	______	______________
192.	trochanter/o-	______	______________
193.	turbin/o-	______	______________
194.	uln/o-	______	______________
195.	-ure	______	______________
196.	vascul/o-	______	______________
197.	-verse	______	______________
198.	vertebr/o-	______	______________
199.	xiph/o-	______	______________
200.	zygomat/o-	______	______________

Symptoms, Signs, and Diseases

True or False

Indicate whether each statement is true or false by writing T or F on the line.

1. ____ An arthroscope and a rongeur are surgical instruments.
2. ____ A sprain is the overstretching or tearing of a ligament.
3. ____ An osteoma is a malignant tumor of the bone.
4. ____ A Colles' fracture is often caused by a car accident.
5. ____ Osteoporosis can occur in both men and women.
6. ____ Scoliosis is an abnormal posterior curvature of the thoracic spine.
7. ____ Blood in the joint is known as hemarthrosis.
8. ____ Osteoarthritis is an autoimmune disease in which the body attacks its own cartilage.
9. ____ Pectus excavatum is another name for clubfoot.

Matching Exercise

Match each numbered word or phrase to its description.

1. comminuted	____ Wear and tear disease of the joints
2. osteomyelitis	____ Screening is done for this deformity in school children
3. spondylolisthesis	____ Pain in the joints
4. arthropathy	____ Infection in the bone and bone marrow
5. compound	____ Malignant tumor of the bone
6. osteoarthritis	____ Fracture where the bone is crushed into several pieces
7. arthralgia	____ Fracture where the bone breaks the overlying skin
8. scoliosis	____ One vertebra slips anteriorly over another due to degeneration
9. osteosarcoma	____ General word for disease of a joint

Word-Building Exercise

Use the combining forms, prefixes, and suffixes given here to build medical words that match the definitions given. Write the word that you build on the blank line. Some word parts may be used more than once. The first one has been done for you.

Word Parts		
-algia (condition of pain)	-itis (inflammation of)	-osis (condition; abnormal condition; process)
arthr/o- (joint)	kyph/o- (bent; humpbacked)	oste/o- (bone)
chondr/o- (cartilage)	-malacia (condition of softening)	-pathy (disease, suffering)
-dactyly (condition of fingers or toes)	-oma (tumor, mass)	poly- (many, much)

1. Disease of the joint arthr/o- + -pathy = arthropathy
2. Condition of pain in the joints ____________________
3. Congenital condition of extra fingers or toes ____________________
4. Tumor of the cartilage ____________________
5. Excessive posterior curvature of the thoracic spine ____________________
6. Abnormal softening of the cartilage ____________________
7. Also known as degenerative joint disease ____________________

Circle Exercise

Circle the correct word from the choices given.

1. Infection in the bone and bone marrow is known as (**osteoarthritis, osteomyelitis, osteoporosis**).
2. An injury that disrupts the blood flow to a bone might cause (**ankylosing spondylitis, avascular necrosis, bone tumor**).
3. (**Demineralization, Levoscoliosis, Malalignment**) is seen in patients with osteoporosis.
4. Trauma or hemophilia can cause (**chondromalacia, hemarthrosis, scoliosis**).
5. A bony abnormality that affects the thorax: (**gout, lordosis, pectus excavatum**).
6. Spondylolisthesis involves slipping of the (**joints, sutures, vertebrae**).
7. A (**comminuted, hairline, transverse**) fracture is when the bone is crushed into several pieces.

Laboratory, Radiology, Surgery, and Drugs

Circle Exercise

Circle the correct word from the choices given.

1. The degree of joint movement is measured with a/an (**arthroscope, goniometer, osteotome**).
2. A patient with an amputated limb would be fitted with a (**brace, cast, prosthesis**).
3. A surgical procedure to fuse a degenerated, unstable joint is known as an (**allograft, arthrocentesis, arthrodesis**).
4. Gold compound drugs are used to treat (**fractures, osteoarthritis, rheumatoid arthritis**).
5. Rheumatoid factor can be identified by (**arthroscopy, a blood test, an x-ray**).
6. A DEXA scan is also known as (**bone densitometry, bone graft, uric acid**).
7. Radiologic procedure that uses contrast dye injected into a joint: (**arthrography, closed reduction, traction**).
8. An orthopedic device like a brace or splint is known as a/an (**cast, external fixation, orthosis**).
9. A transplant of bone from a cadaver is known as a/an (**allograft, arthroscopy, autograft**).
10. To diagnose rheumatoid arthritis, the physician would check the (**bone density, rheumatoid factor, uric acid**).

Abbreviations

Matching Exercise

Match each abbreviation to its description.

1.	NSAID	_____ Uses sound to break up bony spurs in the foot
2.	RLE	_____ An autoimmune disease of the joints
3.	ESWT	_____ Also known as osteoarthritis
4.	ROM	_____ Right leg
5.	DJD	_____ Joint between the metacarpal bone and the phalanx
6.	RA	_____ Drug that treats inflammation
7.	MCP	_____ Ability of a limb to move normally

Applied Skills

Plural Noun and Adjective Spelling

Fill in the blanks with the correct word form. Be sure to check your spelling. The first one has been done for you.

Singular Noun	Plural Noun	Adjective	Singular Noun	Plural Noun	Adjective
1. cranium		cranial	7. clavicle		
2. mandible			8. phalanx		
3. zygoma			9. ilium		
4. thorax			10. fibula		
5. rib			11. patella		
6. vertebra			12. scapula		

English and Medical Word Equivalents

For each English word, write its equivalent medical word. The first one has been done for you.

English Word	Medical Word	English Word	Medical Word
1. top of skull	cranium	12. thigh bone	
2. cheek bone		13. kneecap	
3. soft spot		14. shin bone	
4. upper jaw		15. heel bone	
5. lower jaw		16. hunchback	
6. shoulder blade		17. swayback	
7. breast bone		18. bowleg	
8. collar bone		19. knock-knee	
9. point of the elbow		20. clubfoot	
10. fingers or toes		21. bone spur	
11. tail bone		22. great toe/big toe	

Dictionary Challenge

Some dictionaries prefer the spelling **disk** *and give* **disc** *as acceptable alternative spelling for this structure; other dictionaries do just the opposite! This is because there are two different word origins for this same structure: the Latin word* discus *and the Greek word* diskos. *Practice your medical dictionary skills by looking up both spellings and determine which one is the preferred spelling in your medical dictionary.*

1. Preferred spelling ______________________
2. Acceptable spelling ______________________

Analysis of a Medical Report

This exercise contains a physician's office chart note. Read the report and answer the questions.

CHART NOTE

PATIENT NAME: LOWE, James

RECORD NUMBER: 63-1004

DATE: November 19, 20xx

S: This is a 24-year-old male who has been having problems with intermittent low back pain for several years now. He leads an active lifestyle and his job requires him to do a lot of lifting and walking. The pain is getting worse, and he would like to get some definitive treatment at this time. He has been told in the past by a physician that his pelvis is tilted up on the left. However, he does not believe this was diagnosed as a leg-length discrepancy. He denies any radiation of the pain to his buttocks or legs and he says he has not noticed any tingling in his lower extremities.

O: Left leg: The leg length from the ASIS to the medial malleolus is 106 cm. Right leg: The leg length from the ASIS to the medial malleolus is 103 cm. Examination of his back reveals diffuse tenderness over the spinous processes in the lumbar region. I also noticed a dextroscoliosis in the lower thoracic region, which seemed to be significant. Neurologically, the patient had normal reflexes and normal strength in the lower extremities.

A: Chronic back pain due to a significant leg-length discrepancy. He also has a dextroscoliosis, although the exact number of degrees of the curvature was not measured.

P:

1. Refer to an orthopedist for a definitive diagnosis and measurement of the scoliosis.
2. Prescription for Motrin 600 mg tablets, 1 tablet 3 times a day.

Samantha P. Campbell, M.D.
____
Samantha P. Campbell, M.D.

SPC: lcc
D: 11/19/xx
T: 11/19/xx

WORD ANALYSIS QUESTIONS

1. Divide *dextroscoliosis* into its three word parts and define each word part.

Word Part **Definition**

__________ ______________________________

__________ ______________________________

__________ ______________________________

2. The adjective *spinal* refers to the spine or backbone while the adjective *spinous* refers to a bony process. **True** **False**
3. Divide *orthopedist* into its three word parts and define each word part.

Word Part **Definition**

__________ ______________________________

__________ ______________________________

__________ ______________________________

FACT FINDING QUESTIONS

1. The medial malleolus is located on the distal end of what bone? ____________________
2. Which leg was shorter, the patient's right leg or his left leg? ____________________
3. The spinous processes are located on what bones? ____________________
4. What is the single-letter designation for the bones of the spine in the lumbar region? ____________________
5. What does the abbreviation *ASIS* stand for? ____________________

CRITICAL THINKING QUESTIONS

1. Which way did the patient's spine curve? To the right or to the left? ____________________
2. What category of drugs does Motrin belong to? What drug action does it have? ____________________
3. What will the orthopedist measure that this physician did not measure during the office visit? ____________________

Pronunciation Checklist

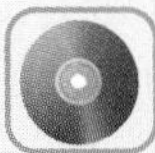

Read each word and its pronunciation. Practice pronouncing each word. Verify your pronunciation by listening to the Pronunciation List on the CD-ROM. Check the box next to the word after you master its pronunciation.

- ❑ acetabular (AS-eh-TAB-yoo-lar)
- ❑ acetabulum (AS-eh-TAB-yoo-lum)
- ❑ acromion (ah-KROM-mee-on)
- ❑ allograft (AL-oh-graft)
- ❑ amputation (AM-pyoo-TAY-shun)
- ❑ amputee (AM-pyoo-tee)
- ❑ analgesic drug (AN-al-JEE-zik DRUHG)
- ❑ ankylosing spondylitis (ANG-kih-LOH-sing SPAWN-dih-LY-tis)
- ❑ appendicular skeleton (AP-en-DIK-yoo-lar SKEL-eh-ton)
- ❑ arthralgia (ar-THRAL-jee-ah)
- ❑ arthritis (ar-THRY-tis)
- ❑ arthrocentesis (AR-throh-sen-TEE-sis)
- ❑ arthrodesis (AR-throh-DEE-sis)
- ❑ arthrogram (AR-throh-gram)
- ❑ arthrography (ar-THRAWG-rah-fee)
- ❑ arthropathy (ah-THRAWP-ah-thee)
- ❑ arthroplasty (AR-throh-PLAS-tee)
- ❑ arthroscope (AR-throh-skohp)
- ❑ arthroscopic (AR-throh-SKAW-pik)
- ❑ arthroscopy (ar-THRAWS-koh-pee)
- ❑ articular (ar-TIK-yoo-lar)
- ❑ articulation (ar-TIK-yoo-LAY-shun)
- ❑ atlas (AT-las)
- ❑ autograft (AW-toh-graft)
- ❑ avascular necrosis (aa-VAS-kyoo-lar neh-KROH-sis)
- ❑ axial skeleton (AK-see-al SKEL-eh-ton)
- ❑ bony (BOH-nee)
- ❑ bunion (BUN-yun)
- ❑ bunionectomy (BUN-yun-EK-toh-mee)
- ❑ calcaneal (kal-KAY-nee-al)
- ❑ calcaneus (kal-KAY-nee-us)
- ❑ cancellous bone (kan-SEL-us BOHN)
- ❑ capsular (KAP-soo-lar)
- ❑ capsule (KAP-sool)
- ❑ carpal (KAR-pal)
- ❑ cartilage (KAR-tih-lij)
- ❑ cartilaginous (KAR-tih-LAJ-ih-nus)
- ❑ cast (KAST)
- ❑ cavity (KAV-ih-tee)
- ❑ cervical (SER-vih-kal)
- ❑ chondroma (con-DROH-mah)
- ❑ chondromalacia (CON-droh-mah-LAY-shee-ah)
- ❑ clavicle (KLAV-ih-kl)
- ❑ clavicular (klah-VIK-yoo-lar)
- ❑ coccygeal (kawk-SIJ-ee-al)
- ❑ coccyx (KAWK-siks)
- ❑ Colles' fracture (KOH-leez FRAK-chur)
- ❑ comminuted fracture (COM-ih-nyoo-ted FRAK-chur)
- ❑ compression (com-PRESH-un)
- ❑ congenital (con-JEN-ih-tal)
- ❑ coracoid (KOR-ah-koyd)
- ❑ coronal suture (kor-OH-nal SOO-chur)
- ❑ corticosteroid drug (KOR-tih-koh-STAIR-oyd DRUHG)
- ❑ cortisone (KOR-tih-zohn)
- ❑ costal (KAW-stal)
- ❑ costochondral (KAWS-toh-CON-dral)
- ❑ cranial (KRAY-nee-al)
- ❑ cranium (KRAY-nee-um)
- ❑ degenerative joint disease (dee-JEN-er-ah-tiv JOYNT dih-ZEEZ)
- ❑ demineralization (dee-MIN-er-al-ih-ZAY-shun)
- ❑ densitometry (DEN-sih-TAWM-eh-tree)
- ❑ depressed fracture (dee-PRESD FRAK-chur)
- ❑ DEXA scan (DEK-sah SKAN)
- ❑ dextroscoliosis (DEKS-troh-SKOH-lee-OH-sis)
- ❑ diaphyses (dy-AF-ih-seez)
- ❑ diaphysial (DY-ah-FIZ-ee-al)
- ❑ diaphysis (dy-AF-ih-sis)
- ❑ digit (DIJ-it)
- ❑ disk, disc (DISK)
- ❑ dislocation (DIS-loh-KAY-shun)
- ❑ displaced fracture (dis-PLAYSD FRAK-chur)
- ❑ epiphyses (eh-PIF-ih-seez)
- ❑ epiphysial (EP-ih-FIZ-ee-al)
- ❑ epiphysis (eh-PIF-ih-sis)
- ❑ ethmoid (ETH-moyd)
- ❑ Ewing's sarcoma (YOO-ingz sar-KOH-mah)
- ❑ external fixation (eks-TER-nal fik-SAY-shun)
- ❑ extracorporeal (EKS-trah-kor-POH-ree-al)
- ❑ extremity (eks-TREM-ah-tee)
- ❑ femora (FEM-oh-rah)
- ❑ femoral (FEM-oh-ral)
- ❑ femur (FEE-mur)
- ❑ fibula (FIB-yoo-lah)
- ❑ fibulae (FIB-yoo-lee)
- ❑ fibular (FIB-yoo-lar)
- ❑ foramen (foh-RAY-min)
- ❑ fracture (FRAK-chur)
- ❑ frontal (FRUN-tal)
- ❑ facial (FAY-shal)
- ❑ fossa (FAW-sah)
- ❑ fontanel (FAWN-tah-NEL)
- ❑ foramen magnum (foh-RAY-min MAG-num)
- ❑ genu valgum (JEE-noo VAL-gum)
- ❑ genu varum (JEE-noo VAR-um)
- ❑ glenoid fossa (GLEH-noyd FAW-sah)
- ❑ goniometer (GOH-nee-AWM-eh-ter)
- ❑ goniometry (GOH-nee-AWM-eh-tree)
- ❑ gout (GOWT)
- ❑ gouty arthritis (GOW-tee ar-THRY-tis)
- ❑ graft (GRAFT)
- ❑ hallux (HAL-uks)
- ❑ hallux valgus (HAL-uks VAL-gus)
- ❑ hemarthrosis (HEE-mar-TROH-sis)
- ❑ humeral (HYOO-mer-al)
- ❑ humeri (HYOO-mer-eye)
- ❑ humerus (HYOO-mer-us)
- ❑ hyoid (HY-oyd)
- ❑ iliac (IL-ee-ak)
- ❑ ilium (IL-ee-um)
- ❑ injection (in-JEK-shun)
- ❑ intervertebral (IN-ter-ver-TEE-bral)
- ❑ intra-articular (IN-trah-ar-TIK-yoo-lar)
- ❑ ischial (IS-kee-al)
- ❑ ischium (IS-kee-um)
- ❑ joint (JOYNT)
- ❑ kyphoscoliosis (KY-foh-SKOH-lee-OH-sis)
- ❑ kyphosis (ky-FOH-sis)
- ❑ kyphotic (ky-FAWT-ik)
- ❑ lacrimal (LAK-rih-mal)
- ❑ lateral (LAT-er-al)
- ❑ levoscoliosis (LEE-voh-SKOH-lee-OH-sis)
- ❑ ligament (LIG-ah-ment)
- ❑ ligamentous (LIG-ah-MEN-tus)
- ❑ lordosis (lor-DOH-sis)
- ❑ lordotic (lor-DAWT-ik)
- ❑ lumbar (LUM-bar)
- ❑ malalignment (MAL-ah-LINE-ment)
- ❑ malleolar (mah-LEE-oh-lar)
- ❑ malleoli (mah-LEE-oh-ligh)
- ❑ malleolus (mah-LEE-oh-lus)
- ❑ mandible (MAN-dih-bl)
- ❑ mandibular (man-DIB-yoo-lar)
- ❑ manubrium (mah-NOO-bree-um)
- ❑ maxilla (mak-SIL-ah)

- ❑ maxillary (MAK-sih-lair-ee)
- ❑ medial (MEE-dee-al)
- ❑ medullary cavity (MED-yoo-lair-ee KAV-ih-tee)
- ❑ meniscal (meh-NIS-kal)
- ❑ menisci (meh-NIS-kigh)
- ❑ meniscus (meh-NIS-kus)
- ❑ metacarpal (MET-ah-KAR-pal)
- ❑ metatarsal (MET-ah-TAR-sal)
- ❑ musculoskeletal (MUS-kyoo-loh-SKEL-eh-tal)
- ❑ nasal (NAY-zal)
- ❑ nondisplaced fracture (non-dis-PLAYSD FRAK-chur)
- ❑ nonsteroidal anti-inflammatory drug (non-stair-OY-dal AN-tee-in-FLAM-ah-TOR-ee DRUHG)
- ❑ nucleus pulposis (NOO-klee-us pul-POH-sis)
- ❑ oblique fracture (awb-LEEK FRAK-chur)
- ❑ obturator foramen (AWB-too-RAY-tor foh-RAY-min)
- ❑ occipital (awk-SIP-ih-tal)
- ❑ olecranon (oh-LEK-rah-non)
- ❑ orthopedics (OR-thoh-PEE-diks)
- ❑ orthopedist (OR-thoh-PEE-dist)
- ❑ orthosis (or-THOH-sis)
- ❑ osseous (AW-see-us)
- ❑ ossicle (AWS-ih-kl)
- ❑ ossicular (aw-SIK-yoo-lar)
- ❑ ossification (AWS-ih-fih-KAY-shun)
- ❑ osteoarthritis (AWS-tee-oh-ar-THRY-tis)
- ❑ osteoblast (AWS-tee-oh-blast)
- ❑ osteoclast (AWS-tee-oh-klast)
- ❑ osteocyte (AWS-tee-oh-site)
- ❑ osteogenic (AWS-tee-oh-JEN-ik)
- ❑ osteoma (AWS-tee-OH-mah)
- ❑ osteomalacia (AWS-tee-oh-mah-LAY-shee-ah)
- ❑ osteomyelitis (AWS-tee-oh-my-LIE-tis)
- ❑ osteophyte (AWS-tee-oh-fite)
- ❑ osteoporosis (AWS-tee-oh-poh-ROH-sis)
- ❑ osteoporotic (AWS-tee-oh-poh-RAWT-ik)
- ❑ osteosarcoma (AWS-tee-oh-sar-KOH-mah)
- ❑ osteotome (AWS-tee-oh-tohm)
- ❑ palatine (PAL-ah-tine)
- ❑ parietal (pah-RY-eh-tal)
- ❑ patella (pah-TEL-ah)
- ❑ patellae (pah-TEL-ee)
- ❑ patellar (pah-TEL-ar)
- ❑ pathologic fracture (PATH-oh-LAWJ-ik FRAK-chur)
- ❑ pectus excavatum (PEK-tus EKS-kah-VAH-tum)
- ❑ pelvic (PEL-vik)
- ❑ pelvis (PEL-vis)
- ❑ periosteal (PAIR-ee-AWS-tee-al)
- ❑ periosteum (PAIR-ee-AWS-tee-um)
- ❑ peroneal (PAIR-oh-NEE-al)
- ❑ phalangeal (fah-LAN-jee-al)
- ❑ phalanx (FAY-langks)
- ❑ physical therapy (FIZ-ih-kal THAIR-ah-pee)
- ❑ physical therapist (FIZ-ih-kal THAIR-ah-pist)
- ❑ popliteal (pop-LIT-ee-al) (pop-lih-TEE-al)
- ❑ process (PRAWS-es)
- ❑ prosthesis (praws-THEE-sis)
- ❑ prosthetic (praws-THET-ik)
- ❑ pubic (PYOO-bik)
- ❑ pubis (PYOO-bis)
- ❑ radial (RAY-dee-al)
- ❑ radii (RAY-dee-eye)
- ❑ radius (RAY-dee-us)
- ❑ reduction (ree-DUK-shun)
- ❑ resorption (ree-SORP-shun)
- ❑ rheumatoid arthritis (ROO-mah-toyd ar-THRY-tis)
- ❑ rongeur (rawn-ZHER)
- ❑ sacral (SAY-kral)
- ❑ sacrum (SAY-krum)
- ❑ sagittal suture (SAJ-ih-tal SOO-chur)
- ❑ sarcoma (sar-KOH-mah)
- ❑ scapula (SKAP-yoo-lah)
- ❑ scapulae (SKAP-yoo-lee)
- ❑ scapular (SKAP-yoo-lar)
- ❑ scintigram (SIN-tih-gram)
- ❑ scintigraphy (sin-TIG-rah-fee)
- ❑ scoliosis (SKOH-lee-OH-sis)
- ❑ scoliotic (SKOH-lee-AWT-ik)
- ❑ skeletal (SKEL-eh-tal)
- ❑ skeletomuscular system (SKEL-eh-toh-MUS-kyoo-lar SIS-tem)
- ❑ skeleton (SKEL-eh-ton)
- ❑ socket (SAWK-et)
- ❑ sphenoid (SFEE-noyd)
- ❑ spinal (SPY-nal)
- ❑ spine (SPYN)
- ❑ spinous process (SPY-nus PRAWS-es)
- ❑ spiral fracture (SPY-ral FRAK-chur)
- ❑ spondylolisthesis (SPAWN-dih-LOH-lis-THEE-sis)
- ❑ sprain (SPRAYN)
- ❑ sternal (STER-nal)
- ❑ sternum (STER-num)
- ❑ suture (SOO-chur)
- ❑ symphysis pubis (SIM-fih-sis PYOO-bis)
- ❑ synovial joint (sih-NOH-vee-al JOYNT)
- ❑ talipes equinovarus (TAY-lih-peez ee-KWY-noh-VAR-us)
- ❑ tarsal (TAR-sal)
- ❑ temporal (TEM-poh-ral)
- ❑ thoracic (thoh-RAS-ik)
- ❑ thorax (THOH-raks)
- ❑ tibia (TIB-ee-ah)
- ❑ tibiae (TIB-ee-ee)
- ❑ tibial (TIB-ee-al)
- ❑ tomography (toh-MAWG-rah-fee)
- ❑ tophi (TOH-fie)
- ❑ tophus (TOH-fus)
- ❑ traction (TRAK-shun)
- ❑ transplant (TRANS-plant)
- ❑ transverse fracture (trans-VERS FRAK-chur)
- ❑ trochanter (troh-KAN-ter)
- ❑ trochanteric (troh-kan-TAIR-ik)
- ❑ turbinate (TUR-bih-nayt)
- ❑ ulna (UL-nah)
- ❑ ulnae (UL-nee)
- ❑ ulnar (UL-nar)
- ❑ uric acid (YOO-rik AS-id)
- ❑ vertebra (VER-teh-brah)
- ❑ vertebrae (VER-teh-bree)
- ❑ vertebral (VER-teh-bral)
- ❑ vomer (VOH-mer)
- ❑ xiphoid (ZY-foyd)
- ❑ x-ray (EKS-ray)
- ❑ zygoma (zy-GOH-mah)
- ❑ zygomatic (ZY-goh-MAT-ik)

Experience Multimedia

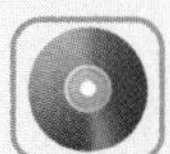

CD-ROM Learning Activities Checklist

Check off the box as you complete each learning activity.

❑ **CD-ROM Learning Activity 8.1: *ANATOMY WORD PARTS FLASHCARDS***

Use flashcards to help you memorize word parts. Make your own flashcards or print out the prepared flashcards. Also see the electronic flashcard game. Time: 20 minutes.

❑ **CD-ROM Learning Activity 8.2: *MEDICINE IN ACTION***

Watch a video clip of an arthroscopy. Time: 5 minutes

❑ **CD-ROM Learning Activity 8.3: *DISEASE AND OTHER WORD PARTS FLASHCARDS***

A continuation of the flashcard learning activity. Time: 20 minutes

❑ **CD-ROM Learning Activity 8.4: *MEMORY AIDS***

Use memory aids to help you memorize medical words and meanings. Time: 5 minutes.

❑ **CD-ROM Learning Activity 8.5: *MEDICAL LANGUAGE SPOKEN HERE***

Listen to actual medical reports and spell the missing medical words. Time: 20 minutes.

❑ **CD-ROM Learning Activity 8.6: *SPELLING CHALLENGE***

Listen to a pronounced medical word and then spell it. Time: 5 minutes.

❑ **CD-ROM Learning Activity 8.7: *MEDICAL LANGUAGE PRONUNCIATION***

Listen to a pronounced medical word and then practice pronouncing it. Time: 30 minutes.

❑ **CD-ROM Learning Activity 8.8: *EDUCATIONAL FUN AND GAMES***

Enjoy these fun activities while reinforcing your knowledge. Time: 15 minutes.

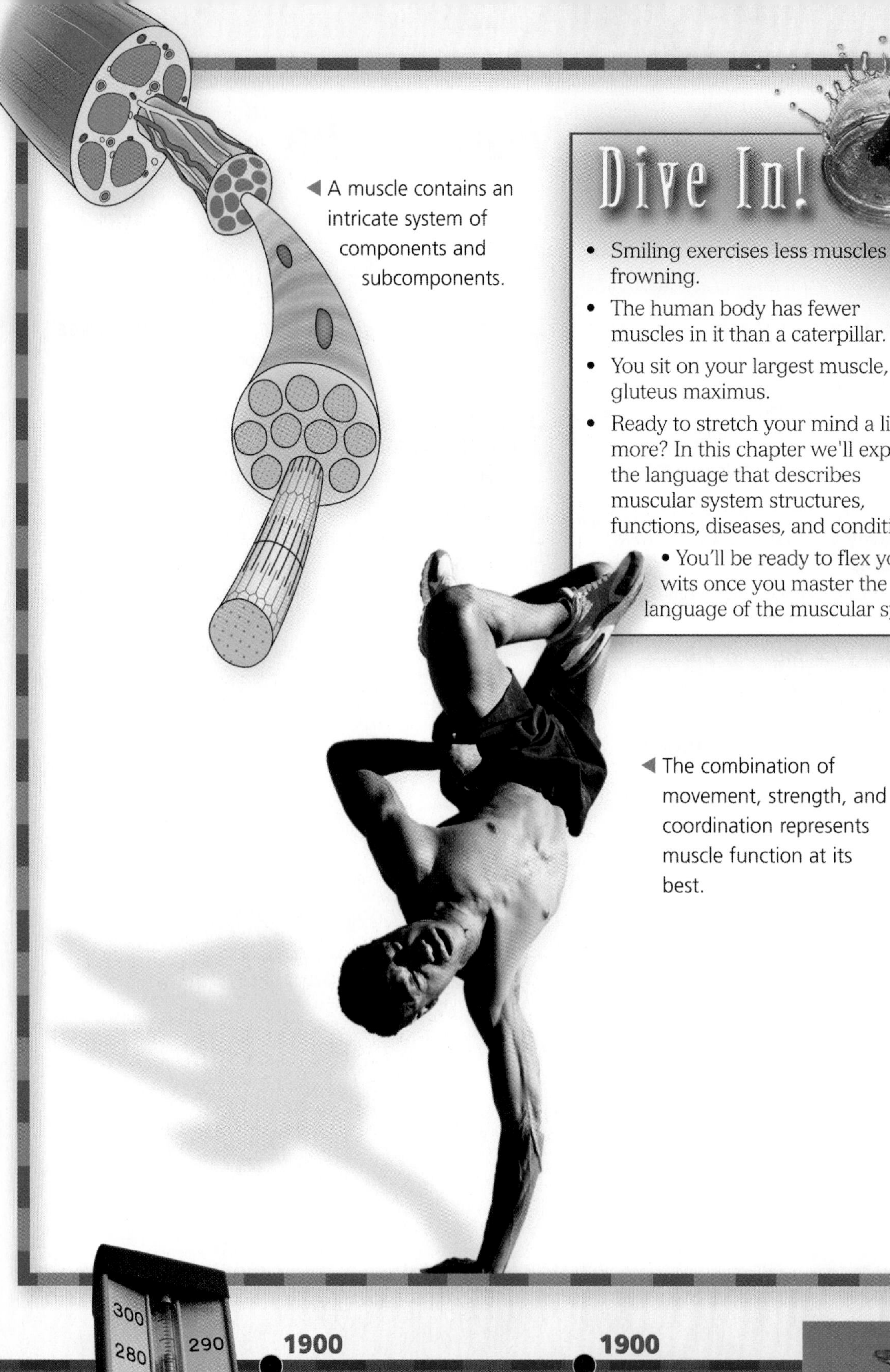

A muscle contains an intricate system of components and subcomponents.

Dive In!

- Smiling exercises less muscles than frowning.
- The human body has fewer muscles in it than a caterpillar.
- You sit on your largest muscle, the gluteus maximus.
- Ready to stretch your mind a little more? In this chapter we'll explore the language that describes muscular system structures, functions, diseases, and conditions.
- You'll be ready to flex your wits once you master the language of the muscular system!

The combination of movement, strength, and coordination represents muscle function at its best.

Medicine Through HISTORY

1900

The sphygmomanometer, a device for measuring the blood pressure, is invented by an Italian physician

1900

Dr. Walter Reed discovers that mosquitos transmit yellow fever

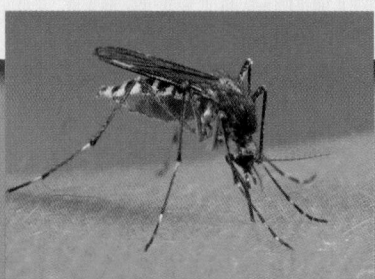

CHAPTER 9

Orthopedics

Muscular System

Orthopedics (OR-thoh-PEE-diks) is the medical specialty that studies the anatomy and physiology of the muscular and skeletal systems and uses diagnostic tests, medical and surgical procedures, and drugs to treat muscular and skeletal diseases. In Chapter 8, you studied orthopedics from the perspective of the skeletal system. In this chapter, you will study the muscular system.

◀ The muscular system is the engine that moves the bony framework of the body.

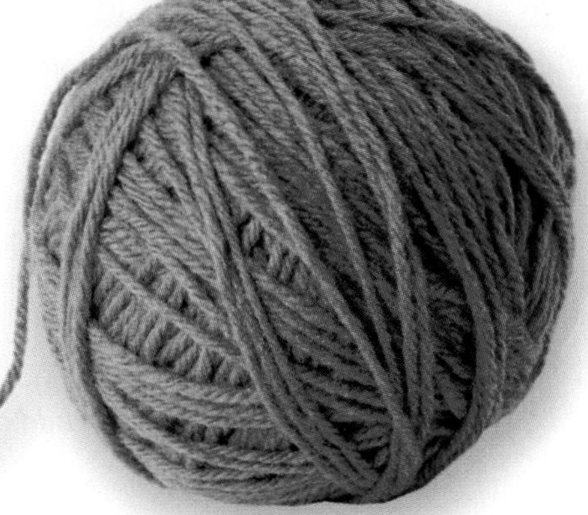

▶ Like yarn, muscles are composed of fibers made up of even thinner strands wrapped around each other.

1904

"An apple a day keeps the doctor away." First uttered by J.T. Stinson while addressing the St. Louis Exposition, it becomes a well-known expression

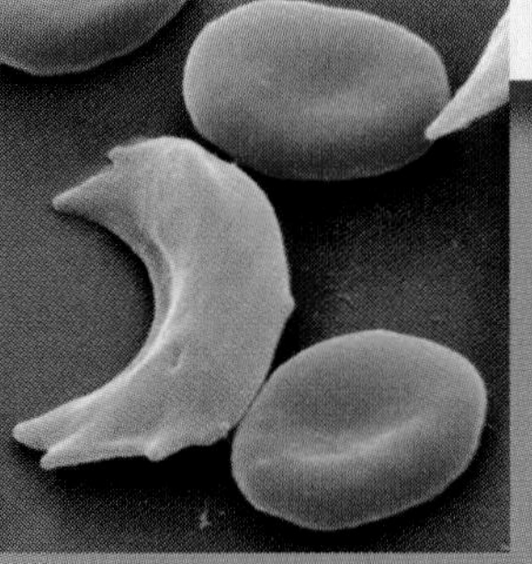

1904

The sickle cells of sickle cell anemia are first seen under the microscope

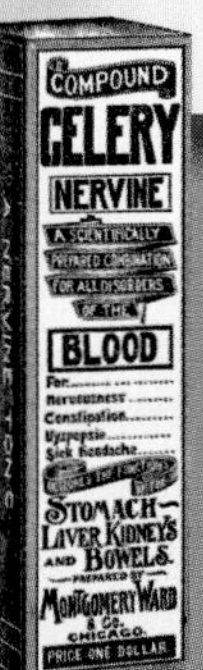

1905

The Food and Drug Act is the first federal drug law. It prohibits mislabeling of the ingredients in drugs

MEASURE YOUR PROGRESS: LEARNING OBJECTIVES

After you study this chapter, you should be able to

1. Identify the anatomical structures of the muscular system by correctly labeling them on anatomical illustrations.
2. Describe how muscles contract and produce movement.
3. Build muscular words from combining forms, prefixes, and suffixes.
4. Describe common muscular diseases.
5. Describe common muscular diagnostic laboratory tests.
6. Describe common muscular medical and surgical procedures and drug categories.
7. Define common muscular abbreviations.
8. Correctly spell and pronounce muscular words.
9. Apply your skills by analyzing an orthopedic (muscular) report.
10. Test your knowledge of orthopedics (muscular) by completing review exercises at the end of the chapter and learning activities on the CD-ROM.

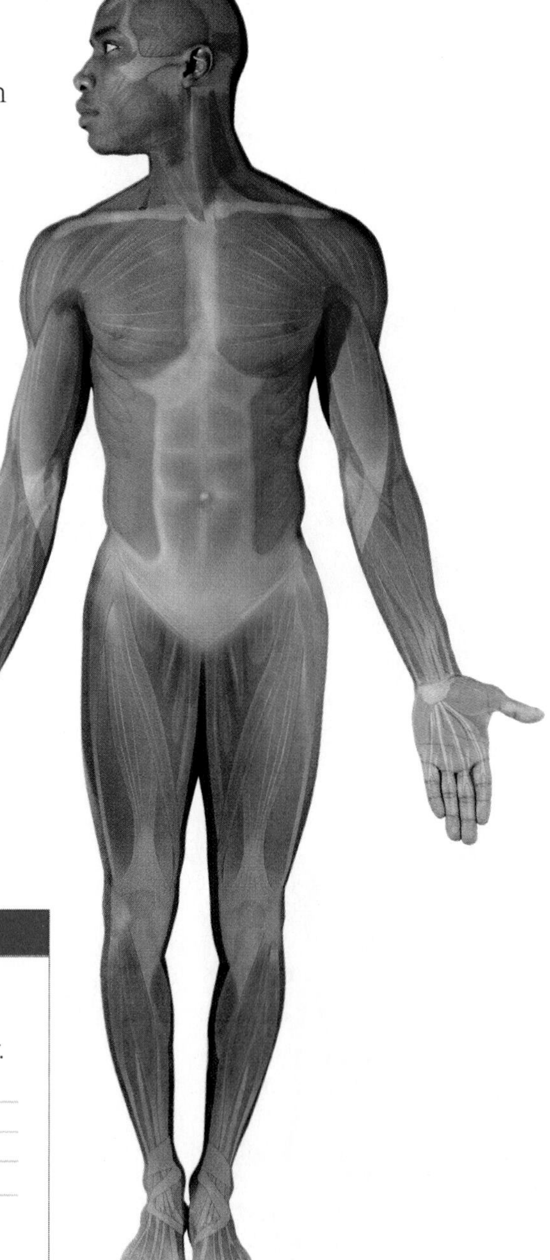

Figure 9-1 ■ The muscular system.

The muscular system is a widespread body system that consists of the voluntary skeletal muscles and other structures throughout the body.

Medical Language Key

To unlock the meaning of a medical word, first define each word part. Then put the word part definitions in order, beginning with the suffix, followed by the first word part, then the other word parts in order.

	Word Part	Word Part Definition
SUFFIX	**-ics**	***knowledge, practice***
COMBINING FORM	**orth/o-**	***straight***
COMBINING FORM	**ped/o-**	***child***

Orthopedics: ***The knowledge and practice of producing straightness in a child or an adult.***

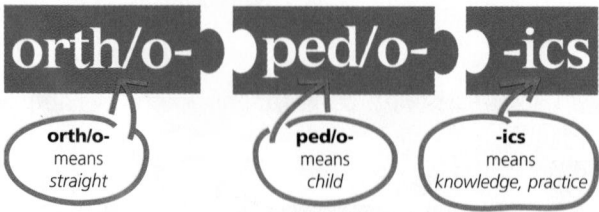

orth/o- means straight
ped/o- means child
-ics means knowledge, practice

www.prenhall.com/turley

For interactive flashcards, real-life video clips, games, exercises, and audio pronunciations please explore the companion CD-ROM in the back of the book. Click on the companion website for bonus chapters, additional resources, and links to on-line learning.

Anatomy and Physiology

The **muscular system** is the engine that moves the bony framework of the body (see Figure 9-1 ■). There are approximately 700 skeletal muscles in the body, as well as tendons and other structures of the muscular system. Some skeletal muscles are readily visible on the surface of the body because of their size and the movement they create when they contract. Others are located more deeply, and their movements are not visible, although they may be felt. All of the muscles of the body (or the muscles in a particular part of the body) are referred to as the **musculature.** The muscular system is often referred to as the **musculoskeletal system** because without the muscles, the bones would not be able to move and without the bones, the muscles would lack support.

muscle (MUS-el)
Muscle is derived from a Latin word meaning *little mouse* because of the movement of muscles under the skin.

muscular (MUS-kyoo-lar)
muscul/o- *muscle*
-ar *pertaining to*

system (SIS-tem)
System is derived from a Greek word meaning *combination of parts to make an organized whole.*

musculature (MUS-kyoo-lah-choor)
muscul/o- *muscle*
-ature *system composed of*

musculoskeletal (MUS-kyoo-loh-SKEL-eh-tal)
muscul/o- *muscle*
skelet/o- *skeleton*
-al *pertaining to*

Anatomy of the Muscular System

Types of Muscles

There are three types of muscles in the body: skeletal muscles, the cardiac muscle, and smooth muscles (see Figure 9-2 ■).

- **Skeletal muscles:** Skeletal muscles provide the means by which the body can move. Skeletal muscles are **voluntary muscles** that contract and relax in response to conscious thought. Skeletal muscles are **striated,** showing bands of color when examined under the microscope.
- **Cardiac muscle:** The heart or cardiac muscle pumps blood through the circulatory system. It is an involuntary muscle that is not under conscious control. The heart was discussed in detail in Cardiology (Chapter 5).
- **Smooth muscles:** Smooth muscles are involuntary, nonstriated muscles. They form a continuous, thin layer in various organs and structures (for example, the blood vessels and intestines). Smooth muscles are discussed in various chapters.

Of the three types of muscles, only skeletal muscles belong to the muscular system. In the rest of this chapter, the word *muscle* should be understood to mean skeletal muscle.

voluntary (VAWL-un-tair-ee)
volunt/o- *done by one's own free will*
-ary *pertaining to*

striated (STRY-aa-ted)
Striate is derived from a Latin word meaning *stripe.*

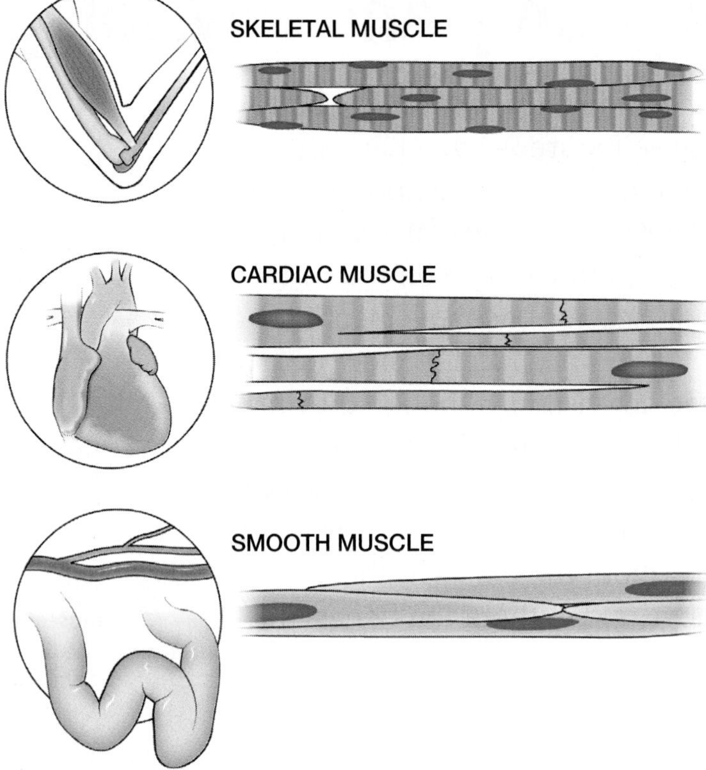

Figure 9-2 ■ Types of muscle.

There are three types of muscles—skeletal muscles, the cardiac muscle, and smooth muscles. Each can be distinguished from the other by its cellular appearance under a microscope. Note the very pronounced color bands (striations) and multiple nuclei in each skeletal muscle cell. Cardiac muscle cells have less pronounced bands, and nonstriated smooth muscle cells have no bands.

Muscle Origins, Insertions, and Related Structures

Each muscle has distinct beginning and ending points. The **origin** or beginning of a muscle is where it is attached to a stationary or nearly stationary bone of the skeleton. The **insertion** or ending point is where the muscle attaches to the bone that it moves when it contracts and relaxes. In traveling from its origin to its insertion, many muscles cross a joint. The belly of the muscle is where the muscle mass is the greatest, which is usually at the center.

origin (OR-ih-jin)

insertion (in-SER-shun)
insert/o- *to put in or introduce*
-ion *action; condition*

The muscle is attached to the bone at its origin or insertion by a **tendon,** a cordlike, nonelastic, white fibrous band of connective tissue (see Figure 9-3 ■). Each muscle is wrapped in **fascia,** a thin connective tissue that also joins to the tendon. An **aponeurosis** is a flat, wide, white fibrous sheet of connective tissue, sometimes composed of several tendons, that attaches a flat muscle to a bone or to other, deeper muscles. A **bursa** is a slender, elongated pocket of synovial membrane that contains synovial fluid. A bursa acts as a cushion to reduce friction in areas where a tendon rubs against a bone. A **retinaculum** is a nearly, translucent band of fibrous tissue and fascia that holds down the extensor and flexor tendons that cross the wrist and ankle (see Figure 9-13).

tendon (TEN-dun)

tendinous (TEN-dih-nus)
tendin/o- *tendon*
-ous *pertaining to*

fascia (FASH-ee-ah)

fascial (FASH-ee-al)
fasci/o- *fascia*
-al *pertaining to*

aponeurosis (AP-oh-nyoo-ROH-sis)

bursa (BER-sah)
bursae (BER-see)
Bursa is a Latin singular feminine noun meaning *a purse.* Form the plural by changing *-a* to *-ae.*

bursal (BER-sal)
burs/o- *bursa*
-al *pertaining to*

retinaculum (RET-ih-NAK-yoo-lum)
Retinaculum is a Latin word that means *a band to hold back.*

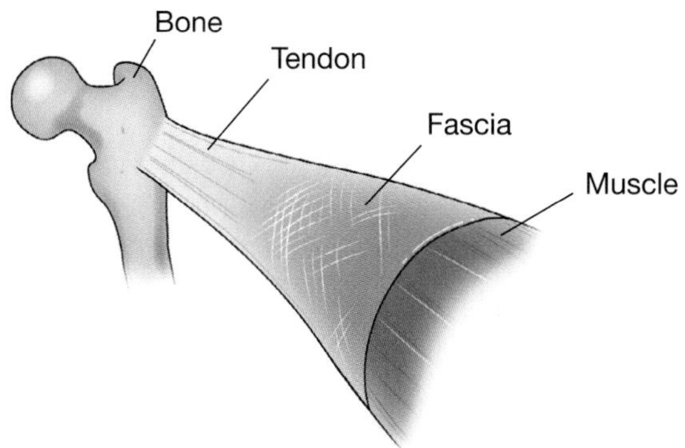

Figure 9-3 ■ The muscle and related structures.
At their origins and insertions, most muscles are attached to the bone by a tendon. In the area where the muscle transitions to the tendon, the red color of the muscle is gradually replaced by the white color of the tendon. The fascia envelops the muscle and also merges with the tendon.

Muscle Names

Muscle names can seem complex because they are in Latin, but you will recognize some of the Latin words because they relate to bones you studied in Chapter 8. Other Latin words become familiar because they consistently describe where the muscle is located, what shape it is, what size it is, or what action it performs (see Figure 9-4 ■ and Table 9-1).

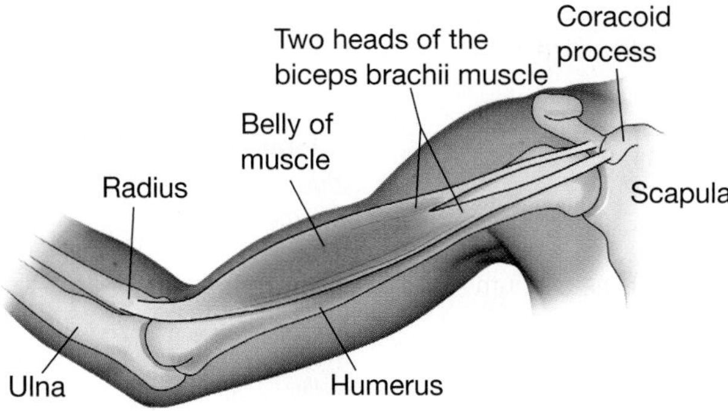

Figure 9-4 ■ Origin and insertion of a muscle.
Every muscle has at least one point of origin on a stationary or nearly stationary bone and an insertion on a bone that moves when the muscle contracts. The biceps brachii muscle has two heads whose origins are on different parts of the scapula. This muscle crosses the elbow joint and ends at its insertion on the radius. When the biceps brachii muscle contracts, the radius is pulled toward the upper arm and the arm flexes.

Table 9-1 Muscle Names and Their Meanings

Muscle Name	What the Muscle Name Tells You		Word Part and Definition
biceps brachii	Shape: Location:	One end divides into two parts or heads (*biceps*) Arm (*brachii*)	**biceps** (BY-seps) **bi-** *two* **-ceps** *head* Every medical word must contain a combining form. The suffix of *biceps* contains a combining form derived from the Latin word *caput* (head). **brachii** (BRAY-kee-eye) *Brachii* is a Latin word meaning *of the arm.*
brachioradialis	Location:	Radial bone in the arm (*brachi/o-)*	**brachioradialis** (BRAY-kee-oh-RAY-dee-AL-is) **brachi/o-** *arm* **radi/o-** *radius (forearm bone); x-rays; radiation* **-alis** *pertaining to*
extensor digitorum	Action: Location:	Extends Digits (digitorum)	**extensor** (eks-TEN-sor) **extens/o-** *straightening* **-or** *person or thing that produces or does* **digitorum** (dij-ih-TOR-um) *Digitorum* is a Latin word meaning *of the digit.*
flexor hallucis brevis	Action: Location: Size:	Flexes Big toe (*hallux*) Short (*brevis*)	**flexor** (FLEK-sor) **flex/o-** *bending* **-or** *person or thing that produces or does* **hallucis** (HAL-yoo-sis) *Hallux* is a Latin word meaning *the big toe.* **brevis** (BREV-is) *Brevis* is a Latin word meaning *short in length.*
gluteus maximus	Location: Size:	Buttocks (*gluteus*) Large (*maximus*)	**gluteus** (gloo-TEE-us) *Gluteus* is a Latin word meaning *the buttocks.* **maximus** (MAK-sih-mus) *Maximus* is a Latin word meaning *the largest one of a group.*
rectus abdominis	Orientation: Location:	Straight up and down (*rectus*) Abdomen	**rectus** (REK-tus) *Rectus* is a Latin word meaning *straight.* **abdominis** (ab-DAWM-ih-nis) *Abdominis* is a Latin word meaning *of the abdomen.*
temporalis	Location:	Temporal bone of the cranium	**temporalis** (TEM-poh-RAY-lis) **tempor/o-** *temple (side of the head)* **-alis** *pertaining to*
triceps brachii	Shape: Location:	One end divides into three parts or heads (*triceps*) Arm (*brachii*)	**triceps** (TRY-seps) **tri-** *three* **-ceps** *head*

Types of Muscle Movement

Muscles function in pairs to produce movement. When the first muscle contracts, the second one relaxes to allow movement. When the second muscle contracts, the first one relaxes to allow movement in the opposite direction. Flexion and extension, abduction and adduction, rotation to the right and to the left, supination and pronation, and eversion and inversion are opposite movements that are controlled by muscle pairs (see Figures 9-5■ through 9-8■ and Table 9-2).

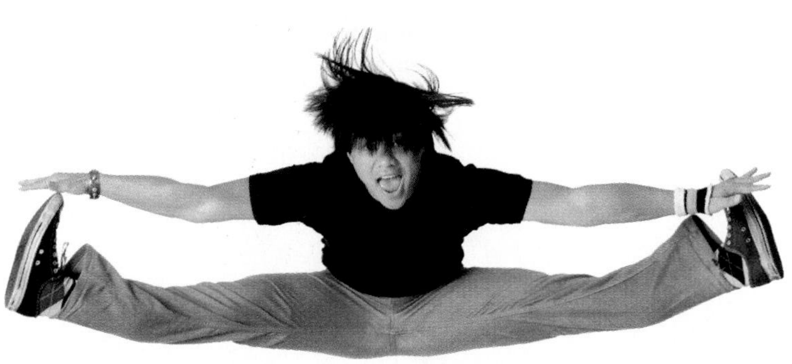

Figure 9-5 ■ Extension, abduction, and dorsiflexion.
This dancer has his arms and legs extended and abducted. His feet are in dorsiflexion.

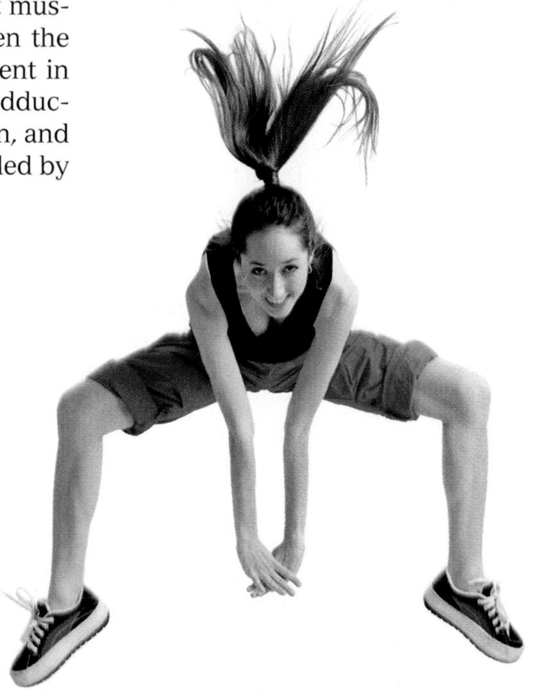

Figure 9-6 ■ Extension, adduction, pronation, abduction, flexion, and dorsiflexion.
This dancer has her arms extended and adducted, her thighs abducted, and her knees flexed. Her feet are in plantar flexion, and her hands are in pronation.

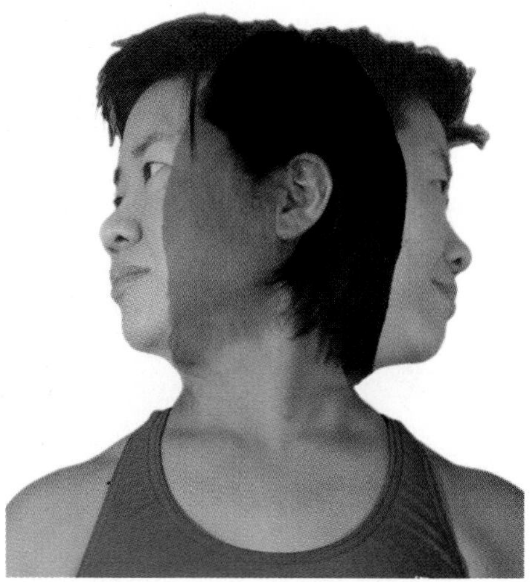

Figure 9-7 ■ Rotation.
The head rotates to the right and left on its axis, the vertebral column.

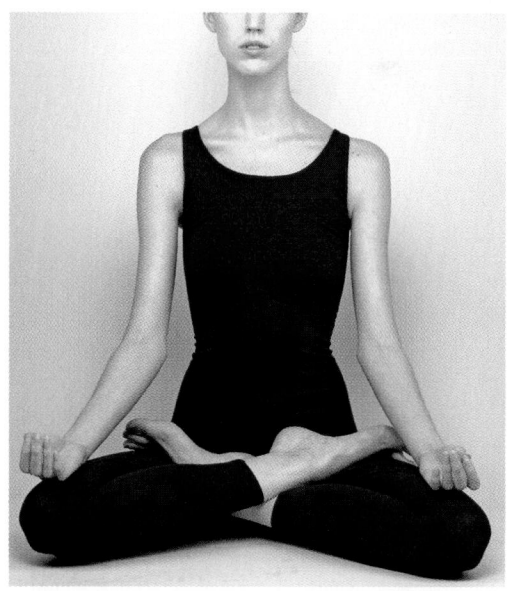

Figure 9-8 ■ Extension, supination, abduction, flexion, and inversion.
This person is in a yoga position with her arms extended, her hands in supination, her thighs abducted, and her knees flexed. Her feet are in inversion.

Table 9-2 Types of Muscle Movement

Movement	Description	Muscle Type	Word Part and Definition
flexion	Bending a joint to decrease the angle between two bones or two body parts. Plantar flexion of the foot causes the toe to point downward. Dorsiflexion of the foot causes the toe to point upward.	**flexor**	**flexion** (FLEK-shun) **flex/o-** *bending* **-ion** *action; condition* **flexor** (FLEK-sor) **flex/o-** *bending* **-or** *person or thing that produces or does*
extension	Straightening and extending a joint to increase the angle between two bones or two body parts	**extensor**	**extension** (eks-TEN-shun) **extens/o-** *straightening* **-ion** *action; condition* **extensor** (eks-TEN-sor) **extens/o-** *straightening* **-or** *person or thing that produces or does*
abduction	Moving a body part away from the midline of the body	**abductor**	**abduction** (ab-DUK-shun) **ab-** *away from* **duct/o-** *bring or move; a duct* **-ion** *action; condition* **abductor** (ab-DUK-tor) **ab-** *away from* **duct/o-** *bring or move; a duct* **-or** *person or thing that produces or does*
adduction	Moving a body part toward the midline of the body	**adductor**	**adduction** (ad-DUK-shun) **ad-** *toward* **duct/o-** *bring or move; a duct* **-ion** *action; condition* **adductor** (ad-DUK-tor) **ad-** *toward* **duct/o-** *bring or move; a duct* **-or** *person or thing that produces or does*

Table 9-2 Types of Muscle Movement (*cont.*)

Movement	Description	Muscle Type	Word Part and Definition
rotation	Moving a body part around its axis	**rotator**	**rotation** (roh-TAY-shun) **rotat/o-** *rotate* **-ion** *action; condition* **rotator** (ROH-tay-tor) **rotat/o-** *rotate* **-or** *person or thing that produces or does*
supination	Turning the palm of the hand upward	**supinator**	**supination** (SOO-pih-NAY-shun) **supinat/o-** *lying on the back* **-ion** *action; condition* **supinator** (SOO-pih-nay-tor) **supinat/o-** *lying on the back* **-or** *person or thing that produces or does*
pronation	Turning the palm of the hand downward	**pronator**	**pronation** (proh-NAY-shun) **pronat/o-** *lying face down* **-ion** *action; condition* **pronator** (proh-NAY-tor) **pronat/o-** *lying face down* **-or** *person or thing that produces or does*
eversion	Turning a body part outward	**evertor**	**eversion** (ee-VER-zhun) **e-** *without, out* **vers/o-** *to travel; to turn* **-ion** *action; condition* **evertor** (ee-VER-tor) **e-** *without, out* **vert/o-** *to travel; to turn* **-or** *person or thing that produces or does*
inversion	Turning a body part inward	**invertor**	**inversion** (in-VER-zhun) **in-** *in; without; not* **vers/o-** *to travel; to turn* **-ion** *action; condition* **invertor** (in-VER-tor) **in-** *in; without; not* **vert/o-** *to travel; to turn* **-or** *person or thing that produces or does*

Muscles of the Head and Neck

The most important muscles of the head and neck are described in this section (see Figure 9-9 ■).

- **frontalis:** Moves the forehead skin to elevate the eyebrows or wrinkle the forehead
- **temporalis:** Moves the mandible upward and backward
- **orbicularis oculi:** Closes the eyelids; presses the eyelids together
- **orbicularis oris:** Closes the lips, presses the lips together
- **masseter:** Moves the mandible upward
- **buccinator:** Moves the cheeks to produce a sucking motion and moves food from the side of the mouth toward the tongue
- **sternocleidomastoid:** Bends the head toward the sternum (flexion) and turns the head to either side (rotation)
- **platysma:** Moves the mandible down

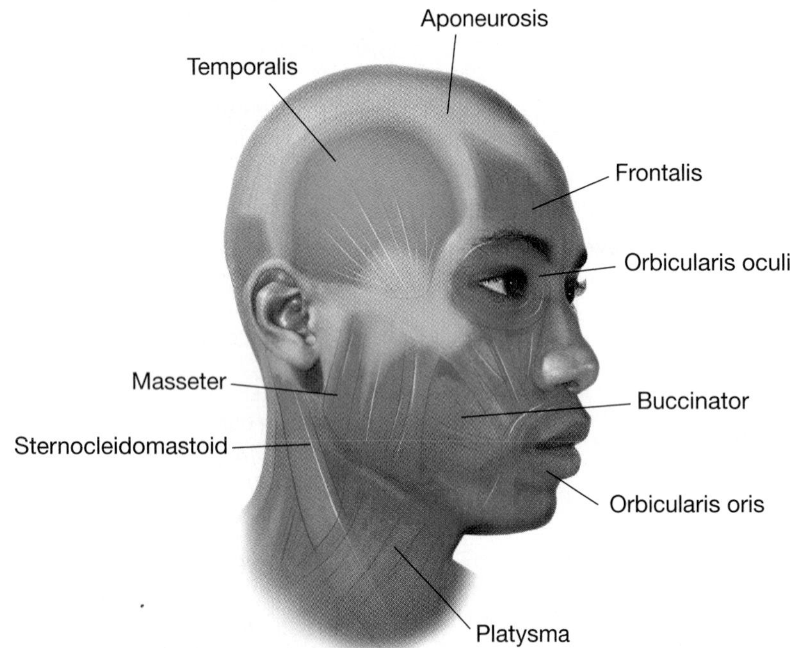

Figure 9-9 ■ Muscles of the head and neck.

These muscles contract and relax when you close your eyes, make facial expressions, chew food, and move your mouth and lips while speaking. They also support your head and move it from side to side or up and down.

frontalis (frun-TAY-lis)
front/o- *front*
-alis *pertaining to*

temporalis (tem-poh-RAY-lis)
tempor/o- *temple (side of the head)*
-alis *pertaining to*

orbicularis (or-BIK-yoo-LAIR-is)
orbicul/o- *small circle*
-aris *pertaining to*

oculi (AWK-yoo-ligh)
Oculi is a Latin word meaning *of the eye.*

oris (OR-is)
Oris is a Latin word meaning *of the mouth.*

masseter (MAS-eh-ter)
masset/o- *chewing*
-er *person or thing that produces or does*

buccinator (BUK-sih-NAY-tor)
buccinat/o- *cheek*
-or *person or thing that produces or does*
Buccinator is derived from a Latin word meaning *someone who plays the trumpet.* The buccinator muscles bulge outward from pressure in the mouth when playing the trumpet.

sternocleidomastoid (STER-noh-KLY-doh-MAS-toyd)
stern/o- *sternum (breast bone)*
cleid/o- *clavicle (collar bone)*
mast/o- *breast; mastoid process*
-oid *resembling*
This muscle is not attached to the breast but to the mastoid process, a bony, rounded prominence behind the ear that resembles the shape of a breast.

platysma (plah-TIZ-mah)
Platysma is a Greek word meaning *a flat plate.*

Muscles of the Shoulders, Chest, and Back

The most important muscles of the shoulders, chest, and back are described in this section (see Figures 9-10 ■ and 9-11 ■).

- **deltoid:** Raises and lowers the arm and moves the arm away from the body (abduction).
- **pectoralis major:** Moves the arm anteriorly and medially across the chest (adduction)
- **intercostals:** Muscle pairs between the ribs; one contracts during inspiration to spread the ribs apart; the other contracts during expiration, coughing, or sneezing.
- **trapezius:** Raises the shoulder, pulls the shoulder blades together, elevates the clavicle. Turns the head from side to side (rotation). Moves the head posteriorly (extension).
- **latissimus dorsi:** Moves the arm posteriorly and medially toward the spinal column (adduction)

deltoid (DEL-toyd)
delt/o- *triangle*
-oid *resembling*
This muscle name is derived from the Greek capital alphabet letter *delta,* which is shaped like a triangle.

pectoralis (PEK-toh-RAY-lis)
pector/o- *chest*
-alis *pertaining to*

intercostal (IN-ter-KAWS-tal)
inter- *between*
cost/o- *rib*
-al *pertaining* to

trapezius (trah-PEE-zee-us)
This muscle resembles a trapezoid, a geometric figure that has two parallel sides and two nonparallel sides.

latissimus (lah-TIS-ih-mus)
Latissimus is a Latin word meaning *the widest.*

dorsi (DOR-see)
Dorsi is a Latin word meaning *of the back.*

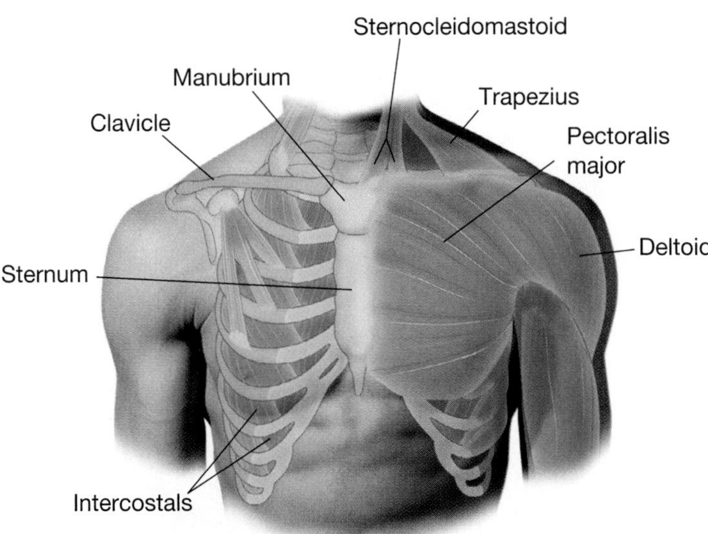

Figure 9-10 ■ Muscles of the shoulder and chest.

These muscles contract and relax when you raise your arms, move your arms and shoulders toward the midline to hug someone you love, or rotate your arms inwardly.

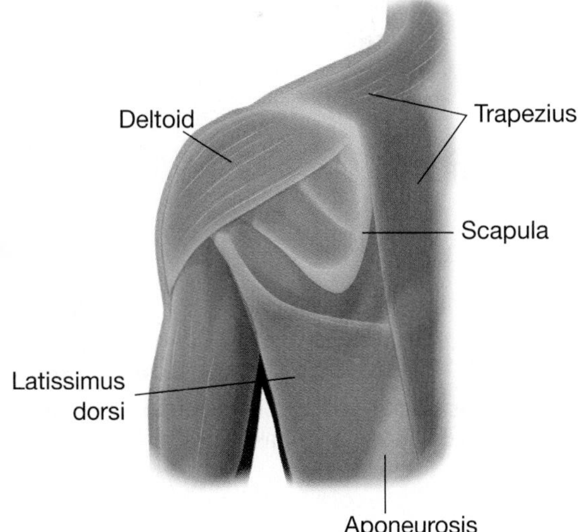

Figure 9-11 ■ Muscles of the shoulder and back.

These muscles contract and relax when you shrug your shoulders or pull your shoulder blades together to sit up straight. They also pull your head backward and to the side, and turn your trunk to the right or left.

Muscles of the Arms and Hands

The most important muscles of the arms and hands are described in this section (see Figures 9-12■ and 9-13■).

- **biceps brachii:** Bends the upper arm toward the shoulder (flexion) and bends the lower arm toward the upper arm (flexion).
- **triceps brachii:** Straightens the lower arm (extension)
- **brachioradialis:** Bends the lower arm toward the upper arm (flexion)
- **thenars:** Bends the thumb (flexion) and moves it toward the palm (adduction)

biceps (BY-seps)
bi- *two*
-ceps *head*

brachii (BRAY-kee-eye)
Brachii is the Latin word meaning *of the arm.*

triceps (TRY-seps)
tri- *three*
-ceps *head*

brachioradialis (BRAY-kee-oh-ray-dee-AL-is)
brachi/o- *arm*
radi/o- *radius (forearm bone); x-rays; radiation*
-alis *pertaining to*

thenar (THEE-nar)
Thenar is a Greek word meaning *palm at the base of the thumb.*

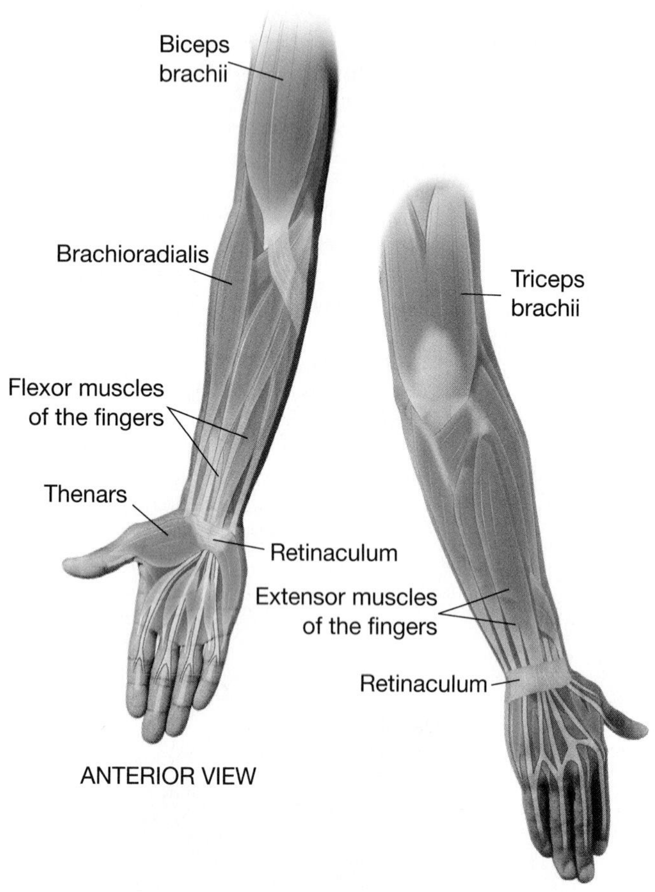

Figure 9-12 ■ Muscles of the arm and hand.
These muscles contract and relax when you lift a heavy box, straighten your arms to do a handstand, shake hands, make a fist, or play the piano.

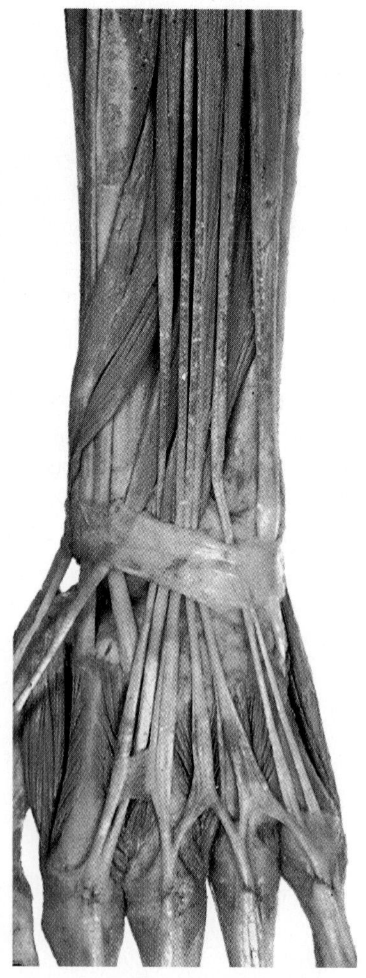

Figure 9-13 ■ Extensor muscles of the forearm and the extensor retinaculum.
There are several long muscles in the forearm that contract to extend and straighten the fingers. Each muscle has a long tendon that travels across the wrist to one or more of the fingers. These tendons are held in place by the extensor retinaculum, a translucent, horizontal band of tissue.

Muscles of the Abdomen

The most important muscles of the abdomen are described in this section (see Figure 9-14■).

- **external oblique:** Bends the upper body forward (flexion) and rotates it medially, and compresses the side of the abdominal wall
- **internal oblique:** Bends the upper body forward (flexion) and rotates it medially and compresses the side of the abdominal wall
- **rectus abdominis:** Bends the upper body forward (flexion) and compresses the anterior abdominal wall

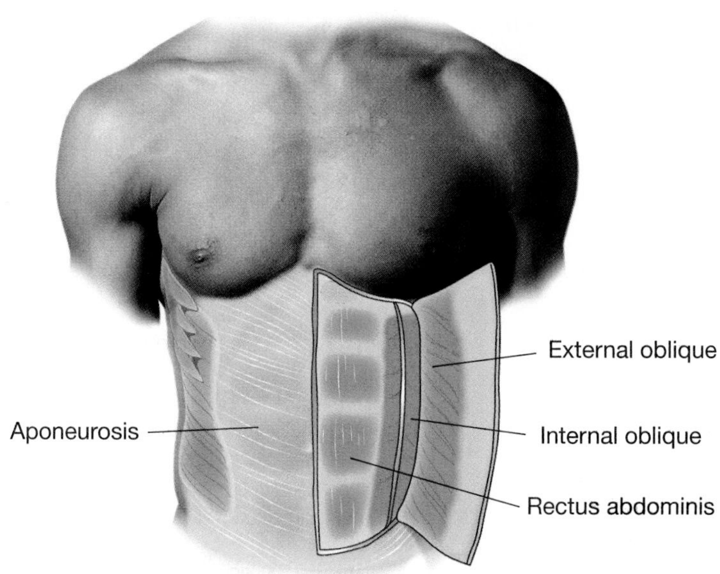

Figure 9-14 ■ Muscles of the abdomen.
These muscles contract and relax when you rotate the trunk of your body from side to side, flatten your abdomen, or bend forward.

Word Alert

SOUND-ALIKE WORDS

rectus (noun) Latin noun for a straight muscle
Example: When the rectus abdominis muscle contracts, it pulls the chest toward the legs.

rectum (noun) Straight part of the distal large intestine that comes after the curving S-shaped sigmoid colon
Example: Digested food travels through the colon, through the rectum, through the anus, and is then expelled from the body.

external (eks-TER-nal)
extern/o- *outside*
-al *pertaining to*

oblique (awb-LEEK)
Oblique is derived from a Latin word meaning *slanted.*

internal (in-TER-nal)
intern/o- *inside*
-al *pertaining to*

rectus (REK-tus)
Rectus is a Latin word meaning *straight.*

abdominis (ab-DAWM-ih-nis)
Abdominis is a Latin word meaning *of the abdomen.*

Muscles of the Legs and Buttocks

The most important muscles of the buttocks and legs are described in this section (see Figure 9-15 ■).

Anterior Leg

- **rectus femoris:** Bends the upper leg toward the abdomen (flexion); straightens the lower leg (extension)
- **quadriceps femoris:** Straightens the lower leg (extension)
- **sartorius:** Bends the upper leg toward the abdomen (flexion) and rotates it laterally
- **peroneus longus:** Raises the lateral edge of the foot (eversion) and bends the foot downward (plantar flexion)
- **tibialis anterior:** Bends the foot up toward the leg (dorsiflexion)

Buttocks and Posterior Leg

- **gluteus maximus:** Moves the upper leg posteriorly and rotates it laterally
- **biceps femoris:** Moves the upper leg posteriorly (extension) and bends the lower leg toward the buttocks (flexion)
- **gastrocnemius:** Bends the foot downward (plantar flexion)

rectus (REK-tus)
Rectus is a Latin word meaning *straight.*

femoris (FEM-oh-ris)
Femoris is a Latin word meaning *of the femur.*

quadriceps (KWAD-rih-seps)
quadri- *four*
-ceps *head*
Quadriceps femoris is a collective phrase for four muscles whose heads join to a single tendon: the rectus femoris, vastus lateralis, vastus medialis, and vastus intermedius (not pictured).

sartorius (sar-TOR-ee-us)
Sartorius is a Latin word meaning *a tailor.* The sartorius muscle contracts for the cross-leg position a tailor used to sit on the floor.

peroneus (PAIR-oh-NEE-us)

longus (LONG-us)
Longus is a Latin word meaning *long.*

peroneal (PAIR-oh-NEE-al)
perone/o- *fibula (lower leg bone)*
-al *pertaining to*
Peroneal is derived from a Greek word meaning *fibula.*

tibialis (TIB-ee-AL-is)
tibi/o- *tibia (shin bone)*
-alis *pertaining to*

anterior (an-TEER-ee-or)
anter/o- *before; front part*
-ior *pertaining to*

gluteus (gloo-TEE-us)
Gluteus is a Latin word meaning *the buttocks.*

maximus (MAK-sih-mus)
Maximus is a Latin word meaning *the largest one of a group.*

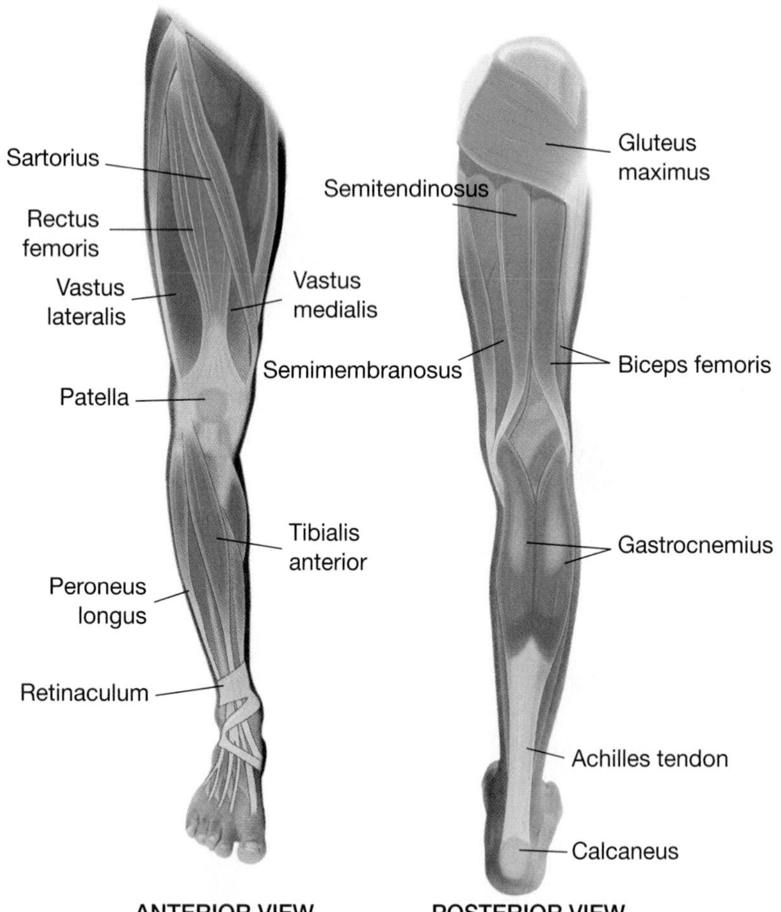

Figure 9-15 ■ Muscles of the leg and buttocks.

The muscles of the legs and buttocks contract and relax when you move your legs in any direction, bend your knees, walk on your toes, climb the stairs, or get up from a sitting position.

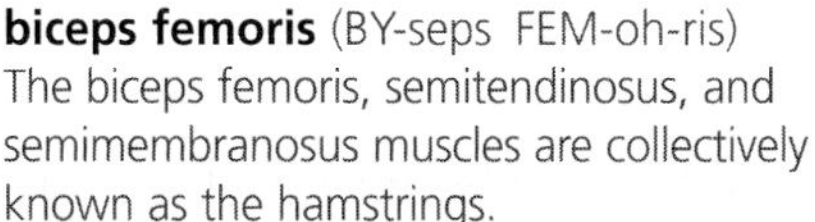

Quadriceps femoris is the collective name for four muscles on the anterior and lateral aspects of the thigh. All of these muscles—the rectus femoris, vastus lateralis, vastus intermedius (beneath the vastus lateralis), and vastus medialis—have tendons that insert at the patella. Contraction of the three vastus muscles straightens the lower leg (extension).

Hamstrings is the collective name for three muscles on the posterior aspect of the thigh. The tendons of all of these muscles—the biceps femoris, semitendinosus, and semimembranosus—form two tendon groups, one on each side of the popliteal space at the back of the knee. Contraction of these muscles moves the upper leg posteriorly and bends the lower leg toward the buttocks (flexion).

biceps femoris (BY-seps FEM-oh-ris)
The biceps femoris, semitendinosus, and semimembranosus muscles are collectively known as the hamstrings.

gastrocnemius (GAS-trawk-NEE-mee-us)
gastr/o- *stomach*
-cnemius *leg*
The gastrocnemius muscle is shaped somewhat like the stomach, which may be how it got its name.

Did You Know?

The gastrocnemius muscle has its insertion through the calcaneal tendon to the calcaneus (heel bone). This tendon is also known as the Achilles tendon in reference to Achilles, the mythical Greek hero of Homer's *Iliad,* who was wounded in the heel, his only vulnerable spot.

Across the Life Span

Throughout life, regular exercise is an important component of wellness and physical fitness. One of the early developmental milestones for an infant is to be able to lift up the head and chest (see Figure 9-16■). Aging and chronic disease can limit mobility and decrease muscle strength. The size and strength of the muscles decrease over time. There is less flexibility because the elastic muscle tissue is replaced by fibrous connective tissue, but active exercise helps maintain muscle strength and flexibility.

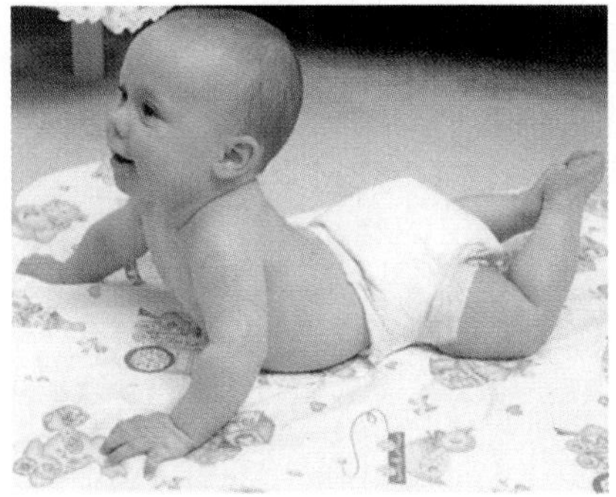

Figure 9-16 ■ Growth and development milestones.

A 1-month-old baby can only lift its head briefly. By 3 months of age, a baby has developed the muscular coordination to turn over in bed. This slightly older baby exhibits the next step in growth and development. He is able to lift his head and support his entire upper body with his arms, an activity that requires strength and coordination in the muscles of the neck, shoulders, and arms.

Physiology of a Muscle Contraction

A muscle is composed of several muscle fascicles, each of which is wrapped in fascia and connected to the tendon (see Figure 9-17■). Each muscle **fascicle** is a bundle of individual muscle fibers. These muscle fibers run parallel to each other so that, when they contract, they all pull in the same direction. A muscle fiber is **multinucleated,** having not just one, but hundreds of nuclei scattered along its length. This speeds up the chemical processes that must occur along the entire length of the muscle fiber before it can contract. Each muscle fiber is composed of myofibrils. Each **myofibril** is composed of thin strands of the protein actin and thick strands of the protein myosin that give skeletal muscle its characteristic striated (striped) appearance. Actin and myosin are the basis of a muscle contraction at the microscopic level.

A muscle contracts in response to an electrical impulse from a nerve. Each muscle fiber is connected to a single nerve cell at a **neuromuscular junction.** The nerve cell releases the **neurotransmitter** acetylcholine. **Acetylcholine** is a chemical messenger that moves across the neuromuscular junction and acts as a key to unlock **receptors** on the muscle fiber. This changes the permeability of the cell membrane and allows calcium ions to flow into the muscle fiber. Calcium ions cause the thin filaments (actin) to slide between the thick filaments (myosin), shortening the muscle and producing a muscle **contraction.** The muscle eventually relaxes when (1) acetylcholine is inactivated by an enzyme at the neuromuscular junction and (2) the calcium ions are pumped out of the cell.

Even when not actively moving, your muscles are in a state of mild, partial contraction because of nerve impulses from the brain and spinal cord. This produces muscle tone that keeps the muscles firm and ready to act. This is the only aspect of the skeletal muscle activity that is not under conscious control.

fascicle (FAS-ih-kl)

multinucleated (MUL-tee-NOO-klee-aa-ted)
multi- *many*
nucle/o- *nucleus*
-ated *pertaining to a condition; composed of*

myofibril (MY-oh-FY-bril)
my/o- *muscle*
fibr/o- *fiber*
-il *a thing*

neuromuscular (NYOOR-oh-MUS-kyoo-lar)
neur/o- *nerve*
muscul/o- *muscle*
-ar *pertaining to*

neurotransmitter (NYOOR-oh-TRANS-mit-er) (NYOOR-oh-trans-MIT-er)
neur/o- *nerve*
trans- *across, through*
mitt/o- *to send*
-er *person or thing that produces or does*

acetylcholine (AS-ee-til-KOH-leen)

receptor (ree-SEP-tor)
recept/o- *receive*
-or *person or thing that produces or does*

contraction (con-TRAK-shun)
contract/o- *pull together*
-ion *action; condition*

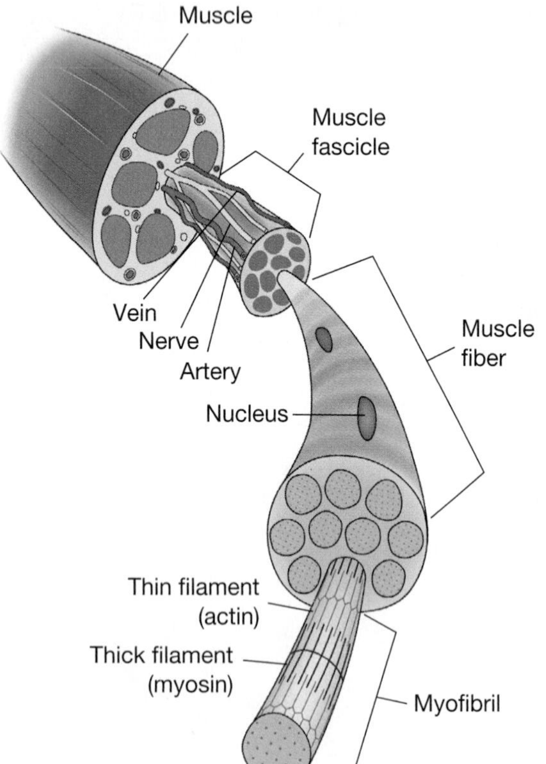

Figure 9-17 ■ Parts of a muscle.

A muscle is composed of many parts. The body of the muscle is composed of muscle fascicles. Around each fascicle are arteries, veins, and nerves. Each fascicle contains bundles of muscle fibers (muscle cells) that contain thin strands of actin and thick strands of myosin.

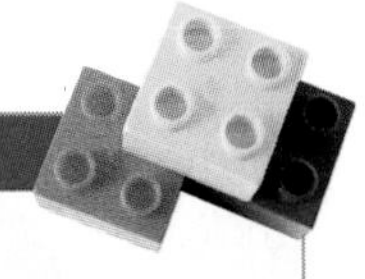

Connections

Sports Medicine. Professional athletes depend on their muscular systems to help them win competitions. The muscle cells/fibers of a marathon runner are different from those of a sprinter. Marathon runners have mostly slow-twitch muscle fibers that contract many times without becoming fatigued. Sprinters have fast-twitch fibers that contract very quickly and with intensity, but soon become tired. Because of the effects of testosterone, a male hormone, men have larger individual muscles than women and a bulkier body musculature, but vigourous weight training can increase the size of a muscle (**muscle hypertrophy**) in either sex. Bodybuilders work to enlarge, define, and sculpt their muscles (see Figure 9-18 ■). Some athletes try to enhance their performance with the use of illicit drugs, particularly anabolic steroids that add bulk to the muscles.

hypertrophy (hy-PER-troh-fee)
hyper- *above; more than normal*
-trophy *process of development*
Every medical word must contain a combining form. The suffix of *hypertrophy* contains the combining form *troph/o-*.

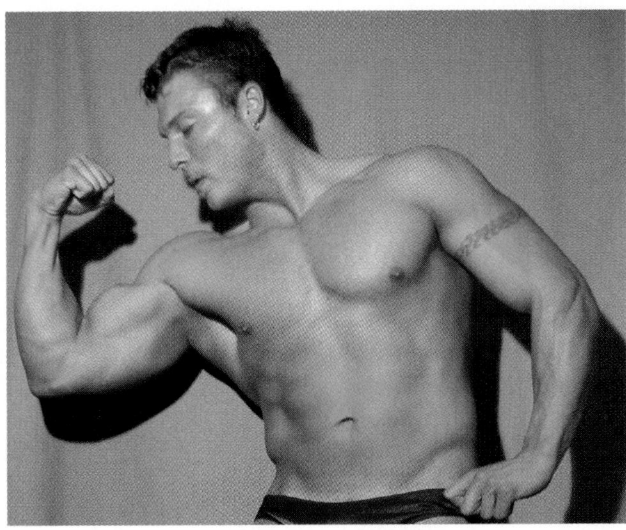

Figure 9-18 ■ Muscle strength and size.
Because of the effects of testosterone, a male hormone, men have larger individual muscles than women. This bodybuilder has highly developed muscles. Even the individual segments of the rectus abdominis muscles can be seen on either side of the umbilicus. The biceps brachii of his flexed right arm is impressive, and the pectoralis major muscles of the chest are enlarged and sculptured.

Vocabulary Review

Anatomy and Physiology

Now that you have studied the anatomy and physiology of the muscular system, take time to review those new words and descriptions. Memorize the combining forms and their definitions before going on to the next section.

Word or Phrase	Combining Form and Definition	Description
abduction	duct/o- *bring or move; a duct*	Moving a body part away from the midline. Opposite of adduction.
abductor	duct/o- *bring or move; a duct*	Muscle that produces abduction when it contracts
acetylcholine		Neurotransmitter that initiates muscle contraction
adduction	duct/o- *bring or move; a duct*	Moving a body part toward the midline. Opposite of abduction.
adductor	duct/o- *bring or move; a duct*	Muscle that produces adduction when it contracts
aponeurosis		Flat, wide, white sheet of fibrous connective tissue that attaches a muscle to a bone or other structure
belly of muscle		Area of greatest mass, usually in the center
biceps brachii muscle		Muscle of the upper arm that bends the upper arm toward the shoulder (flexion) and bends the lower arm toward the upper arm (flexion). One end is divided into two heads.
brachioradialis muscle	brachi/o- *arm* radi/o- *radius (forearm bone); x-rays; radiation*	Muscle of the lower arm that bends the lower arm toward the upper arm (flexion)
buccinator muscle	buccinat/o- *cheek*	Muscle in the cheek that produces sucking and moves food toward the tongue
bursa	burs/o- *bursa*	Fluid-filled sac that decreases friction where a tendon rubs against a bone near a synovial joint. It contains synovial fluid.
contraction	contract/o- *pull together*	Shortening of the length of all the muscle fibers and of the muscle itself. Opposite of relaxation.
deltoid muscle	delt/o- *triangle*	Muscle in the shoulder that raises and lowers the arm and moves the arm away from the body (abduction)
eversion	vers/o- *to travel; to turn*	Turning a body part outward and toward the side. Opposite of inversion.
evertor	vers/o- *to travel; to turn*	Muscle that produces eversion when it contracts
extension	extens/o- *straightening*	Straightening and extending a joint to increase the angle between two bones or two body parts. Opposite of flexion.
extensor	extens/o- *straightening*	Muscle that produces extension when it contracts

Word or Phrase	Combining Form and Definition	Description
extensor digitorum muscle	extens/o- *straightening*	Muscle that extends the fingers or toes
external oblique muscle	extern/o- *outside* intern/o- *inside*	Muscle of the abdomen that bends the upper body forward (flexion) and rotates it medially. Compresses the side of the abdominal wall. The **internal oblique muscle** lies directly beneath it and performs the same movements, but its muscle fibers are oriented in the opposite direction.
fascia	fasci/o- *fascia*	Thin connective tissue sheet around each muscle or groups of muscles. It merges into and becomes part of the tendon.
fascicle		A bundle composed of many muscle fibers surrounded by fascia
flexion	flex/o- *bending*	Bending of a joint to decrease the angle between two bones or two body parts. Opposite of extension.
flexor	flex/o- *bending*	Muscle that produces flexion when it contracts
flexor hallucis brevis muscle	flex/o- *bending*	Muscle that flexes the big toe
frontalis muscle	front/o- *front*	Muscle in the forehead that moves the forehead skin and eyebrows
gastrocnemius muscle		Muscle in the lower leg that bends the foot downward (plantar flexion)
gluteus maximus muscle		Muscle in the buttocks that moves the upper leg posteriorly and rotates it laterally
hamstrings		Group of muscles in the posterior aspect of the upper leg that moves the upper leg posteriorly and bends the lower leg toward the buttocks (flexion). Includes the biceps femoris, semitendinosus, and semimembranous muscles.
hypertrophy	troph/o- *development*	An increase in the size of a muscle
insertion	insert/o- *to put in or introduce*	Where a muscle ends on a bone that moves as the muscle contracts
intercostal muscles	cost/o- *rib*	Muscles of the chest that work in pairs to spread the ribs apart during inspiration and move the ribs together during expiration, coughing, and sneezing
inversion	vers/o- *to travel; to turn*	Turning a body part inward. Opposite of eversion.
invertor	vers/o- *to travel; to turn*	Muscle that produces inversion when it contracts
latissimus dorsi muscle		Muscle of the back that moves the arm posteriorly and medially toward the spinal column (adduction)
masseter muscle	masset/o- *chewing*	Muscle on the side of the face that moves the mandible upward
multinucleated	nucle/o- *nucleus*	Having many nuclei within one cell. A characteristic of skeletal muscle cells.
muscle	muscul/o- *muscle*	Many muscle fascicles grouped together and surrounded by fascia

Word or Phrase	Combining Form and Definition	Description
muscle fiber		One muscle cell. So named because it stretches over a long distance.
muscular system	musculo/o- *muscle*	Provides movement for the body in conjunction with support from the bones. Also known as the **musculoskeletal system.**
musculature	muscul/o- *muscle*	Group of skeletal muscles in one body part or the muscles in the body as a whole
myofibril	my/o- *muscle* fibr/o- *fiber*	Thin filament (actin) and thick filament (myosin) within the muscle fiber that give it its characteristic striated appearance
neuromuscular junction	neur/o- *nerve* muscul/o- *muscle*	Area on a single muscle fiber where a nerve connects to it
neurotransmitter	neur/o- *nerve* mitt/o- *to send*	Chemical messenger between nerves and muscles. Acetylcholine is the neurotransmitter released from a nerve to stimulate a muscle to contract.
orbicularis oculi muscle	orbicul/o- *small circle*	Muscle around the eye that closes the eyelids
orbicularis oris muscle	orbicul/o- *small circle*	Muscle around the mouth that closes the lips
origin		Where a muscle begins and is attached to a stationary or nearly stationary bone
pectoralis major muscle	pector/o- *chest*	Muscle of the chest that moves the arm anteriorly and medially across the chest (adduction)
peroneus longus muscle	perone/o- *fibula (lower leg bone)*	Muscle in the lower leg that moves the foot to the side (eversion) and bends the foot downward (plantar flexion)
platysma muscle		Muscle in the neck that moves the mandible down
pronation	pronat/o- *lying face down*	Turning the palm of the hand down. Opposite of supination.
pronator	pronat/o- *lying face down*	Muscle that produces pronation when it contracts
quadriceps femoris		Group of muscles in the anterior and lateral aspect of the upper leg that straightens the lower leg (extension). Includes the rectus femoris, vastus lateralis, vastus intermedius, and vastus medialis muscles.
receptor	recept/o- *receive*	Structure on the cell membrane of a muscle fiber. It interacts with a neurotransmitter from a nerve.
rectus abdominis muscle		Muscle of the abdomen that bends the upper body forward (flexion) and compresses the anterior abdominal wall
rectus femoris muscle		Muscle of the upper leg that bends the upper leg toward the abdomen (flexion) and straightens the lower leg (extension)
retinaculum		Thin, nearly translucent band of fibrous tissue and fascia that holds down extensor and flexor tendons that cross the wrist and ankle

Word or Phrase	Combining Form and Definition	Description
rotation	rotat/o- *rotate*	Moving a body part around its axis
rotator	rotat/o- *rotate*	Muscle that produces rotation when it contracts
sartorius muscle		Muscle of the upper leg that bends the upper leg toward the abdomen (flexion) and rotates it laterally
skeletal muscles	skelet/o- *skeleton* volunt/o- *done by one's own free will*	One of three types of muscles in the body, but the only muscles that are under **voluntary,** conscious control. Under the microscope, skeletal muscle has a striated appearance.
sternocleido-mastoid muscle	stern/o- *sternum (breast bone)* cleid/o- *clavicle (collar bone)* mast/o- *breast; mastoid process*	Muscle in the neck that bends the head toward the sternum (flexion) and turns the head to either side (rotation). Its origin is at two muscle heads on the sternum and clavicle. Its insertion is at the mastoid process of the temporal bone.
striated		Having stripes. This is a characteristic of skeletal muscle cells at the cellular level. The stripes are alternating strands of **actin** and **myosin.**
supination	supinat/o- *lying on the back*	Turning the palm of the hand upward. Opposite of pronation.
supinator	supinat/o- *lying on the back*	Muscle that produces supination when it contracts
temporalis muscle	tempor/o- *temple (side of the head)*	Muscle on the side of the head that moves the mandible upward and backward
tendon	tendin/o- *tendon*	Cordlike white band of nonelastic fibrous connective tissue that attaches a muscle to a bone
thenar muscles		Group of muscles in the hand that bends the thumb (flexion) and moves it toward the palm (adduction)
tibialis anterior muscle	tibi/o- *tibia (shin bone)*	Muscle in the lower leg that bends the foot up toward the leg (dorsiflexion)
trapezius muscle		Muscle of the shoulder that raises the shoulder, pulls the shoulder blades together, and elevates the clavicle. Turns the head from side to side (rotation). Moves the head posteriorly (extension).
triceps brachii muscle		Muscle of the upper arm that straightens the lower arm (extension). One end is divided into three heads.
voluntary muscle	volunt/o- *done by one's own free will*	Skeletal muscle. It contracts and relaxes in response to conscious thought.

Labeling Exercise

A. *Match each anatomy word or phrase to its numbered structure in Figure 9-19 ■. Write that word or phrase on the blank line next to its number. Use the Answer Key at the end of the book to check your answers.*

abduction and extension	flexion and adduction	slight flexion
flexion	rotation	

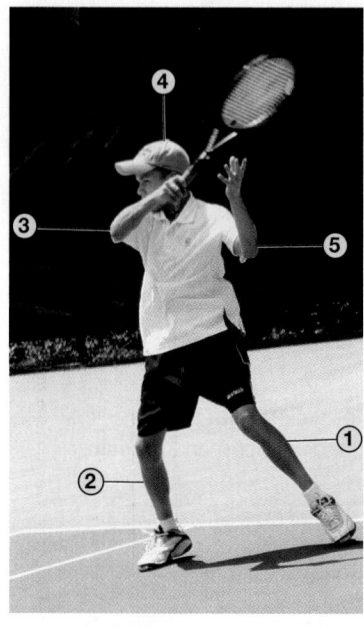

Figure 9-19 ■

1. ______________________
2. ______________________
3. ______________________
4. ______________________
5. ______________________

B. *Match each anatomy word or phrase to its numbered structure in Figure 9-20 ■. Write that word or phrase on the blank line next to its number.*

biceps brachii muscle	gluteus maximus muscle	peroneus longus muscle	tibialis anterior muscle
brachioradialis muscle	latissimus dorsi muscle	rectus abdominis muscle	trapezius muscle
deltoid muscle	masseter muscle	rectus femoris muscle	triceps brachii muscle
frontalis muscle	pectoralis major muscle	temporalis muscle	sternocleidomastoid muscle
gastrocnemius muscle			

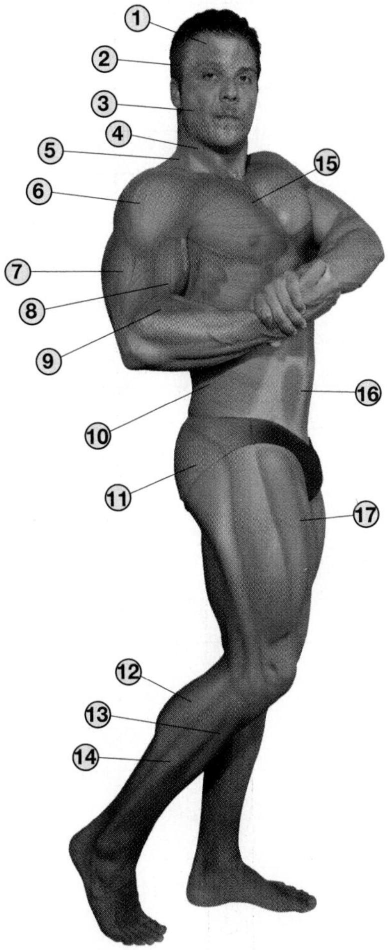

1. ______________________________
2. ______________________________
3. ______________________________
4. ______________________________
5. ______________________________
6. ______________________________
7. ______________________________
8. ______________________________
9. ______________________________
10. ______________________________
11. ______________________________
12. ______________________________
13. ______________________________
14. ______________________________
15. ______________________________
16. ______________________________
17. ______________________________

Figure 9-20 ■

Building Medical Words

Combining Forms

Here are the muscular combining forms you have learned so far. Next to each combining form, write its meaning. Use the Answer Key at the end of the book to check your answers. The first one has been done for you.

	Combining Form	Medical Meaning		Combining Form	Medical Meaning
1.	volunt/o-	done by one's own free will	22.	mitt/o-	
2.	anter/o-		23.	muscul/o-	
3.	brachi/o-		24.	my/o-	
4.	buccinat/o-		25.	neur/o-	
5.	burs/o-		26.	nucle/o-	
6.	cleid/o-		27.	orbicul/o-	
7.	contract/o-		28.	pector/o-	
8.	cost/o-		29.	perone/o-	
9.	delt/o-		30.	pronat/o-	
10.	duct/o-		31.	radi/o-	
11.	extens/o-		32.	recept/o-	
12.	extern/o-		33.	rotat/o-	
13.	fasci/o-		34.	stern/o-	
14.	fibr/o-		35.	supinat/o-	
15.	flex/o-		36.	tempor/o-	
16.	front/o-		37.	tendin/o-	
17.	gastr/o-		38.	tibi/o-	
18.	insert/o-		39.	troph/o-	
19.	intern/o-		40.	vers/o-	
20.	masset/o-		41.	vert/o-	
21.	mast/o-				

Combining Forms and Suffixes

Read the definition hint for the medical word you are to build. Look at the combining form that is given. Write the correct suffix on the blank line. Then write the medical word. (Remember: You may need to remove the combining vowel. Always remove the hyphens and slash.) Use the Answer Key at the end of the book to check your answers. The first one has been done for you.

SUFFIX LIST

-al (pertaining to)	-ature (system composed of)	-oid (resembling)
-ar (pertaining to)	-er (person or thing that produces or does)	-or (person or thing that produces or does)
-aris (pertaining to)	-ion (action; condition)	-ous (pertaining to)
-ary (pertaining to)		

	Definition Hint	Combining Form	Suffix	Write the Medical Word
1.	Thing that produces rotation	rotat/o-	-or	rotator
2.	Pertaining to a tendon	tendin/o-	________	________
3.	Pertaining to a muscle	muscul/o-	________	________
4.	Action of flexing	flex/o-	________	________
5.	Pertaining to the fascia	fasci/o-	________	________
6.	System composed of muscles	muscul/o-	________	________
7.	Resembling a triangle	delt/o-	________	________
8.	Pertaining to one's own free will	volunt/o-	________	________
9.	Thing that does chewing	masset/o-	________	________
10.	Pertaining to a small circle of muscle	orbicul/o-	________	________
11.	Pertaining to the chest muscle	pector/o-	________	________
12.	Thing that receives	recept/o-	________	________
13.	Action of lying the hand on its back	supinat/o-	________	________

Symptoms, Signs, and Diseases

Diseases of the Muscles

Word or Phrase	Word Part and Definition	Description
atrophy	**atrophy** (AT-roh-fee) **a-** *away from, without* **-trophy** *process of development* **atrophic** (ah-TROF-ik) **a-** *away from, without* **troph/o-** *development* **-ic** *pertaining to*	Loss of muscle bulk in one or more muscles. It can be caused by malnutrition or can occur in any part of the body that is paralyzed where the muscles receive no electrical impulses from the nerves. The muscles are said to be **atrophic.** Also known as muscle wasting. Treatment: Correct the underlying cause.
avulsion	**avulsion** (ah-VUL-shun) **a-** *away from, without* **vuls/o-** *to tear away* **-ion** *action; condition*	Muscle tears away from the tendon or the tendon tears away from the bone. Treatment: Surgical repair.
compartment syndrome		A severe blunt or crushing injury to the muscles of the leg can cause this syndrome. The enveloping fascia acts like a compartment, holding in blood as it accumulates. The increased pressure causes cellular death and nerve damage. Treatment: Fasciotomy to allow the blood and fluid to drain.
contracture	**contracture** (con-TRAK-choor) **contract/o-** *pull together* **-ure** *system; result of*	Inactivity or paralysis coupled with continuing nerve impulses causes an arm or leg to be progressively flexed and drawn into a position where it becomes nearly immovable. Treatment: Muscle relaxant drugs, range of motion (ROM) exercises. **Word Alert** **SOUND-ALIKE WORDS** **contraction** (noun) the normal tensing and shortening of a muscle in response to a nerve impulse *Example: After lifting a heavy box with a strong, sustained contraction of the arm muscles, it feels good to let the muscles relax.* **contracture** (noun) abnormal, fixed position in which the muscle is permanently flexed *Example: Contractures of the legs occur in bedridden nursing home patients who are not properly positioned and do not receive regular range of motion exercises.*
fibromyalgia	**fibromyalgia** (FY-broh-my-AL-jah) **fibr/o-** *fiber* **my/o-** *muscle* **alg/o-** *pain* **-ia** *condition, state, thing*	Pain located at specific, small trigger points along the neck, back, and hips. The trigger points are very tender to the touch and feel firm. Caused by injury or trauma. Fibromyalgia is associated with disturbed sleep patterns and sometimes depression. Treatment: Analgesic drugs, massage, and trigger point injections.

Word or Phrase	Word Part and Definition	Description
hyperextension-hyperflexion injury	**hyperextension** (HY-per-eks-TEN-shun) **hyper-** *above; more than normal* **extens/o-** *straightening* **-ion** *action; condition* **hyperflexion** (HY-per-FLEK-shun) **hyper-** *above; more than normal* **flex/o-** *bending* **-ion** *action; condition*	Injury that occurs during a car accident as a person's head snaps backward and then forward. This can cause muscle strain or a muscle tear, as well as damage to the nerves. Also known as acceleration-deceleration injury or whiplash. Treatment: Rest, analgesic drugs, nonsteroidal anti-inflammatory drugs.
muscle contusion	**contusion** (con-TOO-shun) **contus/o-** *bruising* **-ion** *action; condition*	A blunt trauma that causes bleeding in the muscle but does not break the skin. Also known as a bruise. Treatment: Analgesic drugs.
muscle spasm	**spasm** (SPAZM)	Painful but temporary condition with a sudden, severe, involuntary, and prolonged contraction of a muscle, usually in the legs. Often brought on by overexercise. Also known as a muscle cramp. Treatment: None.
muscle strain	**strain** (STRAYN) **inflammation** (IN-flah-MAY-shun) **inflammat/o-** *redness and warmth* **-ion** *action; condition*	Overstretching of a muscle, often due to physical overexertion. This causes **inflammation,** pain, swelling, and bruising as capillaries in the muscle tear. There can be small tears in the muscle fibers. Also known as a pulled muscle. Treatment: Rest, analgesic drugs.
muscular dystrophy	**dystrophy** (DIS-troh-fee) **dys-** *painful, difficult, abnormal* **-trophy** *process of development* Every medical word must contain a combining form. The suffix of *dystrophy* contains the combining form *troph/o-*. **Duchenne** (doo-SHAYN) Named by Guillaume Duchenne (1806–1875), a French neurologist. This is an example of an eponym: a person from whom something takes its name.	Genetic inherited disease due to a mutation of the gene that makes the muscle protein dystrophin. Without dystrophin, the muscles weaken and then atrophy. Symptoms appear in early childhood as weakness in the lower extremities and then in the upper extremities (see Figure 9-21 ■). The most common and most severe form is **Duchenne's muscular dystrophy;** Becker's muscular dystrophy is a milder form. Weakness of the diaphragm muscle and inability to breathe is the most frequent cause of death. Treatment: Supportive care. 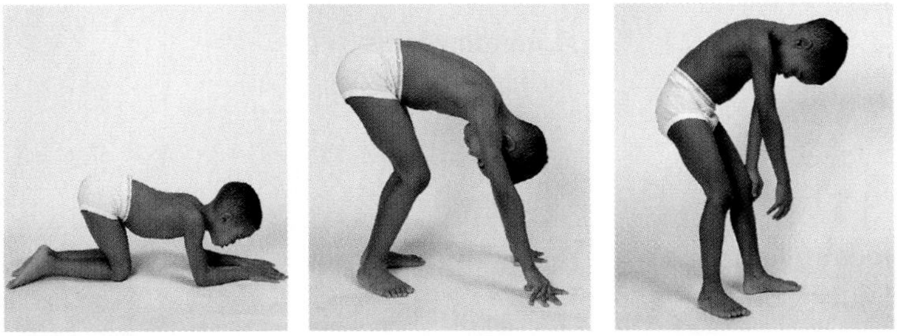 **Figure 9-21 ■ Muscular dystrophy.** Weakness of the muscles in the legs causes this patient with muscular dystrophy to stand up in a way that is characteristic of this disease. The legs and arms must work together to raise the body. Because muscular dystrophy is a progressive disease, this patient soon may not be able to walk at all.

Word or Phrase	Word Part and Definition	Description
myalgia	**myalgia** (my-AL-jee-ah) (my-AL-jah) **my/o-** *muscle* **alg/o-** *pain* **-ia** *condition, state, thing* **polymyalgia** (PAWL-ee-my-AL-jee-ah) (PAWL-ee-my-AL-jah) **poly-** *many, much* **alg/o-** *pain* **-ia** *condition, state, thing*	Pain in one or more muscles due to injury or muscle disease. **Polymyalgia** is pain in several muscle groups. Treatment: Analgesic drugs, massage.
myasthenia gravis	**myasthenia gravis** (MY-as-THEE-nee-ah GRAV-is) **my/o-** *muscle* **a-** *away from, without* **sthen/o-** *strength* **-ia** *condition, state, thing* **ptosis** (TOH-sis) *Ptosis* is a Greek word meaning *a falling.*	Abnormal and rapid fatigue of the muscles, particularly evident in the muscles of the face; there is **ptosis** of the eyelids. Symptoms worsen during the day and can be relieved by rest. The body produces antibodies against its own acetylcholine receptors located on muscle fibers. The antibodies destroy many of the receptors. There are normal levels of acetylcholine, but too few receptors remain to produce sustained muscle contractions. Treatment: Drugs that prolong the action of acetylcholine.
myopathy	**myopathy** (my-AWP-ah-thee) **my/o-** *muscle* **-pathy** *disease, suffering*	Category that includes many different diseases of the muscles. Treatment: Correct the underlying cause.
myositis	**myositis** (MY-oh-SY-tis) **myos/o-** *muscle* **-itis** *inflammation of* **polymyositis** (PAWL-ee-MY-oh-SY-tis) **poly-** *many, much* **myos/o-** *muscle* **-itis** *inflammation of* **dermatomyositis** (DER-mah-toh-MY-oh-SY-tis) **dermat/o-** *skin* **myos/o-** *muscle* **-itis** *inflammation of*	Inflammation of a muscle with localized swelling and tenderness. Can be caused by injury or strain. **Polymyositis** is a chronic, progressive disease that causes widespread inflammation of muscles with weakness and fatigue. The cause is unknown, although it may be an autoimmune disease. **Dermatomyositis** causes a skin rash as well as muscle weakness and inflammation. Treatment: Corticosteroid drugs, analgesic drugs.
repetitive strain injury (RSI)		Condition affecting the muscles, tendons, and sometimes the nerves. It occurs as a result of trauma due to repetitious movements over an extended period of time. Includes tennis elbow, carpal tunnel syndrome, and other disorders. Also known as cumulative trauma disorder (CTD). Treatment: Rest, analgesic drugs, nonsteroidal anti-inflammatory drugs. **Did You Know?** The Occupational Safety and Health Administration (OSHA) educates healthcare professionals about workplace-related injuries, including repetitive strain disorder. The most common causes are muscle overexertion from lifting, carrying, pulling, or pushing something heavy or not using proper body mechanics.

Word or Phrase	Word Part and Definition	Description
rhabdomyoma	**rhabdomyoma** (RAB-doh-my-OH-mah) **rhabd/o-** *rod shaped* **my/o-** *muscle* **-oma** *tumor, mass* The immature muscle cells in this tumor are shaped like a rod. **benign** (bee-NINE) *Benign* is derived from a Latin word meaning *kind, not cancerous.*	**Benign** tumor that arises from striated muscle tissue. Treatment: Surgical excision.
rhabdomyo-sarcoma	**rhabdomyosarcoma** (RAB-doh-MY-oh-sar-KOH-mah) **rhabd/o-** *rod shaped* **my/o-** *muscle* **sarc/o-** *connective tissue* **-oma** *tumor, mass* **malignancy** (mah-LIG-nan-see) **malign/o-** *intentionally causing harm; cancer* **-ancy** *state of*	Cancerous tumor that arises from muscle tissue. This **malignancy** usually occurs in children and young adults. Treatment: Surgical excision, chemotherapy, and radiation therapy.
rotator cuff tear		Tear in the rotator muscles of the shoulder that surround the head of the humerus. These muscles help to abduct the arm. The tear can result from acute or cumulative trauma and overuse. Treatment: Surgical repair.
torticollis	**torticollis** (TOR-tih-KOL-is) **tort/i-** *twisted position* **-collis** *condition of the neck* *Wry* is an English word meaning *distorted or lopsided.*	Painful contraction of the muscles on one side of the neck. It is also known as **wryneck.** Treatment: Massage, muscle relaxant drugs, analgesic drugs.

Connections

rigor mortis (RIG-or MOR-tis)
Rigor is a Latin word meaning *stiffness. Mortis* is a Latin word meaning *of death.*

Forensic Science. Rigor mortis is not a muscle disease of the living, but rather a normal condition of the muscles that occurs several hours after death. As the muscle fibers die, the permeability of the cell membrane changes and calcium ions enter the cells. This causes all the muscles of the body to contract. Because the cell is dead, it can no longer pump out calcium ions and so the muscles remain contracted for about 72 hours until the cell begins to decompose. Forensic scientists use rigor mortis to help determine the time of death.

Movement Disorders

Word or Phrase	Word Part and Definition	Description
ataxia	**ataxia** (ah-TAK-see-ah) a- *away from, without* tax/o- *coordination* -ia *condition, state, thing* **ataxic** (ah-TAK-sik) a- *away from, without* tax/o- *coordination* -ic *pertaining to*	Incoordination of the muscles during movement, particularly the gait. Caused by diseases of the brain or spinal cord, cerebral palsy, or an adverse reaction to a drug. The patient is said to be **ataxic.** Treatment: Correct the underlying cause. Leg braces or crutches, if needed.
bradykinesia	**bradykinesia** (BRAD-ee-kin-EE-zee-ah) brady- *slow* kines/o- *movement* -ia *condition, state, thing*	Abnormally slow muscle movements or a decrease in the number of spontaneous muscle movements. Usually associated with Parkinson's disease, a neurological disease of the brain. Treatment: Drugs for Parkinson's disease.
dyskinesia	**dyskinesia** (DIS-kih-NEE-zee-ah) dys- *painful, difficult, abnormal* kines/o- *movement* -ia *condition, state, thing* **myoclonus** (MY-oh-KLOH-nus) my/o- *muscle* -clonus *condition of rapid contracting and relaxing* **athetoid** (ATH-eh-toyd) athet/o- *without position or place* -oid *resembling*	Abnormal motions due to difficulty controlling the voluntary muscles. Attempts at movement turn into tics, muscle spasms, muscle jerking (**myoclonus**), or slow, wandering, purposeless writhing of the hand, (**athetoid movements**) in which some muscles of the fingers are flexed and others are extended. Associated with neurological disorders (Parkinson's disease, Huntington's chorea, cerebral palsy). Treatment: Correct the underlying cause. **Connections** **Neurology (Chapter 10).** Cerebral palsy is caused by a lack of oxygen to parts of the baby's brain before or during birth. The extent of the symptoms varies, but can include spastic muscles; dyskinesia; lack of coordination in walking, eating, and talking; and even muscle paralysis.
hyperkinesis	**hyperkinesis** (HY-per-kih-NEE-sis) hyper- *above; more than normal* -kinesis *condition of movement*	An abnormally increased amount of muscle movements. Restlessness. Can be a side effect of some drugs. Treatment: Correct the underlying cause.
tremor	**tremor** (TREM-or) *Tremor* is a Latin word meaning *a shaking.* **tremulous** (TREM-yoo-lus) tremul/o- *shaking* -ous *pertaining to*	Small, involuntary, sometimes jerky, back-and-forth movements of the hands, neck, jaw, or extremities. These are continuous movements that cannot be suppressed by the patient. The patient is said to be **tremulous.** Usually associated with essential familial tremor. Treatment: Beta-blocker drugs.

Word or Phrase	Word Part and Definition	Description
restless legs syndrome		Uncomfortable restlessness and twitching of the muscles of the legs, particularly the calf muscles, along with an indescribable tingling, aching, or crawling-insect sensation. The symptoms occur mainly at night and can become severe enough to prevent sleep. The exact cause of this disorder is unknown. Treatment: Tranquilizer drugs, although they are not always effective.
Diseases of the Tendon, Bursa, or Fascia		
bursitis	**bursitis** (ber-SY-tis) **burs/o-** *bursa* **-itis** *inflammation of*	Inflammation of the bursal sac because of repetitive muscular activity or pressure on the bone underneath the bursa. Can occur in any joint that has a bursa, but most often occurs in the shoulders and knees. Prolonged periods of kneeling cause bursitis known as housemaid's knee. Treatment: Rest, analgesic drugs, nonsteroidal anti-inflammatory drugs.
Dupuytren's contracture	**Dupuytren** (DOO-pyoo-tren) Dupuytren's contracture was named for Guillaume Dupuytren (1770–1835), a French surgeon. This is an example of an eponym: a person from whom something takes its name.	Progressive disease in which the fascia of the palm of the hand becomes thickened and shortened, causing a contracture and flexion deformity of the fingers. Treatment: Surgery.
ganglion	**ganglion** (GANG-glee-on) *Ganglion* is a Greek word meaning *swelling or knot.*	Semisolid or fluid-containing cyst that develops on a tendon, often on the wrist, hand, or foot. A ganglion is clearly visible as a rounded lump under the skin that may or may not be painful (see Figure 9-22 ■). Treatment: Needle aspiration of fluid from the ganglion or ganglionectomy. **Figure 9-22 ■ Ganglion.** This patient has a semisolid ganglion on the extensor tendon of the digit. Even after a ganglionectomy to remove it, it may recur.
golfer's elbow		Inflammation and pain of the flexor and pronator muscles of the forearm where their tendons originate on the medial epicondyle of the humerus by the elbow joint. An overuse injury caused by repeated motions where the wrist flexes and the fingers tightly grasp. Also known as pitcher's elbow or medial epicondylitis. Treatment: Rest, analgesic drugs, nonsteroidal anti-inflammatory drugs.

Word or Phrase	Word Part and Definition	Description
shin splints		Pain and inflammation of the tendons of the flexor muscles of the lower leg over the anterior tibia (shin bone). An overuse injury common to athletes who run. Treatment: Rest, analgesic drugs, nonsteroidal anti-inflammatory drugs.
tendonitis	**tendonitis** (TEN-dih-NY-tis) **tendon/o-** *tendon* **-itis** *inflammation of* *Tendinitis* is also an acceptable spelling.	Inflammation of any tendon from injury or overuse. Treatment: Rest, analgesic drugs, nonsteroidal anti-inflammatory drugs.
tennis elbow		Inflammation and pain of the extensor and supinator muscles where their tendons originate on the lateral epicondyle of the humerus by the elbow joint. Also known as lateral epicondylitis. An overuse injury caused by repeated extension and supination of the wrist. Treatment: Rest, analgesic drugs, nonsteroidal anti-inflammatory drugs.
tenosynovitis	**tenosynovitis** (TEN-oh-SIN-oh-VY-tis) **ten/o-** *tendon* **synov/o-** *synovium (membrane)* **-itis** *inflammation of*	Inflammation and pain due to overuse of the tendon and inability of the tendon sheath to produce enough lubricating fluid. Treatment: Rest, analgesic drugs, nonsteroidal anti-inflammatory drugs.

Diagnostic Procedures

Blood Tests

Word or Phrase	Word Part and Definition	Description
acetylcholine receptor antibodies	**antibody** (AN-tee-BAWD-ee) (AN-tih-BAWD-ee) **anti-** *against* **-body** *a structure or thing*	Blood test for myasthenia gravis. It detects antibodies that the body has formed against its own acetylcholine receptors.
creatine phosphokinase (CPK-MM)	**creatine phosphokinase** (KREE-ah-teen FAWS-foh-KY-nays)	Blood test to measure the level of serum CPK-MM, an isoenzyme found in the muscles. High levels of CPK-MM are present in various diseases, particularly muscular dystrophy, in which muscle tissue is being destroyed.

Muscle Tests

Word or Phrase	Word Part and Definition	Description
electromyography (EMG)	**electromyography** (ee-LEK-troh-my-AWG-rah-fee) **electr/o-** *electricity* **my/o-** *muscle* **-graphy** *process of recording* **electromyogram** (ee-LEK-troh-MY-oh-gram) **electr/o-** *electricity* **my/o-** *muscle* **-gram** *a record or picture*	Diagnostic procedure to diagnose muscle disease or nerve damage. A needle electrode inserted into a muscle records electrical activity as the muscle contracts and relaxes. The electrical activity is displayed as waveforms on a screen and permanently recorded on paper as an **electromyogram.**
Tensilon test	**Tensilon** (TEN-sih-lawn)	Diagnostic procedure in which the drug Tensilon is given to confirm a diagnosis of myasthenia gravis. The drug blocks the enzyme that breaks down acetylcholine, and patients with myasthenia gravis show increased muscle strength.

Medical and Surgical Procedures

Medical Procedures

Word or Phrase	Word Part and Definition	Description
braces and adaptive devices		Orthopedic device that supports a body part with weak muscles. It keeps it in anatomical alignment while still permitting movement (see Figure 9-23 ■). An adaptive or assistive device is one that increases mobility or independence by helping the physically challenged patient to perform activities of daily living (ADLs). Examples of adaptive devices include a grasper to extend the reach, spoons that can be attached to the wrist, and pens with extra-large barrels.

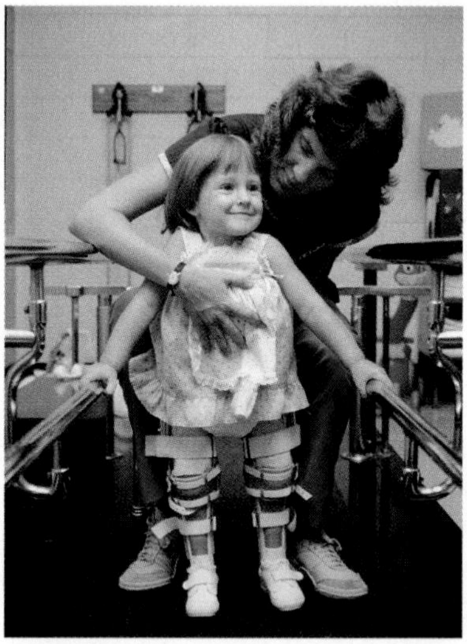

Figure 9-23 ■ Braces.
Braces provide support and stability when the muscles are weak or uncoordinated. The physical therapist is assisting this young child to walk with leg braces that are held on by Velcro straps.

Did You Know?

The Americans with Disabilities Act (ADA) of 1990 is a federal law that prohibits discrimination against disabled persons. It provides guidelines and requirements for accommodating persons with disabilities at work and in public buildings and transportation.

Instead of *handicapped person,* the correct phrase is *physically challenged person.*

Word or Phrase	Word Part and Definition	Description
deep tendon reflexes (DTR)	**reflex** (REE-fleks)	Tapping briskly on a tendon causes an involuntary, automatic contraction of the muscle connected to that tendon (see Figure 9-24 ■). This tests whether the muscular-nervous pathway is functioning normally. This test can be done in several places, but the most common site is at the knee. Also known as the **knee jerk** or **patellar reflex.** **Figure 9-24 ■ Deep tendon reflex.** A percussion hammer with a rubber triangular mallet is used to tap just below the patella on the combined tendons of the quadriceps femoris muscle group. A normal response is a sudden involuntary contraction of the muscles that briskly extends the lower leg. The response in both legs is tested and compared. **Word Alert** **SOUND-ALIKE WORDS** **reflex** (noun) involuntary automatic response of the muscular-nervous pathway *Example: The patient's knee jerk reflexes were equal and symmetrical bilaterally.* **reflux** (noun) backward flowing of fluid *Example: Acid reflux from the stomach can cause inflammation and ulcers in the esophagus.*
muscle strength test	**motor** (MOH-tor) mot/o- *movement* -or *person or thing that produces or does*	Medical procedure used to test the strength of certain muscle groups. For muscles in the legs and feet, the physician presses against the lower leg or foot and asks the patient to extend the leg or flex the foot upward. For shoulder muscles, the physician presses down and the patient tries to shrug the shoulders. For muscles in the hand, the patient grasps two of the physician's fingers and squeezes them as tightly as possible. Muscle strength or **motor strength** is measured on a scale of 5, with 5 being normal strength and 0 being the inability to move the muscles being tested.

Word or Phrase	Word Part and Definition	Description
rehabilitation exercises	**rehabilitation** (REE-hah-BIL-ih-TAY-shun) **re-** *again and again; backward; unable to* **habilitat/o-** *give ability* **-ion** *action; condition* For *rehabilitation,* the best meaning of the prefix *re-* is *again and again.* Rehabilitation is a continuing process of exercises that are repeated again and again.	Physical therapy procedure that includes exercises to increase muscle strength and improve coordination and balance, prescribed as part of a rehabilitation plan. In active exercise, the patient exercises without assistance (see Figure 9-25■). In passive exercise, the physical therapist or nurse performs range of motion (ROM) exercises for a patient who is unable to move. This does not build muscle strength, but it decreases stiffness and spasticity and prevents contractures. 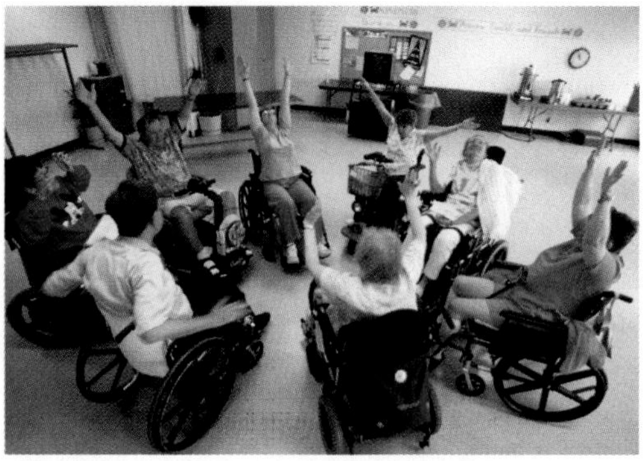 **Figure 9-25 ■ Active exercise.** These patients are part of a friendly and supportive physical therapy group. Even patients confined to wheelchairs benefit from regular exercise.
trigger point injections		Medical procedure to treat fibromyalgia and myofascial pain syndrome. A local anesthetic and a corticosteroid drug are injected into each trigger point to relieve pain and decrease inflammation.
Surgical Procedures		
fasciectomy	**fasciectomy** (FASH-ee-EK-toh-mee) **fasci/o-** *fascia* **-ectomy** *surgical excision*	Surgical procedure to partially or totally remove the fascia causing Dupuytren's contracture.
fasciotomy	**fasciotomy** (FASH-ee-AWT-oh-mee) **fasci/o-** *fascia* **-tomy** *process of cutting or making an incision*	Surgical procedure to cut the fascia and release pressure from built up blood and tissue fluid in patients with compartment syndrome.
ganglionectomy	**ganglionectomy** (GANG-glee-oh-NEK-toh-mee) **ganglion/o-** *ganglion* **-ectomy** *surgical excision*	Surgical procedure to remove a ganglion from a tendon.
muscle biopsy	**biopsy** (BY-awp-see) **bi/o-** *life; living organisms; living tissue* **-opsy** *the process of viewing* **incisional** (in-SIZH-un-al) **incis/o-** *to cut into* **-ion** *action; condition* **-al** *pertaining to*	Surgical procedure that is performed to make a definitive diagnosis when muscle weakness could be caused by many different muscular diseases. An incision is made into the muscle and a piece of tissue is removed; this is known as an **incisional biopsy** or open biopsy. Alternatively, a needle is inserted and some tissue is aspirated through the needle. This is known as a closed biopsy.

Word or Phrase	Word Part and Definition	Description
myorrhaphy	**myorrhaphy** (my-OR-ah-fee) **my/o-** *muscle* **-rrhaphy** *procedure of suturing*	Surgical procedure to suture together the torn ends of a muscle following an injury.
tenorrhaphy	**tenorrhaphy** (teh-NOR-ah-fee) **ten/o-** *tendon* **-rrhaphy** *procedure of suturing*	Surgical procedure to suture together the torn ends of a tendon following an injury.
thymectomy	**thymectomy** (thy-MEK-toh-mee) **thym/o-** *thymus; rage* **-ectomy** *surgical excision* For *thymectomy,* the best meaning of the combining form *thym/o-* is *thymus.*	Surgical excision of the thymus gland. Used to treat patients with myasthenia gravis. After a thymectomy, the patient produces fewer antibodies against acetylcholine receptors.

Drug Categories

Several different categories of drugs are used to treat the symptoms, signs, and diseases of the muscular system. The most common drugs in each category are listed.

Category	Word Part and Definition	Description	Example
analgesic drugs	**analgesic** (AN-al-JEE-zik) **an-** *without, not* **alges/o-** *sensation of pain* **-ic** *pertaining to*	Over-the-counter aspirin and non-aspirin drugs used to decrease inflammation and pain. Used to treat minor injuries, muscle strains, tendonitis, bursitis, and overuse.	Bayer aspirin, Ecotrin, Tylenol
beta-blocker drugs		Block the action of epinephrine to suppress essential familial tremor.	Inderal
chemotherapy drugs	**chemotherapy** (KEE-moh-THAIR-ah-pee) **chem/o-** *chemical, drug* **-therapy** *treatment*	Kill rapidly dividing cancer cells in the muscles.	Adriamycin, VePesid
corticosteroid drugs	**corticosteroid** (KOR-tih-koh-STAIR-oyd) **cortic/o-** *cortex (outer region)* **-steroid** *steroid*	Suppress inflammation. Given orally or intravenously.	hydrocortisone, Medrol, prednisone, Solu-Medrol
muscle relaxant drugs	**relaxant** (ree-LAK-sant) **relax/o-** *relax* **-ant** *pertaining to*	Relieve muscle spasm and stiffness. Used to treat muscle strains. Also used to treat muscle spasms in patients with multiple sclerosis, cerebral palsy, and stroke.	Flexeril, Parafon Forte, Soma

Category	Word Part and Definition	Description	Example
nonsteroidal anti-inflammatory drugs (NSAIDs)	**nonsteroidal** (non-stair-OY-dal) **non-** *not* **steroid/o-** *steroid* **-al** *pertaining to* **anti-inflammatory** (AN-tee-in-FLAM-ah-TOR-ee) **anti-** *against* **inflammat/o-** *redness and warmth* **-ory** *having the function of*	Suppress inflammation and decrease pain. Used to treat minor injuries, muscle strains, tendonitis, bursitis, and overuse.	ibuprofen, Motrin, Orudis KT
neuromuscular blocker drugs	**neuromuscular** (NYOOR-oh-MUS-kyoo-lar) **neur/o-** *nerve* **muscul/o-** *muscle* **-ar** *pertaining to*	Block nerve impulses to muscles. Used during surgery to produce muscle relaxation, particularly during certain kinds of abdominal surgery to provide visualization of the organs in the abdominal cavity.	Tracrium

Across the Life Span

intramuscular (IN-trah-MUS-kyoo-lar)
intra- *within*
muscul/o- *muscle*
-ar *pertaining to*

injection (in-JEK-shun)
inject/o- *insert or put in*
-ion *action; condition*

Some drugs are administered by **intramuscular (IM) injection.** Intramuscular injections are given in a muscle that is large enough that the needle will not accidentally injure a nerve. In adults, these sites include the deltoid muscle (lateral upper arm), the vastus lateralis (anterolateral thigh), the gluteus medius muscle (lateral hip), and the gluteus maximus (upper outer quadrant of the buttocks). In infants, the only suitable site for an intramuscular injection is in the anterolateral thigh (see Figure 9-26■).

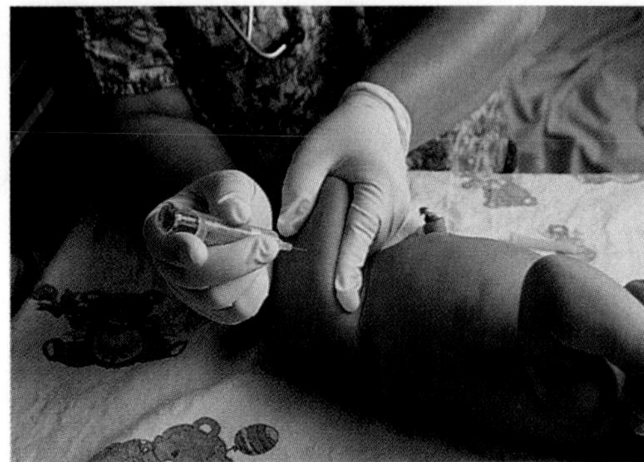

Figure 9-26 ■ Intramuscular injection.
The thigh muscles are the largest muscles in a baby's body, and infant immunizations are injected there.

Abbreviations

ADA	Americans with Disabilities Act
ADLs	activities of daily living
COTA	certified occupational therapy assistant
CPK-MM	creatine phosphokinase (MM bands)
CTD	cumulative trauma disorder
DTRs	deep tendon reflexes
EMG	electromyography
IM	intramuscular
LLE	left lower extremity
LUE	left upper extremity
MD	muscular dystrophy
NSAID	nonsteroidal anti-inflammatory drug
OOB	out of bed
ortho	orthopedics (slang)
OSHA	Occupational Safety and Health Administration
OT	occupational therapy/therapist
PM&R	physical medicine and rehabilitation
PT	physical therapy/therapist
rehab	rehabilitation (slang)
RLE	right lower extremity
ROM	range of motion
RUE	right upper extremity
RSI	repetitive strain injury

Word Alert

ABBREVIATIONS

Abbreviations are commonly used in all types of medical documentation; however, they can mean different things to different people and their meaning can be misinterpreted. Always verify the meaning of an abbreviation.

ADA stands for *Americans with Disabilities Act,* but it can also stand for *American Diabetes Association, American Dental Association,* or *American Dietetic Association.*

MD stands for *muscular dystrophy,* but it can also stand for *macular degeneration* or *doctor of medicine (M.D.).*

ROM stands for *range of motion,* but it can also stand for *rupture of membranes* (prior to delivery of a baby).

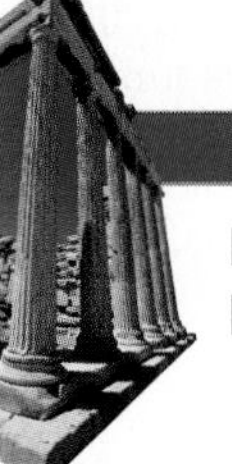

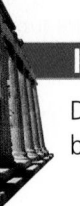

It's Greek to Me!

Did you notice that some muscular words have two different combining forms? Combining forms from both Greek and Latin languages remain a part of medical language today.

English Word	Greek	Latin	Examples of Medical Words
muscle	my/o-	muscul/o-	fibromyalgia, muscular
tendon	ten/o-	tendin/o-	tenorrhaphy, tendinous

Career Focus

Osteopaths, doctors of **osteopathy** (D.O.), can diagnose and treat any patient that an orthopedist with an M.D. can treat, but they base their treatment on osteopathy, the study of how to prevent and treat diseases by using proper nutrition and keeping the body structures in a normal anatomical relationship.

Chiropractors, doctors of **chiropractic** (D.C.), diagnose and treat patients with injuries involving the bones, muscles, and nerves by manipulating the alignment of the vertebral column.

Podiatrists, doctors of **podiatric medicine** (D.P.M.), diagnose and treat medical and surgical conditions of the foot. This medical specialty is known as **podiatry.**

Physiatrists are physicians who specialize in physical medicine and rehabilitation. **Physiatry** is the medical specialty that diagnoses and treats musculoskeletal diseases and acute and chronic pain by using the physical properties of cold, heat, light, and water in conjunction with exercise and some drugs. It is also known as the field of **physical medicine and rehabilitation (PM&R).** Sports medicine encompasses the prevention, treatment, and rehabilitation of musculoskeletal injuries from sports, as well as athletic training and endurance, biomechanics, nutrition, and psychology. A physician (D.O. or M.D.) can take additional training and become board certified in physical medicine and rehabilitation or in sports medicine.

Massage therapists are allied health professionals who use pressure and manipulation of the muscles and soft tissues to relieve stress and prevent or treat muscular injuries. Massage therapists work in athletic clubs, resorts, salons, chiropractic or orthopedic offices or their own private offices.

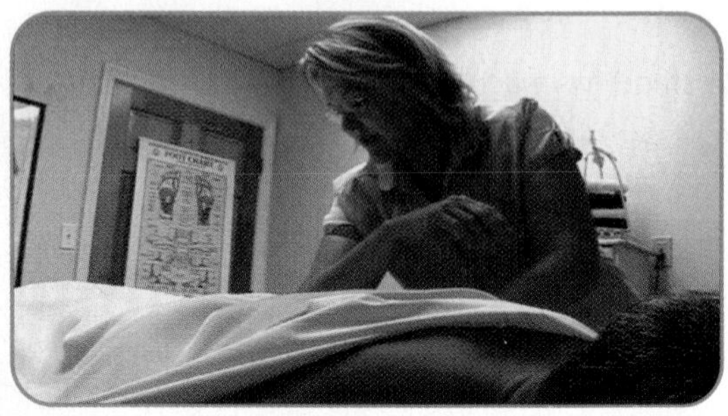

Meet Iris, a massage therapist.

"I became a massage therapist because I wanted to help people. I get to see clients that I can honestly say I enjoy and to see the progress of them, physically—and emotionally, sometimes—is very rewarding. Massage therapy is basically known for its relaxation qualities, but more and more people are understanding that it increases circulation, increases range of motion, and reduces pain. I personally use a lot of medical terminology. I use the names of muscles—origins and insertions. The education involved with massage therapy begins with intense anatomy and physiology. There's a lot of ethics training, a lot of training in dealing with people."

osteopath (AW-stee-oh-path)
oste/o- *bone*
-path *disease, suffering*

osteopathy (AWS-tee-AWP-ah-thee)
oste/o- *bone*
-pathy *disease, suffering*

chiropractor (KY-roh-PRAK-tor)
chir/o- *hand*
pract/o- *medical practice*
-or *person or thing that produces or does*
Add words to make a correct and complete definition of *chiropractor: Person who does [manipulation and alignment of the body by using the] hands [to perform] medical practice.*

chiropractic (KY-roh-PRAK-tic)
chir/o- *hand*
pract/o- *medical practice*
-ic *pertaining to*

podiatrist (poh-DY-ah-trist)
pod/o- *foot*
iatr/o- *physician; treatment*
-ist *one who specializes in*

podiatric (POH-dee-AT-rik)
pod/o- *foot*
iatr/o- *physician; treatment*
-ic *pertaining to*

podiatry (poh-DY-ah-tree)
pod/o- *foot*
-iatry *medical treatment*

physiatrist (fiz-EYE-ah-trist) (FIZ-ee-AT-rist)
physi/o- *physical function*
iatr/o- *physician; medical treatment*
-ist *one who specializes in*

physiatry (fih-ZY-ah-tree) (FIZ-ee-AT-ree)
physi/o- *physical function*
-iatry *medical treatment*

rehabilitation (REE-hah-BIL-ih-TAY-shun)
re- *again and again; backward; unable to*
habilitat/o- *give ability*
-ion *action; condition*

therapist (THAIR-ah-pist)
therap/o- *treatment*
-ist *one who specializes in*

CHAPTER REVIEW EXERCISES

Review all the material in this chapter by completing the review exercises in this section. Use the Answer Key at the end of the book to check your answers.

Anatomy and Physiology

Matching Exercise

Match each muscle to its location in the body. Some locations will be used more than once.

1.	deltoid muscle	_____ Head and neck
2.	biceps brachii muscle	_____ Shoulders
3.	tibialis anterior muscle	_____ Chest
4.	rectus femoris muscle	_____ Abdomen
5.	trapezius muscle	_____ Back
6.	sternocleidomastoid muscle	_____ Arms
7.	biceps femoris muscle	_____ Buttocks
8.	gastrocnemius muscle	_____ Legs
9.	gluteus maximus muscle	
10.	masseter muscle	
11.	pectoralis major muscle	
12.	rectus abdominis muscle	
13.	latissimus dorsi muscle	

Circle Exercise

Circle the correct word from the choices given.

1. The (**belly, insertion, origin**) is where the muscle is attached to a stationary bone.
2. The (**aponeurosis, bursa, fascia**) is a flat, wide, white sheet of fibrous connective tissue that attaches a muscle to a bone.
3. The (**muscle, musculature, musculus**) is a group of muscles in one body part.
4. Skeletal muscle is (**involuntary, nonstriated, striated**).
5. Myofibrils are (**small fibrous muscles, thin and thick filaments, types of nuclei**).
6. Hallux means (**big toe, short in length, three**).
7. The (**deltoid, pectoralis, rectus**) muscle is shaped like a triangle.
8. The prefix (**bi-, quadri-, tri-**) means *three.*

Matching Exercise

Match each numbered word or phrase to its description.

1. striated	_____ Sheet of fibrous tissue that holds muscle to bone
2. muscle fiber	_____ Beginning of a muscle
3. origin	_____ Several muscle fibers
4. tendon	_____ Fibrous cord that holds muscle to bone
5. aponeurosis	_____ A neurotransmitter
6. fascia	_____ A single cell in a muscle
7. fascicle	_____ Thin connective tissue wrapped around a muscle
8. acetylcholine	_____ Characteristic of skeletal muscle

Recall and Describe

In your own words, describe what happens when the stated action occurs to the body part given below.

1. Abduction of the arm ____________________
2. Extension of the knee ____________________
3. Pronation of the hand ____________________
4. Rotation of the head ____________________
5. Flexion of the knee ____________________
6. Dorsiflexion of the foot ____________________

Matching Exercise

Match each numbered word or phrase to its description.

1. acetylcholine	_____ Originates the thought for muscle movement
2. actin and myosin	_____ Carries an electrical impulse from the brain or spinal cord
3. brain	_____ Area where a nerve ends and a muscle begins
4. calcium	_____ Neurotransmitter within the neuromuscular junction
5. contraction	_____ Area on the muscle cell membrane where acetylcholine attaches
6. nerve	_____ Electrolyte that plays a role in muscle contraction
7. neuromuscular junction	_____ Muscle becomes shorter
8. receptor	_____ Thin and thick strands of protein that slide together as a muscle contracts

Medical Language Word Parts

Name That Word Part

Identify each of the word parts given here by writing in the correct letter (P, C, or S) on the line beside it. Then write the definition of the word part on the blank line. The first one has been done for you.

Prefix = P **Combining Form = C** **Suffix = S**

		Word Part	Definition			Word Part	Definition
1.	a-	P	away from, without	35.	cortic/o-	______	______________
2.	ab-	______	______________	36.	cost/o-	______	______________
3.	ad-	______	______________	37.	delt/o-	______	______________
4.	-al	______	______________	38.	dermat/o-	______	______________
5.	alges/o-	______	______________	39.	duct/o-	______	______________
6.	alg/o-	______	______________	40.	dys-	______	______________
7.	-alis	______	______________	41.	e-	______	______________
8.	an-	______	______________	42.	-ectomy	______	______________
9.	-ancy	______	______________	43.	electr/o-	______	______________
10.	-ant	______	______________	44.	-er	______	______________
11.	anter/o-	______	______________	45.	extens/o-	______	______________
12.	anti-	______	______________	46.	extern/o-	______	______________
13.	-ar	______	______________	47.	fasci/o-	______	______________
14.	-aris	______	______________	48.	fibr/o-	______	______________
15.	-ary	______	______________	49.	flex/o-	______	______________
16.	-ated	______	______________	50.	front/o-	______	______________
17.	athet/o-	______	______________	51.	ganglion/o-	______	______________
18.	-ature	______	______________	52.	gastr/o-	______	______________
19.	bi-	______	______________	53.	-gram	______	______________
20.	bi/o-	______	______________	54.	-graphy	______	______________
21.	-body	______	______________	55.	habilitat/o-	______	______________
22.	brachi/o-	______	______________	56.	hyper-	______	______________
23.	brady-	______	______________	57.	-ia	______	______________
24.	buccinat/o-	______	______________	58.	iatr/o-	______	______________
25.	burs/o-	______	______________	59.	-iatry	______	______________
26.	-ceps	______	______________	60.	-ic	______	______________
27.	chem/o-	______	______________	61.	-ics	______	______________
28.	chir/o-	______	______________	62.	-il	______	______________
29.	cleid/o-	______	______________	63.	in-	______	______________
30.	-clonus	______	______________	64.	incis/o-	______	______________
31.	-cnemius	______	______________	65.	inflammat/o-	______	______________
32.	-collis	______	______________	66.	inject/o-	______	______________
33.	contract/o-	______	______________	67.	insert/o-	______	______________
34.	contus/o-	______	______________	68.	inter-	______	______________

		Word Part	Definition
69.	intern/o-		
70.	intra-		
71.	-ion		
72.	-ior		
73.	-itis		
74.	-kinesis		
75.	kines/o-		
76.	malign/o-		
77.	masset/o-		
78.	mast/o-		
79.	mitt/o-		
80.	mot/o-		
81.	multi-		
82.	muscul/o-		
83.	my/o-		
84.	myos/o-		
85.	neur/o-		
86.	non-		
87.	nucle/o-		
88.	-oid		
89.	-oma		
90.	-opsy		
91.	-or		
92.	-ory		
93.	orbicul/o-		
94.	orth/o-		
95.	oste/o-		
96.	-ous		
97.	-path		
98.	-pathy		
99.	pector/o-		
100.	ped/o-		
101.	perone/o-		
102.	physi/o-		
103.	pod/o-		
104.	poly-		
105.	pract/o-		
106.	pronat/o-		

		Word Part	Definition
107.	quadri-		
108.	radi/o-		
109.	re-		
110.	recept/o-		
111.	relax/o-		
112.	rhabd/o-		
113.	rotat/o-		
114.	-rrhaphy		
115.	sarc/o-		
116.	skelet/o-		
117.	sthen/o-		
118.	stern/o-		
119.	-steroid		
120.	steroid/o-		
121.	supinat/o-		
122.	synov/o-		
123.	tax/o-		
124.	tempor/o-		
125.	tendin/o-		
126.	tendon/o-		
127.	ten/o-		
128.	therap/o-		
129.	-therapy		
130.	thym/o-		
131.	tibi/o-		
132.	-tic		
133.	-tomy		
134.	tort/i-		
135.	trans-		
136.	tremul/o-		
137.	tri-		
138.	troph/o-		
139.	-trophy		
140.	vers/o-		
141.	vert/o-		
142.	volunt/o-		
143.	vuls/o-		

Word-Building Exercise

Use the combining forms, prefixes, and suffixes given here to build medical words that match the definitions given. Write the word that you build on the blank line. Some word parts may be used more than once. The first one has been done for you.

Word Parts

a- (away from, without)	-ic (pertaining to)	-pathy (disease; suffering)
-al (pertaining to)	-ion (action; condition)	perone/o- (fibula)
-ature (system composed of)	-itis (inflammation of)	pronat/o- (lying face down)
burs/o- (bursa)	muscul/o- (muscle)	tax/o- (coordination)
delt/o- (triangle)	my/o- (muscle)	tendin/o- (tendon)
flex/o- (bending)	-oid (resembling)	troph/o- (development)
-ia (condition, state, thing)	-ous (pertaining to)	

1. System composed of the body's muscles (You think *muscul/o- + -ature.*) You write musculature
2. Decreasing the angle between two bones or two body parts ______
3. Pertaining to a tendon ______
4. Muscle that resembles a triangle ______
5. Pertaining to the muscle in the lower leg that lies over the fibula bone ______
6. Action to place the palm face down ______
7. Condition of being without coordination ______
8. Pertaining to without muscle development ______
9. Any disease of muscles ______
10. Inflammation of a bursa ______

Symptoms, Signs, and Diseases

Matching Exercise

Match each numbered word or phrase to its description or synonym.

1. polymyalgia	______ Repetitive strain injury
2. atrophy	______ Bruise
3. contusion	______ Pain in many muscle groups
4. cumulative trauma disorder	______ Small, involuntary muscle movements
5. acceleration-deceleration injury	______ Wryneck
6. torticollis	______ Whiplash
7. tremor	______ Muscle wasting
8. muscular dystrophy	______ Duchenne's
9. ataxia	______ Incoordination of muscle movement

True or False

Indicate whether each statement is true or false by writing T or F on the line.

1. ____ *Myalgia* means inflammation in a muscle.
2. ____ Muscular dystrophy and myasthenia gravis are genetic disorders.
3. ____ Involuntary muscle jerking is known as bradykinesia.
4. ____ Muscle wasting is also known as muscle atrophy.
5. ____ The two types of muscular dystrophy are Duchenne's and Dupuytren's.
6. ____ Patients with fibromyalgia may also develop rigor mortis.
7. ____ Myasthenia gravis is caused by antibodies that destroy acetylcholine receptors.
8. ____ Golfer's elbow is the same type of overuse injury as pitcher's elbow.
9. ____ A contracture is a fixed state of inflexible flexion of a muscle.
10. ____ Muscular dystrophy causes pain at certain trigger points.

Circle Exercise

Circle the correct word from the choices given.

1. (**Ataxia, Atrophy, Contracture**) is a type of movement disorder.
2. A ganglion develops on a (**muscle, nerve, tendon**).
3. A slow, writhing movement of the hand is described as (**athetoid, myalgia, tendonitis**).
4. An injury in which the muscle is torn away from the tendon is a/an (**avulsion, compartment syndrome, contusion**).
5. Which is not a type of muscular dystrophy? (**Becker's, Duchenne's, Dupuytren's**)
6. A (**ganglion, rhabdomyosarcoma, tenosynovitis**) is a malignant tumor of the muscle.

Laboratory, Surgery, and Drugs

Multiple Choice

Circle the best answer from those given.

1. A ganglionectomy is a procedure to surgically remove a ____________________.
   a. ganglion
   b. fascia
   c. muscle
   d. tendon

2. All of the following are sports-related injuries EXCEPT ____________________.
   a. shin splints
   b. golfer's elbow
   c. rigor mortis
   d. lateral epicondylitis

3. In which of the following is a piece of muscle tissue removed and examined?
   a. muscle biopsy
   b. serum aldolase
   c. electromyography
   d. CPK-MM

4. Which of the following is a procedure that may need to be performed after a laceration of the hand?
   a. Tensilon test
   b. tenorrhaphy
   c. trigger point injection
   d. muscle biopsy

5. Which of the following is a class of drugs used to relieve muscular spasm?
   a. neuromuscular blockers
   b. muscle relaxants
   c. analgesics
   d. NSAIDs

Circle Exercise

Circle the correct word from the choices given.

1. Trigger point injections are used to treat (**bursitis, fibromyalgia, tendonitis**).
2. Exercises where the therapist moves the extremity for the patient are (**active, passive, rehabilitation**) exercises.
3. A (**muscle biopsy, tenorrhaphy, thymectomy**) is used to treat myasthenia gravis.
4. Surgical procedure to remove a piece of muscle for examination is a/an (**fasciotomy, incisional biopsy, tenorrhaphy**).

Abbreviations

Define and Match Exercise

Give the full meaning for each abbreviation listed below. Then match each to its correct description.

1. EMG	________________	____	Stimulates a muscle with electricity
2. ADLs	________________	____	An arm
3. NSAID	________________	____	Does strengthening exercises and uses assistive devices
4. RUE	________________	____	Progressive muscle weakness beginning in childhood
5. OT	________________	____	Tasks at home and on the job
6. MD	________________	____	A drug route
7. IM	________________	____	Drug for muscle pain and inflammation

Applied Skills

Plural Noun and Adjective Spelling

Fill in the blanks with the correct word form. Be sure to check your spelling. The first one has been done for you.

Singular Noun	Plural Noun	Adjective	Singular Noun	Plural Noun	Adjective
1. muscle	muscles	muscular	3. tendon	________	________
2. fascia		________	4. bursa	________	________

English and Medical Word Equivalents

For each English word, write its equivalent medical word. The first one has been done for you.

English Word	Medical Word	English Word	Medical Word
1. bruise	contusion	4. pulled muscle	________
2. muscle wasting	________	5. whiplash	________
3. wryneck	________		

Dictionary Challenge

1. On the job, you will often encounter new medical words. Practice your medical dictionary skills by looking up *muscle* and *musculus* (the Latin word for *muscle*). Which entry has subentries with full descriptions of each muscle?

   ____

2. Also look up *tendon* and *tendo* (the Latin name for *tendon*). Are these complete lists of all the tendons in the body? **Yes/No** What other anatomical structure might lend its name to a tendon?

   ____

Analysis of a Medical Report

This exercise contains two related reports: a hospital Operative Report and a Pathology Report. Read both reports and answer the questions.

OPERATIVE REPORT

PATIENT NAME: PHELPS, GEORGE R.

HOSPITAL NUMBER: 42-51-55

DATE OF OPERATION: November 19, 20xx

PREOPERATIVE DIAGNOSIS: Myopathy of undetermined etiology.

POSTOPERATIVE DIAGNOSIS: Myopathy of undetermined etiology.

PROCEDURE: Right quadriceps muscle biopsy.

ANESTHESIA: Xylocaine 1% local anesthetic with I.V. sedation.

SPECIMEN: Muscle biopsy x3.

COMPLICATIONS: None.

CLINICAL HISTORY: The patient is a 68-year-old male who has had progressive lower back and right leg weakness for approximately 6 months. He notes difficulty climbing stairs or getting up from a chair or bed. He moves slowly. There is mild eyelid ptosis noted.

OPERATIVE TECHNIQUE: After the induction of I.V. sedation, the right thigh was prepped with Betadine and draped in the usual fashion. After infiltration with local anesthesia, a longitudinal incision was made over the anterolateral aspect of the thigh. The incision was deepened through subcutaneous tissue to the quadriceps fascia, which was incised. Three specimens were obtained for biopsy as per Armed Forces Institute of Pathology (AFIP) protocol. A core of muscle, approximately the thickness of a pencil, was submitted for the first biopsy. Then 2 muscle segments were grasped with biopsy clamps and excised. Pressure was held over the muscle for hemostasis. The wound was irrigated with warm saline solution, and the fascia was reapproximated with 2 interrupted sutures of #2-0 Vicryl. The subcutaneous and subcuticular tissues were approximated with interrupted sutures of #3-0 Vicryl. The skin was approximated with skin staples. A sterile dressing was applied. The patient was transferred to the recovery room in stable condition. Blood loss during the procedure was minimal.

Jamison R. Smith, M.D.

Jamison R. Smith, M.D.

JRS:srd
D: 11/19/xx
T: 11/19/xx

PATHOLOGY REPORT

PATIENT NAME: PHELPS, GEORGE R.

HOSPITAL NUMBER: 42-51-55

DATE: November 19, 20xx

OPERATION PERFORMED: Right quadriceps muscle biopsy.

CLINICAL HISTORY: Myopathy.

GROSS SPECIMEN: Received on ice are 3 specimen jars. One is a porcelain jar labeled "without a clamp, for freezing" and it contains a fragment of red-tan muscle wrapped in gauze, $1.2 \times 1.0 \times 0.7$ cm. There are 2 glass jars. One is labeled "formalin" and within the jar is a large clamp with a fragment of red-tan muscle, $2.2 \times 1.3 \times 1.3$ cm. The other jar is labeled "glutaraldehyde" and contains a small clamp to which is attached a fragment of red-tan muscle measuring about $1.8 \times 2.0 \times 1.3$ cm. All 3 containers are sent to the Armed Forces Institute of Pathology on ice for processing and diagnosis.

MICROSCOPIC SPECIMEN: Biopsy of right quadriceps muscle. Await forthcoming report from the Armed Forces Institute of Pathology.

Ralph A. Stanley, M.D.

Ralph A. Stanley, M.D.

RAS:drc
D: 11/19/xx
T: 11/19/xx

WORD ANALYSIS QUESTIONS

1. Divide *myopathy* into its two word parts and define each word part.

   Word Parts **Definition**

   ________________ ____

   ________________ ____

2. Divide *etiology* into its two word parts and define each word part.

   Word Parts **Definition**

   ________________ ____

   ________________ ____

3. Divide *biopsy* into its two word parts and define each word part.

   Word Parts **Definition**

   ________________ ____

   ________________ ____

4. Use your medical dictionary to look up the definition of these words.

   glutaraldehyde____

   protocol ____

FACT FINDING QUESTIONS

1. What operative procedure was performed?

2. In what muscle group was this procedure done?

3. Where is that muscle group located?

4. How many specimens were taken?

5. What two ADLs does the report specifically mention that the patient had difficulty doing before surgery?

6. What color is the muscle biopsy specimen?

7. What was this patient's postoperative diagnosis?

CRITICAL THINKING SKILLS

1. In what order were these structures encountered when the incision was performed?
   a. Quadriceps muscle, skin, fascia, subcutaneous tissue
   b. Skin, subcutaneous tissue, fascia, quadriceps muscle
   c. Fascia, skin, subcutaneous tissue, quadriceps muscle

2. Formalin and glutaraldehyde are ____________________.
   a. used to prep and drape the skin
   b. used as preservatives for biopsy specimens
   c. local anesthetics

Pronunciation Checklist

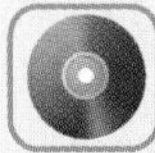

Read each word and its pronunciation. Practice pronouncing each word. Verify your pronunciation by listening to the Pronunciation List on the CD-ROM. Check the box next to the word after you master its pronunciation.

- ❑ abduction (ab-DUK-shun)
- ❑ abductor (ab-DUK-tor)
- ❑ acetylcholine (AS-ee-til-KOH-leen)
- ❑ adduction (ad-DUK-shun)
- ❑ adductor (ad-DUK-tor)
- ❑ analgesic drug (AN-al-JEE-zik DRUHG)
- ❑ antibody (AN-tee-BAWD-ee) (AN-tih-BAWD-ee)
- ❑ aponeurosis (AP-oh-nyoo-ROH-sis)
- ❑ ataxia (ah-TAK-see-ah)
- ❑ ataxic (ah-TAK-sik)
- ❑ athetoid (ATH-eh-toyd)
- ❑ atrophic (aa-TROF-ik)
- ❑ atrophy (AT-roh-fee)
- ❑ avulsion (ah-VUL-shun)
- ❑ benign (bee-NINE)
- ❑ biceps brachii muscle (BY-seps BRAY-kee-eye MUS-el)
- ❑ biopsy (BY-awp-see)
- ❑ brachioradialis muscle (BRAY-kee-oh-RAY-dee-AL-is MUS-el)
- ❑ bradykinesia (BRAD-ee-kin-EE-zee-ah)
- ❑ buccinator muscle (BUK-sih-NAY-tor MUS-el)
- ❑ bursa (BER-sah)
- ❑ bursae (BER-see)
- ❑ bursal (BER-sal)
- ❑ bursitis (ber-SY-tis)
- ❑ chiropractic (KY-roh-PRAK-tic)
- ❑ chiropractor (KY-roh-PRAK-tor)
- ❑ contraction (con-TRAK-shun)
- ❑ contracture (con-TRAK-choor)
- ❑ contusion (con-TOO-shun)
- ❑ corticosteroid drug (KOR-tih-koh-STAIR-oyd DRUHG)
- ❑ creatine phosphokinase (KREE-ah-teen FAWS-foh-KY-nays)
- ❑ deltoid muscle (DEL-toyd MUS-el)
- ❑ dermatomyositis (DER-mah-toh-MY-oh-SY-tis)
- ❑ Duchenne (doo-SHAYN)
- ❑ Dupuytren (DOO-pyoo-tren)
- ❑ dyskinesia (DIS-kih-NEE-zee-ah)
- ❑ dystrophy (DIS-troh-fee)
- ❑ electromyogram (ee-LEK-troh-MY-oh-gram)
- ❑ electromyography (ee-LEK-troh-my-AWG-rah-fee)
- ❑ eversion (ee-VER-zhun)
- ❑ evertor (ee-VER-tor)
- ❑ extension (eks-TEN-shun)
- ❑ extensor digitorum muscle (eks-TEN-sor dij-ih-TOR-um MUS-el)
- ❑ external oblique muscle (eks-TER-nal awb-LEEK MUS-el)
- ❑ fascia (FASH-ee-ah)
- ❑ fascial (FASH-ee-al)
- ❑ fascicle (FAS-ih-kl)
- ❑ fasciectomy (FASH-ee-EK-toh-mee)
- ❑ fasciotomy (FASH-ee-AWT-oh-mee)
- ❑ fibromyalgia (FY-broh-my-AL-jah)
- ❑ flexion (FLEK-shun)
- ❑ flexor hallucis brevis muscle (FLEK-sor HAL-yoo-sis BREV-is MUS-el)
- ❑ frontalis muscle (frun-TAY-lis MUS-el)
- ❑ ganglion (GANG-glee-on)
- ❑ ganglionectomy (GANG-glee-oh-NEK-toh-mee)
- ❑ gastrocnemius muscle (GAS-trawk-NEE-mee-us MUS-el)
- ❑ gluteus maximus muscle (gloo-TEE-us MAK-sih-mus MUS-el)
- ❑ hyperextension (HY-per-eks-TEN-shun)
- ❑ hyperflexion (HY-per-FLEK-shun)
- ❑ hyperkinesis (HY-per-kih-NEE-sis)
- ❑ hypertrophy (hy-PER-troh-fee)
- ❑ incisional (in-SIZH-un-al)
- ❑ injection (in-JEK-shun)
- ❑ intercostal muscle (IN-ter-KAWS-tal MUS-el)
- ❑ internal oblique muscle (in-TER-nal awb-LEEK MUS-el)
- ❑ intramuscular (IN-trah-MUS-kyoo-lar)
- ❑ inversion (in-VER-zhun)
- ❑ invertor (in-VER-tor)
- ❑ latissimus dorsi muscle (lah-TIS-ih-mus DOR-see MUS-el)
- ❑ malignancy (mah-LIG-nan-see)
- ❑ masseter muscle (MAS-eh-ter MUS-el)
- ❑ multinucleated (MUL-tee-NOO-klee-aa-ted)
- ❑ muscle (MUS-el)
- ❑ muscle insertion (MUS-el in-SER-shun)
- ❑ muscle origin (MUS-el OR-ih-jin)
- ❑ muscular (MUS-kyoo-lar)
- ❑ musculature (MUS-kyoo-lah-chur)
- ❑ musculoskeletal (MUS-kyoo-loh-SKEL-eh-tal)
- ❑ myalgia (my-AL-jee-ah) (my-AL-jah)
- ❑ myasthenia gravis (MY-as-THEE-nee-ah GRAV-is)
- ❑ myoclonus (MY-oh-KLOH-nus)
- ❑ myofibril (MY-oh-FY-bril)
- ❑ myopathy (my-AWP-ah-thee)
- ❑ myorrhaphy (my-OR-ah-fee)
- ❑ myositis (MY-oh-SY-tis)
- ❑ neuromuscular (NYOOR-oh-MUS-kyoo-lar)
- ❑ neurotransmitter (NYOOR-oh-TRANS-mit-er) (NYOOR-oh-trans-MIT-er)
- ❑ nonsteroidal anti-inflammatory drug (non-stair-OY-dal AN-tee-in-FLAM-ah-TOR-ee DRUHG)
- ❑ orbicularis oculi muscle (or-BIK-yoo-LAIR-is AWK-yoo-ligh MUS-el)
- ❑ orbicularis oris muscle (or-BIK-yoo-LAIR-is OR-is MUS-el)
- ❑ orthopedics (OR-thoh-PEE-diks)
- ❑ osteopath (AW-stee-oh-path)
- ❑ osteopathy (AWS-tee-AWP-ah-thee)
- ❑ pectoralis major muscle (PEK-toh-RAY-lis MAY-jur MUS-el)
- ❑ peroneal (PAIR-oh-NEE-al)
- ❑ peroneus longus muscle (PAIR-oh-NEE-us LONG-gus MUS-el)
- ❑ physiatrist (fiz-EYE-ah-trist) (FIZ-ee-AT-rist)
- ❑ physiatry (fi-ZY-ah-tree)
- ❑ platysma muscle (plah-TIZ-mah MUS-el)
- ❑ podiatric (POH-dee-AT-rik)
- ❑ podiatrist (poh-DY-ah-trist)
- ❑ podiatry (poh-DY-ah-tree)
- ❑ polymyalgia (PAWL-ee-my-AL-jee-ah) (PAWL-ee-my-AL-jah)
- ❑ polymyositis (PAWL-ee-MY-oh-SY-tis)
- ❑ pronation (proh-NAY-shun)
- ❑ pronator (proh-NAY-tor)
- ❑ ptosis (TOH-sis)
- ❑ quadriceps femoris muscles (KWAD-rih-seps FEM-oh-ris MUS-elz)
- ❑ receptor (ree-SEP-tor)
- ❑ rectus abdominis muscle (REK-tus ab-DAWM-ih-nis MUS-el)

- ❑ rectus femoris muscle (REK-tus FEM-oh-ris MUS-el)
- ❑ rehabilitation (REE-hah-BIL-ih-TAY-shun)
- ❑ relaxant drug (ree-LAK-sant DRUHG)
- ❑ retinaculum (RET-ih-NAK-yoo-lum)
- ❑ rhabdomyoma (RAB-doh-my-OH-mah)
- ❑ rhabdomyosarcoma (RAB-doh-MY-oh-sar-KOH-mah)
- ❑ rigor mortis (RIG-or MOR-tis)
- ❑ rotation (roh-TAY-shun)
- ❑ rotator (ROH-tay-tor)
- ❑ sartorius muscle (sar-TOR-ee-us MUS-el)
- ❑ spasm (SPAZM)
- ❑ sternocleidomastoid muscle (STER-noh-KLY-doh-MAS-toyd MUS-el)
- ❑ strain (STRAYN)
- ❑ striated muscle (STRY-aa-ted MUS-el)
- ❑ supination (SOO-pih-NAY-shun)
- ❑ supinator (SOO-pih-nay-tor)
- ❑ temporalis muscle (TEM-poh-RAY-lis MUS-el)
- ❑ tendinous (TEN-dih-nus)
- ❑ tendon (TEN-dun)
- ❑ tendonitis (TEN-doh-NY-tis)
- ❑ tenorrhaphy (teh-NOR-ah-fee)
- ❑ tenosynovitis (TEN-oh-SIN-oh-VY-tis)
- ❑ Tensilon (TEN-sih-lawn)
- ❑ thenar muscle (THEE-nar MUS-el)
- ❑ therapist (THAIR-ah-pist)
- ❑ thymectomy (thy-MEK-toh-mee)
- ❑ tibialis anterior muscle (TIB-ee-AL-is an-TEER-ee-or MUS-el)
- ❑ torticollis (TOR-tih-KOL-is)
- ❑ trapezius muscle (trah-PEE-zee-us MUS-el)
- ❑ tremor (TREM-or)
- ❑ tremulous (TREM-yoo-lus)
- ❑ triceps brachii muscle (TRY-seps BRAY-kee-eye MUS-el)
- ❑ voluntary muscle (VAWL-an-tair-ee MUS-el)

Experience Multimedia

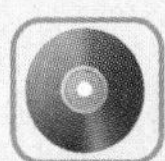

CD-ROM Learning Activities Checklist

Check off the box as you complete each learning activity.

- ❑ **CD-ROM Learning Activity 9.1: *ANATOMY WORD PARTS FLASHCARDS***
  Use flashcards to help you memorize word parts. Make your own flashcards or print out prepared flashcards. Also see the elecronic flashcard games. Time: 20 minutes.
- ❑ **CD-ROM Learning Activity 9.2: *MEDICINE IN ACTION***
  Watch a video clip of a child with muscular dystrophy. Time: 5 minutes.
- ❑ **CD-ROM Learning Activity 9.3: *DISEASE AND OTHER WORD PARTS FLASHCARDS***
  A continuation of the flashcard learning activity. Time: 20 minutes.
- ❑ **CD-ROM Learning Activity 9.4: *MEMORY AIDS***
  Use memory aids to help you memorize medical words and meanings. Time: 5 minutes.
- ❑ **CD-ROM Learning Activity 9.5: *MEDICAL LANGUAGE SPOKEN HERE***
  Listen to actual medical reports and spell the missing medical words. Time: 20 minutes.
- ❑ **CD-ROM Learning Activity 9.6: *SPELLING CHALLENGE***
  Listen to a pronounced medical word and then spell it. Time: 5 minutes.
- ❑ **CD-ROM Learning Activity 9.7: *MEDICAL LANGUAGE PRONUNCIATION***
  Listen to a pronounced medical word and then practice pronouncing it. Time: 30 minutes.
- ❑ **CD-ROM Learning Activity 9.8: *EDUCATIONAL FUN AND GAMES***
  Enjoy these fun activities while reinforcing your knowledge. Time: 15 minutes.

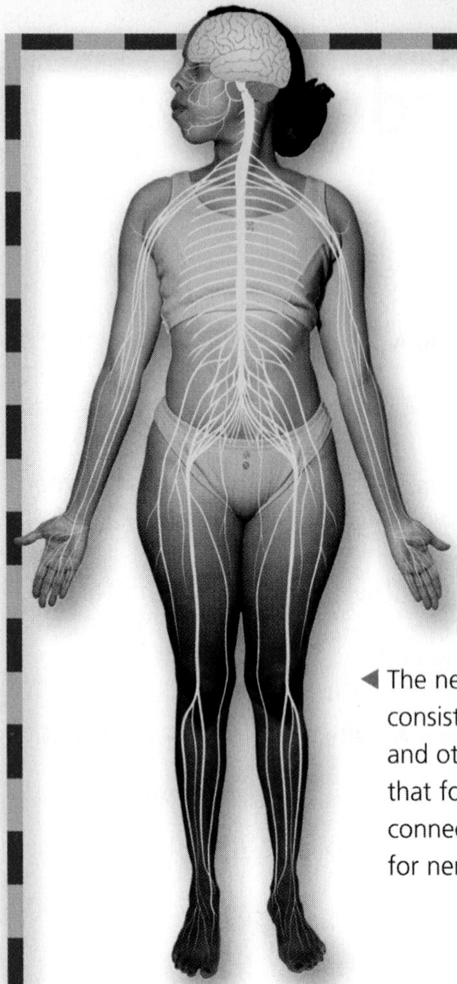

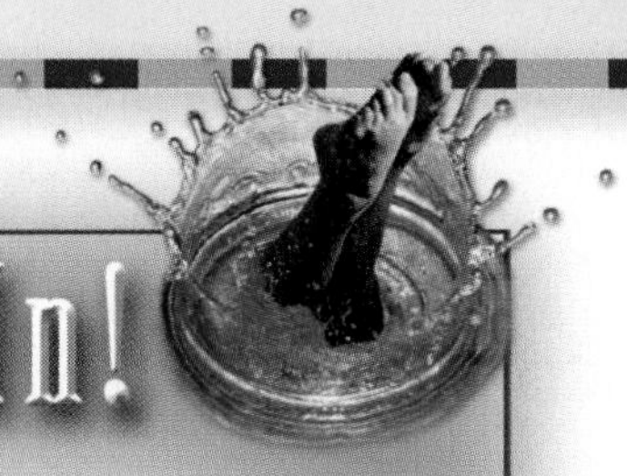

Dive In!

- The brain continues to send out electric wave signals until approximately 37 hours after death.
- There are more nerve cells in the human brain than stars in the Milky Way.
- Albert Einstein's brain was found to be no larger than average.
- Do you have the impulse to learn more? In this chapter we'll explore the language that describes nervous system structures, functions, diseases, and conditions.
- You'll get the message once you master the language of neurology!

◀ The nervous system consists of the brain and other structures that form a connected pathway for nerve impulses.

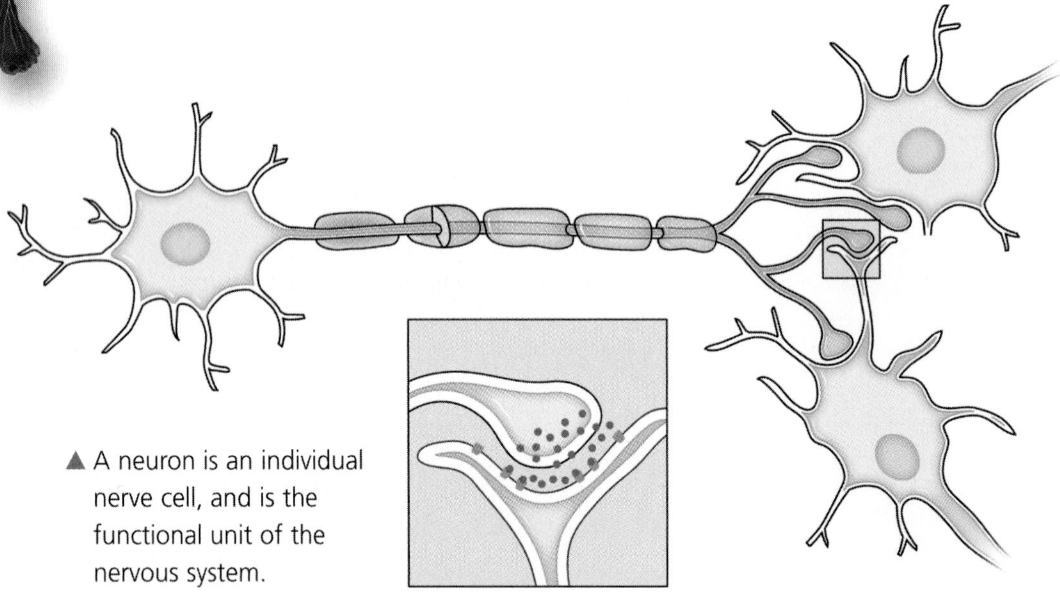

▲ A neuron is an individual nerve cell, and is the functional unit of the nervous system.

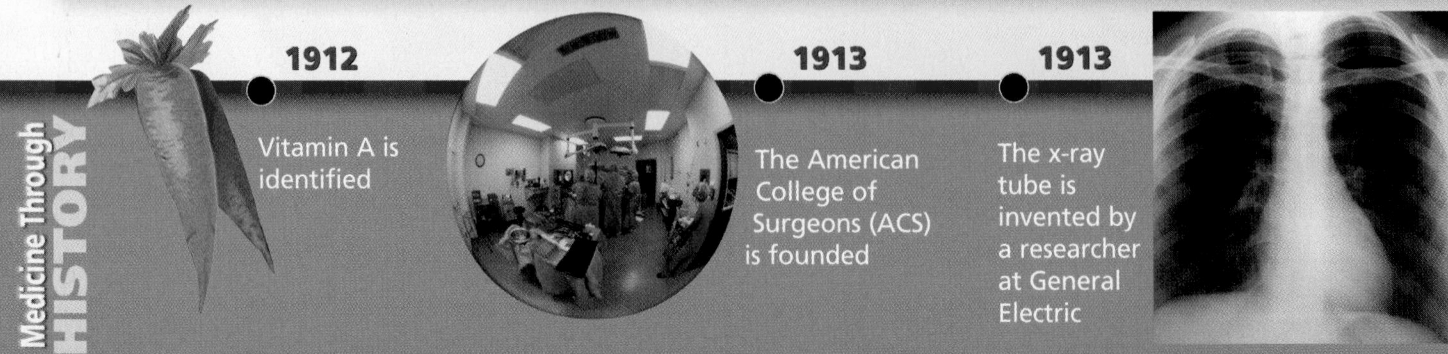

Medicine Through HISTORY
1912
Vitamin A is identified
1913
The American College of Surgeons (ACS) is founded
1913
The x-ray tube is invented by a researcher at General Electric

CHAPTER 10

Neurology

Nervous System

Neurology (nyoo-RAWL-oh-jee) is the medical specialty that studies the anatomy and physiology of the nervous system and uses diagnostic tests, medical and surgical procedures, and drugs to treat nervous system diseases.

▲ Like a computer motherboard, the nervous system processes, interprets, and sends electrical impulses to control body functions.

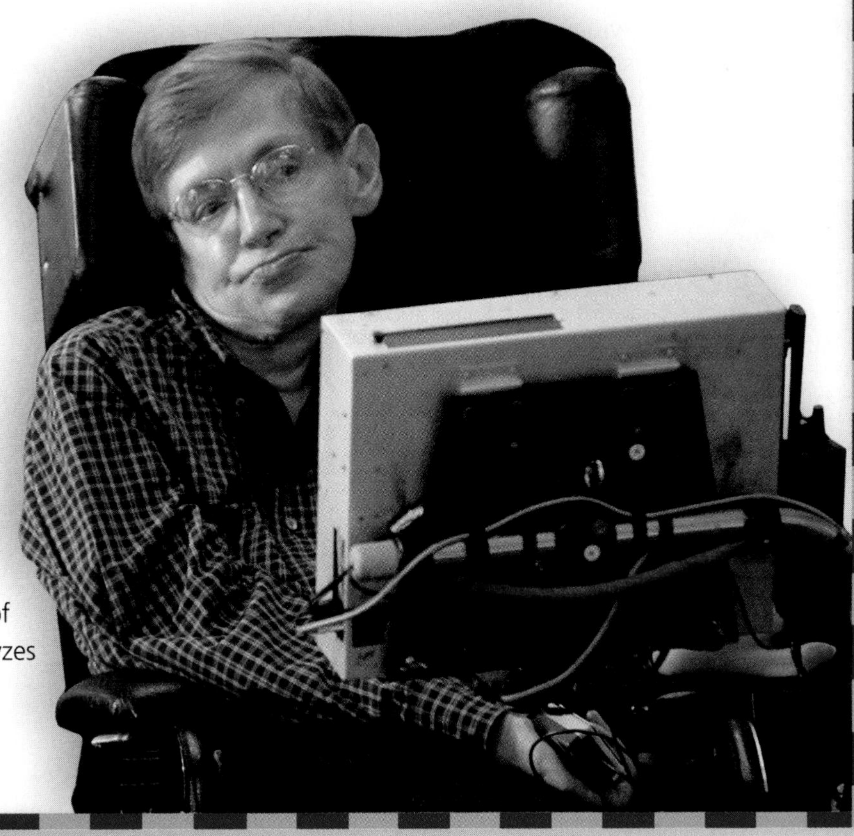

▶ Since 1963, preeminent astronomer Stephen Hawking has lived with ALS, a disease of the nervous system that paralyzes motor functions but does not affect mental capacity.

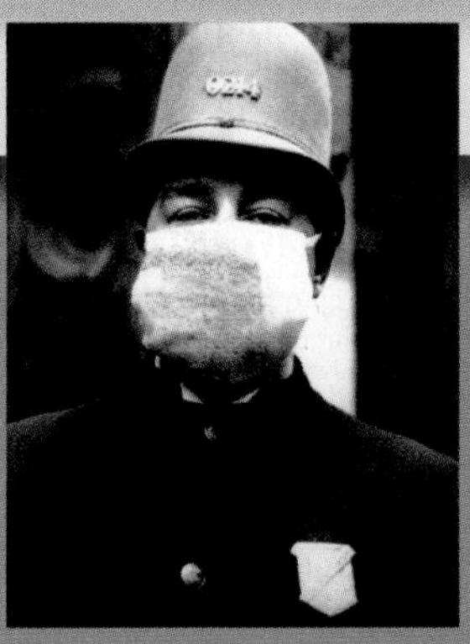

1918

Influenza kills 15 million people around the world

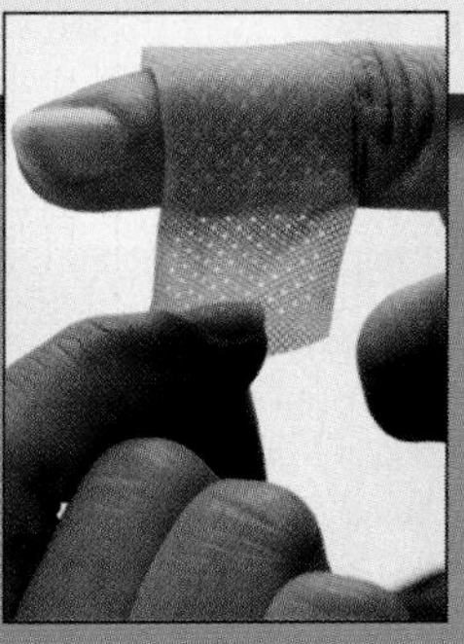

1920

The Band-Aid is invented by an employee of Johnson & Johnson Company

Measure Your Progress: Learning Objectives

After you study this chapter, you should be able to

1. Identify the anatomical structures of the nervous system by correctly labeling them on anatomical illustrations.
2. Describe the process of nerve transmission.
3. Build nervous system words from combining forms, prefixes, and suffixes.
4. Describe common nervous system diseases.
5. Describe common nervous system diagnostic laboratory and radiology tests.
6. Describe common nervous system medical and surgical procedures and drug categories.
7. Define common nervous system abbreviations.
8. Correctly spell and pronounce nervous system words.
9. Apply your skills by analyzing a neurology report.
10. Test your knowledge of neurology by completing review exercises at the end of the chapter and learning activities on the CD-ROM.

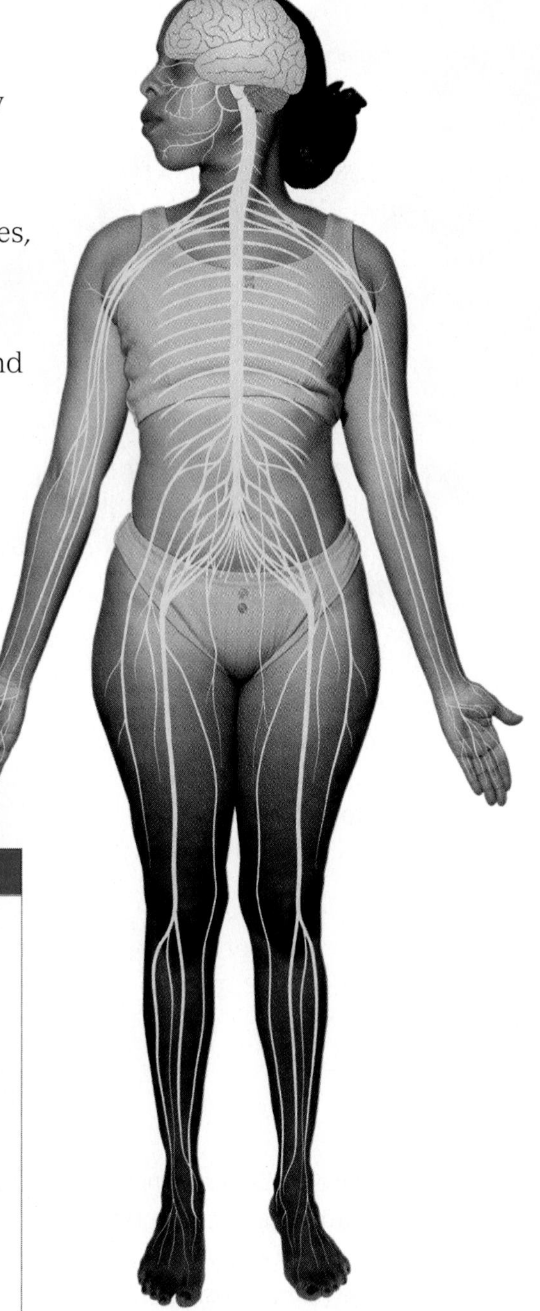

Figure 10-1 ■ The nervous system.
The nervous system is a widespread body system that consists of one main organ (the brain) and other structures that form a connected pathway along which nerve impulses travel throughout the body.

Medical Language Key

To unlock the meaning of a medical word, first define each word part. Then put the word part definitions in order, beginning with the suffix, followed by the first word part.

	Word Part	Word Part Definition
SUFFIX	-logy	*the study of*
COMBINING FORM	neur/o-	*nerve*

Neurology: ***The study of the nerves.***

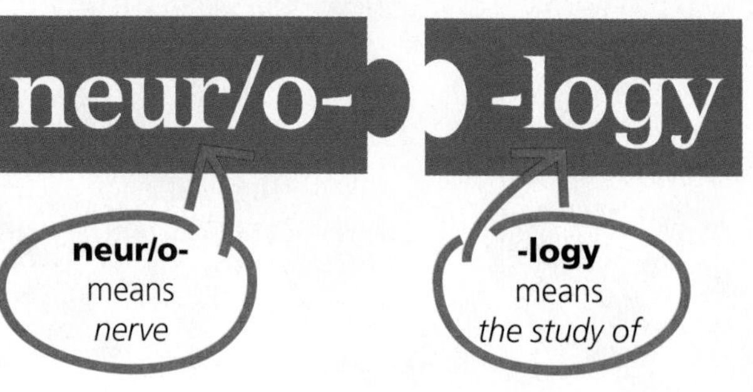

www.prenhall.com/turley

For interactive flashcards, real-life video clips, games, exercises, and audio pronunciations please explore the companion CD-ROM in the back of the book. Click on the companion website for bonus chapters, additional resources, and links to on-line learning.

Anatomy and Physiology

The **nervous system** is a body system that is found in every part of the body from the head to the tips of the fingers and toes (see Figure 10-1 ■). The main organ of the nervous system is the brain. It is located in the cranial cavity. The spinal cord is a vertical structure of the nervous system that connects to the brain. It is located along the back in the spinal cavity. The nerves are slender structures that travel from the brain to the upper body and from the spinal cord to the upper and lower body. The purpose of the nervous system is to receive nerve impulses from the body and the senses. These nerve impulses are processed and interpreted by the brain, which then sends nerve impulses back to the body. The nervous system is also known as the **neuromuscular system** because many nerve impulses initiate movement of muscles.

nervous (NER-vus)
nerv/o- *nerve*
-ous *pertaining to*

system (SIS-tem)
System is derived from a Greek word meaning *combination of parts to make an organized whole.*

neuromuscular (NYOOR-oh-MUS-kyoo-lar)
neur/o- *nerve*
muscul/o- *muscle*
-ar *pertaining to*

Anatomy of the Nervous System

Central and Peripheral Nervous System

The anatomy of the nervous system can be divided into the central nervous system and the peripheral nervous system. The **central nervous system (CNS)** consists of the brain and the spinal cord. The **peripheral nervous system** consists of the cranial nerves (nerves that originate in the brain) and the spinal nerves (nerves that originate in the spinal cord).

central (SEN-tral)
centr/o- *center; dominant part*
-al *pertaining to*

peripheral (peh-RIF-eh-ral)
peripher/o- *outer aspects*
-al *pertaining to*

Brain

The **brain** is the part of the central nervous system that is housed within the bony **cranium.** The brain and its surrounding structures fill the **cranial cavity.** The largest and most obvious part of the brain is the cerebrum. Other parts of the brain include the centrally located ventricles, the thalamus and hypothalamus, the inferior structures of the brainstem, and the posterior cerebellum. Each of these parts performs several specialized functions.

brain (BRAYN)

cranium (KRAY-nee-um)

cranial (KRAY-nee-al)
crani/o- *cranium (skull)*
-al *pertaining to*

cavity (KAV-ih-tee)
cav/o- *hollow space*
-ity *state; condition*

Cerebrum The largest part of the brain is the **cerebrum.** The cerebrum is divided into large sections known as **lobes.** These lobes are separated from each other by large, deep grooves. Each lobe is named for the bone of the cranium that lies next to it (see Figure 10-2 ■).

cerebrum (SER-eh-brum) (seh-REE-brum)
Cerebrum is a Latin word meaning *brain.*

lobe (LOHB)

Frontal Lobe

- Coordinates and analyzes information received by other lobes of the cerebrum to predict future events and the benefits or consequences of actions.
- Exerts conscious, voluntary control over the skeletal muscles.
- Analyzes **sensory** nerve impulses from the tongue and taste receptors. This occurs in a special area of the frontal lobe known as the **gustatory cortex.**

frontal (FRUN-tal)
front/o- *front*
-al *pertaining to*

sensory (SEN-soh-ree)
sens/o- *sensation*
-ory *having the function of*

gustatory (GUS-tah-tor-ee)
gustat/o- *the sense of taste*
-ory *having the function of*

Parietal Lobe

- Analyzes sensory nerve impulses from the skin and the internal organs of the body for temperature, touch, pressure, vibration, and pain.

parietal (pah-RY-eh-tal)
pariet/o- *wall of a cavity*
-al *pertaining to*

Occipital Lobe

- Analyzes sensory nerve impulses from the eyes. This occurs in a special area of the occipital lobe known as the **visual cortex.**

occiptal (awk-SIP-ih-tal)
occipit/o- *occiput (back of the head)*
-al *pertaining to*

visual (VIZ-yoo-al)
vis/o- *sight; vision*
-al *pertaining to*

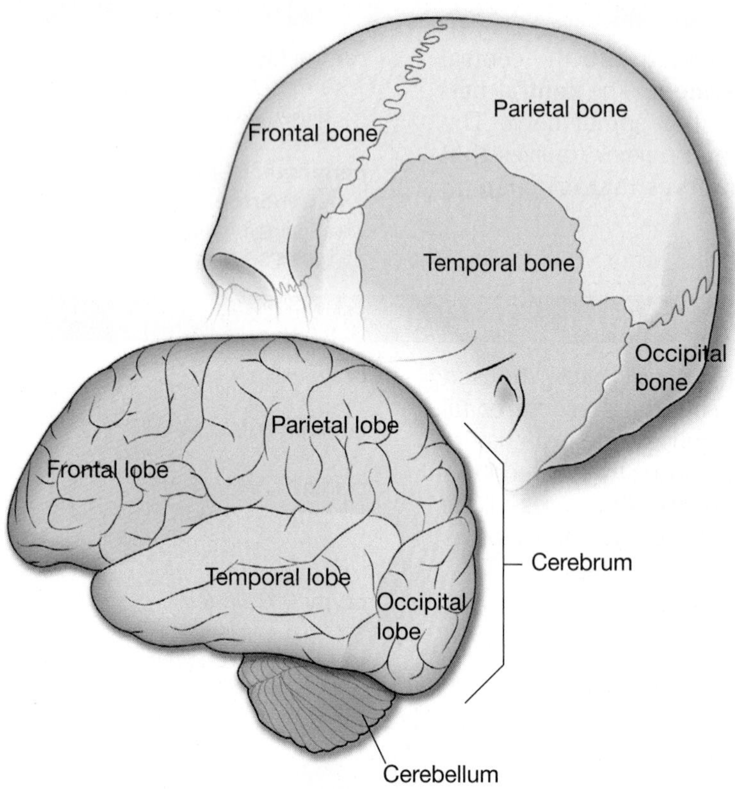

Figure 10-2 ■ Lobes of the cerebrum.
Each lobe of the cerebrum takes its name from the bone of the cranium that lies next to it.

Temporal Lobe

- Analyzes sensory nerve impulses from the ears. This occurs in a special area of the temporal lobe known as the **auditory cortex.**
- Analyzes sensory nerve impulses from the nose. This occurs in a special area of the temporal lobe known as the **olfactory cortex.**

The surface of the cerebrum is notable for striking folds (**gyri**) and deep grooves (**sulci**) (see Figure 10-3■). The **cerebral cortex** or gray matter is the narrow outermost layer of the cerebrum that follows the curves of the gyri and sulci. The white matter of the cerebrum is beneath that (see Figure 10-4■).

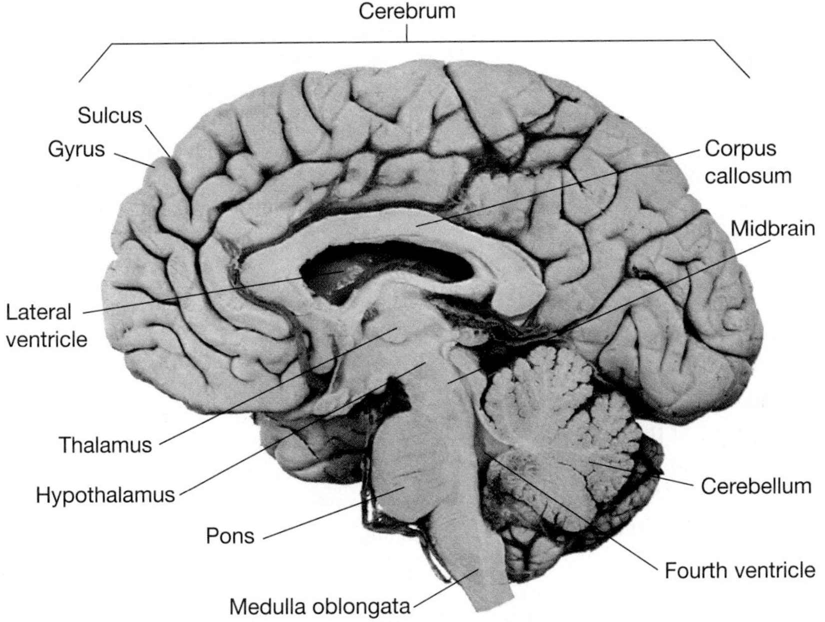

Figure 10-3 ■ Midline cut section of the brain.

This cut section shows the right half of the brain. The large size of the cerebrum is seen in relation to the cerebellum and other structures. Many gyri and sulci are visible on the surface of the cerebrum. The lateral ventricle, thalamus, hypothalamus, midbrain, pons, and medulla oblongata are clearly seen.

temporal (TEM-poh-ral)
tempor/o- *temple (side of the head)*
-al *pertaining to*

auditory (AW-dih-TOR-ee)
audit/o- *the sense of hearing*
-ory *having the function of*

olfactory (ol-FAK-toh-ree)
olfact/o- *the sense of smell*
-ory *having the function of*

gyrus (JY-rus)
gyri (JY-rye)
Gyrus is a Latin singular masculine noun. Form the plural by changing *-us* to *-i.*

sulcus (SUL-kus)
sulci (SUL-sigh)
Sulcus is a Latin singular masculine noun. Form the plural by changing *-us* to *-i.*

cerebral (SER-eh-bral) (seh-REE-bral)
cerebr/o- *cerebrum (largest part of the brain)*
-al *pertaining to*

cortex (KOR-teks)
Cortex is a Latin word meaning *the bark of a tree.*

cortical (KOR-tih-kal)
cortic/o- *cortex (outer region)*
-al *pertaining to*

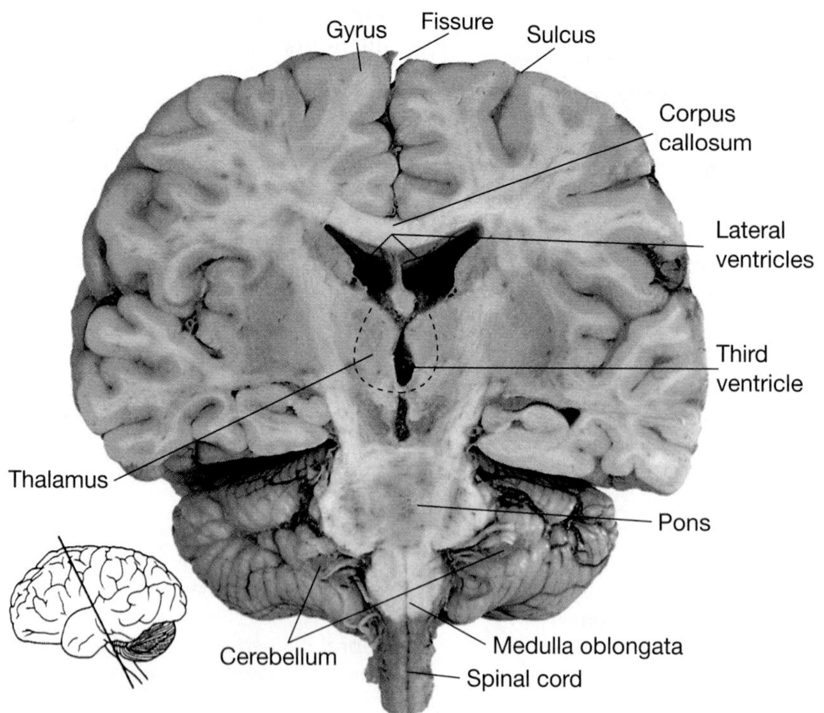

Figure 10-4 ■ Posterior half of the brain.

The anterior part of the cerebrum has been removed. A fissure divides the top of the right and left hemispheres of the cerebrum. The corpus callosum is the white connecting bridge between the hemispheres. The right and left ventricles and the small, central, third ventricle can be seen. The brainstem descends from the brain and merges with the spinal cord.

There is a very deep **fissure** running anterior to posterior that divides the cerebrum into right and left **hemispheres** (see Figure 10-4). The right hemisphere of the brain plays an important role in recognizing faces, patterns, and three-dimensional structures. It also analyzes the emotional content of words but not the actual words. The left hemisphere of the brain performs mathematical and logical reasoning and problem-solving (see Figure 10-5 ■) and analyzes and interprets sights, sounds, words, and sensations. It coordinates the recall of memories. It is active in reading, writing and speaking, and contains the speech center. The two hemispheres are physically separate and their only connection is through the **corpus callosum,** a thick white band of nerves deep within the brain. It allows the two hemispheres to communicate and coordinate their activities (see Figures 10-3 and 10-4).

fissure (FISH-ur)
fiss/o- *splitting*
-ure *system; result of*

hemisphere (HEM-ih-sfeer)
hemi- *one half*
-sphere *sphere or ball*
Every medical word must contain a combining form. The suffix of *hemisphere* contains the combining form *spher/o-*.

corpus callosum
(KOR-pus kah-LOH-sum)
Corpus callosum is a Latin phrase meaning *body of tough fibers.*

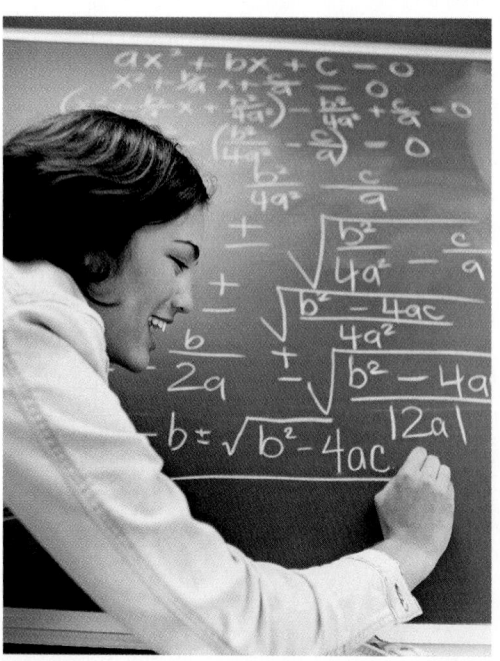

Figure 10-5 ■ Left-brain thinking.

Left-brain thinking uses the left hemisphere, the site of mathematical and logical reasoning.

Ventricles The **ventricles** are four hollow chambers in the brain. There are two large lateral ventricles in the cerebrum, one on either side in the right and left hemispheres (see Figures 10-3 and 10-4). The third ventricle, a narrow, central chamber, connects to the two lateral ventricles above it and to the fourth ventricle beneath it. The fourth ventricle is a narrow chamber that connects to the spinal canal.

The ventricles contain **cerebrospinal fluid (CSF),** a clear, colorless fluid that cushions and protects the brain and contains glucose and other nutrients. Cerebrospinal fluid is produced continuously by special cells that line the ventricles. It flows in a circuit around the ventricles, the spinal canal, then back to the brain and through the subarachnoid space in the meninges where it is absorbed into the blood by large veins.

ventricle (VEN-trih-kl)
Ventricle is a Latin word meaning *little belly.*

ventricular (ven-TRIK-yoo-lar)
ventricul/o- *ventricle (lower heart chamber; chamber in the brain)*
-ar *pertaining to*

cerebrospinal (seh-REE-broh-SPY-nal) (SER-eh-broh-SPY-nal)
cerebr/o- *cerebrum (largest part of the brain)*
spin/o- *spine; backbone*
-al *pertaining to*

Thalamus and Hypothalamus The **thalamus** is located near the center of the cerebrum (see Figures 10-3 and 10-4). It forms the walls of the third ventricle. The thalamus acts as a relay station, sending sensory nerve impulses like pain and touch from the body to the cerebrum. The thalamus is also part of the limbic system that deals with emotions. This is discussed in Psychiatry (Chapter 17). Cranial nerves II through IV (all of which go to the eyes) originate from the thalamus. (The cranial nerves are described later in this chapter.)

The **hypothalamus** is located inferior to the thalamus. It coordinates the activities of the pons and medulla oblongata that control the heart rate, blood pressure, and respiratory rate. The hypothalamus also regulates body temperature, sensations of hunger and thirst, and the circadian (24-hour) rhythm of the body. One thin section of the hypothalamus forms a stalk that connects to the pituitary gland. The hypothalamus also functions as part of the endocrine system because it produces hormones that are stored in and released by the posterior pituitary gland. This is discussed in Endocrinology (Chapter 14).

thalamus (THAL-ah-mus)
Thalamus is a Greek word meaning *an inner chamber.*

thalamic (thah-LAM-ik)
thalam/o- *thalamus*
-ic *pertaining to*

hypothalamus (HY-poh-THAL-ah-mus)

hypothalamic (HY-poh-thah-LAM-ik)
hypo- *below; deficient*
thalam/o- *thalamus*
-ic *pertaining to*

Brainstem The **brainstem** (see Figures 10-3 and 10-4) is a column of tissue composed of the midbrain, the pons, and the medulla oblongata.

The **midbrain** is the most superior part of the brainstem. It keeps the mind conscious. It also contains a gray-to-black pigmented area, the **substantia nigra,** that produces the neurotransmitter dopamine.

The **pons** acts as a relay station for nerve impulses from the body to the cerebellum and cerebrum and back to the body. Within the pons, nerve tracts cross, and nerve impulses from the right side of the body are relayed to the left side of the cerebrum and visa versa. Cranial nerves V through VIII originate in the pons.

The **medulla oblongata** joins the pons to the spinal cord. It relays nerve impulses from the cerebrum to the cerebellum. It also contains the respiratory center that automatically sets the respiratory rate. Cranial nerves IX through XII originate in the medulla oblongata.

brainstem (BRAYN-stem)

substantia nigra (sub-STAN-shee-ah NY-grah)
Substantia nigra is a Latin phrase meaning *structure of black.*

pons (PAWNZ)
Pons is a Latin word meaning *bridge.*

medulla (meh-DUL-ah) (meh-DYOOL-ah) **oblongata** (AWB-long-GAW-tah)
Medulla oblongata is a Latin phrase meaning *soft, marrowlike substance that is long.*

Cerebellum The **cerebellum** is the separate rounded section of the brain that lies inferior and posterior to the cerebrum (see Figures 10-3 and 10-4). The cerebellum monitors muscle tone and body position and adjusts movements of the body that are initiated by other parts of the brain.

cerebellum (SAIR-eh-BEL-um)

cerebellar (SAIR-eh-BEL-ar)
cerebell/o- *cerebellum (posterior part of the brain)*
-ar *pertaining to*

Did You Know?

Although the brain contains millions of neurons, it cannot feel pain. Only the meninges have sensory receptors for pain.

Meninges The entire brain and spinal cord are surrounded by three separate membrane layers that are collectively known as the **meninges** (see Figure 10-6■). The outermost membrane, the **dura mater,** is a tough, fibrous layer that lies directly beneath the cranium and protects the brain. The second layer is the **arachnoid,** a thin membrane. Below the arachnoid is the **subarachnoid space,** which is filled with cerebrospinal fluid and contains fibers from the arachnoid that connect to the pia mater beneath it. The third layer is the **pia mater,** a thin, delicate membrane that contains many small blood vessels. The pia mater follows the contours of the brain, flowing over the gyri and going deep into the sulci.

meninges (meh-NIN-jeez)
Meninx, the singular form, is seldom used.

meningeal
(meh-NIN-jee-al) (MEN-in-JEE-al)
mening/o- *meninges*
-eal *pertaining to*

dura mater (DYOO-rah MAY-ter)
(DYOO-rah MAH-ter)
Dura mater is a Latin phrase meaning *hard mother.*

dural (DYOO-ral)
dur/o- *dura mater*
-al *pertaining to*

arachnoid (ah-RAK-noyd)
arachn/o- *spider, spider web*
-oid *resembling*

subarachnoid (SUB-ah-RAK-noyd)
sub- *below; underneath; less than*
arachn/o- *spider, spider web*
-oid *resembling*

pia mater (PY-ah MAY-ter)
(PEE-ah MAH-ter)
Pia mater is a Latin phrase meaning *tender mother.*

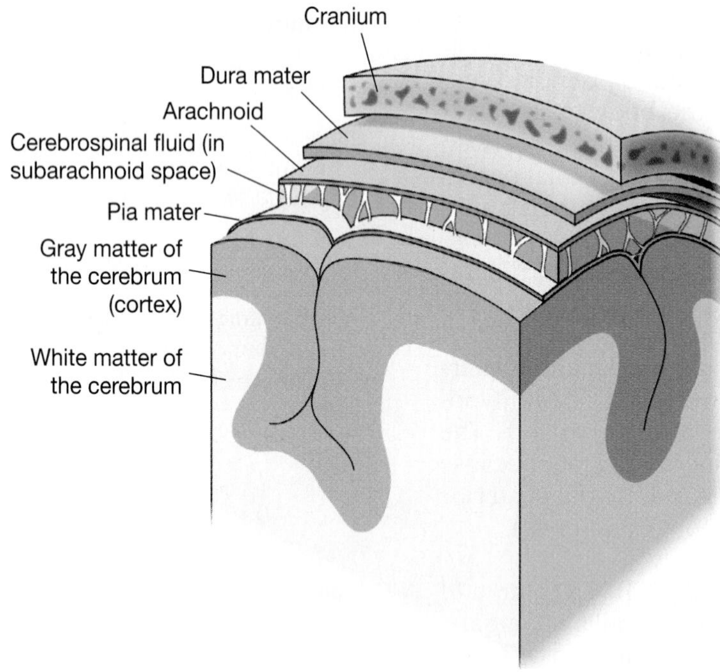

Figure 10-6 ■ Meninges.
The three membrane layers of the dura mater, arachnoid, and pia mater make up the meninges. Between the arachnoid and the pia mater is the subarachnoid space which is filled with cerebrospinal fluid.

Cranial Nerves

The **cranial nerves** are part of the peripheral nervous system (see Table 10-1). These 12 pairs of nerves originate in the brain and carry nerve impulses between the brain and the face, head, neck, and upper back. The only exception is cranial nerve X, which carries nerve impulses between the brain and the organs of the thoracic and abdominal cavities.

Some cranial nerves carry **sensory** information (sensation, pressure, vibration, temperature, pain, and position) from the body to the brain. Other cranial nerves carry sensory information (images, sounds, smells, and tastes) from the eyes, ears, nose, and mouth to the brain. Other cranial nerves carry **motor** commands from the brain to the muscles of the face, head, and neck or to the glands (lacrimal, salivary) in those areas. Some cranial nerves carry a mixture of both sensory and motor nerve impulses.

sensory (SEN-soh-ree)
sens/o- *sensation*
-ory *having the function of*

motor (MOH-tor)
mot/o- *movement*
-or *person or thing that produces or does*

Table 10-1 Cranial Nerves

Cranial Nerve	Areas of Body	Function	
I **olfactory**	nose	sense of smell	
II **optic**	retina of the eye	sense of vision	**optic** (AWP-tik) **opt/o-** *eye; vision* **-ic** *pertaining to*
III **oculomotor**	eye and eyelid	moves the eye and upper eyelid; changes the shape of the pupil and lens	**oculomotor** (AWK-yoo-loh-MOH-tor) **ocul/o-** *eye* **mot/o-** *movement* **-or** *person or thing that produces or does*
IV **trochlear**	eye	moves the eye	**trochlear** (TROHK-lee-ar) **trochle/o-** *structure shaped like a pulley* **-ar** *pertaining to* This cranial nerve goes to an eye muscle that is shaped like a pulley.
V **trigeminal**	eye, eyelid, scalp, face, lips, tongue	moves the eye and lower eyelid; moves the scalp, face, lips, and tongue; sensation in all these areas	**trigeminal** (try-JEM-ih-nal) **tri-** *three* **gemin/o-** *twins; set or group* **-al** *pertaining to* The trigeminal nerve is composed of three different branches: the ophthalmic, maxillary, and mandibular nerves.
VI **abducens**	eye	moves the eye	**abducens** (ab-DOO-senz)
VII **facial**	face and scalp	moves the face and scalp; sense of taste; controls the salivary and lacrimal glands	**facial** (FAY-shal) **faci/o-** *face* **-al** *pertaining to*
VIII **auditory**	ear	sense of hearing; sense of balance (inner ear)	
IX **glossopharyngeal**	mouth	swallowing; controls the salivary glands; sensation in mouth	**glossopharyngeal** (GLAWS-oh-phah-RIN-jee-al) **gloss/o-** *tongue* **pharyng/o-** *pharynx (throat)* **-eal** *pertaining to*
X **vagus**	neck, chest, abdomen	heart beating; breathing (diaphagm); peristalsis in the GI tract; sensation in the throat and ears; sensation in the internal organs	**vagus** (VAY-gus) *Vagus* is a Latin word meaning *wandering.* The vagus nerve travels farther into the body than any of the other cranial nerves.
XI **accessory**	neck, upper back	moves the vocal cords; moves the neck and upper back	**accessory** (ak-SES-oh-ree) **access/o-** *supplemental or contributing part* **-ory** *having the function of* The accessory nerve has two branches that supplement the work of the vagus nerve.
XII **hypoglossal**	tongue	moves the tongue	**hypoglossal** (HY-poh-GLAWS-al) **hypo-** *below; deficient* **gloss/o-** *tongue* **-al** *pertaining to*

Spinal Cord

The **spinal cord** is part of the central nervous system. The spinal cord is a long, narrow column of nerve tissue within the **spinal cavity** or **spinal canal.** At its superior end, the spinal cord is continuous with the medulla oblongata of the brain. At its inferior end, the spinal cord extends to the level of the second lumbar vertebra. There, the spinal cord ends and becomes a group of nerve roots, known as the **cauda equina,** that continues inferiorly in the spinal canal. The spinal cord and spinal cavity pass through the foramen of each protective, bony vertebra (see Figure 10-7 ■). The spinal cord is also protected and nourished by the meninges, which continue in an uninterrupted fashion from around the brain. Cerebrospinal fluid also circulates around the spinal cord. The **epidural space** is an area that is unique to the spinal cord. It lies between the dura mater and the vertebrae and is filled with fatty tissue and blood vessels.

spinal (SPY-nal)
spin/o- *spine; backbone*
-al *pertaining to*

cord (KORD)
Cord is derived from a Latin word meaning *a string.*

cavity (KAV-ih-tee)
cav/o- *hollow space*
-ity *state; condition*

canal (kah-NAL)
Canal is derived from a Latin word meaning *a tubular passageway or channel.*

cauda equina (KAW-dah ee-KWY-nah)
Cauda equina is a Latin phrase meaning *a horse's tail.* The individual nerve roots at the end of the spinal cord resemble the individual hairs in a horse's tail.

epidural (EP-ih-DYOO-ral)
epi- *upon, above*
dur/o- *dura mater*
-al *pertaining to*

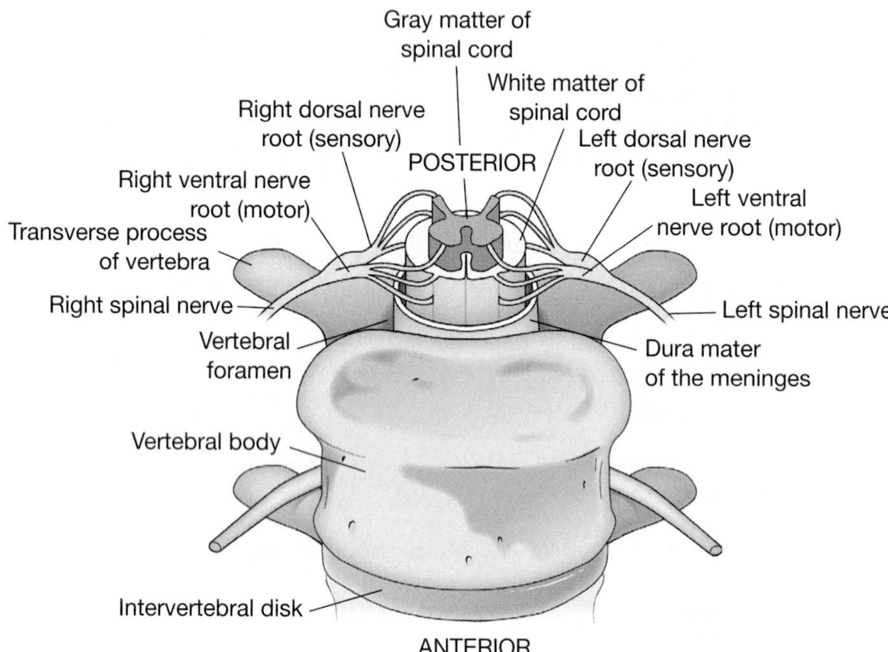

Figure 10-7 ■ Spinal cord and spinal nerves.

The spinal cord passes through the foramen of each vertebra. The spinal nerves originate at regular intervals along the spinal column. Each spinal nerve consists of the ventral nerve roots that carry motor commands to the body and the dorsal nerve roots that receive sensory information from the body.

Spinal Nerves

The **spinal nerves** are part of the peripheral nervous system because they travel toward the periphery, or most distal parts of the body. There are 31 pairs of spinal nerves that originate at regular intervals along the spinal cord. Each pair consists of a spinal nerve to the right side of the body and a spinal nerve to the left side of the body.

Each spinal nerve consists of two groups of nerve roots (see Figure 10-7). The anterior or **ventral nerve roots** carry motor commands from the spinal cord to skeletal muscles and involuntary smooth muscles around organs in the body. These are categorized as **efferent nerves** because they carry nerve impulses away from the spinal cord. The posterior or **dorsal nerve roots** carry sensory information (sensation, pressure, vibration, temperature, pain, and body position) from the skin to the spinal cord and brain. These are categorized as **afferent nerves** because they carry nerve impulses toward the spinal cord and brain.

A **reflex** is an involuntary muscle reaction that is controlled by the spinal cord. The spinal cord reacts immediately to certain types of sensory information (sudden pain, excessive heat, or sudden trauma) without waiting for the brain to consciously think about what is happening. Placing your hand on a hot stove sends sensory information to the spinal cord and the spinal cord immediately sends a motor command to the muscles to move your hand. This entire circuit is known as a reflex arc.

Each group of dorsal nerve roots receives sensory information from a specific area of the skin known as a dermatome, as discussed in Dermatology (Chapter 7). Dermatomes are important in the diagnosis of nerve injuries because they correlate an area of the skin where there is loss of sensation or movement to the spinal nerve for that dermatome.

ventral (VEN-tral)
ventr/o- *front; abdomen*
-al *pertaining to*

efferent (EF-eh-rent)
effer/o- *go out from the center*
-ent *pertaining to*

dorsal (DOR-sal)
dors/o- *back; dorsum; uppermost part*
-al *pertaining to*

afferent (AF-eh-rent)
affer/o- *bring toward the center*
-ent *pertaining to*

reflex (REE-fleks)
Reflex is derived from a Latin word meaning *to bend back.*

Neurons and Neurolgia

Nerves are bundles of individual nerve cells. A **neuron,** an individual nerve cell, is the functional unit of the nervous system. All of the neurons in the nervous system are collectively known as the **parenchyma.** Other cells that create a framework to hold the neurons in place or perform specialized tasks to help the neurons are known as **neuroglia.** Those special cells include the following (see Table 10-2).

nerve (NERV)
Nerve is derived from the Latin word *nervus.*

neuron (NYOOR-on)
Neuron is a Greek word meaning a *nerve.*

parenchyma (pah-RENG-kih-mah)

parenchymal (pah-RENG-kih-mal)
parenchym/o- *parenchyma (functional cells of an organ)*
-al *pertaining to*

neuroglia (nyoo-ROHG-lee-ah)
neur/o- *nerve*
-glia *substance that holds things together*

Table 10-2 Neuroglia

Cell Type	Cell Function	Word Part and Definition
astrocyte	Large cell with radiating branches that support nearby neurons and connect them to capillaries. Astrocytes form the blood-brain barrier that keeps certain substances in the blood from getting to the brain.	**astrocyte** (AS-troh-site) **astr/o-** *starlike structure* **-cyte** *cell* The radiating branches of an astrocyte give it a starlike appearance.
ependymal cell	Cell that lines the ventricles of the brain and the spinal canal and forms cerebrospinal fluid.	**ependymal** (ep-EN-dih-mal) **ependym/o-** *lining membrane* **-al** *pertaining to*
microglia	Cell that can move anywhere in the central nervous system. It engulfs and destroys dead tissue and pathogens (bacteria, viruses, and so forth). Microglia are the smallest of all the neuroglia.	**microglia** (my-KROHG-lee-ah) **micr/o-** *small* **-glia** *substance that holds things together*
oligodendroglia	Cell that forms myelin that covers each axon (a part of the neuron) in the central nervous system (brain and spinal cord).	**oligodendroglia** (OL-ih-goh-den-DROHG-lee-ah) **olig/o-** *scanty* **dendr/o-** *branching structure* **-glia** *substance that holds things together* Add words to make a correct and complete definition of *oligodendroglia: [cell] that holds things together [and has a] scanty, branching structure.*
Schwann cell	Cell that forms myelin that covers each axon in the peripheral nervous system (cranial nerves and spinal nerves).	**Schwann** (SHVAHN) Named by Theodor Schwann (1810–1882), a Germany anatomist. This is an example of an eponym: a person from whom something takes its name. Schwann also discovered pepsin in the stomach and coined the word *metabolism.*

Other Divisions of the Nervous System

The brain and spinal cord send nerve impulses through the cranial and spinal nerves of the central and peripheral nervous systems to make some type of change in the body. If the brain or spinal cord wants a voluntary skeletal muscle to move, this command is transmitted to the muscle by the **somatic nervous system.** If the brain or the spinal cord wants to change the heart rate, wants involuntary smooth muscles around an organ to contract or relax, or wants to stimulate a gland to secrete, this command is transmitted to the heart, smooth muscles, or glands by the **autonomic nervous system.** The autonomic nervous system can be further broken down into two parts: the parasympathetic nervous system and the sympathetic nervous system (see Figure 10-8■).

somatic (soh-MAT-ik)
somat/o- *body*
-ic *pertaining to*

autonomic (AW-toh-NAWM-ik)
autonom/o- *independent, self-governing*
-ic *pertaining to*

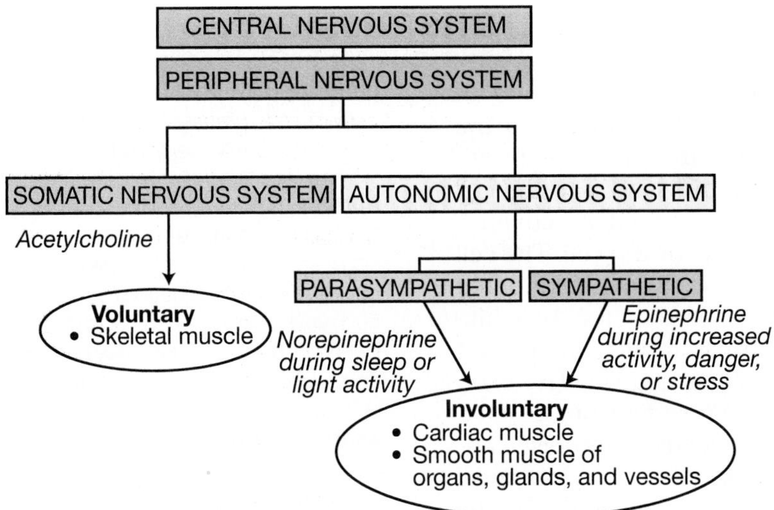

Figure 10-8 ■ Divisions of the nervous system.

The **parasympathetic nervous system** is active while the body is sleeping, resting, eating, or doing light activity. The neurotransmitter of the parasympathetic nervous system is norepinephrine. The parasympathetic nervous system:

- Raises or lowers the heart rate
- Changes the diameter of the pupils in response to changing levels of light
- Produces peristalsis in the gastrointestinal tract
- Stimulates the salivary glands during eating
- Prepares the body for sexual activity.

parasympathetic
(PAIR-ah-SIM-pah-THET-ik)
para- *beside, apart from; two parts of a pair; abnormal*
sym- *together, with*
pathet/o- *suffering*
-ic *pertaining to*
The parasympathetic nervous system works beside the sympathetic nervous system as one part of a pair.

The **sympathetic nervous system** is active when the body is confronted with danger or during times of stress or anxiety. It prepares the body for "fight or flight." The neurotransmitter of the sympathetic nervous system is epinephrine. The sympathetic nervous system:

- Raises the heart rate to prepare for running or fighting
- Dilates the pupils to better visualize danger
- Causes the smooth muscles around the arteries to constrict to raise the blood pressure
- Causes the smooth muscles around the bronchi to dilate to increase air flow to the lungs.

sympathetic (SIM-pah-THET-ik)
sym- *together, with*
pathet/o- *suffering*
-ic *pertaining to*
The sympathetic nervous system is active when the body is suffering from fear.

Physiology of Nerve Transmission

Each neuron consists of three parts: the dendrites, a cell body, and an axon (see Figure 10-9 ■). The **dendrites** are multiple branches at the beginning of a neuron that receive a neurotransmitter from the previous neuron, convert it to an electrical impulse, and send it to the cell body. The cell body contains the **nucleus** that directs cellular activities, produces neurotransmitters, and provides energy for the cell. The cell body sends the electrical impulse to the **axon,** a single, enlongated branch at the end of the neuron. The axon is covered by a fatty, white insulating layer of **myelin** that keeps the electrical impulse intact as it travels. Myelin is only present on the axon of the neuron. The axon does not directly connect to the dendrites of the next neuron. Instead, there is a space or **synapse** between them. The electrical impulse cannot travel across the synapse, and so the axon releases a chemical messenger or **neurotransmitter.** The neurotransmitter crosses the synapse and binds to **receptors** on the dendrites of the next neuron. This creates a new electrical impulse that continues through that neuron, and so forth. These events all happen within a fraction of a second.

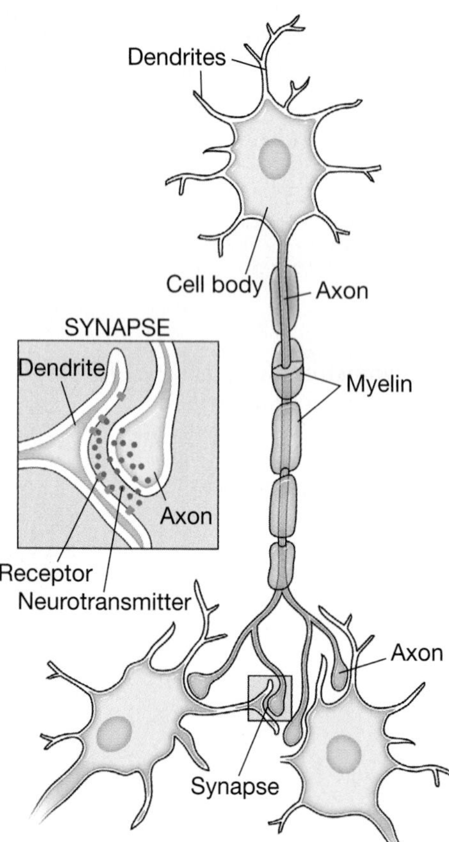

Figure 10-9 ■ A neuron.

A neuron consists of several dendrites, a cell body, and an axon. The dendrites receive nerve impulses from other neurons. The cell body contains the nucleus of the neuron. The axon transmits nerve impulses to other neurons (or to a muscle fiber, to a cell in an organ, or to a cell in a gland).

dendrite (DEN-dryt)
dendr/o- *branching structure*
-ite *thing that pertains to*

nucleus (NYOO-klee-us)
Nucleus is a Latin word meaning *little kernel or stone inside a fruit.* The Romans did not have a microscope to see a cell and its nucleus. However, when microscopes were invented, this Latin word was borrowed and applied to the nucleus inside a cell.

axon (AK-sawn)
Axon is a Greek word meaning *axle* or *axis.* When an axon was first seen with a microscope, this Greek word was used to describe it because the axon appeared as a line around which the other parts of the neuron were arranged.

myelin (MY-eh-lin)

myelinated (MY-eh-lih-NAYT-ed)
myelin/o- *myelin*
-ated *pertaining to a condition; composed of*

synapse (SIN-aps)
Synapse is derived from a Greek word meaning *connection.*

neurotransmitter
(NYOOR-oh-trans-MIT-er)
neur/o- *nerve*
trans- *across, through*
mitt/o- *to send*
-er *person or thing that produces or does*

receptor (ree-SEP-tor)
recept/o- *receive*
-or *person or thing that produces or does*

The **gray matter** of the cerebral cortex, cerebellar cortex, and spinal cord contains the dendrites and bodies of thousands of neurons. These parts are not covered by myelin and so the tissue is gray-tan in color. The **white matter** of the brain and spinal cord contains the axons of thousands of neurons, each of which is covered with **myelin** that gives this tissue its characteristic white color. These areas are said to be **myelinated.**

There are many different neurotransmitters in the nervous system. The most common ones are described in Table 10-3.

Table 10-3 Neurotransmitters

Neurotransmitter	Location	Word Part and Definition
acetylcholine	In the synapse between a neuron and a voluntary skeletal muscle. It is released by the somatic nervous system.	**acetylcholine** (AS-ee-til-KOH-leen)
dopamine	In the synapse between neurons in the limbic system and hypothalamus.	**dopamine** (DOHP-ah-meen)
endorphins	In the synapse between neurons in the hypothalamus, thalamus, and brainstem. Endorphins are the body's own natural pain relievers.	**endorphins** (en-DOR-finz) *Endorphins* is a combination of the words *endogenous* (*produced within*) and *morphine*. Morphine is a pain-relieving drug made from opium. Endorphins are the body's own natural pain relievers.
epinephrine	In the synapse between a neuron and the heart, involuntary smooth muscles, or the adrenal gland. It is released by the sympathetic nervous system during stress or danger.	**epinephrine** (EP-ih-NEF-rin)
norepinephrine	In the synapse between a neuron and the heart, involuntary smooth muscles, or a gland. It is released by the parasympathetic nervous system during sleep and light activity.	**norepinephrine** (NOR-ep-ih-NEF-rin)
serotonin	In the synapse between neurons in the limbic system, hypothalamus, cerebellum, and spinal cord.	**serotonin** (SER-oh-TOH-nin)

Vocabulary Review

Anatomy and Physiology

Now that you have studied the anatomy and physiology of the nervous system, take time to review those new words and descriptions. Memorize the combining forms and their definitions before going on to the next section.

Word or Phrase	Combining Form and Definition	Description
abducens nerve		Cranial nerve VI. Movement of the eyeball.
accessory nerve	access/o- *supplemental or contributing part*	Cranial nerve XI. Movement of the vocal cords and muscles of the neck and upper back. Two of its nerve branches also assist the vagus nerve.
acetylcholine		Neurotransmitter between neurons in the brain and the spinal cord, also between a neuron and a voluntary skeletal muscle
afferent nerves	affer/o- *bring toward the center*	Nerves that carry sensory nerve impulses to the brain or to the spinal cord from the body
arachnoid	arachn/o- *spider, spiderweb*	Thin, middle layer of the meninges
astrocyte	astr/o- *starlike structure*	Star-shaped cell that provides structural support for neurons, connects them to capillaries, and forms the blood-brain barrier
auditory nerve	audit/o- *the sense of hearing*	Cranial nerve VIII. Sense of hearing and maintains the balance
auditory cortex	audit/o- *the sense of hearing*	Area in the temporal lobe of the cerebrum that receives and analyzes nerve impulses from the ears
autonomic nervous system	autonom/o- *independent, self-governing*	Division of the nervous system that carries nerve impulses to the heart, involuntary smooth muscles, and glands. It includes the parasympathetic nervous system and the sympathetic nervous system.
axon		Part of the neuron that is a single, elongated branch at the opposite end from the dendrites. It conducts the electrical impulse and releases neurotransmitters into the synapse. Axons are covered by an insulating layer of myelin.
brain		Largest organ of the nervous system. It is part of the central nervous system and is located in the cranial cavity.
brainstem		Most inferior part of the brain that joins with the spinal cord. It is composed of the midbrain, pons, and medulla oblongata.
cauda equina		Group of nerve roots that begin where the spinal cord ends and continue inferiorly within the spinal cavity. They look like the tail of a horse.
cell body		Part of the neuron that contains the nucleus and produces neurotransmitters
central nervous system	centr/o- *center; dominant part* nerv/o- *nerve*	Division of the nervous system that includes the brain and the spinal cord

Word or Phrase	Combining Form and Definition	Description
cerebellum	cerebell/o- *cerebellum (posterior part of the brain*	Small, rounded structure that is the most posterior part of the brain. It monitors muscle tone and position and coordinates new muscle movements.
cerebral cortex	cortic/o- *cortex (outer region)*	The outermost surface of the cerebrum and cerebellum. It consists of gray matter.
cerebrospinal fluid	cerebr/o- *cerebrum (largest part of the brain)* spin/o- *spine; backbone*	Clear, colorless fluid that circulates through the subarachnoid space, around the brain, through the ventricles, and the spinal cavity. It cushions and protects the brain and contains glucose and other nutrients. It is produced by the ependymal cells that line the ventricles and spinal canal.
cerebrum	cerebr/o- *cerebrum (largest part of the brain)*	The largest and most visible part of the brain. Its surface contains gyri and sulci and it is divided into two hemispheres.
corpus callosum		Thick white band of nerves that connects the two hemispheres of the cerebrum and allows them to communicate and coordinate their activities
cranial cavity	crani/o- *cranium (skull)* cav/o- *hollow space*	Hollow cavity inside the cranium that contains the brain and the origins of the cranial nerves
cranial nerves (I through XII)	crani/o- *cranium (skull)*	Twelve pairs of nerves that originate in the brain. They carry sensory nerve impulses to the brain and motor nerve impulses from the brain.
cranium	crani/o- *cranium (skull)*	Rounded dome of bone at the top of the skull
dendrite	dendr/o- *branching structure*	Multiple branches at the beginning of a neuron that receive a neuro-transmitter and convert it to an electrical impulse
dopamine		Neurotransmitter between neurons in the limbic system or hypo-thalamus
dorsal nerve roots	dors/o- *back; dorsum; uppermost part*	Group of spinal nerve roots that enter the posterior (dorsal) part of the spinal cord and carry sensory nerve impulses from the body to the spinal cord
dura mater	dur/o- *dura mater*	Tough, outermost layer of the meninges. The dura mater lies just beneath the bones of the cranium and within the foramen of each vertebra.
efferent nerves	effer/o- *go out from the center*	Nerves that carry motor nerve impulses from the brain or from the spinal cord to the body
endorphins		Neurotransmitter between neurons in the hypothalamus, thalamus, or brainstem. Endorphins are the body's own natural pain relievers.
ependymal cells	ependym/o- *lining membrane*	Specialized cells that line the walls of the ventricles and spinal canal and produce cerebrospinal fluid
epidural space	dur/o- *dura mater*	Area between the dura mater and the vertebral body
epinephrine		Neurotransmitter for the sympathetic nervous system
facial nerve	faci/o- *face*	Cranial nerve VII. Sense of taste. Control of salivary and lacrimal glands. Movement of face and scalp muscles.

Word or Phrase	Combining Form and Definition	Description
fissure	**fiss/o-** *splitting*	Deep division that runs anteriorly to posteriorly through the cerebrum and divides it into right and left hemispheres
frontal lobe	**front/o-** *front*	Lobe of the cerebrum that predicts future events and consequences. Exerts conscious control over the skeletal muscles. Contains the gustatory cortex for the sense of taste.
glossopharyngeal nerve	**gloss/o-** *tongue* **pharyng/o-** *pharynx (throat)*	Cranial nerve IX. Sensation in the mouth. Movement of the throat muscles for swallowing. Controls the salivary glands.
gray matter		Areas of gray tissue in the brain and spinal cord that are composed of cell bodies and dendrites
gustatory cortex	**gustat/o-** *the sense of taste*	Area in the frontal lobe of the cerebrum that receives and analyzes sensory nerve impulses from the tongue and taste receptors
gyrus		One of many large elevated folds of brain tissue on the surface of the cerebrum with smaller folds on the cerebellum. In between each gyrus is a sulcus (groove). Plural: gyri.
hemisphere		One half of the cerebrum. The right hemisphere recognizes patterns and three-dimensional structures (including faces) and the emotions of words. The left hemisphere deals with mathematical and logical reasoning, analysis, and interpreting sights, sounds, and sensations. The left hemisphere is active in reading, writing, and speaking.
hypoglossal nerve	**gloss/o-** *tongue*	Cranial nerve XII. Movement of the tongue.
hypothalamus	**thalam/o-** *thalamus*	Area in the center of the brain just below the thalamus that coordinates the activities of the pons and medulla oblongata. It also controls heart rate, blood pressure, respiratory rate, body temperature, sensations of hunger and thirst, and the circadian rhythm. It also produces hormones as part of the endocrine system.
lobe		Large area of the cerebrum. Each lobe is named for the bone of the cranium that is next to it: frontal lobe, parietal lobe, temporal lobe, and occipital lobe.
medulla oblongata		Most inferior part of the brainstem that joins to the spinal cord. It relays nerve impulses from the cerebrum to the cerebellum. It contains the respiratory center. Cranial nerves IX through XII originate there.
meninges	**mening/o-** *meninges*	Three separate membranes that envelope and protect the entire brain and spinal cord. The meninges include the dura mater, arachnoid, and pia mater
microglia	**micr/o-** *small*	Cells that move, engulf, and destroy pathogens anywhere in the central nervous system
myelin	**myelin/o-** *myelin*	Fatty sheath around the axon of a neuron. It acts as an insulator to keep the electrical impulse intact. Myelin around the axons of neurons in the brain and spinal cord is produced by oligodendroglia. Myelin around axons of the cranial and spinal nerves is produced by the Schwann cells. An axon with myelin is said to be myelinated.

Word or Phrase	Combining Form and Definition	Description
neuroglia	**neur/o-** *nerve*	Cells that hold neurons in place and perform specialized tasks. Includes astrocytes, ependymal cells, microglia, oligodendroglia, and Schwann cells.
nerve	**nerv/o-** *nerve*	A bundle of individual neurons
nervous system	**nerv/o-** *nerve* **muscul/o-** *muscle*	Body system that consists of the brain, cranial nerves, spinal cord, spinal nerves and other structures. Its purpose is to receive nerve impulses from the body and send nerve impulses to the body. Anatomically, it consists of the central nervous system and the peripheral nervous system. Physiologically, it consists of the somatic nervous system and the autonomic nervous system. Also known as the **neuromuscular system.**
neuron		An individual nerve cell. The functional part of the nervous system.
neurotransmitter	**neur/o-** *nerve* **mitt/o-** *to send*	Chemical messenger that travels across the synapse between neurons
norepinephrine		Neurotransmitter for the parasympathetic nervous system
nucleus		Structure in the cell body of a neuron that directs cellular activities like synthesizing neurotransmitters
occipital lobe	**occipit/o-** *occiput (back of the head)*	Lobe of the cerebrum that receives and analyzes sensory information from the eyes. Contains the visual cortex for the sense of sight.
oculomotor nerve	**ocul/o-** *eye* **mot/o-** *movement*	Cranial nerve III. Movement of the eyeball, upper eyelid, pupil, and lens
oligodendroglia	**olig/o-** *scanty* **dendr/o-** *branching structure*	Cell that forms the myelin sheath around axons of neurons in the brain and spinal cord
olfactory cortex	**olfact/o-** *the sense of smell*	Area in the temporal lobe of the cerebrum that receives and analyzes nerve impulses from the nose
olfactory nerve	**olfact/o-** *the sense of smell*	Cranial nerve I. Sense of smell.
optic nerve	**opt/o-** *eye; vision*	Cranial nerve II. Sense of vision.
parenchyma		All the neurons in the nervous system. The functional units (as opposed to the structural components) of any body system.
parasympathetic nervous system		Division of the autonomic nervous system that uses the neurotransmitter norepinephrine and carries nerve impulses to the heart, involuntary smooth muscles, and glands while the body is at rest
parietal lobe	**pariet/o-** *wall of a cavity*	Lobe of the cerebrum that receives and analyzes sensory information about temperature, touch, pressure, vibration, and pain from the skin and internal organs
peripheral nervous system	**peripher/o-** *outer aspects*	Division of the nervous system that includes the cranial nerves and the spinal nerves

Word or Phrase	Combining Form and Definition	Description
pia mater		Thin, delicate innermost layer of the meninges. It covers the surface of the brain and contains many small blood vessels.
pons		Area of the brainstem that relays nerve impulses from the body to the cerebellum and back to the body. Area where nerve tracts cross from one side of the body to the opposite side of the cerebrum. Cranial nerves V through VIII originate there.
receptor	recept/o- *receive*	Structure on the cell membrane of a dendrite (or organ, muscle, or gland) where a neurotransmitter binds
reflex		Involuntary muscle reaction that is controlled by the spinal cord. In response to pain, the spinal cord immediately sends a command to the muscles of the body to move. All of this takes place without conscious thought or processing by the brain. The entire circuit is also known as a **reflex arc.**
Schwann cell		Cell that forms the myelin sheaths around axons of the cranial and spinal nerves
serotonin		Neurotransmitter between neurons in the limbic system, hypothalamus, cerebellum, and spinal cord
somatic nervous system	somat/o- *body*	Division of the nervous system that uses the neurotransmitter acetylcholine and carries nerve impulses to the voluntary skeletal muscles
spinal cavity	spin/o- *spine; backbone* cav/o- *hollow space*	Hollow cavity inside the vertebral column that contains the spinal cord and the origins of the spinal nerves. Also known as the **spinal canal.**
spinal cord	spin/o- *spine; backbone*	Part of the central nervous system. It joins the medulla oblongata of the brain and extends down the back in the spinal cavity. It ends at lumbar vertebra L2 and separates into individual nerves (cauda equina).
spinal nerves	spin/o- *spine; backbone*	Thirty-one pairs of nerves. Each pair comes out from the spinal cord between two vertebrae. An individual spinal nerve consists of dorsal nerve roots and ventral nerve roots.
subarachnoid space	arachn/o- *spider, spider web*	Space beneath the arachnoid layer of the meninges. It is filled with cerebrospinal fluid.
substantial nigra		A darkly pigmented area in the midbrain of the brainstem that produces the neurotransmitter dopamine
sulcus		One of many large grooves between the gyri in the cerebrum and cerebellum. Plural: sulci.
sympathetic nervous system	pathet/o- *suffering*	Division of the autonomic nervous system that uses the neurotransmitter epinephrine and carries nerve impulses to the heart, involuntary muscles, and glands during times of increased activity, danger, or stress
synapse		Space between the axon of one neuron and the dendrites of the next neuron
temporal lobe	tempor/o- *temple (side of the head)*	Lobe of the cerebrum that receives and analyzes sensory information. Contains the auditory cortex for the sense of hearing and the olfactory cortex for the sense of smell.
thalamus	thalam/o- *thalamus*	Area in the center of the brain that acts as a relay station. It takes sensory nerve impulses from the body and sends them to areas in the cerebrum. Cranial nerves II, III, and IV originate from the thalamus.

Word or Phrase	Combining Form and Definition	Description
trigeminal nerve	gemin/o- *twins; set or group*	Cranial nerve V. Sensation in the eyeball, lower eyelid, scalp, face, lips, and tongue. Movement of the muscles in these areas. Composed of three nerve branches: ophthalmic nerve, maxillary nerve, mandibular nerve.
trochlear nerve	trochle/o- *structure shaped like a pulley*	Cranial nerve IV. Movement of the eyeball.
vagus nerve		Cranial nerve X. Sensation in throat and ears. Beating of the heart. Sensation in internal organs of chest and abdomen. Movement of the muscles of respiration and digestion.
ventral nerve roots	ventr/o- *front; abdomen*	Group of spinal nerve roots that exit from the anterior (ventral) part of the spinal cord and carry motor nerve impulses to the body
ventricles	ventricul/o- *ventricle (lower heart chamber; chamber in the brain)*	Four hollow chambers within the brain that contain cerebrospinal fluid. The two lateral ventricles are within the right and left hemispheres of the cerebrum. The third ventricle is small and connects the lateral ventricles to the fourth ventricle, which is next to the cerebellum.
visual cortex	vis/o- *sight; vision*	Area in the occipital lobe of the cerebrum that receives and analyzes sensory nerve impulses from the eye
white matter		Areas of white tissue in the brain and spinal cord that are composed of axons covered with myelin

Labeling Exercise

A. *Match each anatomy word or phrase to its numbered structure in Figure 10-10■. Write that word or phrase on the blank line next to its number. Use the Answer Key at the end of the book to check your answers.*

cerebellum	frontal lobe	parietal lobe
cerebrum	occipital lobe	temporal lobe

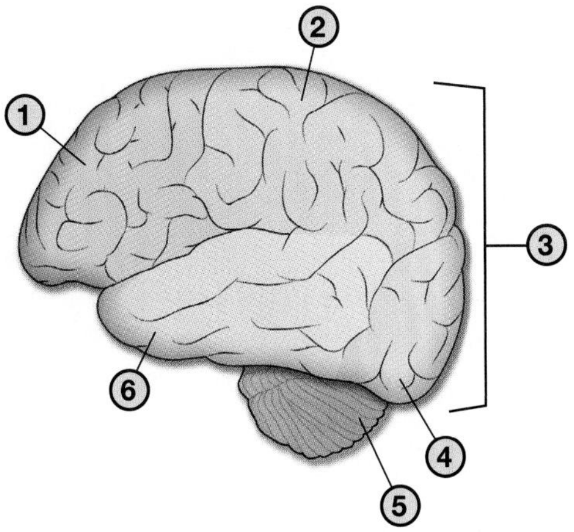

1. ______________________
2. ______________________
3. ______________________
4. ______________________
5. ______________________
6. ______________________

Figure 10-10 ■

B. *Match each anatomy word or phrase to its numbered structure in Figure 10-11■. Write that word or phrase on the blank line next to its number.*

arachnoid cranium dura mater	gray matter of the cerebrum (cortex) subarachnoid space	pia mater white matter of the cerebrum

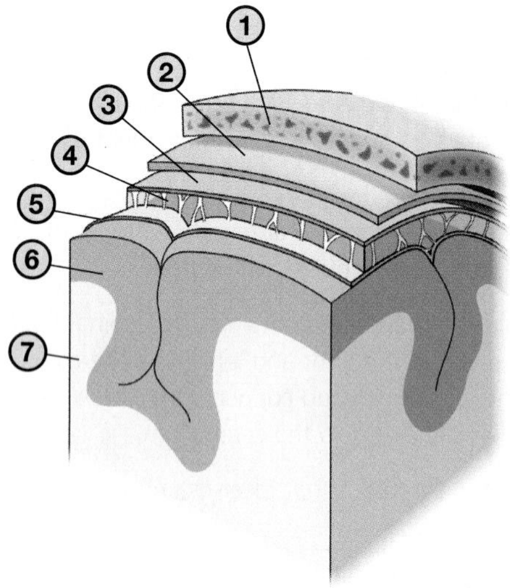

1. ______________________
2. ______________________
3. ______________________
4. ______________________
5. ______________________
6. ______________________
7. ______________________

Figure 10-11 ■

C. *Match each anatomy word or phrase to its numbered structure in Figure 10-12■. Write that word or phrase on the blank line next to its number.*

cerebellum cerebrum corpus callosum	fourth ventricle gyrus hypothalamus	lateral ventricle medulla oblongata midbrain	pons sulcus thalamus

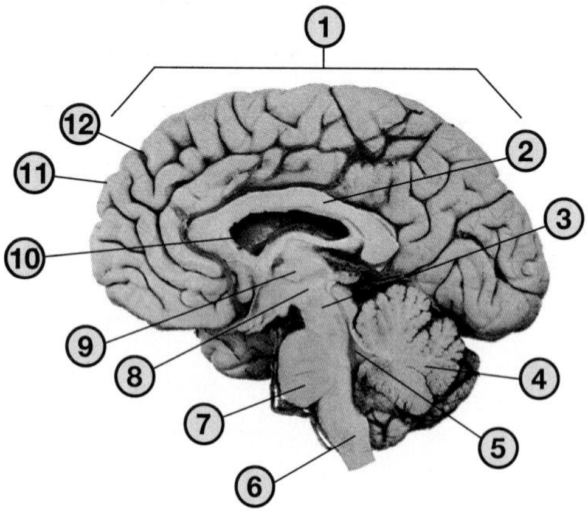

1. ______________________
2. ______________________
3. ______________________
4. ______________________
5. ______________________
6. ______________________
7. ______________________
8. ______________________
9. ______________________
10. ______________________
11. ______________________
12. ______________________

Figure 10-12 ■

Building Medical Words

Combining Forms

Here are the nervous system combining forms you have learned so far. Next to each combining form, write its meaning. Use the Answer Key at the end of the book to check your answers. The first one has been done for you.

	Combining Form	Medical Meaning		Combining Form	Medical Meaning
1.	gemin/o-	twins; a set or group	27.	mot/o-	________
2.	access/o-	________	28.	muscul/o-	________
3.	affer/o-	________	29.	myelin/o-	________
4.	arachn/o-	________	30.	nerv/o-	________
5.	astr/o-	________	31.	neur/o-	________
6.	audit/o-	________	32.	occipit/o-	________
7.	autonom/o-	________	33.	ocul/o-	________
8.	cav/o-	________	34.	olfact/o-	________
9.	centr/o-	________	35.	olig/o-	________
10.	cerebell/o-	________	36.	opt/o-	________
11.	cerebr/o-	________	37.	parenchym/o-	________
12.	cortic/o-	________	38.	pariet/o-	________
13.	crani/o-	________	39.	pathet/o-	________
14.	dendr/o-	________	40.	peripher/o-	________
15.	dors/o-	________	41.	pharyng/o-	________
16.	dur/o-	________	42.	recept/o-	________
17.	effer/o-	________	43.	sens/o-	________
18.	ependym/o-	________	44.	somat/o-	________
19.	faci/o-	________	45.	spin/o-	________
20.	fiss/o-	________	46.	tempor/o-	________
21.	front/o-	________	47.	thalam/o-	________
22.	gloss/o-	________	48.	trochle/o-	________
23.	gustat/o-	________	49.	ventricul/o-	________
24.	mening/o-	________	50.	ventr/o-	________
25.	micr/o-	________	51.	vis/o-	________
26.	mitt/o-	________			

Combining Forms and Suffixes

Read the definition hint for the medical word you are to build. Look at the combining form that is given. Write the correct suffix on the blank line. Then write the medical word. (Remember: You may need to remove the combining vowel. Always remove the hyphens and slash.) Use the Answer Key at the end of the book to check your answers. The first one has been done for you.

SUFFIX LIST

-al (pertaining to)	-eal (pertaining to)	-ite (thing that pertains to)	-ory (having the function of)
-ar (pertaining to)	-ent (pertaining to)	-logy (the study of)	-ous (pertaining to)
-cyte (cell)	-ic (pertaining to)	-oid (resembling)	-ure (system; result of)

	Definition Hint	Combining Form	Suffix	Write the Medical Word
1.	Pertaining to the cerebrum	cerebr/o-	-al	*cerebral*
2.	The study of the nerves	neur/o-	______	______
3.	Pertaining to the top of the skull	crani/o-	______	______
4.	Pertaining to the nerves	nerv/o-	______	______
5.	Having the function of hearing	audit/o-	______	______
6.	Pertaining to the ventricles (in the brain)	ventricul/o-	______	______
7.	Resembling a spider web	arachn/o-	______	______
8.	Pertaining to the meninges	mening/o-	______	______
9.	A cell shaped like a star	astr/o-	______	______
10.	Pertaining to the spine	spin/o-	______	______
11.	Thing that pertains to a branching structure	dendr/o-	______	______
12.	Pertaining to going out from the center	effer/o-	______	______
13.	Something that is the result of splitting	fiss/o-	______	______
14.	Pertaining to the outer aspects of the body	peripher/o-	______	______
15.	Pertaining to the thalamus	thalam/o-	______	______
16.	Having the function of sensation	sens/o-	______	______

Combining Forms and Prefixes

Read the definition hint for the medical word you are to build. Look at the medical word or word part that is given. It already contains a combining form and a suffix. Write the correct prefix on the blank line. Then write the medical word. (Remember: You may need to remove the combining vowel. Always remove the hyphens and slash.) Use the Answer Key at the end of the book to check your answers. The first one has been done for you.

PREFIX LIST		
epi- (upon, above)	hypo- (below; deficient)	sym- (with)
hemi- (one half)	sub- (below; underneath; less than)	tri- (three)

Definition Hint	Prefix	Medical Word or Word Part	Write the Medical Word
1. Pertaining to suffering with	sym-	pathetic	sympathetic
2. Structure beneath the thalamus	________	thalamus	________
3. Pertaining to above the dura mater	________	dural	________
4. Underneath the arachnoid	________	arachnoid	________
5. One half of a ball or sphere	________	sphere	________
6. Cranial nerve composed of three branches	________	geminal	________

Symptoms, Signs, and Diseases

Brain

Word or Phrase	Word Part and Definition	Description
amnesia	**amnesia** (am-NEE-zee-ah) *Amnesia* is a Greek word meaning *forgetfulness.*	Partial or total loss of memory of recent or remote (past) experiences. Often a consequence of brain injury or a stroke that damages the hippocampus where long-term memories are stored and processed. Treatment: None.
anencephaly	**anencephaly** (AN-en-SEF-ah-lee) **an-** *without, not* **-encephaly** *condition of the brain* Every medical word must contain a combining form. The suffix of *anencephaly* contains the combining form *encephal/o-.*	Rare congenital condition in which some or all of the cranium and cerebrum are missing in a newborn. The infant breathes because the respiratory center in the medulla oblongata is intact, but only survives a few hours or days. Treatment: None.
aphasia	**aphasia** (ah-FAY-zee-ah) **a-** *without, not* **phas/o-** *speech* **-ia** *condition, state, thing* **aphasic** (ah-FAY-sik) **a-** *without, not* **phas/o-** *speech* **-ic** *pertaining to* **expressive** (eks-PREH-siv) **express/o-** *communicate* **-ive** *pertaining to* **receptive** (ree-SEP-tiv) **recept/o-** *receive* **-ive** *pertaining to* **global** (GLOH-bal) **glob/o-** *shaped like a globe; comprehensive* **-al** *pertaining to* **dysphasia** (dis-FAY-zee-ah) **dys-** *painful, difficult, abnormal* **phas/o-** *speech* **-ia** *condition, state, thing*	Loss of the ability to communicate verbally or in writing. Aphasia is caused by injury to the areas of the brain that deal with language and the interpretation of sounds and symbols. Patients with aphasia are said to be **aphasic. Expressive aphasia** is the inability to verbally express thoughts. **Receptive aphasia** is the inability to understand the spoken or written word. Patients with both types are said to have **global aphasia.** Impairment that involves some difficulty speaking or understanding words is known as **dysphasia.** Aphasia can be the result of head trauma, a stroke, or Alzheimer's disease. Treatment: Correct the underlying cause, if possible.

Word or Phrase	Word Part and Definition	Description
arteriovenous malformation (AVM)	**arteriovenous** (ar-TEER-ee-oh-VEE-nus) **arteri/o-** *artery* **ven/o-** *vein* **-ous** *pertaining to* **malformation** (MAL-for-MAY-shun) **mal-** *bad, inadequate* **format/o-** *structure; arrangement* **-ion** *action; condition*	Abnormality in which arteries in the brain connect directly to veins (rather than to capillaries), forming a twisted nest of blood vessels. An AVM can rupture and cause a stroke. Treatment: Focused beam radiation to destroy the AVM or embolization to block blood flow to the AVM; surgical excision, if needed.
brain tumor	**benign** (bee-NINE) *Benign* is derived from a Latin word meaning *kind, not cancerous.* **malignant** (mah-LIG-nant) **malign/o-** *intentionally causing harm; cancer* **-ant** *pertaining to* Malignant tumors are cancerous. **intracranial** (IN-trah-KRAY-nee-al) **intra-** *within* **crani/o-** *cranium (skull)* **-al** *pertaining to*	**Benign** or **malignant** tumor of any area of the brain. Brain tumors arise from the neuroglia or meninges, rather than from neurons themselves. They are named according to the type of brain cell from which they originated (see Table 10-3). Malignant brain tumors can also be secondary tumors that metastasized from a primary malignant tumor elsewhere in the body. Because the cranium is rigid, the enlarging bulk of a benign or malignant tumor causes increased **intracranial pressure (ICP)** and cerebral edema (see Figure 10-13 ■). This compresses and destroys brain tissue. Treatment: Surgery to remove or debulk the tumor. Chemotherapy or radiation therapy for malignant tumors. **Figure 10-13 ■ Glioma.** This patient's MRI scan of the brain shows a large glioma that is pressing on the cerebellum.
cephalalgia	**cephalalgia** (SEF-al-AL-jee-ah) **cephal/o-** *head* **alg/o-** *pain* **-ia** *condition, state, thing*	Pain in the head or headache. Headaches can be caused by eyestrain, muscular tension in the face or neck, generalized infections like the flu, migraine headaches, hypertension, or by more serious conditions like head trauma, meningitis, or brain tumors. Treatment: Correct the underlying cause.
cerebral palsy (CP)	**cerebral** (SER-eh-bral) (seh-REE-bral) **cerebr/o-** *cerebrum (largest part of the brain)* **-al** *pertaining to* **palsy** (PAWL-zee) *Palsy* is derived from the word *paralysis.*	Cerebral palsy is caused by a lack of oxygen to parts of the baby's brain during birth. The extent of involvement varies, but can include spastic muscles and lack of coordination in walking, eating, and talking. There can be muscle paralysis, seizures, and mental retardation. Treatment: Braces, muscle relaxant drugs.

Table 10-3 Types of Brain Tumors

Brain Tumor	Characteristic	Originating Cell or Structure	Word Part and Definition
astrocytoma	malignant	astrocyte in the cerebrum	**astrocytoma** (AS-troh-sy-TOH-mah) **astr/o-** *starlike structure* **cyt/o-** *cell* **-oma** *tumor, mass*
ependymoma	benign	ependymal cells that line the ventricles	**ependymoma** (eh-PEN-dih-MOH-mah) **ependym/o-** *lining membrane* **-oma** *tumor, mass*
glioma (see Figure 10-13)	either	any neuroglial cell	**glioma** (gly-OH-mah) **gli/o-** *substance that holds things together* **-oma** *tumor, mass*
glioblastoma multiforme	malignant	immature astrocyte in the cerebrum	**glioblastoma multiforme** (GLY-oh-blas-TOH-mah MUL-tih-FOR-may) **gli/o-** *substance that holds things together* **blast/o-** *immature; embryonic* **-oma** *tumor, mass*
lymphoma	malignant	microglia in the cerebrum	**lymphoma** (lim-FOH-mah) **lymph/o-** *lymph; lymphatic system* **-oma** *tumor, mass*
meningioma	benign	meninges of brain or spinal cord	**meningioma** (meh-NIN-jee-OH-mah) **meningi/o-** *meninges* **-oma** *tumor, mass*
oligodendroglioma	malignant	oligodendroglia in the cerebrum	**oligodendroglioma** (OL-ih-goh-den-DROH-gly-OH-mah) **olig/o-** *scanty* **dendr/o-** *branching structure* **gli/o-** *substance that holds things together* **-oma** *tumor, mass*
schwannoma	benign	Schwann cells near the cranial or spinal nerves	**schwannoma** (shwah-NOH-mah)

Word or Phrase	Word Part and Definition	Description
cerebrovascular accident (CVA)	**cerebrovascular** (SER-eh-broh-VAS-kyoo-lar) **cerebr/o-** *cerebrum (largest part of the brain)* **vascul/o-** *blood vessel* **-ar** *pertaining to* **infarct** (IN-farkt) **infarction** (in-FARK-shun) **infarct/o-** *area of dead tissue* **-ion** *action; condition* **ischemia** (is-KEE-mee-ah) **isch/o-** *keep back; block* **-emia** *condition of the blood; substance in the blood* **ischemic** (is-KEE-mik) **isch/o-** *keep back; block* **-emic** *pertaining to condition of the blood or a substance in the blood* **neurologic** (NYOOR-oh-LAWJ-ik) **neur/o-** *nerve* **log/o-** *the study of* **-ic** *pertaining to* **deficit** (DEF-ih-sit) **hemiparesis** (HEM-ee-pah-REE-sis) (HEM-ee-PAIR-eh-sis) **hemi-** *one half* **-paresis** *weakness*	Disruption or blockage of blood flow to the brain, which causes tissue death and an area of necrosis known as an **infarct**. The blood flow can be disrupted by an embolus, thrombus, arteriosclerosis, or hemorrhage. An embolus is a blood clot or piece of fat that forms in another part of the body, travels through the circulatory system, and becomes lodged in an artery of the brain. A thrombus is a blood clot that forms in an artery of the brain that is already partially occluded by arteriosclerosis. Hemorrhage occurs when high blood pressure causes an artery to rupture or when an aneurysm ruptures. A CVA is also known as a **stroke** or **brain attack**. A **transient ischemic attack (TIA)** is a temporary lack of oxygenated blood to an area of brain. It is like a CVA, but its effects only last 24 hours. A **reversible ischemic neurologic deficit (RIND)** is a TIA whose effects last for several days. TIAs and RINDs are precursors to an impending CVA. A cerebrovascular accident on the left side of the brain affects the right side of the body and visa versa (see Figure 10-14 ■). The severity of the CVA depends on how much brain tissue was damaged. **Hemiparesis** is muscle weakness on one side 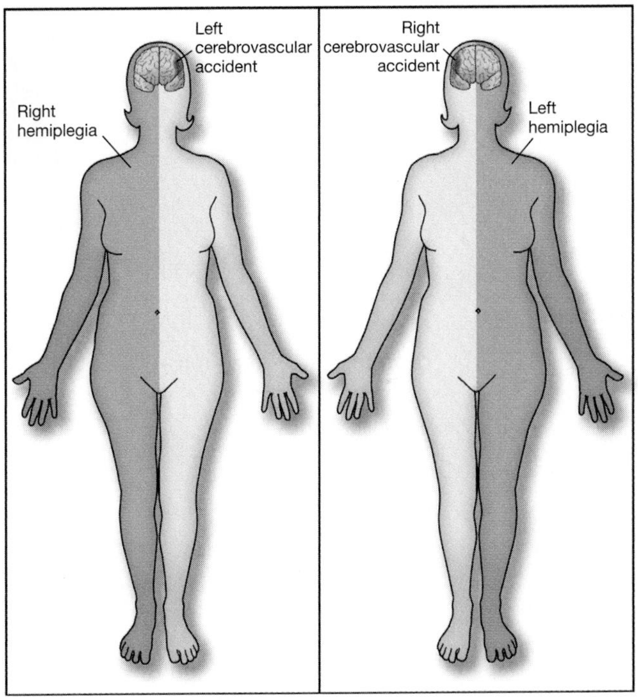 Left cerebrovascular accident Right hemiplegia Right cerebrovascular accident Left hemiplegia **Figure 10-14 ■ Cerebrovascular accident.** A cerebrovascular accident on the left side of the brain affects the right side of the body.

(continued)

Word or Phrase	Word Part and Definition	Description
cerebrovascular accident (CVA) *(continued)*	**hemiplegia** (HEM-ee-PLEE-jee-ah) **hemi-** *one half* **pleg/o-** *paralysis* **-ia** *condition, state, thing* **hemiplegic** (HEM-ee-PLEE-jik) **hemi-** *one half* **pleg/o-** *paralysis* **-ic** *pertaining to*	of the body. **Hemiplegia** is paralysis on one side of the body, and the patient is said to be **hemiplegic** (see Figure 10-15■). A CVA can also cause amnesia, aphasia, dysphasia, or dysphagia (difficulting swallowing). Treatment: Thrombolytic drugs to break up a thrombus or embolus that is occluding the artery. Surgery: Carotid endarterectomy, aneurysm clipping, or aneurysmectomy to prevent a CVA. **Figure 10-15 ■ Cerebrovascular accident.** This patient had a cerebrovascular accident on the left side of her brain that has paralyzed the right side of her body. Notice the drooping of the right side of her mouth and her right shoulder. The elbow and wrist of her right arm are covered with protective padding. She is using her good left hand to hold her right hand in her lap and move her right arm from time to time.
coma	**coma** (KOH-mah) *Coma* is derived from a Latin word meaning *deep sleep.* **comatose** (KOH-mah-tohs) **comat/o-** *deep unconsciousness* **-ose** *full of*	Deep state of unconsciousness and unresponsiveness caused by trauma or disease in the brain, metabolic imbalance with accumulation of waste products (hepatic coma), or a deficiency of sugar in the blood (diabetic coma). The patient is said to be **comatose.** Treatment: Correct the underlying cause. **Brain death** is a condition in which there is irreversible loss of all brain function as confirmed by an electroencephalogram (EEG) that is flat, showing no brain wave activity of any kind for 30 minutes.
concussion	**concussion** (con-KUHSH-un) **concuss/o-** *violent shaking or jarring* **-ion** *action; condition* **contusion** (con-TOO-shun) **contus/o-** *bruising* **-ion** *action; condition*	Traumatic injury to the brain that results in the immediate loss of consciousness for a brief or prolonged period of time. Even after consciousness returns, the patient must be watched closely for signs of sleepiness or irritability that could indicate a slowly enlarging hemorrhage in the brain. A **contusion** is a traumatic injury to the brain or spinal cord. There is no loss of consciousness, but there is bruising with some bleeding in the tissues. **Shaken baby syndrome** is caused by an adult vigorously shaking an infant in anger or to discipline the child. Because the infant's head is large and the neck muscles are weak, severe shaking causes the head to whip back and forth. This can cause a contusion, concussion, hemorrhaging, mental retardation, coma, or even death.

Word or Phrase	Word Part and Definition	Description

Connections

Creutzfeldt-Jakob (KROITS-felt YAH-kohp)
Named by Hans Creutzfeldt (1885–1964) and Alfons Jakob (1884–1931), two German psychiatrists.

Public Health. New variant **Creutzfeldt-Jakob disease,** a fatal neurologic disorder, is caused by a prion (a small infectious protein particle) contracted from cows infected with mad cow disease (bovine spongiform encephalopathy). It was first discovered in British cows. It is transmitted to cows when they eat animal feed contaminated with the processed spinal cords and brains of infected cows. All such animal feed has been banned in the United States. The disease can be transmitted to humans who eat meat from the infected cows. People who have lived or traveled extensively in England are even prohibited from donating blood to prevent possible transmission of this disease.

Word or Phrase	Word Part and Definition	Description
dementia	**dementia** (deh-MEN-shee-ah) **de-** *reversal of; without* **ment/o-** *mind; chin* **-ia** *condition, state, thing* Some word parts have more than one definition. The best definition of *dementia* is *condition [of being] without the mind.* **senile** (SEE-nile) **sen/o-** *old age* **-ile** *pertaining to*	Disease of the brain in which many neurons in the cerebrum die, the cerebral cortex shrinks in size, and there is progressive deterioration in mental function (see Figures 10-16 ■ and 10-17 ■). The initial symptoms include a gradual decline in mental abilities, with forgetfulness, inability to learn new things, inability to perform daily activities, and difficulty making decisions. The patient uses the wrong words and is unable to comprehend what others say. The symptoms become progressively more severe over time and include inability to care for personal needs, inability to recognize friends and family, and complete memory loss. Psychiatric symptoms of depression, anxiety, impulsiveness, and combativeness may also be present. Dementia is most often associated with old age (**senile dementia**) and the cumulative effect of multiple small cerebrovascular accidents (**multi-infarct dementia**). Dementia can also be caused by brain trauma, chronic alcoholism or drug abuse, or chronic neurodegenerative diseases like multiple sclerosis, Parkinson's disease, and Huntington's chorea. However, the most common cause of

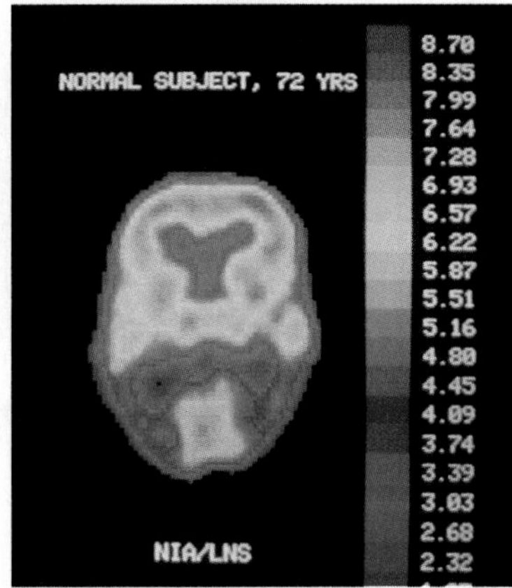

Figure 10-16 ■ PET scan of a normal brain.

A PET scan shows the metabolic activity of the brain. This patient's scan shows large, symmetrical areas of metabolism and active brain cells. The bar at the right correlates colors on the scan with numerical measurements for the amount of metabolic activity. Areas with the highest metabolic activity appear red.

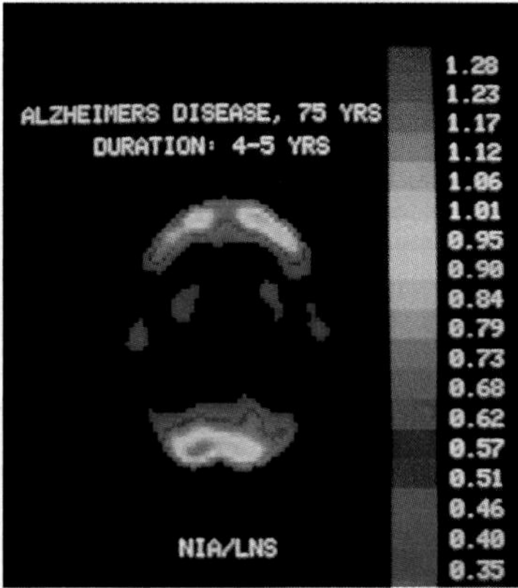

Figure 10-17 ■ PET scan of the brain of a patient with Alzheimer's disease.

Notice the large areas that are without any evidence of metabolism or cellular activity.

(continued)

Word or Phrase	Word Part and Definition	Description
dementia *(continued)*	**Alzheimer** (AWLZ-hy-mer) Alzheimer's disease was named by Alois Alzheimer (1864–1915), a German neurologist. **neurofibrillary** (NYOOR-oh-FIB-rih-LAIR-ee) **neur/o-** *nerve* **fibrill/o-** *muscle fiber; nerve fiber* **-ary** *pertaining to* **plaque** (PLAK) *Plaque* is a French word meaning *plate.* **presenile** (pree-SEE-nile) **pre-** *before; in front of* **sen/o-** *old age* **-ile** *pertaining to*	dementia is Alzheimer's disease. **Alzheimer's disease** is a hereditary dementia that is known to run in families with inherited mutations on chromosomes 1, 14, and 21. At autopsy, the neurons show characteristic **neurofibrillary tangles** that distort the cells. There are also microscopic **senile plaques.** The brain also has decreased levels of the neurotransmitter acetylcholine. Alzheimer's disease usually occurs in late middle age or elderly persons and is a form of senile dementia. Alzheimer's disease that occurs in early middle age is known as early-onset Alzheimer's disease or **presenile dementia.** Treatment: Drugs that increase the level of acetylcholine in the brain or increase blood flow to the brain.
Down syndrome	Down syndrome was named by John Down (1828–1896), an English physician. **mental** (MEN-tal) **ment/o-** *mind; chin* **-al** *pertaining to* **retardation** (REE-tar-DAY-shun) **retard/o-** *to slow down or delay* **-ation** *a process; being or having*	Congenital genetic defect in which there are three of chromosome 21, instead of the normal two. This defect affects every cell in the body, but the most obvious functional limitation is mild-to-severe **mental retardation.** Persons with Down syndrome also have characteristic facial features with a thick, protruding tongue and short fingers with a single transverse palmar crease (see Figure 10-18 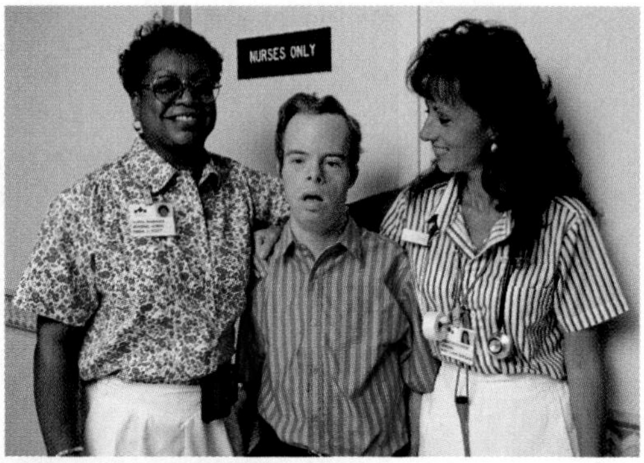 ■). **Figure 10-18 ■ Down syndrome.** This patient with Down syndrome shows the characteristic facial features (eyes and tongue) that accompany mental retardation.

Word or Phrase	Word Part and Definition	Description
dyslexia	**dyslexia** (dis-LEK-see-ah) **dys-** *painful, difficult, abnormal* **lex/o-** *word* **-ia** *condition, state, thing* **dyslexic** (dis-LEK-sik) **dys-** *painful, difficult, abnormal* **lex/o-** *word* **-ic** *pertaining to*	Difficulty reading and writing words even though visual acuity and intelligence are normal. The patient may write particular alphabet letters backwards or may change the order of letters in a word. Dyslexia tends to run in families and is more prevalent in left-handed persons and in males. Dyslexia is caused by an abnormality in the areas of the cerebrum that process visual images, particularly moving images (as the eye moves quickly across the page). A person with dyslexia is said to be **dyslexic.** Treatment: Educational techniques that help a child learn to compensate or overcome this difficulty.
encephalitis	**encephalitis** (en-SEF-ah-LY-tis) **encephal/o-** *brain* **-itis** *inflammation of*	Inflammation of the brain caused by a virus. Herpes simplex virus is the most common cause of encephalitis, but others include herpes zoster virus, West Nile virus, and cytomegalovirus. Initial symptoms include fever, headache, stiff neck, lethargy, vomiting, irritability, and photophobia. Treatment: Only encephalitis caused by the herpesvirus responds to antiviral drugs. Corticosteroid drugs to decrease inflammation of the brain. Antibiotic drugs are not effective against viruses.
epilepsy	**epilepsy** (EP-ih-LEP-see) *Epilepsy* is derived from a Greek word meaning *seizures.* **seizure** (SEE-zher) *Seizure* is derived from an Old French word meaning *to grab.* **convulsion** (con-VUL-shun) **convuls/o-** *seizure* **-ion** *action; condition* *Convulsion* is derived from a Latin word meaning *shatter or tear apart.* **epileptic** (EP-ih-LEP-tik) **epilept/o-** *seizure* **-ic** *pertaining to* **status epilepticus** (STAT-us EP-ih-LEP-tih-kus) *Status epilepticus* is a Latin phrase meaning *a state of being in a seizure.* **aura** (AW-rah) *Aura* is a Latin word meaning *breeze, odor, or gleam of light.* **postictal** (post-IK-tal) **post-** *after, behind* **ict/o-** *seizure* **-al** *pertaining to*	Recurring condition in which a group of neurons in the brain spontaneously sends out electrical impulses in an abnormal, uncontrolled way. These impulses spread from neuron to neuron, causing altered consciousness and abnormal muscle movements. The type and extent of the symptoms depend on the number and location of the affected neurons. Also known as **seizures** or **convulsions.** A patient with epilepsy is said to be **epileptic.** There are four common types of epilepsy (see Table 10-4). With each type of epilepsy, the patient displays a specific EEG pattern during a seizure (see Figures 10-19■ and 10-20■). **Status epilepticus** is a state of prolonged continuous seizure activity or frequently repeated individual seizures that occur without the patient regaining consciousness. Before the onset of a seizure, some epileptics experience an **aura,** a visual, olfactory, sensory, or auditory sign (flashing lights, strange odor, tingling, or buzzing sound) that warns them of an impending seizure. After a tonic-clonic seizure, the patient experiences sleepiness and confusion. This is known as the **postictal state.** Treatment: Antiepileptic drugs. 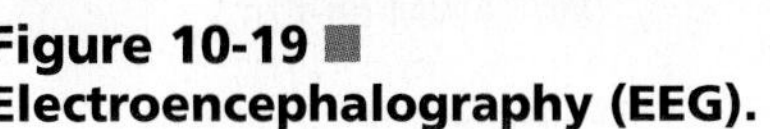 **Figure 10-19 ■ Electroencephalography (EEG).** This boy is having an EEG to diagnose what type of seizures he is having.

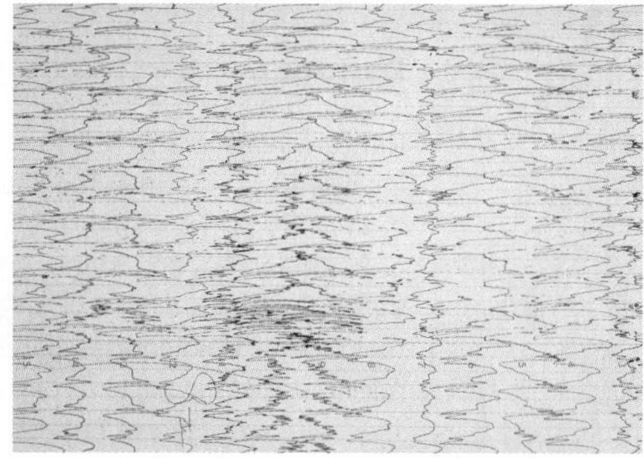

Figure 10-20 ■ Petit mal epilepsy.
This patient's EEG shows the characteristic abnormal brain wave patterns of petit mal epilepsy.

Table 10-4 Seizures

Type of Seizure	Word Part and Definition	Description
tonic-clonic (grand mal)	**tonic** (TAWN-ik) ton/o- *pressure; tone* -ic *pertaining to* **clonic** (CLAWN-ik) clon/o- *rapid contracting and relaxing* -ic *pertaining to* **grand mal** (GRAHN MAWL) *Grand mal* is a French phrase meaning *major disorder.*	Unconsciousness with excessive motor activity. The body alternates between excessive muscle tone with rigidity (tonic) and jerking muscle contractions (clonic) in the extremities, with tongue biting, and sometimes incontinence. Lasts 1–2 minutes.
absence (petit mal)	**absence** (AB-sens) *Absence* is a French word meaning *absent.* **petit mal** (peh-TEE MAWL) *Petit mal* is a French phrase meaning *minor disorder.*	Impaired consciousness with slight or no muscle activity. Muscle tone is retained and the patient does not fall down, but is unable to respond to external stimuli. Sometimes includes vacant staring and repetitive blinking or facial tics. Lasts 10 seconds, after which the patient resumes activities and is unaware of the seizure. Patient may have many absence seizures during the course of a day.
complex partial (psychomotor)	**psychomotor** (SY-koh-MOH-tor) psych/o- *mind* mot/o- *movement* -or *person or thing that produces or does* **automatism** (aw-TAWM-ah-tizm)	Some degree of impairment of consciousness. Involuntary contractions of one or several muscle groups. Obvious **automatisms** like lip smacking and patterns of muscle movement can be present.
simple partial (focal motor)	**focal** (FOH-kal) foc/o- *point of activity* -al *pertaining to*	No impairment of consciousness. The patient is aware of the seizure but is unable to stop the motor activity. Involuntary contractions of one or several muscle groups (jerking of one hand, turning of the head). May also include sensory hallucinations.

Word or Phrase	Word Part and Definition	Description
hematoma	**hematoma** (HEE-mah-TOH-mah) **hemat/o-** *blood* **-oma** *tumor, mass* **intraventricular** (IN-trah-ven-TRIK-yoo-lar) **intra-** *within* **ventricul/o-** *ventricle (lower heart chamber; chamber in the brain)* **-ar** *pertaining to* **subdural** (sub-DYOO-ral) **sub-** *below; underneath; less than* **dur/o-** *dura mater* **-al** *pertaining to*	Localized collection of blood that forms in the brain because of the rupture of an artery or vein. This can be caused by trauma to the cranium or an intracranial aneurysm that ruptures. An **intraventricular hematoma** occurs within one of the ventricles. A **subdural hematoma** forms between the dura mater and the arachnoid (see Figure 10-21■). Treatment: Surgery to remove the hematoma, if needed. **Figure 10-21 ■ Subdural hematoma.** This patient developed a subdural hematoma after trauma to the side of the head. Also notice the hematoma between the cranium and the skin.
Huntington's chorea	**Huntington** (HUN-ting-ton) Huntington's chorea was named by George Huntington (1851–1916), an American neurologist. **chorea** (kor-EE-ah) *Chorea* is derived from a Greek word meaning *a dance.*	Progressive inherited degenerative disease of the brain that begins in middle age. It is characterized by dementia with irregular spasms of the extremities and face (chorea) alternating with slow writhing movements of the hands and feet (athetosis). Treatment: None.
hydrocephalus	**hydrocephalus** (HY-droh-SEF-ah-lus) **hydr/o-** *water; fluid* **-cephalus** *head* **hydrocephalic** (HY-droh-sih-FAL-ik) **hydr/o-** *water; fluid* **cephal/o-** *head* **-ic** *pertaining to*	Condition in which an excessive amount of cerebrospinal fluid is produced or the flow of cerebrospinal fluid is blocked. The intracranial pressure builds up, distends the ventricles in the brain, and compresses the brain tissue. Hydrocephalus is most often associated with the congenital conditions of meningocele or myelomeningocele (see Figure 10-22), although it can occur in adults (normal pressure hydrocephalus) when the cerebrospinal fluid is not absorbed back into the blood. Untreated hydrocephalus causes a grossly enlarged head and mental retardation. The patient is said to be **hydrocephalic.** A layman's phrase for this condition is "water on the brain." Treatment: Placement of a ventriculoperitoneal shunt to move excess cerebrospinal fluid from the cranial cavity to the peritoneal cavity.

Word or Phrase	Word Part and Definition	Description
meningitis	**meningitis** (MEN-in-JY-tis) **mening/o-** *meninges* **-itis** *inflammation of* **nuchal** (NYOO-kal) **nuch/o-** *neck; nape of the neck* **-al** *pertaining to*	Inflammation of the meninges of the brain or spinal cord by a bacterial or viral infection. There is fever, headache, **nuchal rigidity** (stiff neck) lethargy, vomiting, irritability, and photophobia. Treatment: Vaccination to prevent bacterial meningitis in susceptible groups (particularly college students). Antibiotic drugs to treat bacterial meningitis. Corticosteroid drugs to decrease inflammation.
migraine headache	**migraine** (MY-grayn) *Migraine* is derived from a Greek phrase meaning *half of the cranium* because migraines often affect just one side of the head. **photophobia** (FOH-toh-FOH-bee-ah) **phot/o-** *light* **phob/o-** *fear or avoidance* **-ia** *condition, state, thing*	Specific type of recurring headache that has a sudden onset with severe, throbbing pain, often on just one side of the head. This is often accompanied by nausea and vomiting and sensitivity to light (**photophobia**). Migraines are caused by a constriction of the arteries in the brain followed by a sudden dilation. Treatment: Drugs that keep the blood vessels constricted during a migraine.
narcolepsy	**narcolepsy** (NAR-koh-lep-see) **narc/o-** *stupor, sleep* **-lepsy** *seizure*	Brief, involuntary episodes of falling asleep during the daytime while engaged in activity. The patient is not unconscious and can be aroused, but is unable to prevent falling asleep. There is a hereditary component to narcolepsy, and it may be an autoimmune disorder. There is also an underlying abnormality of REM sleep. Treatment: Central nervous system stimulant drugs.
Parkinson's disease	**Parkinson** (PAR-kin-son) Parkinson's disease was named by James Parkinson (1755–1824), an English physician.	Chronic, degenerative disease due to an imbalance in the levels of the neurotransmitters dopamine and acetylcholine in the brain. Early symptoms include muscle rigidity, tremors, and a slowing of voluntary movements. Later, the patient shows a mask-like facial expression, shuffling gait, or inability to ambulate. Treatment: Drugs that increase the amount of dopamine in the brain or drugs that inhibit the action of acetylcholine in the brain.
syncope	**syncope** (SIN-koh-pee) *Syncope* is a Greek word meaning *to faint.* **syncopal** (SIN-koh-pal) **syncop/o-** *fainting* **-al** *pertaining to*	Temporary loss of consciousness. A **syncopal episode** is one in which the patient becomes lightheaded and then faints and briefly remains unconscious. Most often caused by carotid artery stenosis and plaque or cardiac arrhythmias that decrease blood flow to the brain.

Spinal Cord

Word or Phrase	Word Part and Definition	Description
neural tube defect	**neural** (NYOOR-al) **neur/o-** *nerve* **-al** *pertaining to* **spina bifida** (SPY-nah BIF-ih-dah) *Spina bifida* is a Latin phrase meaning *backbone that is split into two parts.* **meningocele** (meh-NING-goh-seel) **mening/o-** *meninges* **-cele** *hernia* **meningomyelocele** (meh-NING-goh-MY-loh-seel) **mening/o-** *meninges* **myel/o-** *bone marrow; spinal cord; myelin* **-cele** *hernia* Some word parts have more than one definition. The best definition of *meningomyelocele* is *hernia of the meninges and spinal cord.* **myelomeningocele** (MY-loh-meh-NING-goh-seel) **myel/o-** *bone marrow; spinal cord; myelin* **mening/o-** *meninges* **-cele** *hernia*	Congenital abnormality of the neural tube (embryonic structure that develops into the fetal brain and spinal cord). The vertebrae form incompletely (**spina bifida**), and there is an abnormal opening in the vertebral column through which the spinal cord and nerves may protrude to the outside of the body. This defect is covered only by the meninges (see Figure 10-22 ■). A **meningocele** is the protrusion of the meninges through the defect. A **meningomyelocele** is the protrusion of the meninges and the spinal cord; it is also known as **myelomeningocele**. Children with meningocele or meningomyelocele may also have hydrocephalus. The amount of spinal cord involvement determines the degree of impairment of muscle control of the legs and bladder and bowel function. Amniotic fluid extracted during the pregnancy shows elevated levels of alpha fetoprotein. Treatment: Surgery to close the defect immediately after birth because of the risk of infection. The surgery is not able to restore function. The hydrocephalus is treated separately.

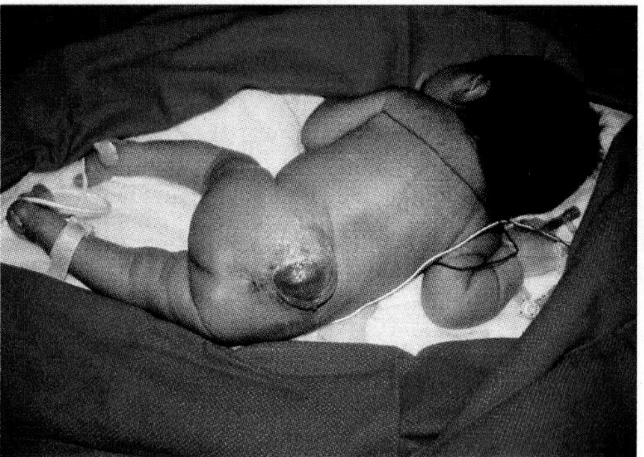

Figure 10-22 ■ Meningomyelocele.
This infant has a meningomyelocele in which there is a protrusion or herniation of the meninges and spinal cord through a defect in the vertebra. The delicate tissues of the meningocele can easily be traumatized, allowing infection to enter and travel to the brain. Therefore, the meningocele is surgically closed shortly after birth.

Connections

Dietetics. Folic acid supplementation taken during pregnancy greatly reduces the risk of neural tube defects. Folic acid is present in prenatal vitamins and in enriched cereals and breads.

Word or Phrase	Word Part and Definition	Description
radiculopathy	**radiculopathy** (rah-DIK-yoo-LAWP-ah-thee) **radicu/lo-** *spinal nerve root* **-pathy** *disease, suffering* **herniated** (HER-nee-aa-ted) **herni/o-** *hernia* **-ated** *pertaining to a condition; composed of* **nucleus pulposus** (NYOO-klee-us pul-POH-sus) The nucleus is the central part of a structure. *Pulposus* refers to the pulpy, gel-like consistency of the contents within the intervertebral disk. **sciatica** (sy-AT-ih-kah) *Sciatica* is derived from a Greek word meaning *related to the ischium (hip bone).* The sciatic nerve passes through a large notch in the ischium.	Acute or chronic condition that occurs when the **herniated nucleus pulposus (HNP)** of an intervertebral disk is forced out through a weak area in the disk wall and presses on adjacent spinal nerve roots. This usually involves a lumbar disk and is often caused by heavy lifting and poor body mechanics. Also known as a slipped disk. Symptoms include pain, numbness, and paresthesias along the dermatome for that spinal nerve. Also known as **sciatica** because the pain is often from compression of several branches of the sciatic nerve whose nerve roots come from L4, L5, and the sacrum. Treatment: Anti-inflammatory drugs, bed rest, traction to the spine, physical therapy. Nerve root injection. Surgery: Rhizotomy, diskectomy, or laminectomy.
spinal cord injury (SCI)	**transection** (tran-SEK-shun) **trans-** *across, through* **sect/o-** *to cut* **-ion** *action; condition* When the word parts are combined, the duplicate *s* is dropped. **paralysis** (pah-RAL-ih-sis) **para-** *beside, apart from; two parts of a pair; abnormal* **-lysis** *abnormal condition or process of breaking down or dissolving* Some word parts have more than one definition. The best definition of *paralysis* is *an abnormal condition of breaking down two parts of a pair.* **paraplegia** (PAIR-ah-PLEE-jee-ah) **para-** *beside, apart from; two parts of a pair; abnormal* **pleg/o-** *paralysis* **-ia** *condition, state, thing*	Trauma to the spinal cord with a partial or complete **transection** of the cord. This interrupts nerve impulses to particular dermatomes, causing partial or complete anesthesia (loss of sensation) and **paralysis** (an inability to voluntarily move the muscles). An injury to the lower spinal cord causes **paraplegia** with paralysis of the legs. A patient with paraplegia is known as a **paraplegic.** An injury to the upper spinal cord causes **quadriplegia** with paralysis of all four extremies. A patient with quadriplegia is known as a **quadriplegic** (see Figure 10-23■). After a suspected spinal cord injury, the patient is carefully transported to the hospital on a rigid spinal board, with a cervical collar in place, and with the head taped to the board to prevent any movement of the head, neck, or back that might further injure the spinal cord. Without nerve impulses, the muscles lose their tone and firmness and eventually atrophy. This is known as **flaccid paralysis.** However, the reflex arc of the lower spinal cord often remains intact and, in response to pain or a full bladder, the spinal cord below the injury will send nerve impulses that cause the muscles to spasm. This is known as **spastic paralysis.** The bladder may also contract spontaneously, causing incontinence. Treatment: Traction to the skull to align the vertebrae. Surgery may be needed to fuse damaged vertebrae. Corticosteroid drugs to decrease spinal cord swelling. Passive range of motion exercises, splints, muscle relaxant drugs. *(continued)*

Word or Phrase	Word Part and Definition	Description
spinal cord injury (SCI) *(continued)*	**paraplegic** (PAIR-ah-PLEE-jik) **para-** *beside, apart from; two parts of a pair; abnormal* **pleg/o-** *paralysis* **-ic** *pertaining to* **quadriplegia** (KWAH-drih-PLEE-jee-ah) **quadri-** *four* **pleg/o-** *paralysis* **-ia** *condition, state, thing* Add words to make a correct and complete definition of *quadriplegia: condition [in which all] four [extremities have] paralysis.* **quadriplegic** (KWAH-drih-PLEE-jik) **quadri-** *four* **pleg/o-** *paralysis* **-ic** *pertaining to* **flaccid** (FLAS-id) (FLAK-sid) **spastic** (SPAS-tic) **spast/o-** *spasm* **-ic** *pertaining to*	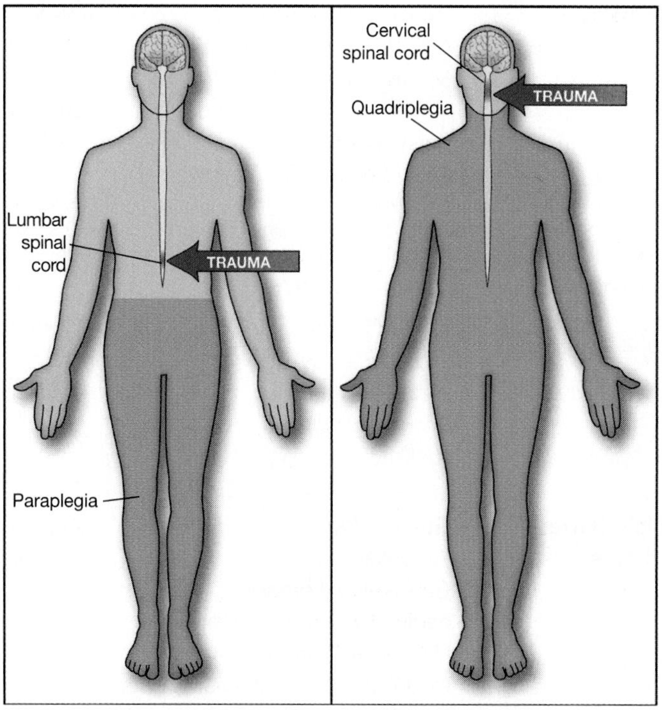 **Figure 10-23 ■ Spinal cord injury.** The level of the spinal cord where an injury occurs and whether the spinal cord was partially or completely transected determines how much of the body is affected and to what extent. Paraplegia affects the lower body and the legs. Quadriplegia affects the body from the neck down and all four extremities.
Nerves		
amyotrophic lateral sclerosis (ALS)	**amyotrophic** (ah-MY-oh-TROH-fik) **a-** *away from, without* **my/o-** *muscle* **troph/o-** *development* **-ic** *pertaining to* **sclerosis** (skleh-ROH-sis) **scler/o-** *hard; sclera (white of the eye)* **-osis** *condition; abnormal condition; process*	Chronic, progressive disease of the motor nerves of the spinal cord. Symptoms include muscle wasting, spasms, and eventual paralysis of all the muscles, including the swallowing and respiratory muscles. There is no damage to the sensory nerves and so sensation remains intact. Some cases of ALS are caused by the lack of an enzyme, which is an inherited defect; but in most cases the cause is not known. Also known as Lou Gehrig's disease after the famous baseball player who developed the disease in the late 1930s. Treatment: Supportive care.
anesthesia	**anesthesia** (AN-es-THEE-zee-ah) **an-** *without, not* **esthes/o-** *sensation, feeling* **-ia** *condition, state, thing* **anesthetic** (AN-es-THET-ik) **an-** *without, not* **esthet/o-** *sensation, feeling* **-ic** *pertaining to*	Condition in which sensation of any type, including touch, pressure, proprioception, or pain, has been completely lost. Local areas of anesthesia can occur temporarily when your hand goes numb from pressing on a nerve in your arm as you sleep. Permanent anesthesia along a dermatome can occur after a spinal cord injury. Unconsciousness is accompanied by an inability to perceive any sensation, and this is the basis for the use of drugs that induce general anesthesia prior to a surgical procedure. Temporary therapeutic anesthesia can also be produced in specific regions by injecting an **anesthetic drug** under the skin, near a nerve root, or into the epidural space in the spinal cavity.

Word or Phrase	Word Part and Definition	Description
Bell's palsy	Bell's palsy was named by Charles Bell (1774–1842), a Scottish surgeon. **palsy** (PAWL-zee) *Palsy* is derived from the word *paralysis*.	Weakness, drooping, or actual paralysis of one side of the face because of inflammation of the facial nerve (cranial nerve VII). Probably due to a viral infection, possibly herpesvirus. The condition usually lasts a month and resolves by itself. Treatment: Corticosteroid drugs.
carpal tunnel syndrome (CTS)	**carpal** (KAR-pal) **carp/o-** *wrist* **-al** *pertaining to*	Chronic condition with tingling in the hand because of inflammation and swelling of the tendons that go through the carpal tunnel of the wrist bones to reach the hand. The swelling compresses the median nerve. Caused by repetitive motions of the hand and wrist, often from constant typing or data entry. Bending the wrist down aggravates the pain and is a positive diagnostic test. Treatment: Rest, splinting the wrist, use of a special split keyboard that positions the wrists differently, physical therapy. Surgery, if needed.
Guillain-Barré syndrome	**Guillain-Barré** (GEE-yah bah-RAY) Guillain-Barré syndrome was named by George Guillian (1876–1961) and Jean Barré (1880–1967), French neurologists.	Autoimmune disorder in which the body makes antibodies against myelin. There is acute inflammation of the peripheral nerves, loss of myelin with interruption of nerve conduction, muscle weakness, and changes in sensation (paresthesias). This disease is caused by a triggering event of an infection (often a viral respiratory illness), stress, or trauma. The muscle weakness begins in the legs and then rapidly involves the entire body. The patient may even temporarily require respiratory support until the inflammation subsides. Guillain-Barré does not recur, and the patient recovers some or all neurologic function over a period of days to months. Treatment: Corticosteroid drugs.
hyperesthesia	**hyperesthesia** (HY-per-es-THEE-zee-ah) **hyper-** *above; more than normal* **esthes/o-** *sensation, feeling* **-ia** *condition, state, thing*	Condition in which there is an abnormally heightened awareness and sensitivity to touch and increased response to painful stimuli. Treatment: A variety of drugs (antidepressants, tranquilizers) are used and are somewhat effective.
multiple sclerosis (MS)	**sclerosis** (skleh-ROH-sis) **scler/o-** *hard; sclera (white of the eye)* **-osis** *condition; abnormal condition; process* Some word parts have more than one definition. The best definition of *sclerosis* is *an abnormal condition of hardness.*	Chronic, progressive, degenerative autoimmune disease in which the body makes antibodies against myelin. There is acute inflammation of the nerves and loss of myelin (demyelinization) with interruption of nerve conduction in the brain and spinal cord. The areas of demyelinization eventually become scar tissue that is hard. These areas are known as plaque and can be seen on MRI scans of the brain. This disease may be caused by a triggering event such as a viral infection. Patients are typically in their 20s to early middle age. Early symptoms include double vision, nystagmus, large muscle weakness, uncoordinated gait, spasticity, incoordination, early fatigue after repeated muscle contractions, tremors, and paresthesias. Patients with MS experience periodic remissions in which their symptoms become slightly better, followed by exacerbations or flare-ups with worsening of symptoms over time. Heat, stress, and fatigue temporarily worsen the symptoms. Late symptoms include inability to walk and sometimes dementia. Treatment: Anti-inflammatory drugs, corticosteroid drugs for flare-ups, muscle relaxant drugs.

Word or Phrase	Word Part and Definition	Description
neuralgia	**neuralgia** (nyoo-RAL-jee-ah) **neur/o-** *nerve* **alg/o-** *pain* **-ia** *condition, state, thing* **trigeminal** (try-JEM-ih-nal) **tri-** *three* **gemin/o-** *twins; set or group* **-al** *pertaining to* The trigeminal nerve is composed of a group of three different branches: the ophthalmic nerve, the maxillary nerve, and the mandibular nerve. **tic douloreux** (TIK DOO-LOO-reh) **causalgia** (kaw-ZAL-jee-ah) **caus/o-** *burning* **alg/o-** *pain* **-ia** *condition, state, thing*	Pain along the path of a nerve and its branches caused by an injury. Neuralgia can be mild to severe in nature. **Trigeminal neuralgia,** also known as **tic douloreux,** is characterized by stabbing pain for a few seconds on one side of the face or jaw along the distribution of the trigeminal nerve (cranial nerve V). **Causalgia** is severe, burning pain along a nerve and its branches. **Complex regional pain syndrome (CRPS)** involves causalgia, with hyperesthesia, changes in skin color and temperature, and swelling. Treatment: A variety of different drugs have been tried with varying levels of success: Anti-inflammatory drugs, topical anesthetic drugs, corticosteroid drugs, antidepressant drugs, anticonvulsant drugs, skeletal muscle relaxant drugs. Also nerve blocks, TENS unit, and physical therapy. **Connections** **Dermatology (Chapter 7).** Shingles is a painful skin condition caused by the herpes zoster virus, the virus that causes chicken-pox in children. The virus remains dormant in the body until later in life when a stress triggers it to erupt. It affects nerves and the skin in the distribution of the dermatomes of those nerves and causes redness, pain, and vesicles. Lingering, chronic pain from shingles is known as postherpetic neuralgia. Treatment: Antiviral drugs.
neuritis	**neuritis** (nyoo-RY-tis) **neur/o-** *nerve* **-itis** *inflammation of* **polyneuritis** (PAWL-ee-nyoo-RY-tis) **poly-** *many, much* **neur/o-** *nerve* **-itis** *inflammation of*	Inflammation or infection of a nerve. **Polyneuritis** is a generalized inflammation of many nerves in one part of the body or all the nerves in the body. Treatment: Correct the underlying cause; analgesic drugs, anti-inflammatory drugs, corticosteroid drugs, or antibiotic drugs.

Word or Phrase	Word Part and Definition	Description
neurofibromatosis	**neurofibromatosis** (NYOOR-oh-fy-BROH-mah-TOH-sis) **neur/o-** *nerve* **fibr/o-** *fiber* **-omatosis** *abnormal condition of muliple tumors or masses* **neurofibroma** (NYOOR-oh-fy-BROH-mah) **neur/o-** *nerve* **fibr/o-** *fiber* **-oma** *tumor, mass* *Neurofibroma* is a Greek singular noun. Form the plural by changing *-oma* to *-omata.* **von Recklinghausen** (vawn REK-ling-HOW-sen) This disease was named for Friedrich von Recklinghausen (1833–1910), a German pathologist.	Hereditary disease with multiple benign tumors (**neurofibromata**) that arise from the peripheral nerves. These are most noticeable on the skin, but they can also be present anywhere in the body—on the internal organs and even in the eye. They range in size from small-to-medium nodules to large tumors. Also known as **von Recklinghausen's disease.**
neuroma	**neuroma** (nyoo-ROH-mah) **neur/o-** *nerve* **-oma** *tumor, mass*	Benign tumor of a nerve or any of the specialized cells of the nervous system. A **Morton's neuroma** specifically forms from repetitive damage to the nerve around the metatarsophalangeal joint between the ball of the foot and the toes. Treatment: Surgical excision, if desired.
neuropathy	**neuropathy** (nyoo-RAWP-ah-thee) **neur/o-** *nerve* **-pathy** *disease, suffering*	General category for any type of disease or injury to a nerve. Treatment: Correct the underlying cause.

Connections

diabetic (DY-ah-BET-ik)
diabet/o- *diabetes*
-ic *pertaining to*

neuropathy (nyoo-RAWP-ah-thee)
neur/o- *nerve*
-pathy *disease, suffering*

Endocrinology (Chapter 14). Diabetic neuropathy is a chronic, slowly progressive condition that affects the peripheral nerves in diabetic patients. The symptoms, which include severe pain and a loss of sensation and sense of position, are caused by a lack of blood flow to the nerves (from arteriosclerosis).

Word or Phrase	Word Part and Definition	Description
paresthesia	**paresthesia** (PAIR-es-THEE-zee-ah) **para-** *beside, apart from; two parts of a pair; abnormal* **esthes/o-** *sensation, feeling* **-ia** *condition, state, thing* The last *a* in the prefix *para-* is dropped in *paresthesia.*	Condition in which abnormal sensations like tingling, burning, or pinpricks are felt on the skin. Paresthesias are often the result of chronic nerve damage from pinched nerves or diabetic neuropathy. Treatment: Correct the underlying cause.

Diagnostic Procedures

Laboratory Tests

Word or Phrase	Word Part and Definition	Description
alpha fetoprotein (AFP)	**alpha fetoprotein** (AL-fah FEE-toh-PROH-teen)	Chemistry test performed on amniotic fluid extracted from the uterus via amniocentesis during pregnancy. Used to diagnose a neural tube defect in the fetus before birth. The fetal liver makes alpha fetoprotein, and small amounts are normally present in the amniotic fluid. However, increased levels indicate that alpha fetoprotein is leaking into the amniotic fluid from a myelocele or meningomyelocele.
cerebrospinal fluid (CFS) examination		Laboratory test that examines the CSF macroscopically for clarity and color, microscopically for cells, and chemically for proteins and other substances. Normal CSF is clear and colorless. Large numbers of red blood cells cause the CSF to have a pink or reddish tint. Red blood cells indicate bleeding in the brain from a stroke or trauma. Large numbers of white blood cells cause the CSF to appear cloudy. White blood cells indicate an infection like meningitis or encephalitis. Elevated protein levels indicate infection or the presence of a tumor. The presence of oligoclonal bands points to multiple sclerosis. Myelin-basic protein is elevated in multiple sclerosis and amyotrophic lateral sclerosis.

Radiologic and Nuclear Medicine Procedures

Word or Phrase	Word Part and Definition	Description
carotid duplex scan	**carotid** (kah-ROT-id) **duplex** (DOO-pleks)	Radiologic procedure that uses ultrasound (high-frequency sound waves) to produce a two-dimensional image to visualize areas of stenosis and plaque in the carotid arteries.
cerebral angiography	**angiography** (AN-jee-AWG-rah-fee) **angi/o-** *blood vessel; lymphatic vessel* **-graphy** *process of recording* **angiogram** (AN-jee-oh-gram) **angi/o-** *blood vessel; lymphatic vessel* **-gram** *a record or picture* **arteriography** (ar-TEER-ee-AWG-rah-fee) **arteri/o-** *artery* **-graphy** *process of recording* **arteriogram** (ar-TEER-ee-oh-gram) **arteri/o-** *artery* **-gram** *a record or picture*	Radiologic procedure in which a radiopaque contrast dye is injected into the carotid arteries, and an x-ray is taken to visualize the arterial circulation in the brain (see Figure 10-24 ■). This shows an aneurysm, stenosis, or plaque in the arteries. A tumor can be seen as an interwoven collection of new blood vessels, or it can be seen indirectly when it distorts normal anatomy and forces arteries into abnormal positions. Also known as **arteriography.** The x-ray image is known as an **angiogram** or an **arteriogram.**

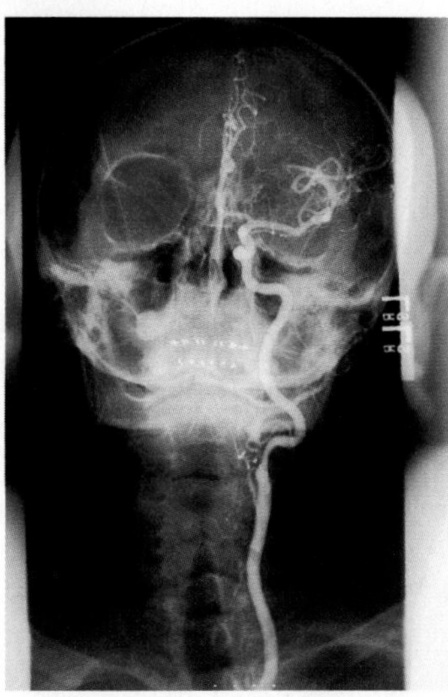

Figure 10-24 ■ Arteriogram of the left carotid artery and cerebral arteries.
This procedure is also known as a cerebral angiography or carotid arteriography. The injected dye clearly outlines the carotid artery and its many smaller branches within the cranial cavity. There is no evidence of carotid artery plaques or cerebral aneurysm.

Word or Phrase	Word Part and Definition	Description
computed axial tomography (CAT, CT)	**axial** (AK-see-al) **axi/o-** *axis* **-al** *pertaining to* The x-ray emitter and detector rotate around the axis of the body to produce an axial (transverse) plane image. **tomography** (toh-MAWG-rah-fee) **tom/o-** *a cut, slice, or layer* **-graphy** *process of recording*	Radiologic procedure that uses x-rays to create many individual, closely spaced images ("slices"). The computer can combine these into one three-dimensional image. CT scans are used to view the skull, brain, vertebral column, and spinal cord. Radiopaque contrast dye can be injected to provide more detail.
magnetic resonance imaging (MRI)	**magnetic** (mag-NET-ik) **magnet/o-** *magnet* **-ic** *pertaining to* **resonance** (REZ-oh-nans)	Radiologic procedure that uses a magnetic field and radiowaves to align the protons in the body and cause them to emit signals. The signals are used to construct an image. Magnetic resonance imaging is a type of tomography that creates many individual "slice" images. MRI scans are used to view the skull, brain, vertebral column, and spinal cord (see Figure 10-13). Radiopaque contrast dye can be injected to provide more detail.
myelography	**myelography** (MY-eh-LAWG-rah-fee) **myel/o-** *bone marrow; spinal cord; myelin* **-graphy** *process of recording* **myelogram** (MY-eh-loh-gram) **myel/o-** *bone marrow; spinal cord; myelin* **-gram** *a record or picture*	Radiologic procedure in which a radiopaque contrast dye is injected into the subarachnoid space at the level of the L3 and L4 vertebrae. The contrast dye outlines the spinal cavity and shows spinal nerves, nerve roots, and intervertebral disks, plus any tumors, herniated disks, or obstructions within the cavity. The x-ray image is known as a **myelogram**. Because myelograms can have a side effect of severe headache, they are not used as often as MRI scans of the spine.
positron emission tomography (PET) scan	**positron** (PAWZ-ih-trawn) **emission** (ee-MISH-un) **emiss/o-** *to send out* **-ion** *action; condition* **tomography** (toh-MAWG-rah-fee) **tom/o-** *a cut, slice, or layer* **-graphy** *process of recording*	Nuclear medicine procedure that uses a radioactive substance that emits positrons. This substance is combined with glucose molecules and injected intravenously. As the glucose is metabolized, the radioactive substance emits positrons, and these form gamma rays that are detected by a gamma camera. The camera produces an image that reflects the amount of metabolism in that area (see Figure 10-16). PET scans show areas of increased metabolism due to cancerous tumors. PET scans also show areas of abnormally increased or decreased metabolism in the brains of patients with Alzheimer's disease, Parkinson's disease, epilepsy, and schizophrenia (see Figure 10-17).
skull x-ray		Radiologic procedure in which a plain film (without contrast dye) is taken of the skull. An x-ray can show fractures of the bones of the skull but cannot clearly show the soft tissues of the brain or blood vessels.
Other Diagnostic Tests		
electroencephalography (EEG)	**electroencephalography** (ee-LEK-troh-en-SEF-ah-LAWG-rah-fee) **electr/o-** *electricity* **encephal/o-** *brain* **-graphy** *process of recording*	Diagnostic procedure to record the electrical activity of the brain (see Figure 10-19). Multiple electrodes are placed on the scalp overlying the specific lobes of the brain. The electrodes are attached to lead wires that go to the **electroencephalograph,** the machine that records the brain waves. The computerized or paper recording of the brain waves is an **electroencephalogram.** There are four types of normal brain waves (named for letters of the Greek alphabet: alpha, beta, delta, and theta). *(continued)*

Word or Phrase	Word Part and Definition	Description
electroencephalography (EEG) *(continued)*	**electroencephalograph** (ee-LEK-troh-en-SEF-ah-loh-graf) **electr/o-** *electricity* **encephal/o-** *brain* **-graph** *instrument used to record* **electroencephalogram** (ee-LEK-troh-en-SEF-ah-loh-gram) **electr/o-** *electricity* **encephal/o-** *brain* **-gram** *a record or picture*	The patterns of brain waves in each of the two hemispheres of the cerebrum are compared for symmetry. Differences between the two hemispheres suggest a tumor or injury. The presence of abnormal waves suggests encephalopathy or dementia. Brain waves during an epileptic seizure show specific patterns that are used to diagnose the particular type of epilepsy. In order to induce an epileptic seizure during the EEG, the patient may look at flashing lights or have a sleep-deprived EEG recording. An EEG is also done as a polysomnography to diagnose sleep disorders and also as part of evoked potential testing.
evoked potential testing	**evoked** (ee-VOKED) *Evoke* is an English word meaning *to draw forth or provoke.* **potential** (poh-TEN-shal) **potent/o-** *being capable of doing* **-al** *pertaining to* **somatosensory** (soh-MAH-toh-SEN-soh-ree) **somat/o-** *body* **sens/o-** *sensation* **-ory** *having the function of*	Diagnostic procedure in which an EEG is used to record changes in brain waves that occur following various stimuli. Used to evaluate the potential ability of a particular nervous pathway to conduct nerve impulses. A stimulus is presented to evoke a response, which is why this procedure is also called an evoked response. For a **visual evoked potential (VEP)** or **visual evoked response (VER),** the patient watches a TV monitor that displays rapidly alternating checkerboard patterns. This evaluates the condition of nerve pathways from the eye to the cerebrum. For a **brainstem auditory evoked potential (BAEP)** or **brainstem auditory evoked response (BAER),** the patient has on headphones and listens to a series of clicks in one ear and then the other. This evaluates the nerve pathways from the ears to the cerebrum. For a **somatosensory evoked potential (SSEP)** or **somatosensory evoked response (SSER),** a small electrical impulse is administered to the arm or leg. This test evaluates the nerve pathways from the limbs to the cerebrum. These tests are particularly helpful with patients who are too young or too incapacitated to respond to standard vision and hearing tests. These tests are also used to detect subtle abnormalities in patients with multiple sclerosis, head trauma, or spinal cord injury. The patient cannot voluntarily alter the response to these tests.
nerve conduction study	**conduction** (con-DUK-shun) **conduct/o-** *carrying, conveying* **-ion** *action; condition*	Medical procedure to measure the speed at which an electrical impulse travels along a nerve. An electrode is used to stimulate a peripheral nerve with an electrical impulse. Another electrode a measured distance away records how long it takes for the electrical impulse to reach it. This test is usually performed in conjunction with electromyography to help differentiate between weakness due to nerve disorders versus muscle disorders.
polysomnography	**polysomnography** (PAWL-ee-sawm-NAWG-rah-fee) **poly-** *many, much* **somn/o-** *sleep* **-graphy** *process of recording* Add words to make a correct and complete definition of *polysomnography: The process of recording many [of the body's activities that occur during] sleep.*	Multifaceted test to diagnose the underlying conditions that can cause insomnia, sleep disruption, sleep apnea, or narcolepsy. Electrodes on the face and head and various other monitors are applied to the patient. During sleep, the patient's EEG, eye movements, muscle activity, heartbeat, and respirations are monitored. Also known as a sleep study.

Medical and Surgical Procedures

Medical Procedures

Word or Phrase	Word Part and Definition	Description
Babinski's sign	**Babinski** (bah-BIN-skee) Babinski's sign was named by Joseph Babinski (1857–1932), a French neurologist.	Neurologic test in which the end of the metal handle of the percussion hammer is used to firmly stroke the lateral sole of the foot from the heel to the toes. A normal test or negative Babinski shows downward curling of the toes. An abnormal test or positive Babinski shows upward extension of the great toe and lateral fanning of the other toes (see Figure 10-25 ■). A positive Babinski indicates injury to the parietal lobe or to the spinal nerves. **Figure 10-25 ■ Positive Babinski's sign.** This patient has a positive (abnormal) Babinski sign with extension of the great toe and fanning of the other toes laterally.
Glasgow Coma Scale (GCS)	**Glasgow** (GLAS-goh)	Numerical scale that measures the depth of a coma. The scores range from 3 to 15 and are the sum of individual scores for eye opening, motor response, and verbal response following a painful stimulus such as pressure on the nailbed or on the supraorbital ridge over the eye. For example, if a patient opens his eyes to a verbal command, has confused answers, and withdraws from the painful stimulus, his GCS would be E(3) + V (4) + M (4) = 11.

Word or Phrase	Word Part and Definition	Description
lumbar puncture (LP)	**lumbar** (LUM-bar) lumb/o- *lower back; area between the ribs and pelvis* -ar *pertaining to* **puncture** (PUNGK-chur) punct/o- *hole, perforation* -ure *system; result of* **manometer** (mah-NAWM-eh-ter) man/o- *thin* -meter *instrument used to measure* A manometer is a thin, calibrated tube.	Medical procedure to obtain cerebrospinal fluid (CSF) for testing. Also known as a **spinal tap.** The patient is positioned on the side with the chest flexed toward the thighs. This curves the spine and widens the space between the spinous processes of two vertebrae, allowing accurate positioning of the spinal needle (see Figure 10-26 ■). A needle is inserted in the space between the L3–4 or L4–5 vertebrae and into the subarachnoid space. Cerebrospinal fluid flows through the needle and is collected and sent to the laboratory. Before the spinal needle is removed, a calibrated **manometer** may be attached to the needle to measure the intracranial pressure as the CSF rises in the manometer. 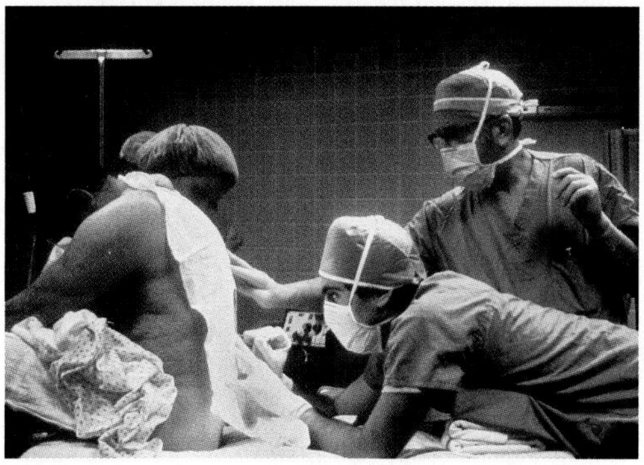 **Figure 10-26 ■ Lumbar puncture.** The patient is positioned with the spine flexed. This older patient does not have much flexibility of the spine and is only able to flex the head and shoulders forward. One physician is helping the patient to maintain this position while the other physician inserts the spinal needle. A white sterile drape covers the patient's back except for a round opening in the drape where the needle is inserted.
mini mental status examination (MMSE)	**mental** (MEN-tal) ment/o- *mind; chin* -al *pertaining to*	Tests the patient's concrete and abstract thought processes and long- and short-term memory. The patient is asked to state his/her name, the date, and where he/she is. If the answers are all correct, the patient is said to be oriented to person, time, and place or oriented x3. The patient is asked to perform simple mental arithmetic, recall objects or words, name the current and recent past presidents, spell a word backwards, and give the meaning of a proverb. A full mental status examination is used for psychiatric evaluations.

Word or Phrase	Word Part and Definition	Description
neurologic examination	**proprioception** (PROH-pree-oh-SEP-shun) *Proprioception* is derived from the combining form *propri/o-* (*one's own self*); part of the word *receptor,* and the suffix *-tion* (*a process; being or having*). **Romberg** (RAWM-berg) The Romberg test is named for Moritz Romberg (1795–1873), a German physician.	Tests coordination, sensation, balance, and gait. *Coordination.* Rapid alternating movements: Tap the tip of the index finger against the thumb many times as rapidly as possible. Finger-to-nose test: Touch the tip of the index finger to the nose with the eyes closed. Touch the nose, then the examiner's finger as it moves around, then the nose. Heel-to-shin test: Put the heel of one foot onto the opposite leg and then run it from the knee down the shin to the toes. *Sensation.* With the patient's eyes closed, the skin is touched in various places with a cotton swab (to test light touch), a vibrating tuning fork (to test vibration), the point of a pin (pinprick to test pain). One or two pins are used to see if the patient can distinguish the number of things touching the skin (2-point discrimination). The patient's toe or finger is moved up and down and the patient is asked to identify the direction (to test body position and **proprioception**). *Balance.* **Romberg test** in which the patient stands with the feet together and the eyes closed. In a normal test, the patient does not sway excessively or lose balance. The Romberg test is also known as the station test. *Gait.* The manner of walking is assessed for a normal arm swing and stride. The patient is asked to walk across the room in a heel-to-toe fashion, then on the toes, on the heels, and then hop in place on each foot.
spinal traction	**traction** (TRAK-shun) **tract/o-** *pulling* **-ion** *action; condition*	Medical procedure in which a fracture of the vertebra is immobilized while it heals. Two metal pins are surgically inserted into the cranium and attached to a set of tongs (see Figure 10-27■) with a rope and pulley and 7–10 pounds of weight. A patient with a partially healed fracture of the vertebra can be fitted for a halo vest with pins in the cranium attached to a metal ring (halo). 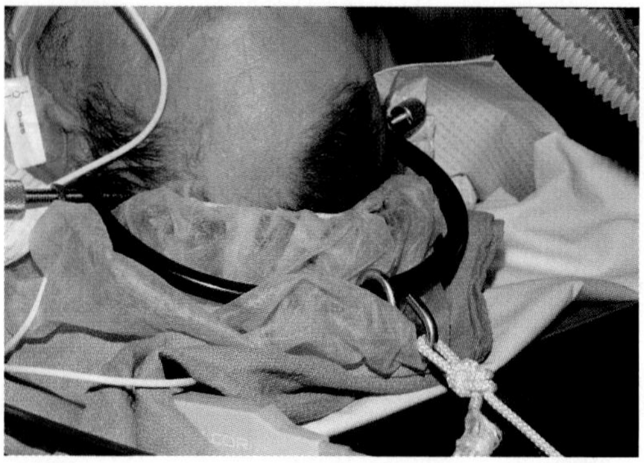 **Figure 10-27 ■ Spinal traction with tongs.** This patient's spine is immobilized while a fractured vertebra heals. Notice the pins inserted into the cranium, tongs, and the rope that is connected to weights to exert steady and constant traction.
transcutaneous electrical nerve stimulation (TENS) unit	**transcutaneous** (TRANS-kyoo-TAY-nee-us) **trans-** *across, through* **cutane/o-** *skin* **-ous** *pertaining to*	Medical procedure that uses an electrical device to control chronic pain. A battery produces regular, preset electrical impulses that travel through wires to electrodes on the skin. These impulses block the transmission of pain sensations to the brain. The impulses also stimulate the body to produce its own natural pain-relieving endorphins.

Surgical Procedures

Word or Phrase	Word Part and Definition	Description
biopsy	**biopsy** (BY-awp-see) **bi/o-** *life; living organisms; living tissue* **-opsy** *process of viewing* **excisional** (ek-SIHZ-un-al) **excis/o-** *to cut out* **-ion** *action; condition* **-al** *pertaining to*	Surgical procedure to remove a tumor or mass from the brain or other part of the nervous system. This is an **excisional biopsy** because the entire tumor or mass is removed and sent to the laboratory for microscopic examination to determine if it is benign or malignant. Even a benign tumor must be totally removed because it causes increasing pressure within the inflexible bony cranium.
carotid endarterectomy	**endarterectomy** (END-ar-ter-EK-toh-mee) **endo-** *innermost, within* **arter/o-** *artery* **-ectomy** *surgical excision*	Surgical procedure to remove plaque from the carotid artery. This opens up the lumen of the artery, restores blood flow to the brain, and decreases the possibility of a stroke.
craniotomy	**craniotomy** (KRAY-nee-AWT-oh-mee) **crani/o-** *cranium (skull)* **-tomy** *process of cutting or making an incision*	Surgical incision into the cranium to expose the brain tissue. A craniotomy is the first phase of any type of brain surgery (i.e., evacuation of a subdural hematoma or excising a brain tumor).
diskectomy	**diskectomy** (dis-KEK-toh-mee) **disk/o-** *disk* **-ectomy** *surgical excision*	Surgical excision of part or all of the herniated nucleus pulposus from an intervertebral disk. This relieves pressure on the adjacent dorsal nerve roots and relieves the pain.
laminectomy	**laminectomy** (LAM-ih-NEK-toh-mee) **lamin/o-** *lamina (flat area on the vertebra)* **-ectomy** *surgical excision*	Surgical excision of the lamina (the flat area of the arch of the vertebra). Removal of this bony segment relieves pressure on the dorsal nerve roots and relieves pain from a herniated nucleus pulposus.

Connections

rhizotomy (ry-ZAWT-oh-mee)
rhiz/o- *spinal nerve root*
-tomy *process of cutting or making an incision*

Pain Management. This subspecialty for treating chronic or severe pain is shared by both neurology and anesthesiology. Pain mangement procedures include a dorsal nerve root injection into an area where a nerve is compressed. Surgical treatment includes a **rhizotomy,** an incision to cut spinal nerve roots. The dorsal (sensory) nerve roots can be cut to relieve severe pain. The ventral (motor) nerve roots can be cut to relieve severe muscle spasticity and spasm.

Word or Phrase	Word Part and Definition	Description
stereotactic neurosurgery	**stereotactic** (STAIR-ee-oh-TAK-tik) **stere/o-** *three dimensions* **tact/o-** *touch* **-ic** *pertaining to* **neurosurgery** (NYOO-roh-SER-jer-ee) **neur/o-** *nerve* **surg/o-** *operative procedure* **-ery** *process of*	Surgical procedure that uses three-dimensional excision of a deep tumor within the cerebrum. A CT or MRI scan is used to show the tumor in three dimensions and obtain its precise coordinates. The patient's head is fixed in a stereotactic apparatus that acts as a guidance system to position an electrode within the brain. Then heat, cold, or high-energy gamma rays are used to destroy the tumor.

Word or Phrase	Word Part and Definition	Description
ventriculo-peritoneal shunt	**ventriculoperitoneal** (ven-TRIK-yoo-loh-PAIR-ih-toh-NEE-al) **ventricul/o-** *ventricle (lower heart chamber; chamber in the brain)* **peritone/o-** *peritoneum* **-eal** *pertaining to* **shunt** (SHUNT) *Shunt* is derived from an Old English word meaning *to turn away from the path.*	Surgical procedure to insert a plastic tube to connect the ventricles of the brain to the peritoneal cavity. The shunt continuously removes excess cerebrospinal fluid associated with hydrocephalus.

Drug Categories

Several different categories of drugs are used to treat the symptoms, signs, and diseases of the nervous system. The most common drugs in each category are listed.

Category	Word Part and Definition	Description	Examples
analgesic drugs	**analgesic** (AN-al-JEE-zik) **an-** *without, not* **alges/o-** *sensation of pain* **-ic** *pertaining to* **narcotic** (nar-KAWT-ik) **narc/o-** *stupor, sleep* **-tic** *pertaining to*	Over-the-counter aspirin and nonaspirin drugs used to decrease inflammation and pain. **Narcotic** drugs are another type of analgesic drugs that are addicting and used to treat severe, chronic pain.	Nonnarcotic drugs: acetaminophen, Bayer aspirin, ibuprofen, Motrin, Tylenol Narcotic drugs: Darvon, Demerol, morphine, OxyContin
antiepileptic drugs	**antiepileptic** (AN-tee-EP-ih-LEP-tik) (AN-tih-EP-ih-LEP-tik) **anti-** *against* **epilept/o-** *seizure* **-ic** *pertaining to* **anticonvulsant** (AN-tee-con-VUL-sant) (AN-tih-con-VUL-sant) **anti-** *against* **convuls/o-** *seizure* **-ant** *pertaining to*	Prevent the seizures of epilepsy. Also known as **anticonvulsant drugs.**	Depakene, Dilantin, Tegretol, Zarontin
chemotherapy drugs	**chemotherapy** (KEE-moh-THAIR-ah-pee) **chem/o-** *chemical, drug* **-therapy** *treatment*	Kill rapidly dividing cancer cells in the brain.	Cytoxan, Gliadel, Myleran

Category	Word Part and Definition	Description	Examples
COMT inhibitor drugs	**inhibitor** (in-HIB-ih-tor) **inhibit/o-** *block; hold back* **-or** *person or thing that produces or does*	Treat Parkinson's disease by inhibiting the enzyme that metabolizes the drug levodopa. This allows more levodopa to reach the brain.	Comtan, Tasmar
corticosteroid drugs	**corticosteroid** (KOR-tih-koh-STAIR-oyd) **cortic/o-** *cortex (outer region)* **-steroid** *steroid*	Used to suppress inflammation in chronic pain conditions and multiple sclerosis. Used to treat swelling and edema in the brain or spinal cord following traumatic injury or stroke.	hydrocortisone, Medrol, prednisone
drugs for Alzheimer's disease		Treat the lack of acetylcholine in the brain by inhibiting the enzyme that breaks down acetylcholine.	Aricept, Cognex, Exelon, Reminyl
drugs for myasthenia gravis		Treat the lack of acetylcholine in the muscles by inhibiting the enzyme that breaks down acetylcholine.	Mestinon, Prostigmin
drugs for Parkinson's disease		Treat the imbalance in the brain between dopamine and acetylcholine by supplying dopamine or inhibiting acetylcholine.	Cogentin,levodopa (L-dopa), Permax, Symmetrel

Connections

tardive (TAR-dive)
tard/o- *late, slow*
-ive *pertaining to*

dyskinesia (DIS-kih-NEE-zee-ah)
dys- *painful, difficult, abnormal*
kines/o- *movement*
-ia *condition, state, thing*

Pharmacology. Patients who take drugs to treat Parkinson's disease can develop a serious adverse effect known as **tardive dyskinesia.** This occurs only after the patient has been on the drug for some time. It manifests as involuntary chewing movements, blinking, grimacing, and athetoid movements of the hands.

Category	Word Part and Definition	Description	Examples
general anesthetic drugs	**anesthetic** (AN-es-THET-ik) **an-** *without, not* **esthet/o-** *sensation, feeling* **-ia** *condition, state, thing*	Produces unconsciousness. Used during surgery.	Pentothal (intravenous), nitrous oxide (inhaled gas)

Abbreviations

AFP	alpha fetoprotein
ALS	amyotrophic lateral sclerosis
AVM	arteriovenous malformation
BAEP	brainstem auditory evoked potential
BAER	brainstem auditory evoked response
CNS	central nervous system
COMT	catechol-*O*-methyltransferase
CP	cerebral palsy
CRPS	chronic regional pain syndrome
CSF	cerebrospinal fluid
CT	computed tomography
CTS	carpal tunnel syndrome
CVA	cerebrovascular accident
EEG	electroencephalography
END	electroneurodiagnostic (technician)
GCS	Glasgow Coma Scale (or Score)
HNP	herniated nucleus pulposus
ICP	intracranial pressure
LP	lumbar puncture
MRI	magnetic resonance imaging
MS	multiple sclerosis
NICU	neurologic intensive care unit
PET	positron emission scan
RIND	reversible ischemic neurological deficit
SCI	spinal cord injury
SSEP	somatosensory evoked potential
SSER	somatosensory evoked response
TENS	transcutaneous electrical nerve stimulation (unit)
TIA	transient ischemic attack
VEP	visual evoked potential
VER	visual evoked response

Word Alert

MEDICAL ABBREVIATIONS

Abbreviations are commonly used in all types of medical documents; however, they can mean different things to different people and their meaning can be misinterpreted. Always verify the meaning of an abbreviation.

CP stands for *cerebral palsy,* but it can also stand for *cardiopulmonary.*

CNS stands for *central nervous system,* but it can be confused with the sound-alike abbreviation *C&S,* which stands for *culture and sensitivity.*

HNP stands for *herniated nucleus pulposus,* but it can be confused with the sound-alike abbreviation *H&P,* which stands for *history and physical examination.*

MS stands for *multiple sclerosis,* but it can also stand for the drug *morphine sulfate.*

NICU stands for *neurologic intensive care unit,* but it can also stand for *neonatal intensive care unit.*

Career Focus

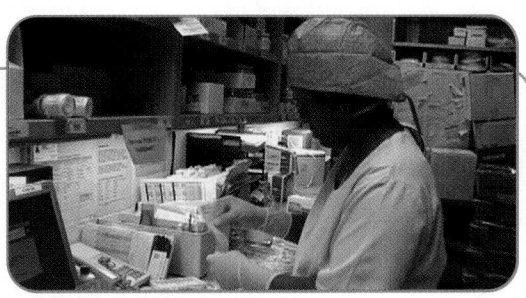

Meet Amelia, a pharmacy technician.

"Here in the hospital pharmacy, I have the responsibility of making IVs and filling orders. I deliver med carts; I deliver patient meds. I do expiration dates—pulling all expired drugs off the shelf, and I also get to work with wonderful pharmacists. Even though I initial my orders, they cannot leave the pharmacy until the pharmacist has checked off on them. The best part of my job is meeting different people. I enjoy helping people and making someone's day a little better."

Pharmacy technicians are allied health professionals who assist pharmacists in their work. Pharmacy technicians provide pharmacy services to home health, long-term care, and outpatient facilities, and to hospitals. They also work in retail pharmacies (drug stores).

Neurologists are physicians who practice in the medical specialty of neurology. They diagnose and treat patients with diseases of the nervous system. **Neurosurgeons** perform surgery on the brain, spinal cord, and nerves. Physicians can take additional training and become board certified in the subspecialty of pediatric neurology.

Malignancies of the nervous system are treated medically by an oncologist or surgically by a neurosurgeon.

pharmacy (FAR-mah-see)

technician (tek-NISH-un)
techn/o- *technical skill*
-ician *a skilled professional or expert*

neurologist (nyoo-RAWL-oh-jist)
neur/o- *nerve*
log/o- *the study of*
-ist *one who specializes in*

neurosurgeon (NYOOR-oh-SER-jun)
neur/o- *nerve*
surg/o- *operative procedure*
-eon *one who performs*
Surgeon is derived from a Latin word meaning *hand work.*

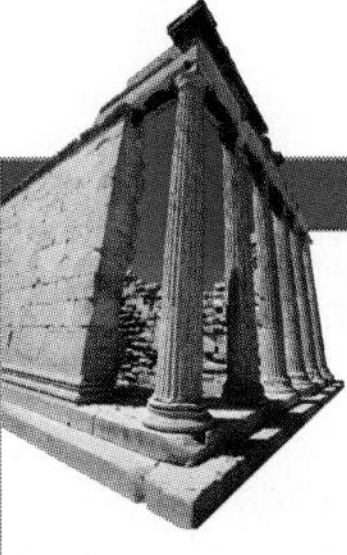

It's Greek To Me!

Did you notice that some neurology words have two different combining forms? Combining forms from both Greek and Latin languages remain a part of medical language today.

English Word	Greek	Latin	Examples of Medical Words
mind	psych/o-	ment/o-	psychomotor, dementia
nerve	neur/o-	nerv/o-	neuron, nervous system
nerve root	rhiz/o-	radicul/o-	rhizotomy, radiculopathy
seizure	epilept/o-	convuls/o-	epileptic, convulsion
		ict/o-	postictal
sensation	esthes/o-	sens/o-	paresthesia, sensory nerve
spine, spinal cord	myel/o-	spin/o-	myelomeningocele, spinal

CHAPTER REVIEW EXERCISES

Review all the material in this chapter by completing the review exercises in this section. Use the Answer Key at the end of the book to check your answers.

Anatomy and Physiology

Matching Exercise

Match each numbered word or phrase to its description.

1. axon	_____	Neurotransmitter of the sympathetic nervous system
2. cauda equina	_____	Four hollow chambers within the brain that contain CSF
3. corpus callosum	_____	Joins the pons to the spinal cord
4. cranial nerves	_____	Cell that makes the myelin sheath around axons
5. cranium	_____	Involuntary muscle reaction controlled by the spinal cord
6. dermatome	_____	There are 12 pairs of them
7. epinephrine	_____	Nerves that come out of the end of the spinal cord
8. gustatory cortex	_____	Part of the neuron that may be myelinated
9. medulla oblongata	_____	Space between the axon of one neuron and the dendrites of the next neuron
10. neurotransmitter	_____	Area that contains cerebrospinal fluid around the brain
11. oligodendroglia	_____	Area of the cerebrum that receives sensory impulses from the taste receptors
12. reflex	_____	Area of the skin that supplies sensory information to a specific spinal nerve
13. subarachnoid space	_____	Dome-shaped bone of the skull
14. synapse	_____	Chemical messenger
15. ventricles	_____	Band of nerve fibers that connects the two hemispheres of the cerebrum

Circle Exercise

Circle the correct word from the choices given.

1. The (**axon, cerebellum, cerebrum**) is divided into two hemispheres.
2. The olfactory cortex receives sensory impulses from the (**ears, eyes, nose**).
3. The most delicate of the meninges and the one that is closest to the brain is the (**arachnoid, dura mater, pia mater**).
4. The functional unit of the nervous system is the (**nephron, nerve, neuron**).
5. In the majority of people, the (**cerebellum, gyrus, left hemisphere of the cerebrum**) performs math, analysis, and logical thinking.
6. The hypothalamus is located (**above, below, beside**) the thalamus.
7. The (**auditory, oculomotor, trigeminal**) cranial nerve controls eye movements.
8. The neurotransmitter that goes between a neuron and a voluntary skeletal muscle is (**acetylcholine, dopamine, endorphins**).

True or False

Indicate whether each statement is true or false by writing T or F on the line.

1. ____ The autonomic nervous system is composed of the central nervous system and the peripheral nervous system.
2. ____ Efferent nerves carry nerve impulses away from the brain or spinal cord.
3. ____ After a nerve impulse passes through the cell body, it then goes to the dendrites.
4. ____ The occipital lobe is a lobe of the cerebellum that is directly beneath the occipital skull bone.
5. ____ The peripheral nervous system consists of the cranial nerves and spinal nerves.
6. ____ The hypothalamus functions as part of the nervous system and endocrine system.
7. ____ Cranial nerve X (vagus nerve) is the only cranial nerve that goes into the thoracic and abdominal cavities.
8. ____ Endorphins are the body's own natural pain relievers.

Recall and Relate

Write the correct answers in the blanks provided.

1. Name the three layers that comprise the meninges.
   ____
   ____
   ____
2. Rounded tissue folds in the cerebral cortex are known as ____________ and the deep grooves between the folds are known as ____________.
3. Medical name for one half of the cerebrum. ____________
4. The ____________ cells that line the ventricles produce cerebrospinal fluid.
5. The ____________ regulates sensations of hunger and thirst as well as the body's 24-hour circadian rhythm.

Multiple Choice

Circle the best answer from the choices given.

1. Sensory information consists of all of the following EXCEPT ____________.
   a. pain
   b. sounds
   c. motor commands
   d. temperature
2. All of the neurons in the nervous system are collectively known as the ____________ or functional units of the nervous system.
   a. dermatomes
   b. parenchyma
   c. cranial cavity
   d. neurotransmitters
3. The type of nervous system cell that can move anywhere to engulf and destroy dead tissue and pathogens is the ____________.
   a. microglia
   b. axon
   c. cerebrospinal fluid
   d. dorsal nerve root
4. The division of the nervous system that is active in the "fight or flight" response is the ____________.
   a. central nervous system
   b. peripheral nervous system
   c. brain
   d. sympathetic nervous system

Medical Language Word Parts

Name That Word Part

Identify each of the word parts given here by writing in the correct letter (P, C, or S) on the line beside it. Then write the definition of the word part on the blank line. The first one has been done for you.

Prefix = P **Combining Form = C** **Suffix = S**

		Word Part	Definition
1.	-al	S	pertaining to
2.	a-	______	______________
3.	access/o-	______	______________
4.	affer/o-	______	______________
5.	alges/o-	______	______________
6.	alg/o-	______	______________
7.	an-	______	______________
8.	angi/o-	______	______________
9.	-ant	______	______________
10.	anti-	______	______________
11.	-ar	______	______________
12.	arachn/o-	______	______________
13.	arteri/o-	______	______________
14.	arter/o-	______	______________
15.	-ary	______	______________
16.	astr/o-	______	______________
17.	-ated	______	______________
18.	-ation	______	______________
19.	audit/o-	______	______________
20.	autonom/o-	______	______________
21.	axi/o-	______	______________
22.	bi/o-	______	______________
23.	blast/o-	______	______________
24.	carp/o-	______	______________
25.	caus/o-	______	______________
26.	cav/o-	______	______________
27.	-cele	______	______________
28.	centr/o-	______	______________
29.	cephal/o-	______	______________
30.	-cephalus	______	______________
31.	cerebell/o-	______	______________
32.	cerebr/o-	______	______________
33.	chem/o-	______	______________
34.	clon/o-	______	______________
35.	comat/o-	______	______________
36.	concuss/o-	______	______________
37.	conduct/o-	______	______________
38.	contus/o-	______	______________
39.	convuls/o-	______	______________
40.	cortic/o-	______	______________
41.	crani/o-	______	______________
42.	cutane/o-	______	______________
43.	-cyte	______	______________
44.	cyt/o-	______	______________
45.	de-	______	______________
46.	dendr/o-	______	______________
47.	diabet/o-	______	______________
48.	disk/o-	______	______________
49.	dors/o-	______	______________
50.	dur/o-	______	______________
51.	dys-	______	______________
52.	-eal	______	______________
53.	-ectomy	______	______________
54.	effer/o-	______	______________
55.	electr/o-	______	______________
56.	-emia	______	______________
57.	-emic	______	______________
58.	emiss/o-	______	______________
59.	encephal/o-	______	______________
60.	-encephaly	______	______________
61.	endo-	______	______________
62.	-ent	______	______________
63.	-eon	______	______________
64.	ependym/o-	______	______________
65.	epi-	______	______________
66.	epilept/o-	______	______________
67.	-er	______	______________
68.	-ery	______	______________
69.	esthes/o-	______	______________
70.	excis/o-	______	______________

		Word Part	Definition
71.	express/o-	______	________________
72.	faci/o-	______	________________
73.	fibrill/o-	______	________________
74.	fibr/o-	______	________________
75.	fiss/o-	______	________________
76.	foc/o-	______	________________
77.	format/o-	______	________________
78.	front/o-	______	________________
79.	gemin/o-	______	________________
80.	-glia	______	________________
81.	gli/o-	______	________________
82.	glob/o-	______	________________
83.	gloss/o-	______	________________
84.	-gram	______	________________
85.	-graph	______	________________
86.	-graphy	______	________________
87.	gustat/o-	______	________________
88.	hemat/o-	______	________________
89.	hemi-	______	________________
90.	herni/o-	______	________________
91.	hydr/o-	______	________________
92.	hyper-	______	________________
93.	hypo-	______	________________
94.	-ia	______	________________
95.	-ic	______	________________
96.	ict/o-	______	________________
97.	-ile	______	________________
98.	infarct/o-	______	________________
99.	inhibit/o-	______	________________
100.	intra-	______	________________
101.	-ion	______	________________
102.	isch/o-	______	________________
103.	-ist	______	________________
104.	-ite	______	________________
105.	-itis	______	________________
106.	-ity	______	________________
107.	-ive	______	________________
108.	kines/o-	______	________________
109.	lamin/o-	______	________________
110.	-lepsy	______	________________
111.	lex/o-	______	________________

		Word Part	Definition
112.	log/o-	______	________________
113.	-logy	______	________________
114.	lumb/o-	______	________________
115.	lymph/o-	______	________________
116.	-lysis	______	________________
117.	magnet/o-	______	________________
118.	mal-	______	________________
119.	malign/o-	______	________________
120.	meningi/o-	______	________________
121.	mening/o-	______	________________
122.	ment/o-	______	________________
123.	micr/o-	______	________________
124.	mitt/o-	______	________________
125.	mot/o-	______	________________
126.	muscul/o-	______	________________
127.	myelin/o-	______	________________
128.	myel/o-	______	________________
129.	my/o-	______	________________
130.	narc/o-	______	________________
131.	nerv/o-	______	________________
132.	neur/o-	______	________________
133.	nuch/o-	______	________________
134.	occipit/o-	______	________________
135.	ocul/o-	______	________________
136.	-oid	______	________________
137.	olfact/o-	______	________________
138.	olig/o-	______	________________
139.	-oma	______	________________
140.	-omatosis	______	________________
141.	-opsy	______	________________
142.	opt/o-	______	________________
143.	-or	______	________________
144.	-ory	______	________________
145.	-ose	______	________________
146.	-osis	______	________________
147.	-ous	______	________________
148.	para-	______	________________
149.	parenchym/o-	______	________________
150.	-paresis	______	________________
151.	pariet/o-	______	________________
152.	pathet/o-	______	________________

		Word Part	Definition
153.	-pathy	______	________________
154.	peripher/o-	______	________________
155.	peritone/o-	______	________________
156.	pharyng/o-	______	________________
157.	phas/o-	______	________________
158.	phob/o-	______	________________
159.	phot/o-	______	________________
160.	pleg/o-	______	________________
161.	poly-	______	________________
162.	potent/o-	______	________________
163.	pre-	______	________________
164.	psych/o-	______	________________
165.	punct/o-	______	________________
166.	quadri-	______	________________
167.	radicul/o-	______	________________
168.	recept/o-	______	________________
169.	retard/o-	______	________________
170.	rhiz/o-	______	________________
171.	scler/o-	______	________________
172.	sect/o-	______	________________
173.	sen/o-	______	________________
174.	sens/o-	______	________________
175.	somat/o-	______	________________
176.	somn/o-	______	________________
177.	spast/o-	______	________________
178.	-sphere	______	________________
179.	spin/o-	______	________________
180.	stere/o-	______	________________
181.	-steroid	______	________________
182.	sub-	______	________________
183.	surg/o-	______	________________
184.	sym-	______	________________
185.	syncop/o-	______	________________
186.	tact/o-	______	________________
187.	tard/o-	______	________________
188.	tempor/o-	______	________________
189.	thalam/o-	______	________________
190.	-therapy	______	________________
191.	-tic	______	________________
192.	tom/o-	______	________________
193.	-tomy	______	________________
194.	ton/o-	______	________________
195.	tract/o-	______	________________
196.	trans-	______	________________
197.	tri-	______	________________
198.	trochle/o-	______	________________
199.	troph/o-	______	________________
200.	-ure	______	________________
201.	vascul/o-	______	________________
202.	ven/o-	______	________________
203.	ventricul/o-	______	________________
204.	ventr/o-	______	________________
205.	vis/o-	______	________________

Symptoms, Signs, and Diseases

True or False

Indicate whether each statement is true or false by writing T or F on the line.

1. ____ Causalgia is a severe type of neuralgia.
2. ____ A neural tube defect can result in multiple sclerosis.
3. ____ A hematoma is a type of brain tumor.
4. ____ Presenile dementia is another name for early-onset Alzheimer's disease.
5. ____ Photophobia and throbbing pain are symptoms of migraine headaches.
6. ____ A TIA and a RIND are types of cerebrovascular accidents.
7. ____ Mad cow disease can be transmitted to humans as new variant Creutzfeldt-Jakob disease.
8. ____ The incidence of myelomeningocele can be greatly decreased if the mother takes folic acid supplements while she is pregnant.

Circle Exercise

Circle the correct word from the choices given.

1. (**Amnesia, Myelomeningocele, Shingles**) is a painful skin condition caused by herpes zoster infection of a nerve.
2. Prior to the onset of a seizure, a patient may experience a/an (**aura, coma, polyneuritis**).
3. (**Dyslexia, Status epilepticus, Subdural hematoma**) is caused by trauma to the head.
4. An imbalance of dopamine and acetylcholine in the brain is associated with (**Down syndrome, multiple sclerosis, Parkinson's disease**).
5. Abnormal burning or tingling sensations on the skin are (**neuritis, paralysis, paresthesias**).

Matching Exercise

Match each numbered word or phrase to its description.

1.	amnesia	_____	Symptoms caused by progressive demyelinization
2.	aphasia	_____	Head trauma with loss of consciousness
3.	concussion	_____	Involuntary falling asleep during the day
4.	hydrocephalus	_____	Enlarged head because of excess CSF
5.	mental retardation	_____	Continuous seizure activity
6.	multiple sclerosis	_____	Partial or total loss of memory
7.	narcolepsy	_____	Radiculopathy in the lumbar area
8.	nuchal rigidity	_____	Down syndrome
9.	sciatica	_____	Stiff neck associated with meningitis
10.	status epilepticus	_____	Inability to communicate verbally or in writing
11.	syncope	_____	Temporary loss of consciousness with fainting

Multiple Choice

Circle the correct word from the choices given.

1. All of the following are congenital disorders EXCEPT ______________________.
   a. cerebral palsy c. myelomeningocele
   b. hemiplegia d. anencephaly
2. Alzheimer's disease is diagnosed at autopsy by the presence of ______________________.
   a. demyelinization c. hydrocephalus
   b. coma d. neurofibrillary tangles
3. All of the following are types of epilepsy EXCEPT ______________________.
   a. petit mal c. absence
   b. complex partial d. aura
4. Neurofibromatosis is also known as ______________________.
   a. Lou Gehrig's disease c. von Recklinghausen's disease
   b. Down syndrome d. Parkinson's disease

Word-Building Exercise

Use the combining forms, prefixes, and suffixes here to build medical words that match the definitions given. Write the word that you build on the blank line. Some word parts may be used more than once. The first one has been done for you.

Word Parts

-al (pertaining to)	crani/o- (cranium)	-ic (pertaining to)	-oma (tumor, mass)
alg/o- (pain)	cyt/o- (cell)	intra- (within)	-ose (full of)
astr/o- (starlike structure)	de- (reversal of, without)	-ion (action; condition)	-pathy (disease, suffering)
cephal/o- (head)	hemat/o- (blood)	-itis (inflammation of)	pleg/o- (paralysis)
comat/o- (deep unconsciousness)	hemi- (one half)	mening/o- (meninges)	quadri- (four)
concuss/o- (violent shaking or jarring)	hydr/o- (water; fluid)	ment/o- (mind; chin)	
contus/o- (bruising)	-ia (condition, state, thing)	neur/o- (nerve)	

1. Pertaining to within the cranium (You think *intra-* + *crani/o-* + *-al*) You write intracranial
2. Malignant tumor whose cells have a star shape ______
3. Headache ______
4. Pertaining to paralysis of the right or left side of the body ______
5. Describes a patient who is in a state of deep unconsciousness ______
6. Condition of bruising ______
7. Pertaining to four limbs being paralyzed ______
8. State of being without a mind ______
9. Condition resulting from the action of violent jarring ______
10. Benign tumor on a nerve ______
11. Collection of blood when an artery ruptures ______
12. Inflammation of the membranes around the brain ______
13. Pertaining to excess CSF in the head ______
14. Pain along the path of a nerve ______
15. Disease of the nerves ______

Laboratory, Radiology, Surgery, Drugs

True or False

Indicate whether each statement is true or false by writing T or F on the line.

1. ____ Antiepileptic drugs are also known as anticonvulsant drugs.
2. ____ A halo vest is used to provide spinal traction.
3. ____ A laminectomy is a surgical procedure to remove plaque from a carotid artery.
4. ____ A TENS unit is used during a sleep study.

Matching Exercise

Match each numbered word or phrase to its description.

1. DTRs	_____	Tests patient's balance with the eyes closed
2. vision test	_____	Passing this test shows normal function of cranial nerve II (optic nerve)
3. hearing test	_____	Patient's manner of walking
4. Babinski's sign	_____	Tested by briskly tapping on a tendon to elicit a knee jerk
5. cranial nerve XII	_____	Passing this test shows normal function of the cranial nerve VIII (auditory nerve)
6. mental status exam	_____	Abnormal upward extension of big toe and fanning of other toes
7. gait	_____	The ability to stick out the tongue and move it back and forth shows normal function of this cranial nerve
8. pinprick	_____	Test to detect numbness on the skin
9. Romberg test	_____	Proverbs, counting backwards, recall of objects, names of presidents

Matching Exercise

Match each numbered word or phrase to its description.

1. spinal tap	_____	Used to treat edema of the brain or spinal cord after injury
2. EEG	_____	Uses dye to outline the spinal cord and nerves
3. myelography	_____	Indicates the presence of a neural tube defect
4. PET scan	_____	Surgical procedure to cut spinal nerve roots
5. alpha fetoprotein	_____	Used to diagnose the type of epilepsy
6. polysomnography	_____	Shows patterns of metabolism in the brain
7. corticosteroid drug	_____	Sleep study
8. rhizotomy	_____	Lumbar puncture

Abbreviations

Matching Exercise

Match each abbreviation to its definition.

1.	ALS	_____ Presses on spinal nerve roots
2.	CP	_____ Congenital disorder from lack of oxygen to the fetal brain
3.	CSF	_____ Lou Gehrig's disease
4.	CVA	_____ Can result in paraplegia or quadriplegia
5.	EEG	_____ Also known as a spinal tap
6.	HNP	_____ Circulates through the subarachnoid space
7.	LP	_____ Test that records brain wave patterns
8.	SCI	_____ A stroke

Applied Skills

Plural Noun and Adjective Spelling

Fill in the blanks with the correct word form. Be sure to check your spelling. The first one has been done for you.

Singular Noun	Plural Noun	Adjective	Singular Noun	Plural Noun	Adjective
1. thalamus		thalamic	7. gyrus	_____	_____
2. astrocyte	_____		8. meninx	_____	_____
3. cerebellum		_____	9. nerve	_____	_____
4. cerebrum		_____	10. spine		_____
5. cortex	_____	_____	11. sulcus	_____	_____
6. cranium		_____	12. ventricle	_____	_____

Analysis of a Medical Report

This exercise contains a neurologic office consultation. Read the report and answer the questions that follow.

Neurologic Associates
Centennial Medical Building, Suite 312
5005 Frankstown Road
Pittsburgh, PA 15237

November 19, 20xx

Marshall Gibbons, M.D.
Primary Care Associates
19 Walker Avenue
Middletown, PA 15222

Re: JENCKS, Justine

Dear Dr. Gibbons:

I saw your patient, Justine Jencks, in neurologic consultation on November 19, 20xx. She is a 38-year-old, right-handed Caucasian female who has complained of intermittent dizziness and other symptoms for the past year. She reports temporary dizziness with hyperextension of the neck when raising her hands above her head to reach a high shelf or hang drapes. Two months ago, the patient had an acute episode in which she awoke with a sense of doom, headache, profuse perspiration, nausea, paresthesias of the fingers, dizziness, tachycardia, and felt the room was spinning. On the way to the emergency room, her husband commented about their dogs, but she could only remember her older dog and had no recollection of having another dog. In the emergency room, she commented to the nurse that she felt like her "blood pressure was zero." When asked about her last menstrual period, she felt that she might be pregnant but could not explain why she felt this way. On the mental status exam, she could not name the current and most recent presidents but was otherwise oriented x3. She was able to count back by serial 7s. The physical examination in the emergency room was essentially negative. Her blood pressure and blood sugar results were normal.

The patient has a past history that is significant for possible MS. This was tentatively diagnosed 10 years ago. At that time, laboratory test results were inconclusive: visual evoked responses were abnormal, but the CFS showed no oligoclonal bands and an MRI scan of the brain was read as negative. At that time, her symptoms included extreme muscle weakness. She could only walk a short distance by using a wide-based gait for stability. This initial episode lasted 2 months and then the symptoms gradually resolved.

She does not routinely have headaches. She denies ever having had seizures. She denies any smell or taste disturbances. She denies difficulty swallowing. She has no speech difficulties and is able to relate her medical history easily.

(*continued*)

Examination of cranial nerves V through XII was normal. Examination of the motor system revealed normal muscle strength. Babinski was negative. Sensory examination to light touch, pinprick, vibration, position, and 2-point discrimination was normal. Cerebellar functions in the form of finger-to-nose and heel-to-shin tests were normal. Gait was normal. Romberg's sign was negative. There was marked muscle spasm of the trapezius muscles bilaterally and limitation of neck motion laterally to the right and rotationally to the left.

Several of the patient's complaints could be due to a vestibular migraine, but the episode with the 2-hour alteration in memory is problematic and may suggest a TIA. She has some typical migraine symptoms, but the dizziness points to a vestibular focus to the migraine. Because of the past history of possible MS, I will have her undergo an MRI scan with contrast to pinpoint any demyelinization that has occurred since her last MRI. I have also ordered a carotid arteriography to rule out blockage of the carotid arteries.

After these tests are obtained, I will follow up with her in about 3 weeks to review the test results.

Thank you for referring this interesting and delightful patient to me.

Sincerely yours,

Renworth R. Pitman, M.D.

Renworth R. Pitman, M.D.

RRP: sct
D: 11/19/xx
T: 11/19/xx

WORD ANALYSIS QUESTIONS

1. Divide *neurologic* into its three word parts and define each word part.

Word Part	**Definition**
________________	________________________________
________________	________________________________
________________	________________________________

2. Divide *paresthesia* into its three word parts and define each word part.

Word Part	**Definition**
________________	________________________________
________________	________________________________
________________	________________________________

3. What is the abbreviation for *visual evoked response?* ________________

4. Divide *arteriography* into its two word parts and define each word part.

Word Part	**Definition**
________________	________________________________
________________	________________________________

FACT FINDING QUESTIONS

1. Two months ago, what symptom did the patient experience in her fingers? ____________________
2. Define these neurologic abbreviations.

   MS ____________________

   TIA ____________________

   CFS ____________________
3. The sensory examination consisted of five separate tests. Name them.

   a. ____________________

   b. ____________________

   c. ____________________

   d. ____________________

   e. ____________________
4. The mental status examination mentions what three mental status tests?

   a. ____________________

   b. ____________________

   c. ____________________
5. Which test showed that the patient's balance was intact? (**Babinski, Romberg, serial 7s**)
6. Which of the patient's symptoms is directly related to the nervous system? (**nausea, paresthesias, tachycardia**)
7. The carotid arteriography will be done to look for evidence of what disease? (**blockage of the artery, demyelinization, muscle weakness**)
8. If present, oligoclonal bands are found in what body fluid? ____________________

CRITICAL THINKING QUESTIONS

1. When the patient could remember the name of her older dog but not the name of her newest dog, this would be described as which of the following?
   a. Impairment of both remote and recent memory
   b. Impairment of remote memory; recent memory intact
   c. Remote memory intact; impairment of recent memory
2. A specimen of the patient's CSF was tested in the laboratory. What medical procedure was done to obtain that specimen?

   ____
3. The finger-to-nose and heel-to-shin tests are used to test what function? (**coordination, eye sight, memory**)
4. If the carotid arteriography showed a blockage of those arteries, this would relate to which of the patient's symptoms? (**alteration in memory, multiple sclerosis, wide-based gait**)
5. If the MRI with contrast does show areas of demyelinization, what diagnosis would that confirm?

   ____

Pronunciation Checklist

Read each word and its pronunciation. Practice pronouncing each word. Verify your pronunciation by listening to the Pronunciation List on the CD-ROM. Check the box next to each word after you master its pronunciation.

- ❑ abducens nerve (ab-DOO-senz NERV)
- ❑ absence seizure (AB-sens SEE-zher)
- ❑ accessory nerve (ak-SES-oh-ree NERV)
- ❑ acetylcholine (AS-ee-til-KOH-leen)
- ❑ afferent nerve (AF-eh-rent NERV)
- ❑ alpha fetoprotein (AL-fah FEE-toh-PROH-teen)
- ❑ Alzheimer's disease (AWLZ-hy-merz dih-ZEEZ)
- ❑ amnesia (am-NEE-zee-ah)
- ❑ amyotrophic lateral sclerosis (ah-MY-oh-TROH-fik LAT-eh-ral SKLEH-roh-sis)
- ❑ analgesic drug (AN-al-JEE-zik DRUHG)
- ❑ anencephaly (AN-en-SEF-ah-lee)
- ❑ anesthesia (AN-es-THEE-zee-ah)
- ❑ anesthetic drug (AN-es-THET-ik DRUHG)
- ❑ angiogram (AN-jee-oh-gram)
- ❑ angiography (AN-jee-AWG-rah-fee)
- ❑ anticonvulsant drug (AN-tee-con-VUL-sant DRUHG) (AN-tih-con-VUL-sant)
- ❑ antiepileptic drug (AN-tee-EP-ih-LEP-tik DRUHG) (AN-tih-EP-ih-LEP-tik)
- ❑ aphasia (ah-FAY-zee-ah)
- ❑ aphasic (ah-FAY-sik)
- ❑ arachnoid membrane (ah-RAK-noyd MEM-brayn)
- ❑ arteriogram (ar-TEER-ee-oh-gram)
- ❑ arteriography (ar-TEER-ee-AWG-rah-fee)
- ❑ arteriovenous malformation (ar-TEER-ee-oh-VEE-nus MAL-for-MAY-shun)
- ❑ astrocyte (AS-troh-site)
- ❑ astrocytoma (AS-troh-sy-TOH-mah)
- ❑ auditory cortex (AW-dih-TOR-ee KOR-teks)
- ❑ auditory nerve (AW-dih-TOR-ee NERV)
- ❑ aura (AW-rah)
- ❑ automatism (aw-TAWM-ah-tizm)
- ❑ autonomic nervous system (AW-toh-NAWM-ik NER-vus SIS-tem)
- ❑ axon (AK-sawn)
- ❑ Babinski's sign (bah-BIN-skeez SIGHN)
- ❑ benign (bee-NINE)
- ❑ biopsy (BY-awp-see)
- ❑ brain (BRAYN)
- ❑ brainstem (BRAYN-stem)
- ❑ carotid duplex scan (kah-ROT-id DOO-pleks SKAN)
- ❑ carotid endarterectomy (kah-ROT-id END-ar-ter-EK-toh-mee)
- ❑ carpal (KAR-pal)
- ❑ cauda equina (KAW-dah ee-KWY-nah)
- ❑ causalgia (kaw-ZAL-jee-ah)
- ❑ central nervous system (SEN-tral NER-vus SIS-tem)
- ❑ cephalalgia (SEF-al-AL-jee-ah)
- ❑ cerebellar (SAIR-eh-BEL-ar)
- ❑ cerebellum (SAIR-eh-BEL-um)
- ❑ cerebral hemisphere (SER-eh-bral HEM-is-feer)
- ❑ cerebral palsy (SER-eh-bral PAWL-zee) (seh-REE-bral PAWL-see)
- ❑ cerebrospinal fluid (seh-REE-broh-SPY-nal FLOO-id) (SER-eh-broh-SPY-nal)
- ❑ cerebrovascular accident (SER-eh-broh-VAS-kyoo-lar AK-sih-dent)
- ❑ cerebrum (SER-eh-brum) (seh-REE-brum)
- ❑ chemotherapy drug (KEE-moh-THAIR-ah-pee DRUHG)
- ❑ coma (KOH-mah)
- ❑ comatose (KOH-mah-tohs)
- ❑ computed axial tomography (com-PYOO-ted AK-see-al toh-MAWG-rah-fee)
- ❑ concussion (con-KUHSH-shun)
- ❑ contusion (con-TOO-shun)
- ❑ convulsion (con-VUL-shun)
- ❑ corpus callosum (KOR-pus kah-LOH-sum)
- ❑ cortex (KOR-teks)
- ❑ cortical (KOR-tih-kal)
- ❑ corticosteroid drug (KOR-tih-koh-STAIR-oyd DRUHG)
- ❑ cranial cavity (KRAY-nee-al KAV-ih-tee)
- ❑ craniotomy (KRAY-nee-AWT-oh-mee)
- ❑ cranium (KRAY-nee-um)
- ❑ Creutzfeldt-Jakob disease (KROITS-felt YAH-kohp dih-ZEEZ)
- ❑ dementia (deh-MEN-shee-ah)
- ❑ dendrite (DEN-dryt)
- ❑ diabetic neuropathy (DY-ah-BET-ik nyoo-RAWP-ah-thee)
- ❑ diskectomy (dis-KEK-toh-mee)
- ❑ dopamine (DOHP-ah-meen)
- ❑ dorsal (DOR-sal)
- ❑ dural membrane (DYOO-ral MEM-brayn)
- ❑ dura mater (DYOO-rah MAY-ter) (DYOO-rah MAH-ter)
- ❑ dyslexia (dis-LEK-see-ah)
- ❑ dyslexic (dis-LEK-sik)
- ❑ dysphasia (dis-FAY-zee-ah)
- ❑ efferent nerve (EF-eh-rent NERV)
- ❑ electroencephalogram (ee-LEK-troh-en-SEF-ah-loh-gram)
- ❑ electroencephalograph (ee-LEK-troh-en-SEF-ah-loh-graf)
- ❑ electroencephalography (ee-LEK-troh-en-SEF-ah-LAWG-rah-fee)
- ❑ encephalitis (en-SEF-ah-LY-tis)
- ❑ endorphins (en-DOR-finz)
- ❑ ependymal (ep-EN-dih-mal)
- ❑ ependymal cell (ep-EN-dih-mal SELL)
- ❑ ependymoma (eh-PEN-dih-MOH-mah)
- ❑ epidural (EP-ih-DYOO-ral)
- ❑ epilepsy (EP-ih-LEP-see)
- ❑ epileptic (EP-ih-LEP-tic)
- ❑ epinephrine (EP-ih-NEF-rin)
- ❑ evoked potential (ee-VOKED poh-TEN-shal)
- ❑ excisional biopsy (ek-SIHZ-un-al BY-awp-see)
- ❑ expressive aphasia (eks-PREH-siv ah-FAY-zee-ah)
- ❑ facial nerve (FAY-shall NERV)
- ❑ fissure (FISH-ur)
- ❑ flaccid paralysis (FLAS-id) (FLAK-sid pah-RAL-ih-sis)
- ❑ focal seizure (FOH-kal SEE-zher)
- ❑ frontal lobe (FRUN-tal LOHB)
- ❑ Glasgow Coma Scale (GLAS-goh KOH-mah SKAYL)
- ❑ glioblastoma multiforme (GLY-oh-blas-TOH-mah MUL-tih-FOR-may)
- ❑ glioma (gly-OH-mah)
- ❑ global aphasia (GLOH-bal ah-FAY-zee-ah)
- ❑ glossopharyngeal nerve (GLAWS-oh-phah-RIN-jee-al NERV)
- ❑ grand mal seizure (GRAHN MAWL SEE-zher)
- ❑ Guillain-Barré syndrome (GEE-yah bah-RAY SIN-drohm)

- ❑ gustatory cortex (GUS-tah-tor-ee KOR-teks)
- ❑ gyri (JY-rye)
- ❑ gyrus (JY-rus)
- ❑ hematoma (HEE-mah-TOH-mah)
- ❑ hemiparesis (HEM-ee-pah-REE-sis) (HEM-ee-PAIR-eh-sis)
- ❑ hemiplegia (HEM-ee-PLEE-jee-ah)
- ❑ hemiplegic (HEM-ee-PLEE-jik)
- ❑ hemisphere (HEM-ih-sfeer)
- ❑ herniated nucleus pulposus (HER-nee-aa-ted NYOO-klee-us pul-POH-sus)
- ❑ hippocampus (HIP-oh-KAM-pus)
- ❑ Huntington's chorea (HUN-ting-tonz kor-EE-ah)
- ❑ hydrocephalic (HY-droh-sih-FAL-ik)
- ❑ hydrocephalus (HY-droh-SEF-ah-lus)
- ❑ hyperesthesia (HY-per-es-THEE-zee-ah)
- ❑ hypoglossal nerve (HY-poh-GLAWS-al)
- ❑ hypothalamic (HY-poh-thah-LAM-ik)
- ❑ hypothalamus (HY-poh-THAL-ah-mus)
- ❑ infarct (IN-farkt)
- ❑ inhibitor (in-HIB-ih-tor)
- ❑ intracranial (IN-trah-KRAY-nee-al)
- ❑ intraventricular (IN-trah-ven-TRIK-yoo-lar)
- ❑ ischemia (is-KEE-mee-ah)
- ❑ ischemic (is-KEE-mik)
- ❑ laminectomy (LAM-ih-NEK-toh-mee)
- ❑ lobe (LOHB)
- ❑ lumbar puncture (LUM-bar PUNGK-chur)
- ❑ lymphoma (lim-FOH-mah)
- ❑ magnetic resonance imaging (mag-NET-ik REZ-oh-nans IM-ah-jing)
- ❑ malignant (mah-LIG-nant)
- ❑ medulla oblongata (meh-DYOO-lah AWB-long-GAW-tah)
- ❑ meningeal (meh-NIN-jee-al) (MEN-in-JEE-al)
- ❑ meninges (meh-NIN-jeez)
- ❑ meningioma (meh-NIN-jee-OH-mah)
- ❑ meningitis (MEN-in-JY-tis)
- ❑ meningocele (meh-NING-goh-seel)
- ❑ meningomyelocele (meh-NING-goh-MY-loh-seel)
- ❑ mental retardation (MEN-tal REE-tar-DAY-shun)
- ❑ mental status (MEN-tal STAT-us)
- ❑ microglia (my-KROHG-lee-ah)
- ❑ migraine (MY-grayn)
- ❑ motor nerve (MOH-tor NERV)
- ❑ multiple sclerosis (MUL-tih-pl skleh-ROH-sis)
- ❑ myelin (MY-eh-lin)
- ❑ myelinated (MY-eh-lih-NAYT-ed)
- ❑ myelogram (MY-eh-loh-gram)
- ❑ myelography (MY-eh-LAWG-rah-fee)
- ❑ myelomeningocele (MY-loh-meh-NING-goh-seel)
- ❑ narcolepsy (NAR-koh-lep-see)
- ❑ narcotic drug (nar-KAWT-ik DRUHG)
- ❑ nerve (NERV)
- ❑ nerve conduction (NERV con-DUK-shun)
- ❑ nervous system (NER-vus SIS-tem)
- ❑ neural (NYOOR-al)
- ❑ neuralgia (nyoo-RAL-jee-ah)
- ❑ neuritis (nyoo-RY-tis)
- ❑ neurofibrillary (NYOOR-oh-FIB-rih-LAIR-ee)
- ❑ neurofibroma (NYOOR-oh-fy-BROH-mah)
- ❑ neurofibromatosis (NYOOR-oh-fy-BROH-mah-TOH-sis)
- ❑ neuroglia (nyoo-ROHG-lee-ah)
- ❑ neurologic (NYOOR-oh-LAWJ-ik)
- ❑ neurologic deficit (NYOOR-oh-LAWJ-ik DEF-ih-sit)
- ❑ neurologist (nyoo-RAWL-oh-jist)
- ❑ neurology (nyoo-RAWL-oh-jee)
- ❑ neuroma (nyoo-ROH-mah)
- ❑ neuromuscular system (NYOOR-oh-MUS-kyoo-lar SIS-tem)
- ❑ neuron (NYOOR-on)
- ❑ neuropathy (nyoo-RAWP-ah-thee)
- ❑ neurosurgeon (NYOOR-oh-SER-jun)
- ❑ neurotransmitter (NYOOR-oh-trans-MIT-er)
- ❑ norepinephrine (NOR-ep-ih-NEF-rin)
- ❑ nuchal rigidity (NYOO-kal rih-GID-ih-tee)
- ❑ nucleus pulposus (NYOO-klee-us pul-POH-sus)
- ❑ occipital lobe (awk-SIP-ih-tal LOHB)
- ❑ oculomotor nerve (AWK-yoo-loh-MOH-tor NERV)
- ❑ olfactory cortex (ol-FAK-toh-ree KOR-teks)
- ❑ olfactory nerve (ol-FAK-toh-ree NERV)
- ❑ oligodendroglia (OL-ih-goh-den-DROHG-lee-ah)
- ❑ oligodendroglioma (OL-ih-goh-den-DROH-gly-OH-mah)
- ❑ optic nerve (AWP-tik NERV)
- ❑ palsy (PAWL-see)
- ❑ paralysis (pah-RAL-ih-sis)
- ❑ paraplegia (PAIR-ah-PLEE-jee-ah)
- ❑ paraplegic (PAIR-ah-PLEE-jik)
- ❑ parasympathetic nervous system (PAIR-ah-SIM-pah-THET-ik NER-vus SIS-tem)
- ❑ parenchyma (pah-RENG-kih-mah)
- ❑ parenchymal (pah-RENG-kih-mal)
- ❑ paresthesia (PAIR-es-THEE-zee-ah)
- ❑ parietal lobe (pah-RY-eh-tal LOHB)
- ❑ Parkinson's disease (PAR-kin-sonz dih-ZEEZ)
- ❑ peripheral nervous system (peh-RIF-eh-ral NER-vus SIS-tem)
- ❑ petit mal seizure (peh-TEE MAWL SEE-zher)
- ❑ photophobia (FOH-toh-FOH-bee-ah)
- ❑ pia mater (PY-ah MAY-ter) (PEE-ah MAH-ter)
- ❑ plaque (PLAK)
- ❑ polyneuritis (PAWL-ee-nyoo-RY-tis)
- ❑ polysomnography (PAWL-ee-sawm-NAWG-rah-fee)
- ❑ pons (PAWNZ)
- ❑ positron emission tomography (PAWZ-ih-trawn ee-MISH-un toh-MAWG-rah-fee)
- ❑ postictal (post-IK-tal)
- ❑ presenile dementia (pree-SEE-nile deh-MEN-shee-ah)
- ❑ proprioception (PROH-pree-oh-SEP-shun)
- ❑ psychomotor seizure (SY-koh-MOH-tor SEE-zher)
- ❑ quadriplegia (KWAH-drih-PLEE-jee-ah)
- ❑ quadriplegic (KWAH-drih-PLEE-jik)
- ❑ radiculopathy (rah-DIK-yoo-LAWP-ah-thee)
- ❑ receptive aphasia (ree-SEP-tiv ah-FAY-zee-ah)
- ❑ receptor (ree-SEP-tor)
- ❑ reflex (REE-fleks)
- ❑ rhizotomy (ry-ZAWT-oh-mee)
- ❑ Romberg test (RAWM-berg TEST)
- ❑ Schwann cell (SHVAHN SELL)
- ❑ schwannoma (shwah-NOH-mah)
- ❑ sciatica (sy-AT-ih-kah)
- ❑ seizure (SEE-zher)
- ❑ senile dementia (SEE-nile deh-MEN-shee-ah)
- ❑ sensory nerve (SEN-soh-ree NERV)
- ❑ serotonin (SER-oh-TOH-nin)
- ❑ somatic nervous system (soh-MAT-ik NER-vus SIS-tem)
- ❑ somatosensory (soh-MAH-toh-SEN-soh-ree)
- ❑ spastic (SPAS-tik)
- ❑ spina bifida (SPY-nah BIF-ih-dah)
- ❑ spinal canal (SPY-nal kah-NAL)
- ❑ spinal cavity (SPY-nal KAV-ih-tee)
- ❑ spinal cord (SPY-nal KORD)
- ❑ spinal nerve (SPY-nal NERV)
- ❑ spinal traction (SPY-nal TRAK-shun)

- ❑ status epilepticus (STAT-us EP-ih-LEP-tih-kus)
- ❑ stereotactic neurosurgery (STAIR-ee-oh-TAK-tik NYOO-roh-SER-jer-ee)
- ❑ subarachnoid (SUB-ah-RAK-noyd)
- ❑ subdural hematoma (sub-DYOO-ral HEE-mah-TOH-mah)
- ❑ substantia nigra (sub-STAN-shee-ah NY-grah)
- ❑ sulci (SUL-sigh)
- ❑ sulcus (SUL-kus)
- ❑ sympathetic nervous system (SIM-pah-THET-ik NER-vus SIS-tem)
- ❑ synapse (SIN-aps)
- ❑ syncopal (SIN-koh-pal)
- ❑ syncope (SIN-koh-pee)
- ❑ tardive dysinesia (TAR-dive DIS-kih-NEE-zee-ah)
- ❑ temporal lobe (TEM-poh-ral LOHB)
- ❑ thalamic (thah-LAM-ik)
- ❑ thalamus (THAL-ah-mus)
- ❑ tic douloreux (TIK DOO-LOO-reh)
- ❑ tonic-clonic seizure (TAWN-ik CLAWN-ik SEE-zher)
- ❑ transcutaneous (TRANS-kyoo-TAY-nee-us)
- ❑ transection (tran-SEK-shun)
- ❑ trigeminal nerve (tri-JEM-ih-nal NERV)
- ❑ trochlear nerve (TROHK-lee-ar NERV)
- ❑ vagus nerve (VAY-gus NERV)
- ❑ ventral (VEN-tral)
- ❑ ventricle (VEN-trih-kl)
- ❑ ventricular (ven-TRIK-yoo-lar)
- ❑ ventriculoperitoneal shunt (ven-TRIK-yoo-loh-PAIR-ih-toh-NEE-al SHUNT)
- ❑ visual cortex (VIZ-yoo-al KOR-teks)
- ❑ von Recklinghausen's disease (vawn REK-ling-HOW-senz dih-ZEEZ)

Experience Multimedia

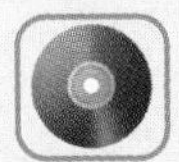

CD-ROM Learning Activities Checklist

Check off the box as you complete each learning activity.

❑ **CD-ROM Learning Activity 10.1: *ANATOMY WORD PARTS FLASHCARDS***
Use flashcards to help you memorize word parts. Make your own flashcards or print out prepared flashcards. Also see the electronic flashcard game. Time: 20 minutes.

❑ **CD-ROM Learning Activity 10.2: *MEDICINE IN ACTION***
Watch a video clip about epilepsy (seizures). Time: 5 minutes.

❑ **CD-ROM Learning Activity 10.3: *DISEASE AND OTHER WORD PART FLASHCARDS***
A continuation of the flashcard learning activity. Time: 20 minutes.

❑ **CD-ROM Learning Activity 10.4: *MEMORY AIDS***
Use memory aids to help you memorize medical words and their meanings. Time: 5 minutes.

❑ **CD-ROM Learning Activity 10.5: *MEDICAL LANGUAGE SPOKEN HERE***
Listen to actual medical reports and spell the missing medical words. Time: 20 minutes.

❑ **CD-ROM Learning Activity 10.6: *SPELLING CHALLENGE***
Listen to a pronounced medical word and then spell it. Time: 5 minutes.

❑ **CD-ROM Learning Activity 10.7: *MEDICAL LANGUAGE PRONUNCIATION***
Listen to a pronounced medical word and then practice pronouncing it. Time: 30 minutes.

❑ **CD-ROM Learning Activity 10.8: *EDUCATIONAL FUN AND GAMES***
Enjoy these fun activities while reinforcing your knowledge. Time: 15 minutes.

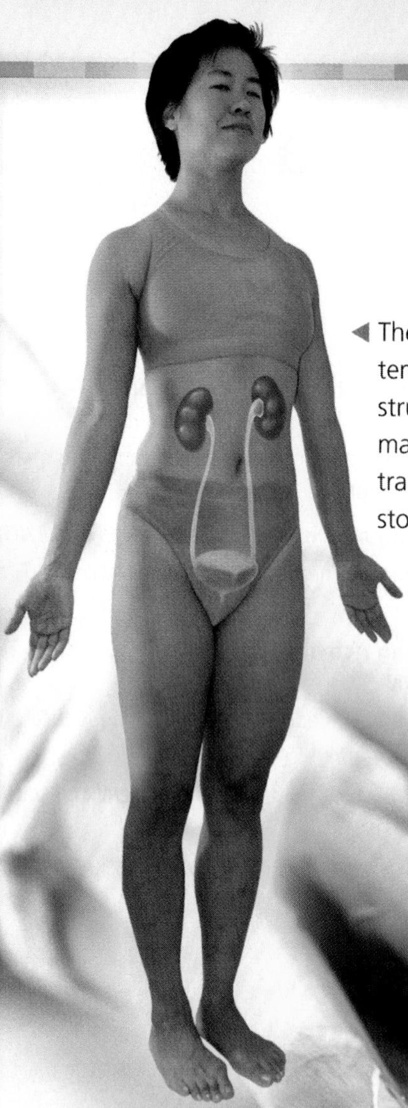

Dive In!

- Urine is odorless inside the body.
- Drinking urine is part of many non-traditional remedies used today, especially in Ayurvedic medicine.
- Don Winfield of Ontario, Canada has produced and passed over 4,500 kidney stones since his condition began in 1986.
- Don't let these facts go to waste. In this chapter we'll explore the language that describes urinary system structures, functions, diseases, and conditions.
- You'll be relieved once you master the language of urology!

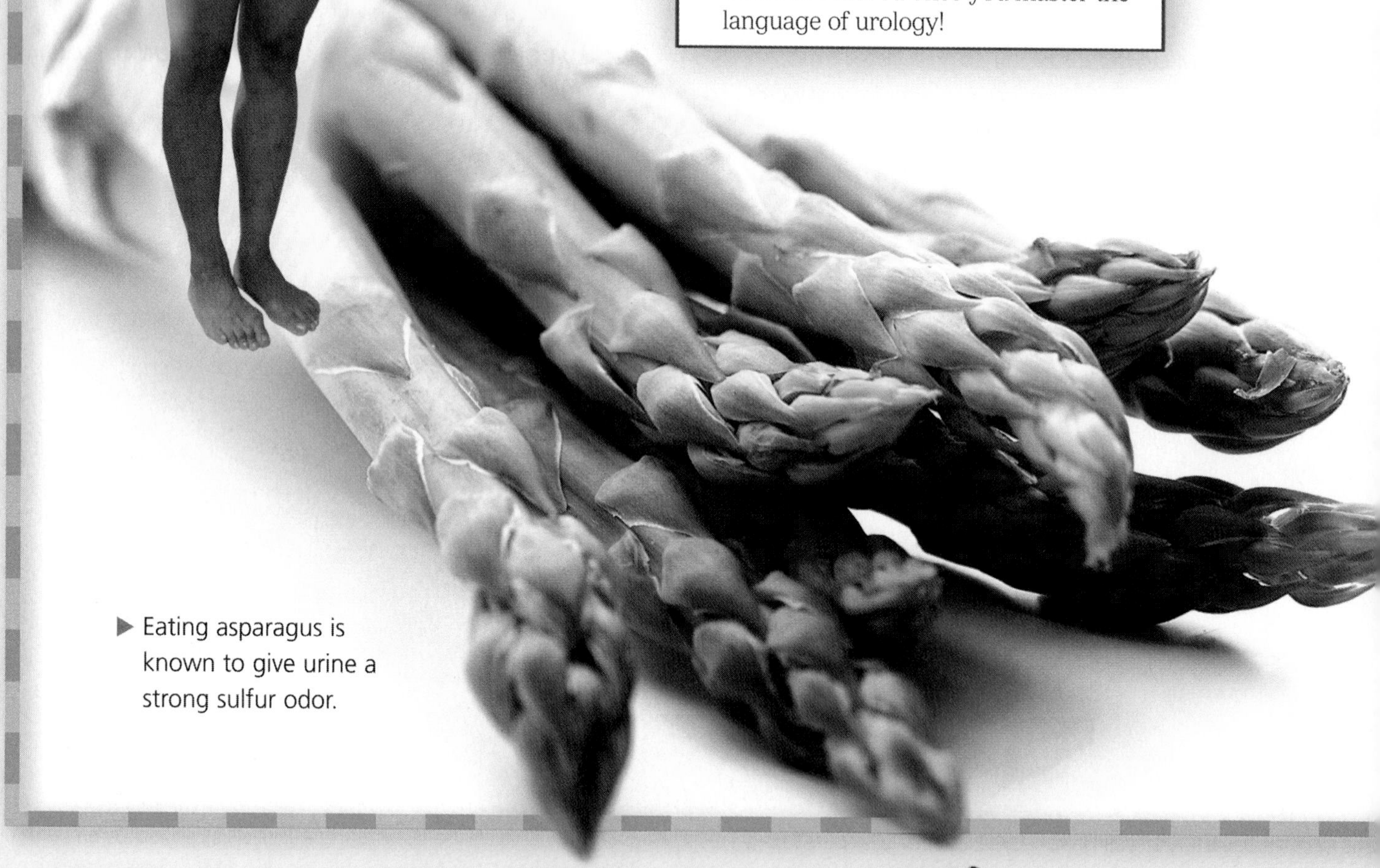

◀ The urinary system consists of structures that manufacture, transport, and store urine.

▶ Eating asparagus is known to give urine a strong sulfur odor.

Medicine Through HISTORY

1921

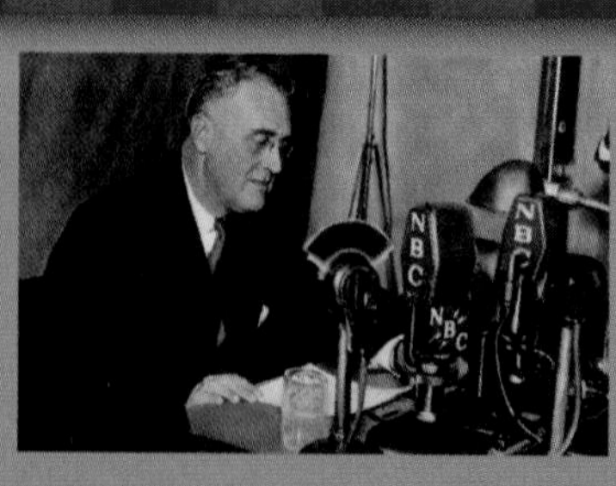

Franklin Delano Roosevelt, age 39, contracts polio and is partially paralyzed from the waist down. He goes on to become the 32nd President from 1933–1945, but conceals his illness because of societal views of the handicapped

1921

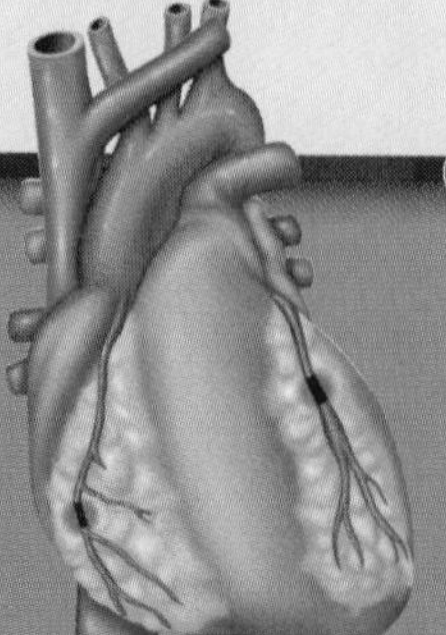

Heart disease becomes the number one cause of death in the United States

CHAPTER 11
Urology
Urinary System

Urology (yoo-RAWL-oh-jee) is the medical specialty that studies the anatomy and physiology of the urinary system and uses diagnostic tests, medical and surgical procedures, and drugs to treat urinary diseases.

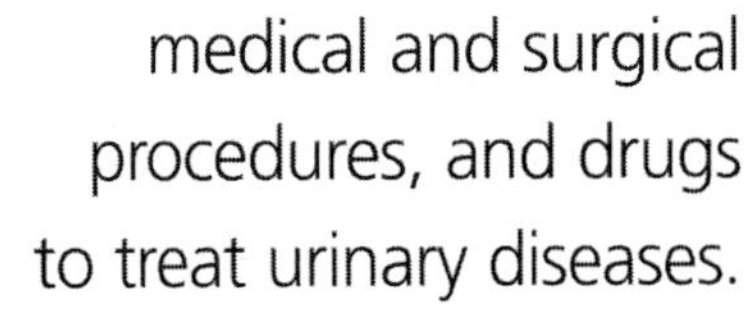

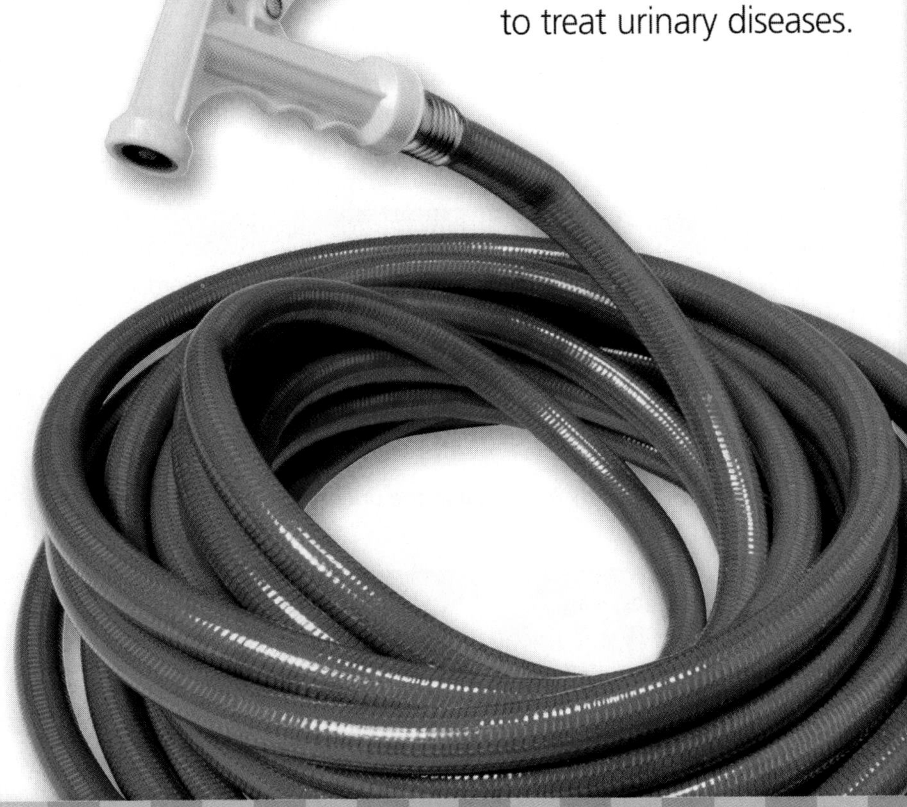

▲ The nephron is a microscopic structure that is the site of urine production in the kidney.

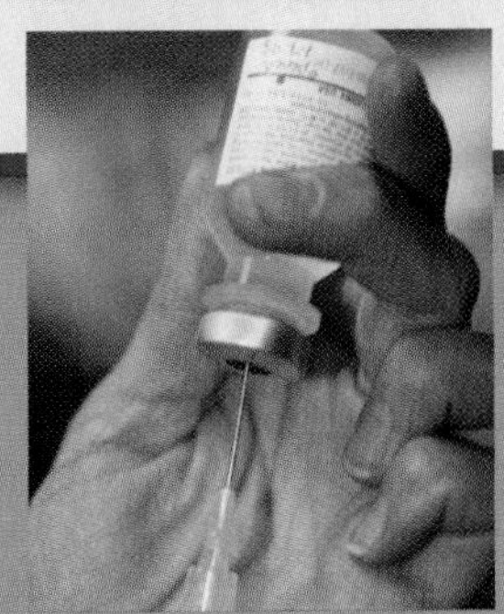

1922

Researchers Frederick Banting and Charles Best extract insulin and inject it to treat a patient with diabetes mellitus

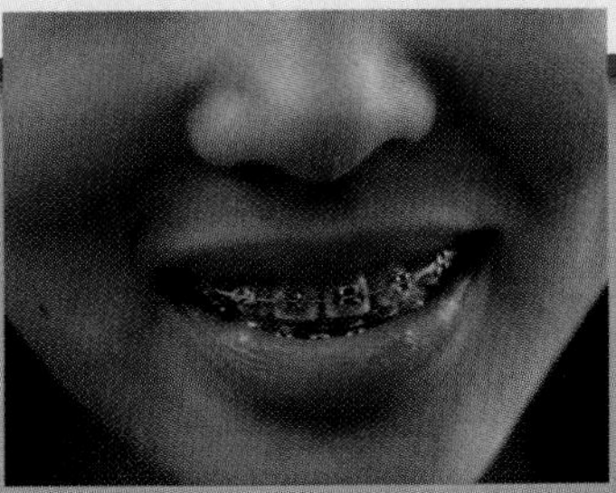

1922

Dr. Edward Angle invents the bracket system for braces to straighten teeth

Measure Your Progress: Learning Objectives

After you study this chapter, you should be able to

1. Identify the anatomical structures of the urinary system by correctly labeling them on anatomical illustrations.
2. Describe the process of the production of urine.
3. Build urinary words from combining forms, prefixes, and suffixes.
4. Describe common urinary diseases.
5. Describe common urinary diagnostic laboratory and radiology tests.
6. Describe common urinary medical and surgical procedures and drug categories.
7. Define common urinary abbreviations.
8. Correctly spell and pronounce urinary words.
9. Apply your skills by analyzing a urology report.
10. Test your knowledge of urology by completing the review exercises at the end of the chapter and learning activities on the CD-ROM.

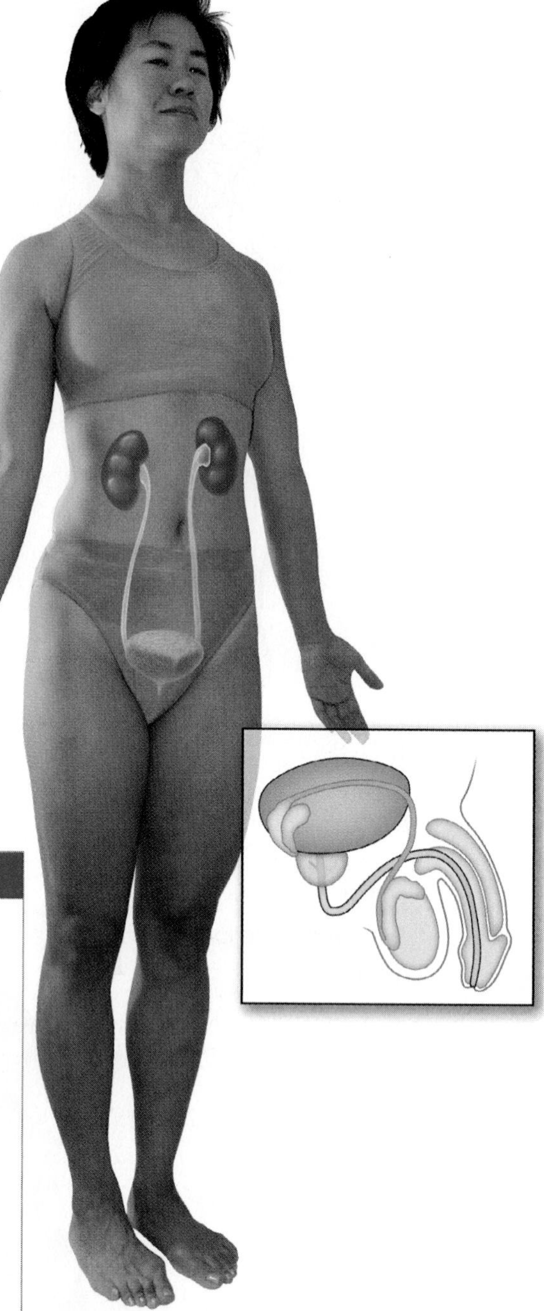

Figure 11-1 ■ The urinary system.
The urinary system consists of the kidneys (in the retroperitoneal space) that manufacture urine, and other structures in the pelvic cavity that transport or store urine.

Medical Language Key

To unlock the meaning of a medical word, first define each word part. Then put the word part definitions in order, beginning with the suffix, followed by the first word part.

	Word Part	Word Part Definition
SUFFIX	-logy	*the study of*
COMBINING FORM	ur/o-	*urine; urinary system*

Urology: ***The study of urine and the urinary system***

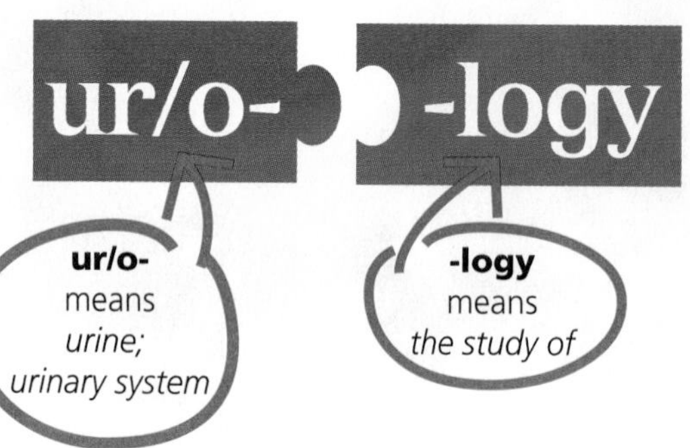

www.prenhall.com/turley

For interactive flashcards, real-life video clips, games, exercises, and audio pronunciations please explore the companion CD-ROM in the back of the book. Click on the companion website for bonus chapters, additional resources, and links to on-line learning.

Anatomy and Physiology

The **urinary system** is a body system that begins with the kidneys. They are located in the **retroperitoneal space,** a small area behind the peritoneum of the abdominal cavity that is filled with fatty tissues that cushion the kidneys. The superior ends of the kidneys are actually positioned up under the lower edge of the posterior rib cage. This area of the back is known as the **flank.** The other structures of the urinary system are located within the abdominopelvic cavity. The male ureter is located within the male penis (see Figure 11-1 ■). The purpose of the urinary system is to remove the waste products of metabolism from the blood and maintain the body's internal environment by excreting urine.

urinary (YOO-rih-nair-ee)
urin/o- *urine; urinary system*
-ary *pertaining to*

system (SIS-tem)
System is derived from a Greek word meaning *combination of parts to make an organized whole.*

retroperitoneal (REH-troh-PAIR-ih-toh-NEE-al)
retro- *behind, backward*
peritone/o- *peritoneum*
-al *pertaining to*

Flank is derived from an Old English word meaning *side between the ribs and pelvis.*

Anatomy of the Urinary System

Kidneys

The **kidney** is reddish-brown in color, shaped like (of all things!) a kidney bean, measuring four inches long and two inches wide and weighing less than 1/2 pound (see Figure 11-2 ■). The adrenal gland sits on top of each kidney like a cap. The adrenal gland is part of the endocrine system and will be discussed in Endocrinology (Chapter 14). The upper end of the kidney is known as the superior pole, and the lower end as the inferior pole. The **hilum** (an indentation in the medial surface of the kidney) is where branches of the **renal artery** enter and branches of the renal vein and the ureter exit the kidney.

kidney (KID-nee)

hilum (HY-lum)
hila (HY-lah)
Hilum is a Latin singular neuter noun meaning *a little mark.* Form the plural by changing *-um* to *-a.*

hilar (HY-lar)
hil/o- *hilum (indentation in an organ)*
-ar *pertaining to*

renal (REE-nal)
ren/o- *kidney*
-al *pertaining to*
Renal is the adjective form for *kidney.*

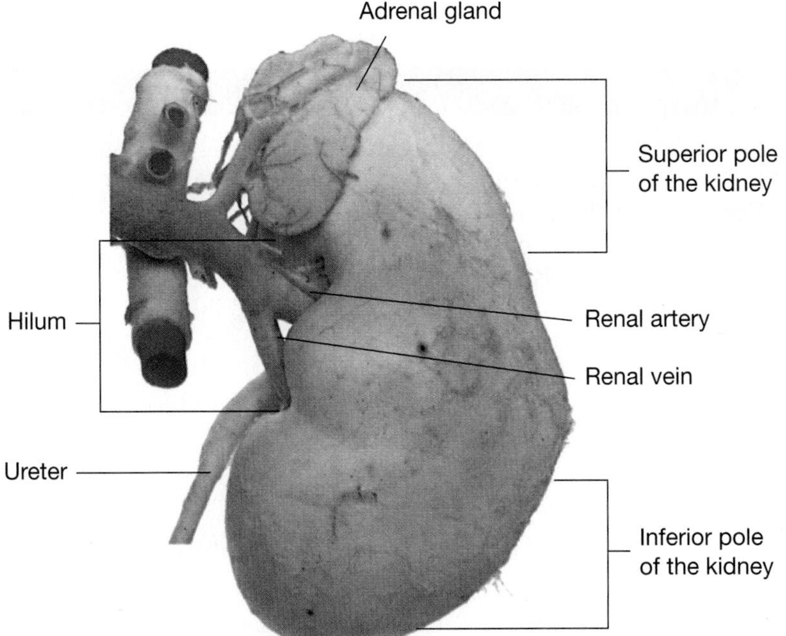

Figure 11-2 ■ Left kidney.
The kidney is shaped like a kidney bean. The adrenal gland of the endocrine system sits on top of the kidney but is not part of the urinary system. Notice the hilum where the renal artery enters and the renal veins and ureter exit the kidney.

The renal **capsule,** a layer of fibrous connective tissue, surrounds the kidney (see Figure 11-3 ■). The renal **cortex** is the thin layer of tissue just beneath the renal capsule. The renal **medulla** is the rest of the tissue beneath the cortex. The medulla contains the triangular-shaped renal pyramids. The tip of each renal pyramid connects to a **minor calix,** a duct that drains urine. Several minor calices drain into a **major calix.** The major calices drain into the **renal pelvis,** the large, funnel-shaped cavity on the medial side of the kidney. The inferior part of the renal pelvis narrows and becomes the ureter.

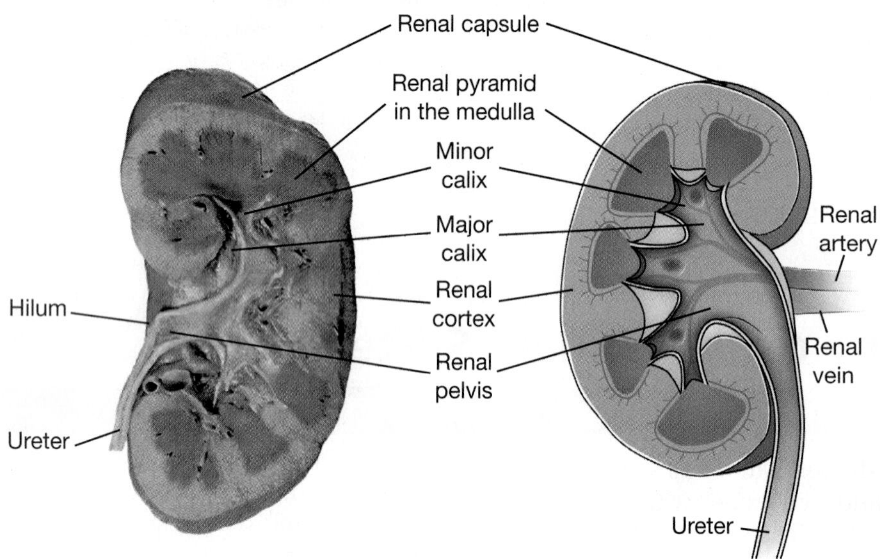

Figure 11-3 ■ Cut section of a kidney.

The internal structures of the kidney include the cortex, medulla, renal pyramids, calices, and renal pelvis. The renal pelvis narrows to become the ureter. The minor and major calices and the pelvis are known as the collecting system because they collect the urine as it is produced.

capsule (KAP-sool)
Capsule is derived from a Latin word meaning *little box.*

cortex (KOR-teks)
cortices (KOR-tih-seez)
Cortex is a Latin noun meaning *bark*. Form the plural by changing *-ex* to *-ices.*

cortical (KOR-tih-kal)
cortic/o- *cortex (outer region)*
-al *pertaining to*

medulla (meh-DOOL-ah)
medullae (meh-DOOL-ee)
Medulla is a Latin singular feminine noun meaning *marrow.* Form the plural by changing *-a* to *-ae.*

medullary (MED-yoo-lair-ee)
medull/o- *medulla (inner region)*
-ary *pertaining to*

calix (KAY-liks)
calices (KAL-ih-seez)
Calix is a Latin singular noun meaning *cup of a flower.* Form the plural by changing *-ix* to *-ices. Calyx* is an alternate spelling.

caliceal (KAL-ih-see-al)
calic/o- *calix*
-eal *pertaining to*

pelvis (PEL-vis)
pelves (PEL-vees)
Pelvis is a Latin noun meaning *basin.*

pelvic (PEL-vik)
pelv/o- *pelvis (hip bone; renal pelvis)*
-ic *pertaining to*

Ureters

The **ureter** is a 12-inch tube that extends from the renal pelvis of the kidney to the bladder (see Figures 11-3 and 11-5). The openings where the ureters join the bladder are the **ureteral orifices.** The walls of the ureters are composed of smooth muscle that contracts every 30 seconds to propel urine into the bladder, a process known as **peristalsis.**

ureter (YOO-ree-ter) (yoo-REE-ter)
Ureter is derived from a Greek noun meaning *urinary canal.*

ureteral (yoo-REE-teh-ral)
ureter/o- *ureter*
-al *pertaining to*

orifice (OR-ih-fis)
Orifice is derived from a Latin word meaning *an opening.*

peristalsis (PAIR-ih-STAL-sis)
peri- *around*
-stalsis *process of contraction*

Bladder

The **bladder,** a reservoir for storing urine, is located in the pelvic cavity (see Figure 11-4 ■). The rounded top of the bladder is called the dome or **fundus.** The inside of the bladder is lined with **mucosa,** a mucous membrane. When the bladder is empty, the mucosa collapses into folds called **rugae.** The triangular area between the two ureteral orifices and the opening to the urethra is known as the **trigone.** The base of the bladder where it connects to the urethra is called the bladder neck. When the bladder is full, the bladder wall contracts to expel urine. At the base of the bladder, in the bladder neck is a sphincter, a muscular ring that opens so that urine can flow into the urethra. This is an involuntary reflex that cannot be consciously controlled.

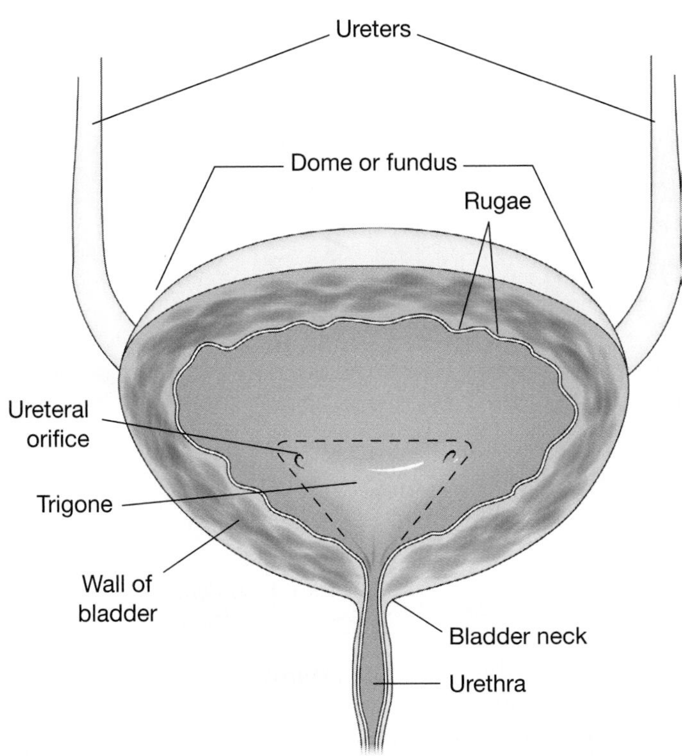

Figure 11-4 ■ Bladder.

The bladder is a hollow cavity that collects urine. Rugae are mucous membrane folds in the bladder wall that allow it to expand as it fills.

bladder (BLAD-er)

vesical (VES-ih-kal)
vesic/o- *bladder; fluid-filled sac*
-al *pertaining to*
Vesical is the adjective form for *bladder.*

fundus (FUN-dus)
Fundus is a Latin word meaning *part farthest away from the opening.*

mucosa (myoo-KOH-sah)
Mucosa is a Latin word meaning *mucus.*

mucosal (myoo-KOH-sal)
mucos/o- *mucous membrane*
-al *pertaining to*

rugae (ROO-gee)
Ruga is a Latin singular feminine noun meaning *a wrinkle.* Form the plural by changing *-a* to *-ae.* Because there are so many rugae in the bladder, the singular form is seldom used.

trigone (TRY-gohn)

Word Alert

SOUND-ALIKE WORDS

ureter (noun) tube that connects the kidney to the bladder

ureteral (adjective)

Example: The ureters carry urine between the kidneys and the bladder, and the ureteral orifices open into the bladder cavity.

urethra (noun) tube that connects the bladder to the outside of the body

urethral (adjective)

Example: The urethra carries urine between the bladder and the outside of the body, and the urethral meatus opens to the outside of the body.

vesical (adjective) descriptive word for the bladder

Example: Intravesical chemotherapy drugs are instilled into the bladder cavity to treat bladder cancer.

vesicle (noun) small fluid-filled blister on the skin

Example: Herpes zoster causes vesicles on the skin.

Urethra

The **urethra** is a tube that carries urine from the bladder to the outside of the body. At the end of the urethra is the **external urethral sphincter,** a ring of voluntary muscles that can be consciously controlled to release or hold back urine. The **urethral meatus** is where the urethra opens to the outside of the body.

In men, the urethra is 7 to 8 inches long. As the urethra leaves the bladder, it travels though the **prostate gland,** a spherical gland at the base of the bladder. The prostate gland completely surrounds the first part of the male urethra. This part is known as the prostatic urethra. The prostate gland is not part of the urinary system, however, enlargement of the prostate gland can affect the urinary system by pressing on and narrowing the urethra. The prostate gland is discussed in Male Reproductive Medicine (Chapter 12). The urethra is part of both the urinary and the male reproductive system because it transports both urine and semen. The urethra travels through the length of the **penis** until it reaches the external surface of the body (see Figure 11-5■). This part is known as the **penile urethra.** In men, the urethral meatus is located at the tip of the penis. If the male is uncircumcised, the urethral meatus is covered by the foreskin of the penis.

In women, the urethra is much shorter, traveling only 1 to 2 inches from the bladder to the external surface of the body (see Figure 11-6■). The urethral meatus is located just anterior to the opening to the vagina.

urethra (yoo-REE-thrah)
Urethra is derived from a Greek word meaning *passage for urine.*

urethral (yoo-REE-thrawl)
urethr/o- *urethra*
-al *pertaining to*

external (eks-TER-nal)
extern/o- *outside*
-al *pertaining to*

sphincter (SFINGK-ter)
Sphincter is derived from a Greek word meaning *a band.*

meatus (mee-AA-tus)
Meatus is derived from a Latin word meaning *a passage.*

prostate (PRAWS-tayt)

prostatic (praws-TAT-ik)
prostat/o- *prostate gland*
-ic *pertaining to*

penis (PEE-nis)

penile (PEE-nile)
pen/o- *penis*
-ile *pertaining to*

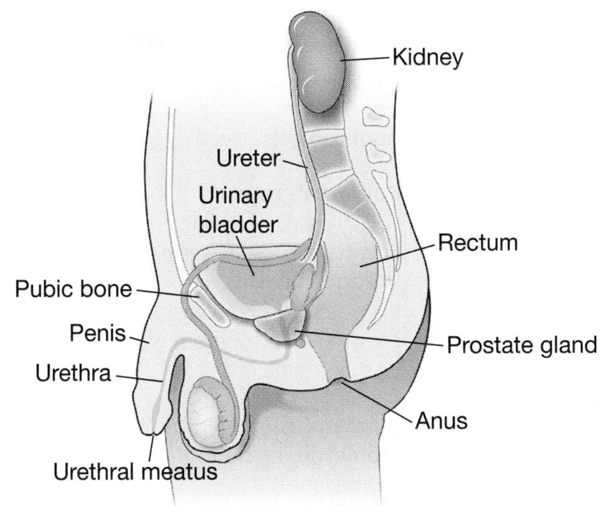

Figure 11-5 ■ Male urinary system.

The male urethra is long and travels through the prostate gland and the penis before opening to the outside of the body.

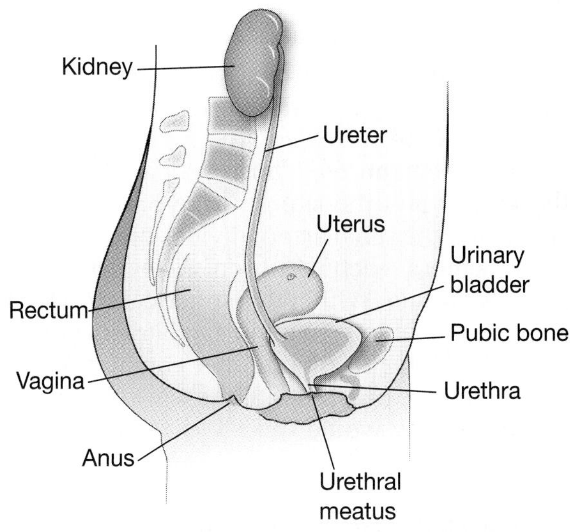

Figure 11-6 ■ Female urinary system.

The female urethra is short and straight. Notice how the bladder is just below the uterus. During pregnancy, the bladder is often compressed by the expanding uterus and fetus inside it.

Word Alert

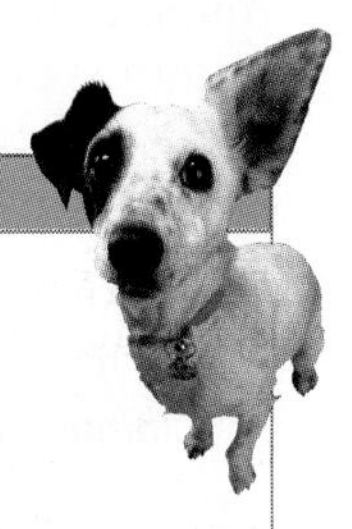

ALTERNATE NAMES

The urinary system is known by several different names: the urinary tract, the **genitourinary (GU) system,** the genitourinary (GU) tract, the **urogenital system,** the urogenital tract, and the **excretory system.** Why are there so many different names? Because each name highlights a different characteristic of this body system.

1. Genitourinary and urogenital refer to the close proximity or shared structures of the two systems.
2. Tract: a continuous pathway.
3. Excretory: describes the purpose of the system (to excrete urine).

genitourinary
(JEN-ih-toh-YOO-rih-nair-ee)
genit/o- *genitalia*
urin/o- *urine; urinary system*
-ary *pertaining to*

urogenital (YOO-roh-JEN-ih-tal)
ur/o- *urine; urinary system*
genit/o- *genitalia*
-al *pertaining to*

excretory (EKS-kreh-tor-ee)
(eks-KREE-toh-ree)
excret/o- *removing from the body*
-ory *having the function of*

Physiology of the Formation of Urine

The **parenchyma** is the functional or working area of any organ (as opposed to the organ's structural framework). The renal parenchyma is made up of the cortex and the medulla because these areas contain nephrons. The **nephron,** a microscopic structure, is the functional unit of the kidney and the site of urine production (see Figure 11-7 ■). It begins when the renal artery divides into small arterioles, and a single arteriole enters each nephron. The first part of the nephron is **Bowman's capsule.** Within this spherical structure, the arteriole divides into a network of intertwining capillaries known as a **glomerulus.**

The blood in the glomerulus contains waste products from the body's metabolic processes. If these waste products were not excreted in the urine, they would quickly reach toxic levels in the blood. They include

- **urea** (from protein metabolism)
- **creatinine** (from muscle contraction)
- **uric acid** (from purine metabolism to construct cellular DNA and RNA)
- inactive chemicals (from drug metabolism).

The blood in the glomerulus also contains substances that are not waste products, for example electrolytes, glucose, amino acids, vitamins, and so forth. **Electrolytes** are chemicals that have a positive or negative electrical charge: sodium (Na^+), potassium (K^+), chloride (Cl^-),

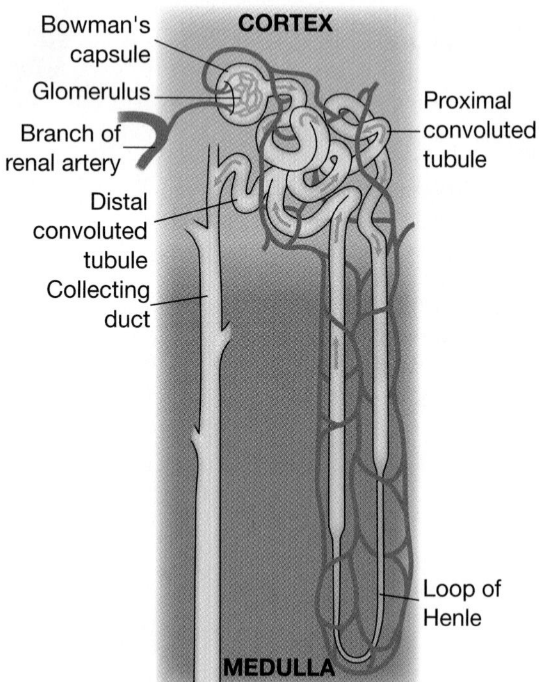

Figure 11-7 ■ Nephron.

The functional unit of the kidneys is composed of many smaller structures that filter substances and water out of the blood, then help certain substances and some water return to the blood, and finally send the remaining fluid and substances (urine) to the collecting ducts.

parenchyma (pah-RENG-kih-mah)

nephron (NEF-rawn)

Bowman's capsule (BOH-manz KAP-sool)
Bowman's capsule was named by Sir William Bowman (1816–1892), an English physician. This is an example of an eponym: a person from whom something takes its name.

glomerulus (gloh-MAIR-yoo-lus)
glomeruli (gloh-MAIR-yoo-lie)
Glomerulus is a Latin singular masculine noun meaning *ball of yarn.* Form the plural by changing *-us* to *-i.*

glomerular (gloh-MAIR-yoo-lar)
glomerul/o- *glomerulus*
-ar *pertaining to*

urea (yoo-REE-ah)

creatinine (kree-AT-ih-neen)

uric acid (YOO-rik AS-id)

electrolyte (ee-LEK-troh-lite)
electr/o- *electricity*
-lyte *dissolved substance*
Add word parts to make a correct and complete definition of *electrolyte: a dissolved substance [that can conduct] electricity [through a solution].*

and bicarbonate (HCO_3^-). Glucose is the simple sugar that the body uses for energy. Amino acids are the building blocks of proteins.

In the glomerulus, the pressure of the blood pushes water, waste products, electrolytes, glucose, and other substances through pores and out into Bowman's capsule. This process is known as **filtration.** Other substances in the blood (red blood cells, white blood cells, platelets, and albumin molecules) are too large to pass through pores, and so these substances remain in the blood. The network of capillaries that makes up the glomerulus then combines into a single arteriole that leaves Bowman's capsule and travels along the tubular parts of the nephron (see Figure 11-7).

The **filtrate** or solution of water, waste products, and non-waste substances in Bowman's capsule then flows into the **proximal convoluted tubule** of the nephron. In the proximal convoluted tubule, some of the water and non-waste substances move out of the tubule and into the blood in a nearby capillary. This process is known as **reabsorption.** How much water and non-waste substances are reabsorbed depends on the composition of the blood. If the blood is low in a particular substance (for example, glucose), then almost all of the glucose is reabsorbed. If the blood has normal or excessive amounts of glucose, then almost none of the glucose in the proximal convoluted tubule is reabsorbed.

The proximal convoluted tubule becomes a U-shaped tubule known as the loop of Henle. In the **loop of Henle,** more water and electrolytes are reabsorbed. The loop of Henle widens to become the distal convoluted tubule. In the **distal convoluted tubule,** more water and electrolytes as well as amino acids and other non-waste substances are reabsorbed. The distal convoluted tubules from many nephrons empty into a common **collecting duct.** Some reabsorption takes place in the collecting duct. The fluid is now known as **urine.** Urine flows continuously from the collecting duct into the minor calices, then the major calices, renal pelvis, and so forth (see Figure 11-8■).

The process of eliminating urine from the body is described in several ways: **urination, micturition, voiding,** or passing water (a layperson's word).

Across the Life Span

Each kidney contains more than 1 million individual nephrons. If laid end to end, these nephrons would be 80 miles in length.

The kidneys of a fetus begin to produce urine by about the twelfth week of life. The urine is excreted and becomes part of the amniotic fluid around the fetus. Infants ages 1 to 3 produce about 400–600 cc (about a pint) of urine each day. Children ages 3 to 8 produce about 600–1000 cc (about a quart) of urine daily. Adults produce about 1200–1500 cc (1 to 3 quarts) of urine each day.

As a person ages, some nephrons deteriorate and die. Because the body does not repair or replace nephrons, the total number of nephrons in the kidneys continues to decline with age, and kidney function decreases proportionately.

filtration (fil-TRAY-shun)
filtrat/o- *filtering; straining*
-ion *action; condition*

filtrate (FIL-trayt)
filtr/o- *filter*
-ate *composed of, pertaining to*

proximal (PRAWK-sih-mal)
proxim/o- *near the center or point of origin*
-al *pertaining to*
The proximal tubule is the part closest to the glomerulus.

convoluted (CON-voh-LOO-ted)
Convoluted is derived from a Latin word meaning *rolled together on itself.*

tubule (TOO-byool)
tub/o- *tube*
-ule *small thing*

tubular (TOO-byoo-lar)
tubul/o- *tube, small tube*
-ar *pertaining to*

reabsorption (REE-ab-SORP-shun)
re- *again and again; backward; unable to*
absorpt/o- *absorb or take in*
-ion *action; condition*

Henle (HEN-lee)
The loop of Henle was named by Friedrich Henle (1809–1885), a German anatomist.

distal (DIS-tal)
dist/o- *away from the center or point of origin*
-al *pertaining to*

urine (YOO-rin)

urination (YOO-rih-NAY-shun)
urin/o- *urine; urinary system*
-ation *a process; being or having*

micturition (MIK-choo-RISH-un)
mictur/o- *making urine*
-ition *a process; being or having*

void (VOYD)
Void is an Old English word meaning *to excrete.*

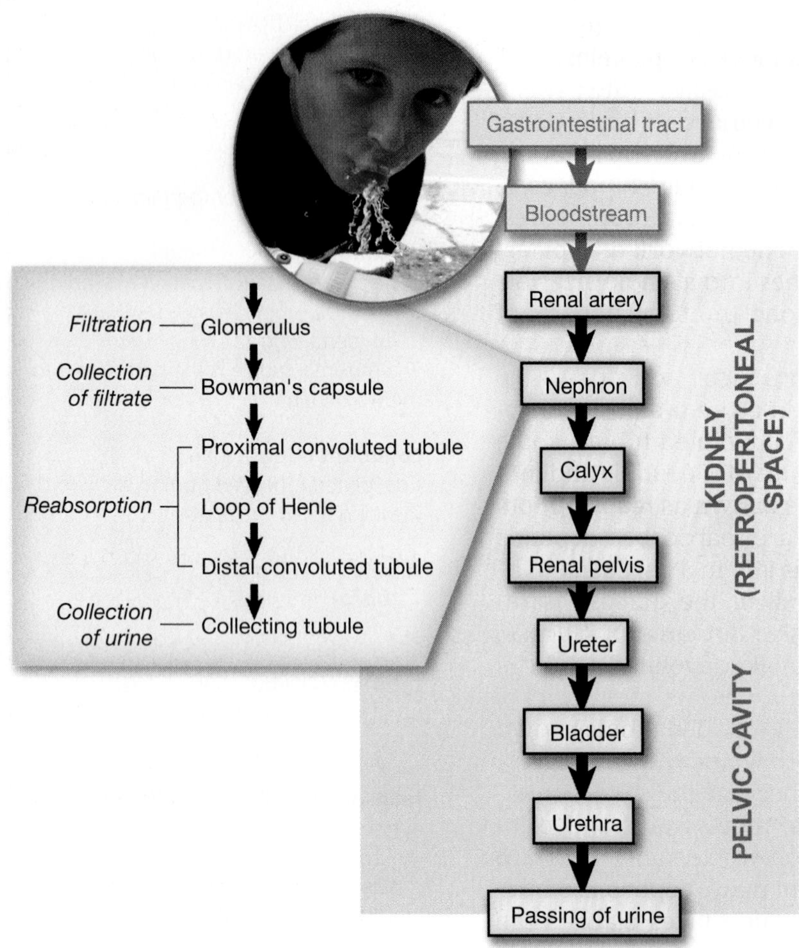

Figure 11-8 ■ Pathway of urine production.

Physiology of Other Functions of the Kidneys

Besides producing and excreting urine, the kidneys also help the body maintain a normal and constant internal environment.

1. If the blood pressure decreases, the kidneys
   - Produce concentrated urine with less water in it. The hormone aldosterone (from the adrenal gland) and antidiuretic hormone (from the posterior pituitary gland in the brain) act on the distal convoluted tubule to cause more sodium and water to be reabsorbed. This increases the blood volume and the blood pressure.
   - Secrete the enzyme **renin** from special cells located beside the nephrons. Renin stimulates the production of angiotensin, a powerful vasoconstrictor that causes blood vessels to constrict and this increases the blood pressure.
2. If the pH of the blood decreases, the kidneys cause bicarbonate (an electrolyte) to be reabsorbed and this increases the pH of the blood.
3. If the number of red blood cells decreases, the kidneys secrete the hormone **erythropoietin** to stimulate the bone marrow to produce more red blood cells.

renin (REE-nin)
ren/o- *kidney*
-in *a substance*

erythropoietin (eh-RITH-roh-POY-eh-tin)
erythr/o- *red*
-poietin *a substance that forms*

Vocabulary Review

Anatomy and Physiology

Now that you have studied the anatomy and physiology of the urinary system, take time to review those new words and descriptions. Memorize the combining forms and their definitions before going on to the next section.

Word or Phrase	Combining Form and Definition	Description
bladder	vesic/o- *bladder; fluid-filled sac*	Expandable reservoir for storing urine
Bowman's capsule		Sphere-shaped structure that surrounds the glomerulus and collects filtrate
calix	calic/o- *calix*	Ducts at the tip of each renal pyramid. The minor calices take urine to the major calices.
collecting duct		Common passageway that collects fluid from many nephrons. The final step of reabsorption takes place there and the fluid is known as urine.
cortex	cortic/o- *cortex (outer region)*	Tissue layer of the kidney just beneath the renal capsule
creatinine		Waste product from muscle contractions. It is removed from the blood by the kidneys.
distal convoluted tubule	dist/o- *away from the center or point of origin*	Tubule of the nephron that begins at the loop of Henle. It empties into the collecting duct. Reabsorption takes place there.
electrolytes	electr/o- *electricity*	Substances that have a positive or negative charge and conduct electricity when dissolved in a solution. Excess amounts in the blood are removed by the kidneys. Examples: Sodium, potassium, chloride, bicarbonate.
erythropoietin	erythr/o- *red*	Hormone secreted by the kidneys when the number of red blood cells decreases. It stimulates the bone marrow to produce more red blood cells.
filtration	filtrat/o- *filtering; straining* filtr/o- *filter*	Process in which water and substances in the blood are pushed through the pores of the glomerulus. The resulting fluid is known as **filtrate.**
flank		Area of the back between the ribs and the pelvis that overlies the kidneys
fundus		Dome-shaped top of the bladder
glomerulus	glomerul/o- *glomerulus*	Network of intertwining capillaries within Bowman's capsule in the nephron. Filtration takes place in the glomerulus.
hilum	hil/o- *indentation in an organ*	Indentation in the medial side of each kidney where the renal artery enters and the renal vein and the ureter leave
kidney	ren/o- *kidney*	Organ of the urinary system that produces urine

Word or Phrase	Combining Form and Definition	Description
loop of Henle		Tubule of the nephron that is U-shaped. It begins at the proximal convoluted tubule and ends at the distal convoluted tubule. Reabsorption takes place there.
medulla	**medull/o-** *medulla (inner region)*	Area of kidney tissue beneath the cortex. It contains the renal pyramids.
mucosa	**mucos/o-** *mucous membrane*	Mucous membrane lining the inside of the bladder
nephron	**nephr/o-** *nephron*	Microscopic functional unit of the kidney
parenchyma		Functional area of the kidney that is made up of the cortex and medulla and contains the nephrons
pelvis	**pelv/o-** *pelvis (hip bone; renal pelvis)*	Large, funnel-shaped cavity within each kidney that collects urine from the major calices and sends it to the ureter
penis	**pen/o-** *penis*	Structure that is part of the male reproductive system. In a man, the inferior part of the urethra passes through the center of the penis.
peristalsis		Process of smooth muscle contractions that propel urine through the ureter
prostate gland	**prostat/o-** *prostate gland*	Gland that is part of the male reproductive system. In a man, the superior part of the urethra passes through the center of the prostate gland.
proximal convoluted tubule	**proxim/o-** *near the center or point of origin*	Tubule of the nephron that begins at Bowman's capsule and ends at the loop of Henle in the nephron. Reabsorption takes place there.
reabsorption	**absorpt/o-** *absorb or take in*	Process by which water and substances in the filtrate move out of the tubule and into the blood in a nearby capillary
renal capsule	**ren/o-** *kidney*	Tough outer layer that surrounds the kidney
renal pyramids	**ren/o-** *kidney*	Triangular-shaped areas of tissue in the medulla of the kidney
renin	**ren/o-** *kidney*	Enzyme secreted by special cells near the nephron when the blood pressure decreases. Renin stimulates the production of angiotensin, a powerful vasoconstrictor.
retroperitoneal space	**peritone/o-** *peritoneum*	Area behind the peritoneum that lines the abdominal cavity. The retroperitoneal space contains the kidneys and fatty tissue.
rugae		Folds in the mucosa of the bladder that disappear as the bladder fills with urine
sphincter		Muscular ring around a tube. The sphincter in the bladder neck is not under conscious control. The external urethral sphincter at the end of the urethra is under voluntary, conscious control.
trigone		Triangular-shaped area in the bladder that is formed by the two ureteral orifices and the opening to the urethra
tubules	**tubul/o-** *tube, small tube*	Small tubes within the nephron

Word or Phrase	Combining Form and Definition	Description
urea		Waste product from protein metabolism. It is removed from the blood by the kidneys.
ureter	ureter/o- *ureter*	Tube that carries urine from the pelvis of the kidney to the bladder
ureteral orifice	ureter/o- *ureter*	Opening at the end of the ureter as it enters the bladder
urethra	urethr/o- *urethra*	Tube that carries urine from the bladder to the outside of the body
urethral meatus	urethr/o- *urethra*	The opening to the outside of the body that is at the end of the urethra
uric acid		Waste product from purine metabolism. It is removed from the blood by the kidneys.
urinary system	urin/o- *urine; urinary system* genit/o- *genitalia* excret/o- *removing from the body*	Body system that includes the kidneys, ureters, bladder, and urethra. Its function is to produce urine. It also helps regulate the internal environment of the body by secreting the enzyme renin and the hormone erythropoietin. Also known as the urinary tract, **genitourinary system** or tract, **urogenital system** or tract, or the **excretory system.**
urination	urin/o- *urine; urinary system* mictur/o- *making urine*	The process of producing urine and expelling it from the body. Also known as **voiding** and **micturition.**
urine		Water, waste products, and other substances excreted by the kidneys

Labeling Exercise

A. *Match each anatomy word or phrase to its numbered structure in Figure 11-9 ■. Write that word or phrase on the blank line next to its number. Use the Answer Key at the end of the book to check your answers.*

hilum	major calix	renal cortex	renal pyramid
minor calix	renal capsule	renal pelvis	ureter

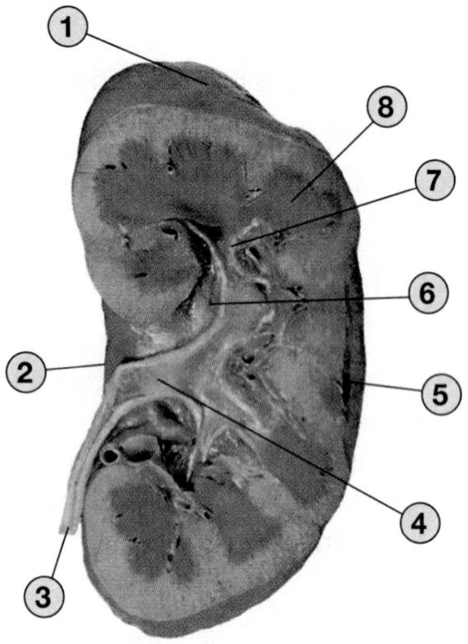

1. ______________________
2. ______________________
3. ______________________
4. ______________________
5. ______________________
6. ______________________
7. ______________________
8. ______________________

Figure 11-9 ■

B. *Match each anatomy word or phrase to its numbered structure in Figure 11-10 ■.*

anus	prostate gland	ureter	urethral meatus
kidney	pubic bone	urethra	urinary bladder
penis	rectum		

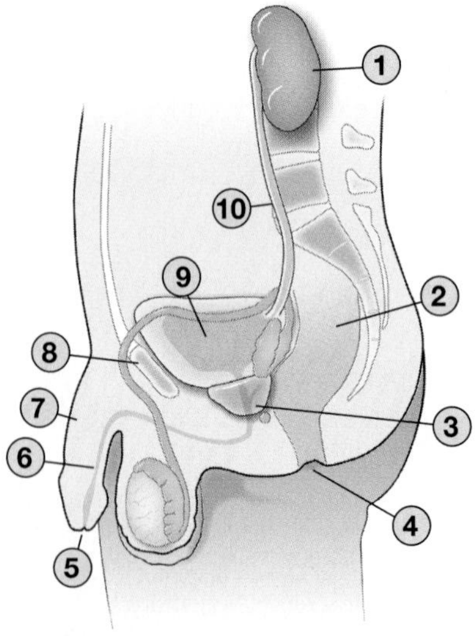

1. ______________________
2. ______________________
3. ______________________
4. ______________________
5. ______________________
6. ______________________
7. ______________________
8. ______________________
9. ______________________
10. ______________________

Figure 11-10 ■

C. *Match each anatomy word or phrase to its numbered structure in Figure 11-11 ■.*

Bowman's capsule	distal convoluted tubule	proximal convoluted tubule
branch of renal artery	glomerulus	
collecting duct	loop of Henle	

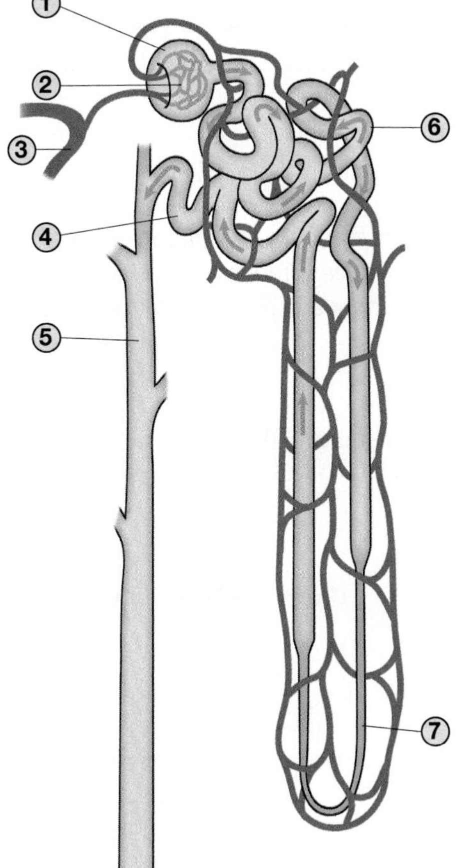

1. ____________________
2. ____________________
3. ____________________
4. ____________________
5. ____________________
6. ____________________
7. ____________________

Figure 11-11 ■

Building Medical Words

Combining Forms

Here are the urinary combining forms you have learned so far. Next to each combining form, write its meaning. Use the Answer Key at the end of the book to check your answers. The first one has been done for you.

	Combining Form	Medical Meaning		Combining Form	Medical Meaning
1.	absorpt/o-	*absorb or take in*	9.	filtrat/o-	
2.	calic/o-		10.	filtr/o-	
3.	cortic/o-		11.	genit/o-	
4.	dist/o-		12.	glomerul/o-	
5.	electr/o-		13.	hil/o-	
6.	erythr/o-		14.	medull/o-	
7.	excret/o-		15.	mictur/o-	
8.	extern/o-		16.	mucos/o-	

Combining Form	Medical Meaning	Combining Form	Medical Meaning
17. pelv/o-	______	24. tubul/o-	______
18. pen/o-	______	25. ureter/o-	______
19. peritone/o-	______	26. urethr/o-	______
20. prostat/o-	______	27. urin/o-	______
21. proxim/o-	______	28. ur/o-	______
22. ren/o-	______	29. vesic/o-	______
23. tub/o-	______		

Combining Forms and Suffixes

Read the definition hint for the medical word you are to build. Look at the combining form that is given. Write the correct suffix on the blank line. Then write the medical word. (Remember: You may need to remove the combining vowel. Always remove the hyphens and slash.) Use the Answer Key at the end of the book to check your answers. The first one has been done for you.

SUFFIX LIST

-al (pertaining to)	-ate (composed of, pertaining to)	-eal (pertaining to)	-ory (having the function of)
-ar (pertaining to)	-ation (a process; being or having)	-ic (pertaining to)	-ule (small thing)
-ary (pertaining to)			

Definition Hint	Combining Form	Suffix	Write the Medical Word
1. Pertaining to the hilum	hil/o-	-ar	hilar
2. Pertaining to the medulla	medull/o-	______	______
3. The process of expelling urine from the body	urin/o-	______	______
4. Pertaining to the calix	calic/o-	______	______
5. Pertaining to the kidney	ren/o-	______	______
6. Pertaining to the bladder	vesic/o-	______	______
7. Pertaining to the prostate gland	prostat/o-	______	______
8. Pertaining to the glomerulus	glomeru/o-	______	______
9. Small tube	tub/o-	______	______
10. Having the function of removing waste from the body	excret/o-	______	______
11. Composed of a substance that has been filtered	filtr/o-	______	______

Symptoms, Signs, and Diseases

Kidneys and Ureters

Word or Phrase	Word Part and Definition	Description
glomerulonephritis	**glomerulonephritis** (gloh-MAIR-yoo-loh-neh-FRY-tis) **glomerul/o-** *glomerulus* **nephr/o-** *kidney; nephron* **-itis** *inflammation of*	Complication that develops following an acute infection with streptococcus bacteria or viruses. The original infection, which is in the throat, causes the immune system to produce antibodies. Antibodies combine with bacteria or viruses to form antigen-antibody complexes that clog the pores of the glomeruli. The kidney becomes inflamed and urine production decreases. Treatment: Corticosteroid drugs to decrease inflammation. Renal dialysis, if necessary.
hydronephrosis	**hydronephrosis** (HY-droh-neh-FROH-sis) **hydr/o-** *water; fluid* **nephr/o-** *kidney; nephron* **-osis** *condition; abnormal condition; process* **caliectasis** (KAY-lee-EK-tah-sis) **cali/o-** *calix* **-ectasis** *condition of dilation* **hydroureter** (HY-droh-YOO-ree-ter) (HY-droh-yoo-REE-ter) *Hydroureter* is a combination of the combining form *hydro-* (water; fluid) and the word *ureter.*	Enlargement of the kidney due to constant pressure from backed-up urine in the ureter because of an obstructing stone or stricture. In **caliectasis,** the calices of the kidney are grossly enlarged. In **hydroureter,** only the ureter is grossly enlarged. Treatment: Removal of the stone or stricture.
nephrolithiasis	**nephrolithiasis** (NEF-roh-lih-THY-ah-sis) **nephr/o-** *kidney; nephron* **lith/o-** *stone* **-iasis** *state of; process of* **calculus** (KAL-kyoo-lus) **calculi** (KAL-kyoo-lie) *Calculus* is a Latin singular masculine noun meaning *pebble.* Form the plural by changing *-us* to *-i.*	Kidney stone or **calculus** formation in the urinary system. Kidney stones can vary in size from microscopic (often referred to as sand or gravel) (see Figure 11-12 ■) to large enough to block the ureter or fill the renal 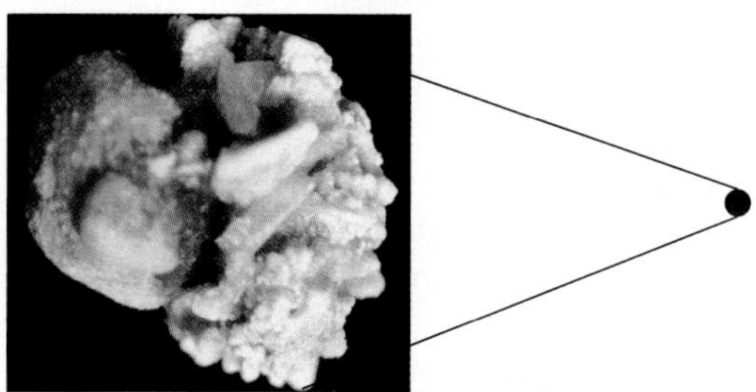 **Figure 11-12 ■ Kidney stone.** A kidney stone no bigger than this dot caused hematuria, vomiting, renal colic, and such severe pain that the patient had to be given several doses of morphine in the emergency department. Under the microscope, the many sharp, jagged edges of the kidney stone can be seen.

(continued)

Word or Phrase	Word Part and Definition	Description
nephrolithiasis *(continued)*	**calculogenesis** (KAL-kyoo-loh-JEN-eh-sis) **calcul/o-** *stone* **gen/o-** *arising from; produced by* **-esis** *condition* **lithogenesis** (LITH-oh-JEN-eh-sis) **lith/o-** *stone* **gen/o-** *arising from; produced by* **-esis** *condition* **colic** (KAWL-ik) **col/o-** *colon* **-ic** *pertaining to* Colic is a spasm of the smooth muscles of the intestine that causes abdominal pain. Renal colic is also a spasm of the smooth muscle, but of the bladder and ureters, not the colon.	pelvis (see Figure 11-13 ■). They are composed of magnesium, calcium, or uric acid crystals. **Calculogenesis** or **lithogenesis** is the process of forming stones. Many stones pass out of the body spontaneously, although in the process they can cause nausea and vomiting, hematuria, and renal colic. **Renal colic** is a spasm of the smooth muscle of the ureters or bladder as the kidney stone's jagged edges scrape the mucosa and cause pain. Stones that do not pass spontaneously can be removed surgically or destroyed by lithotripsy. Treatment: Analgesic drugs, lithotripsy, or the surgical procedures of stone basketing or percutaneous nephrolithotomy. 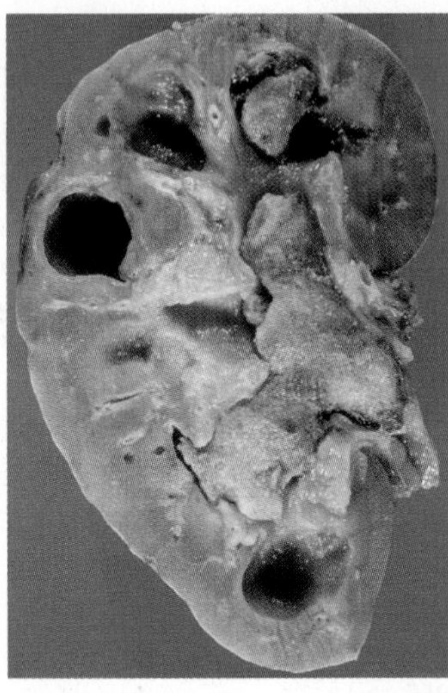 **Figure 11-13 ■ Nephrolithiasis.** These multiple large kidney stones in the calices and pelvis of the kidney have become so large that they cannot pass spontaneously. They disrupt the caliceal structure and leave little room in the pelvis for urine. **Did You Know?** Egyptian mummies have been found to have kidney stones.
nephropathy	**nephropathy** (neh-FRAWP-ah thee) **nephr/o-** *kidney; nephron* **-pathy** *disease, suffering* **diabetic** (DY-ah-BET-ik) **diabet/o-** *diabetes* **-ic** *pertaining to* **glomerulosclerosis** (gloh-MAIR-yoo-loh-skleh-ROH-sis) **glomerul/o-** *glomerulus* **scler/o-** *hard; sclera (white of the eye)* **-osis** *condition; abnormal condition; process* Some word parts have more than one definition. The best definition of *glomerulosclerosis* is *abnormal condition or process of the glomerulus becoming hard.*	General word for any disease process involving the kidney. **Diabetic nephropathy** involves progressive damage to the glomeruli because of diabetes mellitus. The tiny arteries of the glomerulus harden (**glomerulosclerosis**) because of accelerated arteriosclerosis throughout the body. Treatment: Correct the underlying cause; manage the diabetes mellitus.

Word or Phrase	Word Part and Definition	Description
nephroptosis	**nephroptosis** (NEF-rawp-TOH-sis) **nephr/o-** *kidney; nephron* **-ptosis** *state of prolapse or drooping; falling*	Abnormally low position of a kidney. It sometimes requires surgery, but more often is mentioned as an incidental finding seen on an x-ray.
nephrotic syndrome	**nephrotic** (nef-RAWT-ik) **nephr/o-** *kidney; nephron* **-tic** *pertaining to* **ascites** (ah-SIGH-teez) *Ascites* is a Greek word meaning *bag or belly.*	Damage to the pores of the glomeruli allows large amounts of albumin (protein) to leak into the urine, decreasing the amount of blood proteins. This changes the osmotic pressure of the blood and allows fluid to go into the tissues, producing edema in the extremities, and into the abdominal cavity, producing **ascites** (a grossly enlarged, fluid-distended abdomen). Treatment: Diuretic drugs to decrease edema. Correct the underlying cause. **Connections** **Dietetics.** In the nutritional disease kwashiorkor (protein malnutrition), patients have grossly distended abdomens. The lack of dietary protein causes low blood protein, and fluid moves from the blood into the abdominal cavity. At the same time, their bodies break down muscle tissue to meet the protein needs of the rest of the body. This results in thin extremities (muscle wasting).
polycystic kidney disease	**polycystic** (PAWL-ee-SIS-tik) **poly-** *many, much* **cyst/o-** *bladder; fluid-filled sac; semisolid cyst* **-ic** *pertaining to* Some word parts have more than one definition. The best definition of *polycystic* is *pertaining to many semisolid cysts.* **congenital** (con-JEN-ih-tal) **congenit/o-** *present at birth* **-al** *pertaining to*	**Congenital** disease characterized by cysts in the kidney that eventually obliterate the nephrons, causing kidney failure (see Figure 11-14 ■). The early stage of this progressive degenerative disease shows few symptoms and is not detected until hypertension and already-enlarged kidneys are detected on physical examination. Treatment: Dialysis or kidney transplanation. 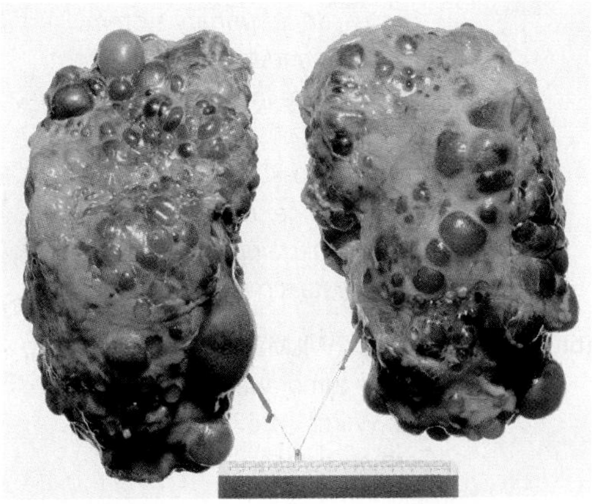 **Figure 11-14 ■ Polycystic kidney disease.** Nonfunctioning cysts replace large numbers of nephrons, and the patient's kidney function slowly declines.

Word or Phrase	Word Part and Definition	Description
pyelonephritis	**pyelonephritis** (PY-eh-loh-neh-FRY-tis) **pyel/o-** *renal pelvis* **nephr/o-** *kidney; nephron* **-itis** *inflammation of* **nephritis** (neh-FRY-tis) **nephr/o-** *kidney; nephron* **-itis** *inflammation of*	Inflammation and infection of the pelves of the kidneys. Infection of the kidneys (**nephritis**) would also involve the renal pelves. Caused by a bacterial infection of the bladder that ascends the ureters to the kidneys.
renal cell cancer	**cancerous** (KAN-ser-us) **cancer/o-** *cancer* **-ous** *pertaining to* **carcinoma** (KAR-sih-NOH-mah) **carcin/o-** *cancer* **-oma** *tumor, mass*	**Cancerous** tumor (**carcinoma**) that arises from tubules in the nephrons. Treatment: Surgical removal of the kidney.
renal failure	**acute** (ah-KYOOT) *Acute* is derived from a Latin word meaning *sharp, sudden.* **necrosis** (neh-KROH-sis) **necr/o-** *death* **-osis** *condition; abnormal condition; process* **chronic** (KRAWN-ik) **chron/o-** *time* **-ic** *pertaining to*	Disease in which the kidneys progressively decrease and then stop producing urine. Symptoms do not appear until 80 percent of kidney function has been lost. **Acute renal failure (ARF)** occurs suddenly and is usually due to trauma, severe blood loss, or overwhelming infection. It is accompanied by **acute tubular necrosis,** the sudden destruction of large numbers of nephrons and their tubules. **Chronic renal failure (CRF)** begins with renal insufficiency, followed by gradual worsening with progressive damage to the kidneys from diabetes mellitus, hypertension, or glomerulonephritis. **End-stage renal disease (ESRD)** is the final, irreversible stage of chronic renal failure in which there is little or no remaining kidney function. Treatment: Treat the underlying cause. Treat end-stage failure with dialysis.
uremia	**uremia** (yoo-REE-mee-ah) **ur/o-** *urine; urinary system* **-emia** *condition of the blood; substance in the blood* **uremic** (yoo-REE-mik) **ur/o-** *urine; urinary system* **-emic** *pertaining to blood or a substance in the blood*	Excessive amounts of urea in the blood because of renal failure. The kidneys are unable to remove the waste product urea. It reaches toxic levels in the blood and is excreted through the sweat glands, making white deposits on the skin that look like ice (uremic frost). Treatment: Dialysis.
Wilms' tumor	**Wilms'** (WILMZ) Wilms' tumor was named by Max Wilms (1867–1918), a German surgeon. **nephroblastoma** (NEF-roh-blas-TOH-mah) **nephr/o-** *kidney; nephron* **blast/o-** *immature; embryonic* **-oma** *tumor, mass*	Cancerous tumor of the kidney that occurs in children and arises from residual embryonic or fetal tissue. Also known as a **nephroblastoma.** Treatment: Surgery, radiation therapy, chemotherapy.

Bladder

Word or Phrase	Word Part and Definition	Description
bladder cancer		Cancerous tumor (carcinoma) of the epithelium of the bladder, most commonly seen in men over age 60. Hematuria is often a presenting sign. Treatment: Transurethral resection of the bladder tumor (TURBT), surgical excision of the bladder (cystectomy), radiation therapy, or intravesical instillation of chemotherapy drugs.
cystitis	**cystitis** (sis-TY-tis) cyst/o- *bladder; fluid-filled sac; semisolid cyst* -itis *inflammation of* Some word parts have more than one definition. The best definition of *cystitis* is *inflammation of the bladder.* **interstitial** (IN-ter-STISH-al) interstiti/o- *spaces within tissue* -al *pertaining to* **radiation** (RAY-dee-AA-shun) radi/o- *radius (forearm bone); x-rays; radiation* -ation *a process; being or having* Some word parts have more than one meaning. The best definition of *radiation* is *being or having x-rays or radiation.*	Inflammation or infection of the bladder (see Figure 11-15 ■). This is commonly caused by a bacterial infection of the urethra that ascends into the bladder, particularly in women because of the short length of the urethra. **Interstitial cystitis** is a chronic and progressive infection in which the mucosal lining becomes extremely irritated and red, with bleeding. **Radiation cystitis** is caused by the irritating effects of radiation therapy given to treat bladder cancer. Treatment: Correct the underlying condition. 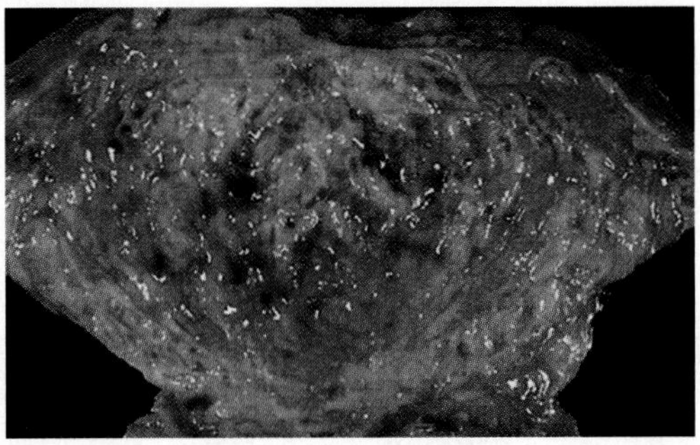 **Figure 11-15 ■ Acute cystitis.** This opened bladder from a cadaver shows severe irritation and infection of the mucosa with areas of hemorrhage.
cystocele	**cystocele** (SIS-toh-seel) cyst/o- *bladder; fluid-filled sac; semisolid cyst* -cele *hernia* **vesicocele** (VES-ih-koh-seel) vesic/o- *bladder; fluid-filled sac* -cele *hernia*	Hernia in which the bladder bulges through a weakness in the muscular wall of the vagina or rectum. This causes urinary retention in the part of the bladder that pouches into the vagina or rectum. Also known as a **vesicocele.** Treatment: Surgical repair of the vagina or rectum, if severe.
neurogenic bladder	**neurogenic** (NYOOR-oh-JEN-ik) neur/o- *nerve* gen/o- *arising from; produced by* -ic *pertaining to*	Urinary retention due to a lack of innervation of the nerves of the bladder. Caused by a spinal cord injury, spina bifida, multiple sclerosis, or Parkinson's disease. The bladder must be catheterized intermittently because it does not contract to expel urine. Treatment: Catheterization.

Word or Phrase	Word Part and Definition	Description
overactive bladder		Urinary urgency and frequency due to involuntary contractions of the bladder wall as the bladder fills with urine. This sometimes causes incontinence. Treatment: Antispasmodic drugs to decrease bladder wall contractions.
urinary retention	**retention** (ree-TEN-shun) **retent/o-** *keep, hold back* **-ion** *action; condition* **postvoid** (POST-voyd) *Postvoid* is a combination of the prefix *post-* (after, behind) and the word *void* (urinate).	Inability to empty the bladder because of an obstruction (enlargement of the prostate gland, kidney stone), nerve damage (neurogenic bladder), or as a side effect of certain types of drugs. Even when the bladder contracts, a large amount of **postvoid residual** remains in the bladder. Treatment: Correct the underlying cause.
vesicovaginal fistula	**vesicovaginal** (VES-ih-koh-VAJ-ih-nal) **vesic/o-** *bladder; fluid-filled sac* **vagin/o-** *vagina* **-al** *pertaining to* **fistula** (FIS-tyoo-lah) *Fistula* is a Latin word meaning *tube or pipe.*	Formation of an abnormal passageway connecting the bladder to the vagina. Urine flows from the bladder into the vagina and is excreted through the vagina. Treatment: Surgical correction.
	Urethra	
epispadias	**epispadias** (EP-ih-SPAY-dee-as) *Epispadias* is a combination of the prefix *epi-* (upon, above), the Greek word *spadon* (a tear), and the suffix *-ias* (condition). **hypospadias** (HY-poh-SPAY-dee-as) *Hypospadias* is a combination of the prefix *hypo-* (below; deficient), the Greek word *spadon* (a tear), and the suffix *-ias* (condition).	Congenital condition in which the female urethral meatus is incorrectly located near the clitoris or the male urethral meatus is incorrectly located on the upper surface of the shaft of the penis rather than at the tip of the glans penis. **Hypospadias** is when the male urethral meatus is incorrectly located on the underside of the shaft of the penis rather than at the tip of the glans penis. Treatment: Surgery to reposition the urethral meatus.
urethritis	**urethritis** (YOO-ree-THRY-tis) **urethr/o-** *urethra* **-itis** *inflammation of*	Inflammation or infection of the urethra. Gonococcal urethritis is a symptom of the sexually transmitted disease gonorrhea caused by the bacterium *Neisseria gonorrhoeae.* Nongonococcal urethritis is a sexually transmitted disease caused by the bacterium *Chlamydia trachomatis.* Nonspecific urethritis is an inflammation or infection of the urethra from bacteria, chemicals, or trauma; it is not a sexually transmitted disease. Treatment: Antibiotic drugs for bacterial infections.

Urine and Urination

Word or Phrase	Word Part and Definition	Description
albuminuria	**albuminuria** (AL-byoo-mih-NYOO-ree-ah) **albumin/o-** *albumin* **ur/o-** *urine; urinary system* **-ia** *condition, state, thing* **proteinuria** (PROH-tee-NYOO-ree-ah) **protein/o-** *protein* **ur/o-** *urine; urinary system* **-ia** *condition, state, thing*	Presence of albumin in the urine. Albumin is the major protein in the blood. Normally there is none in the urine because albumin molecules are too large to pass through the pores in the glomerulus; but if the membrane is damaged by kidney disease or infection, albumin passes through and is excreted in the urine. Albuminuria is an important first sign of kidney disease. It is also present in pregnant women who are developing preeclampsia. Also called **proteinuria.** Treatment: Correct the underlying cause.
anuria	**anuria** (an-YOO-ree-ah) **an-** *without, not* **ur/o-** *urine; urinary system* **-ia** *condition, state, thing*	Absence of urine production by the kidney. The underlying cause is acute or chronic renal failure. Treatment: Diuretic drugs or renal dialysis.
bacteriuria	**bacteriuria** (BAK-teer-ee-YOO-ree-ah) **bacteri/o-** *bacterium* **ur/o-** *urine; urinary system* **-ia** *condition, state, thing*	Presence of bacteria in the urine. Normally, urine is sterile. Bacteria indicate a urinary tract infection. Treatment: Antibiotic drugs.
dysuria	**dysuria** (dis-YOO-ree-ah) **dys-** *painful, difficult, abnormal* **ur/o-** *urine; urinary system* **-ia** *condition, state, thing*	Difficult or painful urination. It can be due to many factors (kidney stone, cystitis, and so forth). Treatment: Correct the underlying cause.
enuresis	**enuresis** (EN-yoo-REE-sis) **enur/o-** *to urinate in* **-esis** *condition* Add words to make a correct and complete definition of *enuresis: condition [that causes the patient] to urinate in [the bed during sleep].*	Involuntary urination during sleep. Also known as **nocturnal enuresis** or bedwetting. It is only considered a disease in older children or adults who should have voluntary bladder control. Treatment: Antidiuretic hormone (ADH), a pituitary gland hormone; psychological therapy.
frequency		Urinating often, usually in small amounts. Can be caused by a kidney stone, enlargement of the prostate gland, or a urinary tract infection. Treatment: Correct the underlying cause. Frequency is also present during pregnancy when the enlarging uterus limits the capacity of the bladder; however, this is not considered a disease.
glycosuria	**glycosuria** (GLY-kohs-YOO-ree-ah) **glycos/o-** *glucose* **ur/o-** *urine; urinary system* **-ia** *condition, state, thing*	Glucose in the urine, an indication of elevated blood sugar levels seen in diabetes mellitus. Treatment: Correct the underlying cause.

Word or Phrase	Word Part and Definition	Description
hematuria	**hematuria** (HEE-mah-TYOO-ree-ah) **hemat/o-** *blood* **ur/o-** *urine; urinary system* **-ia** *condition, state, thing* **microscopic** (MY-kroh-SKAWP-ik) **micr/o-** *small* **scop/o-** *examine with an instrument* **-ic** *pertaining to* Add words to make a correct and complete definition of *microscopic: pertaining to small [things] examined with an instrument.* **hemoglobinuria** (HEE-moh-GLOH-bih-NYOO-ree-ah) **hemoglobin/o-** *hemoglobin* **ur/o-** *urine; urinary system* **-ia** *condition, state, thing*	Blood in the urine. This may be gross or frank blood (easily seen with the naked eye) or **microscopic** blood (**hemoglobinuria**). Can be caused by a kidney stone, cystitis, bladder cancer, and so forth. In addition, menstrual blood can contaminate a urine specimen. Treatment: Correct the underlying cause.
hesitancy		Inability to initiate a normal stream of urine. There is dribbling, and the urinary stream has a decreased **caliber.** The volume of urine passed is less, and urine may remain in the bladder. Can be caused by blockage of the urethra by a kidney stone, a urinary tract infection, or an enlarged prostate gland. Treatment: Correct the underlying cause.
hypokalemia	**hypokalemia** (HY-poh-kay-LEE-mee-ah) **hypo-** *below; deficient* **kal/i-** *potassium* **-emia** *condition of the blood; substance in the blood*	Decreased amounts of potassium in the blood. Can be caused by diuretic drugs that cause the kidney to excrete excessive amounts of urine (and potassium). Treatment: Adjust the dose of the diuretic drug.
incontinence	**incontinence** (in-CON-tih-nens) **in-** *in; within; not* **contin/o-** *hold together* **-ence** *state of* Some word parts have more than one definition: The best definition of *incontinence* is *state of not [being able] to hold [all urine] together [in the bladder].*	Inability to voluntarily keep urine in the bladder. Can be caused by a spinal cord injury, surgery on the prostate gland, unconsciousness, or mental conditions such as dementia. Treatment: Correct the underlying cause. **Across the Life Span** Incontinence of urine is normal in babies because the nerve connections to the external urethral sphincter do not develop until about two years of age—about the time that parents begin toilet training. Incontinence in middle-aged and postmenopausal women is due to relaxation of the muscles of the pelvic floor. When the patient laughs, coughs, or sneezes, the increased intra-abdominal pressure causes urine to pass. This is known as **stress incontinence.** Muscle tone may be improved by doing Kegel exercises (the perineum is alternatively tensed and relaxed), or surgery may be needed. Incontinence in the geriatric population is due to a loss of muscle tone in the bladder and sphincters or to dementia.

Word or Phrase	Word Part and Definition	Description
ketonuria	**ketonuria** (KEE-toh-NYOO-ree-ah) **keton/o-** *ketones* **ur/o-** *urine; urinary system* **-ia** *condition, state, thing*	Ketone bodies in the urine. Ketones are waste products produced when fat is metabolized. Patients with diabetes mellitus metabolize fat for energy because they cannot metabolize glucose; they have ketonuria. Also seen in malnourished patients. Treatment: Correct the underlying cause.
nocturia	**nocturia** (nawk-TYOO-ree-ah) **noct/o-** *night* **ur/o-** *urine; urinary system* **-ia** *condition, state, thing*	Increased frequency and urgency of urination during the night. It can be due to cystitis, an enlarged prostate gland, or decreased capacity of the bladder due to aging. Expressed as the number of times the patient voids each night (example: nocturia x3). Treatment: Correct the underlying cause.
oliguria	**oliguria** (OL-ih-GYOO-ree-ah) **olig/o-** *scanty* **ur/o-** *urine; urinary system* **-ia** *condition, state, thing*	Decreased production of urine associated with kidney failure, although dehydration can cause temporary oliguria. Treatment: Correct the underlying cause.
polyuria	**polyuria** (PAWL-ee-YOO-ree-ah) **poly-** *many, much* **ur/o-** *urine; urinary system* **-ia** *condition, state, thing*	Excessive production of urine associated with diabetes mellitus and diabetes insipidus. Treatment: Correct the underlying cause.
pyuria	**pyuria** (py-YOO-ree-ah) **py/o-** *pus* **ur/o-** *urine; urinary system* **-ia** *condition, state, thing*	White blood cells (WBCs) in the urine, indicating a urinary tract infection. Pyuria can be seen with the naked eye when the urine is cloudy or milky, or the number of white blood cells may be so few that only microscopic examination during urinalysis reveals them. Treatment: Antibiotic drugs.
urgency		Strong urge to urinate and a sense of pressure in the bladder. It is caused by obstruction from an enlarged prostate gland or a kidney stone or inflammation from a urinary tract infection. Treatment: Correct the underlying cause.
urinary tract infection (UTI)	**infection** (in-FEK-shun) **infect/o-** *disease within* **-ion** *action; condition*	General category of an infection anywhere in the urinary tract. Urinary tract infections are caused by bacteria, most often by *Escherichia coli* (*E. coli*), which is commonly found in the intestines and rectum. When the infection is only in the urethra, it is called urethritis. When the infection is in the bladder, it is called cystitis. When the infection is in the kidney, it is called pyelonephritis. Because of the short length of the urethra in women and its location close to the anus, women are more prone than men to develop urinary tract infections. Catheterization can also introduce bacteria into the urinary tract. Treatment: Antibiotic drugs.

Diagnostic Procedures

Blood Tests

Word or Phrase	Word Part and Definition	Description
blood urea nitrogen (BUN)		Blood test that measures the amount of urea. Used to monitor kidney function and the progression of kidney disease or watch for signs of nephrotoxicity in patients taking aminoglycoside antibiotic drugs.
creatinine		Blood test that measures the amount of creatinine. Used to monitor kidney function and the progression of kidney disease. Creatinine is measured in conjunction with the BUN to give a comprehensive picture of kidney function.

Urine Tests

Word or Phrase	Word Part and Definition	Description
culture and sensitivity (C&S)	**culture** (KUL-chur) **sensitivity** (SEN-sih-TIV-ih-tee) **sensitiv/o-** *affected by, sensitive to* **-ity** *state; condition*	Urine test that puts urine onto culture medium in a Petri dish to identify the cause of a urinary tract infection (see Figure 11-16 ■). Microorganisms present in the urine grow into colonies. The specific disease-causing microorganism is identified and tested to determine its sensitivity to various antibiotic drugs. **Figure 11-16 ■ Culture and sensitivity testing.** These Petri dishes grew colonies of the bacterium *E. coli,* the most common cause of urinary tract infections. Antibiotic disks were placed in the Petri dishes. The antibiotic drugs that are most effective against *E. coli* show a large zone of inhibition (clear ring) around the disk where the bacterium could not grow. Those are the antibiotic drugs that could be prescribed to treat this patient's urinary tract infection.
drug screening		Urine test performed on a group of employees or athletes to detect any individual who is using illegal, addictive, or performance-enhancing drugs.
leukocyte esterase	**leukocyte** (LOO-koh-site) **leuk/o-** *white* **-cyte** *cell* **esterase** (ES-ter-ace)	Urine test to detect esterase, an enzyme associated with leukocytes and a urinary tract infection. This dipstick test gives a quick result so that antibiotic drugs can be started immediately. At the same time, a urine specimen is sent for C&S.

Word or Phrase	Word Part and Definition	Description
24-hour creatinine clearance		Urine test that collects all urine for 24 hours to measure the total amount of creatinine "cleared" (excreted) by the kidneys. The result is compared to the level of creatinine in the blood to determine the level of kidney function.
urinalysis (UA)	**urinalysis** (YOO-rih-NAL-ih-sis) *Urinalysis* is a combination of the combining form *urin/o-* (urine; urinary system) plus a shortened form of *analysis*.	Urine test to describe the characteristics of the urine and detect substances in it. A quick urinalysis can be done with a dipstick test (see Figure 11-17 ■) or the urine specimen can be sent to the laboratory for a full analysis. **Figure 11-17 ■ A urine dipstick.** This plastic strip with chemical-impregnated pads can perform several different laboratory tests (pH, protein, glucose, blood, and ketone bodies) at one time with a single dip in a urine specimen. The pads change color over the two-minute waiting period. The final color of each pad is compared to a chart on the back of the container that gives a range of colors for each test and the associated test result numbers.
color	**turbid** (TUR-bid) *Turbid* is derived from a Latin word meaning *muddy or confused.*	Normal urine is light yellow to amber in color, depending on its concentration. Pink or smoky-colored urine indicates red blood cells from bleeding. **Turbid** (cloudy or milky) urine indicates white blood cells and a urinary tract infection. The urinary antispasmodic drug Pyridium turns the urine bright orange.
odor		Urine has a faint odor due to the waste products in it. The urine of patients with uncontrolled diabetes mellitus has a fruity smell because of the glucose in it. When urine stands at room temperature, bacteria from the air grow in it, breaking down the urea into ammonia; this gives old urine its characteristic smell.
pH	**pH** (pee-H) **acidic** (ah-SID-ik) **acid/o-** *acid (low pH)* **-ic** *pertaining to* **alkaline** (AL-kah-line) **alkal/o-** *base (high pH)* **-ine** *pertaining to*	A test of how **acidic** or **alkaline** the urine is. Urine is normally slightly alkaline. Bacteria grow quickly and some types of kidney stones form readily in alkaline urine. Patients with urinary tract infections or kidney stones may be told to drink cranberry juice to make their urine more acidic.
protein	**protein** (PROH-teen)	Protein (or albumin) is not normally found in the urine. Its presence (proteinuria or albuminuria) indicates damage to the glomerulus.
glucose	**glucose** (GLOO-kohs)	Glucose is not normally found in the urine. Its presence (glycosuria) indicates uncontrolled diabetes mellitus with excess glucose in the blood "spilling" over into the urine.

Word or Phrase	Word Part and Definition	Description
red blood cells (RBCs)	**occult** (oh-KULT) *Occult* is derived from a Latin word meaning *hidden.*	Microscopic examination of the urine under high-power magnification to count the number of erythrocytes (red blood cells). Even clear urine can contain **occult blood.** This microscopic hematuria is reported as the number of RBCs per high-power field (hpf). If the urine has visible blood, the red blood cell count is reported as "TNTC" (too numerous to count).
white blood cells (WBCs)		Microscopic examination of the urine under high-power magnification to count the number of leukocytes (white blood cells) to identify a urinary tract infection. If the specimen is milky or cloudy, the white blood cell count is reported as "TNTC."
ketones	**ketones** (KEE-tohnz)	Ketones are not normally found in the urine. They are produced when the body cannot use or does not have enough glucose and instead metabolizes fat. Seen in patients with uncontrolled diabetes mellitus, malnutrition, or in marathon runners.
specific gravity (SG)	**urinometer** (YOO-rih-NAWM-eh-ter) **urin/o-** *urine; urinary system* **-meter** *instrument used to measure* **refractometer** (REE-frak-TAWM-eh-ter) **refract/o-** *bend or deflect* **-meter** *instrument used to measure*	Measurement of the concentration of the urine as compared to that of water (specific gravity 1.000). Dilute (not concentrated) urine has a specific gravity of 1.005, while concentrated urine is 1.030. Above 1.030 means the patient is dehydrated. Instruments used to measure specific gravity include a **urinometer** (see Figure 11-18 ■) or a **refractometer,** a handheld instrument that uses light rays bent (refracted) by a thin layer of urine on glass. 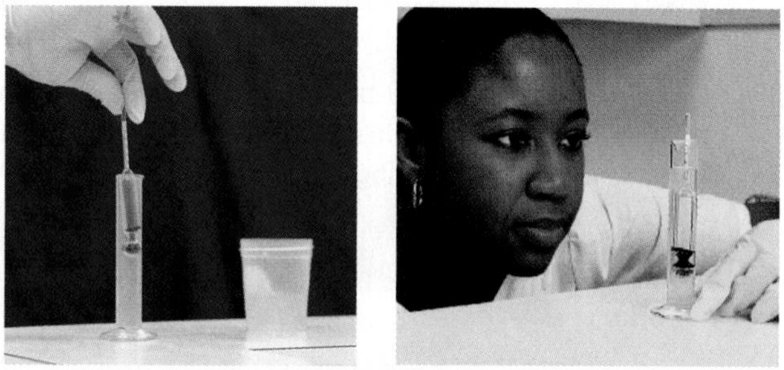 **Figure 11-18 ■ Urinometer.** This test tube-like container holds the urine. A calibrated glass weight floats in the urine. The specific gravity is measured where the surface of the urine touches the calibrated scale.
sediment	**hyaline** (HY-ah-lin) **hyal/o-** *clear glass-like substance* **-ine** *pertaining to*	There are several types of sediment in the urine. Crystals (calcium oxalate, uric acid, and so forth) may become a kidney stone. Casts are protein molecules (**hyaline casts**) or blood (red cell casts) that have been molded by the cylindrical shape of the tubules before they enter the bladder. Epithelial cells are normal in the urine as they are shed continuously from the lining of the urinary tract.
other substances		Chemical compounds whose presence helps to diagnose certain disease conditions. Bence Jones protein is seen in multiple myeloma (cancer of the bone marrow), vanillylmandelic acid (VMA) is seen in pheochromocytoma and neuroblastoma, and 5-HIAA is seen in carcinoid syndrome.

Radiology and Nuclear Medicine Procedures

Word or Phrase	Word Part and Definition	Description
intravenous pyelography (IVP)	**intravenous** (IN-trah-VEE-nus) intra- *within* ven/o- *vein* -ous *pertaining to* **pyelography** (PY-eh-LAWG-rah-fee) pyel/o- *renal pelvis* -graphy *process of recording* **excretory** (EKS-kreh-toh-ree) (eks-KREE-toh-ree) excret/o- *removing from the body* -ory *having the function of* **urography** (yoo-RAWG-rah-fee) ur/o- *urine; urinary system* -graphy *process of recording* **pyelogram** (PY-eh-loh-gram) pyel/o- *renal pelvis* -gram *a record or picture* **urogram** (YOO-roh-gram) ur/o- *urine; urinary system* -gram *a record or picture* **retrograde** (RET-roh-grayd) retro- *behind, backward* -grade *going* Every medical word must contain a combining form. The suffix of *retrograde* contains the combining form *grad/o-*.	Radiologic procedure that uses x-rays and radiopaque contrast dye (see Figure 11-19 ■). The dye is injected intravenously and flows through the blood and into the kidneys. It outlines the renal pelves, ureters, bladder, and urethra. It shows any obstruction, blockage, kidney stone, or abnormal anatomy in the urinary tract. Also known as **excretory urography**. The x-ray image is known as a **pyelogram** or **urogram.** Alternatively, **retrograde pyelography** can be done in which a cystoscopy is performed first, and then a catheter is advanced into the ureter and dye is injected. The dye outlines the ureter, as well as the pelvis and calices of the kidney. 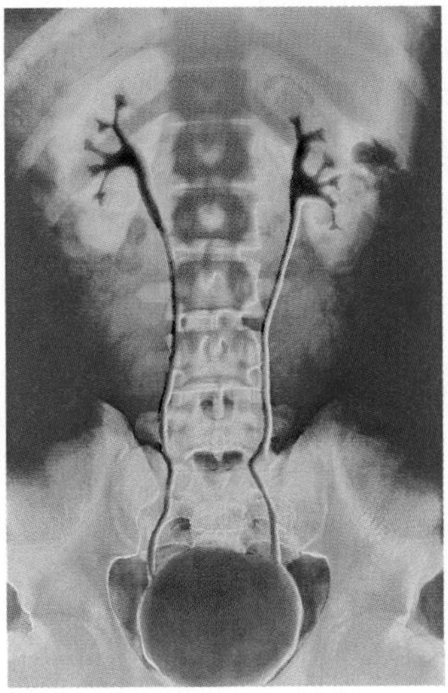 **Figure 11-19 ■ Color-enhanced intravenous pyelogram.** The contrast dye has outlined the structures of the urinary tract from the kidneys to the urethra. This is a normal pyelogram with no evidence of tumor, obstruction, or kidney stone.
kidneys, ureters, bladder (KUB) x-ray		Radiologic procedure that uses x-rays of the kidneys, ureters, and bladder (KUB) without contrast dye. It is used to find kidney stones or as a preliminary x-ray (scout film) before performing a pyelogram.
nephrotomography	**nephrotomography** (NEF-roh-toh-MAWG-rah-fee) nephr/o- *kidney; nephron* tom/o- *a cut, slice, or layer* -graphy *process of recording*	Radiologic procedure that uses a computerized axial tomography (CT) scan and radiopaque contrast dye injected intravenously. It takes x-ray images as multiple slices through the kidneys. The images can be examined layer by layer to show the exact location of tumors.

Word or Phrase	Word Part and Definition	Description
renal angiography	**angiography** (AN-jee-AWG-rah-fee) **angi/o-** *blood vessel; lymphatic vessel* **-graphy** *process of recording* **arteriography** (ar-TEER-ee-AWG-rah-fee) **arteri/o-** *artery* **-graphy** *process of recording* **angiogram** (AN-jee-oh-gram) **angi/o-** *blood vessel; lymphatic vessel* **-gram** *a record or picture* **arteriogram** (ar-TEER-ee-oh-gram) **arteri/o-** *artery* **-gram** *a record or picture*	Radiologic procedure that uses x-rays and radiopaque contrast dye. The dye is injected intravenously and flows through the blood into the renal artery. It outlines the renal artery and shows any obstruction or blockage. Also known as **renal arteriography.** The x-ray image is known as a **renal angiogram** or **renal arteriogram.**
renal scan		Nuclear medicine procedure that uses a radioactive isotope injected intravenously. It is taken up by the kidney and emits radioactive particles that are captured by a scanner and made into an image. Used after a kidney transplant to look for signs of organ rejection.
ultrasonography	**ultrasonography** (UL-trah-soh-NAWG-rah-fee) **ultra-** *beyond; higher* **son/o-** *sound* **-graphy** *process of recording* **sonogram** (SAWN-oh-gram) **son/o-** *sound* **-gram** *a record or picture*	Radiologic procedure that uses ultra high-frequency sound waves emitted by a transducer or probe to produce an image of the kidneys, ureters, or bladder. The ultrasound image is known as a **sonogram.**

Other Laboratory Tests

Word or Phrase	Word Part and Definition	Description
voiding cystourethrography (VCUG)	**cystourethrography** (SIS-toh-YOO-ree-THRAWG-rah-fee) **cyst/o-** *bladder; fluid-filled sac; semisolid cyst* **urethr/o-** *urethra* **-graphy** *process of recording* **cystourethrogram** (SIS-toh-yoo-REE-throh-gram) **cyst/o-** *bladder; fluid-filled sac; semisolid cyst* **urethr/o-** *urethra* **-gram** *a record or picture*	Radiologic procedure that uses x-rays and radiopaque contrast dye. The dye is inserted into the bladder through a cystoscope. It outlines the bladder and urethra. The x-ray image, taken while the patient is urinating, is known as a **voiding cystourethrogram.**
cystometry	**cystometry** (sis-TAWM-eh-tree) **cyst/o-** *bladder; fluid-filled sac; semisolid cyst* **-metry** *process of measuring* **cystometer** (sis-TAWM-eh-ter) **cyst/o-** *bladder; fluid-filled sac; semisolid cyst* **-meter** *instrument used to measure* **cystometrogram** (SIS-toh-MET-roh-gram) **cyst/o-** *bladder; fluid-filled sac; semisolid cyst* **metr/o-** *measurement* **-gram** *a record or picture*	Diagnostic procedure that evaluates the function of the nerves to the bladder. A catheter is used to inflate the bladder with liquid (or gas). A **cystometer** attached to the catheter measures the amount of liquid and the pressure in the bladder. The patient indicates when the first urge to urinate occurs. At that time, the cystometer makes a graphic recording known as a **cystometrogram (CMG).**

Medical and Surgical Procedures

Medical Procedures

Word or Phrase	Word Part and Definition	Description
catheterization	**catheterization** (KATH-eh-ter-ih-ZAY-shun) **catheter/o-** *catheter* **-ization** *process of making, creating, or inserting* **catheter** (KATH-eh-ter) *Catheter* is derived from a Greek word meaning *to send down.* **Foley** (FOH-lee) **suprapubic** (SOO-prah-PYOO-bik) **supra-** *above* **pub/o-** *pubis (hip bone)* **-ic** *pertaining to* **condom** (CON-dom) *Condom* is derived from an Italian word meaning *glove.*	Medical procedure in which a **catheter** (flexible tube) is inserted through the urethra and into the bladder to drain urine (see Figure 11-20■). A straight catheter is inserted each time the bladder becomes full, or it can also be used to obtain a single urine specimen for testing. A **Foley catheter** is an indwelling catheter that drains urine continuously. It has an expandable balloon tip that keeps it positioned in the bladder. A **suprapubic catheter** is inserted through the abdominal wall (just above the pubic bone) and into the bladder. It is sometimes inserted after bladder or prostate gland surgery. A **condom catheter** is shaped like a condom (male contraceptive device). It fits snugly over the male penis and collects the urine as it leaves the urethra meatus. 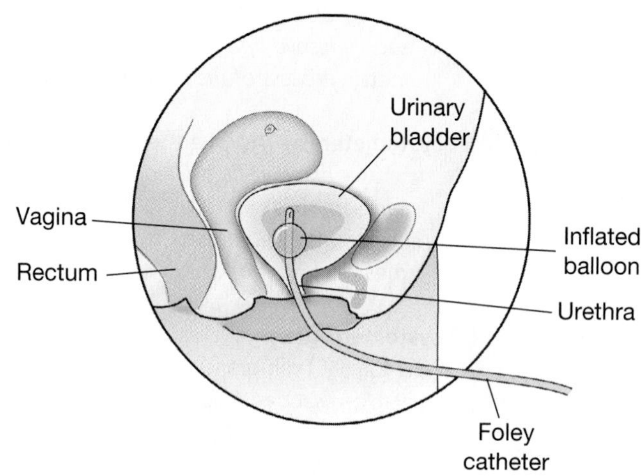 **Figure 11-20 ■ Foley catheter.** The inflated balloon at the tip of the catheter holds the Foley catheter in place in the bladder. The catheter drains urine from the bladder continuously as the kidneys produce urine. The urine is collected in a drainage bag that must be emptied periodically.

Word or Phrase	Word Part and Definition	Description
dialysis	**dialysis** (dy-AL-ih-sis) **dia-** *complete; completely through* **-lysis** *process of breaking down or dissolving* Every medical word must contain a combining form. The suffix of *dialysis* contains the combining form *lys/o-*. **hemodialysis** (HEE-moh-dy-AL-ih-sis) **hem/o-** *blood* **dia-** *complete; completely through* **-lysis** *process of breaking down or dissolving* **peritoneal** (PAIR-ih-toh-NEE-al) **peritone/o-** *peritoneum* **-al** *pertaining to* **dialysate** (dy-AL-ih-sayt) **dia-** *complete; completely through* **lys/o-** *break down or dissolve* **-ate** *composed of, pertaining to* **ambulatory** (AM-byoo-lah-TOR-ee) **ambulat/o-** *walking* **-ory** *having the function of*	Medical procedure to remove waste products from the blood of patients in renal failure. There are two types of dialysis: hemodialysis and peritoneal dialysis. **Hemodialysis** uses a fistula or a shunt in the patient's arm. A fistula is created by surgically joining an artery and vein. Over a few weeks, the vein enlarges enough to accommodate two needles, one that removes blood and sends it to the dialysis machine and another that receives purified blood from the dialysis machine and returns it to the body. In patients whose blood vessels are small, an external shunt (loop of tubing) is used instead to join the artery to the vein (see Figure 11-21■). **Peritoneal dialysis** uses a permanent catheter inserted through the abdominal wall. **Dialysate fluid** flows through the catheter and remains in the abdominal cavity for several hours. During that time, the fluid pulls body wastes from the blood. Then the fluid is removed, carrying waste products with it. In **continuous ambulatory peritoneal dialysis (CAPD),** the patient is able to walk around between the three or four daily episodes of dialysis. In **continuous cycling peritoneal dialysis (CCPD),** a machine inserts and removes dialysate fluid several times a night while the patient sleeps. (a) 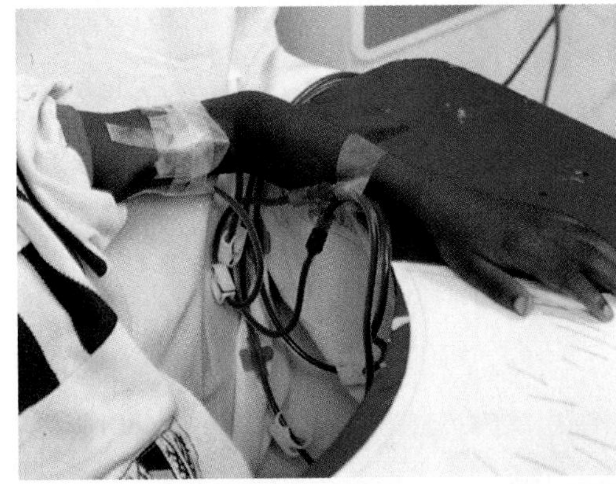 (b) 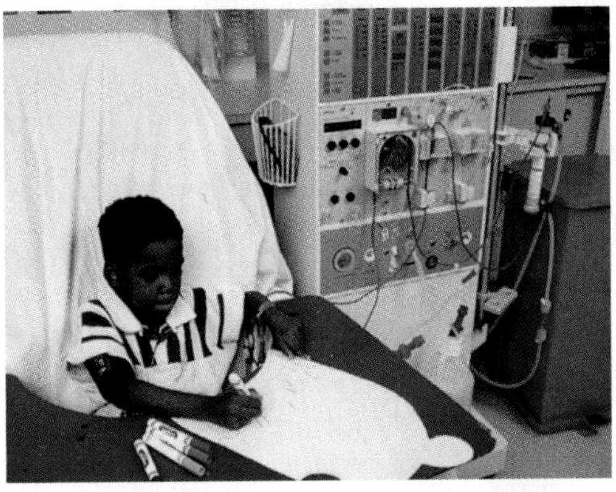 **Figure 11-21 ■ Hemodialysis.** This young patient is undergoing hemodialysis. (a) The shunt was placed in his upper arm where the arteries and veins are larger. It was placed in his left arm because he is right handed. (b) During dialysis he is able to color and read to pass the time while his blood is cleansed of wastes. His blood pressure is checked frequently during dialysis and so the blood pressure cuff is allowed to remain on his right upper arm.

Word or Phrase	Word Part and Definition	Description
intake and output (I&O)		Nursing procedure that documents the total amount of fluid intake (oral, nasogastric tube, intravenous line, and so forth) and the total amount of fluid output (urine, wound drainage, and so forth) (see Figure 11-22■). Used to monitor the body's fluid balance in patients with renal failure, burns, congestive heart failure, large draining wounds, dehydration, overdose of diuretic drugs, and so forth. 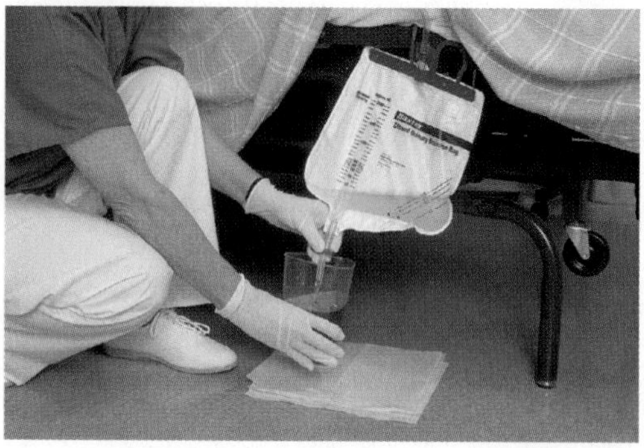 **Figure 11-22 ■ Urine output.** This nurse is measuring the urine output from a patient who has an indwelling Foley catheter that continuously drains urine into a collecting bag.
urine specimens		Medical procedure to obtain a urine specimen for testing. A clean-caught specimen (the urethral meatus is first cleansed) or a catheterized specimen (obtained directly from a catheter) is placed in a sterile container and used for culture and sensitivity testing.
Surgical Procedures		
bladder neck suspension	**suspension** (sus-PEN-shun) **suspens/o-** *hanging* **-ion** *action; condition*	Surgical procedure to correct stress incontinence. A supportive sling of muscle tissue or synthetic material is inserted around the base of the bladder and the urethra to elevate them to a normal position.
cystectomy	**cystectomy** (sis-TEK-toh-mee) **cyst/o-** *bladder; fluid-filled sac; semisolid cyst* **-ectomy** *surgical excision* **radical** (RAD-ih-kal) **radic/o-** *all parts including the root* **-al** *pertaining to*	Surgical procedure to remove the bladder because of bladder cancer. A **radical cystectomy** removes the bladder, surrounding tissues, and lymph nodes.

Word or Phrase	Word Part and Definition	Description
cystoscopy	**cystoscopy** (sis-TAWS-koh-pee) **cyst/o-** *bladder; fluid-filled sac; semisolid cyst* **-scopy** *process of using an instrument to examine* **cystoscope** (SIS-toh-skohp) **cyst/o-** *bladder; fluid-filled sac; semisolid cyst* **-scope** *instrument used to examine*	Surgical procedure that uses a rigid or flexible **cystoscope** inserted through the urethra in order to examine the bladder (see Figure 11-23■). A wide-angle lens and a light allow a full view of the bladder. A video attachment can be used to create a permanent visual record. 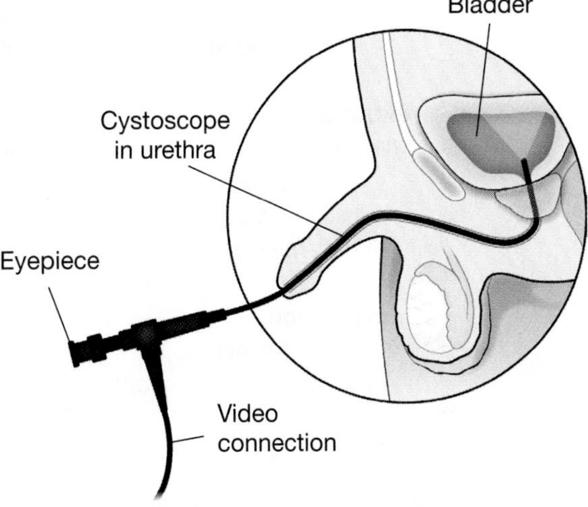 **Figure 11-23 ■ Cystoscopy.** The cystoscope is a flexible tube that has a viewing eyepiece and a light to illuminate the inside of the bladder. The cystoscope is inserted through the urethra and into the bladder. **Did You Know?** Cystoscopes have been used since the early 1800s. Because this was before the invention of the light bulb, early cystoscopes used a platinum wire that glowed when an electrical current ran through it to illuminate the inside the bladder.
kidney transplantation	**transplantation** (TRANS-plan-TAY-shun) **transplant/o-** *move something to another place* **-ation** *a process; being or having* **donor** (DOH-nor) *Donor* is derived from a Latin word meaning *one who gives.*	Surgical procedure to remove a severely damaged kidney from a patient with end-stage kidney failure and insert a new kidney from a donor. The patient (the recipient) is matched by blood type and tissue type to the **donor.** The patient's diseased kidney is removed and the donor kidney is sutured in place. Kidney transplantation patients must take immunosuppressant drugs for the rest of their lives to keep their bodies from rejecting the foreign tissue that is their new kidney. Patients continue to undergo dialysis while waiting for a donor kidney. **Did You Know?** The first successful kidney transplant occurred in 1954 in the United States between identical twins. It was not until FDA approval of the antirejection immunosuppressant drug cyclosporine in 1984 that transplantation of kidneys from cadavers or unrelated living donors could be performed successfully. There are approximately 13,000 kidney transplants performed each year in the United States. However, there are over 47,000 patients currently waiting for a suitable donor kidney to become available.

Word or Phrase	Word Part and Definition	Description
lithotripsy	**lithotripsy** (LITH-oh-trip-see) **lith/o-** *stone* **-tripsy** *process of crushing* **lithotriptor** (LITH-oh-TRIP-tor) **lith/o-** *stone* **-triptor** *thing that crushes* **extracorporeal** (EKS-trah-kohr-POH-ree-al) **extra-** *outside of* **corpor/o-** *body* **-eal** *pertaining to* **percutaneous** (PER-kyoo-TAY-nee-us) **per-** *through, throughout* **cutane/o-** *skin* **-ous** *pertaining to* **ultrasonic** (UL-trah-SAWN-ik) **ultra-** *beyond; higher* **son/o-** *sound* **-ic** *pertaining to* Ultrasonic waves have a higher frequency than the human ear can hear.	Medical or surgical procedure that uses sound waves to break up a kidney stone (see Figure 11-24■). After an x-ray pinpoints the location of the stone, a **lithotriptor** generates sound waves that break up the stone. Because the sound waves are generated by a source outside the body, the procedure is known as **extracorporeal shock wave lithotripsy (ESWL)**. Alternatively, the surgical procedure **percutaneous ultrasonic lithotripsy** may be used. An endoscope is inserted through the flank skin and into the kidney. A lithotriptor probe is inserted through the endoscope and into the kidney to break up large stones. Sometimes a holmium laser that generates a laser beam is used to break up very hard kidney stones. 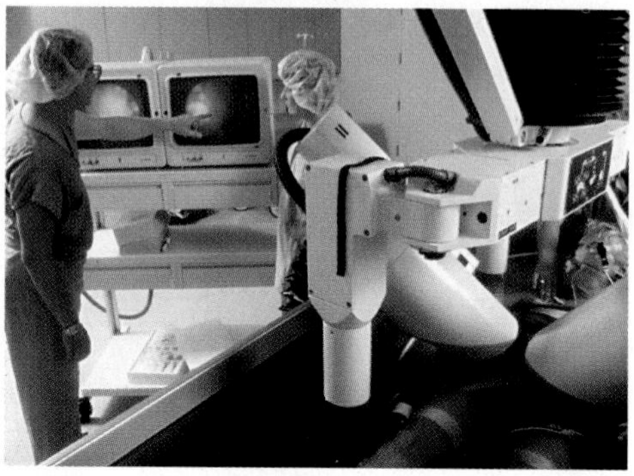 **Figure 11-24 ■ Lithotripsy.** The patient lies on a table or is immersed in a tank of water. The lithotriptor emits sound at a frequency that creates shock waves to break up a kidney stone.
nephrectomy	**nephrectomy** (neh-FREK-toh-mee) **nephr/o-** *kidney; nephron* **-ectomy** *surgical excision*	Surgical procedure to remove a diseased or cancerous kidney. Alternatively, a healthy kidney may be removed from a donor so that it can be transplanted into a patient with renal failure.
nephrolithotomy	**nephrolithotomy** (NEF-roh-lih-THAWT-oh-mee) **nephr/o-** *kidney; nephron* **lith/o-** *stone* **-tomy** *process of cutting or making an incision*	Surgical procedure in which a small incision is made in the skin and an endoscope is inserted in a percutaneous approach into the kidney to remove a kidney stone embedded in the pelvis or calices.
nephropexy	**nephropexy** (NEF-roh-pek-see) **nephr/o-** *kidney; nephron* **-pexy** *process of surgically fixing in place*	Surgical procedure to correct a kidney that is in an abnormally low position (nephroptosis) by suturing it back into anatomical position.

Word or Phrase	Word Part and Definition	Description
renal biopsy	**biopsy** (BY-awp-see) **bi/o-** *life; living organisms; living tissue* **-opsy** *process of viewing*	Surgical procedure in which a small piece of kidney is excised for microscopic analysis. This is done to confirm or exclude a diagnosis of cancer or kidney disease.
stone basketing		Surgical procedure in which a cystoscope is inserted into the bladder. A stone basket (a long-handled instrument with several interwoven wires at its end) is then passed through the cystoscope to snare a kidney stone and remove it.
transurethral resection of a bladder tumor (TURBT)	**transurethral** (TRANS-yoo-REE-thral) **trans-** *across, through* **urethr/o-** *urethra* **-al** *pertaining to* **resection** (ree-SEK-shun) **resect/o-** *to cut out and remove* **-ion** *action; condition* **resectoscope** (ree-SEK-toh-skohp) **resect/o-** *to cut out and remove* **-scope** *instrument used to examine*	Surgical procedure to remove a bladder tumor from inside the bladder. A special cystoscope known as a **resectoscope** is inserted through the urethra into the bladder. It has built-in cutting instruments and cautery to resect the bladder tumor and cauterize bleeding blood vessels. Pieces of tissue are then irrigated out of the bladder.
urethroplasty	**urethroplasty** (yoo-REE-throh-PLAS-tee) **urethr/o-** *urethra* **-plasty** *process of reshaping by surgery*	Surgical procedure that involves plastic surgery to reposition the urethra. Used to correct congenital hypospadias or epispadias.

Drug Categories

Several different categories of drugs are used to treat the symptoms, signs, and diseases of the urinary system. The most common drugs in each category are listed.

Category	Word Part and Definition	Description	Examples
antibiotic drugs	**antibiotic** (AN-tee-by-AWT-ik) (AN-tih-by-AWT-ik) **anti-** *against* **bi/o-** *life; living organisms; living tissue* **-tic** *pertaining to*	Used to treat urinary tract infections. Urinary antibiotics have a special affinity for the urinary tract, although other types of antibiotics are also used to treat urinary tract infections.	Gantrisin, Macrobid, Macrodantin

Connections

nephrotoxic (NEF-roh-TAWK-sik)
nephr/o- *kidney; nephron*
tox/o- *poison*
-ic *pertaining to*
Add words to make a correct and complete definition of *nephrotoxic: pertaining to [a substance that acts on the] kidney [as a] poison.*

Pharmacology. Aminoglycoside antibiotic drugs can cause a severe, **nephrotoxic** effect on the kidneys. Patients receiving aminoglycoside antibiotics have their kidney function monitored by periodic BUN and creatinine tests.

Category	Word Part and Definition	Description	Examples
chemotherapy drugs	**chemotherapy** (KEE-moh-THER-ah-pee) **chem/o-** *chemical, drug* **-therapy** *treatment* **intravesical** (IN-trah-VES-ih-kal) **intra-** *within* **vesic/o-** *bladder; fluid-filled sac* **-al** *pertaining to*	Kill rapidly dividing cancer cells in the bladder or kidney. **Intravesical** chemotherapy drugs are instilled into the bladder to treat bladder cancer.	Adriamycin, Vincasar
diuretic drugs	**diuretic** (DY-yoo-RET-ik) **dia-** *complete; completely through* **ur/o-** *urine; urinary system* **-etic** *pertaining to* The *a* is dropped from the prefix *dia-* when the word parts are combined to form *diuretic.*	Block sodium from being absorbed from the tubule back into the blood. As the sodium is excreted in the urine, it brings water and potassium with it because of osmotic pressure. This process is known as diuresis. This decreases the volume of blood and is useful in the treatment of hypertension, congestive heart failure, and nephrotic syndrome.	Aldactone, Esidrix, Hygroton, Lasix, Zaroxolyn
potassium supplements		Used as a replacement for potassium lost due to diuretics. Diuretics increase sodium excretion but also potassium excretion because they are both positively charged electrolytes. The presence of *K* in the drug name refers to the chemical symbol for potassium (K^+).	K-Dur

Category	Word Part and Definition	Description	Examples
urinary analgesic drugs	**analgesic** (AN-al-JEE-zik) **an-** *without, not* **alges/o-** *sensation of pain* **-ic** *pertaining to*	Exert a pain-relieving effect on the mucosa of the urinary tract.	Pyridium, Urogesic
antispasmodic drugs	**antispasmodic** (AN-tee-spaz-MAWD-ik) **anti-** *against* **spasmod/o-** *spasm* **-ic** *pertaining to*	Relax the smooth muscle in the walls of the ureter, bladder, and urethra. Used to treat spasm from cystitis and overactive bladder.	Cystospaz, Detrol, Urispas

Abbreviations

ARF	acute renal failure
BUN	blood urea nitrogen
CAPD	continuous ambulatory peritoneal dialysis
cath	catheterize or catheterization (slang)
cc	cubic centimeter (measure of volume)
CCPD	continuous cycling peritoneal dialysis
C&S	culture and sensitivity
CRF	chronic renal failure
cysto	cystoscopy (slang)
epi	epithelial cells (in the urine specimen) (slang)
ESWL	extracorporeal shock wave lithotripsy
ESRD	end-stage renal disease
GU	genitourinary gonococcal urethritis
hpf	high-power field
I&O	intake and output
IVP	intravenous pyelogram
K or K$^+$	potassium
KUB	kidneys, ureters, bladder
mL	milliliter (measure of volume)
pH	potential of hydrogen (acidity or alkalinity)
RBC	red blood cell
SG, sp gr	specific gravity
TNTC	too numerous to count
TURBT	transurethral resection of bladder tumor
UA	urinalysis
UTI	urinary tract infection
VMA	vanillylmandelic acid
WBC	white blood cell

Word Alert

MEDICAL ABBREVIATIONS

Abbreviations are commonly used in all types of medical documentation; however, they can mean different things to different people and their meaning can be misinterpreted. Always verify the meaning of an abbreviation.

ARF stands for *acute renal failure,* but it can also stand for *acute respiratory distress* or *acute rheumatic fever.*

C&S stands for *culture and sensitivity,* but the sound-alike word *CNS* stands for *central nervous system.*

CRF stands for *chronic renal failure,* but it can also stand for *cardiac risk factors.*

GU stands for *genitourinary,* but it can also stand for *gonococcal urethritis.*

Career Focus

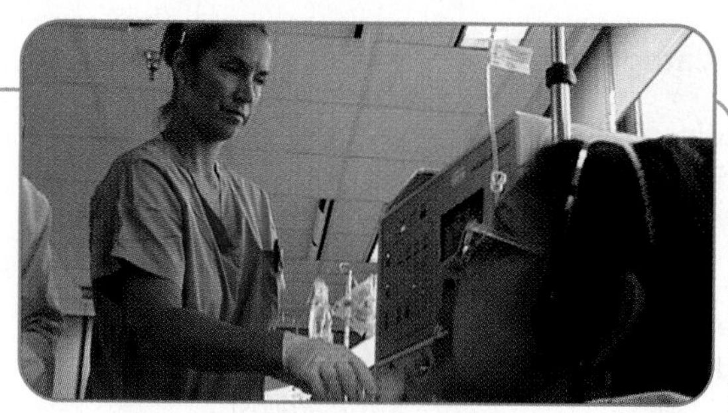

Meet Cindy, a dialysis nurse.

"I came into dialysis because my brother actually was on dialysis for a very long time, and it was something I thought would be interesting. The dialysis center let me come in and let me observe for a few hours, and I found that was also very fascinating. I had already been a nurse for over eight years. This dialysis center gave me all the on-the-job training. It was just a whole different field. You really get to know your patients. You do have the time to actually sit down and talk to them. The majority of our patients have hypertension or they have diabetes, so we do a lot of diabetic teaching."

Dialysis nurses are allied health professionals who work in dialysis centers. They specialize in caring for patients with end-stage kidney disease who are receiving dialysis.

Urologists are physicians who practice in the specialty of urology. They diagnose and treat patients with diseases of the urinary tract. Some urologists further specialize and become **nephrologists** who only treat patients with diseases of the kidney. Physicians can take additional training and become board certified in the subspecialty of pediatric nephrology. Cancerous tumors of the urinary tract are treated medically by an oncologist or surgically by a urologist or a general surgeon.

urologist (yoo-RAWL-oh-jist)
ur/o- *urine; urinary system*
log/o- *the study of*
-ist *one who specializes in*

nephrologist (neh-FRAWL-oh-jist)
nephr/o- *kidney; nephron*
log/o- *the study of*
-ist *one who specializes in*

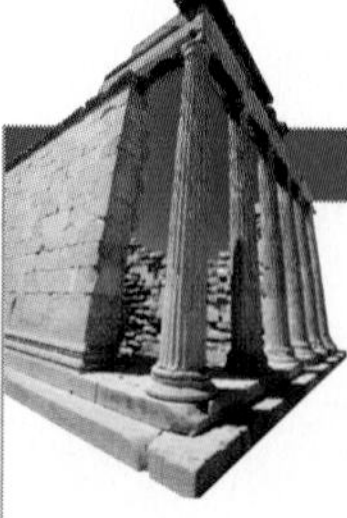

It's Greek to Me!

Did you notice that some urologic words have two different combining forms? Combining forms from both Greek and Latin languages remain a part of medical language today.

English Word	Greek	Latin	Examples of Medical Words
bladder	cyst/o-	vesic/o-	cystitis, vesicovaginal
kidney	nephr/o-	ren/o-	nephritis, renal
make urine	urin/o-	mictur/o-	urination, micturition
renal pelvis	pyel/o-	pelv/o-	pyelonephritis, pelvic
stone	lith/o-	calcul/o-	lithotripsy, calculogenesis

CHAPTER REVIEW EXERCISES

Review all of the material in this chapter by completing the review exercises in this section. Use the Answer Key at the end of the book to check your answers.

Anatomy and Physiology

Unscramble and Match

Unscramble the medical word and write the correct spelling of the word in the blank provided, then match each word with its description. The first one has been done for you.

	Scrambled	Answer		Description
1.	beddrla	bladder	____	Tube from renal pelvis to bladder
2.	deiykns	______________________	____	Proximal and distal convoluted
3.	hulmi	______________________	____	Triangular area in bladder
4.	lbeuut	______________________	____	Contains renal pyramids
5.	eprhstnic	______________________	____	Ball of yarn
6.	gearu	______________________	____	Paired organs shaped like beans
7.	rlelguosum	______________________	____	Ring of muscles around tube
8.	lepscau	______________________	____	Tube from bladder to outside the body
9.	irntgoe	______________________	1	Holds urine
10.	aotestrp	______________________	____	Male gland around urethra
11.	rteeur	______________________	____	Major and minor
12.	claxi	______________________	____	Fibrous layer around kidney
13.	ulameld	______________________	____	Indentation in an organ
14.	rthurae	______________________	____	Folds in the bladder mucosa

Sequencing Exercise

Beginning with blood entering the kidney, write each structure of the urinary system in order. Use the list of anatomical structures to help you sequence the structures in their correct order.

Structure	**Correct Order**
bladder	1. ______________________
Bowman's capsule	2. ______________________
calix	3. ______________________
collecting duct	4. ______________________
distal convoluted tubule	5. ______________________
glomerulus	6. ______________________
loop of Henle	7. ______________________
proximal convoluted tubule	8. ______________________
renal artery	9. ______________________
renal pelvis	10. ______________________
ureter	11. ______________________
urethra	12. ______________________
urethral meatus	13. ______________________

Medical Language Word Parts

Name that Word Part

Identify each of the word parts given here by writing in the correct letter (P, C, or S) on the line beside it. Then write the definition of the word part on the blank line. The first one has been done for you.

Prefix = P **Combining Form = C** **Suffix = S**

		Word Part	Definition			Word Part	Definition
1.	-al	S	pertaining to	36.	dia-		
2.	absorpt/o-			37.	diabet/o-		
3.	acid/o-			38.	dist/o-		
4.	albumin/o-			39.	dys-		
5.	alges/o-			40.	-eal		
6.	alkal/o-			41.	-ectasis		
7.	ambulat/o-			42.	-ectomy		
8.	an-			43.	electr/o-		
9.	angi/o-			44.	-emia		
10.	anti-			45.	-emic		
11.	-ar			46.	-ence		
12.	arteri/o-			47.	enur/o-		
13.	-ary			48.	epi-		
14.	-ate			49.	erythr/o-		
15.	-ation			50.	-esis		
16.	bacteri/o-			51.	-etic		
17.	bi/o-			52.	excret/o-		
18.	blast/o-			53.	extern/o-		
19.	calcul/o-			54.	extra-		
20.	calic/o-			55.	filtrat/o-		
21.	cali/o-			56.	filtr/o-		
22.	cancer/o-			57.	genit/o-		
23.	carcin/o-			58.	gen/o-		
24.	catheter/o-			59.	glomerul/o-		
25.	-cele			60.	glycos/o-		
26.	chem/o-			61.	-grade		
27.	chron/o-			62.	-gram		
28.	col/o-			63.	-graphy		
29.	congenit/o-			64.	hemat/o-		
30.	contin/o-			65.	hem/o-		
31.	corpor/o-			66.	hemoglobin/o-		
32.	cortic/o-			67.	hil/o-		
33.	cutane/o-			68.	hyal/o-		
34.	cyst/o-			69.	hydr/o-		
35.	-cyte			70.	hypo-		

	Word Part	Definition
71. -ia	______	______________
72. -iasis	______	______________
73. -ic	______	______________
74. ile-	______	______________
75. -in	______	______________
76. -ine	______	______________
77. infect/o-	______	______________
78. interstiti/o-	______	______________
79. intra-	______	______________
80. -ion	______	______________
81. -ist	______	______________
82. -ition	______	______________
83. -itis	______	______________
84. -ity	______	______________
85. -ization	______	______________
86. kal/i-	______	______________
87. keton/o-	______	______________
88. leuk/o-	______	______________
89. lith/o-	______	______________
90. log/o-	______	______________
91. -logy	______	______________
92. -lysis	______	______________
93. lys/o-	______	______________
94. -lyte	______	______________
95. medull/o-	______	______________
96. -meter	______	______________
97. metr/o-	______	______________
98. -metry	______	______________
99. micr/o-	______	______________
100. mictur/o-	______	______________
101. mucos/o-	______	______________
102. necr/o-	______	______________
103. nephr/o-	______	______________
104. neur/o-	______	______________
105. noct/o-	______	______________
106. olig/o-	______	______________
107. -oma	______	______________
108. -opsy	______	______________
109. -ory	______	______________
110. -osis	______	______________
111. -ous	______	______________
112. -pathy	______	______________

	Word Part	Definition
113. pelv/o-	______	______________
114. pen/o-	______	______________
115. per-	______	______________
116. peri-	______	______________
117. peritone/o-	______	______________
118. -pexy	______	______________
119. -plasty	______	______________
120. -poietin	______	______________
121. poly-	______	______________
122. post-	______	______________
123. prostat/o-	______	______________
124. protein/o-	______	______________
125. proxim/o-	______	______________
126. -ptosis	______	______________
127. pub/o-	______	______________
128. pyel/o-	______	______________
129. py/o-	______	______________
130. radic/o-	______	______________
131. radi/o-	______	______________
132. re-	______	______________
133. refract/o-	______	______________
134. ren/o-	______	______________
135. resect/o-	______	______________
136. retent/o-	______	______________
137. retro-	______	______________
138. scler/o-	______	______________
139. -scope	______	______________
140. scop/o-	______	______________
141. -scopy	______	______________
142. sensitiv/o-	______	______________
143. son/o-	______	______________
144. spasmod/o-	______	______________
145. -stalsis	______	______________
146. supra-	______	______________
147. suspens/o-	______	______________
148. -therapy	______	______________
149. -tic	______	______________
150. tom/o-	______	______________
151. -tomy	______	______________
152. tox/o-	______	______________
153. trans-	______	______________
154. transplant/o-	______	______________

	Word Part	Definition
155. -tripsy	______	______________
156. -triptor	______	______________
157. tub/o-	______	______________
158. tubul/o-	______	______________
159. -ule	______	______________
160. ultra-	______	______________
161. ureter/o-	______	______________
162. urethr/o-	______	______________
163. urin/o-	______	______________
164. ur/o-	______	______________
165. vagin/o-	______	______________
166. ven/o-	______	______________
167. vesic/o-	______	______________

Word-Building Exercise

Use the combining forms, prefixes, and suffixes given here to build medical words that match the definitions given. Write the word that you build on the blank line. Some word parts may be used more than once. The first one has been done for you.

Word Parts

-ary (pertaining to)
-cele (hernia)
cyst/o- (bladder; fluid-filled sac; semisolid cyst)
dys- (painful, difficult, abnormal)
glomerul/o- (glomerulus)
hemat/o- (blood)
-ia (condition, state, thing)
-iasis (abnormal condition, condition)
-itis (inflammation of)
lith/o- (stone)
nephr/o- (kidney; nephron)
-osis (condition; abnormal condition; process)
poly- (many, much)
py/o- (pus)
scler/o- (hard; white of the eye)
-scope (instrument used to examine)
-tomy (process of cutting or making an incision)
-tripsy (process of crushing)
urin/o- (urine; urinary system)
ur/o- (urine; urinary system)

1. Pertaining to the urine (You think *urin/o-* + *-ary*) You write urinary
2. Condition of blood in the urine ______________
3. Condition of hardness of the glomeruli ______________
4. Hernia of the bladder ______________
5. Condition of painful urine ______________
6. Inflammation or infection of the bladder ______________
7. Condition of much urine ______________
8. Instrument used to examine the bladder ______________
9. Abnormal condition of kidney stones ______________
10. Process of crushing a (kidney) stone ______________
11. Process of making an incision to remove a kidney stone ______________
12. Condition of pus in the urine ______________

Symptoms, Signs, and Diseases

Matching Exercise

Match each numbered word to its description.

1.	anuria	____	Bedwetting
2.	dysuria	____	Excessive urine
3.	enuresis	____	Difficult urination
4.	glycosuria	____	Voiding at night
5.	incontinence	____	WBCs in the urine
6.	nocturia	____	No urine production
7.	oliguria	____	Sugar in the urine
8.	polyuria	____	Bladder distended with urine
9.	pyuria	____	Scanty urine production
10.	retention	____	Inability to hold urine in the bladder

Antonyms Exercise

For each medical word given, write the antonym (opposite word) in the blank provided.

Medical Word	Antonym
1. acute	____________
2. anuria	____________
3. epispadias	____________
4. gross blood	____________
5. urinary retention	____________

Synonyms Exercise

For each medical word given, write the synonym (similar word) in the blank provided.

Medical Term	Synonym
1. albuminuria	____________
2. cystocele	____________
3. enuresis	____________
4. gross blood	____________
5. nephroblastoma	____________

True or False

Indicate whether each statement is true or false by writing T or F on the line.

1. ____ Wilms' tumor is cancer of the kidney in children.
2. ____ Glomerulonephritis can develop following a strep throat.
3. ____ Albumin and protein are normally found in the urine.
4. ____ Glycosuria is a symptom of diabetes insipidus.
5. ____ A spinal cord injury can result in polycystic kidneys.
6. ____ Pyelonephritis is an infection of the renal pelvis and kidney.
7. ____ A vesicovaginal fistula is an abnormal passage between the ureter and vagina.
8. ____ Renal colic is caused by a kidney stone in the intestines.
9. ____ Hydroureter develops because of an obstructing kidney stone.
10. ____ Bacteriuria is a symptom of a urinary tract infection.
11. ____ Calculogenesis is another name for lithogenesis.

Laboratory, Radiology, Surgery, and Drugs

Laboratory Test Exercise

Review this form for ordering laboratory tests (see Figure 11-25■). Find each of the following tests related to urology and put a checkmark in the box next to it.

albumin	creatinine clearance	gonococcus, urethra	urea nitrogen
creatinine	culture, urine	UA (dipstick & microscopic)	uric acid

PANELS AND PROFILES			TESTS		
968T		Lipid Panel	19687W		Bilirubin (Direct)
315F		Electrolyte Panel	265F		HBsAg
10256F		Hepatic Function Panel	51870R		HB Core Antibody
10165F		Basic Metabolic Panel	1012F		Cardio CRP
10231A		Comprehensive Metabolic Panel	23242E		GGT
10306F		Hepatitis Panel, Acute	28852E		Protein, Total
182Aaa		Obstetric Panel	141A		CBC Hemogram
18T		Chem-Screen Panel (Basic)	21105R		hCG, Qualitative, Serum
554T		Chem-Screen Panel (Basic with HDL)	10321A		ANA
7971A		Chem-Screen Panel (Basic with HDL, TIBC)	80185		Cardio CRP with Lipid Profile
TESTS			26F		PT with INR
56713E		Lead, Blood	232Aaa		UA, Dipstick
2782A		Antibody Screen	42A		CBC with Diff
3556F		Iron, TIBC	20867W		HDL Cholesterol
20933E		Cholesterol	31732E		PTT
3084111E		Uric Acid	34F		UA, Dipstick and Microscopic
53348W		Rubella Antibody	20396R		CEA
27771E		Phosphate	45443E		Hematocrit
2111600E		Creatinine	28571E		PSA, Total
29868W		Testosterone, Total	66902E		WBC count
9704F		Creatinine Clearance	20750E		Chloride
19752E		Bilirubin (Total)	7187W		Hemoglobin
30536Rrr		T3, Total	4259T		HIV-1 Antibody
687T		Protein Electrophoresis	45484R		Hemoglobin A1c
3563444R		Digoxin	67868R		Alk Phosphatase
15214R		Glucose, 2-Hour Postprandial	24984R		Iron
30502E		T3, Uptake	28512E		Sodium
7773E		Platelet Count	17426R		ALT
39685R		Dilantin (phenytoin)	MICROBIOLOGY		
30494R		Triglycerides	112680E		Group A Beta Strep Culture, Throat
26013E		Magnesium	5827W		Group B Beta Strep Culture, Genitals
15586R		Glucose, Fasting	49932E		Chlamydia, Endocervix/Urethra
30237W		T4, Free	6007W		Culture, Blood
28233E		Potassium	2692E		Culture, Genitals
19208W		AST	2649T		Culture, HSV
30163E		TSH	612A		Culture, Sputum
22764R		Ferritin	6262E		Culture, Throat
20008W		Calcium	6304R		Culture, Urine
54726F		Occult Blood, Stool	50286R		Gonococcus, Endocervix/Urethra
51839W		HAV Antibody, Total	6643E		Gram Stain
430A		Blood Group and Rh Type	STOOL PATHOGENS		
28399W		Progesterone	10045F		Culture, Stool
30262E		T4, Total	4475F		Culture, Campylobacter
20289W		Carbon Dioxide	10018T		Culture, Salmonella
1156F		RPR	86140A		E. coli Toxins
30940E		Urea Nitrogen	1099T		Ova and Parasites
17417W		Albumin	VENIPUNCTURE		
28423E		Prolactin	63180		Venipuncture

Figure 11-25 ■

Circle Exercise

Circle the correct word from the choices given.

1. Ultrasonography uses (**radiation, sound waves, x-rays**) to produce an image.
2. To detect the presence of a kidney stone, a/an (**cystometrogram, IVP, KUB**) is performed after contrast dye is injected into a vein.
3. After the diagnosis of renal cell carcinoma was made, a (**biopsy, nephrectomy, nephropexy**) was performed to remove the entire kidney.
4. A (**catheter, cystoscope, shunt**) is permanent tubing that is surgically inserted in the arm in order to perform hemodialysis.
5. The (**BUN, KUB, UA**) results showed that the urine had TNTC WBC.
6. Urine specific gravity is measured with all of these instruments EXCEPT (**dialysis, refractometer, urinometer**).
7. Intravenous pyelography uses (**a CT scan, contrast dye, sound waves**) to produce an image.

Multiple Choice

Select the best answer for the question from the answers provided.

1. A culture and sensitivity test on a urine specimen shows the ______________________.
   a. color and odor of the urine.
   b. amount of urea and creatinine.
   c. microorganism present and its response to antibiotic drugs.
   d. specific gravity, pH, and sediment.

2. Which procedure uses a special solution and machine to remove waste products from the blood?
   a. catheterization c. lithotripsy
   b. cystoscopy d. hemodialysis

3. Which drug is used to increase urine output?
   a. diuretic c. analgesic
   b. antispasmodic d. chemotherapy

Abbreviations

Define and Match Exercise

Give the definition for each abbreviation listed below, then match it to its description.

1. BUN	______________________	_____	X-ray after injection of dye
2. cc	______________________	_____	Test to determine what is causing an infection and how to treat it
3. CRF	______________________	_____	Long-term decrease in kidney function
4. C&S	______________________	_____	Presence of this cell in the urine means infection
5. ESWL	______________________	_____	X-ray of the kidneys, ureters, and bladder
6. I&O	______________________	_____	Unit of measurement of volume of liquid
7. IVP	______________________	_____	Used when there are too many cells to count
8. K	______________________	_____	Blood test that measures kidney function
9. KUB	______________________	_____	Measures consumption and excretion of fluids
10. TNTC	______________________	_____	Multiple tests done on one urine specimen
11. UA	______________________	_____	An electrolyte
12. WBC	______________________	_____	Shock waves dissolve kidney stones

Applied Skills

Plural Noun and Adjective Spelling

Fill in the blanks with the correct word form. Be sure to check your spelling. The first one has been done for you.

Singular Noun	Plural Noun	Adjective
1. cortex	cortices	cortical
2. glomerulus	________	________
3. hilum	________	________
4. kidney	________	________
5. medulla	________	________

Singular Noun	Plural Noun	Adjective
6. pelvis	________	________
7. tubule	________	________
8. ureter	________	________
9. urethra		________
10. urine		________

Dictionary Challenge

On the job, you will often encounter new medical words. Practice your medical dictionary skills by looking up the medical word in bold and writing its definition on the blank line.

OFFICE CHART NOTE

The patient presented with **strangury** and dysuria. A urinalysis showed both WBCs and RBCs. A diagnosis of cystitis was made, and the patient was given Cipro 250 mg b.i.d. and Pyridium 200 mg q.8h.

Strangury: ____

Analysis of a Medical Report

This exercise contains an emergency department report. Read the report and answer the questions.

EMERGENCY DEPARTMENT REPORT

PATIENT NAME: NGUYEN, Li

HOSPITAL NUMBER: 082-344-8463

DATE: November 19, 20xx

CHIEF COMPLAINT
This 40-year-old female presented to the emergency department with complaints of abdominal pain, nausea, and vomiting.

HISTORY OF PRESENT ILLNESS
The patient had been seen 3 days earlier in the office of her primary care physician for a complaint of pressure and pain in the urethra. She was given a tentative diagnosis of urinary tract infection. The physician ordered a clean-catch urine specimen, and the patient provided this to the office lab. The patient was given a prescription for the antibiotic Bactrim and the urinary antiseptic Pyridium. She was told to call the office in 3 days for the result of the urine culture.

The patient states that, even though she was on the antibiotic, her symptoms worsened over the next 48 hours. She was taking Pyridium regularly, as well as Extra Strength Tylenol, and using a heating pad. She was drinking fluids, including cranberry juice as recommended by her primary care physician to acidify the urine to decrease the growth of bacteria.

This evening, when her pain became acute, with pressure in the bladder area, a sense of urgency to urinate, spasm, renal colic, and nausea and vomiting, she presented to the emergency department.

PAST MEDICAL HISTORY
Appendectomy in the remote past. She has a history of kidney stones x2, the last episode being several years ago.

SOCIAL HISTORY
She is married and sexually active in a monogamous relationship. Her husband had a vasectomy several years ago.

PHYSICAL EXAMINATION
Vital signs: Temperature 98.8, pulse 120, respirations 28, blood pressure 140/100; normal blood pressure for her is 116/90. There is tenderness to palpation over the right lumbar and flank areas. There is tenderness to palpation over the suprapubic area. There is no tenderness to palpation elsewhere in the abdomen. Vaginal examination revealed no vaginal discharge or tenderness.

LABORATORY DATA
A catheterized urine specimen was obtained. It showed no bacteria, no gross blood, and no white blood cells. There was, however, microscopic hematuria. A KUB x-ray revealed no abnormalities; however, a subsequent CT scan revealed a moderately sized stone at the bladder neck.

DIAGNOSIS
Solitary kidney stone at the bladder neck.

TREATMENT
The patient was given a urine strainer and will strain all urine. She will call to schedule an appointment with a urologist next week so that these multiple episodes of kidney stones can be investigated. If she passes the stone, the patient will bring it to the hospital laboratory for analysis.

In the emergency department, the patient was given pain medication and hydrated with I.V. fluids. When her pain had subsided, she was released. She will follow up as described above.

Alfred J. Stansbury, M.D.

Alfred J. Stansbury, M.D.

AJS:ljs
D: 11/19/xx
T: 11/19/xx

WORD ANALYSIS QUESTIONS

1. Divide *urologist* into its three word parts and define each word part.

   Word Part **Definition**

   ______________ ______________________________

   ______________ ______________________________

   ______________ ______________________________

2. Divide *suprapubic* into its three word parts and define each word part.

   Word Part **Definition**

   ______________ ______________________________

   ______________ ______________________________

   ______________ ______________________________

3. Divide *hematuria* into its three word parts and define each word part.

   Word Part **Definition**

   ______________ ______________________________

   ______________ ______________________________

   ______________ ______________________________

4. Divide *antibiotic* into its three word parts and define each word part.

   Word Part **Definition**

   ______________ ______________________________

   ______________ ______________________________

   ______________ ______________________________

5. Define these abbreviations.

   KUB ______________________________

   I.V. ______________________________

6. The phrase "tentative diagnosis of urinary tract infection" could be written with an abbreviation as "tentative diagnosis of a __________."

FACT FINDING QUESTIONS

1. What type of urine specimen was obtained by the physician's office lab? ______________
2. What was the purpose of drinking cranberry juice? ______________
3. Define these words.

   renal colic ______________________________

   suprapubic pain ______________________________
4. What type of urine specimen was obtained in the emergency department? ______________
5. Why was the patient given a urine strainer? ______________

CRITICAL THINKING QUESTIONS

1. Why was it important to note that the patient has had an appendectomy? ______________
2. Why was it important to note that the patient's husband has had a vasectomy? ______________
3. Why were the patient's pulse, respirations, and blood pressure elevated on admission to the emergency department, but not her temperature? ______________
4. What did the results of the vaginal examination mean? ______________
5. What is the most likely explanation for the microscopic hematuria? ______________

Pronunciation Checklist

Read each word and its pronunciation. Practice pronouncing each word. Verify your pronunciation by listening to the Pronunciation List on the CD-ROM. Check the box next to the word after you master its pronunciation.

- ❑ acidic (ah-SID-ik)
- ❑ acute renal failure (ah-KYOOT REE-nal FAYL-yoor)
- ❑ acute tubular necrosis (ah-KYOOT TOO-byoo-lar neh-KROH-sis)
- ❑ albuminuria (AL-byoo-mih-NYOO-ree-ah)
- ❑ alkaline (AL-kah-line)
- ❑ ambulatory (AM-byoo-lah-TOR-ee)
- ❑ analgesic drug (AN-al-JEE-zik DRUHG)
- ❑ antibiotic drug (AN-tee-by-AWT-ik DRUHG) (AN-tih-by-AWT-ik)
- ❑ antispasmodic drug (AN-tee-spaz-MAWD-ik DRUHG)
- ❑ anuria (an-YOO-ree-ah)
- ❑ ascites (ah-SIGH-teez)
- ❑ bacteriuria (BAK-teer-ee-YOO-ree-ah)
- ❑ biopsy (BY-awp-see)
- ❑ bladder (BLAD-er)
- ❑ bladder neck suspension (BLAD-er NEK sus-PEN-shun)
- ❑ Bowman's capsule (BOH-manz KAP-sool)
- ❑ calculogenesis (KAL-kyoo-loh-JEN-eh-sis)
- ❑ calculus (KAL-kyoo-lus)
- ❑ caliceal (KAL-ih-see-al)
- ❑ calices (KAL-ih-seez)
- ❑ caliectasis (KAY-lee-EK-tah-sis)
- ❑ calix (KAY-liks)
- ❑ cancerous (KAN-ser-us)
- ❑ carcinoma (KAR-sih-NOH-mah)
- ❑ catheter (KATH-eh-ter)
- ❑ catheterization (KATH-eh-ter-ih-ZAY-shun)
- ❑ chemotherapy (KEE-moh-THAIR-ah-pee)
- ❑ chronic renal failure (KRAWN-ic REE-nal FAYL-yoor)
- ❑ condom catheter (CON-dom KATH-eh-ter)
- ❑ congenital (con-JEN-ih-tal)
- ❑ cortex (KOR-teks)
- ❑ cortical (KOR-tih-kal)
- ❑ cortices (KOR-tih-seez)
- ❑ creatinine (kree-AT-ih-neen)
- ❑ culture and sensitivity (KUL-chur and SEN-sih-TIV-ih-tee)
- ❑ cystectomy (sis-TEK-toh-mee)
- ❑ cystitis (sis-TY-tis)
- ❑ cystocele (SIS-toh-seel)
- ❑ cystometer (sis-TAWM-eh-ter)
- ❑ cystometrogram (SIS-toh-MET-roh-gram)
- ❑ cystometry (sis-TAWM-eh-tree)
- ❑ cystoscope (SIS-toh-skohp)
- ❑ cystoscopy (sis-TAWS-koh-pee)
- ❑ diabetic nephropathy (DY-ah-BET-ik neh-FRAWP-ah-thee)
- ❑ dialysate (dy-AL-ih-sayt)
- ❑ dialysis (dy-AL-ih-sis)
- ❑ distal convoluted tubule (DIS-tal CON-voh-LOO-ted TOO-byool)
- ❑ diuretic drug (DY-yoo-RET-ik DRUHG)
- ❑ dysuria (dis-YOO-ree-ah)
- ❑ electrolyte (ee-LEK-troh-lite)
- ❑ enuresis (EN-yoo-REE-sis)
- ❑ epispadias (EP-ih-SPAY-dee-as)
- ❑ erythropoietin (eh-RITH-roh-POY-eh-tin)
- ❑ excretory system (EKS-kree-toh-ree SIS-tem)
- ❑ excretory urogram (EKS-kree-toh-ree YOO-roh-gram)
- ❑ excretory urography (EKS-kree-toh-ree yoo-RAWG-rah-fee)
- ❑ extracorporeal lithotripsy (EKS-trah-kohr-POH-ree-al LITH-oh-trip-see)
- ❑ filtrate (FIL-trayt)
- ❑ filtration (fil-TRAY-shun)
- ❑ Foley catheter (FOH-lee KATH-eh-ter)
- ❑ fundus (FUN-dus)
- ❑ genitourinary system (JEN-ih-toh-YOO-rih-nair-ee SIS-tem)
- ❑ glomerular (gloh-MAIR-yoo-lar)
- ❑ glomeruli (gloh-MAIR-yoo-lie)
- ❑ glomerulonephritis (gloh-MAIR-yoo-loh-neh-FRY-tis)
- ❑ glomerulosclerosis (gloh-MAIR-yoo-loh-skleh-ROH-sis)
- ❑ glomerulus (gloh-MAIR-yoo-lus)
- ❑ glucose (GLOO-kohs)
- ❑ glycosuria (GLY-kohs-YOO-ree-ah)
- ❑ hematuria (HEE-mah-TYOO-ree-ah)
- ❑ hemodialysis (HEE-moh-dy-AL-ih-sis)
- ❑ hemoglobinuria (HEE-moh-GLOH-bih-NYOO-ree-ah)
- ❑ hila (HY-lah)
- ❑ hilar (HY-lar)
- ❑ hilum (HY-lum)
- ❑ hyaline cast (HY-ah-lin KAST)
- ❑ hydronephrosis (HY-droh-neh-FROH-sis)
- ❑ hydroureter (HY-droh-YOO-ree-ter)
- ❑ hypokalemia (HY-poh-kay-LEE-mee-ah)
- ❑ hypospadias (HY-poh-SPAY-dee-as)
- ❑ incontinence (in-CON-tih-nens)
- ❑ interstitial cystitis (IN-ter-STISH-al sis-TY-tis)
- ❑ intravenous pyelogram (IN-trah-VEE-nus PY-eh-loh-gram)
- ❑ intravenous pyelography (IN-trah-VEE-nus PY-eh-LAWG-rah-fee)
- ❑ intravesical chemotherapy (IN-trah-VES-ih-kal KEE-moh-THAIR-ah-pee)
- ❑ ketones (KEE-tohnz)
- ❑ ketonuria (KEE-toh-NYOO-ree-ah)
- ❑ kidney (KID-nee)
- ❑ kidney donor (KID-nee DOH-nor)
- ❑ kidney transplantation (KID-nee TRANS-plan-TAY-shun)
- ❑ leukocyte (LOO-koh-site)
- ❑ leukocyte esterase (LOO-koh-site ES-ter-ace)
- ❑ lithogenesis (LITH-oh-JEN-eh-sis)
- ❑ lithotripsy (LITH-oh-trip-see)
- ❑ lithotriptor (LITH-oh-trip-tor)
- ❑ loop of Henle (LOOP of HEN-lee)
- ❑ meatus (mee-AA-tus)
- ❑ medulla (meh-DOOL-ah)
- ❑ medullae (meh-DOOL-ee)
- ❑ medullary (MED-yoo-lair-ee)
- ❑ microscopic hematuria (MY-kroh-SKAWP-ik HEE-mah-TYOO-ree-ah)
- ❑ micturition (MIK-choo-RISH-un)
- ❑ mucosa (myoo-KOH-sah)
- ❑ mucosal (myoo-KOH-sal)
- ❑ nephrectomy (neh-FREK-toh-mee)
- ❑ nephritis (neh-FRY-tis)
- ❑ nephroblastoma (NEF-roh-blas-TOH-mah)
- ❑ nephrolithiasis (NEF-roh-lih-THY-ah-sis)
- ❑ nephrolithotomy (NEF-roh-lih-THAWT-oh-mee)
- ❑ nephrologist (neh-FRAWL-oh-jist)
- ❑ nephron (NEF-rawn)
- ❑ nephropathy (neh-FRAWP-ah-thee)

- ❑ nephropexy (NEF-roh-pek-see)
- ❑ nephroptosis (NEF-rawp-TOH-sis)
- ❑ nephrotic syndrome (nef-RAWT-ik SIN-drohm)
- ❑ nephrotomography (NEF-roh-toh-MAWG-rah-fee)
- ❑ nephrotoxic (NEF-roh-TAWK-sik)
- ❑ neurogenic bladder (NYOOR-oh-JEN-ik BLAD-er)
- ❑ nocturia (nawk-TYOO-ree-ah)
- ❑ occult blood (oh-KULT blud)
- ❑ oliguria (OL-ih-GYOO-ree-ah)
- ❑ parenchyma (pah-RENG-kih-mah)
- ❑ penile (PEE-nile)
- ❑ penis (PEE-nis)
- ❑ percutaneous nephrolithotomy (PER-kyoo-TAY-nee-us NEF-roh-lih-THAWT-oh-mee)
- ❑ percutaneous ultrasonic lithotripsy (PER-kyoo-TAY-nee-us UL-trah-SAWN-ik LITH-oh-trip-see)
- ❑ peristalsis (PAIR-ih-STAL-sis)
- ❑ peritoneal dialysis (PAIR-ih-toh-NEE-al dy-AL-ih-sis)
- ❑ pH (pee-H)
- ❑ polycystic kidney disease (PAWL-ee-SIS-tik KID-nee dih-ZEEZ)
- ❑ polyuria (PAWL-ee-YOO-ree-ah)
- ❑ postvoid residual (POST-voyd ree-ZID-yoo-al)
- ❑ prostate gland (PRAWS-tayt GLAND)
- ❑ prostatic (praws-TAT-ik)
- ❑ protein (PROH-teen)
- ❑ proteinuria (PROH-tee-NYOO-ree-ah)
- ❑ proximal convoluted tubule (PRAWK-sih-mal CON-voh-LOO-ted TOO-byool)
- ❑ pyelonephritis (PY-eh-loh-neh-FRY-tis)
- ❑ pyuria (py-YOO-ree-ah)
- ❑ radiation cystitis (RAY-dee-AA-shun sis-TY-tis)
- ❑ radical cystectomy (RAD-ih-kal sis-TEK-toh-mee)
- ❑ reabsorption (REE-ab-SORP-shun)
- ❑ refractometer (REE-frak-TAWM-eh-ter)
- ❑ renal (REE-nal)
- ❑ renal angiogram (REE-nal AN-jee-oh-gram)
- ❑ renal angiography (REE-nal AN-jee-AWG-rah-fee)
- ❑ renal arteriogram (REE-nal ar-TEER-ee-oh-gram)
- ❑ renal arteriography (REE-nal ar-TEER-ee-AWG-rah-fee)
- ❑ renal capsule (REE-nal KAP-sool)
- ❑ renal colic (REE-nal KAWL-ik)
- ❑ renal cortex (REE-nal KOR-teks)
- ❑ renal pelves (REE-nal PEL-veez)
- ❑ renal pelvic area (REE-nal PEL-vik AIR-ee-ah)
- ❑ renal pelvis (REE-nal PEL-vis)
- ❑ renal pyramid (REE-nal PEER-ah-mid)
- ❑ renin (REE-nin)
- ❑ resectoscope (ree-SEK-toh-skohp)
- ❑ retrograde pyelography (RET-roh-grayd PY-eh-LOG-rah-fee)
- ❑ retroperitoneal space (REH-troh-PAIR-ih-toh-NEE-al SPAYS)
- ❑ rugae (ROO-gee)
- ❑ sonogram (SAWN-oh-gram)
- ❑ sphincter (SFINGK-ter)
- ❑ suprapubic catheter (SOO-prah-PYOO-bik KATH-eh-ter)
- ❑ transurethral resection (TRANS-yoo-REE-thral ree-SEK-shun)
- ❑ trigone (TRY-gohn)
- ❑ tubular (TOO-byoo-lar)
- ❑ tubule (TOO-byool)
- ❑ turbid urine (TUR-bid YOO-rin)
- ❑ ultrasonography (UL-trah-soh-NAWG-rah-fee)
- ❑ urea (yoo-REE-ah)
- ❑ uremia (yoo-REE-mee-ah)
- ❑ uremic (yoo-REE-mik)
- ❑ ureter (YOO-ree-ter) (yoo-REE-ter)
- ❑ ureteral (yoo-REE-teh-ral)
- ❑ ureteral orifice (yoo-REE-teh-ral OR-ih-fis)
- ❑ urethra (yoo-REE-thrah)
- ❑ urethral (yoo-REE-thrawl)
- ❑ urethritis (YOO-ree-THRY-tis)
- ❑ urethroplasty (yoo-REE-throh-plas-tee)
- ❑ uric acid (YOO-rik AS-id)
- ❑ urinalysis (YOO-rih-NAL-ih-sis)
- ❑ urinary retention (YOO-rih-nair-ee ree-TEN-shun)
- ❑ urinary system (YOO-rih-nair-ee SIS-tem)
- ❑ urinary tract infection (YOO-rih-nair-ee TRAKT in-FEK-shun)
- ❑ urination (YOO-rih-NAY-shun)
- ❑ urine (YOO-rin)
- ❑ urinometer (YOO-rih-NAWM-eh-ter)
- ❑ urogenital system (YOO-roh-JEN-ih-tal SIS-tem)
- ❑ urologist (yoo-RAWL-oh-jist)
- ❑ urology (yoo-RAWL-oh-jee)
- ❑ vesical (VES-ih-kal)
- ❑ vesicocele (VES-ih-koh-seel)
- ❑ vesicovaginal fistula (VES-ih-koh-VAJ-ih-nal FIS-tyoo-lah)
- ❑ void (VOYD)
- ❑ voiding cystourethrogram (VOY-ding SIS-toh-yoo-REE-throh-gram)
- ❑ voiding cystourethrography (VOY-ding SIS-toh-YOO-ree-THRAWG-rah-fee)
- ❑ Wilms' tumor (WILMZ TOO-mor)

Experience Multimedia

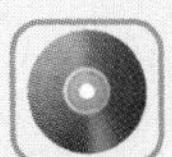

CD-ROM Learning Activities Checklist

Check off the box as you complete each learning activity.

❑ **CD-ROM Learning Activity 11.1: *ANATOMY WORD PARTS FLASHCARDS***
Use flashcards to help you memorize word parts. Make your own flashcards or print out prepared flashcards. Also see the electronic flashcard game. Time: 20 minutes.

❑ **CD-ROM Learning Activity 11.2: *MEDICINE IN ACTION***
Watch a video clip of how a urinalysis is performed. Time: 5 minutes.

❑ **CD-ROM Learning Activity 11.3: *DISEASE AND OTHER WORD PARTS FLASHCARDS***
A continuation of the flashcard learning activity. Time: 20 minutes.

❑ **CD-ROM Learning Activity 11.4: *MEMORY AIDS***
Use memory aids to help you memorize medical words and meanings. Time: 5 minutes.

❑ **CD-ROM Learning Activity 11.5: *MEDICAL LANGUAGE SPOKEN HERE***
Listen to actual medical reports and spell the missing medical words. Time: 20 minutes.

❑ **CD-ROM Learning Activity 11.6: *SPELLING CHALLENGE***
Listen to a pronounced medical word and then spell it. Time: 5 minutes.

❑ **CD-ROM Learning Activity 11.7: *MEDICAL LANGUAGE PRONUNCIATION***
Listen to a pronounced medical word and then practice pronouncing it. Time: 30 minutes.

❑ **CD-ROM Learning Activity 11.8: *EDUCATIONAL FUN AND GAMES***
Enjoy these fun activities while reinforcing your knowledge. Time: 15 minutes.

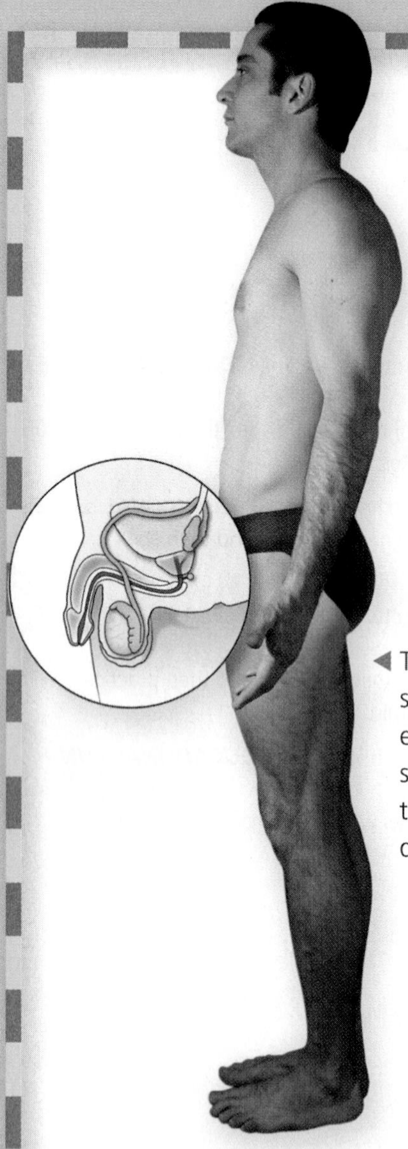

The male reproductive system consists of external and internal structures designed to produce and deposit sperm.

Dive In!

- The sperm of a man is half the size of that of a mouse.
- Viagra was initially used as a treatment for high blood pressure.
- Ready to multiply your odds for success? In this chapter we'll explore the language that describes the genitourinary system structures, functions, diseases, and conditions.
- You'll plant the seeds of knowledge once you master the language of male reproduction!

A spermatozoon is nearly 100,000 times smaller than the ovum.

Medicine Through HISTORY

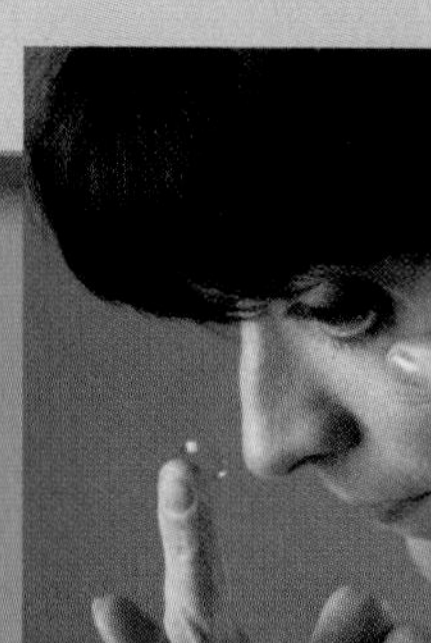

1936

The hard contact lens is invented by an optometrist in New York

1938

The March of Dimes begins to raise money for polio research

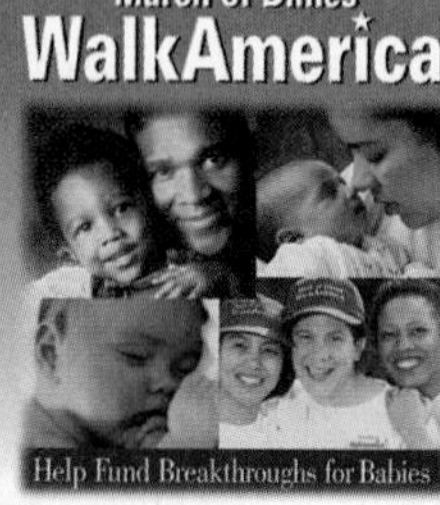

CHAPTER 12

Male Reproductive Medicine

Male Genitourinary System

Male reproductive (RE-proh-DUK-tive) medicine is the medical specialty that studies the anatomy and physiology of the male genitourinary system and uses diagnostic tests, medical and surgical procedures, and drugs to treat male reproductive diseases.

▶ Roosters are male chickens and they showcase their colorful feathers to attract mates for reproduction.

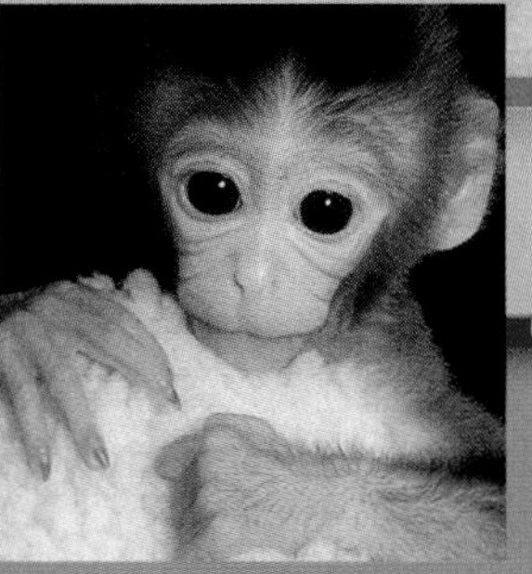

1940

The Rh blood group (first discovered in the Rhesus monkey) is identified by Dr. Karl Landsteiner of Austria

1941

The first commercial batches of the antibiotic drug penicillin became available

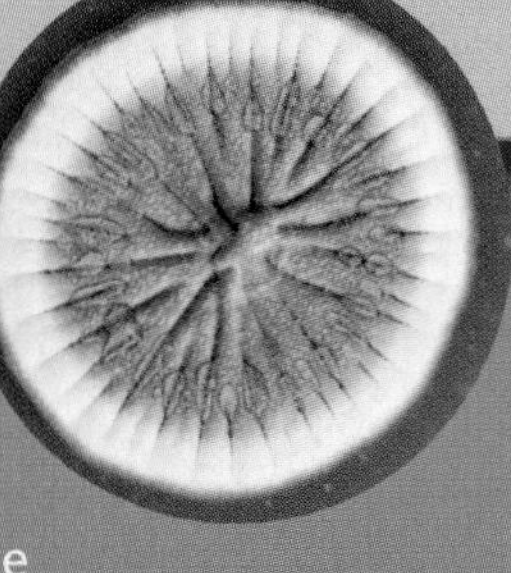

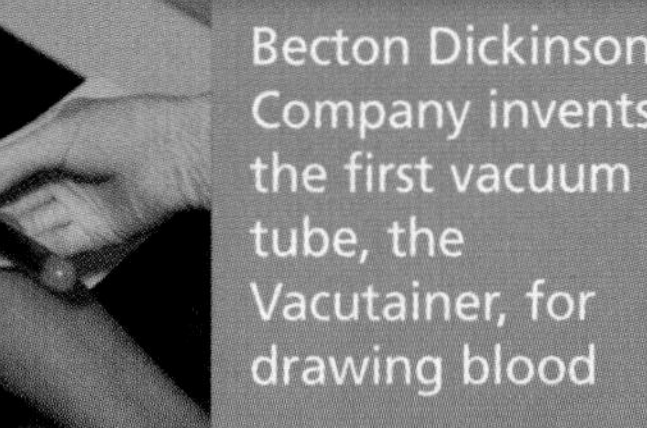

1943

Becton Dickinson Company invents the first vacuum tube, the Vacutainer, for drawing blood

Measure Your Progress: Learning Objectives

After you study this chapter, you should be able to

1. Identify the anatomical structures of the male genitourinary system by correctly labeling them on an anatomical illustration.
2. Describe the processes of spermatogenesis and ejaculation.
3. Build male genitourinary words from combining forms, prefixes, and suffixes.
4. Describe common male genitourinary diseases.
5. Describe common male genitourinary diagnostic laboratory and radiology tests.
6. Describe common male genitourinary medical and surgical procedures and drug categories.
7. Define common male genitourinary abbreviations.
8. Correctly spell and pronounce male genitourinary words.
9. Apply your skills by analyzing a male reproductive medicine report.
10. Test your knowledge of male reproductive medicine by completing review exercises at the end of the chapter and learning activities on the CD-ROM.

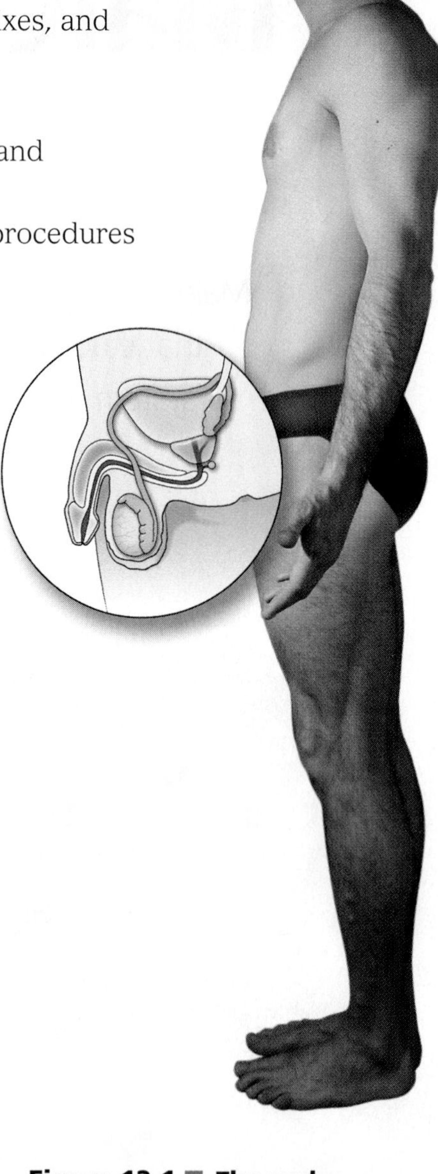

Figure 12-1 ■ The male genitourinary system.

The male genitourinary system is located in the pelvic cavity and outside the body in the area below the pelvic cavity.

Medical Language Key

To unlock the meaning of a medical word, first define each word part. Then put the word part definitions in order, beginning with the suffix, followed by the first word part, then the other word parts in order.

	Word Part	Word Part Definition
SUFFIX	-ive	*pertaining to*
PREFIX	re-	*again and again; backward; unable to*
COMBINING FORM	product/o-	*produce*

Reproductive Medicine: *Medical field pertaining to the continuing function of producing children.*

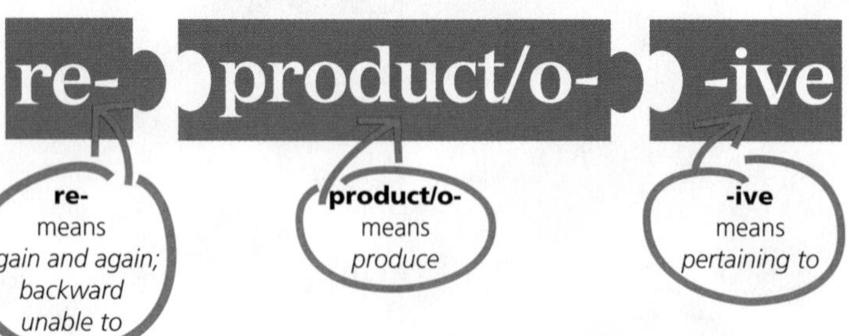

www.prenhall.com/turley

For interactive flashcards, real-life video clips, games, exercises, and audio pronunciations please explore the companion CD-ROM in the back of the book. Click on the companion website for bonus chapters, additional resources, and links to on-line learning.

Anatomy and Physiology

The **male genitourinary (GU) system** is a body system that is composed of the external and internal genitalia or **genital organs** (see Figure 12-1 ■). The **external genitalia** on the outside of the body include the scrotum, testes, epididymis, penis, and urethra. The **internal genitalia** in the pelvic cavity include the vas deferens, seminal vesicle, ejaculatory duct (one of each on both sides), and prostate gland. The male genitourinary system shares the urethra with the urinary system and is known as the urogenital system because of the close proximity and shared structures of these two body systems. The function of the male genitourinary system is to display the male secondary sex characteristics, produce sperm, and, when appropriate, deposit sperm inside the female.

genitourinary
(JEN-ih-toh-YOO-rih-nair-ee)
genit/o- *genitalia*
urin/o- *urine; urinary system*
-ary *pertaining to*

system (SIS-tem)
System is derived from a Greek word meaning *combination of parts to make an organized whole.*

genital (JEN-ih-tal)
genit/o- *genitalia*
-al *pertaining to*

external (eks-TER-nal)
extern/o- *outside*
-al *pertaining to*

genitalia (JEN-ih-TAY-lee-ah)
Genitalia is a Latin word meaning *generation and birth.*

internal (in-TER-nal)
intern/o- *inside*
-al *pertaining to*

Anatomy of the Male Genitourinary System

Scrotum

The **scrotum** is a soft pouch of skin behind the penis and in front of the legs (see Figure 12-2 ■). The scrotum is always a few degrees cooler than the core body temperature. This temperature difference is necessary for the proper development of spermatozoa. Muscles in the wall of the scrotum contract or relax to move the pouch closer to or farther away from the body to adjust to temperature changes in the environment. The **perineum** is the area between the anus and where the scrotum attaches to the body.

scrotum (SKROH-tum)
Scrotum is a Latin word meaning *a bag.*

scrotal (SKROH-tal)
scrot/o- *a bag; scrotum*
-al *pertaining to*

perineum (PAIR-ih-NEE-um)
Perineum is a Latin word meaning *the area between the vulva or scrotum and the anus.*

perineal (PAIR-ih-NEE-al)
perine/o- *perineum*
-al *pertaining to*

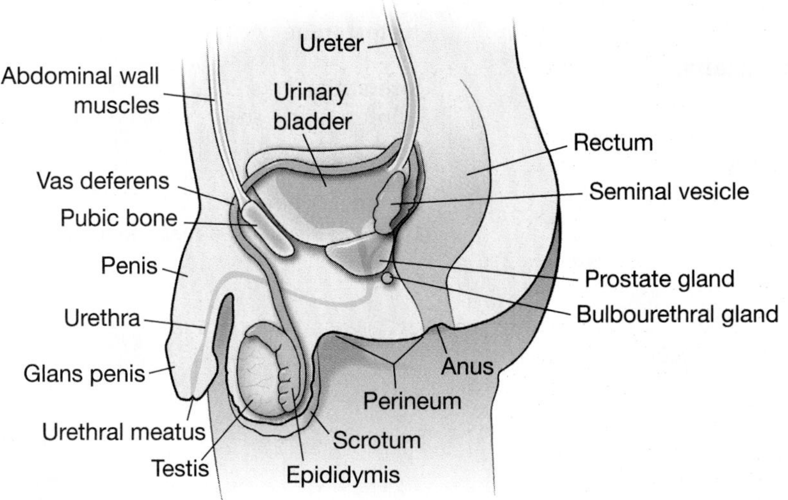

Figure 12-2 ■ External and internal male genitalia.
This midsagittal view shows the interconnected relationship of the external and internal male genitalia. The urinary bladder is in the area of the internal male genitalia. The urethra is shared by the male genitourinary system and the urinary system.

Testis and Epididymis

The scrotum contains the **testes** or **testicles.** Each testis is a flat, oval-shaped gland about 2 inches in length (see Figures 12-2 and 12-3■). The testes are the male **gonads** or sex glands. They function as part of both the male genitourinary system and the endocrine system.

As part of the male genitourinary system, the testes contain the **seminiferous tubules,** a series of compartmentalized, tightly coiled tubules that produce **spermatozoa** or **sperm.** As part of the endocrine system, the testes act as glands that secrete testosterone when stimulated by hormones from the anterior pituitary gland in the brain. The hormone **testosterone,** the most abundant and biologically active of all the male sex hormones, is secreted by the **interstitial cells** (between the seminiferous tubules). The testes also secrete a small amount of the female hormone estradiol. Testosterone also stimulates the maturation of spermatozoa. Mature spermatozoa are continuously released into the **lumen** of the seminiferous tubules and carried by fluid into the epididymis.

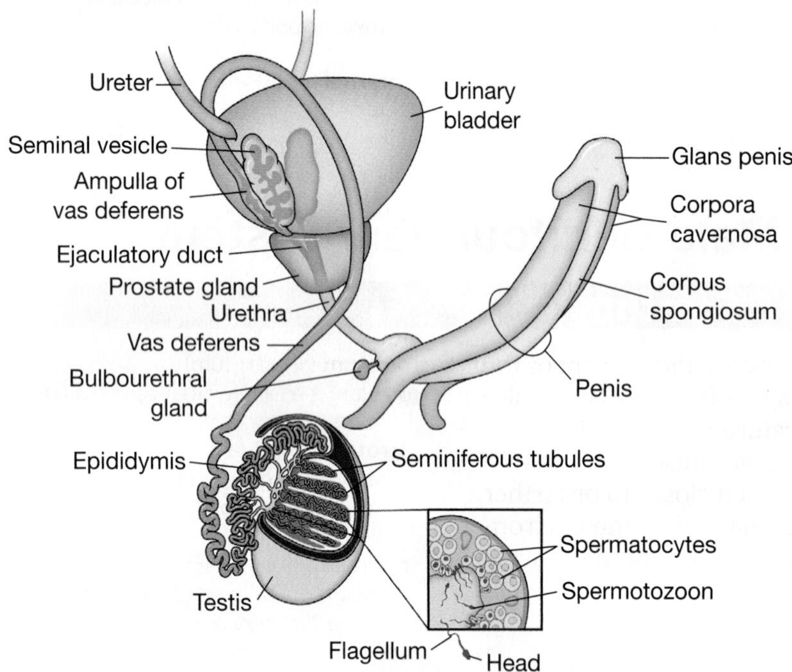

Figure 12-3 ■ External and internal male genitalia.

Notice the tightly coiled seminiferous tubules and epididymis that become the single tubule of the vas deferens that connects the external genitalia to the internal genitalia. The three columns of erectile tissue in the penis can be seen clearly.

testis (TES-tis)
testes (TES-teez)
Testis means *a witness.* The testes in the scrotum were a visible witness of manhood. *Testis* is a Latin singular noun. Form the plural by changing *-is* to *-es.*

testicle (TES-tih-kl)
Testicle is a combination of *testis* and the suffix *-cle* (small thing). *Testis* and *testicle* are used interchangeably (like *drop* and *droplet*), without implying any difference in their sizes.

testicular (tes-TIK-yoo-lar)
testicul/o- *testis; testicle*
-ar *pertaining to*

gonad (GOH-nad)
gon/o- *seed (ovum or spermatozoon)*
-ad *toward, in the direction of*
The gonads include the testes in men that produce spermatozoa and the ovaries in women that produce ova.

seminiferous (SEM-ih-NIF-er-us)
semin/i- *spermatozoon; sperm*
fer/o- *to bear*
-ous *pertaining to*

tubule (TOO-byool)
tub/o- *tube*
-ule *small thing*

spermatozoon (SPER-mah-toh-ZOH-on)
spermatozoa (SPER-mah-toh-ZOH-ah)
spermat/o- *spermatozoon; sperm*
-zoon *animal; living thing*
Spermatozoon is a Greek noun. Form the plural by changing *-on* to *-a.*

sperm (SPERM)
Sperm is derived from a Greek word meaning *seed.*

testosterone (tes-TAWS-teh-rohn)

interstitial (IN-ter-STISH-al)
interstiti/o- *spaces within tissue*
-al *pertaining to*

lumen (LOO-men)
Lumen is a Latin word meaning *a window.*

The **epididymis** is a long, coiled tube (over 20 feet in length) that is attached to the outer wall of each testis (see Figures 12-2 and 12-3). The epididymis is a storage and processing area for spermatozoa. Here, the head of each spermatozoon is given a cap, a layer of enzymes that will help it penetrate and fertilize the ovum of the female. The epididymis also destroys defective spermatozoa. Spermatozoa in the epididymis are mature but not yet **motile.** The inferior section of the epididymis makes a U-turn, and the tubules in the epididymis become one large duct known as the ductus deferens or vas deferens.

epididymis (EP-ih-DID-ih-mis)
epididymides (EP-ih-dih-DIM-ih-deez)
epi- *upon, above*
-didymis *testes (twin structures)*
Epididymis is a Greek singular noun. Form the plural by changing *-is* to *-ides.*

epididymal (EP-ih-DID-ih-mal)
epi- *upon, above*
didym/o- *testes (twin structures)*
-al *pertaining to*
Didym/o- is a Greek combining form meaning *the twins.* The testes are the twin structures in the scrotum.

motile (MOH-til)
mot/o- *movement*
-ile *pertaining to*

Across the Life Span

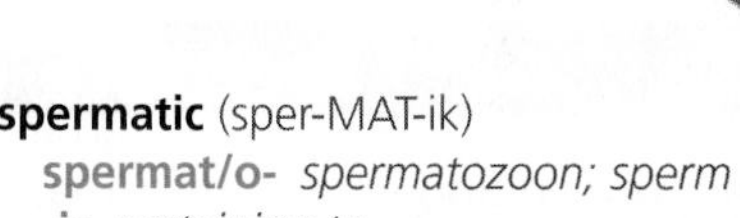

Before birth, the fetal testes develop in the abdominal cavity, not in the scrotum. Two months before birth, both testes move through the pelvic cavity into the scrotum. Each testis has an accompanying spermatic cord that descends with it. The **spermatic cord** is a muscular tube that contains arteries, veins, nerves, and the vas deferens (the tube that will carry sperm in the adult male). Each testis with its spermatic cord enters the **inguinal canal,** a passageway that goes through abdominal muscles, over the pubic bone, through the groin (area of the skin crease at the top of the leg), to the scrotum (see Figure 12-4 ■). At birth or before 2 years of age, the inguinal canal closes. If the inguinal canal fails to close, a loop of intestine can go through the inguinal canal and create a bulge in the groin or in the scrotum. This is known as an indirect inguinal hernia. It can occur in childhood or any time in adulthood.

spermatic (sper-MAT-ik)
spermat/o- *spermatozoon; sperm*
-ic *pertaining to*

inguinal (ING-gwih-nal)
inguin/o- *groin*
-al *pertaining to*

canal (kah-NAL)
A canal is a tubular channel.

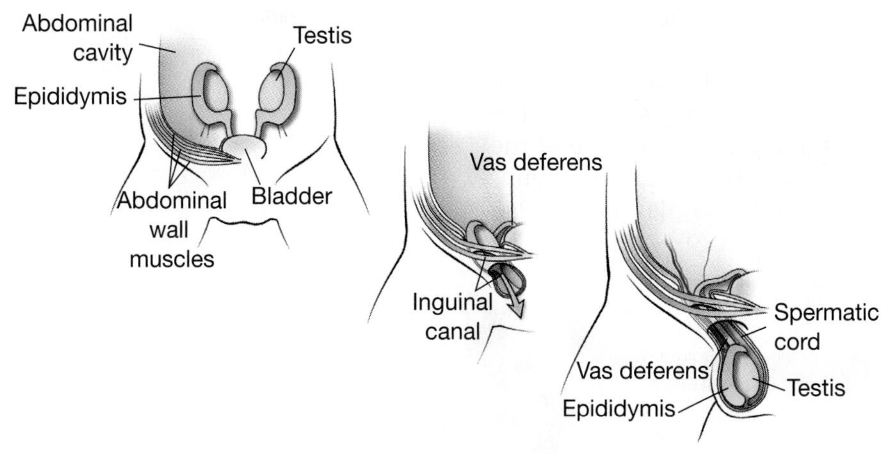

Figure 12-4 ■ Testes.
Before birth, the testes and their spermatic cords move from the abdominal cavity, through the inguinal canals, and into the scrotum.

Vas Deferens, Seminal Vesicles, and Ejaculatory Duct

The **vas deferens,** also known as the **ductus deferens,** is a very long, narrow tube that receives spermatozoa from the epididymis (see Figures 12-2 and 12-3). Spermatozoa can be stored in the vas deferens for several months in an inactive state. From the epididymis, the vas deferens continues superiorly through the inguinal canal as part of the spermatic cord. At the superior end of the inguinal canal, however, the vas deferens continues on alone and goes behind the urinary bladder. There, the vas deferens merges with the duct of a seminal vesicle. The **seminal vesicles** are two elongated glands that form a *V* along the posterior wall of the urinary bladder. The seminal vesicles produce **seminal fluid,** which makes up most of the volume of **semen.** The **ejaculatory duct** is a large collecting area for spermatozoa from each vas deferens and seminal fluid from the seminal vesicles. The ejaculatory duct goes into the superior aspect of the prostate gland and empties into the urethra within the prostate gland.

vas deferens (VAS DEF-er-enz)
Vas is a Latin word meaning *a vessel. Deferens* is derived from a Latin word meaning *to carry away.*

ductus (DUK-tus)
Ductus is a Latin word meaning *to lead.*

seminal (SEM-ih-nal)
semin/o- *spermatozoon; sperm*
-al *pertaining to*

vesicle (VES-ih-kl)
Vesicle is derived from a Latin word meaning *little fluid-filled sac.*

semen (SEE-men)
Semen is a Latin word meaning *seed.*

ejaculatory (ee-JAK-yoo-lah-tohr-ree)
ejaculat/o- *to expel suddenly*
-ory *having the function of*

Prostate Gland and Bulbourethral Glands

The **prostate gland** is a round gland at the base of the bladder (see Figures 12-2 and 12-3). It completely surrounds the first part of the urethra (the prostatic urethra). The prostate gland is not part of the urinary system, however. The prostate gland produces **prostatic fluid,** a milky substance that makes up some of the volume of semen. Prostatic fluid is secreted into the urethra through many tiny ducts. This fluid contains an antibiotic that acts against bacteria in the woman's vagina, as well as a substance that activates enzymes in the head of a spermatozoon so that it can penetrate the woman's ovum to fertilize it. Prostatic fluid also contains acid phosphatase, an enzyme that breaks the deposit of semen apart and releases the spermatozoa in the woman's vagina.

The **bulbourethral glands** are small, bulblike glands about the size of peas that are located on either side of the urethra just below the prostate gland. They produce thick mucus that makes up some of the volume of the semen and neutralizes the acidity of any urine remaining in the urethra at the time of ejaculation. These glands are also known as Cowper's glands.

prostate (PRAWS-tayt)
Prostate is derived from a Greek word meaning *one who stands before.*

prostatic (praws-TAT-ik)
prostat/o- *prostate gland*
-ic *pertaining to*

bulbourethral (BUL-boh-yoo-REE-thral)
bulb/o- *like a bulb*
urethr/o- *urethra*
-al *pertaining to*

Word Alert

SOUND-ALIKE WORDS

prostate (noun) gland that surrounds the urethra in men
Example: When the prostate gland is enlarged, it interferes with urination in men.

prostrate (adjective) descriptive word for *lying in a face-down position from humility or exhaustion*
Example: After the marathon race, the exhausted winner lay prostrate on the track.

Penis

The **penis** functions as an organ of the male genitourinary system and the urinary system (see Figures 12-2 and 12-3). The urethra of the urinary system passes through the length of the penis. The urethral meatus is located at the tip of the **glans penis.** In uncircumcised men, the urethral meatus is covered by the **prepuce** or foreskin of the penis. The urethra is also part of the male genitourinary system and serves as a passageway for semen.

Three columns of erectile tissue run the length of the penis. Two of the columns, the **corpora cavernosa,** are located along the upper surface of the penis. The third column, the **corpus spongiosum,** is centered along the underside of the penis. The urethra is located within the corpus spongiosum. These three columns are composed of **erectile tissue** that fills with blood during sexual arousal, causing the penis to become firm and erect (an **erection**).

penis (PEE-nis)
Penis is a Latin word meaning *a tail.*

penile (PEE-nile)
pen/o- *penis*
-ile *pertaining to*

glans penis (GLANZ PEE-nis)
Glans is a Latin word meaning *acorn,* a reference to the shape of the head of the penis.

prepuce (PREE-poos)
Prepuce is a combination of the prefix *pre-* (before, in front of) and the Latin word *putos* (penis).

corpora cavernosa
(KOR-por-ah KAV-er-NOH-sah)
Corpus is a Latin singular masculine noun meaning *body.* Form the plural by changing *-us* to *-ora.*

corpus spongiosum
(KOR-puhs SPUN-jee-OH-sum)
There is one corpus spongiosum, but two corpora cavernosa.

erectile (ee-REK-tile)
erect/o- *to stand up*
-ile *pertaining to*

erection (ee-REK-shun)
erect/o- *to stand up*
-ion *action; condition*

Physiology of Spermatogenesis and Ejaculation

Spermatogenesis

During childhood, the outer walls of the seminiferous tubules contain immature cells known as **spermatocytes.** These cells are round and each contains 46 chromosomes. At the onset of **puberty** or **adolescence,** the anterior pituitary gland of the endocrine system, discussed in Endocrinology (Chapter 14), begins to secrete hormones to stimulate the testes. **Follicle-stimulating hormone (FSH)** causes the seminiferous tubules to enlarge. Because these tubules comprise 80% of the structure of the testes, the testes themselves enlarge significantly during puberty. FSH also stimulates the spermatocytes to begin to divide. **Luteinizing hormone (LH)** causes the interstitial cells to begin to produce testosterone.

During puberty, testosterone causes the development of the male sex characteristics: enlargement of the external genitalia; development of large body muscles; deepening of the voice (as the larynx widens); growth of body hair on the face, axillary, and genital areas; and development of the sexual drive (see Figure 12-5■).

spermatocyte (SPER-mah-toh-site)
spermat/o- *spermatozoon; sperm*
-cyte *cell*

puberty (PYOO-ber-tee)
puber/o- *growing up*
-ty *quality or state*
Puberty is derived from a Greek word meaning *grown up.* Puberty is a series of physical events of growth and the development of sexual maturity.

adolescence (AD-oh-LES-ens)
adolesc/o- *the beginning of being an adult*
-ence *state of*
Adolescence is a life stage that begins with puberty and ends with physical maturity.

follicle (FAWL-ih-kl)
FSH is so named because it stimulates both spermatocytes as well as follicles in the female ovaries that contain immature eggs.

luteinizing (LOO-tee-ih-ny-zing)
Luteinizing hormone is so named because it stimulates interstitial cells of the testes as well as the corpus luteum of the ovary.

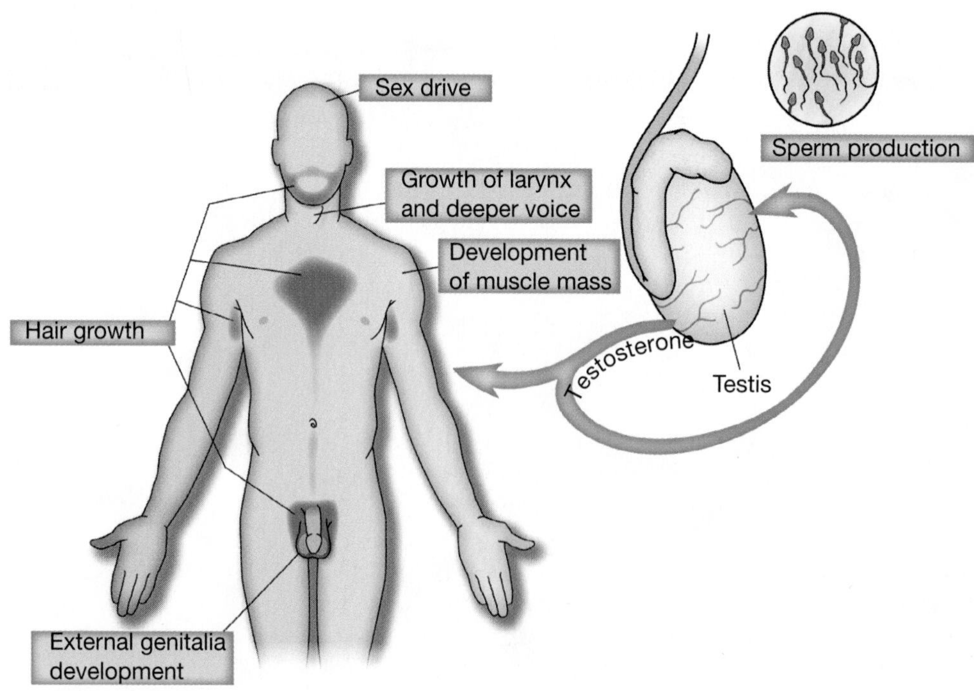

Figure 12-5 ■ Testosterone.

Testosterone is secreted by interstitial cells between the seminiferous tubules of the testes. Testosterone causes the development of the male sex characteristics during puberty. It also causes spermatozoa to develop and mature.

A Closer Look

Most cells in the body divide by the process of **mitosis,** in which the 46 chromosomes in the nucleus duplicate and then split, creating two identical cells each with 46 chromosomes. However, the spermatozoon is different from other cells in the body. It is created by mitosis and **meiosis.** First, the 46 chromosomes in the immature spermatocyte duplicate by mitosis, and the duplicated chromosomes group together and randomly exchange genetic material. This is how different combinations of genes from previous generations are passed on to offspring. Then the spermatocyte divides two more times into four individual spermatozoon, each with 23 chromosomes or half the usual number. Each spermatozoon is composed of a head that contains the 23 chromosomes and a tail or **flagellum** that propels it. The process of forming mature spermatozoa is known as **spermatogenesis.**

Spermatozoa (and ova from the female) that have only half of the usual number of chromosomes are known as **gametes.**

mitosis (my-TOH-sis)
mit/o- *threadlike structure*
-osis *condition; abnormal condition; process*
When a cell is not dividing, the chromosomes appear as loosely arranged threads in the nucleus.

meiosis (my-OH-sis)
Meiosis is a Greek word meaning *lessening.*

flagellum (flah-JEL-um)
Flagellum is a Latin word meaning *a little whip.* A spermatozoon is the only cell in the human body that has a flagellum.

spermatogenesis (SPER-mah-toh-JEN-eh-sis)
spermat/o- *spermatozoon; sperm*
gen/o- *arising from; produced by*
-esis *condition*

gamete (GAM-eet)
Gamete is derived from two closely related Greek words, one of which means *husband* and the other means *wife.* A gamete can be either the spermatozoon or the ovum (*egg*).

Ejaculation

The process of ejaculation begins in response to thoughts or sensations that initiate sexual arousal. Smooth muscles in the walls of arteries in the penis relax, allowing increased blood flow into the penis. The corpora cavernosa and the corpus spongiosum distend with blood and produce an erection.

Stimulation from the sympathetic nervous system causes muscles in the perineum at the base of the penis to contract. Spermatozoa in the vas deferens move into the ejaculatory duct, where they are mixed with fluid from the seminal vesicles. This fluid has a high level of sugar, a source of energy for the spermatozoa. It is at this point that the spermatozoa become active. Then the spermatozoa move into the urethra. The prostate gland contracts, forcing prostatic fluid through ducts into the urethra. As the spermatozoa move through the urethra, they are mixed with thick mucus from the bulbourethral glands. Semen is a combination of spermatozoa and secretions from the seminal vesicles, prostate gland, and the bulbourethral glands. A series of contractions of the muscles around the penis and pelvic area cause 2 to 5 mL of semen to be expelled from the penis through the urethral meatus. This process is known as **ejaculation.** Within this small volume of semen are 100 to 500 million spermatozoa! Sugar and other nutrients in the semen keep the spermatozoa motile and strong as they travel through the female cervix, uterus, and fallopian tube to fertilize an ovum.

ejaculation (ee-JAK-yoo-LAY-shun)
ejaculat/o- *to expel suddenly*
-ion *action; condition*

Vocabulary Review

Anatomy and Physiology

Now that you have studied the anatomy and physiology of the male genitourinary system, take time to review those new words and descriptions. Memorize the combining forms and their definitions before going on to the next section.

Word or Phrase	Combining Form and Definition	Description
bulbourethral glands	bulb/o- *like a bulb* urethr/o- *urethra*	Small, bulblike glands below the prostate that secrete mucus into the urethra during ejaculation. Also known as Cowper's glands.
ejaculation	ejaculat/o- *to expel suddenly*	Sudden expulsion of semen from the penis during sexual arousal of the male
ejaculatory duct	ejaculat/o- *to expel suddenly*	Duct that collects semen from both the vas deferens and the seminal vesicles and empties into the urethra during ejaculation
epididymis	didym/o- *testes (twin structures)*	Long, coiled tube on the outer wall of each testis. It receives spermatozoa from the seminiferous tubules, stores them, and destroys defective spermatozoa.
external genitalia	extern/o- *outside*	Scrotum, testes, epididymides, penis, and urethra.
flagellum	mot/o- *movement*	The long tail on a spermatozoon that propels it and makes it **motile**
FSH		**Follicle-stimulating hormone** from the anterior pituitary gland. It causes the seminiferous tubules of the testes to enlarge during puberty.
gamete		A cell (ovum or spermatozoon) that has 23 chromosomes instead of the usual 46 chromosomes like other cells of the body
genital organs	genit/o- *genitalia*	Male internal and external **genitalia**
genitourinary system	genit/o- *genitalia* urin/o- *urine; urinary system* ur/o- *urine; urinary system*	Two closely related body systems that share some of the same structures: the male genital system and the urinary system. Also known as the **urogenital system.**
gonads	gon/o- *seed (ovum or spermatozoon)*	The male sex glands (i.e., the testes)
inguinal canal	inguin/o- *groin*	Passageway in the groin area through which the testes travel as they descend from the abdomen to the scrotum. The open canal closes snugly around the spermatic cord at birth or shortly thereafter.
internal genitalia	intern/o- *inside*	Vas deferens, seminal vesicals, ejaculatory ducts, and prostate gland in the pelvic cavity
interstitial cells	interstiti/o- *spaces within tissue*	Special cells between the seminiferous tubules of the testes. These cells secrete testosterone when stimulated by luteinizing hormone (LH).
LH		**Luteinizing hormone** from the anterior pituitary gland. It causes the interstitial cells of the testes to secrete testosterone.

Word or Phrase	Combining Form and Definition	Description
lumen		Central open area throughout the length of a tube or duct (such as the seminiferous tubule, vas deferens, ejaculatory duct, or urethra)
meiosis		Process by which a spermatocyte reduces the number of chromosomes in its nucleus to 23, or half the normal number, to create gametes
mitosis	**mit/o-** *threadlike structure*	Process by which most body cells reproduce. The 46 chromosomes in the nucleus duplicate, and then split, creating two identical cells each with 46 chromosomes.
penis	**pen/o-** *penis* **erect/o-** *to stand up*	Organ of **erectile tissue** that fills with blood during male sexual arousal. The **corpora cavernosa** are two columns of tissue that fill with blood along the upper surface of the penis. The **corpus spongiosum** is a column of tissue that fills with blood on the underside of the penis. The urethra travels through the corpus spongiosum. During sexual arousal, the penis becomes firm and erect (an erection).
perineum	**perine/o-** *perineum*	Area of skin between the anus and where the scrotum attaches to the body
prostate gland	**prostat/o-** *prostate gland*	Round gland at the base of the bladder. It surrounds the first part of the urethra. It produces **prostatic fluid** that contributes to the volume of semen.
puberty	**puber/o-** *growing up*	Period of time when FSH and LH from the anterior pituitary gland first begin to stimulate the testes. The male sexual characteristics develop, and there is a growth spurt. Also known as **adolescence.**
scrotum	**scrot/o-** *scrotum*	Pouch of skin that holds the two testes
semen		Fluid expelled from the penis during ejaculation. Semen contains spermatozoa, seminal fluid, prostatic fluid, and mucus from the bulbourethral glands.
seminal vesicles	**semin/o-** *spermatozoon; semen*	Glands along the posterior wall of the bladder that secrete **seminal fluid,** a source of energy for the spermatozoa and the main component of semen
seminiferous tubules	**semin/i-** *spermatozoon; semen* **fer/o-** *to bear* **tub/o-** *tube*	Tubules within each testis where spermatozoa develop
spermatic cord	**spermat/o-** *spermatozoon; sperm*	Muscular tube that contains arteries, veins, and nerves for each testis as well as the vas deferens. It passes through the inguinal canal.
spermatocyte	**spermat/o-** *spermatozoon; sperm*	Immature spermatozoon in the wall of the seminiferous tubule.
spermatogenesis	**spermat/o-** *spermatozoon; sperm*	Process of producing a mature spermatozoon through the processes of mitosis and meiosis
spermatozoon	**spermat/o-** *spermatozoon; sperm*	An individual mature sperm. It contains 23 chromosomes and is known as a gamete. Also known as sperm.
testes	**testicul/o-** *testis; testicle*	Small, egg-shaped glands in the scrotum. Also known as the **testicles.** They contain interstitial cells that secrete testosterone. They also contain the seminiferous tubules that produce spermatozoa.

Word or Phrase	Combining Form and Definition	Description
testosterone		Most abundant and most biologically active of the male sex hormones secreted by the testes. It causes the development of the male sex characteristics during puberty. Testosterone produces mature spermatozoa.
vas deferens		Long tube that receives spermatozoa from the epididymis and carries them to the seminal vesicles. Also known as the **ductus deferens.**

Labeling Exercise

Match each anatomy word or phrase to its numbered structure in Figure 12-6 ■. Write that word or phrase on the blank line next to its number. Use the Answer Key at the end of the book to check your answers.

abdominal wall muscles	epididymis	pubic bone	ureter
anus	glans penis	rectum	urethra
bulbourethral gland	inguinal canal	scrotum	urethral meatus
corpus cavernosum	penis	seminal vesicle	urinary bladder
corpus spongiosum	perineum	testis	vas deferens
ejaculatory duct	prostate gland		

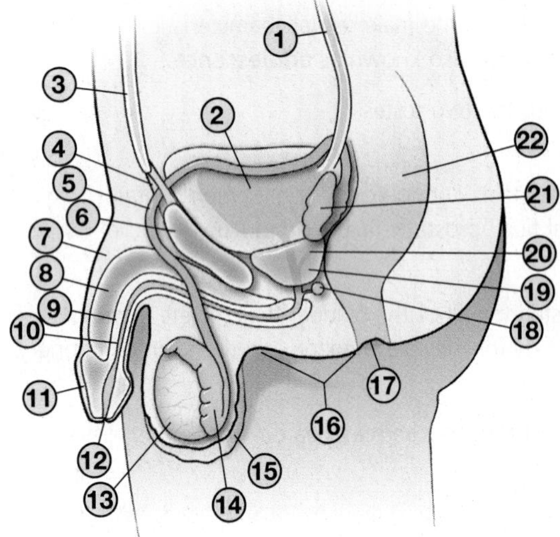

Figure 12-6 ■

1. ____________________
2. ____________________
3. ____________________
4. ____________________
5. ____________________
6. ____________________
7. ____________________
8. ____________________
9. ____________________
10. ____________________
11. ____________________
12. ____________________
13. ____________________
14. ____________________
15. ____________________
16. ____________________
17. ____________________
18. ____________________
19. ____________________
20. ____________________
21. ____________________
22. ____________________

Building Medical Words

Combining Forms

Here are the combining forms you have learned so far. Next to each combining form, write its meaning. Use the Answer Key at the end of the book to check your answers. The first one has been done for you.

	Combining Form	Medical Meaning		Combining Form	Medical Meaning
1.	adolesc/o-	the beginning of being an adult	15.	mot/o-	________
2.	bulb/o-	________	16.	pen/o-	________
3.	didym/o-	________	17.	perine/o-	________
4.	ejaculat/o-	________	18.	product/o-	________
5.	erect/o-	________	19.	prostat/o-	________
6.	extern/o-	________	20.	puber/o-	________
7.	fer/o-	________	21.	scrot/o-	________
8.	genit/o-	________	22.	semin/i-	________
9.	gen/o-	________	23.	semin/o-	________
10.	gon/o-	________	24.	spermat/o-	________
11.	inguin/o-	________	25.	testicul/o-	________
12.	intern/o-	________	26.	tub/o-	________
13.	interstiti/o-	________	27.	urethr/o-	________
14.	mit/o-	________	28.	urin/o-	________

Combining Forms and Suffixes

Read the definition hint for the medical word you are to build. Look at the combining form that is given. Write the correct suffix on the blank line. Then write the medical word. (Remember: You may need to remove the combining vowel. Always remove the hyphens and slash.) Use the Answer Key at the end of the book to check your answers. The first one has been done for you.

SUFFIX LIST

-ar (pertaining to)	-ence (state of)	-ion (action; condition)	-ty (quality or state)
-al (pertaining to)	-ic (pertaining to)	-ory (having the function of)	-ule (small thing)
-cyte (cell)	-ile (pertaining to)		

	Definition Hint	Combining Form	Suffix	Write the Medical Word
1.	Pertaining to the cavity within the hip bones	pelv/o-	-ic	pelvic
2.	Pertaining to the scrotum	scrot/o-	______	______
3.	State of growing up	puber/o-	______	______
4.	Immature cell that will produce sperm	spermat/o-	______	______
5.	Pertaining to a small tube	tub/o-	______	______
6.	An action of standing up	erect/o-	______	______
7.	State of the beginning of being an adult	adolesc/o-	______	______
8.	Pertaining to the genitalia	genit/o-	______	______
9.	Pertaining to the testes	testicul/o-	______	______
10.	Pertaining to the penis	pen/o-	______	______
11.	Pertaining to the prostate	prostat/o-	______	______
12.	Having the function of expelling suddenly	ejaculat/o-	______	______
13.	Pertaining to movement	mot/o-	______	______
14.	Pertaining to the groin	inguin/o-	______	______

Symptoms, Signs, and Diseases

Testis and Epididymis

Word or Phrase	Word Part and Definition	Description
cryptorchism	**cryptorchism** (krip-TOHR-kiz-em) crypt/o- *hidden* orch/o- *testis* -ism *process; disease from a specific cause*	Failure of one or both of the testicles to descend through the inguinal canal into the scrotum. This causes a low sperm count and male infertility. Also known as cryptorchidism. Treatment: Orchiopexy.
epididymitis	**epididymitis** (EP-ih-DID-ih-MY-tis) epi- *upon, above* didym/o- *testes (twin structures)* -itis *inflammation of*	Inflammation and infection of the epididymis. Caused by a bacterial urinary tract infection or sexually transmitted diseases like gonorrhea or Chlamydia. Treatment: Antibiotic drugs.
infertility	**infertility** (IN-fer-TIL-ih-tee) in- *in; within; not* fertil/o- *able to conceive a child* -ity *state; condition*	Failure to conceive after at least one year of regular intercourse. Can be caused by hormonal imbalance involving FSH or LH, undescended testicles, genetic abnormalities, damage to the testes from mumps, infection, abnormalities of the spermatozoa, and other causes. Treatment: Correct the underlying cause.
oligospermia	**oligospermia** (OHL-ih-goh-SPER-mee-ah) olig/o- *scanty* sperm/o- *spermatozoon; sperm* -ia *condition, state, thing*	Less than normal amount of spermatozoa produced by the testes. This results in male infertility. Caused by a hormone imbalance or an undescended testicle. Treatment: Correct the underlying cause.
orchitis	**orchitis** (or-KY-tis) orch/o- *testis* -itis *inflammation of*	Inflammation or infection of the testes. Caused by a bacterium, the mumps virus, or trauma. Treatment: Antibiotic drugs for a bacterial infection. An antibiotic drug is not effective against a virus.
testicular cancer	**seminoma** (SEM-ih-NOH-mah) semin/o- *spermatozoon; semen* -oma *tumor, mass*	Cancerous tumor of one of the testes. Almost all of these arise from abnormal spermatocytes, not from the tubules or connective tissue of the testes. Also known as a **seminoma.** Treatment: Chemotherapy and orchiectomy.
varicocele	**varicocele** (VAR-ih-koh-SEEL) varic/o- *varix; varicose vein* -cele *hernia*	Varicose vein in the spermatic cord to the testis. The valves in the vein leak, allowing blood to back up in them. This causes pooling of the blood. The vein becomes distended and painful. A varicocele can cause a low sperm count and infertility. Treatment: Varicocelectomy.

Prostate Gland

Word or Phrase	Word Part and Definition	Description
benign prostatic hypertrophy (BPH)	**benign** (bee-NINE) *Benign* is derived from a Latin word meaning *kind, not cancerous.* **hypertrophy** (hy-PER-troh-fee) hyper- *above; more than normal* -trophy *process of development*	**Benign,** gradual enlargement of the prostate gland that normally occurs as a man ages. The enlarged prostate compresses the urethra and causes the bladder to retain urine. Symptoms include hesitancy and dribbling on urination and a weak urine stream. Treatment: Drugs to decrease the size of the prostate. Surgery: Transurethral resection of the prostate (TURP).

Word or Phrase	Word Part and Definition	Description
cancer of the prostate gland	**cancerous** (KAN-ser-us) cancer/o- *cancer* -ous *pertaining to* **malignancy** (mah-LIG-nan-see) malign/o- *intentionally causing harm; cancer* -ancy *state of*	**Cancerous** tumor of the prostate gland. This **malignancy** is the most common cancer in men. There are few early symptoms, but the cancer grows slowly. Later the cancer makes the prostate feel hard or nodular on digital rectal examination. Treatment: Radiation therapy, chemotherapy, or prostatectomy.
prostatitis	**prostatitis** (PRAWS-tah-TY-tis) prostat/o- *prostate gland* -itis *inflammation of*	Acute or chronic bacterial infection of the prostate gland. Caused by a urinary tract infection or a sexually transmitted disease. Treatment: Antibiotic drug.
		Penis
balanitis	**balanitis** (BAL-ah-NY-tis) balan/o- *glans penis* -itis *inflammation of* *Balanos* is a Greek word meaning *acorn*. The glans penis is shaped somewhat like an acorn.	Inflammation and infection of the glans penis caused by bacteria. Often associated with phimosis and inadequate hygiene of the prepuce. Treatment: Antibiotic drug.
chordee	**chordee** (kor-DEE) *Chordee* is derived from a French word meaning *having a cord.*	Downward curvature of the penis during erection. Caused by a constricting, cordlike band of tissue along the underside of the penis. Congenital abnormality often associated with hypospadias. Treatment: Surgical correction.
dyspareunia	**dyspareunia** (DIS-pah-ROO-nee-ah) dys- *painful, difficult, abnormal* pareun/o- *sexual intercourse* -ia *condition, state, thing* **postcoital** (post-KOH-ih-tal) post- *after, behind* coit/o- *sexual intercourse* -al *pertaining to* *Coitus* is a Latin word meaning *sexual intercourse.*	Painful or difficult sexual intercourse or **postcoital** pain. Caused by a penile or prostatic infection, chordee of the penis, or phimosis. Treatment: Correct the underlying cause.
erectile dysfunction (ED)	**erectile** (ee-REK-tile) erect/o- *to stand up* -ile *pertaining to* **dysfunction** (dis-FUNK-shun) *Dysfunction* is a combination of the prefix *dys-* (painful, difficult, abnormal) and the word *function.* **impotence** (IM-poh-tens) *Impotence* is derived from a Latin word meaning *inability.*	Inability to achieve or sustain an erection of the penis. Can be caused by cardiovascular disease that impedes blood flow to the penis, neurological disease (such as spinal cord injury) that impairs sensory stimuli and innervation, a low level of testosterone, the side effects of drugs, or psychological factors. Also known as **impotence.** Treatment: Drugs to stimulate an erection, penile implant.

Word or Phrase	Word Part and Definition	Description
phimosis	**phimosis** (fy-MOH-sis) *Phimosis* is a combination of a Greek word meaning *a muzzle* and the suffix *-osis* (condition; abnormal condition; process). **smegma** (SMEG-mah) *Smegma* is a Greek word meaning *soap*.	Congenital condition in which the opening of the foreskin is too small to allow the foreskin to pull back over the glans penis. This traps **smegma** (a white, cheesy, discharge of skin cells and oil) and can cause an infection. Treatment: Circumcision.
premature ejaculation	**premature** (pree-mah-CHUR) *Premature* is a combination of the prefix *pre-* (before, in front of) and the word *mature* (fully developed).	Ejaculation of semen that often occurs with minimal stimulation and before the penis becomes fully erect to penetrate the vagina. This lessens the enjoyment of sexual intercourse and decreases the chance of conception. Can be caused by a hormonal imbalance but more often by stress or a psychological reason. Treatment: Correct the underlying cause.
priapism	**priapism** (PRY-ah-pizm) Priapus was the mythical Roman god of procreation.	Continuing erection of the penis with pain and tenderness. Caused by spinal cord injury or a side effect of drugs to treat erectile dysfunction. Treatment: Correct the underlying cause.
sexually transmitted disease (STD)	**venereal** (veh-NEER-ee-al) **venere/o-** *sexual intercourse* **-al** *pertaining to* *Venereal* is derived from the Latin word *Venus* (the mythical goddess of love).	Contagious disease that is contracted during sexual intercourse with an infected individual (see Table 12-1). A positive test for a sexually transmitted disease means that the patient and all sexual partners need to be treated. Sexually transmitted diseases, which can also be passed to the newborn infant in utero or as it travels through the birth canal, can cause serious illness, blindness, and even death. Also known as **venereal disease (VD).** Treatment: Antibiotic drugs or antiviral drugs.

Table 12-1 Sexually Transmitted Diseases (STDs)

Physicians are required to report all cases of sexually transmitted diseases to the state health department, which, in turn, reports all cases to the Centers for Disease Control and Prevention (CDCP).

Chlamydia		**Chlamydia** (klah-MID-ee-ah)
Pathogen	*Chlamydia trachomatis,* a gram-negative coccus (sphere-shaped) bacterium	
Symptoms	Men: Painful urination with burning and itching. Thin, watery discharge from the urethra. May have no symptoms. Women: Frequently have no symptoms or slight vaginal discharge	
Diagnosis	Smear of discharge from urethra (men) or cervix (women)	
Treatment	Oral antibiotic drugs	
Other	Most common sexually transmitted disease. Also known as *nongonococcal urethritis.*	
genital herpes		**herpes** (HER-peez)
Pathogen	Herpes simplex virus (HSV), type 2	
Symptoms	Men: Vesicular lesions (blisters) on the penis, scrotum, perineum, or anus. When the blisters break, they become skin ulcers. There may be flu-like symptoms or no symptoms at all. Women: Same, on the vulva, perineum, anus, or vagina	
Diagnosis	Culture grown from swab of lesion, polymerase chain reaction test	
Treatment	Topical and oral antiviral drugs shorten the duration of each outbreak	

Table 12-1 Sexually Transmitted Diseases (*continued*)

genital warts (condylomata acuminata), see Figure 12-7 ■)

Pathogen	Human papillomavirus (HPV) Certain strains cause genital warts; other strains cause dysplasia of the cervix which can lead to cervical cancer in women
Symptoms	Men: Itching, flesh-colored, irregular lesions that are raised and cauliflower-like Women: Same, with vaginal discharge
Diagnosis	Visual examination of the skin of the genital area. In women, a Pap smear examined under the microscope.
Treatment	Topical chemicals or cryosurgery, cautery, or laser to remove warts
Other	Also known as *venereal warts*

condylomata acuminata
(CON-dih-LOH-mah-tah ah-KOO-mih-NAH-tah)
Condylomata acuminata is a Latin phrase meaning *knoblike tumors with sharp points.*

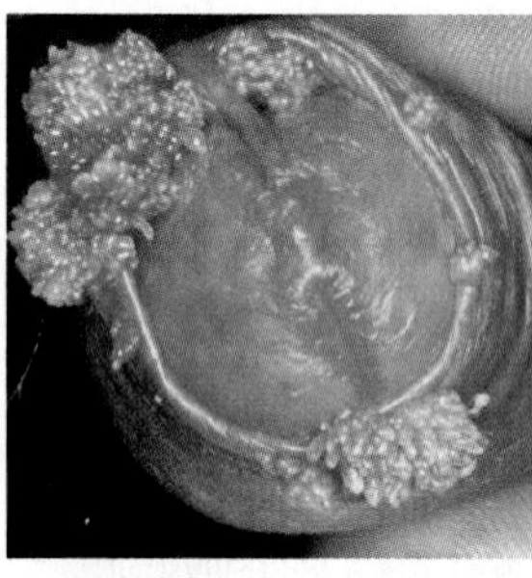
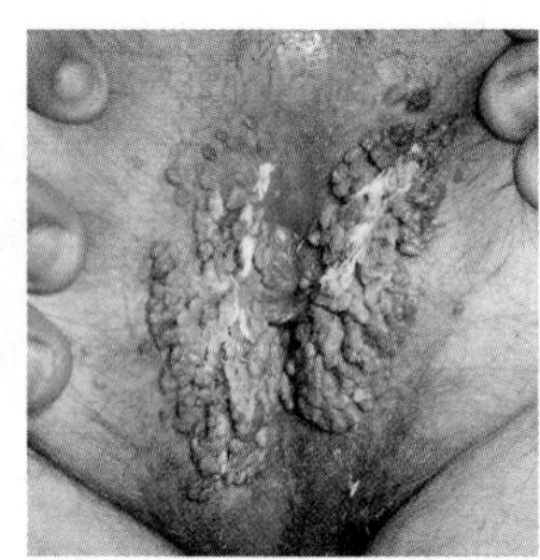

Figure 12-7 ■ Genital warts in a male and female.
These raised, irregular, flesh-colored lesions are caused by the human papillomavirus (HPV). Some strains of this virus are associated with cancer of the cervix in women.

gonorrhea

Pathogen	*Neisseria gonorrhoeae,* a gram-negative diplococcus (double sphere) bacterium. Also known as gonococcus (GC).
Symptoms	Men: Painful urination. Thick yellow urethral discharge (gonococcal urethritis). Some men have no symptoms. Women: Painful urination. Thick yellow vaginal discharge. Half of infected women have no symptoms.
Diagnosis	Gram-stained smear of discharge shows characteristic intracellular diplococci under the microscope Culture grown from a swab of discharge from urethra (men) or cervix (women)
Treatment	Oral antibiotic drug

gonorrhea (GAWN-oh-REE-ah)
gon/o- *seed (ovum or spermatozoon)*
-rrhea *flow, discharge*

acquired immunodeficiency syndrome (AIDS)

Pathogen	Human immunodeficiency virus (HIV), a retrovirus
Symptoms	Men: Fever, night sweats, weight loss, fatigue Women: Same
Diagnosis	Blood test for antibodies to HIV
Treatment	Oral antiviral drugs taken in combination
Other	Treatment can only slow the progress of this fatal disease

immunodeficiency
(IM-yoo-noh-dee-FISH-en-see)
immun/o- *immune response*
defici/o- *lacking, inadequate*
-ency *condition of being*

syphilis

Pathogen	*Treponema pallidum,* a spirochete (spiral) bacterium
Symptoms	Men: Single, painless **chancre** (lesion that ulcerates, forms a crust, and then heals) on the penis. Later symptoms include fever, rash, and various symptoms that mimic other diseases. Women: Same, with chancre on female genitalia
Diagnosis	Fluid from a lesion viewed with special illumination under darkfield microscopy shows the spiral bacterium Blood tests for antibodies (RPR, VDRL)
Treatment	Oral antibiotic drug

syphilis (SIF-ih-lis)
Syphilis is a Latin word. It was the name of a character in a poem called *Syphilis: A Poetical History of the French Disease,* written in 1530. The character, a shepherd, was portrayed as the first person to have the disease. It was called the French disease because, at that time, all sexual diseases supposedly originated with the French. *Lues,* another Latin word for *syphilis,* means *pestilence.*

chancre (SHANG-ker)

Male Breast

Word or Phrase	Word Part and Definition	Description
gynecomastia	**gynecomastia** (GY-neh-koh-MAS-tee-ah) **gynec/o-** *female, woman* **mast/o-** *breast; mastoid process* **-ia** *condition, state, thing*	Enlargement of the male breast. Caused by an imbalance of testosterone and estradiol because of puberty, aging, surgical removal of the testes, or estrogen drug treatment for prostate cancer. Treatment: Androgen drug. Plastic surgery to decrease breast size.

Diagnostic Procedures

Blood Tests

Word or Phrase	Word Part and Definition	Description
acid phosphatase	**acid phosphatase** (AS-id FAWS-fah-tays) So named because it is most active in a low pH (acidic) environment.	Blood test for an enzyme found mostly in the prostate gland (small amounts are found in some other body structures as well). Prostatic acid phosphatase (PAP) only measures acid phosphatase from the prostate gland as opposed to the total acid phosphatase level. Increased levels in the blood indicate cancer of the prostate that has metastasized to the body.
hormone testing	**hormone** (HOR-mohn) A hormone is a chemical messenger.	Blood test to determine the levels of FSH and LH from the anterior pituitary gland and testosterone from the testes. Used to diagnose infertility problems.
prostate-specific antigen (PSA)	**antigen** (AN-tih-jen) **anti-** *against* **-gen** *that which produces* The prefix *anti-* is actually a shortened form of the word *antibody.*	Blood test that detects a glycoprotein in cells of the prostate gland. PSA is increased in men with prostate cancer. The higher the level, the more advanced the cancer. PSA levels fall after successful treatment of the cancer.

Semen Tests

Word or Phrase	Word Part and Definition	Description
acid phosphatase		There are concentrated levels of acid phosphatase in semen. The presence of acid phosphatase in the vagina indicates intercourse and is used in rape investigations.
DNA analysis		DNA analysis of semen from a crime scene or rape victim can be compared to the samples of known DNA in a criminal database.

Word or Phrase	Word Part and Definition	Description
semen analysis	**motility** (moh-TIL-ih-tee) mot/o- *movement* -ility *having the quality of* **morphology** (mor-FAWL-oh-jee) morph/o- *shape* -logy *the study of* **aspermia** (aa-SPER-mee-ah) a- *away from, without* sperm/o- *spermatozoon; sperm* -ia *condition, state, thing*	Microscopic examination of the spermatozoa (see Figure 12-8 ■). A semen analysis is done as part of a workup for infertility. After not ejaculating for 36 hours, the man gives a semen specimen. A normal **sperm count** is greater than 50 million/mL. The **motility** (forward movement) and **morphology** (normal shape) of the spermatozoa are evaluated. A semen analysis is also done after a vasectomy to verify **aspermia** and a successful sterilization. **Figure 12-8 ■ Spermatozoon.** This sperm shows normal morphology. Under the microscope, the back-and-forth movement of its flagellum would indicate normal motility.
Radiologic Tests		
ProstaScint scan		Nuclear medicine procedure that uses ProstaScint to detect areas of metastasis from a primary site of prostate cancer. ProstaScint is a combination of a radioactive tracer (indium-111) and a monoclonal antibody that binds to receptors on cancer cells in the prostate gland and elsewhere in the body. The radioactive tracer emits gamma rays that are detected by a gamma scintillation camera and made into an image.
ultrasonography	**ultrasonography** (UL-trah-sah-NAWG-rah-fee) ultra- *beyond; higher* son/o- *sound* -graphy *process of recording* **transrectal** (trans-REK-tal) trans- *across, through* rect/o- *rectum* -al *pertaining to* **ultrasound** (UL-trah-sound) *Ultrasound* is a combination of the prefix *ultra-* (beyond; higher) and the word *sound.* **sonogram** (SAWN-oh-gram) son/o- *sound* -gram *a record or picture*	Radiologic procedure that uses ultra high-frequency sound waves emitted by a transducer or probe to produce an image. Ultrasonography of the testis uses an ultrasound transducer that is moved across the scrotum to detect a hydrocele or varicocele. **Transrectal ultrasonography (TRUS)** uses an ultrasound probe inserted into the rectum to obtain an image of the prostate gland or help guide a needle biopsy of the prostate gland. The **ultrasound** image is known as a **sonogram.**

Medical and Surgical Procedures

Medical Procedures

Word or Phrase	Word Part and Definition	Description
digital rectal examination (DRE)	**digital** (DIJ-ih-tal) digit/o- *digit (finger or toe)* -al *pertaining to*	Medical procedure to palpate the prostate gland. A gloved finger inserted through the rectum is used to feel for tenderness, nodules, hardness, or enlargement. This examination should be done yearly in men over age 40.
newborn genital examination		The newborn's genitalia are examined for any evidence of hypospadias, epispadias, phimosis, ambiguous genitalia, or undescended testicles (see Figure 12-9 ■). **Figure 12-9 ■ Newborn scrotal examination.** The scrotum is palpated during the initial physical assessment of a newborn. Both testes should be descended and present in the scrotum at birth.
testicular self-examination (TSE)		Systematic palpation of the testes and scrotum to detect lumps, masses, or enlarged lymph nodes. TSE should be done monthly to detect early signs of testicular cancer.

Surgical Procedures

Word or Phrase	Word Part and Definition	Description
biopsy	**biopsy** (BY-awp-see) bi/o- *life; living organisms; living tissue* -opsy *process of viewing* **aspiration** (AS-pih-RAY-shun) aspir/o- *to breathe in; to suck in* -ation *a process; being or having* **incisional** (in-SIZH-un-al) incis/o- *to cut into* -ion *action; condition* -al *pertaining to*	Surgical procedure to remove tissue from the prostate to diagnose prostatic cancer. A large-bore needle is inserted through the rectum or urethra to take a core of prostatic tissue. **Fine-needle aspiration biopsy** of the testis is performed to investigate a low sperm count. A very fine needle is inserted and a syringe is used to aspirate tissue. An **incisional biopsy** (open biopsy) is performed when a mass is felt in a testis.

Word or Phrase	Word Part and Definition	Description
circumcision	**circumcision** (SER-kum-SIZH-un) **circum-** *around* **cis/o-** *to cut* **-ion** *action; condition*	Surgical procedure to remove the prepuce (foreskin). This can be done to correct a tight prepuce and allow better hygiene of the glans penis. The foreskin is often removed because of social customs or religious requirements.
orchiectomy	**orchiectomy** (OR-kee-EK-toh-mee) **orchi/o-** *testis* **-ectomy** *surgical excision*	Surgical procedure to remove a testis because of testicular cancer.
orchiopexy	**orchiopexy** (OR-kee-oh-PEK-see) **orchi/o-** *testis* **-pexy** *process of surgically fixing in place*	Surgical procedure to reposition an undescended testicle and fix it within the scrotum.
penile implant	**prosthesis** (praws-THEE-sis) *Prosthesis* is a Greek word meaning *an addition to; a putting on*	Surgical procedure to implant an inflatable penile **prosthesis** for patients with erectile dysfunction.
prostatectomy	**prostatectomy** (PRAWS-tah-TEK-toh-mee) **prostat/o-** *prostate gland* **-ectomy** *surgical excision*	Surgical procedure to remove the entire prostate gland, lymph nodes, seminal vesicles, and vas deferens because of prostate cancer. A retropubic or a suprapubic surgical approach can be used.
transurethral resection of the prostate (TURP)	**transurethral** (TRANS-yoo-REE-thral) **trans-** *across, through* **urethr/o-** *urethra* **-al** *pertaining to* **resection** (ree-SEK-shun) **resect/o-** *to cut out and remove* **-ion** *action; condition* **resectoscope** (ree-SEK-toh-skohp) **resect/o-** *to cut out and remove* **-scope** *instrument used to examine*	Surgical procedure to reduce the size of the prostate gland. A special cystoscope known as a **resectoscope** is inserted through the urethra. It has built-in cutting instruments and cautery to resect pieces of the prostate and cauterize bleeding vessels. Chips of prostatic tissue are then irrigated out.
vasectomy	**vasectomy** (vah-SEK-toh-mee) **vas/o-** *blood vessel; vas deferens* **-ectomy** *surgical excision* **vasovasostomy** (VAY-soh-vah-SAWS-toh-mee) **vas/o-** *blood vessel; vas deferens* **vas/o-** *blood vessel; vas deferens* **-stomy** *surgically created opening*	Surgical procedure in the male to prevent pregnancy in the female. Through a small incision at the base of the scrotum, both vas deferens are divided, a length of each tube is removed, and the cut ends are sutured and crushed or electrocoagulated. Spermatozoa continue to be produced by the testes, but they are absorbed back into the body. A **vasovasostomy** is a reversal of a vasectomy. The cut ends of the vas deferens are rejoined so that spermatozoa are again present in the ejaculate and the woman can become pregnant.

Drug Categories

Several different categories of drugs are used to treat the symptoms, signs, and diseases of the genitourinary system. The most common drugs in each category are listed.

Category	Word Part and Definition	Description	Example
androgen drugs	**androgen** (AN-droh-jen) andr/o- *male* -gen *that which produces*	Treat a lack of production of testosterone by the testes because of cryptorchidism, surgical removal of the testes, or decreased levels of LH from the anterior pituitary gland. *Androgen* refers to testosterone produced by the testes, other testosterone-like hormones, or manufactured testosterone used in drugs.	Virilon
antibiotic drugs	**antibiotic** (AN-tee-by-AWT-ik) (AN-tih-by-AWT-ik) anti- *against* bi/o- *life; living organisms; living tissue* -tic *pertaining to*	Treat infections of the male genitourinary system and sexually transmitted diseases caused by bacteria. Antibiotic drugs are not effective against viral infections.	ampicillin, amoxicillin, erythromycin, Vibramycin
antiviral drugs	**antiviral** (AN-tee-VY-ral) (AN-tih-VY-ral) anti- *against* vir/o- *virus* -al *pertaining to*	Treat viral infections that cause genital herpes and condylomata acuminata. These drugs are applied topically to the affected areas; oral antiviral drugs are used to treat HIV and AIDS.	Aldara, Condylox, Zovirax Combivir, Hivid, Retrovir (for HIV or AIDS)
chemotherapy drugs	**chemotherapy** (KEE-moh-THAIR-ah-pee) chem/o- *chemical, drug* -therapy *treatment*	Kill rapidly dividing cancer cells in the testes or prostate gland. Other drugs block testosterone or are estrogen drugs; both produce an unfavorable hormonal environment for cancer.	Bleomycin, cisplatin, VePesid, Velban Estrogen, Eulexin, Taxol, Zoladex (for prostatic cancer)
drugs for benign prostatic hypertrophy		Inhibit the enzyme that causes the prostate gland to enlarge. Other drugs relax the smooth muscle in the prostate gland and urethra and allow urine to flow more freely.	Proscar Flomax, Hytrin
drugs that produce an erection		Inhibit a substance that would limit blood flow into the penis for an erection.	Cialis, Levitra, Viagra

Did You Know?

Proscar for benign prostatic hypertrophy is also marketed under the trade name Propecia. Propecia comes in a lower dosage and is prescribed specifically to treat male-pattern baldness.

Abbreviations

AIDS	acquired immunodeficiency syndrome
BPH	benign prostatic hypertrophy
CDCP	Centers for Disease Control and Prevention
DRE	digital rectal examination
ED	erectile dysfunction
FSH	follicle-stimulating hormone
GC	gonococcus (*Neisseria gonorrhoeae*)
GU	genitourinary
HIV	human immunodeficiency virus
HPV	human papillomavirus
HSV	herpes simplex virus
LH	luteinizing hormone
PAP	prostatic acid phosphatase
PSA	prostate-specific antigen
RPR	rapid plasma reagin (test for syphilis)
STD	sexually transmitted disease
TRUS	transrectal ultrasound
TSE	testicular self-examination
TURP	transurethral resection of the prostate
VD	venereal disease
VDRL	Venereal Disease Research Laboratory (test for syphilis)

Word Alert

ABBREVIATIONS

Abbreviations are commonly used in all types of medical documents; however, they can mean different things to different people and their meanings can be misinterpreted. Always verify the meaning of an abbreviation.

ED stands for *erectile dysfunction,* but it can also stand for *emergency department.*

PAP stands for *prostatic acid phosphatase,* but *Pap* is a short form for *Papanicolau smear.*

Career Focus

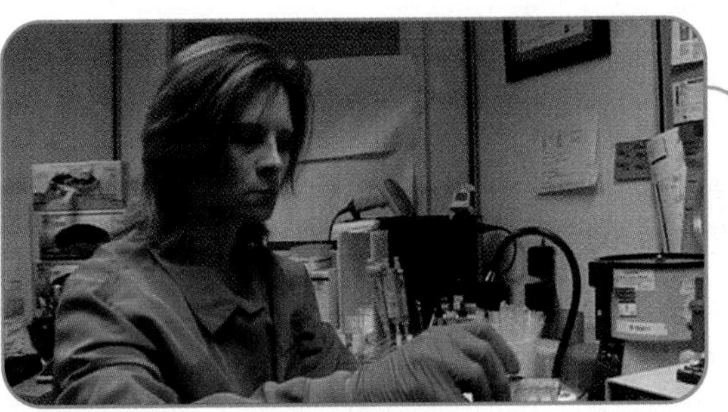

Meet Mindy, a clinical laboratory scientist and blood bank supervisor.

"Clinical laboratory scientist is the newer name, but we know ourselves as medical technologists. In college, I took a microbiology class. I enjoyed it so much that I pursued that as my major. A technologist performs the testing, whether it's hematology, chemistry, blood bank, or microbiology. I have to communicate with the doctors and nurses. I have to have an understanding of medical terminology to be able to communicate clearly with them. When we can interact with the nurses and the doctors, to give them the answers they need to care for the patients, that's what's rewarding."

Clinical laboratory scientists are allied health professionals who work in a hospital or large commercial medical laboratories. They perform all types of laboratory tests on blood, urine, and other body fluids and tissues. They work with microscopes and computerized equipment.

Reproductive medicine physicians treat male (and female) patients who have difficulty conceiving a child because of infertility.

Endocrinologists treat patients with disorders of the endocrine system, including hormonal disorders that affect men, such as infertility. Cancerous tumors of the male genitourinary system are treated medically by an oncologist and surgically by a general surgeon.

clinical (KLIN-ih-kal)
clinic/o- *medicine*
-al *pertaining to*

laboratory (LAB-oh-rah-TOH-ree)
laborat/o- *workplace; testing place*
-ory *having the function of*

scientist (SY-en-tist)
scient/o- *science; knowledge*
-ist *one who specializes in*

reproductive (REE-proh-DUK-tiv)
re- *again and again; backward; unable to*
product/o- *produce*
-ive *pertaining to*

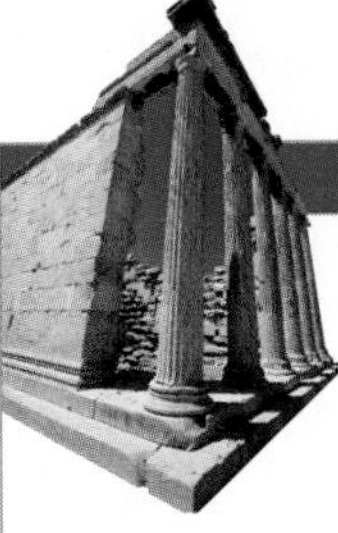

It's Greek to Me!

Did you notice that some male reproductive words have two different combining forms? Combining forms from both Greek and Latin languages remain a part of medical language today.

English Word	Greek	Latin	Examples of Medical Words
penis	balan/o-	pen/o-	balanitis, penile
sexual intercourse	pareun/o-	venere/o-	dyspareunia, venereal disease
		coit/o-	postcoital
testis	orchi/o-	test/o-	orchiectomy, testosterone
	didym/o-	testicul/o-	epididymis, testicular

Chapter Review Exercises

Review all the material in this chapter by completing the review exercises in this section. Use the Answer Key at the end of the book to check your answers.

Anatomy and Physiology

Matching Exercise

Match each numbered word or phrase to its description.

1. ductus deferens	____	Process of making mature sperm
2. ejaculatory duct	____	Internal and external reproductive organs
3. epididymis	____	Contain the seminiferous tubules that make spermatozoa
4. flagellum	____	Area between the anus and scrotum
5. genitals	____	Opening in the center of a tube or duct
6. interstitial	____	Synonym for spermatozoa
7. lumen	____	Tubule on top of the testis
8. perineum	____	Cells that secrete testosterone
9. prepuce	____	Contains arteries, veins, nerves, and vas deferens
10. prostate gland	____	Immature cells in the seminiferous tubules
11. sperm	____	Tail of a sperm
12. spermatic cord	____	Causes the development of sexual characteristics during puberty
13. spermatocyte	____	Also known as the vas deferens
14. spermatogenesis	____	Vas deferens and seminal vesicles empty into this structure
15. testes	____	Spherical gland at the base of the bladder
16. testosterone	____	Structure that is still present in an uncircumcised male

True or False

Indicate whether each statement is true or false by writing T or F on the line.

1. ____ The bulbourethral glands are also known as Cowper's glands.
2. ____ The external male genitalia are located within the pelvic cavity.
3. ____ *Testicles* is a synonym for *testes.*
4. ____ The prostate gland secretes most of the fluid that makes up the volume of an ejaculation.
5. ____ The glans penis is a structure that fills with blood and becomes erect.
6. ____ The flagellum makes a sperm motile.
7. ____ The inguinal canal is a passageway from the pelvic cavity to the scrotum.
8. ____ The penis contains erectile tissue.
9. ____ Gametes are cells that are unique because they have a flagellum.

Circle Exercise

Circle the correct word from the choices given.

1. The (**bladder, penis, scrotum**) is a soft sac of skin that holds the testes.
2. The internal male genitalia includes all of the following EXCEPT the (**epididymis, prostate gland, vas deferens**).
3. Spermatozoa are produced in the (**scrotum, seminal vesicles, seminiferous tubules**).
4. The spermatic cord contains all of the following EXCEPT (**arteries, ejaculatory duct, vas deferens**).
5. The process by which a cell divides to end up with 23 chromosomes is known as (**meiosis, mitosis, puberty**).

Sequencing Exercise

Beginning with the spermatozoon in the lumen of the seminiferous tubules, use the list of anatomical structures given here to help you arrange the structures through which a spermatozoon moves in the correct order.

ejaculatory duct	prostatic urethra	urethral meatus
epididymis	urethra in the penis	vas deferens

1. ______________ → 2. ______________ → 3. ______________ →
4. ______________ → 5. ______________ → 6. ______________

Medical Language Word Parts

Name that Word Part

Identify each of the word parts given here by writing the correct letter (P, C, or S) on the line beside it. Then write the definition of the word part on the blank line. The first one has been done for you.

Prefix = P **Combining form = C** **Suffix = S**

	Word Part	Definition		Word Part	Definition
1. -al	S	pertaining to	17. chem/o-	____	____________
2. a-	____	____________	18. circum-	____	____________
3. adolesc/o-	____	____________	19. cis/o-	____	____________
4. -ad	____	____________	20. clinic/o-	____	____________
5. -ancy	____	____________	21. coit/o-	____	____________
6. andr/o-	____	____________	22. crypt/o-	____	____________
7. anti-	____	____________	23. -cyte	____	____________
8. -ar	____	____________	24. defici/o-	____	____________
9. -ary	____	____________	25. didym/o-	____	____________
10. aspir/o-	____	____________	26. -didymis	____	____________
11. -ation	____	____________	27. digit/o-	____	____________
12. balan/o-	____	____________	28. dys-	____	____________
13. bi/o-	____	____________	29. -ectomy	____	____________
14. bulb/o-	____	____________	30. ejaculat/o-	____	____________
15. cancer/o-	____	____________	31. -ence	____	____________
16. -cele	____	____________	32. -ency	____	____________

	Word Part	Definition		Word Part	Definition
33. epi-	______	______	75. -ory	______	______
34. erect/o-	______	______	76. -osis	______	______
35. -esis	______	______	77. -ous	______	______
36. extern/o-	______	______	78. pareun/o-	______	______
37. fer/o-	______	______	79. pen/o-	______	______
38. fertil/o-	______	______	80. perine/o-	______	______
39. -gen	______	______	81. -pexy	______	______
40. genit/o-	______	______	82. post-	______	______
41. gen/o-	______	______	83. pre-	______	______
42. gon/o-	______	______	84. product/o-	______	______
43. -gram	______	______	85. prostat/o-	______	______
44. -graphy	______	______	86. puber/o-	______	______
45. gynec/o-	______	______	87. re-	______	______
46. hyper-	______	______	88. rect/o-	______	______
47. -ia	______	______	89. resect/o-	______	______
48. -ic	______	______	90. -rrhea	______	______
49. -ile	______	______	91. scient/o-	______	______
50. -ility	______	______	92. -scope	______	______
51. immun/o-	______	______	93. scrot/o-	______	______
52. in-	______	______	94. semin/i-	______	______
53. incis/o-	______	______	95. semin/o-	______	______
54. inguin/o-	______	______	96. son/o-	______	______
55. intern/o-	______	______	97. spermat/o-	______	______
56. interstiti/o-	______	______	98. sperm/o-	______	______
57. -ion	______	______	99. -stomy	______	______
58. -ism	______	______	100. testicul/o-	______	______
59. -ist	______	______	101. -therapy	______	______
60. -itis	______	______	102. -tic	______	______
61. -ity	______	______	103. trans-	______	______
62. -ive	______	______	104. -trophy	______	______
63. laborat/o-	______	______	105. tub/o-	______	______
64. -logy	______	______	106. -ty	______	______
65. malign/o-	______	______	107. -ule	______	______
66. mast/o-	______	______	108. ultra-	______	______
67. mit/o-	______	______	109. urethr/o-	______	______
68. morph/o-	______	______	110. urin/o-	______	______
69. mot/o-	______	______	111. ur/o-	______	______
70. olig/o-	______	______	112. varic/o-	______	______
71. -oma	______	______	113. vas/o-	______	______
72. -opsy	______	______	114. venere/o-	______	______
73. orchi/o-	______	______	115. vir/o-	______	______
74. orch/o-	______	______	116. -zoon	______	______

Word-Building Exercise

Use the combining forms, prefixes, and suffixes given here to build medical words that match the definitions given. Write the word that you build on the blank line. Some word parts may be used more than once. The first one has been done for you.

Word Parts

-ary (pertaining to)	genit/o- (genitalia)	olig/o- (scanty)
-cele (hernia)	gen/o- (arising from; produced by)	orch/o- (testis)
crypt/o- (hidden)	gynec/o- (female, woman)	pareun/o- (sexual intercourse)
didym/o- (testes)	-ia (condition, state, thing)	spermat/o- (spermatozoon; sperm)
dys- (painful, difficult, abnormal)	-ism (process; disease from a specific cause)	sperm/o- (spermatozoon; sperm)
epi- (upon, above)	-itis (inflammation of)	urin/o- (urine; urinary system)
-esis (condition)	mast/o- (breast; mastoid process)	varic/o- (varix; varicose vein)

1. Varicose vein of the spermatic cord that bulges like a hernia (You think *varic/o-* + *-cele*) You write *varicocele*
2. Pertaining to the genitals and urinary system ____________
3. Condition of undescended testes ____________
4. Enlarged breasts on a man ____________
5. Painful or difficult sexual intercourse ____________
6. Scanty amount of sperm in semen ____________
7. Inflammation of the structure located upon the testes ____________
8. Condition of sperm being produced by the testes ____________

Symptoms, Signs, and Diseases

Circle Exercise

Circle the correct word from the choices given.

1. Gynecomastia is a disease that affects the (**breasts, penis, scrotum**).
2. Inflammation of the glans penis is known as (**balanitis, gynecomastia, phimosis**).
3. A low number of sperm on a semen analysis is known as (**cryptorchism, oligospermia, varicocele**).
4. Postcoital pain is also known as (**dyspareunia, impotence, venereal disease**).
5. A chancre is seen with the sexually transmitted disease (**genital warts, gonorrhea, syphilis**).
6. HIV is a (**bacterium, retrovirus, virus**).
7. All of these diseases can be caused by a sexually transmitted disease EXCEPT (**epididymitis, phimosis, prostatitis**).
8. Postcoital pain occurs after (**ejaculation, sexual intercourse, spermatogenesis**).
9. (**Aspermia, Chordee, Phimosis**) is a congenital condition in which the opening of the foreskin is too small to pull it over the glans penis.
10. AIDS is caused by the (**herpes simplex virus, human immunodeficiency virus, human papillomavirus**).

Matching Exercise

Match each numbered word or phrase to its description.

1.	chancre	_____ Caused by *Treponema pallidum*
2.	chordee	_____ Failure to conceive
3.	condylomata acuminata	_____ Enlargement of the male breasts
4.	dyspareunia	_____ Fewer than the normal number of sperm
5.	erectile dysfunction	_____ Can be caused by a mumps infection
6.	gonorrhea	_____ Painful sexual intercourse
7.	gynecomastia	_____ Skin lesion of syphilis
8.	herpes simplex virus	_____ Downward curve of the penis during erection
9.	infertility	_____ Inability to sustain an erection
10.	oligospermia	_____ Genital warts
11.	orchitis	_____ Vesicular lesions like blisters on the skin
12.	syphilis	_____ Intracellular diplococci under the microscope

Laboratory, Radiology, Surgery, and Drugs

Circle Exercise

Circle the correct word from the choices given.

1. The (**acid phosphatase, prostate-specific antigen, sperm count**) is not increased in patients with cancer of the prostate.
2. This procedure can be performed by the patient on himself: (**biopsy, circumcision, testicular self-examination**).
3. An (**incisional biopsy, orchiectomy, orchiopexy**) is performed to reposition an undescended testicle.
4. Antibiotic drugs are effective against (**genital warts, gonorrhea, HIV**).
5. A penile implant is used to treat patients with (**aspermia, erectile dysfunction, prostate cancer**).
6. Patients with cancer of the prostate are given (**androgen, antibiotic, estrogen**) drugs.

Fill-in-the-Blank Exercise

Fill in the blank with the correct word from the word list.

acid phosphatase	digital rectal exam	resectoscope	varicocelectomy
circumcision	morphology	ultrasonography	vasovasostomy

1. Surgical excision of a varicose vein of the spermatic cord ______________________
2. Sperm shape that is checked on sperm analysis ______________________
3. Enzyme found mainly in the prostate gland ______________________
4. Uses sound waves to create an image ______________________
5. Should be done yearly for men over age 40 ______________________
6. Instrument used to perform a TURP ______________________
7. Procedure to reverse a vasectomy ______________________
8. Removal of the foreskin of the penis ______________________

Abbreviations

Definition Exercise

Write the definition of the following abbreviations.

1. BPH ______________________
2. ED ______________________
3. GC ______________________
4. HSV ______________________
5. PSA ______________________
6. STD ______________________
7. TURP ______________________
8. VD ______________________

Applied Skills

Plural Noun and Adjective Spelling

Fill in the blanks with the correct word form. Be sure to check your spelling. The first one has been done for you.

Singular Noun	Plural Noun	Adjective
1. tubule	tubules	tubular
2. testicle	________	________
3. perineum		________
4. spermatozoon	________	
5. epididymis	________	________
6. prostate		________
7. penis		________

Proofreading and Spelling Exercise

Read the following paragraph and identify any misspelled medical words. Write the correct spelling of the word in the blank at the right.

The mail anatomy is located in the pelvic area. It shares the urithra with the urinary system, and this exits from the glands penis or tip of the penis. The peroneal area is the the skin between the anus and skrotum. The testes produce spermatozon if they have descended through the inguinel canal. The The epidydimis holds sperm or gameetes. Then sperm travel through the vas deference and ejaculatory duct. The seminole vesicles add fluid, as does the prostrate gland, to make semen. This briefly describes the male reproducktive anatomy.

1. ________
2. ________
3. ________
4. ________
5. ________
6. ________
7. ________
8. ________
9. ________
10. ________
11. ________
12. ________
13. ________

English and Medical Word Equivalents

For each English word or phrase, write its equivalent medical word. The first one has been done for you.

English Word	Medical Word
1. testicular cancer	seminoma
2. pain during intercourse	________
3. impotence	________
4. sexually transmitted disease	________
5. undescended testicle	________
6. genital warts	________
7. enlarged prostate	________

Analysis of a Medical Report

This exercise contains an operative report. Read the report and answer the questions.

OPERATIVE REPORT

PATIENT: JENKINS, Daniel

MEDICAL RECORD NUMBER: 206-47-5869

DATE OF SURGERY: November 19, 20xx

PREOPERATIVE DIAGNOSES

1. Undescended left testis.
2. Left indirect inguinal hernia

POSTOPERATIVE DIAGNOSES

1. Undescended left testis, corrected.
2. Left indirect inguinal hernia, repaired.

PROCEDURES

1. Left orchiopexy.
2. Left inguinal herniorrhaphy.

DESCRIPTION OF OPERATIVE PROCEDURE

The patient was placed in the dorsal supine position, and general anesthesia was induced via mask anesthesia. The pubic region and external genitalia were prepped and draped with Betadine antibacterial scrub. A transverse incision was made in the suprapubic skin fold on the left side. It was carried down through subcutaneous tissue and fat. Bleeding was controlled with the electrocautery. The left testis was identified in the operative field and was noted to be lying just within the external inguinal ring. The external oblique fascia was incised with a #15 scalpel and Metzenbaum scissors. The left testis was grasped and freed from its surrounding structures up to the level of the internal inguinal ring. This maneuver freed up the cord so that adequate cord length was obtained. The hernia sac was then opened and dissected up to the level of the inguinal ring, where it was closed with 4-0 Vicryl suture. Then we again turned our attention to the undescended left testis. A scrotal incision was made and a subcutaneous pouch created. The left testis was then brought down into the pouch, and a 3-0 silk suture was placed in the lower pole of the testis, brought out through the scrotal skin, and tied over a cotton pledget to secure the testis in place. A careful search detected no bleeding in the scrotal or groin incisions. The scrotal incision was closed with 5-0 Vicryl. The external oblique fascia was closed with a running 4-0 Vicryl suture. The subcutaneous tissue was closed with 4-0 Vicryl. The skin was closed with a running subcuticular 3-0 Prolene suture, and the child was discharged from the operating room in satisfactory condition.

James R. Bentley, M.D.

James R. Bentley, M.D.

JRB:btg
D: 11/19/xx
T: 11/19/xx

WORD ANALYSIS QUESTIONS

1. Divide *orchiopexy* into its two word parts and define each word part.

Word Part	**Definition**
______________	____
______________	____

2. An incision in the suprapubic skin fold would be located ________________.
   a. below the pubic bone
   b. around the pubic bone
   c. above the pubic bone

FACT FINDING QUESTIONS

1. In the dorsal supine position, the patient is placed on his (**abdomen, back, side**).
2. In a male, the external genitalia include what five structures?

   ______________________ ______________________

   ______________________ ______________________

   ____

3. Incisions were made in what two areas? ______________________ ______________________
4. The hernia sac was closed with sutures. **True** **False**
5. *Subcutaneous* means (**around the testis, inside the scrotum, under the skin**).
6. The left testis was not descended. What operative procedure was performed to correct this? ______________

CRITICAL THINKING QUESTIONS

1. A preoperative diagnosis represents the patient's condition (**before, during, after**) surgery.
2. "The maneuver freed up the cord . . ." What *cord* does this refer to? **spinal cord** **spermatic cord** **umbilical cord**

Pronunciation Checklist

Read each word and its pronunciation. Practice pronouncing each word. Verify your pronunciation by listening to the Pronunciation List on the CD-ROM. Check the box next to the word after you master its pronunciation.

- ❑ acid phosphatase (AS-id FAWS-fah-tays)
- ❑ acquired immunodeficiency syndrome (ah-KWY-erd IM-yoo-noh-dee-FISH-en-see SIN-drohm)
- ❑ adolescence (AD-oh-LES-ens)
- ❑ androgen drug (AN-droh-jen DRUHG)
- ❑ antibiotic drug (AN-tee-by-AWT-ik) (AN-tih-by-AWT-ik DRUHG)
- ❑ antiviral drug (AN-tee-VY-ral DRUHG) (AN-tih-VY-ral)
- ❑ aspermia (aa-SPER-mee-ah)
- ❑ aspiration biopsy (AS-pih-RAY-shun BY-awp-see)
- ❑ balanitis (BAL-ah-NY-tis)
- ❑ benign prostatic hypertrophy (bee-NINE praws-TAT-ik hy-PER-troh-fee)
- ❑ biopsy (BY-awp-see)
- ❑ bulbourethral gland (BUL-boh-yoo-REE-thral GLAND)
- ❑ cancerous (KAN-ser-us)
- ❑ chancre (SHANG-ker)
- ❑ chemotherapy drug (KEE-moh-THAIR-ah-pee DRUHG)
- ❑ Chlamydia (klah-MID-ee-ah)
- ❑ chordee (kor-DEE)
- ❑ circumcision (SER-kum-SIZH-un)
- ❑ clinical laboratory scientist (KLIN-ih-kal LAB-oh-rah-TOH-ree SY-en-tist)
- ❑ condylomata acuminata (CON-dih-LOH-mah-tah ah-KOO-mih-NAH-tah)
- ❑ corpora cavernosa (KOR-por-ah KAV-er-NOH-sah)
- ❑ corpus spongiosum (KOR-puhs SPUN-jee-OH-sum)
- ❑ cryptorchism (krip-TOHR-kiz-em)
- ❑ ductus deferens (DUK-tus DEF-er-enz)
- ❑ dyspareunia (DIS-pah-ROO-nee-ah)
- ❑ ejaculation (ee-JAK-yoo-LAY-shun)
- ❑ ejaculatory duct (ee-JAK-yoo-lah-tohr-ee DUKT)
- ❑ epididymal (EP-ih-DID-ih-mal)
- ❑ epididymides (EP-ih-dih-DIM-ih-deez)
- ❑ epididymis (EP-ih-DID-ih-mis)
- ❑ epididymitis (EP-ih-DID-ih-MY-tis)
- ❑ erectile dysfunction (ee-REK-tile dis-FUNK-shun)
- ❑ erection (ee-REK-shun)
- ❑ external genitalia (eks-TER-nal JEN-ih-TAY-lee-ah)
- ❑ flagellum (flah-JEL-um)
- ❑ follicle-stimulating hormone (FAWL-ih-kl STIM-yoo-lay-ting HOR-mohn)
- ❑ gamete (GAM-eet)
- ❑ genitalia (JEN-ih-TAY-lee-ah)
- ❑ genital (JEN-ih-tal)
- ❑ genital herpes (JEN-ih-tal HER-peez)
- ❑ genitourinary system (JEN-ih-toh-YOO-rih-nair-ee SIS-tem)
- ❑ glans penis (GLANZ PEE-nis)
- ❑ gonad (GOH-nad)
- ❑ gonorrhea (GAWN-oh-REE-ah)
- ❑ gynecomastia (GY-neh-koh-MAS-tee-ah)
- ❑ hormone (HOR-mohn)
- ❑ human immunodeficiency virus (HYOO-man IM-yoo-noh-dee-FISH-en-see VY-rus)
- ❑ hydrocele (HY-droh-seel)
- ❑ impotence (IM-poh-tens)
- ❑ incisional biopsy (in-SIZH-un-al BY-awp-see)
- ❑ infertility (IN-fer-TIL-ih-tee)
- ❑ inguinal canal (ING-gwih-nal kah-NAL)
- ❑ internal genitalia (in-TER-nal JEN-ih-TAY-lee-ah)
- ❑ interstitial cell (IN-ter-STISH-al SELL)
- ❑ lumen (LOO-men)
- ❑ luteinizing hormone (LOO-tee-ih-ny-zing HOR-mohn)
- ❑ malignancy (mah-LIG-nan-see)
- ❑ meiosis (my-OH-sis)
- ❑ mitosis (my-TOH-sis)
- ❑ motile (MOH-til)
- ❑ oligospermia (OHL-ih-goh-SPER-mee-ah)
- ❑ orchiectomy (OR-kee-EK-toh-mee)
- ❑ orchiopexy (OR-kee-oh-PEK-see)
- ❑ orchitis (or-KY-tis)
- ❑ pelvic cavity (PEL-vik CAV-ih-tee)
- ❑ penile (PEE-nile)
- ❑ penile implant (PEE-nile IM-plant)
- ❑ penile prosthesis (PEE-nile praws-THEE-sis)
- ❑ penis (PEE-nis)
- ❑ perineal (PAIR-ih-NEE-al)
- ❑ perineum (PAIR-ih-NEE-um)
- ❑ phimosis (fy-MOH-sis)
- ❑ postcoital (post-KOH-ih-tal)
- ❑ premature (pree-mah-CHUR)
- ❑ prepuce (PREE-poos)
- ❑ priapism (PRY-ah-pizm)
- ❑ prostate gland (PRAWS-tayt GLAND)
- ❑ prostatectomy (PRAWS-tah-TEK-toh-mee)
- ❑ prostate-specific antigen (PRAWS-tayt speh-SIF-ik AN-tih-jen)
- ❑ prostatic fluid (praws-TAT-ik FLOO-id)
- ❑ prostatitis (PRAWS-tah-TY-tis)
- ❑ puberty (PYOO-ber-tee)
- ❑ pubic (PYOO-bik)
- ❑ receptor (ree-SEP-tor)
- ❑ reproductive medicine (REE-proh-DUK-tiv MED-ih-sin)
- ❑ reproductive system (REE-proh-DUK-tiv SIS-tem)
- ❑ resectoscope (ree-SEK-toh-skohp)
- ❑ scrotal (SKROH-tal)
- ❑ scrotum (SKROH-tum)
- ❑ semen (SEE-men)
- ❑ seminal fluid (SEM-in-nal FLOO-id)
- ❑ seminal vesicle (SEM-ih-nal VES-ih-kl)
- ❑ seminiferous tubule (SEM-ih-NIF-er-us TOO-byool)
- ❑ seminoma (SEM-ih-NOH-mah)
- ❑ sonogram (SAWN-oh-gram)
- ❑ sperm (SPERM)
- ❑ sperm morphology (SPERM mor-FAWL-oh-jee)
- ❑ sperm motility (SPERM moh-TIL-ih-tee)
- ❑ spermatic cord (sper-MAT-ik KORD)
- ❑ spermatocele (SPER-mah-toh-seel)
- ❑ spermatocyte (SPER-mah-toh-SITE)
- ❑ spermatogenesis (SPER-mah-toh-JEN-eh-sis)
- ❑ spermatozoa (SPER-mah-toh-ZOH-ah)
- ❑ spermatozoon (SPER-mah-toh-ZOH-on)
- ❑ syphilis (SIF-ih-lis)
- ❑ testes (TES-teez)

- ❑ testicle (TES-tih-kl)
- ❑ testicular (tes-TIK-yoo-lar)
- ❑ testis (TES-tis)
- ❑ testosterone (tes-TAWS-teh-rohn)
- ❑ transrectal ultrasonography (trans-REK-tal UL-trah-sah-NAWG-rah-fee)
- ❑ transurethral resection (TRANS-yoo-REE-thral ree-SEK-shun)
- ❑ tubule (TOO-byool)
- ❑ ultrasonography (UL-trah-sah-NAWG-rah-fee)
- ❑ ultrasound (UL-trah-sound)
- ❑ urogenital (YOO-roh-JEN-ih-tal)
- ❑ varicocele (VAR-ih-koh-SEEL)
- ❑ vas deferens (VAS DEF-er-enz)
- ❑ vasectomy (vah-SEK-toh-mee)
- ❑ vasovasostomy (VAY-soh-vah-SAWS-toh-mee)
- ❑ venereal disease (veh-NEER-ee-al dih-ZEEZ)

Experience Multimedia

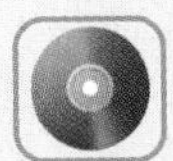

CD-ROM Learning Activities Checklist

Check off the box as you complete each learning activity.

- ❑ **CD-ROM Learning Activity 12.1: *ANATOMY WORD PARTS FLASHCARDS***
  Use flashcards to help you memorize word parts. Make your own flashcards or print out prepared flashcards. Also see the electronic flashcard game. Time: 20 minutes.
- ❑ **CD-ROM Learning Activity 12.2: *MEDICINE IN ACTION***
  Watch a video clip of a vasectomy. Time: 5 minutes.
- ❑ **CD-ROM Learning Activity 12.3: *DISEASE AND OTHER WORD PARTS FLASHCARDS***
  A continuation of the flashcard learning activity. Time: 20 minutes.
- ❑ **CD-ROM Learning Activity 12.4: *MEMORY AIDS***
  Use memory aids to help you memorize medical words and meanings. Time: 5 minutes.
- ❑ **CD-ROM Learning Activity 12.5: *MEDICAL LANGUAGE SPOKEN HERE***
  Listen to actual medical reports and spell the missing medical words. Time: 20 minutes.
- ❑ **CD-ROM Learning Activity 12.6: *SPELLING CHALLENGE***
  Listen to a pronounced medical word and then spell it. Time: 5 minutes.
- ❑ **CD-ROM Learning Activity 12.7: *MEDICAL LANGUAGE PRONUNCIATION***
  Listen to a pronounced medical word and then practice pronouncing it. Time: 30 minutes.
- ❑ **CD-ROM Learning Activity 12.8: *EDUCATIONAL FUN AND GAMES***
  Enjoy these fun activities while reinforcing your knowledge. Time: 15 minutes.

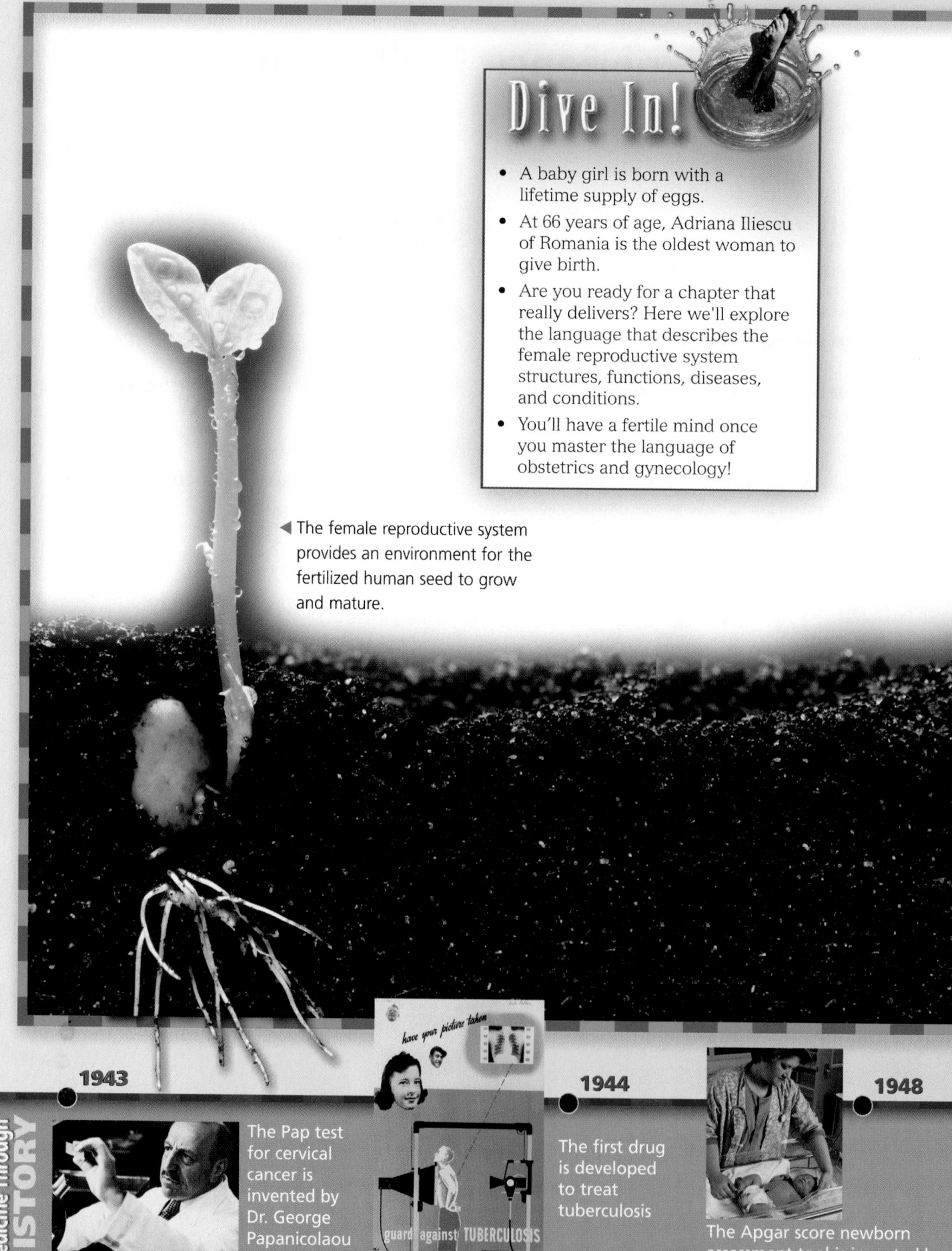

have your picture taken
guard against TUBERCULOSIS

Dive In!

- A baby girl is born with a lifetime supply of eggs.
- At 66 years of age, Adriana Iliescu of Romania is the oldest woman to give birth.
- Are you ready for a chapter that really delivers? Here we'll explore the language that describes the female reproductive system structures, functions, diseases, and conditions.
- You'll have a fertile mind once you master the language of obstetrics and gynecology!

◀ The female reproductive system provides an environment for the fertilized human seed to grow and mature.

Medicine Through HISTORY

1943 The Pap test for cervical cancer is invented by Dr. George Papanicolaou

1944 The first drug is developed to treat tuberculosis

1948 The Apgar score newborn assessment tool is invented by Dr. Virginia Apgar

CHAPTER 13

Gynecology and Obstetrics

Female Genital and Reproductive System

Gynecology (GY-neh-KAWL-oh-jee) is the medical specialty that studies the anatomy and physiology of the female genital system and uses diagnostic tests, medical and surgical procedures, and drugs to treat female genital diseases.

Obstetrics (awb-STET-riks) is the medical specialty that studies the anatomy and physiology of the female reproductive system and uses diagnostic tests, medical and surgical procedures, and drugs to monitor normal pregnancy and childbirth and treat diseases.

◀ Like a bird egg, the womb houses the gestation process.

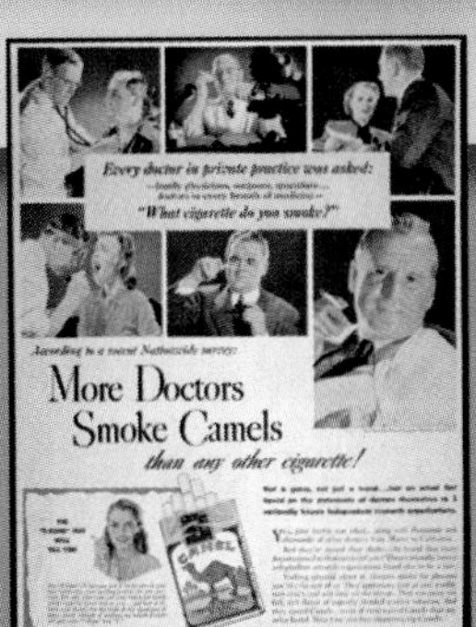

1950

The first scientific research studies are published that link smoking to cancer

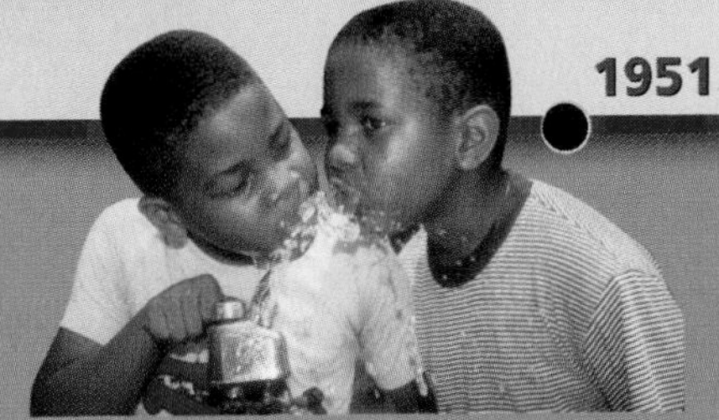

1951

Fluoride is added to public drinking water to prevent dental cavities

1951

Prescription drugs are defined by law as those drugs that must be ordered by a physician and dispensed by a pharmacist

Measure Your Progress: Learning Objectives

After you study this chapter, you should be able to

1. Identify the anatomical structures of the female genital and reproductive system by correctly labeling them on anatomical illustrations.
2. Describe the processes of oogenesis, menstruation, and conception.
3. Describe the process of labor and delivery.
4. Describe normal and abnormal findings in the neonate.
5. Build female genital and reproductive words from combining forms, prefixes, and suffixes.
6. Describe common female genital and reproductive diseases.
7. Describe common female genital and reproductive diagnostic laboratory and radiology tests.
8. Describe common female genital and reproductive medical and surgical procedures and drug categories.
9. Define common female genital and reproductive abbreviations.
10. Correctly spell and pronounce female genital and reproductive words.
11. Apply your skills by analyzing a gynecology report.
12. Test your knowledge of gynecology and obstetrics by completing review exercises at the end of the chapter and learning activities on the CD-ROM.

Medical Language Key

To unlock the meaning of a medical word, first define each word part. Then put the word part definitions in order, beginning with the suffix, followed by the first word part.

	Word Part	Word Part Definition
SUFFIX	-logy	*the study of*
COMBINING FORM	gynec/o-	*female, woman*

Gynecology: ***The study of women.***

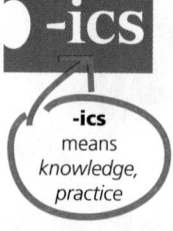

	Word Part	Word Part Definition
SUFFIX	-ics	*knowledge, practice*
COMBINING FORM	obstetr/o-	*pregnancy and childbirth*

Obstetrics: ***The practice pertaining to pregnancy and childbirth.***

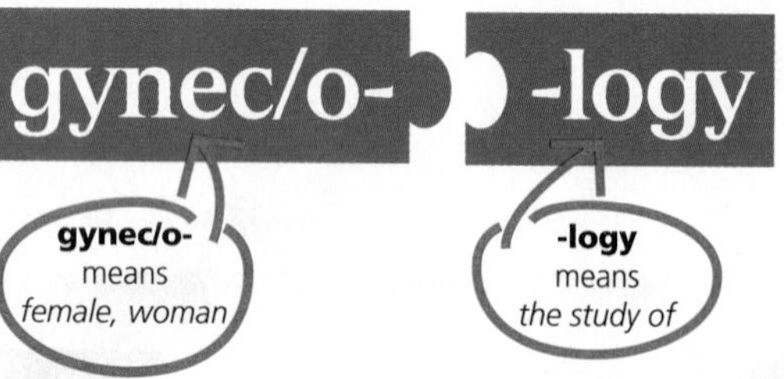

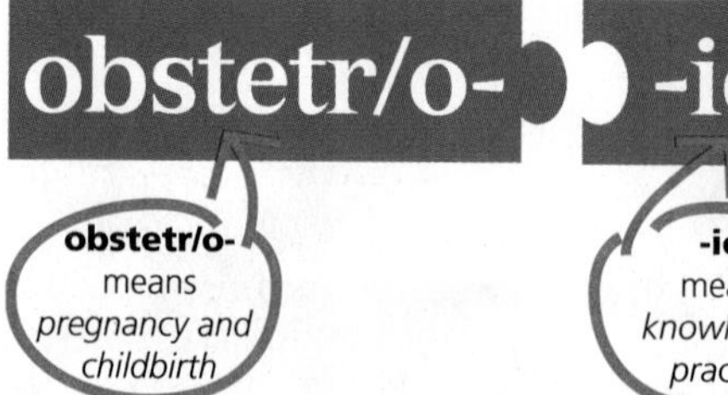

www.prenhall.com/turley

For interactive flashcards, real-life video clips, games, exercises, and audio pronunciations please explore the companion CD-ROM in the back of the book. Click on the companion website for bonus chapters, additional resources, and links to on-line learning.

Anatomy and Physiology

The **female genital and reproductive system** is a body system that is composed of the internal and external genitalia or genital organs (see Figure 13-1 ■). The **internal genitalia** in the pelvic cavity include the ovaries, fallopian tubes, uterus, and vagina. The **external genitalia** include the area of the vulva, which is composed of several structures. The

genital (JEN-ih-tal)
  genit/o- *genitalia*
  -al *pertaining to*

reproductive (REE-proh-DUK-tiv)
  re- *again and again; backward; unable to*
  product/o- *produce*
  -ive *pertaining to*

system (SIS-tem)
System is derived from a Greek word meaning *combination of parts to make an organized whole.*

internal (in-TER-nal)
  intern/o- *inside*
  -al *pertaining to*

external (eks-TER-nal)
  extern/o- *outside*
  -al *pertaining to*

genitalia (JEN-ih-TAY-lee-ah)
Genitalia is a Latin word meaning *pertaining to generation and birth.*

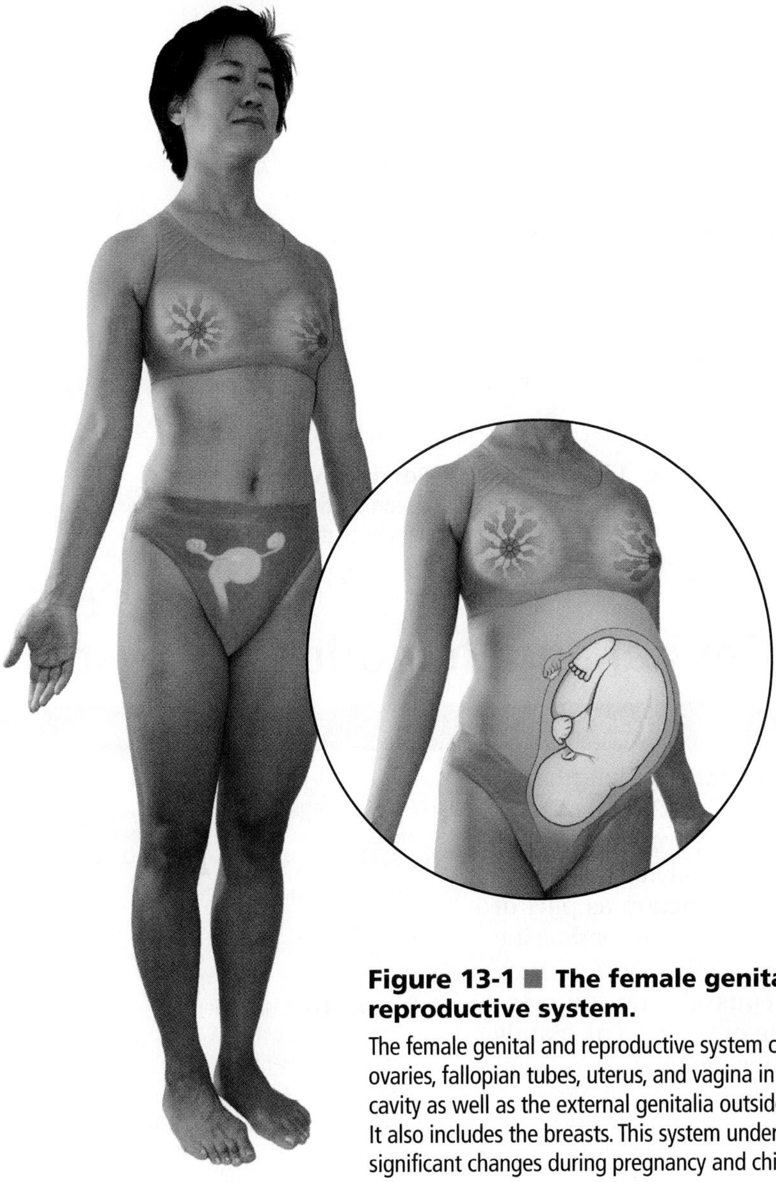

Figure 13-1 ■ The female genital and reproductive system.

The female genital and reproductive system consists of the ovaries, fallopian tubes, uterus, and vagina in the pelvic cavity as well as the external genitalia outside of the body. It also includes the breasts. This system undergoes significant changes during pregnancy and childbirth.

breasts or mammary glands also play a role in the female reproductive system. The female genital and reproductive system together with the urinary system is known as the genitourinary (GU) system or urogenital system because of the close proximity, internally and externally, of these two body systems (see Figure 13-2 ■). The function of the female genital and reproductive system is to display the female secondary sex characteristics, produce eggs, and, when appropriate, conceive and bear children.

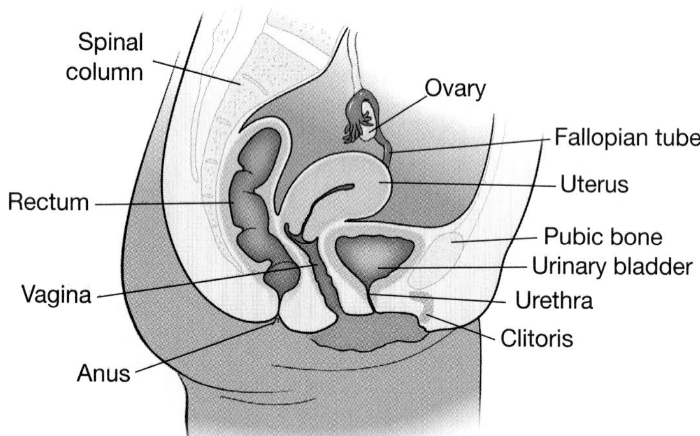

Figure 13-2 ■ Pelvic cavity.
The female genital and reproductive organs in the pelvic cavity lie in close proximity to the organs of the urinary system.

Anatomy of the Female Genital and Reproductive System

Ovaries

Each **ovary** is a flat, oval-shaped gland about two inches in length that is near the end of each fallopian tube (see Figure 13-3 ■). The ovaries are held in place by the **broad ligament,** a folded sheet of peritoneum, and other ligaments that extend to the walls of the pelvic cavity. The ovaries are the female **gonads** or sex glands. They function as part of both the female genital and reproductive system and the endocrine system. As part of the female genital and reproductive system, they contain **follicles** that rupture and release **ova** (eggs) during the menstrual cycle. As part of the endocrine system, the ovaries act as glands that secrete three hormones (estradiol, progesterone, and androgen) that affect puberty, menstruation, and pregnancy.

ovary (OH-vah-ree)
Ovary is derived from a Latin word meaning *egg.*

ovarian (oh-VAIR-ee-an)
ovari/o- *ovary*
-an *pertaining to*

ligament (LIG-ah-ment)

gonad (GOH-nad)
gon/o- *seed (ovum or spermatozoon)*
-ad *toward, in the direction of*

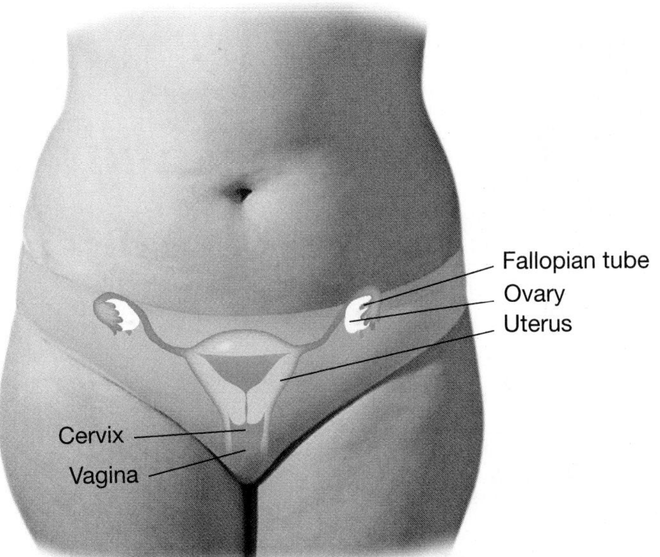

Figure 13-3 ■ The ovaries and fallopian tubes.

The ovaries and fallopian tubes lie on either side of the uterus in the abdominopelvic cavity. Each ovary releases eggs (ova) and secretes hormones into the blood. The fallopian tube carries an ovum from the ovary to the uterus.

follicle (FAWL-ih-kl)
Follicle is derived from a Latin word meaning *little bag.*

ovum (OH-vum)
ova (OH-vah)
Ovum is a Latin singular noun meaning *egg.* Form the plural by changing *-um* to *-a.*

1. **Estradiol.** The most abundant and most biologically active of the female hormones. It is secreted by the follicles. Estradiol causes the development of female sex characteristics: enlargement of the external genitalia, development of the breasts, widening of the pelvis, growth of body hair in the axillary and genital areas, and development of the sexual drive (see Figure 13-4■). Estradiol also stimulates growth of the endometrium (lining of the uterus). Estradiol is metabolized into two less active forms (estrone and estriol) that are found in the blood and urine.
2. **Progesterone.** Hormone secreted by the ruptured follicle (corpus luteum) after ovulation. It further stimulates the endometrium of the uterus to nourish the ovum, if it is fertilized.
3. **Androgen.** A male hormone secreted by cells around the follicle. It plays a role in the female sexual drive.

estradiol (ES-trah-DY-awl)
estr/a- *female*
di- *two*
-ol *chemical substance*
A molecule of estradiol contains two atoms of oxygen.

progesterone (proh-JES-ter-ohn)
Progesterone is a combination of the prefix *pro-* (before), the combining form *gest/o-* (from conception to birth), the letters *er* from *sterol* (a category of chemicals), and the suffix *-one* (chemical substance).

androgen (AN-droh-jen)
andr/o- *male*
-gen *that which produces*

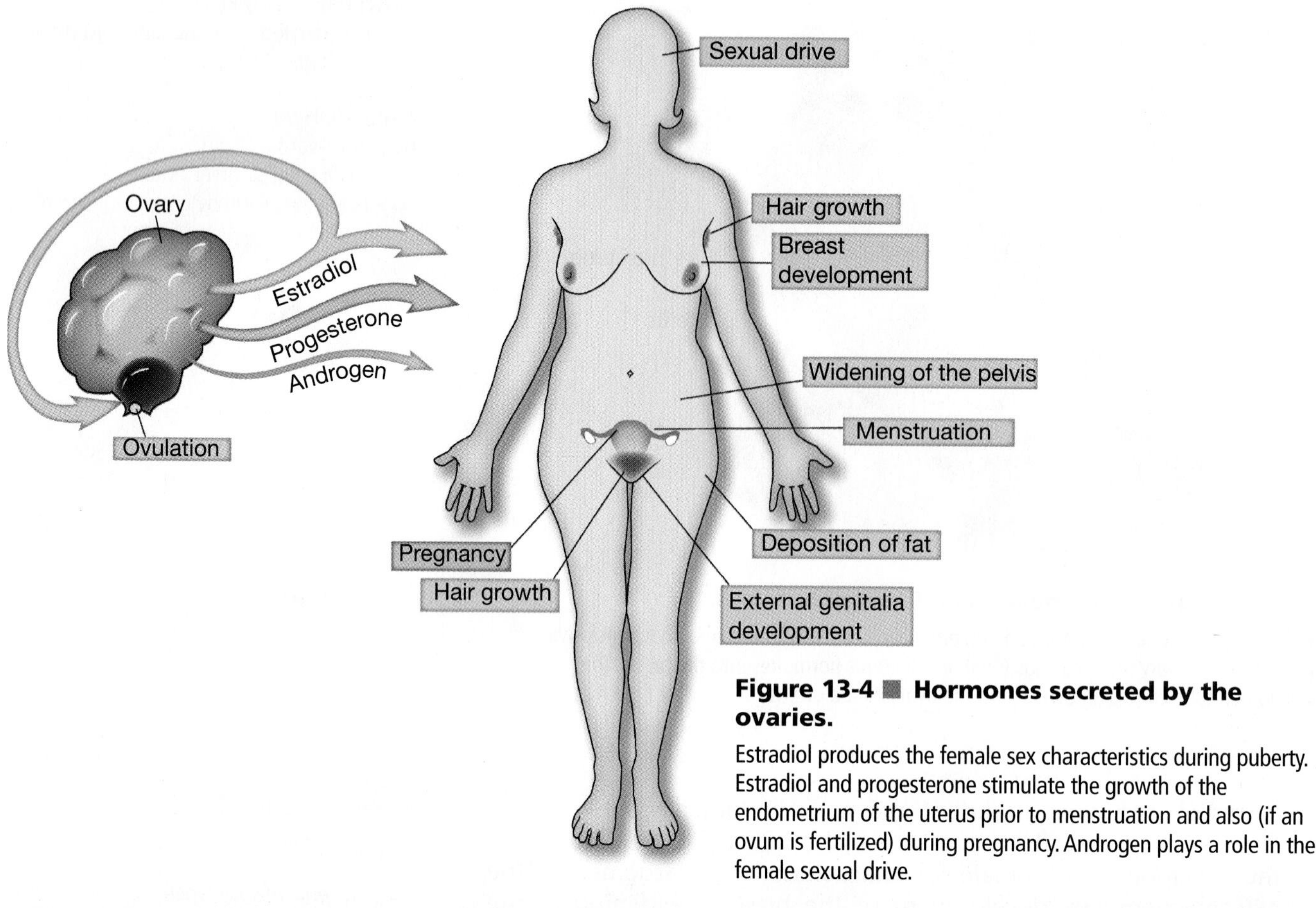

Figure 13-4 ■ Hormones secreted by the ovaries.

Estradiol produces the female sex characteristics during puberty. Estradiol and progesterone stimulate the growth of the endometrium of the uterus prior to menstruation and also (if an ovum is fertilized) during pregnancy. Androgen plays a role in the female sexual drive.

Fallopian Tubes

Each **fallopian tube** is about 5 inches in length and is held in place by the broad ligament. Its medial end is connected to the uterus, but its lateral end is not connected directly to the ovary (see Figure 13-5 ■). There is an open space there that is actually part of the abdominopelvic cavity. The function of the fallopian tube is to transport an ovum from the ovary to the uterus. **Fimbriae,** moving fingerlike projections on the lateral end of the fallopian tube, create currents that carry the ovum toward the **infundibulum,** a funnel-shaped structure that captures the ovum and directs it into the **lumen** of the fallopian tube. There, **cilia,** tiny hairs inside the fallopian tube, beat in waves while **peristalsis** (a coordinated contraction of smooth muscle) propels the ovum toward the uterus. Fluid inside the fallopian tube contains nutrients to nourish the ovum on its three-day journey to the uterus. The fallopian tube is also known as an **oviduct.** Collectively, the ovaries and the fallopian tubes are known as the **adnexa.**

fallopian (fah-LOH-pee-an)
fallopi/o- *fallopian tube*
-an *pertaining to*
The fallopian tubes were named by Gabriele Fallopius (1523–1562), an Italian anatomist. This is an example of an eponym: a person from whom something takes its name.

fimbriae (FIM-bree-ee)
Fimbria is a Latin singular feminine noun meaning *fringe.* Form the plural by changing *-a* to *-ae.* Because the fallopian tube has so many fimbriae, the singular form is seldom used.

infundibulum (IN-fun-DIB-yoo-lum)
Infundibulum is a Latin word meaning *a funnel.*

lumen (LOO-men)
Lumen is a Latin word meaning *window.*

cilia (SIL-ee-ah)
Cilium is a Latin singular neuter noun. Form the plural by changing *-um* to *-a.* Because there are thousands of cilia in the fallopian tubes, the singular form is seldom used.

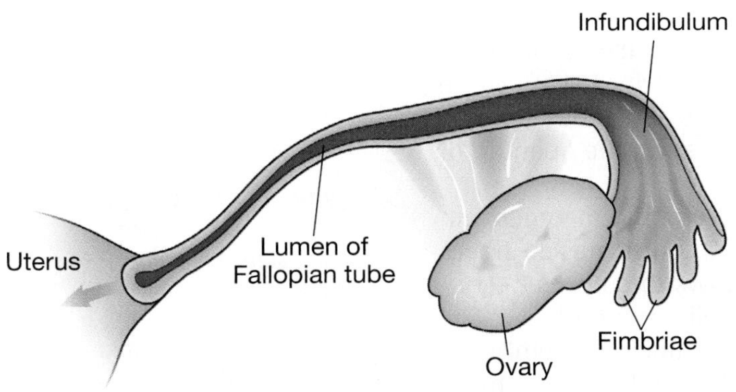

Figure 13-5 ■ Fallopian tube.

The fallopian tube is not directly connected to the ovary. Movements of the fimbriae draw the egg from the ovary into the lumen of the fallopian tube.

peristalsis (PAIR-ih-STAL-sis)
peri- *around*
-stalsis *process of contraction*
Every medical word must contain a combining form. The suffix of *peristalsis* contains the combining form *stal/o-*.

oviduct (OH-vih-dukt)
ov/i- *ovum (egg)*
-duct *duct (tube)*
Duct is derived from a Latin word meaning *to lead.*

adnexa (ad-NEK-sah)
Adnexa is a Latin word meaning *connected parts.*

adnexal (ad-NEK-sal)
adnex/o- *accessory connecting parts*
-al *pertaining to*

Uterus

The **uterus** is an inverted pear-shaped organ about 3 inches in length (see Figure 13-3). It is suspended within the abdominopelvic cavity by the broad ligament and other ligaments that go to the sacrum and to the walls of the pelvic cavity. The broad ligament also creates a small pouch, the cul-de-sac, between the uterus and the rectum. The superior portion of the uterus is tipped anteriorly and rests on the urinary bladder (see Figure 13-2); this normal position is known as **anteflexion.** The uterus connects to the vagina inferiorly.

The **fundus** of the uterus is the round, domelike part above the fallopian tubes (see Figure 13-6 ■). The **corpus** or body of the uterus is its

uterus (YOO-ter-us)
Uterus is a Latin word meaning *womb.*

uterine (YOO-ter-in) (YOO-ter-ine)
uter/o- *uterus (womb)*
-ine *pertaining to*

anteflexion (AN-tee-FLEK-shun)
ante- *forward, before*
flex/o- *bending*
-ion *action; condition*

fundus (FUN-dus)
Fundus is a Latin word meaning *part farthest from the opening.*

fundal (FUN-dal)
fund/o- *fundus (part farthest from the opening)*
-al *pertaining to*

corpus (KOR-pus)
Corpus is a Latin word meaning *body.*

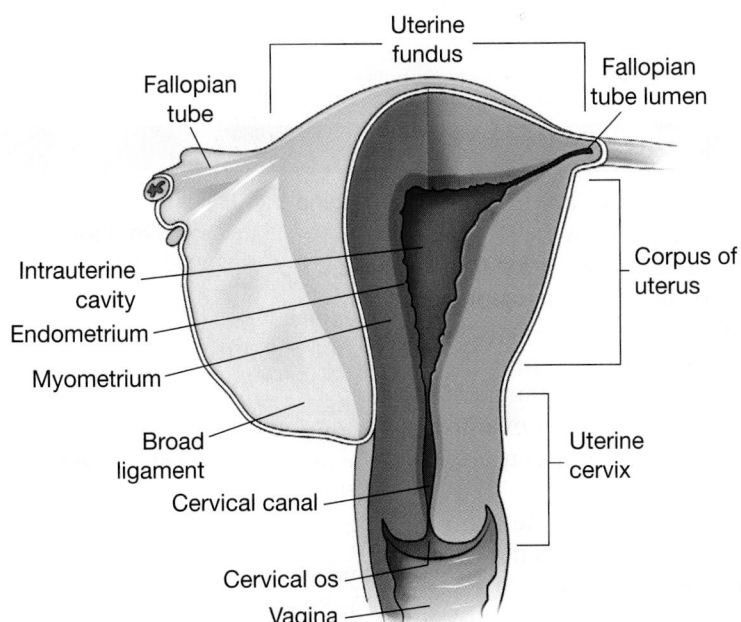

Figure 13-6 ■ The uterus.

The fundus, corpus or body, and cervix are the regions of the uterus. The myometrium is the layer of smooth muscle that makes up the uterine wall. The endometrium is the layer of glands and tissue that lines the intrauterine cavity.

widest part. Inside the body of the uterus is the hollow **intrauterine cavity.** As the uterine body continues inferiorly, it narrows into the **cervix** or neck of the uterus, and the intrauterine cavity becomes the **cervical canal.** The rounded tip of the cervix projects about 1/2 inch into the vagina. In the center of the cervix is the **cervical os,** the opening of the cervical canal.

The wall of the uterus is composed of two layers: the myometrium and endometrium. The **myometrium** contains smooth muscle fibers that are oriented in different directions. This allows the uterus to contract strongly from all sides during labor and delivery of a baby. The inner layer, the **endometrium,** is a specialized mucous membrane that contains glands that build the endometrial lining during the menstrual cycle. If an ovum is not fertilized, this lining is shed during menstruation.

intrauterine (IN-trah-YOO-ter-in) (IN-trah-YOO-ter-ine)
intra- *within*
uter/o- *uterus (womb)*
-ine *pertaining to*

cavity (KAV-ih-tee)
cav/o- *hollow space*
-ity *state; condition*

cervix (SER-viks)
Cervix is a Latin word meaning *neck.*

cervical (SER-vih-kal)
cervic/o- *neck; cervix*
-al *pertaining to*

canal (kah-NAL)
Canal is derived from a Latin word meaning *tubular channel.*

os (AWS)
Os is a Latin word meaning *an opening into a canal or into the hollow part of an organ.*

myometrium (MY-oh-MEE-tree-um)

myometrial (MY-oh-MEE-tree-al)
my/o- *muscle*
metri/o- *uterus (womb)*
-al *pertaining to*

endometrium (EN-doh-MEE-tree-um)

endometrial (EN-doh-MEE-tree-al)
endo- *innermost, within*
metri/o- *uterus (womb)*
-al *pertaining to*

Vagina

The **vagina** is a short, tubelike structure about 3 inches in length (see Figures 13-2 and 13-6). Inside is a slender channel known as the **vaginal canal.** The cervix of the uterus protrudes into the superior end of the vaginal canal. The part of the vagina that lies behind and around the cervix is known as the **fornix.** At the inferior end of the vaginal canal is the **hymen,** an elastic membrane that partially or completely covers the opening, although it is sometimes absent. The hymen, if present, is easily torn by the insertion of a tampon, a vaginal examination, or sexual intercourse. The **introitus** is the external opening of the vagina.

The vagina has three functions. It transports the shed endometrium from menstruation to the outside of the body. It holds the penis during sexual intercourse, collecting the ejaculate that contains spermatozoa. During birth, the vagina is part of the birth canal that takes the baby to the outside of the mother's body.

vagina (vah-JY-nah)
Vagina is a Latin word meaning *a sheath (a long enveloping structure).*

vaginal (VAJ-ih-nal)
vagin/o- *vagina*
-al *pertaining to*

fornix (FOR-niks)
Fornix is a Latin word meaning *the arched part of a roofed space.* The fornix is also known as the vaginal vault.

hymen (HY-men)
Hymen is a Greek word meaning *membrane.*

introitus (in-TROH-ih-tus)
Introitus is a Latin word meaning *entrance.*

External Genitalia

The external genitalia include the labia majora, labia minora, clitoris, vaginal introitus, and several glands that provide lubricating secretions (see Figure 13-7 ■). The **vulva** is the area that includes all of these structures as well as the urethral meatus and the **mons pubis** (the rounded, fleshy pad with pubic hair that overlies the **pubic** bone). The area between the edge of the vulva and the anus is known as the **perineum.**

The labia consist of two sets of lip-shaped structures that run anteriorly to posteriorly and partially cover the urethral meatus and vaginal introitus. The thicker, outermost lips, the **labia majora,** are fleshy and covered with pubic hair on their outer surface. The smooth, thin, inner lips, the **labia minora,** lie beneath the labia majora. The **clitoris** is the organ of sexual response in the female. Its tip is located above the urethral meatus. With sexual stimulation, the clitoris enlarges with blood and becomes firmer. The vaginal introitus (entrance to the vagina), is located below the urethral meatus. **Bartholin's glands,** the **urethral glands,** and **Skene's glands** (abbreviated as *BUS*) near the vaginal introitus secrete mucus during sexual arousal.

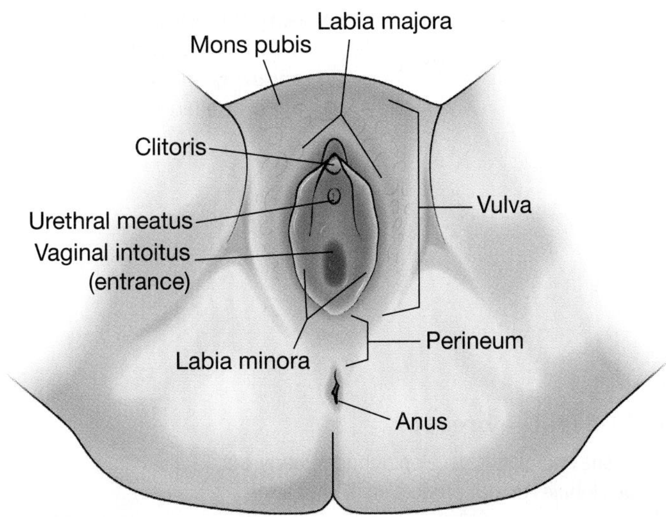

Figure 13-7 ■ The external female genitalia.

The labia majora and labia minora protect and partially cover the clitoris, vaginal introitus, and the glands that secrete mucus. The vulva includes all these structures but also includes the urinary meatus and mons pubis.

vulva (VUL-vah)
Vulva is a Latin word meaning *a covering for the womb.* The female external genitalia are also known as the *pudendum. Pudendum* is derived from a Latin word meaning *to feel ashamed.*

vulvar (VUL-var)
vulv/o- *vulva*
-ar *pertaining to*

mons pubis (MAWNZ PYOO-bis)
Mons is a Latin word meaning *mountain. Pubis* means *of the pubic bone.*

pubic (PYOO-bik)
pub/o- *pubis (hip bone)*
-ic *pertaining to*

perineum (PAIR-ih-NEE-um)
Perineum is a Latin word meaning *the area between the vulva (or scrotum) and the anus.*

perineal (PAIR-ih-NEE-al)
perine/o- *perineum*
-al *pertaining to*

labia majora (LAY-bee-ah mah-JOR-ah)
labia minora (LAY-bee-ah my-NOR-ah)
Labium is a Latin singular neuter noun meaning *a lip.* Form the plural by changing *-um* to *-a.*

labial (LAY-bee-al)
labi/o- *lip; labium*
-al *pertaining to*

clitoris (KLIT-oh-ris)
Clitoris is a Greek word meaning *little hill.*

Bartholin (BAR-thoh-lin)
Named by Casper Bartholin (1655–1738), a Danish anatomist.

urethral (yoo-REE-thral)
urethr/o- *urethra*
-al *pertaining to*

Skene (SKEEN)
Named by Alexander Skene (1838–1900), an American gynecologist.

Breasts

The breasts or **mammary glands** are located on the chest. They are considered accessory glands of the integumentary system because of their structure, but they function as part of the female reproductive system. The breasts develop at puberty in response to estradiol secreted by the ovaries. They are one of the female sex characteristics, and they also provide milk to nourish a baby after birth. The breasts are composed of adipose (fatty) tissue and **lactiferous lobules** (see Figure 13-8■); these lobules produce milk when stimulated by the hormone prolactin from the anterior pituitary gland. During breastfeeding, milk flows through the lactiferous ducts to the nipple. The pigmented area around the nipple is known as the **areola.** The surface of the areola is covered with small, elevated areas that secrete oil to protect the nipple when the baby nurses. The **inframammary crease** is the skin fold beneath each breast.

mammary (MAM-ah-ree)
mamm/o- *breast*
-ary *pertaining to*

lactiferous (lak-TIF-er-us)
lact/i- *milk*
fer/o- *to bear*
-ous *pertaining to*

lobule (LAWB-yool)
lob/o- *lobe of an organ*
-ule *small thing*

areola (ah-REE-oh-lah)

areolae (ah-REE-oh-lee)
Areola is a Latin singular feminine noun meaning *small area.* Form the plural by changing *-a* to *-ae.*

areolar (ah-REE-oh-lar)
areol/o- *small area around the nipple*
-ar *pertaining to*

inframammary (IN-frah-MAM-ah-ree)
infra- *below, beneath*
mamm/o- *breast*
-ary *pertaining to*

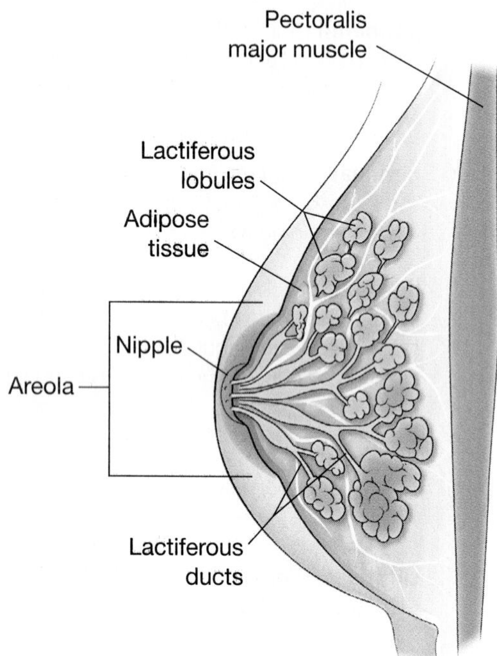

Figure 13-8 ■ The breast.
The breast tissue and glands develop during puberty, but the lactiferous lobules do not produce milk until after childbirth.

Physiology of Menstruation and Conception

Before birth, the fetal ovaries contain many **oocytes** (immature eggs) within follicles. At the onset of puberty or adolescence, the anterior pituitary gland of the endocrine system begins to secrete two hormones to stimulate the ovaries.

1. **Follicle-stimulating hormone (FSH).** FSH stimulates the follicles to produce mature ova. Like a spermatozoon, a mature ovum is created by mitosis and meiosis. However, unlike spermatozoa, only a single, large ovum is produced. It contains 23 chromosomes, and the remaining chromosomes are discarded in small packets of cytoplasm known as polar bodies. The process of forming a mature ovum is known as **oogenesis.** The mature ovum, like a spermatozoon, is known as a gamete. FSH also stimulates the follicles to secrete estradiol, which causes the development of the female sex characteristics.
2. **Luteining hormone (LH).** LH stimulates a single follicle each month to rupture and release its mature ovum. This process known as **ovulation.**

oocyte (OH-oh-site)
o/o- *ovum (egg)*
-cyte *cell*

oogenesis (oh-oh-JEN-eh-sis)
o/o- *ovum (egg)*
gen/o- *arising from; produced by*
-esis *condition*

luteinizing (LOO-tee-ih-ny-zing)
Luteinizing hormone is so named because it stimulates the corpus luteum of the ovary (as well as the interstitial cells of the testis).

ovulation (AWV-yoo-LAY-shun)
ovul/o- *ovum (egg)*
-ation *a process; being or having*

Did You Know?

While a female fetus is still in the mother's uterus, the fetal ovary forms about 2 million oocytes or immature eggs. These are all the eggs that female will ever have, as no more are produced after she is born. By puberty only about 25% of these remain and, of those, only about 400 to 500 are released during ovulation during her lifetime.

In the 1800s, the average age for menarche (the onset of menstruation) was 18 years old. Now the average age for menarche is 12 years old.

The Menstrual Cycle

With the onset of puberty, the female begins to ovulate and menstruate. The beginning of **menstruation** with the first menstrual period or **menses** is known as **menarche.**

Each menstrual cycle takes 28 days, on average, and includes four phases: the menstrual phase, the proliferative phase, the secretory phase, and the ischemic phase (see Figure 13-9■).

1. **Menstrual phase** (Days 1–6)
Menstruation begins. Approximately 30 mL of blood, endometrial tissue, and mucus is shed from the uterus and passes through the vagina. All that remains of the endometrium is a thin layer of glands. At the same time, several follicles are enlarging and their ova are maturing in preparation for one of them to be released during ovulation on day 14.

menstruation (MEN-stroo-AA-shun)
menstru/o- *monthly discharge of blood*
-ation *a process; being or having*

menses (MEN-seez)
Menses is a Latin plural noun for *mensis* (a month).

menarche (meh-NAR-kee)
men/o- *month*
-arche *a beginning*

menstrual (MEN-stroo-al)
menstru/o- *monthly discharge of blood*
-al *pertaining to*

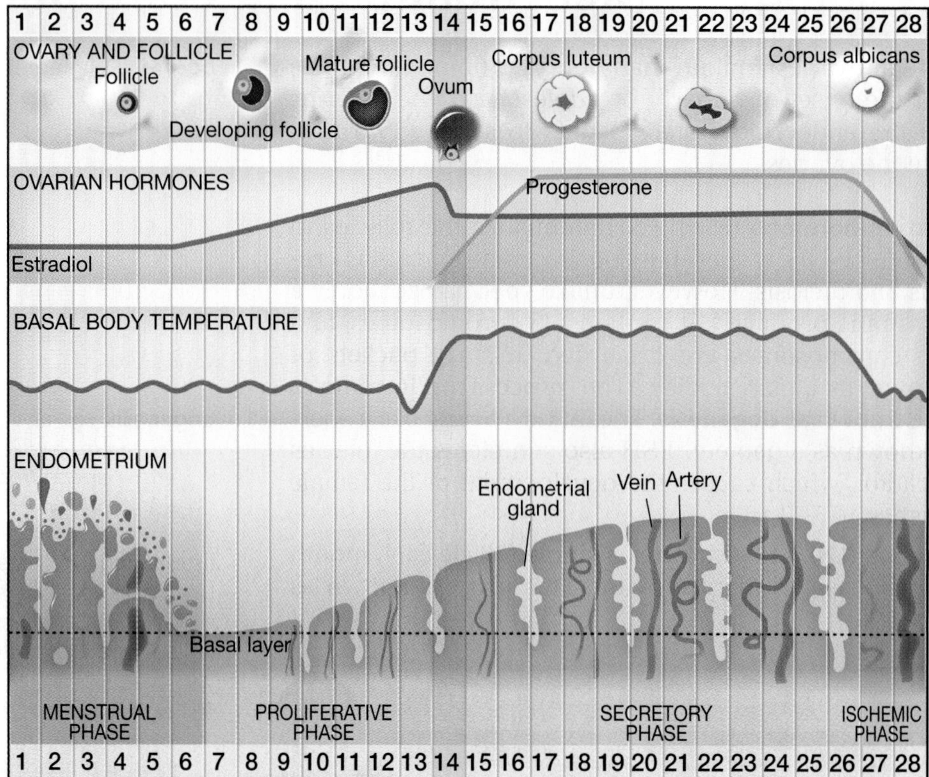

Figure 13-9 ■ The menstrual cycle.

Activities in the ovary are intricately related to activities in the uterus during the menstrual cycle. Hormones (estradiol and progesterone) produced by the follicle and corpus luteum of the ovary cause the endometrium to proliferate in time to receive and nourish the ovum. If the ovum is not fertilized, the declining levels of the hormones cause the endometrium to slough off in menstruation.

2. **Proliferative phase** (Days 7–13)
   Follicle-stimulating hormone (FSH) from the anterior pituitary gland stimulates the ovarian follicles to secrete estradiol. One follicle becomes greatly enlarged and produces a mature ovum. The thickness of the endometrial tissue in the uterus increases under the influence of estradiol. At the end of the proliferative phase, mucus in the cervical canal thins to allow spermatozoa to pass through it, and the **basal (baseline) body temperature** dips slightly.
3. **Ovulation** (Day 14)
   Luteinizing hormone (LH) from the anterior pituitary gland causes the enlarged ovarian follicle to rupture, releasing a mature ovum. The basal body temperature rises sharply at the time of ovulation.
4. **Secretory phase** (Days 15–26)
   The ruptured ovarian follicle fills with yellow fat and becomes the **corpus luteum,** which secretes estradiol and progesterone. Progesterone causes the endometrial glands of the uterus to enlarge, and the endometrium becomes thicker. Small arteries grow to the edge of the endometrium, ready to nourish a fertilized ovum. The basal body temperature continues to be elevated due to progesterone. At the end of the secretory phase, if the ovum is not fertilized, the corpus luteum begins to degenerate.

proliferative (proh-LIF-er-ah-tiv)
Proliferate means *to increase in number by producing more of the same.*

basal (BAY-sal)
bas/o- *base*
-al *pertaining to*

secretory (SEE-kreh-toh-ree)
secret/o- *produce; secrete*
-ory *having the function of*

corpus luteum (KOR-pus LOO-tee-um)
Corpus is a Latin word meaning *body.* The corpus or body can be as large as in the uterine corpus or as small as the corpus luteum. *Luteum* is a Latin word meaning *yellow.* Lutein is a yellow pigment that gives the corpus luteum (and the yolk in a chicken egg) its yellow color.

5. **Ischemic phase** (Days 27–28)
   The corpus luteum degenerates into scar tissue and stops making estradiol and progesterone. The abrupt decrease in these hormones causes the small arteries in the endometrium to contract. This stops the flow of blood and causes ischemia of the tissue. The endometrium begins to slough off, and menstruation (the first phase) begins again.

ischemic (is-KEE-mik)
isch/o- *keep back; block*
-emic *pertaining to blood or a substance in the blood*

Conception

Of the 100 to 500 million spermatozoa deposited in the vagina during sexual intercourse, only some are able to reach the ovum in the fallopian tube; this occurs 24 to 48 hours after sexual intercourse.

In the fallopian tube, chemicals secreted by the ovum attract the spermatozoa. Enzymes in the head of each spermatozoon begin to dissolve the layer of cells around the ovum (see Figure 13-10 ■). Many spermatozoa attach to the ovum, but only one penetrates the ovum. This is the moment of **fertilization** or **conception.** After that, the surface of the ovum changes and actually repels the other spermatozoa. When a spermatozoon unites with an ovum, the resulting cell has 46 chromosomes and is known as a **zygote. Pregnancy** begins at the moment of conception.

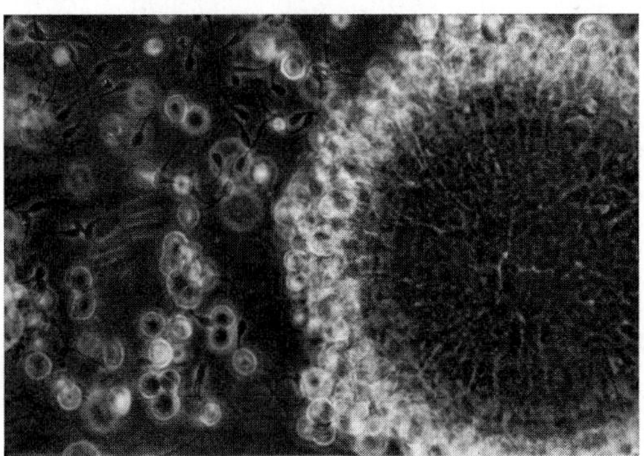

Figure 13-10 ■ An ovum and spermatozoa.
The ovum is nearly 100,000 times larger than a spermatozoon. An ovum and a spermatozoon are gametes and contain only 23 chromosomes. The fertilized cell or zygote contains 46 chromosomes.

fertilization (FER-til-ih-ZAY-shun)
fertil/o- *able to conceive a child*
-ization *process of making, creating, or inserting*

conception (con-SEP-shun)
concept/o- *to conceive or form*
-ion *action; condition*

zygote (ZY-goht)
Zygote is derived from a Greek word meaning *joined together.*

pregnancy (PREG-nan-see)
pregn/o- *being with child*
-ancy *state of*
Pregnancy is derived from a Latin word meaning *before being born.*

pregnant (PREG-nant)
pregn/o- *being with child*
-ant *pertaining to*

Connections

Genetics. The sex chromosomes are one of the chromosome pairs in the nucleus of each cell. A female's sex chromosome pair consists of two X chromosomes. A male's sex chromosome pair consists of an X and a Y chromosome.

A spermatozoon only contains one sex chromosome, either the X chromosome or the Y chromosome. The ovum always contains an X chromosome. An X chromosome from the spermatozoan and an X chromosome from the ovum unite to create a zygote that is a female. A Y chromosome from the spermatozoan and an X chromosome from the ovum unite to create a zygote that is a male. **Fraternal** twins occur when the ovary releases two ova that are fertilized by different spermatozoa. Identical twins occur when one developing zygote splits to create two separate but identical zygotes. Multiple zygotes can be present if the ovary releases multiple ova; this can occur in patients taking ovulation-stimulating drugs for infertility.

fraternal (frah-TER-nal)
fratern/o- *close association or relationship*
-al *pertaining to*
Although a fraternity usually is an association of all male members, fraternal twins can be two males, one male and one female, or two females.

The fertilized ovum immediately begins to divide as it moves through the fallopian tube. Inside the intrauterine cavity, it sinks into the thick endometrium. At this point, it is a hollow ball with an outer layer and an inner mass of cells. The outer layer or **chorion** sends fingerlike projections into the endometrium to absorb nutrients and oxygen. The chorion produces the hormone **human chorionic gonadotropin (HCG).** HCG stimulates the corpus luteum to keep producing estradiol and progesterone, and this prevents menstruation from occurring for the duration of the pregnancy. The inner mass of cells forms the amnion and what will become the embryo. The **amnion** is a membrane that surrounds the **amniotic cavity** which is filled with **amniotic fluid.** The amnion is also known as the bag of waters. The developing embryo floats in and is cushioned by the amniotic fluid. After four days of development, the fertilized ovum is known as an **embryo.** After eight weeks, it is known as a **fetus** (see Figure 13-11 ■).

The chorion develops into the **placenta,** a pancake-like structure that is attached to the endometrium and is about 7 inches in diameter and 1 to 2 inches thick. The placenta is also known as the afterbirth. Other structures form the **umbilical cord** that connects the placenta to the fetus. The fetus, placenta, and all fluids and tissue in the uterus are known as the products of conception. During the pregnancy, the job of the corpus luteum in secreting estradiol and progesterone is taken over by the placenta. The umbilical cord and placenta also bring oxygen, nutrients, and antibodies from the mother to the fetus and remove carbon dioxide and waste products.

The moment of conception to the moment of birth is known as the **gestation.** The gestational period is approximately nine months (38 to 42 weeks), the average being 40 weeks (see Figure 13-12 ■). Gestation can be divided into three equal sections or trimesters. Each **trimester** contains three months. For the fetus, the period of time

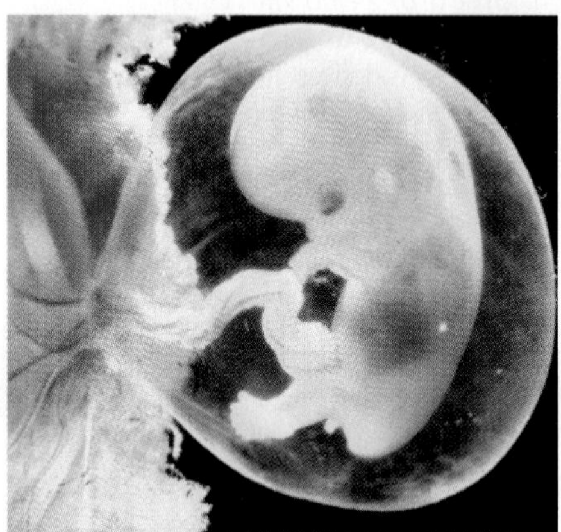

Figure 13-11 ■ A fetus at 9 weeks' gestation.

This fetus would be approximately 1 inch in length. It is floating in clear amniotic fluid in the amniotic sac. The beginnings of the eyes, ears, ribs, fingers, and toes are clearly visible. The heart has been beating since the third week of life. The arteries bringing red, oxygenated blood to the fetus are clearly visible in the umbilical cord.

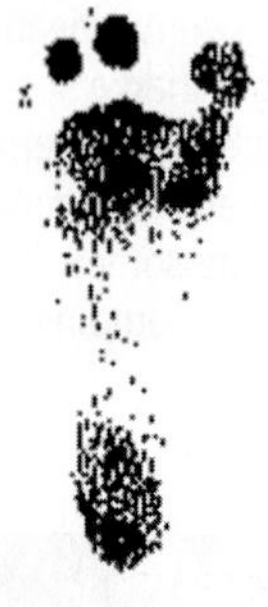

Figure 13-12 ■ Fetal footprint.

This is the actual footprint that appeared on the delivery room record of a fetus who was born prematurely at 23 weeks' gestation.

chorion (KOH-ree-on)

chorionic (KOH-ree-ON-ik)
chorion/o- *chorion (fetal membrane)*
-ic *pertaining to*

gonadotropin (GOH-nah-doh-TROH-pin)
gonad/o- *gonads (ovaries and testes)*
trop/o- *having an affinity for; stimulating; turning*
-in *a substance*

amnion (AM-nee-on)
Amnion is a Greek word meaning *membrane surrounding the fetus.*

amniotic (AM-nee-AWT-ik)
amni/o- *amnion (fetal membrane)*
-tic *pertaining to*

embryo (EM-bree-oh)
Embryo is a Greek word meaning *that which swells and grows within.*

embryonic (EM-bree-ON-ik)
embryon/o- *embryo; immature form*
-ic *pertaining to*

fetus (FEE-tus)
Fetus is a Latin word meaning *offspring.*

fetal (FEE-tal)
fet/o- *fetus*
-al *pertaining to*

placenta (plah-SEN-tah)
Placenta is a Latin word meaning *flat cake.*

placental (plah-SEN-tal)
placent/o- *placenta*
-al *pertaining to*

umbilicus
(um-BIL-ih-kus) (UM-bih-LIE-kus)
Umbilicus is a Latin word meaning *the navel.*

umbilical (um-BIL-ih-kal)
umbilic/o- *umbilicus, navel*
-al *pertaining to*

gestation (jes-TAY-shun)
gestat/o- *from conception to birth*
-ion *action; condition*

trimester (TRY-mes-ter) (try-MES-ter)
Trimester is derived from a Latin word meaning *a three-month duration.* The prefix *tri-* means *three.*

from conception to birth is known as the **prenatal period.** For the mother, the period of time from conception to birth is known as **antepartum.**

prenatal (pree-NAY-tal)
pre- *before; in front of*
nat/o- *birth*
-al *pertaining to*

antepartum (AN-tee-PAR-tum)
ante- *forward, before*
-partum *childbirth*
Every medical word must contain a combining form. The suffix of *antepartum* contains the combining form *part/o-*.

Did You Know?

The fetus swallows amniotic fluid each day. This is absorbed from the intestines into the fetal bloodstream. The fetal kidneys excrete small amounts of urine into the amniotic fluid. The amniotic fluid contains urea and creatinine (waste products in the urine), skin cells and hair shed by the fetus, and two important substances (lecithin and sphingomyelin) that can be used to determine the maturity of the fetal lungs when the amniotic fluid is tested.

Physiology of Labor and Delivery

As the fetus grows, the uterus expands, taking up more of the abdominal cavity and displacing the abdominal organs of the mother. This causes symptoms of constipation, urinary frequency, and shortness of breath in the mother. During the last trimester of pregnancy, the uterus contracts irregularly to strengthen in preparation for childbirth. These are known as **Braxton Hicks contractions** or false labor. Progesterone produced by the placenta keeps the contractions from progressing into labor. The cervical os remains closed (not dilated), and the cervical walls are thick (not effaced). A thick mucus plug occludes the cervical os to keep out microorganisms. Late in the pregnancy, the uterine fundus descends as the fetal head drops into the birth position within the mother's pelvis. This process is known as **engagement** or lightening. The fetus usually assumes a head-down position. The head becomes the presenting part (part of the body that will go first through the birth canal). This is known as a **cephalic presentation.** Any part of the head can be the presenting part, but most commonly it is the top of the head. This is known as a **vertex presentation.**

Sometime between 38 to 42 weeks' gestation, labor begins. The placenta produces more estradiol, which stimulates the release of oxytocin from the posterior pituitary gland. **Oxytocin** causes the uterus to begin to contract regularly. The cervix softens as collagen fibers in its tissues are broken down. This process is known as cervical ripening.

The process of labor and childbirth is known as **parturition.** It is divided into three stages.

1. **First stage of labor.** Uterine contractions occur about every 30 minutes, becoming greater in intensity and duration. Cervical **dilation** (widening of the cervical os) progresses from 0 to 5 cm, and **effacement** (thinning of the cervical wall) progresses from 0 to 50%. **Rupture of membranes (ROM)** occurs and releases amniotic fluid. As the uterine contractions intensify, the mother may receive epidural anesthesia to help control the pain. After 8 to 20 hours of labor, the cervix is completely dilated at 10 cm and 100% effaced (see Figure 13-13■), and the mother is transferred to the delivery room.

Braxton Hicks (BRAK-ston HIKS)
Braxton Hicks contractions were named by John Braxton Hicks (1823–1897), a British gynecologist.

contraction (con-TRAK-shun)
contract/o- *pull together*
-ion *action; condition*

cephalic (seh-FAL-ik)
cephal/o- *head*
-ic *pertaining to*

vertex (VER-teks)
Vertex is a Latin word meaning *top or crown.*

oxytocin (AWK-see-TOH-sin)
ox/y- *oxygen; quick*
toc/o- *labor and childbirth*
-in *a substance*
Some word parts have more than one definition. The best definition of *oxytoxin* is *a substance [that causes] quick labor and childbirth.*

parturition (PAR-tyoo-RIH-shun)
parturit/o- *to be in labor*
-ion *action; condition*

dilation (dy-LAY-shun)
dilat/o- *dilate, widen*
-ion *action; condition*

effacement (eh-FAYS-ment)
efface/o- *do away with; obliterate*
-ment *action; state*

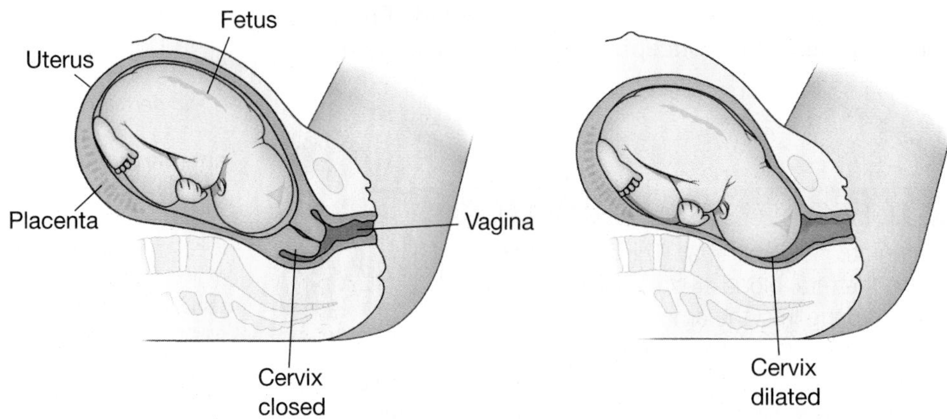

Figure 13-13 ■ Dilation and effacement.

With the cervix 10 cm dilated and 100% effaced, the fetal head is able to pass through the birth canal (cervix and vagina), and the fetus is ready to be born. This fetus is in the vertex position.

2. **Second stage of labor.** The uterine contractions have brought the head of the fetus into the vagina. The mother is encouraged to push by holding her breath to raise the intra-abdominal pressure. **Crowning** occurs when most of the top of the baby's head is visible at the vaginal introitus (see Figure 13-14■). The head of the newborn is delivered, and after several more uterine contractions, the shoulders and the rest of the body are delivered. The newborn is placed on the mother's abdomen while the umbilical cord is clamped and cut (see Figure 13-15■).

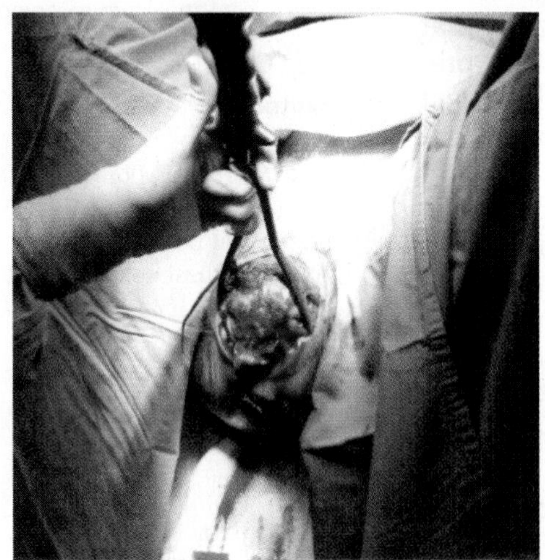

Figure 13-14 ■ Crowning of the fetal head.

The hair on the baby's head is visible. The top of the head bulges outwardly with each contraction, as the mother pushes. The irregular edges of the vagina indicate that an episiotomy has been performed to prevent spontaneous tearing of the vaginal tissues. The obstetrician is using obstetrical forceps to assist in the delivery of the head.

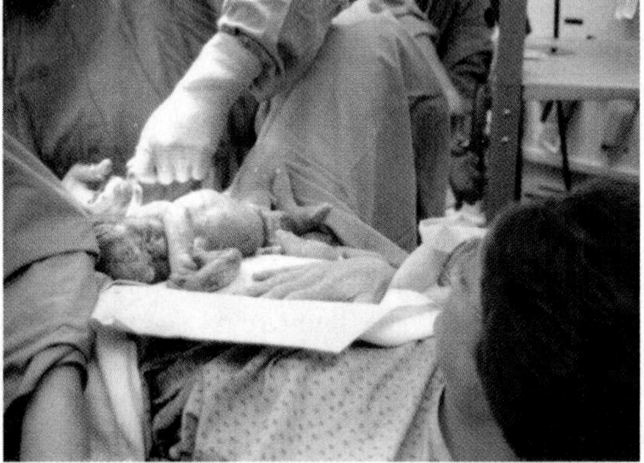

Figure 13-15 ■ Cutting the umbilical cord.

The obstetrician clamps the umbilical cord while the new mother sees her baby for the first time. Notice the length of the umbilical cord as it travels from its attachment to the baby's umbilicus, beneath his body, to the obstetrician. Later, the obstetrician will shorten the stump of the umbilical cord and apply a plastic clamp.

3. **Third stage of labor.** The placenta is delivered about 30 minutes after the birth. Oxytocin causes the uterus to contract to stop blood flow from the raw surfaces where the placenta pulled away. The obstetrician sutures up the episiotomy, if one was performed. The placenta and umbilical cord are sent to pathology for examination. Blood in the umbilical cord is rich in stem cells and can be used for stem cell transplantation in cancer patients.

For the newborn, the period of time after birth is known as the **postnatal period.** For the mother, the period of time after birth is known as **postpartum.** The uterus gradually shrinks in size, a process known as **involution.** Small amounts of blood, tissue, and fluid, known as **lochia,** continue to be discharged from the uterus for a week until all of the endometrial lining is shed.

Lactation is the production of breast milk by the mammary glands after childbirth. Oxytocin from the mother's posterior pituitary gland causes her breasts to release milk for breastfeeding whenever the newborn cries or sucks. This is known as the let-down reflex. The first milk, **colostrum,** is a thick, yellowish fluid. By the third day, the colostrum is replaced by regular breast milk that is thin and white.

Connections

Immunology (Chapter 6). Colostrum is rich in nutrients and contains maternal antibodies. For the first few days of life, the newborn's intestinal tract is more permeable and allows these antibodies to be absorbed from the intestine directly into the blood. These maternal antibodies provide passive immunity to common diseases that the mother has already had. This immunity lasts until the infant begins to make its own antibodies at about 18 months of age.

postnatal (post-NAY-tal)
post- *after, behind*
nat/o- *birth*
-al *pertaining to*

postpartum (post-PAR-tum)
post- *after, behind*
-partum *childbirth*

involution (IN-voh-LOO-shun)
involut/o- *enlarged organ returns to normal size*
-ion *action; condition*

lochia (LOH-kee-ah)
Lochia is derived from a Greek word meaning *relating to childbirth.*

lactation (lak-TAY-shun)
lact/o- *milk*
-ation *a process; being or having*

colostrum (koh-LAWS-trum)

The Newborn

A newborn who is born between 38 and 42 weeks' gestation is a **term neonate.** A newborn between 28 and 37 weeks' gestation is preterm or premature, a reference to the maturity of the internal organs and their ability to function. Because the date of conception is not always known, the gestational age of a newborn is an estimate.

The skin of the neonate is covered with **vernix caseosa,** a thick, white, cheesy substance that protects the skin from amniotic fluid in the uterus (see Figure 13-16 ■). The head can exhibit **molding,** an elongated temporary reshaping of the cranium that occurs as the head passes through the mother's bony pelvis. The bones of the cranium may actually overlap each other slightly. On the top of the head, there is a large area known as the **anterior fontanel** or soft spot. It is soft and flexible and bulges when the newborn cries because it is only covered by the dura mater, not by cranial bone. There is also a smaller posterior fontanel at the back of the head. The fontanels allow the cranium to expand as the brain grows. The neonate's head, hands, and feet are often bluish, a temporary condition known as **acrocyanosis** that disappears over the first few days of life. The first stool is a greenish-black, thick, sticky substance known as **meconium.** It contains mucus and bile (from the fetal digestive tract) and skin cells (that were floating in amniotic fluid swallowed by the fetus).

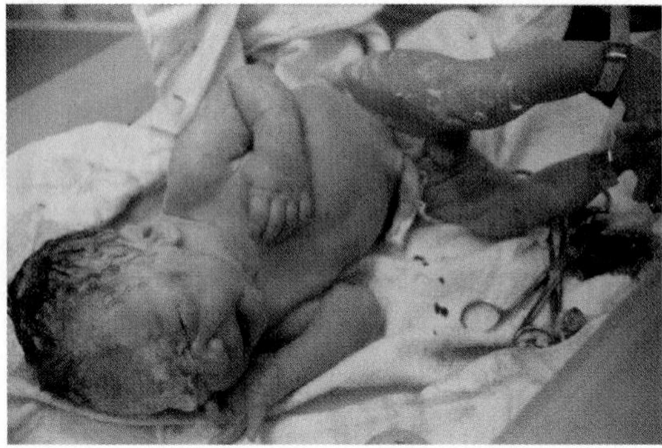

Figure 13-16 ■ A term neonate.

This male newborn is on the warming table in the delivery room. The vernix caseosa has been partially cleaned off of his trunk and arms. His eyes are swollen from the pressure of the birth canal, and there is slight molding of his cranium. Despite the fact that he is crying vigorously, the distal extremities still exhibit acrocyanosis (note the bluish color of the right hand and both legs). There is a plastic clamp on the stump of the umbilical cord. There are identification bracelets on both legs.

neonate (NEE-oh-nayt)
ne/o- *new*
-nate *born*

neonatal (NEE-oh-NAY-tal)
ne/o- *new*
nat/o- *birth*
-al *pertaining to*

vernix caseosa
(VER-niks KAY-see-OH-sah)
Vernix caseosa is a Latin phrase meaning *cheesy varnish.*

acrocyanosis (AK-roh-SY-ah-NOH-sis)
acr/o- *extremity; highest point*
cyan/o- *blue*
-osis *condition; abnormal condition; process*

fontanel (FAWN-tah-NEL)
Also spelled *fontanelle. Fontanel* is derived from a Latin word meaning *fountain* because sometimes a pulse (thought to be the fountain or spring of life) can be felt there.

meconium (meh-KOH-nee-um)
Meconium is a Latin word meaning *waste from a newborn child.*

Vocabulary Review

Anatomy and Physiology

Now that you have studied the anatomy and physiology of the female genital and reproductive system, take time to review those new words and descriptions. Memorize the combining forms and their definitions before going on to the next section.

Female Genital and Reproductive System

Word or Phrase	Combining Form and Definition	Description
adnexa	adnex/o- *accessory connecting parts*	Accessory organs (the ovaries and fallopian tubes) that are connected to the main organ (the uterus)
androgen	andr/o- *male*	Male hormone secreted by cells around the follicles in the ovary. It plays a role in female sexual drive.
anteflexion	flex/o- *bending*	Normal position of the uterus in which the superior portion is tipped anteriorly on top of the bladder
areola	areol/o- *areola*	Pigmented area around the nipple of the breast
broad ligament		Double layer of peritoneum that supports and suspends the uterus, fallopian tubes, and ovaries within the pelvic cavity
BUS	urethr/o- *urethra*	**Bartholin's glands, urethral glands,** and **Skene's glands** are located in or near the vaginal introitus. They secrete mucus during sexual arousal. They are part of the external female genitalia.
cervix	cervic/o- *neck; cervix*	Narrow, most inferior part of the uterus. It contains the **cervical canal.** Part of the cervix protrudes into the vagina. The **cervical os** is the small central opening in the cervix.
cilia		Tiny hairs inside the fallopian tube that beat in waves to propel an ovum toward the uterus
clitoris		Organ of sexual response in the female that enlarges and becomes engorged with blood. It is part of the female external genitalia.
corpus		Body or widest part of the uterus
corpus luteum		The remains of a ruptured follicle. The corpus luteum is filled with yellow fat and secretes estradiol and progesterone during the menstrual cycle. This continues after the ovum is fertilized until the placenta begins to secrete these hormones. Then the corpus luteum becomes white scar tissue.
endometrium	metri/o- *uterus*	Innermost layer of the uterine wall. Composed of a specialized mucous membrane that contains many glands. It lines the uterine cavity.
estradiol	estr/a- *female*	Most abundant and biologically active of the female sex hormones. It is secreted by the follicles of the ovary. During puberty, it causes the development of the female sex characteristics. It causes the endometrium to thicken during the menstrual cycle. After ovulation, it is secreted by the corpus luteum. During pregnancy, it is secreted by the placenta.
external genitalia	extern/o- *outside*	Labia majora, labia minora, clitoris, vaginal introitus, Bartholin's glands, urethral glands, and Skene's glands

Word or Phrase	Combining Form and Definition	Description
fallopian tube	fallopi/o- *fallopian tube*	Narrow tube that is connected at one end to the uterus. The other end, which is not directly connected to the ovary, has a funnel-shaped infundibulum and fingerlike fimbriae that draw an ovum into its lumen.
fimbriae		Fingerlike projections on the end of the fallopian tube that create currents to draw an ovum into the fallopian tube
follicle		Mass of cells with a hollow center. It holds an oocyte before puberty and a maturing ovum after puberty. The follicle ruptures at the time of ovulation and becomes the corpus luteum.
fornix		Area of the superior part of the vagina that lies behind and around the cervix
FSH		**Follicle-stimulating hormone** from the anterior pituitary gland. It causes a follicle in the ovary to enlarge and produce a mature ovum. FSH also stimulates the follicles to secrete estradiol, which causes the development of the female sex characteristics.
fundus	fund/o- *fundus (part farthest away from the opening)*	Round, domelike part of the top of the uterus above the fallopian tubes
gamete		A cell (ovum or spermatozoon) that has 23 chromosomes instead of the usual 46 chromosomes like other cells of the body
genital	genit/o- *genitalia*	Pertaining to the female internal and external genitalia
genitalia		External and internal organs and structures of the female genital and reproductive system
genitourinary system	genit/o- *genitalia* ur/o- *urine; urinary system*	Female internal and external genitalia which are in close proximity to the urinary system. Also known as the urogenital system.
gonads	gon/o- *seed (ovum or spermatozoon)*	The female sex glands (i.e., the ovaries)
hymen		Elastic membrane that partially or completely covers the inferior end of the vaginal canal
infundibulum		Funnel-shaped part of the fallopian tube. It collects an ovum from the ovary and channels it into the fallopian tube.
internal genitalia	intern/o- *inside*	Ovaries, fallopian tubes, uterus, cervix, and vagina
intrauterine cavity	uter/o- *uterus* cav/o- *hollow space*	Hollow cavity inside the uterus. It is lined with endometrium.
introitus		The entrance to the vagina from the outside of the body
ischemic phase	isch/o- *keep back; block*	Days 27–28 of the menstrual cycle when the corpus luteum degenerates into a white scar and progesterone production ceases. The endometrium sloughs off to begin menstruation.

Word or Phrase	Combining Form and Definition	Description
labia	labi/o- *lip; labium*	A pair of fleshy lips covered with pubic hair (the **labia majora**) and a small, thin, inner pair of lips (the **labia minora**) that partially cover the clitoris, urethral meatus, and vaginal introitus. Part of the external female genitalia.
lactiferous lobules	lact/i- *milk* fer/o- *to bear*	Clusters of milk-producing glands throughout the breast that produce and secrete milk after the birth of a baby. The milk flows through the **lactiferous ducts** to the nipple.
LH		**Luteinizing hormone** from the anterior pituitary gland. It causes a follicle to rupture and release a mature ovum.
lumen		Central open area throughout the length of a fallopian tube
mammary glands	mamm/o- *breast*	The breasts. A female sex characteristic that develops during puberty. The breasts contain fatty tissue and lactiferous glands and ducts. The breasts provide milk to nourish the baby after birth. The skin fold beneath each breast is known as the **inframammary crease.**
menarche	men/o- *month*	The first monthly menstruation at the onset of puberty
menses		A monthly menstrual period
menstrual cycle	menstru/o- *monthly discharge of blood*	A 28-day cycle that consists of the menstrual phase, proliferative phase, secretory phase, ovulation, and ischemic phase
menstrual phase	menstru/o- *monthly discharge of blood*	Days 1–6 of the menstrual cycle when the endometrial lining of the uterus is shed
menstruation	menstru/o- *monthly discharge of blood*	Process in which the endometrium of the uterus is shed each month, causing a flow of blood and tissue through the vagina. Under the influence of estradiol, the endometrium thickens in preparation to receive a fertilized ovum. If the ovum is not fertilized, the endometrium is again shed to begin another menstrual cycle.
mons pubis	pub/o- *pubis (hip bone)*	Rounded, fatty pad of tissue covered with pubic hair that lies on top of the pubis (anterior hip bone)
myometrium	metri/o- *uterus*	Smooth muscle layer of the uterine wall. It contracts during menstruation to expel the endometrial lining. It contracts during labor and delivery of the newborn.
nipple		Projecting point of the breast where the lactiferous ducts converge. It is surrounded by the pigmented areola.
oocyte	o/o- *ovum (egg)*	Immature egg in the fetal ovary
oogenesis	o/o- *ovum (egg)* gen/o- *arising from; produced by*	Production of a mature ovum from an oocyte through the processes of mitosis and then meiosis
ovary	ovari/o- *ovary*	Small, oval gland near the end of the fallopian tube. The follicles of the ovary secrete estradiol. The corpus luteum of the ovary secretes estradiol and progesterone. The ovary also secretes androgen.
oviduct	ov/i- *ovum (egg)*	Another name for the fallopian tube

Word or Phrase	Combining Form and Definition	Description
ovulation	ovul/o- *ovum (egg)*	Day 14 of the menstrual cycle when LH from the anterior pituitary gland causes the ovarian follicle to rupture, releasing the mature ovum
ovum		An egg within a follicle in the ovary. A mature ovum is released during ovulation. An ovum is a gamete because it has only 23 chromosomes.
perineum	perine/o- *perineum*	Area of skin between the edge of the vulva and the anus
peristalsis		Coordinated contractions of the smooth muscles in the wall of the fallopian tube to move an ovum toward the uterus.
progesterone		Female sex hormone secreted by the corpus luteum of the ovary after ovulation. It causes the uterine lining to thicken to prepare for a possible fertilized ovum. During pregnancy, it is secreted by the placenta.
proliferative phase		Days 7–13 of the menstrual cycle when a follicle matures in the ovary and the thickness of the endometrium increases.
reproductive system	product/o- *produce*	The other role of the female genital system in conceiving, carrying, and giving birth to a child
secretory phase	secret/o- *produce; secrete*	Days 15–26 of the menstrual cycle when the ruptured follicle becomes the corpus luteum and secretes progesterone to increase the thickness of the endometrium. If the ovum is not fertilized, the corpus luteum begins to disintegrate.
uterus	uter/o- *uterus*	Internal female organ of menstruation and pregnancy. Also known as the womb.
vagina	vagin/o- *vagina*	Short tubular structure connected at its superior end to the cervix and at its inferior end to the outside of the body. It contains the **vaginal canal.** The external entrance is known as the **vaginal introitus.** The vagina is where semen is deposited during sexual intercourse.
vulva	vulv/o- *vulva*	Area between the inner thighs that includes the external genitalia as well as the mons pubis and urethral meatus

Conception and Fetal Development

Word or Phrase	Combining Form and Definition	Description
amnion	amni/o- *amnion (fetal membrane)*	Part of the zygote that becomes a membrane and holds amniotic fluid. Also known as the bag of waters.
amniotic fluid	amni/o- *amnion (fetal membrane)*	Fluid produced by the amnion. It surrounds and cushions the developing embryo and fetus.
antepartum		From the mother's standpoint, the period of time from conception until labor and delivery
chorion	chorion/o- *chorion (fetal membrane)*	Cellular area in a zygote that penetrates the endometrium to bring nutrients and oxygen to the embryo. It later develops into the placenta.
embryo	embryon/o- *embryo; immature form*	The fertilized ovum is an embryo from 4 days after fertilization through 8 weeks of gestation. Then it becomes a fetus.
fertilization	fertil/o- *able to conceive a child* concept/o- *to conceive or form*	The act of a spermatozoon uniting with an ovum. Also known as **conception.**
fetus	fet/o- *fetus*	The embryo becomes a fetus beginning at 9 weeks of gestation. It is called a fetus until the moment of birth.

Word or Phrase	Combining Form and Definition	Description
fraternal twins	fratern/o- *close association or relationship*	The ovary releases two ova that are fertilized by different spermatozoa
gestation	gestat/o- *from conception to birth*	Period of time from the moment of fertilization until birth
HCG	gonad/o- *gonads (ovaries and testes)* trop/o- *having an affinity for; stimulating; turning*	**Human chorionic gonadotropin,** a hormone secreted by the chorion area of the fertilized ovum. It stimulates the corpus luteum of the ovary to keep producing estradiol and progesterone, and this causes menstruation to cease for the duration of the pregnancy.
identical twins		The initial division of a zygote creates two separate but identical developing embryos
placenta	placent/o- *placenta*	Large, pancake-like organ that develops from the chorion. It provides nutrients and oxygen to the developing fetus and removes carbon dioxide and waste products. It assumes the job of the corpus luteum and secretes estradiol and progesterone to maintain the endometrium during pregnancy. Also known as the afterbirth.
pregnancy	pregn/o- *being with child*	State of being with child. It begins at the moment of conception and ends with delivery of the newborn.
prenatal period	nat/o- *birth*	From the fetus' standpoint, the period of time from conception to birth
products of conception	concept/o- *to conceive or form*	The fetus, placenta, and all fluids and tissue in the pregnant uterus
trimester		A period of three months. The time of gestation is divided into three equal trimesters.
umbilical cord	umbilic/o- *umbilicus, (navel)*	Rubbery cord that connects the placenta to the umbilicus (navel) of the fetus. It contains two arteries and one vein.
zygote		Cell that is the product of the union of a spermatozoon and an ovum. This cell has 46 chromosomes.

Labor, Delivery, and Postpartum

Word or Phrase	Combining Form and Definition	Description
Braxton Hicks contractions	contract/o- *pull together*	Irregular uterine contractions during the last trimester. These strengthen the uterine muscle in preparation for labor. Also known as false labor.
cephalic presentation	cephal/o- *head*	Position of the fetus in which the head is the presenting part that is first to go through the birth canal. **Vertex presentation** is a type of cephalic presentation in which the top of the head is the presenting part.
colostrum		First milk from the breasts. It is rich in nutrients and contains maternal antibodies to give the newborn passive immunity to common diseases.
crowning		A large portion of the top of the fetal head is visible at the vaginal introitus
dilation	dilat/o- *dilate, widen*	Widening of the cervical os from 0 to 10 cm during labor to allow passage of the fetal head
effacement	efface/o- *do away with; obliterate*	Thinning of the cervical wall, measured in percentages from 0 to 100%

Word or Phrase	Combining Form and Definition	Description
engagement		Top of the uterine fundus lowers as the fetal head drops into position within the mother's pelvis in anticipation of birth. Also known as **lightening.**
involution	involut/o- *enlarged organ returns to normal size*	Process by which the uterus gradually shrinks in size after childbirth
lactation	lact/o- *milk*	Production of colostrum and then breast milk by the mammary glands after childbirth. The let-down reflex is the release of milk from the breasts in response to crying or sucking by the newborn.
lochia		Small amounts of blood, tissue, and fluid that are discharged from the uterus after childbirth
oxytocin	ox/y- *oxygen; quick* toc/o- *labor and childbirth*	Hormone released by the posterior pituitary gland. It stimulates the uterus to contract and begin labor. It stimulates the let-down reflex to get milk flowing for breastfeeding.
parturition	parturit/o- *to be in labor*	The process of labor and delivery. There are three stages: dilation and effacement of the cervix, delivery of the newborn, delivery of the placenta.
postnatal period	nat/o- *birth*	From the newborn's standpoint, the period of time after birth
postpartum		From the mother's standpoint, the period of time after delivery
rupture of membranes (ROM)		Rupture of the amniotic sac during the first stage of labor, and the release of amniotic fluid that flows out of the vagina.
The Newborn Infant		
acrocyanosis	acr/o- *extremity; highest point* cyan/o- *blue*	Temporary bluish coloration of the skin of the head, hands, and feet after birth
fontanels		Soft, flexible areas on the head between the bones of the cranium. In these areas, the brain is only covered with dura mater. The largest is the anterior fontanel on the top of the head. There is a smaller posterior fontanel on the back of the head. Fontanels allow the cranium to expand as the baby's brain grows. Also known as the soft spot.
meconium		The first stool passed by the neonate. It is a greenish-black, thick, sticky substance.
molding		Reshaping of the fetal cranium as it passes through the mother's pelvic bones
neonate	ne/o- *new*	Newborn from the time of birth until 1 year of age
term neonate		Newborn who is born between 38 and 42 weeks' gestational age. A preterm neonate is one who is born between 28 and 37 weeks' gestational age; also known as a premature baby.
vernix caseosa		Thick, white, cheesy substance that covers the skin of the fetus to protect it from amniotic fluid in the uterus

Labeling Exercise

A. *Match each anatomy word or phrase to its numbered structure in Figure 13-17 ■. Write that word or phrase on the blank line next to its number. Use the Answer Key at the end of the book to check your answers.*

anus	labia minora	urethral meatus
clitoris	mons pubis	vaginal introitus
labia majora	perineum	vulva

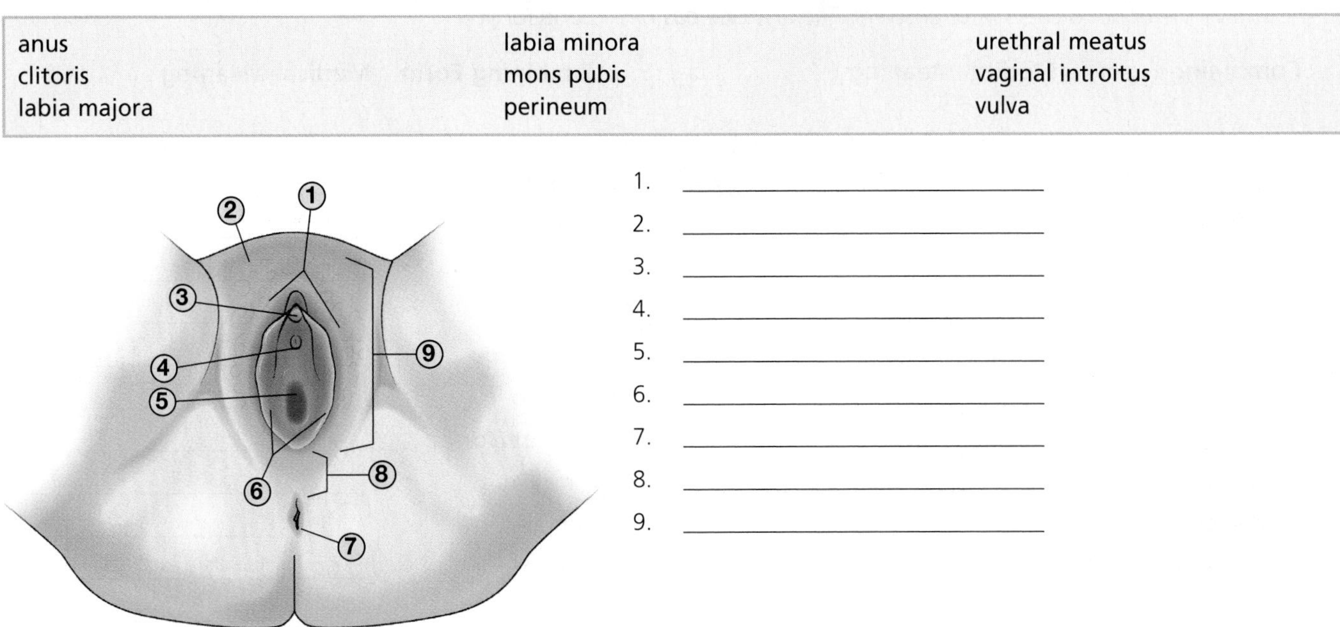

1. ______________________
2. ______________________
3. ______________________
4. ______________________
5. ______________________
6. ______________________
7. ______________________
8. ______________________
9. ______________________

Figure 13-17 ■

B. *Match each anatomy word or phrase to its numbered structure in Figure 13-18 ■.*

broad ligament	corpus luteum	fimbriae	ovary
cervical canal	endometrium	follicle at time of ovulation	uterine cervix
cervical os	fallopian tube	intrauterine cavity	uterine fundus
corpus of uterus	fallopian tube lumen	myometrium	vagina

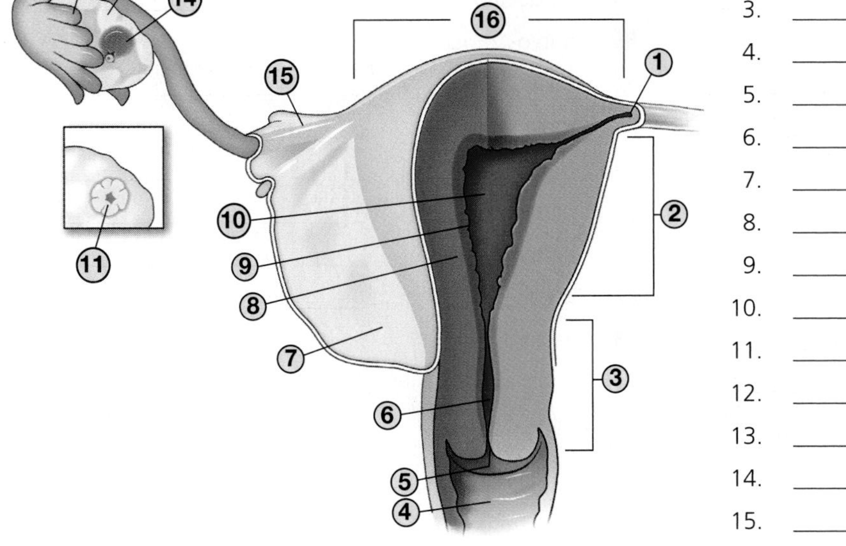

1. ______________________
2. ______________________
3. ______________________
4. ______________________
5. ______________________
6. ______________________
7. ______________________
8. ______________________
9. ______________________
10. ______________________
11. ______________________
12. ______________________
13. ______________________
14. ______________________
15. ______________________
16. ______________________

Figure 13-18 ■

Building Medical Words

Combining Forms

Here are the combining forms you have learned so far. Next to each combining form, write its meaning. Use the Answer Key at the end of the book to check your answers. The first one has been done for you.

	Combining Form	Medical Meaning		Combining Form	Medical Meaning
1.	gon/o-	seed (spermatozoon or ovum)	33.	isch/o-	
2.	acr/o-		34.	labi/o-	
3.	adnex/o-		35.	lact/i-	
4.	amni/o-		36.	lact/o-	
5.	andr/o-		37.	lob/o-	
6.	areol/o-		38.	mamm/o-	
7.	cav/o-		39.	men/o-	
8.	cephal/o-		40.	menstru/o-	
9.	cervic/o-		41.	metri/o-	
10.	chorion/o-		42.	my/o-	
11.	concept/o-		43.	nat/o-	
12.	contract/o-		44.	ne/o-	
13.	cyan/o-		45.	obstetr/o-	
14.	dilat/o-		46.	o/o-	
15.	efface/o-		47.	ovari/o-	
16.	embryon/o-		48.	ov/i-	
17.	estr/a-		49.	ovul/o-	
18.	extern/o-		50.	ox/y-	
19.	fallopi/o-		51.	parturit/o-	
20.	fer/o-		52.	perine/o-	
21.	fertil/o-		53.	placent/o-	
22.	fet/o-		54.	pregn/o-	
23.	flex/o-		55.	product/o-	
24.	fratern/o-		56.	pub/o-	
25.	fund/o-		57.	secret/o-	
26.	genit/o-		58.	toc/o-	
27.	gen/o-		59.	trop/o-	
28.	gestat/o-		60.	umbilic/o-	
29.	gonad/o-		61.	urethr/o-	
30.	gynec/o-		62.	uter/o-	
31.	intern/o-		63.	vagin/o-	
32.	involut/o-		64.	vulv/o-	

Combining Forms and Suffixes

Read the definition hint for the medical word you are to build. Look at the combining form that is given. Write the correct suffix on the blank line. Then write the medical word. (Remember: You may need to remove the combining vowel. Always remove the hyphens and slash.) Use the Answer Key at the end of the book to check your answers. The first one has been done for you.

SUFFIX LIST

-al (pertaining to)	-ary (pertaining to)	-ics (knowledge, practice)	-ity (state; condition)
-an (pertaining to)	-ation (a process; being or having)	-ine (pertaining to)	-ment (action; state)
-ar (pertaining to)	-cyte (cell)	-ion (action; condition)	-tic (pertaining to)
-arche (a beginning)	-duct (duct, tube)		

	Definition Hint	Combining Form	Suffix	Write the Medical Word
1.	Pertaining to the vagina	vagin/o-	-al	vaginal
2.	Pertaining to the breasts	mamm/o-	______	______
3.	Pertaining to the uterus	uter/o-	______	______
4.	An immature ovum	o/o-	______	______
5.	Pertaining to the ovary	ovari/o-	______	______
6.	Pertaining to the areola	areol/o-	______	______
7.	Process of an ovum being released from the follicle	ovul/o-	______	______
8.	Beginning of monthly periods	men/o-	______	______
9.	Pertaining to the cervix	cervic/o-	______	______
10.	Having monthly menses	menstru/o-	______	______
11.	Pertaining to the amnion	amni/o-	______	______
12.	Process of being or having milk	lact/o-	______	______
13.	Action of doing away with	efface/o-	______	______
14.	Pertaining to the fetus	fet/o-	______	______
15.	Action of pulling together	contract/o-	______	______
16.	Knowledge and practice of childbirth, labor	obstetr/o-	______	______
17.	Pertaining to the cord between the placenta and fetus	umbilic/o-	______	______
18.	Another name for the fallopian tube	ov/i-	______	______
19.	Condition of a hollow space	cav/o-	______	______
20.	Pertaining to a lip	labi/o-	______	______

Two Combining Forms and Suffixes

Read the definition hint for the medical word you are to build. Look at the suffix that is given. Write the correct combining forms on the blank lines. Then write the medical word. (Remember: You may need to remove the combining vowel. Always remove the hyphens and slash.) Use the Answer Key at the end of the book to check your answers. The first one has been done for you.

COMBINING FORM LIST

acr/o- (extremity; highest point)	lact/i- (milk)	ne/o- (new)
cynan/o- (blue)	metri/o- (uterus)	o/o- (ovum, egg)
fer/o- (to bear)	my/o- (muscle)	ox/y- (oxygen; quick)
gen/o- (arising from; produced by)	nat/o- (birth)	toc/o- (labor and childbirth)

Definition Hint	Combining Form	Combining Form	Suffix	Write the Medical Word
1. Pertaining to bear or carry milk	lact/i-	fer/o-	-ous	lactiferous
2. Pertaining to the uterine muscle	______	______	-al	______
3. Process by which an ovum is produced	______	______	-esis	______
4. Pertaining to a newborn	______	______	-al	______
5. Hormone that makes a quick labor and childbirth	______	______	-in	______
6. Condition of peripheral body parts being blue	______	______	-osis	______

Combining Forms and Prefixes

Read the definition hint for the medical word you are to build. Look at the medical word or word part that is given. Write the correct prefix on the blank line. Then write the medical word. (Remember: Always remove the hyphens.) Use the Answer Key at the end of the book to check your answers. The first one has been done for you.

PREFIX LIST

ante- (forward, before)	intra- (within)	pre- (before; in front of)
endo- (innermost, within)	peri- (around)	re- (again and again; backward; unable to)
infra- (below, beneath)	post- (after, behind)	tri- (three)

Definition Hint	Prefix	Medical Word or Word Part	Write the New Medical Word
1. Pertaining to producing again and again	re-	productive	reproductive
2. Pertaining to after the birth	______	natal	______
3. Pertaining to within the uterus	______	uterine	______
4. Pertaining to the lining within the uterus	______	-metrial	______
5. Action or condition of bending forward	______	flexion	______
6. Pertaining to below the breast	______	mammary	______
7. Action of contraction around a structure	______	-stalsis	______
8. Pertaining to before birth	______	natal	______
9. A three-month period of time	______	-mester	______

Symptoms, Signs, and Diseases

Ovaries and Fallopian Tubes

Word or Phrase	Word Part and Definition	Description
anovulation	**anovulation** (AN-awv-yoo-LAY-shun) an- *without, not* ovul/o- *ovum (egg)* -ation *a process; being or having*	Failure of the ovaries to release a mature ovum at the time of ovulation, although the menstrual cycle and flow are normal. This results in infertility. Anovulation is a normal condition prior to menarche and during menopause. Treatment: Follicle-stimulating hormone (FSH) and luteinizing hormone (LH) drugs.
ovarian cancer	**cancerous** (KAN-ser-us) cancer/o- *cancer* -ous *pertaining to* **malignancy** (mah-LIG-nan-see) malign/o- *intentionally causing harm; cancer* -ancy *state of*	**Cancerous** tumor of an ovary. This **malignancy** often does not cause symptoms until it is quite large and has already metastasized. Treatment: Surgical excision and chemotherapy.
polycystic ovary syndrome	**polycystic** (PAWL-ee-SIS-tik) poly- *many, much* cyst/o- *bladder; fluid-filled sac; semisolid cyst* -ic *pertaining to*	Ovaries contain multiple cysts. A follicle matures and enlarges, but fails to rupture to release an ovum; it then becomes a cyst. This happens month after month until the ovaries are filled with multiple cysts. The cysts enlarge each month in response to LH, and this causes pain. This syndrome is associated with amenorrhea or menometrorrhagia, infertility, obesity, and insulin resistance syndrome with the development of type 2 diabetes mellitus. Treatment: Oral contraceptive pill (to correct hormone levels), weight control, oral antidiabetic drug.
salpingitis	**salpingitis** (SAL-pin-JY-tis) salping/o- *fallopian tube* -itis *inflammation of* **hydrosalpinx** (HY-droh-SAL-pinks) hydr/o- *water; fluid* -salpinx *fallopian tube* *Salpinx* is a Greek word meaning *a trumpet.* It refers to the trumpet shape of the tube and infundibulum. **pyosalpinx** (PY-oh-SAL-pinks) py/o- *pus* -salpinx *fallopian tube*	Inflammation or infection of the fallopian tube. This is caused by endometriosis or pelvic inflammatory disease that can narrow or block the lumen of the tube. With **hydrosalpinx,** inflammation fills the tube with tissue fluid. With **pyosalpinx,** infection fills the tube with pus. Treatment: Treat the underlying cause.

Uterus

Word or Phrase	Word Part and Definition	Description
endometrial cancer		Cancerous tumor of the endometrium of the uterus. The earliest symptom is abnormal bleeding. Also known as uterine cancer. Treatment: Hysterectomy.

Word or Phrase	Word Part and Definition	Description
endometriosis	**endometriosis** (EN-doh-MEE-tree-OH-sis) **endo-** *innermost, within* **metri/o-** *uterus (womb)* **-osis** *condition; abnormal condition; process*	Endometrial tissue in abnormal places. The endometrium sloughs off during menstruation but is forced upward through the fallopian tubes and out into the pelvic cavity because the uterus is in retroflexion. The endometrial tissue implants itself on the walls of the ovaries, uterus, and pelvic cavity. These tissue implants remain alive and sensitive to hormones. During each menstrual cycle, they thicken and slough off, forming more implants with old blood and tissue debris in the pelvic cavity (see Figure 13-19 ■). They also form adhesions between the internal organs. Endometriosis on the ovary can form "chocolate cysts" that contain old, dark blood. Endometrial implants in the fallopian tubes cause blockage, scarring, and infertility. Endometriosis causes pelvic inflammation, pelvic pain, and pain during sexual intercourse. Treatment: Hormone drugs to suppress the menstrual cycle (to make the implants shrivel up) or laparoscopic surgery to destroy the implants. **Figure 13-19 ■ Endometriosis.** The cul-de-sac outside of the uterus shows many endometrial implants with evidence of new and old blood.
hydatidiform mole	**hydatidiform** (HY-dah-TID-ih-form) **hydatidi/o-** *fluid-filled vesicles* **-form** *having the form of* *Hydatid* is derived from a Greek word meaning *a drop of water.* **mole** (MOHL) *Mole* is derived from a Latin word meaning *a mass.*	Abnormal union of an ovum and spermatozoon that produces hundreds of small, fluid-filled sacs but no embryo. The chorion produces HCG, so the patient has early signs of pregnancy. The hydatiform mole grows more rapidly than a normal pregnancy, and the uterus is much larger than expected for the gestational age. Surgery: Removal of the hydatidiform mole or hysterectomy.

Word or Phrase	Word Part and Definition	Description
leiomyoma	**leiomyoma** (LIE-oh-my-OH-mah) lei/o- *smooth* my/o- *muscle* -oma *tumor, mass* *Leiomyoma* is a Greek singular noun. Form the plural by changing *-oma* to *-omata.* **leiomyomata** (LIE-oh-my-OH-mah-tah)	Benign tumor of the myometrium (see Figure 13-20 ■). It can be small or as large as a soccer ball. There is pelvic pain, excessive uterine bleeding, and painful intercourse. Also known as a uterine fibroid. Treatment: Hysterectomy, myomectomy, or uterine artery embolization, depending on the size of the tumor. 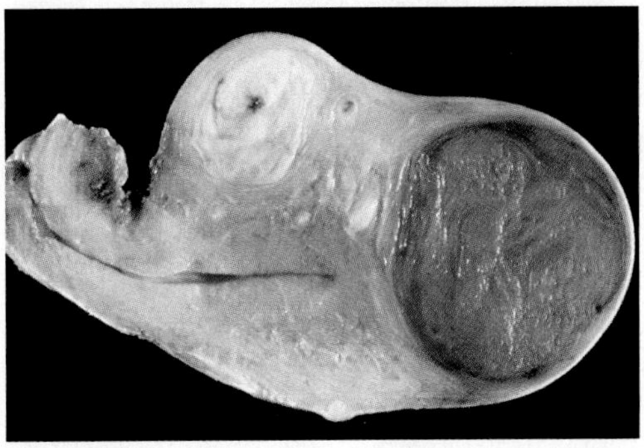 **Figure 13-20 ■ Leiomyoma.** This pathology specimen of a section of a uterus contains a large, benign, red leiomyoma.
leiomyosarcoma	**leiomyosarcoma** (LIE-oh-MY-oh-sar-KOH-mah) lei/o- *smooth* my/o- *muscle* sarc/o- *connective tissue* -oma *tumor, mass*	Cancerous tumor that arises from the myometrium of the uterus. Treatment: Hysterectomy and chemotherapy or radiation therapy.
myometritis	**myometritis** (MY-oh-mee-TRY-tis) my/o- *muscle* metr/o- *uterus (womb)* -itis *inflammation of* **pyometritis** (PY-oh-mee-TRY-tis) py/o- *pus* metr/o- *uterus (womb)* -itis *inflammation of*	Inflammation or infection of the myometrium. Associated with pelvic inflammatory disease. **Pyometritis** is an infection of the myometrium that creates pus in the intrauterine cavity. Treatment: Antibiotic drug.
pelvic inflammatory disease (PID)	**inflammatory** (in-FLAM-ah-tor-ee) inflammat/o- *redness and warmth* -ory *having the function of*	Infection of the cervix that ascends to the uterus, fallopian tubes, and ovaries. Often caused by a sexually transmitted disease. There is pelvic pain, fever, and vaginal discharge. If untreated, it can cause scars in the fallopian tubes and infertility. Treatment: Antibiotic or anti-infective drug.
retroflexion of the uterus	**retroflexion** (RET-roh-FLEK-shun) retro- *behind, backward* flex/o- *bending* -ion *action; condition* **retroversion** (RET-roh-VER-shun) retro- *behind, backward* vers/o- *to turn; to travel* -ion *action; condition*	Abnormal position in which the entire uterus is bent backward while the cervix is in a normal position. Associated with the development of endometriosis. Also known as **retroversion** of the uterus.

Word or Phrase	Word Part and Definition	Description
uterine prolapse	**prolapse** (PROH-laps) *Prolapse* is derived from a Latin word meaning *a falling down.* **descensus** (dee-SEN-sus) *Descensus* is a Latin word meaning *falling from a higher position.*	Descent of the uterus from its normal position. This is caused by stretching of ligaments and weakness in the muscles of the floor of the pelvic cavity. Occurs after childbirth or because of age. The cervix may be visible at the vaginal introitus. Severe prolapse affects urination and bowel movements. Also known as **uterine descensus.** Treatment: Hysterectomy or uterine suspension.
Menstrual Disorders		
amenorrhea	**amenorrhea** (AH-meh-noh-REE-ah) **a-** *away from, without* **men/o-** *month* **-rrhea** *flow, discharge*	Absence of monthly menstrual periods. (This is normal before puberty, during pregnancy, and after menopause.) Caused by hormone imbalance, thyroid disease, or tumors of the uterus or ovaries. Poor nutrition, stress, chronic disease, constant, intense exercise, or the psychiatric illness of anorexia nervosa can also cause amenorrhea. Treatment: Correct the underlying cause.
dysfunctional uterine bleeding (DUB)	**dysfunctional** (dis-FUNK-shun-al) *Dysfunctional* is a combination of the prefix *dys-* (painful, difficult, abnormal), the English word *function* (physiologic working), and the suffix *-al* (pertaining to).	Sporadic menstrual bleeding without a true menstrual period. Occurs in conjunction with anovulation. Estradiol causes the endometrium to thicken and slough off from time to time, but it never reaches its full thickness because there is no ovulation and no corpus luteum to make progesterone. Treatment: Hormone therapy to restore normal menstruation.
dysmenorrhea	**dysmenorrhea** (DIS-men-oh-REE-ah) **dys-** *painful, difficult, abnormal* **men/o-** *month* **-rrhea** *flow, discharge* **prostaglandin** (PRAWS-tah-GLAN-din) Prostaglandin was first isolated from the prostate gland in men, although it is present in many different tissues of the body.	Painful menstruation. During menstruation, the uterus releases **prostaglandin** to constrict blood vessels in the uterine wall and prevent excessive bleeding. Abnormally high levels of prostaglandin cause cramping and temporary ischemia of the myometrium, both of which cause pain. There is also nausea, dizziness, backache, and diarrhea. Pelvic inflammatory disease, endometriosis, or uterine fibroids can also cause dysmenorrhea. Treatment: Nonsteroidal anti-inflammatory drugs to block the action of prostaglandin. Correct the underlying cause.
menopause	**menopause** (MEN-oh-pawz) **men/o-** *month* **-pause** *cessation* The suffix *-pause* is derived from a Greek word meaning *cessation,* not the English word *pause* meaning *a temporary rest.* **perimenopausal** (PAIR-ee-MEN-oh-PAW-zal) **peri-** *around* **men/o-** *month* **paus/o-** *cessation* **-al** *pertaining to*	Normal cessation of menstrual periods, occurring around middle age. The **perimenopausal period** is the time around menopause when menstrual periods first become irregular and menstrual flow is light. Menopause is also known as **climacteric** or the change of life. Treatment: Hormone replacement therapy (HRT). *(continued)*

Word or Phrase	Word Part and Definition	Description
menopause (*continued*)	**climacteric** (kly-MAK-ter-ik) (KLY-mak-TER-ik) *Climacteric* is derived from a Greek word meaning *the rungs of a ladder.* Menopause represents progressive movement toward the next stage of life.	**A Closer Look** As a woman ages, the follicles deteriorate and stop secreting estradiol. Ovulation and menstruation cease. Decreased estradiol causes vaginal dryness, vaginal atrophy, and dryness of the skin. The breasts decrease in size. The anterior pituitary gland responds to low estradiol levels in the blood by secreting more follicle-stimulating hormone (FSH). This causes occasional ovulation and menstruation during the perimenopausal period. These bursts of FSH (which often occur at night) produce vasodilation. As arteries in the skin dilate, the patient experiences hot flashes with perspiration and flushing. Frequent hot flashes throughout the night cause sleeplessness and fatigue during menopause.
menorrhagia	**menorrhagia** (MEN-oh-RAY-jee-ah) **men/o-** *month* **rrhag/o-** *excessive flow or discharge* **-ia** *condition, state, thing*	An excessive amount of menstrual flow or menstrual flow that lasts longer than 7 days. Caused by a hormone imbalance, uterine fibroids, or endometriosis. **Menometrorrhagia** is excessive menstrual flow during menstruation as well as at other times of the month. Both menorrhagia and menometrorrhagia can cause anemia. **Metrorrhagia** is excessive bleeding at a time other than menstruation. This can be caused by a ing at a time other than menstruation. This can be caused by a tubal pregnancy or uterine cancer. Treatment: Hormone therapy or correct the underlying cause.
oligomenorrhea	**oligomenorrhea** (OL-ih-goh-MEN-oh-REE-ah) **olig/o-** *scanty* **men/o-** *month* **-rrhea** *flow, discharge*	Very light menstrual flow or infrequent menstrual cycles (longer than 35 days between the end of one cycle and the beginning of the next cycle) in a woman who previously had normal menstruation. It is caused by a hormone imbalance. Treatment: Hormone therapy.
premenstrual syndrome (PMS)	**premenstrual** (pree-MEN-stroo-al) **pre-** *before; in front of* **menstru/o-** *monthly discharge of blood* **-al** *pertaining to*	Breast tenderness, fluid retention, bloating, and mild mood changes (irritability, anger, sadness) a few days before the onset of menstruation. It is caused by the high levels of estradiol and progesterone just prior to menstruation. These affect the levels of neurotransmitters like serotonin and norepinephrine in the brain. Treatment: Over-the-counter drugs that relieve pain and fluid retention.
premenstrual dysphoric disorder (PMDD)	**dysphoric** (dis-FOR-ik) **dys-** *painful, difficult, abnormal* **phor/o-** *to bear, to carry* **-ic** *pertaining to*	Symptoms of PMS plus feelings of depression, anxiety, tearfulness, mood shifts, difficulty concentrating, sleep and eating disturbances, as well as breast, joint, and muscle pains. It is a psychiatric mood disorder caused by an alteration in the level of neurotransmitters in the brain. Treatment: Antianxiety drugs, antidepressant drugs, and pain relievers.
		Cervix
cervical cancer	**carcinoma** (KAR-sih-NOH-mah) **carcin/o-** *cancer* **-oma** *tumor, mass* **in situ** (IN SY-too) *In situ* is a Latin phrase meaning *in one site or location.*	Cancerous tumor of the cervix. If the cancer is still localized, it is referred to as **carcinoma in situ (CIS).** There is severe dysplasia of the cells seen on the Pap smear. Later there is ulceration and bleeding. Infection with human papillomavirus (HPV) (genital warts, a sexually transmitted disease) predisposes to the development of cervical cancer. Treatment: Conization or hysterectomy.

Word or Phrase	Word Part and Definition	Description
cervical dysplasia	**dysplasia** (dis-PLAY-zee-ah) dys- *painful, difficult, abnormal* plas/o- *growth, formation* -ia *condition, state, thing* Some word parts have more than one definition. The best definition of *dysplasia* is *condition of abnormal growth.* **dysplastic** (dis-PLAS-tik) dys- *painful, difficult, abnormal* plas/o- *growth, formation* -tic *pertaining to*	Abnormal growth of squamous cells that make up the epithelium (surface layer) of the cervix (see Figure 13-21 ■). Cervical dysplasia is seen on abnormal Pap smears and severe dysplasia is a precancerous or cancerous condition. Treatment: Treat the underlying infection or cancer. 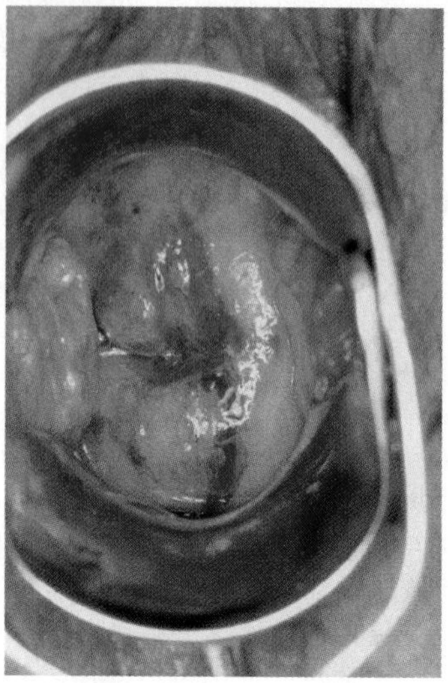 **Figure 13-21 ■ Cervical dysplasia.** A plastic speculum is used to visualize the cervix. The cervix shows a high degree of cervical dysplasia (classified as CIN II on a Pap smear). These areas of redness are abnormal cells that may develop into cancer.
incompetent cervix	**incompetent** (in-COM-peh-tent) *Incompetent means not competent, unable to perform its function.*	Spontaneous dilation of the cervix during the second trimester of pregnancy, but without uterine contractions. This can result in spontaneous abortion of the fetus. Treatment: Bed rest and placement of a cerclage.
Vagina and Perineum		
bacterial vaginosis	**vaginosis** (VAJ-ih-NOH-sis) vagin/o- *vagina* -osis *condition; abnormal condition; process*	Bacterial infection of the vagina due to *Gardnerella vaginalis.* There is a white or grayish vaginal discharge that has a fishy odor. Treatment: Antibiotic drug.
candidiasis	**candidiasis** (KAN-dih-DY-ah-sis) candid/o- *Candida (a yeast)* -iasis *state of, process of* **leukorrhea** (LOO-koh-REE-ah) leuk/o- *white* -rrhea *flow, discharge*	Yeast infection of the vagina due to *Candida albicans.* There is vaginal itching and **leukorrhea,** a cheesy, white discharge. Candidiasis usually occurs after taking an antibiotic drug for a bacterial infection; the drug kills the pathogen but also kills the normal bacterial flora of the vagina. Then yeast, which is unharmed by an antibiotic drug, flourishes without competition from other microorganisms. Treatment: Antiyeast drug applied topically in the vagina.
cystocele	**cystocele** (SIS-toh-seel) cyst/o- *bladder; fluid-filled sac; semisolid cyst* -cele *hernia*	Herniation of the bladder into the vagina because of a weakness in the vaginal wall. It is caused by childbirth or age. It can result in urinary retention. Treatment: Colporrhaphy.
dyspareunia	**dyspareunia** (DIS-pah-ROO-nee-ah) dys- *painful, difficult, abnormal* pareun/o- *sexual intercourse* -ia *condition, state, thing*	Painful or difficult sexual intercourse. This can be caused by the hymen being across the vaginal introitus; infections of the vagina, cervix, or uterus; pelvic inflammatory disease; endometriosis; or retroflexion of the uterus. Treatment: Correct the underlying cause.

Word or Phrase	Word Part and Definition	Description
rectocele	**rectocele** (REK-toh-seel) **rect/o-** *rectum* **-cele** *hernia*	Herniation of the rectum into the vagina because of a weakness in the vaginal wall. It is caused by childbirth or age. It can interfere with bowel movements. Treatment: Colporrhaphy.
vaginitis	**vaginitis** (VAJ-ih-NY-tis) **vagin/o-** *vagina* **-itis** *inflammation of*	Vaginal inflammation or infection. It can be caused by irritation from the chemicals in spermicidal jelly or douches. It can also be caused by candidiasis (yeast infection), trichomonas (parasite infection), bacterial infection, or a sexually transmitted disease. Treatment: Treat the underlying cause.

Connections

toxic (TAWK-sik)
tox/o- *poison*
-ic *pertaining to*

tampon (TAM-pawn)
Tampon is a French word meaning *to stop up.*

Public Health. The first cases of **toxic shock syndrome** were seen in women in 1980. There was a high fever, vomiting, diarrhea, and hypotension (shock). Physicians interviewed patients and family members to discover a common link. All of the patients had used super-absorbant **tampons** during their menstrual period. The normally harmless vaginal bacterium *Staphylococcus aureus* multiplied in the old blood in the tampon and released toxins. The tampon itself created small tears in the vaginal wall that allowed the toxins to enter the blood.

Breasts

Word or Phrase	Word Part and Definition	Description
breast cancer	**adenocarcinoma** (AD-eh-noh-KAR-sih-NOH-mah) **aden/o-** *gland* **carcin/o-** *cancer* **-oma** *tumor, mass* **peau d' orange** (poh-deh-RAHNJ) *Peau d' orange* is a French word meaning *peel of the orange.*	**Cancerous** tumor, usually an **adenocarcinoma** of the lactiferous glands of the breast. A lump is detected on breast self-examination or mammography. There may also be swelling in the area, enlarged lymph nodes, and nipple discharge. Advanced breast cancer manifests as **peau d'orange,** dimpling of the breast skin, and nipple retraction. Long-term hormone replacement therapy with estrogen increases the risk of breast cancer. Treatment: Lumpectomy or mastectomy, chemotherapy, radiation therapy.
failure of lactation	**lactation** (lak-TAY-shun) **lact/o-** *milk* **-ation** *a process; being or having*	Lack of production of milk in the breasts following pregnancy. It is caused by hyposecretion of prolactin from the anterior pituitary gland. The breasts do not produce milk or produce insufficient milk to breastfeed the baby. Treatment: Switch to bottle feeding.
fibrocystic disease	**fibrocystic** (FY-broh-SIS-tik) **fibr/o-** *fiber* **cyst/o-** *bladder; fluid-filled sac; semisolid cyst* **-ic** *pertaining to*	Benign condition in which numerous, fluid-filled cysts of various sizes form in one or both breasts. The sizes of the cysts can change, probably in response to hormone levels. The cysts are painful and tender. Severe fibrocystic disease makes it difficult to detect a cancerous tumor on mammography. Treatment: Hormone therapy. Elimination of certain foods (chocolate, caffeine) from the diet sometimes helps.
galactorrhea	**galactorrhea** (gah-LAK-toh-REE-ah) **galact/o-** *milk* **-rrhea** *flow, discharge*	Discharge of milk from the breasts when the patient is not pregnant or breastfeeding. Caused by increased levels of prolactin from an adenoma (benign tumor) of the anterior pituitary gland in the brain. Treatment: Drug to decrease prolactin production or surgery to remove the adenoma from the anterior pituitary gland.

Pregnancy and Labor and Delivery

Word or Phrase	Word Part and Definition	Description
abnormal presentation	**breech** (BREECH) *Breech* is an Old English word meaning *buttocks.* **malpresentation** (MAL-pree-sen-TAY-shun) The prefix *mal-* means *bad, inadequate.*	Birth position in which the presenting part of the fetus is not the head. In a **breech** presentation, the presenting part is the buttocks, buttocks and the feet, or just the feet (see Figure 13-22 ■). If the fetus is in a transverse lie (the fetal vertebral column is perpendicular to the mother's vertebral column), the shoulder or arm is the presenting part. Also known as **malpresentation** of the fetus. Treatment: Version maneuver to turn the fetus or delivery by cesarean section. 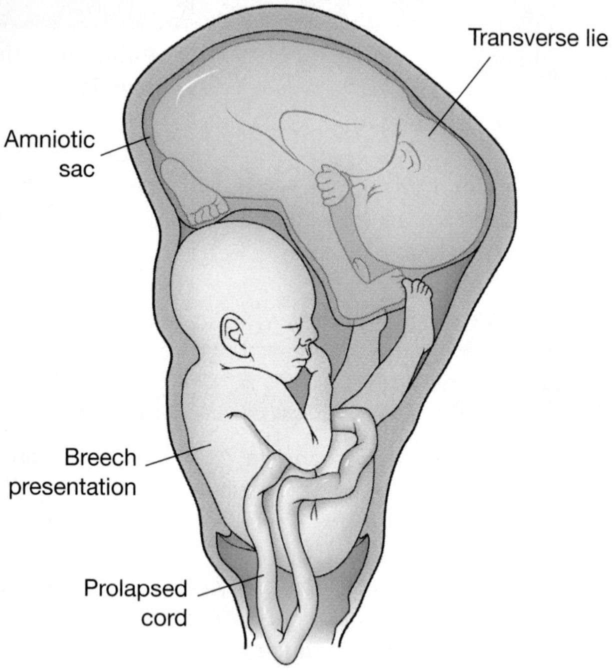 Transverse lie Amniotic sac Breech presentation Prolapsed cord **Figure 13-22 ■ Malpresentation of fraternal twins.** One twin is in the breech position with the buttocks as the presenting part. The amniotic sac has ruptured and the umbilical cord has prolapsed into the vaginal cavity. The second twin, still in its amniotic sac, is in a transverse lie position.
abruptio placentae	**abruptio placentae** (ab-RUP-shee-oh plah-SEN-tee) *Abruptio placentae* is a Latin phrase meaning *a breaking off of the placenta.*	Complete or partial separation of the placenta from the uterine wall before the third stage of labor. This results in uterine hemorrhage that threatens the life of the mother as well as disruption of blood flow and oxygen through the umbilical cord which threatens the life of the fetus. Treatment: Emergency cesarean section.
arrest of labor		Cessation of or prolonging of labor. The cervix does not dilate and efface, and the head of the fetus does not progress through the birth canal. Also known as failure to progress. This can be caused by cephalopelvic disproportion or a malpresentation of the fetus. Treatment: Cesarean section for cephalopelvic disproportion. Version or cesearean section for malpresentation.

Word or Phrase	Word Part and Definition	Description
cephalopelvic disproportion (CPD)	**cephalopelvic** (SEF-ah-loh-PEL-vik) cephal/o- *head* pelv/o- *pelvis (hip bone; renal pelvis)* -ic *pertaining to* **disproportion** (DIS-proh-POR-shun) *Disproportion* is a combination of the prefix *dis-* (away from) and the word *proportion* (a proper relationship between two things).	The size of the fetal head exceeds the size of the opening in the mother's pelvic bones. Treatment: Cesarean section. **Did You Know?** Skeletons of prehistoric women have been discovered that show cephalopelvic disproportion with the skull of the baby still tightly wedged in the mother's pelvic bones.
dystocia	**dystocia** (dis-TOH-see-ah) dys- *painful, difficult, abnormal* toc/o- *labor and childbirth* -ia *condition, state, thing*	Any type of difficult or abnormal labor and delivery. Treatment: Correct the underlying cause.
ectopic pregnancy	**ectopic** (ek-TOP-ik) ectop/o- *outside of a place* -ic *pertaining to* **tubal** (TOO-bal) tub/o- *tube* -al *pertaining to* **hemosalpinx** (HEE-moh-SAL-pinks) hem/o- *blood* -salpinx *fallopian tube*	Implantation of a fertilized ovum in the fallopian tube. Also known as a **tubal pregnancy.** This occurs more readily if the fallopian tube has scar tissue or a blockage in it. The patient has a positive pregnancy test, but there is abdominal tenderness as the fallopian tube swells from the developing embryo. The tube can bleed, a condition known as **hemosalpinx.** The tube can suddenly rupture, causing severe blood loss and shock. Treatment: Salpingectomy to remove the embryo and fallopian tube.
gestational diabetes mellitus	**gestational** (jes-TAY-shun-al) gestat/o- *from conception to birth* -ation *a process; being or having* -al *pertaining to* **diabetes** (DY-ah-BEE-teez) **mellitus** (MEL-ih-tus) *Mellitus* means *honeyed* because of the large amounts of glucose (sugar) present in the urine.	Temporary disorder of glucose metabolism that occurs only during pregnancy. Increased levels of estradiol and progesterone block the action of insulin from the pancreas. The function of insulin is to metabolize glucose. Low levels of insulin lead to high levels of unmetabolized glucose in the mother's blood. These high levels of glucose cross the placenta and cause the fetus to grow too rapidly (as its pancreas produces insulin that can metabolize the glucose). Treatment: Dietary management, oral antidiabetic drug during pregnancy. This condition ceases with childbirth, but the mother often develops type 2 diabetes mellitus later in life.
mastitis	**mastitis** (mas-TY-tis) mast/o- *breast; mastoid process* -itis *inflammation of*	Inflammation or infection of the breast. Caused by milk engorgement in the breast or an infection, usually *Staphylococcus aureus* from the infant's mouth or the mother's skin. The affected breast is red and swollen and the mother has a fever. Treatment: Pumping of breast milk. Antibiotic drug to treat the infection.

Word or Phrase	Word Part and Definition	Description
morning sickness	**hyperemesis** (HY-per-EM-eh-sis) **hyper-** *above; more than normal* **-emesis** *vomiting* Every medical word must contain a combining form. The suffix *-emesis* contains the combining form *eme/o-*. **gravidarum** (GRAV-ih-DAIR-um) *Gravidarum* is a Latin word meaning *of pregnancy.*	Nausea and vomiting during the first trimester of pregnancy. Thought to be due to elevated estradiol and progesterone levels. **Hyperemesis gravidarum** is excessive vomiting that causes weakness, dehydration, and fluid and electrolyte imbalance. Treatment: Intravenous fluids for severe hyperemesis gravidarum.
oligohydramnios	**oligohydramnios** (OL-ih-goh-hy-DRAM-nee-ohs) **olig/o-** *scanty* **hydr/o-** *water; fluid* **-amnios** *amniotic fluid* **in utero** (IN YOO-ter-oh) *In utero* is a Latin phrase meaning *in the uterus.*	Decreased volume of amniotic fluid. The fetus swallows amniotic fluid but does not excrete a similar volume in its urine because of a congenital abnormality of the fetal kidneys. Treatment: Surgery to the fetus while **in utero** or after birth.
placenta previa	**placenta previa** (plah-SEN-tah PREE-vee-ah) *Placenta previa* is a Latin phrase meaning *the placenta is before [the fetus].*	Incorrect placement of the placenta with its edge partially or completely covering the cervical canal (see Figure 13-23 ■). During labor when the cervix dilates, the connection between the placenta and uterus is disrupted. This causes moderate-to-severe bleeding in the mother and disrupts the flow of blood to the fetus. Treatment: Cesarean section. 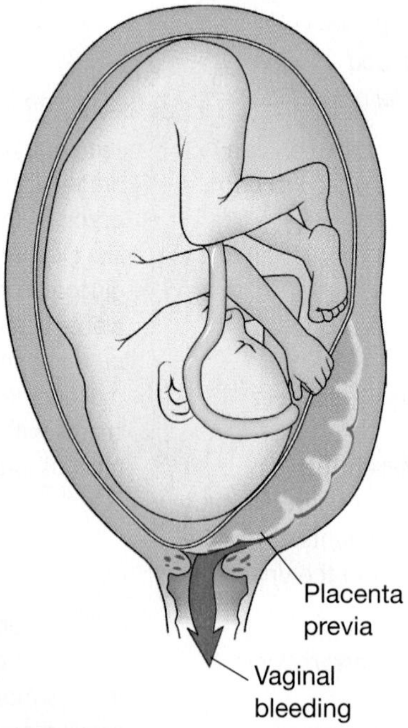 Placenta previa Vaginal bleeding **Figure 13-23 ■ Placenta previa.** A low position of the placenta can cause bleeding when the cervix dilates during labor and delivery.
polyhydramnios	**polyhydramnios** (PAWL-ee-hy-DRAM-nee-ohs) **poly-** *many, much* **hydr/o-** *water; fluid* **-amnios** *amniotic fluid*	Increased volume of amniotic fluid. Caused by maternal diabetes mellitus, twin gestation, and different types of fetal abnormalities. Treatment: Correct the underlying cause.

Word or Phrase	Word Part and Definition	Description
postpartum hemorrhage	**hemorrhage** (HEM-oh-rij) **hem/o-** *blood* **-rrhage** *excessive flow or discharge*	Continual bleeding from the uterus at the site where the placenta separated after a normal birth. The empty uterus is boggy and does not become firm. Caused by hyposecretion of oxytocin from the posterior pituitary gland in the brain. Treatment: Manual massage of the uterus. Intravenous drug therapy with an oxytocin drug.
preeclampsia	**preeclampsia** (PREE-ee-KLAMP-see-ah) **pre-** *before; in front of* **eclamps/o-** *a seizure* **-ia** *condition, state, thing* **eclampsia** (ee-KLAMP-see-ah) *Eclampsia* is derived from a Greek word meaning *a sudden development.*	Hypertensive disorder of pregnancy with increased blood pressure, edema, weight gain, and protein in the urine (proteinuria). The nephrons of the kidneys allow large protein molecules from the blood to be lost in the urine. A low level of protein changes the osmotic pressure of the blood and allows fluid to move into the tissues where it collects as edema. Preeclampsia can progress to **eclampsia** in which the patient has seizures. Treatment: Bed rest, antihypertensive and antiseizure drugs.
premature labor		Regular uterine contractions that occur before the fetus is mature (before full-term gestation of 38 to 42 weeks). The cervix may dilate and small amounts of blood or amniotic fluid may leak out. Treatment: Bed rest, tocolytic drug.
premature rupture of membranes (PROM)		Spontaneous rupture of the amniotic sac and loss of amniotic fluid before labor begins. The mother must deliver or risk the development of infection within 24 hours. Treatment: Induction of labor.
prolapsed cord	**prolapse** (PROH-laps) *Prolapse* is derived from a Latin word meaning *falling down.*	A loop of umbilical cord becomes caught between the presenting part of the fetus and the birth canal (see Figure 13-22). This occurs if the membranes rupture before the fetal head (or other presenting part) is fully engaged in the pelvis. With each uterine contraction, the umbilical cord is compressed, causing decreased blood flow to the fetus and fetal distress. Treatment: Change the mother's position to move the position of the cord, give oxygen to the mother. Surgery: Cesarean section.
spontaneous abortion (SAB)	**abortion** (ah-BOR-shun) **abort/o-** *stop prematurely* **-ion** *action; condition*	Loss of a pregnancy. An early spontaneous abortion usually occurs because of a genetic abnormality or poor implantation of theembryo within the endometrium. A later spontaneous abortion can occur because of preterm labor or an incompetent cervix. In an abortion, the embryo or fetus is expelled but the placenta and other tissue remain in the uterus. Also known as a **miscarriage.**
uterine inertia	**inertia** (in-ER-shah) (in-ER-shee-ah) *Inertia* is a Latin word meaning *inactivity or laziness.*	Weak or uncoordinated contractions during labor. Caused by decreased levels of oxytocin from the posterior pituitary gland. Can also occur if the uterus is very distended and unable to contract normally because of multiple fetuses. Treatment: Intravenous oxytocin drug.

Connections

depression (dee-PRESH-un)
depress/o- *press down*
-ion *action; condition*

involution (IN-voh-LOO-shun-al)
involut/o- *enlarged organ returns to normal size*
-ion *action; condition*
-al *pertaining to*

melancholia (MEL-an-KOH-lee-ah)
melan/o- *black*
chol/o- *bile, gall*
-ia *condition, state, thing*
Ancient Greek physicians believed that the body had four humors, one of which—black bile—was related to a sad or melancholy personality.

Psychiatry (Chapter 17). Postpartum depression is a mood disorder with symptoms of mild-to-moderate depression, anxiousness, irritability, tearfulness, and fatigue. It is caused by hormonal changes after birth and by feelings of overwhelming responsibility and fatigue. Formerly known as **involutional melancholia** because it occurs at the time of involution of the uterus.

Connections

pica (PY-kah) (PEE-kah)
Pica is a Latin word meaning *magpie.* Magpies are birds that will look for all kinds of materials—metal, plastic, and so forth—to use in their nests.

Dietetics. A lack of folic acid during pregnancy can cause neural tube defects in the fetus. Prenatal vitamins for pregnant women and enrichment of cereals and other grain products with added folic acid have greatly decreased the incidence of neural tube defects.

There are many stories about the food cravings of pregnant women: pickles, ice cream, and so forth. Some pregnant women experience **pica,** an unnatural craving for and compulsive eating of substances with no nutritional value, such as clay, chalk, starch, or dirt.

Fetus and Neonate

Word or Phrase	Word Part and Definition	Description
apnea	**apnea** (AP-nee-ah) a- *away from, without* -pnea *breathing* **apneic** (AP-nee-ik) a- *away from, without* pne/o- *breathing* -ic *pertaining to*	Temporary or permanent cessation of breathing after birth. The newborn is said to be **apneic.** The immature central nervous system of a newborn fails to maintain a consistent respiratory rate, and there are occasional long pauses between periods of regular breathing. Treatment: Apnea monitor in the hospital and at home.
fetal distress		Lack of oxygen to the fetus because of decreased blood flow through the placenta or umbilical cord. The fetus has bradycardia and passes meconium. Treatment: Mother is given oxygen. Possible cesarean section.

Word or Phrase	Word Part and Definition	Description
growth abnormalities		Many factors affect the growth rate of the embryo and fetus. Maternal illness, malnutrition, and smoking can make the fetus **small for gestational age (SGA).** This is known as **intrauterine growth retardation (IUGR).** Diabetes mellitus in the mother can make the fetus **large for gestational age (LGA).** A fetus within the normal growth range for weight and height is said to be **appropriate for gestational age (AGA).** Treatment: Correct the underlying cause.
jaundice	**jaundice** (JAWN-dis) *Jaundice* is derived from a French word meaning *yellow.* **hyperbilirubinemia** (HY-per-BIL-ih-ROO-bih-NEE-mee-ah) **hyper-** *above; more than normal* **bilirubin/o-** *bilirubin* **-emia** *condition in the blood; substance in the blood* **phototherapy** (FOH-toh-THAIR-ah-pee) **phot/o-** *light* **-therapy** *treatment*	Yellowish discoloration of the skin. During gestation, the fetus has extra red blood cells that are no longer needed at birth. Their destruction releases hemoglobin which is converted into unconjugated bilirubin. The immature newborn liver is not able to conjugate this much bilirubin, and it builds up in the blood (**hyperbilirubinemia**), moves into the tissues, and causes yellowish discoloration of the skin known as jaundice. The more premature the infant, the greater the chance of developing jaundice. Treatment: **Phototherapy** with bililights, special fluorescent lights that break down bilirubin in the skin to make it water soluble so it can be excreted by the kidneys.
meconium aspiration	**aspiration** (AS-pih-RAY-shun) **aspir/o-** *to breathe in; to suck in* **-ation** *a process; being or having*	Fetal distress causes the fetus to pass meconium into the amniotic fluid. This gets in the mouth and nose of the fetus and is inhaled at birth. This causes severe respiratory distress. Treatment: Suctioning of the newborn's nose and mouth. Use of oxygen and a ventilator to aid respirations after birth.
nuchal cord	**nuchal** (NOO-kal) **nuch/o-** *neck; nape of neck* **-al** *pertaining to*	Umbilical cord is wrapped around the neck of the fetus. A loose nuchal cord can be an incidental finding that causes no problems. A tight nuchal cord with one or more loops around the neck can impair blood flow to the brain, causing brain damage or fetal death. Treatment: Emergency cesarean section.
respiratory distress syndrome (RDS)	**respiratory** (RES-pih-rah-TOR-ee) (reh-SPYR-ah-tor-ee) **re-** *again and again; backward; unable to* **spir/o-** *breathe* **-atory** *pertaining to*	Difficulty inflating the lungs to breathe because of a lack of surfactant. This occurs mainly in premature newborns. Also known as hyaline membrane disease (HMD). Treatment: Surfactant drug given through the endotracheal tube; oxygen therapy or ventilator support.

Diagnostic Procedures

Gynecologic Diagnostic Procedures

Word or Phrase	Word Part and Definition	Description
BRCA1 or BRCA2 gene	**gene** (JEEN) *Gene* is a Greek word meaning *to produce.* **genetic** (jeh-NET-ik) **gene/o-** *gene* **-tic** *pertaining to*	Blood test that shows if a patient has inherited the BRCA1 or BRCA2 gene, **genetic** mutations that significantly increase the risk of developing breast or ovarian cancer. BRCA stands for **br**east **ca**ncer.
biopsy	**biopsy** (BY-awp-see) **bi/o-** *life; living organisms; living tissue* **-opsy** *process of viewing* **aspiration** (AS-pih-RAY-shun) **aspir/o-** *to breathe in; to suck in* **-ation** *a process; being or having* **stereotactic** (STAIR-ee-oh-TAK-tic) **stere/o-** *three dimensions* **tact/o-** *touch* **-ic** *pertaining to* **incisional** (in-SIZH-un-al) **incis/o-** *to cut into* **-ion** *action; condition* **-al** *pertaining to* **excisional** (ek-SIZH-un-al) **excis/o-** *to cut out* **-ion** *action; condition* **-al** *pertaining to*	Diagnostic procedure to remove a small piece of tissue for examination to look for abnormal or cancerous cells. A breast biopsy can be done by **fine-needle aspiration** (a very fine needle is inserted into the mass and a syringe is used to aspirate tissue) or by **vacuum-assisted biopsy** (a Mammotome probe with a cutting device is inserted through the skin and rotated to take multiple specimens). For an endometrial biopsy (EMB), a speculum is used to visualize the cervix and dilators are used to expand the cervical os. A pipette or catheter is inserted into the uterus and rotated while suction pulls in tissue. Used to diagnose abnormal uterine bleeding and uterine cancer. For larger specimens, a surgical procedure is performed. First mammography or ultrasound is used to identify the location of the mass, and a needle or wire marker is inserted to pinpoint the site. A **stereotactic biopsy** uses three different angles of mammography to precisely locate the mass. For an **incisional biopsy,** an incision is made in the skin overlying the mass and a large part (but not all) of the mass is removed. For an **excisional biopsy,** the entire mass is removed along with a surrounding margin of normal tissue.
estrogen receptor assay	**receptor** (ree-SEP-tor) **recept/o-** *receive* **-or** *person or thing that produces or does* **assay** (AS-say) *Assay* is derived from an Old French word meaning *to weigh.*	Cytology test performed on breast tissue that has already been diagnosed as malignant. This test looks for a large number of estrogen receptors on the tumor cell membranes. If present, this means that the tumor requires estrogen (estradiol) in order to grow and that chemotherapy drugs that block estrogen would cause the tumor cells to die.

Word or Phrase	Word Part and Definition	Description
Pap smear	**Pap smear** Named by George Papanicolaou (1883–1962), an American physician. **exfoliative** (eks-FOH-lee-ah-tiv) *Exfoliative* is derived from a Latin word meaning *falling off of* the *leaves.* **cytology** (sy-TAWL-oh-jee) cyt/o- *cell* -logy *the study of* **ectocervical** (EK-toh-SER-vih-kal) ecto- *outermost, outside* cervic/o- *neck; cervix* -al *pertaining to* **endocervical** (EN-doh-SER-vih-kal) endo- *innermost, within* cervic/o- *neck; cervix* -al *pertaining to*	Cytology test used as a screening test to detect abnormal cells or carcinoma in situ (CIS) in the cervix. Also known as a Pap test. This type of test is known as **exfoliative cytology** because it examines cells that have been scraped off of the cervix. A small plastic or wooden spatula is used to obtain **ectocervical cells.** Then a **cytobrush** is inserted into the cervical os to obtain **endocervical cells** (see Figure 13-24 ■). A cervical broom (Papette™) can obtain both types of cells at the same time and also test for HPV. The cell specimen is transferred to a glass slide and sprayed with a fixative. Alternatively, with **liquid cytology,** the specimen is rinsed in a vial of fixative. This captures all the cells, prevents cell drying, and gives a more accurate result. The slides or vials are sent to the laboratory where the cells are examined under the microscope for abnormalities. The Bethesda System is used to report Pap smear results. Cervical broom (Papette™) / Cytobrush / Spatula **Figure 13-24 ■ Pap smear.** Cells from the ectocervix and cells from the endocervix are obtained using a wooden spatula and a cytobrush or by using a cervical broom (Papette™). A microscope is used to examine the cells and detect cells that are precancerous or cancerous. *(continued)*

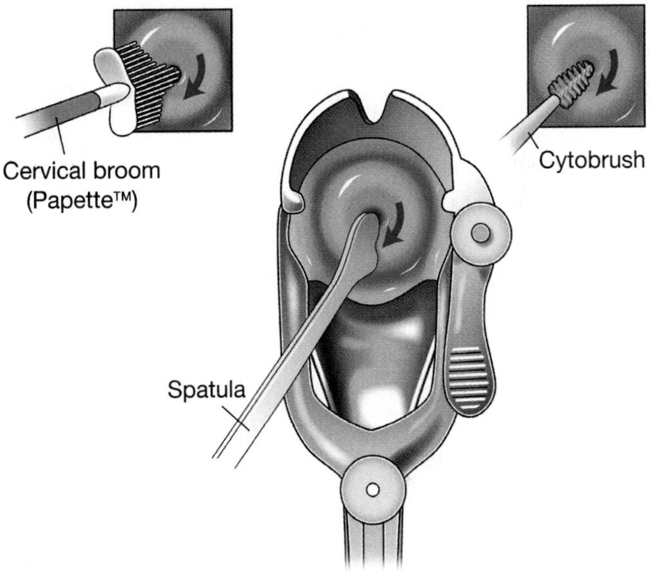

Word or Phrase	Word Part and Definition	Description
Pap smear (*continued*)		**A Closer Look** **Pap Smear Terminology** (Bethesda System Guidelines) **Specimen Adequacy** • Satisfactory (enough cells were collected; cell quality was sufficient for diagnosis) • Unsatisfactory (enough cells were not collected; cell quality was poor) **Normal Pap Smear** Findings are reported as: Negative for intraepithelial lesion or malignancy (The presence of infectious organisms [Trichomonas, herpes, HPV] would also be reported.) **Abnormal Pap Smear** Findings are reported as one of the following: ASC-US Atypical squamous cells of unknown significance ASC-H Atypical squamous cells of unknown significance, cannot exclude HSIL LSIL* Low-grade squamous intraepithelial lesion HSIL** High-grade squamous intraepithelial lesion SCC Squamous cell carcinoma *LSIL includes different levels that are classified according to cervical intraepithelial neoplasia (CIN I) with and without HPV present. **HSIL includes several levels that are classified according to CIN II through III with and without HPV present.
wet mount		Cytology test for yeasts, parasites, or bacteria. A swab is taken of the area of vaginitis. The cells are sent to the laboratory where they are placed on a slide, mixed with saline solution, and examined under the microscope. Also known as a wet prep.
Infertility Diagnostic Tests		
antisperm antibody test	**antibody** (AN-tee-BAWD-ee) (AN-tih-BAWD-ee) **anti-** *against* **-body** *a structure or thing*	Cervical mucus test that detects antibodies against sperm in the woman's cervical mucus. Some antibodies attack the tail of the spermatozoon so that it cannot swim; others prevent the spermatozoon from penetrating cervical mucus. Men can produce antibodies to their own spermatozoa when the spermatozoa must be absorbed by the body after a vasectomy. These antibodies remain even after reversal of the vasectomy.
hormone testing		Blood test to determine the levels of FSH and LH from the anterior pituitary gland and estradiol and progesterone from the ovaries. Used to diagnose menstruation and infertility problems.

Pregnancy and Neonatal Diagnostic Tests

Word or Phrase	Word Part and Definition	Description
amniocentesis	**amniocentesis** (AM-nee-oh-sen-TEE-sis) **amni/o-** *amnion (fetal membrane)* **-centesis** *procedure to puncture* **chromosome** (KROH-moh-sohm) **chrom/o-** *color* **-some** *a body* Add words to make a correct and complete definition of *chromosome: a body [within the nucleus that takes on] color [when stained].* **alpha fetoprotein** (AL-fah FEE-toh-PROH-teen) **lecithin** (LES-ih-thin) **sphingomyelin** (SFING-goh-MY-eh-lin)	Amniotic fluid test. With ultrasound guidance a needle is inserted through the abdominal wall and into the uterus to withdraw amniotic fluid (see Figure 13-25 ■). The test is done between 15 to 18 weeks' gestation. 1. **Chromosome studies** on fetal skin cells can determine the sex of the fetus and identify genetic abnormalities like Down syndrome. 2. **Alpha fetoprotein (AFP).** Increased levels indicate a neural tube defect (myelomeningocele or anencephaly). 3. **L/S ratio** (lecithin/sphingomyelin). **Lecithin** is a component of surfactant that keeps the alveoli from collapsing with each breath. **Sphingomyelin** levels are higher until the fetal lungs are mature, and then lecithin levels become higher than sphingomyelin by 2:1. This test is also done later in pregnancy to determine the maturity of the fetal lungs. **Figure 13-25 ■ Amniocentesis.** The obstetrician is withdrawing amniotic fluid through a needle inserted into the uterus. The position of the needle was verified by ultrasound (on the monitor screen). The technician is holding the ultrasound transducer that is emitting sound waves to produce the image.
chorionic villus sampling (CVS)	**chorionic** (KOH-ree-ON-ik) **chorion/o-** *chorion (fetal membrane)* **-ic** *pertaining to* **villus** (VIL-us) Villi are the fingerlike projections that the chorion sends out to implant in the endometrium.	Genetic test of the chorionic villi from the placenta. A needle is inserted through the abdomen or a catheter is inserted through the cervix to aspirate tissue. This test is performed when a fetal genetic defect is suspected. It can be performed at 12 weeks, which is earlier than an amniocentesis, but it cannot detect neural tube defects in the fetus.
pregnancy test		Blood test to detect human chorionic gonadotropin (HCG) secreted by the fertilized ovum. Serum HCG is positive just nine days after conception. Home pregnancy tests that detect HCG in the urine are easy to use but are not always accurate. Only a positive blood test (serum beta HCG) is diagnostic of pregnancy. The presence of HCG does not indicate that the pregnancy is normal because HCG is also produced in an ectopic pregnancy and hydatidiform mole.

Radiologic Procedures

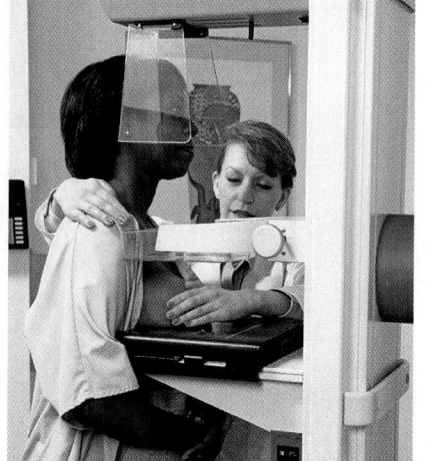

Word or Phrase	Word Part and Definition	Description
hysterosalpingography	**hysterosalpingography** (HIS-ter-oh-SAL-ping-GAWG rah-fee) **hyster/o-** *uterus (womb)* **salping/o-** *fallopian tube* **-graphy** *process of recording* **hysterosalpingogram** (HIS-ter-oh-sal-PING-goh-gram) **hyster/o-** *uterus (womb)* **salping/o-** *fallopian tube* **-gram** *a record or picture*	Radiologic procedure in which radiopaque contrast dye is injected through the cervix into the uterus. It coats and outlines the uterus and fallopian tubes and shows narrowing, scarring, and blockage. The x-ray image is known as a **hysterosalpingogram.** This test is done as part of an infertility workup.
mammography	**mammography** (mah-MAWG-rah-fee) **mamm/o-** *breast* **-graphy** *process of recording* **mammogram** (MAM-oh-gram) **mamm/o-** *breast* **-gram** *a picture or record* **xeromammography** (ZEER-oh-mah-MAWG-rah-fee) **xer/o-** *dry* **mamm/o-** *breast* **-graphy** *process of recording* **xeromammogram** (ZEER-oh-MAM-oh-gram) **xer/o-** *dry* **mamm/o-** *breast* **-gram** *a picture or record*	Radiologic procedure that uses x-rays to create an image of the breast. The breast is compressed and slightly flattened (see Figure 13-26 ■). Mammography is used to detect areas of microcalcification, infection, cysts, and tumors, many of which cannot be felt on a breast examination. The x-ray image is known as a **mammogram.** **Xeromammography** uses a special plate instead of an x-ray plate, and the image is developed with dry powder rather than liquid chemicals. The image is printed on paper and is known as a **xeromammogram.**  **Figure 13-26 ■ Mammography.** A mammogram is the image obtained when an x-ray beam passes through the breast to an x-ray plate. The breast is compressed because the less distance the x-ray travels the sharper the image that is obtained.

Word or Phrase	Word Part and Definition	Description
ultrasonography	**ultrasonography** (UL-trah-soh-NAWG-rah-fee) **ultra-** *beyond; higher* **son/o-** *sound* **-graphy** *process of recording* **ultrasound** (UL-trah-sound) *Ultrasound* is a combination of the prefix *ultra-* (beyond; higher) and the word *sound.* **sonogram** (SAWN-oh-gram) **son/o-** *sound* **-gram** *a record or picture* **biparietal** (BY-pah-RY-eh-tal) **bi-** *two* **pariet/o-** *wall of a cavity* **-al** *pertaining to* **transvaginal** (trans-VAJ-ih-nal) **trans-** *across, through* **vagin/o-** *vagina* **-al** *pertaining to*	Radiologic procedure that uses ultra high-frequency sound waves emitted by a transducer (see Figure 13-25) or probe to produce a somewhat grainy image on a computer screen. Three-dimensional ultrasonography couples the ultrasound with a position sensor to generate a high-resolution image in three dimensions (see Figure 13-27 ■). The **ultrasound** image is known as a **sonogram.** Ultrasonography of the breast or uterus can differentiate between benign, fluid-filled tumors (cysts) and solid tumors that need to be biopsied. A pelvic ultrasound can be used to diagnose a normal pregnancy versus a hydatidiform mole or ectopic pregnancy. In early pregnancy, the beating heart is seen. The image can show multiple fetuses and the sex of the fetus. An ultrasound is done routinely at 16–20 weeks in a normal pregnancy to estimate the gestational age. Serial ultrasounds can be done over time if there is a question of intrauterine growth retardation. The length of the femur, the **biparietal diameter (BPD)** (distance between the two parietal bones of the cranium), and the crown-to-rump length are used to calculate the gestational age. The image can show the position of the placenta to diagnose placenta previa. Pelvic ultrasound is used during amniocentesis to locate a large area of amniotic fluid in which to insert the needle (see Figure 13-25). A **transvaginal ultrasound** uses an ultrasound probe inserted into the vagina to determine the thickness of the endometrium in patients with abnormal uterine bleeding. 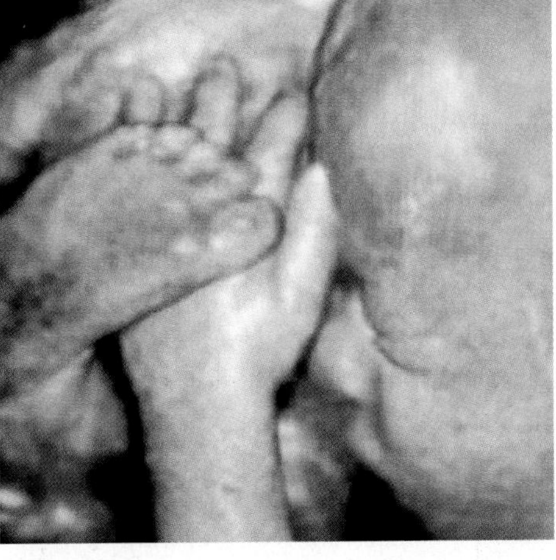 **Figure 13-27 ■** **Three-dimensional ultrasonography.** Sound waves generated by a transducer bounce off the uterus and are captured to create a computer image. The fine details of the fetus are clearly visible in this type of ultrasound.

Medical and Surgical Procedures

Medical Procedures of the Internal Genitalia

Word or Phrase	Word Part and Definition	Description
colposcopy	**colposcopy** (kohl-PAWS-koh-pee) **colp/o-** *vagina* **-scopy** *process of using an instrument to examine*	Medical procedure that uses a magnifying, lighted scope to visually examine the vagina and cervix.
cryosurgery	**cryosurgery** (KRY-oh-SER-jer-ee) **cry/o-** *cold* **surg/o-** *operative procedure* **-ery** *process of* **cryoprobe** (KRY-oh-prohb) **cry/o-** *cold* **-probe** *rodlike instrument*	Medical procedure to destroy small areas of abnormal tissue on the cervix. Colposcopy is used to visualize the cervical lesions to be destroyed. A **cryoprobe** containing extremely cold liquid nitrogen is touched to the areas to freeze and destroy the tissues.
gynecologic examination	**gynecologic** (GY-neh-koh-LAW-jik) **gynec/o-** *female, woman* **log/o-** *the study of* **-ic** *pertaining to* **dorsal** (DOR-sal) **dors/o-** *back; dorsum; uppermost part* **-al** *pertaining to* **lithotomy** (lih-THAWT-oh-mee) **lith/o-** *stone* **-tomy** *process of cutting or making an incision* The lithotomy position was originally used to treat patients who had stones in the bladder. **speculum** (SPEK-yoo-lum) *Speculum* is a Latin word meaning *to behold.* **bimanual** (by-MAN-yoo-al) **bi-** *two* **manu/o-** *hand* **-al** *pertaining to*	Medical procedure to physically examine the external and internal genitalia. This is performed with the patient supine in the **dorsal lithotomy position**. The hips and knees are flexed, and the feet are held up in stirrups. The external genitalia are examined visually for any skin lesions, rashes, or discharge from the vagina. A **speculum** is inserted into the vagina and a Pap smear is performed. The cervix is examined visually for abnormalities. The internal genitalia are examined using a **bimanual examination** (see Figure 13-28 ■). A mass, enlargement of the uterus or ovaries, cystocele, or rectocele can be palpated. Tenderness to palpation can indicate infection or endometriosis. 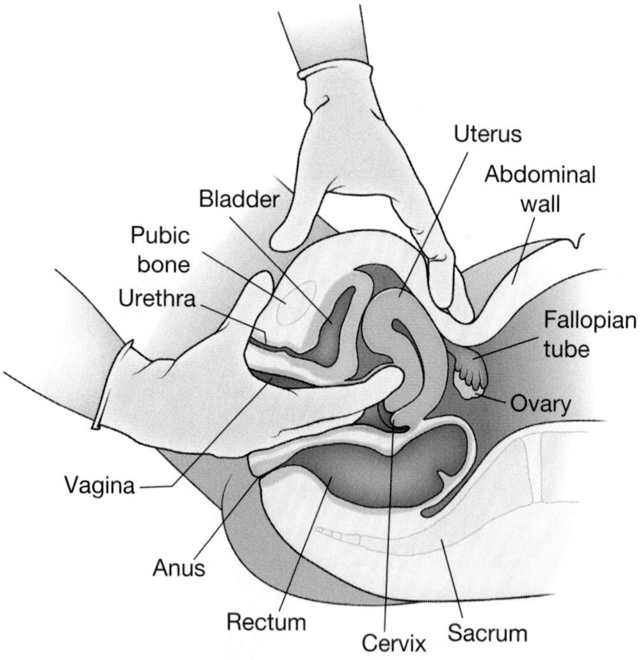 Uterus / Abdominal wall / Bladder / Pubic bone / Urethra / Fallopian tube / Ovary / Vagina / Anus / Rectum / Cervix / Sacrum **Figure 13-28 ■ Bimanual examination.** By using both hands, the physician is able to examine the shape of the uterus and detect tenderness and masses.

Medical Procedures of the Breast

Word or Phrase	Word Part and Definition	Description
breast self-examination (BSE)		Systematic palpation of all areas of the breast and under the arm to detect lumps, masses, or enlarged lymph nodes. BSE should be done monthly to detect early signs of breast cancer.
Tanner staging		System used to describe the development of the female breasts from childhood through puberty. There are five different stages, from Tanner stage 1 (nipple and areola are flat against the chest wall) to Tanner stage 5 (enlargement of the entire breast). The Tanner system is also used to describe the development of the female external genitalia.

Medical Procedures for Obstetrics

Word or Phrase	Word Part and Definition	Description
amniotomy	**amniotomy** (AM-nee-AWT-oh-mee) **amni/o-** *amnion (fetal membrane)* **-tomy** *process of cutting or making an incision*	Medical procedure in which a hook is inserted into the cervix to rupture the amniotic sac and induce labor.
Apgar score	**Apgar** (AP-gar) Named by Virginia Apgar (1909–1974), an American anesthesiologist.	Medical procedure that assigns a score to a newborn at one and five minutes after birth. Points (0–2) are given for the heart rate, respiratory rate, muscle tone, response to stimulation, and skin color.
assisted delivery		Procedure in which obstetrical forceps or a vacuum extractor is used to facilitate delivery of the head of the fetus (see Figure 13-14).
epidural anesthesia	**epidural** (EP-ih-DYOO-ral) **epi-** *upon, above* **dur/o-** *dura mater* **-al** *pertaining to* **anesthesia** (AN-es-THEE-zee-ah) **an-** *without, not* **esthes/o-** *sensation, feeling* **-ia** *condition, state, thing*	Local anesthesia produced by injecting an anesthetic drug into the epidural space between vertebrae in the lower back. This numbs the abdomen, perineum, and legs and decreases labor pain. Epidural anesthesia is not given until the cervix is more than 4 cm dilated to prevent from prolonging labor.
fundal height	**fundal** (FUN-dal) **fund/o-** *fundus (part farthest from the opening)* **-al** *pertaining to*	The distance in centimeters from the top of the symphysis pubis to the top of the uterine fundus. It is a general indication of fetal growth.
induction of labor	**induction** (in-DUK-shun) **induct/o-** *a leading in* **-ion** *action; condition*	Medical procedure to begin labor by administering an oxytocin drug. This is done when the mother is past her estimated due date or when the health of the mother or fetus necessitates delivery.

Word or Phrase	Word Part and Definition	Description
Nägele's rule	**Nägele** (NAY-gel) This rule was developed by Franz Nägele (1777–1851), a German obstetrician. *Estimated date of confinement (EDC)* is an older phrase that indicated when a woman was to be confined to her home around her due date.	Used to calculate the patient's due date, which is also known as the estimated date of birth (EDB) or the estimated date of confinement (EDC). Often the patient does not remember the date of the first day of her last menstrual period (LMP), so the EDB is just an approximate date.
nonstress test (NST)	**biophysical** (BY-oh-FIZ-ih-kal) **bi/o-** *life; living organisms; living tissue* **physic/o-** *body* **-al** *pertaining to*	An external monitor on the mother's abdomen prints out the fetal heart rate. A normal test (reactive test) will show at least two fetal heart rate accelerations associated with fetal movement. A nonreactive test is abnormal. It is followed up by a **biophysical profile (BPP)** that combines a nonstress test with an ultrasound to rate fetal movement, fetal heart rate, and amniotic fluid volume.
pelvimetry	**pelvimetry** (pel-VIM-ih-tree) **pelv/i-** *pelvis (hip bone; renal pelvis)* **-metry** *process of measuring*	Medical procedure to determine the dimensions of the maternal bony pelvis to see if its size is adequate for a vaginal delivery. The measurement can be estimated by feel during a bimanual examination or measured on an x-ray of the pelvis.
obstetrical history	**nulligravida** (NUL-ih-GRAV-ih-dah) **null/i-** *none* **-gravida** *pregnancy* **primigravida** (PRY-mih-GRAV-ih-dah) **prim/i-** *first* **-gravida** *pregnancy* **multigravida** (MUL-tih-GRAV-ih-dah) **mult/i-** *many* **-gravida** *pregnancy* **multiparous** (mul-TIP-ah-rus) **mult/i-** *many* **par/o-** *birth* **-ous** *pertaining to* **gravida** (GRAV-ih-dah) *Gravida* is a Latin word meaning *pregnant woman or pregnancy.* **para** (PAIR-ah) *Para* is derived from a Latin word meaning *to bring forth.* **abortion** (ah-BOR-shun) **abort/o-** *stop prematurely* **-ion** *action; condition*	Good prenatal care includes documentation of past pregnancies and deliveries. A **nulligravida** is a woman who has never been pregnant and is not pregnant now. A **primigravida** is a woman who is pregnant for the first time. A **multigravida** is a woman who has been pregnant many times. If she has born many children, she is said to be **multiparous.** In the past, documentation of the number of pregnancies, deliveries, and abortions was done using **gravida (G), para (P),** and **abortion (Ab).** A woman who was G3, P3, Ab 0 had been pregnant three times and given birth three times. A woman who had had twins would be G1, P2. G/TPAL is a more detailed system to keep track of each pregnancy and its outcome. G = Number of times pregnant T = Number of term births P = Number of premature births A = Number of abortions (spontaneous or induced) L = Number of living children

Word or Phrase	Word Part and Definition	Description
therapeutic abortion (TAB)	**therapeutic** (THAIR-ah-PYOO-tik) **therapeut/o-** *treatment* **-ic** *pertaining to* **abortion** (ah-BOR-shun) **abort/o-** *stop prematurely* **-ion** *action; condition* **elective** (ee-LEK-tiv) *Elective* means *pertaining to something that is subject to choice, not required.*	Medical procedure for planned termination of a pregnancy at any time during gestation. All products of conception are removed from the uterus with suction. Also known as an **elective abortion.**
version	**version** (VER-zhun) **vers/o-** *to turn; to travel* **-ion** *action; condition*	Medical procedure to manually correct a breech or other malpresentation prior to delivery. The physician puts his/her hands on the mother's abdominal wall and manipulates the position of the fetus.

A Closer Look

in vitro (IN VEE-troh)
In vitro is a Latin phrase meaning *in glass* (i.e., in a test tube or culture dish).

intrafallopian (IN-trah-fah-LOH-pee-an)
intra- *within*
fallopi/o- *fallopian tube*
-an *pertaining to*

insemination (in-SEM-ih-NAY-shun)
insemin/o- *plant a seed*
-ation *a process; being or having*

intracytoplasmic (IN-trah-SY-toh-PLAS-mik)
intra- *within*
cyt/o- *cell*
plasm/o- *plasma; formed substance*
-ic *pertaining to*

injection (in-JEK-shun)
inject/o- *insert or put in*
-ion *action; condition*

Assisted reproduction encompasses many different procedures that use technology to assist the process of conception. For ***in vitro* fertilization (IVF),** the woman receives ovulation-stimulating drugs, mature ova are harvested via a needle inserted into the ovary, and some of the ova are combined with spermatozoa and allowed to grow from two to five days in a culture medium. Then the fertilized ovum is transferred into the uterus. This was the first procedure of its type and the newborns were known as test tube babies. For **zygote intrafallopian transfer (ZIFT),** the same procedure is followed but the fertilized ovum (zygote) is grown outside the mother for several days and then transferred into the fallopian tube. For **gamete intrafallopian transfer (GIFT),** the ova and spermatozoa are collected, but then both are transferred to the fallopian tube.

When the man has a low sperm count or the woman's cervical mucus contains antibodies against sperm, the man's sperm may be collected, concentrated, and inserted directly into the uterus, a procedure known as **intrauterine insemination.** In men with very low sperm counts, sperm can be taken from the testis or epididymis and, using a micropipette, a single sperm can be injected into one ovum (see Figure 13-29 ■), a procedure known as **intracytoplasmic sperm injection (ICSI).**

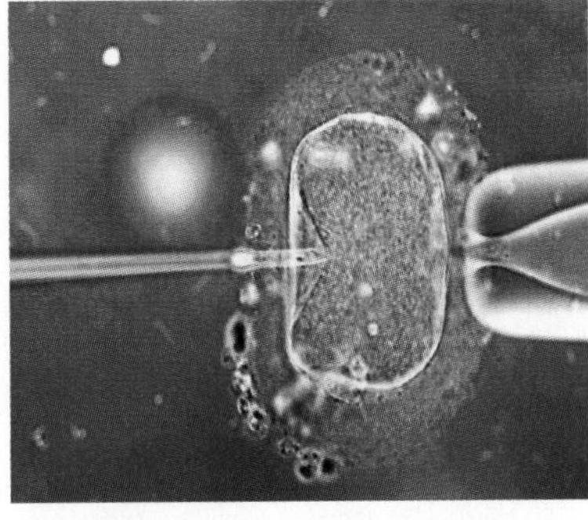

Figure 13-29 ■ Intracytoplasmic sperm injection (ICSI).
A type of assisted reproduction. Under the microscope, a micropipette (on the left) is used to penetrate an ovum and insert a single spermatozoon to fertilize it.

Surgical Procedures of the Cervix and Vagina

Word or Phrase	Word Part and Definition	Description
colporrhaphy	**colporrhaphy** (kol-POR-ah-fee) colp/o- *vagina* -rrhaphy *procedure of suturing*	Surgical procedure to suture a weakness in the vaginal wall. This procedure is done to correct a cystocele or a rectocele.
conization	**conization** (KOH-nih-ZAY-shun) con/o- *cone* -ization *the process of making, creating, or inserting*	Surgical procedure to remove a large, cone-shaped section of tissue that includes the cervical os and part of the cervical canal. Used to diagnosis a lesion or excise an abnormal area identified by a Pap smear. A laser knife or a loop electrosurgical excision procedure (LEEP) with a hot wire loop is used to burn and cut away the tissue. Alternately, a scalpel (cold knife conization) can be used so that no cells are damaged by heat.
culdoscopy	**culdoscopy** (kul-DAWS-koh-pee) culd/o- *cul-de-sac* -scopy *process of using an instrument to examine*	Surgical procedure in which an endoscope is inserted into the vagina, penetrates the posterior wall of the vagina, and enters the pelvic cavity. This procedure is performed under local anesthesia and leaves no abdominal scars. Used to examine the cul-de-sac and the external surfaces of the uterus, fallopian tubes, and ovaries for signs of endometriosis or adhesions.

Surgical Procedures of the Uterus, Fallopian Tubes, and Ovaries

Word or Phrase	Word Part and Definition	Description
dilation and curettage (D&C)	**dilation** (dy-LAY-shun) dilat/o- *dilate, widen* -ion *action; condition* **curettage** (kyoo-reh-TAHZH) *Curettage* is a French word meaning *a scraping.* **tenaculum** (teh-NAK-yoo-lum) *Tenaculum* is derived from a Latin word meaning *to hold.* **curet** (kyoo-RET) *Curet* is a French word meaning *a scraper.* Also spelled *curette.*	Surgical procedure to remove abnormal tissue from inside the uterus. The cervix is dilated with progressively larger dilators inserted into the cervical os. A **tenaculum** (long scissors-like instrument with two curved, pointed ends) is used to grasp and hold the cervix. Then a **curet** (rod with a sharp-edged circular or oval ring at one end) is inserted to scrape the endometrium. Alternatively, a vacuum aspirator is inserted to suction out pieces of endometrium. This procedure is performed for abnormal uterine bleeding or suspected uterine cancer. Also used to perform a therapeutic abortion or remove the products of conception following a spontaneous but incomplete abortion.
endometrial ablation	**ablation** (ab-LAY-shun) ablat/o- *take away; destroy* -ion *action; condition*	Surgical procedure that uses heat or cold to destroy the endometrium. A laser, hot fluid in a balloon, or an electrode with electrical current is inserted into the uterus. Alternatively, a cryoprobe is inserted to freeze the endometrium. Used to treat dysfunctional uterine bleeding.
hysterectomy	**hysterectomy** (HIS-ter-EK-toh-mee) hyster/o- *uterus (womb)* -ectomy *surgical excision* *Hyster/o-* is derived from a Greek word meaning *uterus.* It was later used in the word *hysteria,* to describe an emotional disorder of women thought to be centered in the uterus.	Surgical procedure to remove the uterus. An **abdominal hysterectomy** is performed with a laparoscope through an abdominal incision. A **vaginal hysterectomy (TVH)** is performed through the vagina. A total hysterectomy involves removing both the uterus and cervix. A **TAH-BSO** is a total abdominal hysterectomy and bilateral salpingo-oophorectomy (removal of both fallopian tubes and ovaries). A hysterectomy is done because of uterine fibroids, endometriosis, uterine prolapse, abnormal uterine bleeding, or uterine or cervical cancer. A radical hysterectomy, done for cancer of the uterus, involves removal of the uterus, cervix, upper vagina, and pelvic lymph nodes.

Word or Phrase	Word Part and Definition	Description
laparoscopy	**laparoscopy** (LAP-ah-RAWS-koh-pee) **lapar/o-** *abdomen* **-scopy** *process of using an instrument to examine* **laparoscope** (LAP-ah-roh-skohp) **lapar/o-** *abdomen* **-scope** *instrument used to examine* **endoscope** (EN-doh-skohp) **endo-** *innermost, within* **-scope** *instrument used to examine* **laparoscopic** (LAP-ah-roh-SKAWP-ik) **lapar/o-** *abdomen* **scop/o-** *examine with an instrument* **ic-** *pertaining to*	Surgical procedure to visualize the pelvic cavity, uterus, fallopian tubes, and ovaries for diagnosis, biopsy, or surgery. A small incision is made near the umbilicus, and carbon dioxide gas is used to inflate the abdominal cavity. Then a **laparoscope,** a fiberoptic **endoscope,** is inserted through the incision (see Figure 13-30 ■). Grasping and cutting instruments are inserted through other abdominal incisions. Pelvic adhesions, pelvic inflammatory disease, and endometriosis can be treated and a **laparoscopic** hysterectomy can be done, if needed. 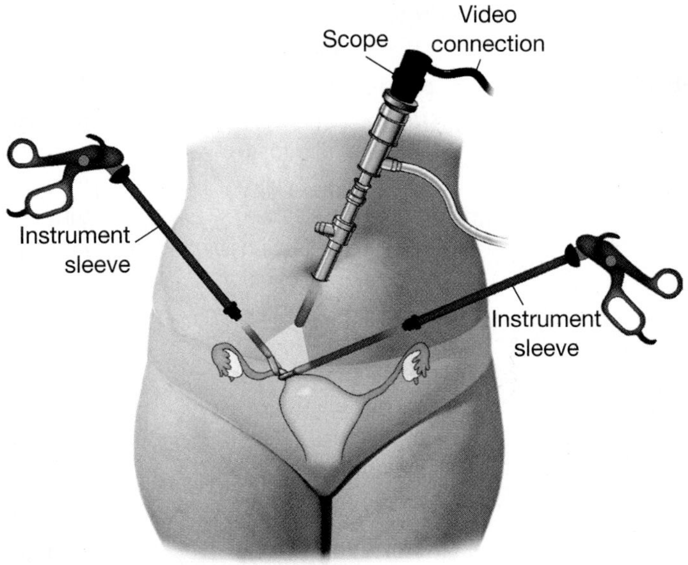 Scope; Video connection; Instrument sleeve; Instrument sleeve **Figure 13-30 ■ Laparoscopy.** Three small incisions allow visualization of the uterus, fallopian tubes, and ovaries during laparoscopic surgery.
myomectomy	**myomectomy** (MY-oh-MEK-toh-mee) **my/o-** *muscle* **om/o-** *tumor, mass* **-ectomy** *surgical excision*	Surgical procedure to remove leiomyomata or fibroids from the uterus. This procedure can be done vaginally or through a laparoscope in the abdomen.
oophorectomy	**oophorectomy** (OH-of-or-EK-toh-mee) **oophor/o-** *ovary* **-ectomy** *surgical excision* *Oophor/o-* is composed of *o/o-* (egg) and *phor/o-* (to carry or bear). The ovary carries or bears the eggs. **bilateral** (by-LAT-er-al) **bi-** *two* **later/o-** *side* **-al** *pertaining to*	Surgical procedure to remove an ovary because of large ovarian cysts or ovarian cancer. A **bilateral oophorectomy** removes both ovaries.

Word or Phrase	Word Part and Definition	Description
salpingectomy	**salpingectomy** (SAL-pin-JEK-toh-mee) **salping/o-** *fallopian tube* **-ectomy** *surgical excision* **salpingo-oophorectomy** (sal-PING-goh-OH-of-or-EK-toh-mee) **salping/o-** *fallopian tube* **oophor/o-** *ovary* **-ectomy** *surgical excision*	Surgical procedure to remove a fallopian tube because of ovarian cancer or an ectopic pregnancy in the tube. A bilateral salpingectomy removes both fallopian tubes. A **bilateral salpingo-oophorectomy (BSO)** removes both fallopian tubes and both ovaries.
tubal ligation	**tubal** (TOO-bal) **tub/o-** *tube* **-al** *pertaining to* **ligation** (ly-GAY-shun) **ligat/o-** *to tie up or bind* **-ion** *action; condition* **anastomosis** (ah-NAS-toh-MOH-sis) **anastom/o-** *unite two tubular structures* **-osis** *condition; abnormal condition; process*	Surgical procedure to prevent pregnancy. A short segment of each fallopian tube is removed. The cut ends are sutured and then crushed or cauterized. The woman continues to ovulate, but the ovum cannot travel through the blocked fallopian tube. Also known as "getting your tubes tied." A **tubal anastomosis** is the procedure to rejoin the fallopian tube segments so that the woman can get pregnant again.
uterine artery embolization	**embolization** (EM-bol-ih-ZAY-shun) **embol/o-** *embolus (occluding plug)* **-ization** *process of making, creating, or inserting*	Surgical and radiologic procedure used to treat uterine fibroids. A catheter is inserted into the femoral artery in the groin and threaded to the uterine artery. Radiopaque contrast dye is injected to identify the smaller artery that supplies blood to a fibroid. Tiny particles are injected to block that artery. Without a blood supply, the fibroid shrinks in size.
uterine suspension	**suspension** (sus-PEN-shun) **suspens/o-** *hanging* **-ion** *action; condition* **hysteropexy** (HIS-ter-oh-pek-see) **hyster/o-** *uterus (womb)* **-pexy** *process of surgically fixing in place*	Surgical procedure to suspend and fix the uterus into an anatomically correct position. Used to correct a retroverted uterus or uterine prolapse. The uplift procedure uses sutures inserted through the abdomen and into the round ligament. Then the suture ends are pulled to shorten the round ligaments, which pulls the uterus up into a normal position. Also known as a **hysteropexy.**
Surgical Procedures of the Breast		
lumpectomy	**lumpectomy** (lum-PEK-toh-mee) *Lumpectomy* is a combination of the English word *lump* and the suffix *-ectomy* (surgical excision).	Surgical procedure to excise a small malignant tumor of the breast. Adjacent normal breast tissue and the axillary lymph nodes are also removed in case any cancerous cells have already spread to them.

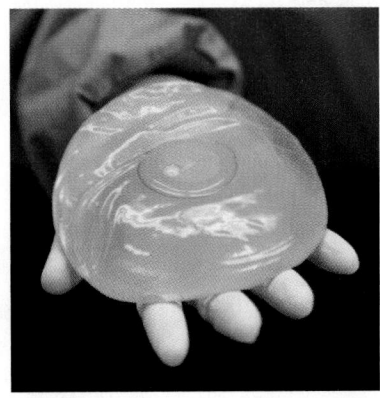

Word or Phrase	Word Part and Definition	Description
mammaplasty	**mammaplasty** (MAM-ah-plas-tee) **mamm/a-** *breast* **-plasty** *process of reshaping by surgery* **mammoplasty** (MAM-oh-plas-tee) **mamm/o-** *breast* **-plasty** *process of reshaping by surgery* **augmentation** (AWG-men-TAY-shun) **augment/o-** *increase in size or degree* **-ation** *a process; being or having* **prosthesis** (praws-THEE-sis) *Prosthesis* is a Greek word meaning *an addition.* **reduction** (re-DUK-shun) **reduct/o-** *to bring back; decrease* **-ion** *action; condition* **pendulous** (PEN-dyoo-lus) **pendul/o-** *hanging down* **-ous** *pertaining to* **mastopexy** (MAS-toh-pek-see) **mast/o-** *breast; mastoid process* **-pexy** *process of surgically fixing in place* **reconstructive** (REE-con-STRUK-tiv) **re-** *again and again; backward; unable to* **construct/o-** *to build* **-ive** *pertaining to*	Surgical procedure to change the size, shape, or position of the breast. Also known as a **mammoplasty.** An **augmentation mammaplasty** enlarges the size of a small breast by inserting a breast **prosthesis** or implant under the skin or chest muscles (see Figure 13-31 ■). A **reduction mammaplasty** reduces the size of a large, **pendulous** breast. The procedure can be performed in conjunction with a **mastopexy** or breast lift to reposition a sagging breast. A **reconstructive mammaplasty** is done to reconstruct a breast after a mastectomy. **Figure 13-31 ■ Breast implant.** A breast implant is a soft container filled with silicone gel or saline (salt water). It is placed beneath the skin or beneath the pectoralis major muscle.

Word or Phrase	Word Part and Definition	Description
mastectomy	**mastectomy** (mas-TEK-toh-mee) mast/o- *breast; mastoid process* -ectomy *surgical excision* **radical** (RAD-ih-kal) radic/o- *all parts including the root* -al *pertaining to* **dissection** (dih-SEK-shun) dissect/o- *to cut apart* -ion *action; condition* **prophylactic** (PROH-fih-LAK-tik) pro- *before* phylact/o- *guarding or protecting* -ic *pertaining to*	Surgical resection of all or part of the breast to excise a malignant tumor. In a **simple** or **total mastectomy,** the entire breast, the overlying skin, and nipple are removed, but not the chest muscle or axillary nodes. In a **modified radical mastectomy,** an **axillary node dissection** is also performed and some of the axillary lymph nodes are removed. In a **radical mastectomy,** the pectoralis major and minor muscles of the chest wall are also removed; this procedure is performed infrequently. A **prophylactic mastectomy** can be performed for women who have a strong family history of breast cancer to prevent breast cancer from occurring.
reconstructive breast surgery	**reconstructive** (REE-con-STRUK-tiv) re- *again and again; backward; unable to* construct/o- *to build* -ive *pertaining to* Some word parts have more than one definition. The best definition of *reconstructive* is *pertaining to again building [the breast].* **transverse** (trans-VERS) trans- *across, through* -verse *to travel; to turn*	Surgical procedure to rebuild a breast after a mastectomy. This can be performed at the same time as a mastectomy or in a later, separate operation. A breast prosthesis or a TRAM flap (see Figure 13-32 ■) is used to recreate the fullness of the breast. With a breast prosthesis procedure, a tissue expander (a saline-filled silicone bag) is first inserted to stretch the skin to accommodate a breast prosthesis, which is later inserted. For a **TRAM (transverse rectus abdominis muscle) flap,** an incision is made around a transverse area of the abdomen. Skin, fat and muscle are excised, except for one end that is left attached to blood vessels (pedicle graft). Alternatively, the latissimus dorsi muscle of the back can be used. Then the flap is tunneled under the skin of the upper abdomen to the site of the previous mastectomy. Later, a tattoo can be done on the skin to create an areola and nipple.

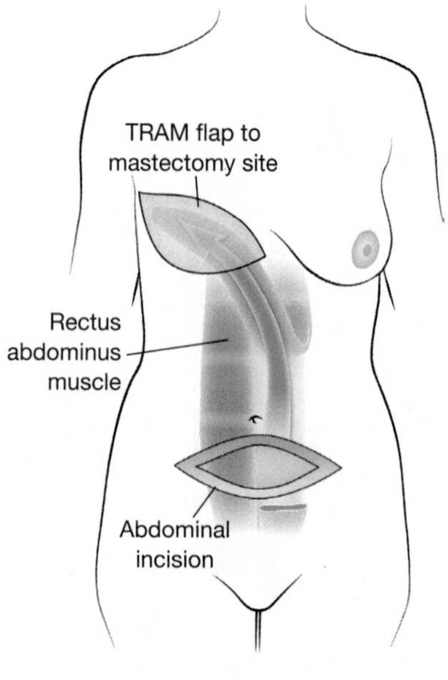

Figure 13-32 ■ TRAM flap reconstruction.

This reconstructive surgery uses a skin, fat, and muscle flap from the abdomen to reconstruct the breast following a mastectomy. The fat and muscle (rectus abdominis muscle) provide a natural feel to the reconstructed breast and take the place of a synthetic breast implant.

Surgical Procedures in Obstetrics

Word or Phrase	Word Part and Definition	Description
cerclage	**cerclage** (sir-CLAWJ) *Cerclage* is a French word meaning *encircling loop.*	Surgical procedure to place a purse-string suture around the cervix to prevent it from dilating prematurely. The sutures are removed prior to delivery.
cesarean section	**cesarean** (seh-ZAY-ree-an) So named because of a Roman law at the time of the caesars. It read "The law of the kings forbids the burial of a woman who died pregnant until her offspring has been excised from her body." The cesarean section was performed to see if the fetus had survived when the mother died.	Surgical procedure to deliver a fetus. It is done because of cephalopelvic disproportion, failure to progress during labor, the mother being past the due date, or health problems in the mother or fetus. The fetus is delivered through an incision in the abdominal wall and uterus. Also known as a C-section. A vaginal birth after a prior cesarean section is abbreviated as VBAC.
episiotomy	**episiotomy** (eh-PIS-ee-AWT-oh-mee) **episi/o-** *vulva* **-tomy** *process of cutting or making an incision*	Surgical incision in the posterior edge of the vagina to prevent a spontaneous tear during delivery of the baby's head. Spontaneous vaginal tears usually have ragged tissue edges that are difficult to suture and can extend into the rectum, causing incontinence.

Drug Categories

Several different categories of drugs are used to treat the symptoms, signs, and diseases of the female genital and reproductive system. The most common drugs in each category are listed.

Category	Word Part and Definition	Description	Example
antibiotic drugs	**antibiotic** (AN-tee-by-AWT-ik) (AN-tih-by-AWT-ik) **anti-** *against* **bi/o-** *life; living organisms; living tissue* **-tic** *pertaining to*	Treat infections of the female genitalia and breasts and sexually transmitted diseases that are caused by bacteria. Antibiotic drugs are not effective against viral infections.	ampicillin, amoxicillin, erythromycin, Vibramycin
chemotherapy drugs	**chemotherapy** (KEE-moh-THAIR-ah-pee) **chem/o-** *chemical, drug* **-therapy** *treatment*	Kill rapidly dividing cancer cells in the ovaries, uterus, or breasts that arise from tissue that is responsive to estradiol. These drugs include androgens (male sex hormones) as well as estrogen-blocking drugs that alter the hormonal environment.	Arimidex, Femara, Megace, Nolvadex, tamoxifen
drugs for amenorrhea and abnormal uterine bleeding		Correct hormone imbalances of FSH, LH, estradiol, or progesterone.	Follistim, Hylutin, Lutrepulse, Prempro, Provera

Category	Word Part and Definition	Description	Example
drugs for contraception	**contraception** (CON-trah-SEP-shun) *Contraception* is a combination of the prefix *contra-* (against) and a shortened form of the word *conception.*	Prevent ovulation. The combination of estrogen and progestin suppresses the release of FSH and LH from the anterior pituitary gland.	oral contraceptive pill (OCP): Demulen, Ortho-Novum, Ortho Tri-Cyclen, Ovral transdermal patch: Ortho Evra vaginal ring: NuvaRing Intrauterine unit: Mirena Injection: Depo-Provera
drugs for dysmenorrhea		Treat the pain associated with dysmenorrhea. These are nonsteroidal anti-inflammatory drugs (NSAIDs).	Motrin, Ponstel
drugs for endometriosis		Suppress the menstrual cycle for several months and cause endometrial implants in the pelvic cavity to atrophy.	Lupron, Zoladex
drugs for premature labor	**tocolytic** (TOH-koh-LIT-ik) **toc/o-** *labor and childbirth* **ly/o-** *break down, separate, dissolve* **-tic** *pertaining to*	Treat premature contractions by relaxing the smooth muscle of the uterine wall. Also known as **tocolytic drugs.**	ritodrine (Yutopar)
drugs for premenstrual syndrome (PMS)		Treat breast tenderness, fluid retention, and mild mood changes. These are over-the-counter drugs.	Midol, Pamprin
drugs for premenstrual dysphoric disorder (PMDD)		Treat the depression associated with this mood disorder. Other drugs are used to relieve the PMS-like physical symptoms.	Paxil, Sarafem, Zoloft
drugs for vaginal yeast infections		Topical drugs used to treat *Candida albicans* infection of the vagina.	Gyne-Lotrimin, Monistat
drugs used to dilate the cervix		Prostaglandin drug applied topically to the cervix to cause dilation and effacement. **Did You Know?** Laminaria is a drug made from dried sea kelp (seaweed). It is placed in the cervix and, as it absorbs moisture, it expands and gently dilates the cervix to induce labor.	Cervidil, Prepidil
drugs used to induce labor		Stimulate the uterus and increase the strength and frequency of contractions of the smooth muscle of the uterine wall.	oxytocin (Pitocin)

Category	Word Part and Definition	Description	Example
hormone replacement therapy (HRT) drugs	**estrogen** (ES-troh-jen) estr/o- *female* -gen *that which produces* Estrogen refers to estradiol produced by the ovary, estrone and estriol (metabolites of estradiol) or manufactured estradiol used in drugs. **progestin** (proh-JES-tin) pro- *before* gest/o- *from conception to birth* -in *a substance* Progestin refers to progesterone produced by the ovary or manufactured progesterone used in drugs.	Treat the symptoms of menopause (hot flashes, vaginal dryness) caused by decreased levels of estradiol. Some combination drugs contain estrogen, progestin, and testosterone. Long-term estrogen use has been associated with an increased risk of breast cancer, endometrial cancer, and thrombophlebitis.	Estraderm, Estratest, Premarin, Prempro, Vivelle
ovulation-stimulating drugs		Stimulate the anterior pituitary gland to release FSH and LH to cause ovulation. Used to treat infertility. These drugs cause several mature ova to be released at the same time for *in vitro* fertilization.	Clomid, Pergonal, Profasi

Did You Know?

On November 20, 1997, a mother in Iowa gave birth to the world's only surviving set of septuplets. The four boys and three girls were born prematurely at only 30 weeks' gestation. The mother was taking ovulation-stimulating drugs for infertility at the time.

Abbreviations

AB, Ab	abortion
AFP	alpha fetoprotein
AGA	appropriate for gestational age
ASC-H	atypical squamous cells, cannot exclude HSIL
ASC-US	atypical squamous cells of undetermined significance
BBT	basal body temperature
BPD	biparietal diameter (of fetal head)
BPP	biophysical profile
BRCA	breast cancer (gene)
BSE	breast self-examination
BSO	bilateral salpingo-oophorectomy
Bx	biopsy
Ca	cancer, carcinoma
CIN	cervical intraepithelial neoplasia (grading system on Pap smear)
CIS	carcinoma in situ
CNM	certified nurse midwife
CPD	cephalopelvic disproportion
CS	cesarean section ("C-section")
CVS	chorionic villus sampling
D&C	dilation and curettage
DUB	dysfunctional uterine bleeding
EDB	estimated date of birth
EDC	estimated date of confinement
EGA	estimated gestational age

(continued)

EMB	endometrial biopsy
FHR	fetal heart rate
FSH	follicle-stimulating hormone
G	gravida
GIFT	gamete intrafallopian transfer
G/TPAL	see *G* and *TPAL*
GYN	gynecology
HCG, hCG	human chorionic gonadotropin
HPV	human papillomavirus
HRT	hormone replacement therapy
HSG	hysterosalpingography
HSIL	high-grade squamous intraepithelial lesion
ICSI	intracytoplasmic sperm injection
IUGR	intrauterine growth retardation
IVF	*in vitro* fertilization
L&D	labor and delivery
LEEP	loop electrocautery excision procedure
LGA	large for gestational age
LH	luteinizing hormone
LMP	last menstrual period
L/S	lecithin/sphingomyelin (ratio)
LSIL	low-grade squamous intraepithelial lesion
NB	newborn
NICU	neonatal intensive care unit
NST	nonstress test
NSVD	normal spontaneous vaginal delivery
OB	obstetrics
OCP	oral contraceptive pill
P	para
Pap	Papanicolaou (smear or test)
PID	pelvic inflammatory disease
PMDD	premenstrual dysphoric disorder
PMS	premenstrual syndrome
PROM	premature rupture of membranes
ROM	rupture of membranes
SAB	spontaneous abortion
SCC	squamous cell carcinoma
SGA	small for gestational age
STD	sexually transmitted disease
TAB	therapeutic abortion
TAH-BSO	total abdominal hysterectomy and bilateral salpingo-oophorectomy
TPAL	term newborns, premature newborns, abortions, living children
TRAM	transverse rectus abdominis muscle (flap)
TVH	total vaginal hysterectomy
VBAC	vaginal birth after ceserean section ("V-back")
ZIFT	zygote intrafallopian transfer

Word Alert

ABBREVIATIONS

Abbreviations are commonly used in all types of medical documentation; however, they can mean different things to different people and their meaning can be misinterpreted. Always verify the meaning of an abbreviation.

AI stands for *artificial insemination,* but it can also stand for *apical impulse, aortic insufficiency,* and *artificial intelligence.*

Ca stands for *cancer,* but it can also stand for the mineral *calcium.*

D&C stands for *dilation and curettage,* but it can be confused with *D/C (discontinued* or *discharge).*

EDC stands for *estimated date of confinement,* but it can also stand for *extensor digitorum communis* (a muscle).

G stands for *gravida,* but it can also stand for *gauge (of a needle).*

P stands for *para,* but it can also stand for the mineral *phosphorus.*

ROM stands for *rupture of membranes,* but it can also stand for *range of motion.*

Career Focus

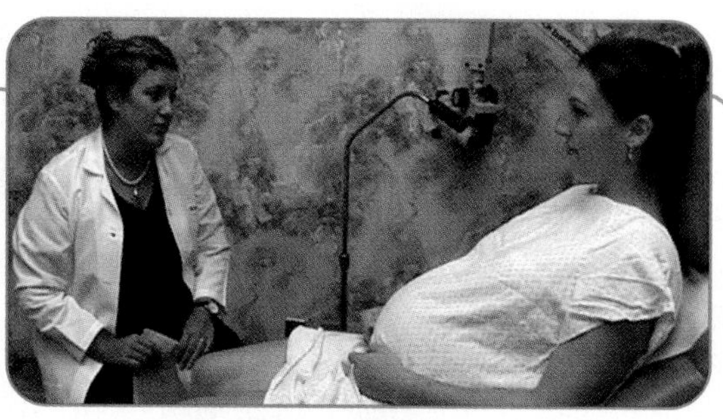

Meet Michele, a nurse midwife.

"I think the role of the nurse midwife differs from that of a physician in that you're more holistically focused on the whole person. You look at psychological factors, social factors. You provide more support and more education. I work in an outpatient setting, providing GYN services. I do labor and delivery in the hospital. I have many clients that I'm seeing for their second and third babies. So that's kind of nice to see growing families. It's a very rewarding career because you get to see new families blossoming."

Nurse midwives are allied health professionals who (with the supervision of a physician) manage a patient's prenatal care, delivery, and postpartum care. They are employed in hospitals, obstetrician offices, and birthing centers. They also manage home births.

Gynecologists are physicians who practice in the medical specialty of gynecology. They diagnose and treat patients with diseases of the female genital and reproductive system. Most gynecologists are also obstetricians who continue to care for their patients during pregnancy and childbirth. **Obstetricians** are physicians who practice in the medical specialty of obstetrics. Obstetricians deliver babies and perform cesarean sections. **Neonatologists** are physicians who practice in the medical specialty of neonatology. They diagnose and treat the fetus during pregnancy and labor; they diagnose and treat the newborn infant after birth. Most neonatologists work in the neonatal intensive care unit (NICU) in a hospital. **Pediatricians** are physicians who practice in the medical specialty of pediatrics. They diagnose and treat newborns, infants, children, and adolescents. Endocrinologists treat patients with disorders of the endocrine system, including hormonal disorders that affect menstruation. Cancerous tumors of the female and genital reproductive system are treated medically by an oncologist and surgically by a general surgeon.

nurse midwife (NURS MID-wyfe)
Midwife is an Old English word meaning *with the wife.* Originally, midwives were birth assistants who were trained at the bedside.

gynecologist (GY-neh-KAWL-oh-jist)
gynec/o- *female, woman*
log/o- *the study of*
-ist *one who specializes in*

obstetrician (AWB-steh-TRISH-an)
obstetr/o- *pregnancy and childbirth*
-ician *a skilled professional or expert*

neonatologist (NEE-oh-nay-TAWL-oh-jist)
ne/o- *new*
nat/o- *birth*
log/o- *the study of*
-ist *one who specializes in*

pediatrician (PEE-dee-ah-TRISH-an)
ped/o- *child*
iatr/o- *physician; medical treatment*
-ician *a skilled professional or expert*

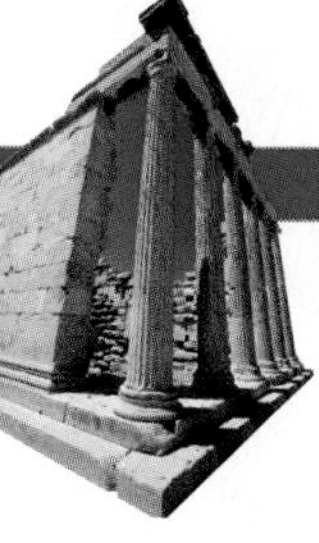

It's Greek to Me!

Did you notice that some gynecologic and obstetrical words have two different combining forms? Combining forms from both Greek and Latin languages remain a part of medical language today.

English Word	Greek	Latin	Examples of Medical Words
birth	par/o-	nat/o-	multiparous, prenatal
bear or carry	phor/o-	fer/o-	oophorectomy, lactiferous
egg	o/o-	ov/i-, ovul/o-	oocyte, oviduct, ovulation
female, woman	gynec/o-	estr/a-, estr/o-	gynecology, estradiol, estrogen
milk	galact/o-	lact/o-	galactorrhea, lactation
ovary	oophor/o-	ovari/o-	oophorectomy, ovarian
vagina	colp/o-	vagin/o-	colposcopy, vaginal
vulva	episi/o-	vulv/o-	episiotomy, vulvar
womb	hyster/o-	uter/o-	hysterectomy, uterine
	metri/o-, metr/o-		endometriosis, metrorrhagia

CHAPTER REVIEW EXERCISES

Review all the material in this chapter by completing the review exercises in this section. Use the Answer Key at the end of the book to check your answers.

Anatomy and Physiology

Matching Exercise

Match each numbered word or phrase to its description. Some may be used more than once.

1. breasts	_____ Gonads or female reproductive organs
2. uterus	_____ Parts of this organ are the fundus and the body
3. fallopian tubes	_____ Follicles in these glands rupture to release a mature ovum
4. ovaries	_____ Also known as the mammary glands
5. cervix	_____ Area between the lower edge of the vulva and the anus
6. vagina	_____ Has a lumen and a fimbriated end
7. vulva	_____ Has a muscular layer known as the myometrium
8. perineum	_____ Also known as the oviduct
	_____ Contains the fornix
	_____ The labia are located within this area
	_____ The fallopian tubes and these are collectively known as the adnexa
	_____ The hymen sometimes covers the inferior end of this structure
	_____ Contain the lactiferous glands
	_____ Contains an os
	_____ Normal position is anteflexion

Matching Exercise

Match each numbered word or phrase to its description.

1. amnion	_____ Fertilized ovum with 46 chromosomes
2. embryo	_____ Also known as conception
3. engagement	_____ Part of fetus that will go first through the birth canal
4. false labor	_____ Inner mass of cells that forms the amniotic cavity
5. fertilization	_____ A spermatozoon or an ovum with 23 chromosomes
6. fetus	_____ Source of nutrients and oxygen for the fetus
7. gamete	_____ Connects the placenta to the fetus
8. gestation	_____ Developmental stage before fetus
9. placenta	_____ After week 8, the embryo is known as this
10. presenting part	_____ Time from conception to birth
11. trimester	_____ Equals three months' time
12. umbilical cord	_____ Fetal head drops into position in mother's pelvis
13. zygote	_____ Also known as Braxton Hicks contractions

Matching Exercise

Match each numbered word or phrase to its description.

1. Apgar	_____ Newborn cries and breasts release milk
2. colostrum	_____ Widening of the diameter of the cervical os
3. crowning	_____ Release of amniotic fluid
4. dilation	_____ Time period after birth
5. effacement	_____ Thinning of the cervical wall
6. lactation	_____ Fetal scalp visible at vaginal introitus
7. let-down reflex	_____ Production of breast milk after childbirth
8. postpartum	_____ Quick scoring system to assess newborn well-being.
9. rupture of membranes	_____ First milk from the breast, contains maternal antibodies

Sequencing Exercise

Beginning with the fetal head moving into the mother's pelvis, write each event in the order in which it occurs. Use the list to help you sequence the events in their correct order.

Event	**Correct Order**
birth of the newborn	1. ______________
dilation and effacement	2. ______________
crowning	3. ______________
engagement	4. ______________
involution	5. ______________
epidural anesthesia	6. ______________
newborn becomes an infant	7. ______________
placenta delivered	8. ______________

True or False

Indicate whether each statement is true or false by writing T or F on the line.

1. ____ A newborn is also known as a neonate.
2. ____ The Bartholin's and Skene's glands secrete mucus during menstruation.
3. ____ The cervical canal is a continuation of the intrauterine cavity.
4. ____ The uterus is suspended within the pelvic cavity by the broad ligament.
5. ____ The funnel-like widening at the end of the fallopian tube is known as the infundibulum.
6. ____ FSH and LH are secreted by the ovary.
7. ____ The onset of menstruation is known as menarche.
8. ____ Ovulation occurs on the first day of the menstrual cycle.
9. ____ Human chorionic gonadotropin is secreted by the vagina.
10. ____ The prenatal period is the period of time before conception.
11. ____ A vertex presentation is the presence of lochia after delivery.
12. ____ Oxytocin causes the uterus to contract.
13. ____ Acrocyanosis is a bluish discoloration of a baby's head and extremities.

Medical Language Word Parts

Name that Word Part

Identify each of the word parts given here by writing the correct letter (P, C, or S) on the line beside it. Then write the definition of the word part on the blank line. The first one has been done for you.

Prefix = P **Combining Form = C** **Suffix = S**

		Word Part	Definition			Word Part	Definition
1.	-al	S	pertaining to	36.	-cele		
2.	a-			37.	-centesis		
3.	ablat/o-			38.	cephal/o-		
4.	abort/o-			39.	cervic/o-		
5.	acr/o-			40.	chem/o-		
6.	-ad			41.	chol/o-		
7.	aden/o-			42.	chorion/o-		
8.	adnex/o-			43.	chrom/o-		
9.	amni/o-			44.	colp/o-		
10.	-amnios			45.	concept/o-		
11.	an-			46.	con/o-		
12.	-an			47.	construct/o-		
13.	anastom/o-			48.	contra-		
14.	-ancy			49.	contract/o-		
15.	andr/o-			50.	cry/o-		
16.	-ant			51.	culd/o-		
17.	ante-			52.	cyan/o-		
18.	anti-			53.	cyst/o-		
19.	-ar			54.	-cyte		
20.	-arche			55.	cyt/o-		
21.	areol/o-			56.	depress/o-		
22.	-ary			57.	di-		
23.	aspir/o-			58.	dilat/o-		
24.	-ate			59.	dissect/o-		
25.	-ation			60.	dors/o-		
26.	-atory			61.	-duct		
27.	augment/o-			62.	dur/o-		
28.	bi-			63.	dys-		
29.	bilirubin/o-			64.	eclamps/o-		
30.	bi/o-			65.	ecto-		
31.	-body			66.	-ectomy		
32.	cancer/o-			67.	ectop/o-		
33.	candid/o-			68.	efface/o-		
34.	carcin/o-			69.	embol/o-		
35.	cav/o-			70.	embryon/o-		

		Word Part	Definition
71.	-emesis	______	______________
72.	-emia	______	______________
73.	-emic	______	______________
74.	endo-	______	______________
75.	epi-	______	______________
76.	epsi/o-	______	______________
77.	-ery	______	______________
78.	-esis	______	______________
79.	esthes/o-	______	______________
80.	estr/a-	______	______________
81.	estr/o-	______	______________
82.	excis/o-	______	______________
83.	extern/o-	______	______________
84.	fallopi/o-	______	______________
85.	fer/o-	______	______________
86.	fertil/o-	______	______________
87.	fet/o-	______	______________
88.	fibr/o-	______	______________
89.	flex/o-	______	______________
90.	-form	______	______________
91.	fratern/o-	______	______________
92.	fund/o-	______	______________
93.	galact/o-	______	______________
94.	-gen	______	______________
95.	gene/o-	______	______________
96.	genit/o-	______	______________
97.	gen/o-	______	______________
98.	gestat/o-	______	______________
99.	gest/o-	______	______________
100.	gonad/o-	______	______________
101.	gon/o-	______	______________
102.	-gram	______	______________
103.	-graphy	______	______________
104.	-gravida	______	______________
105.	gynec/o-	______	______________
106.	hem/o-	______	______________
107.	hydatidi/o-	______	______________
108.	hydr/o-	______	______________
109.	hyper-	______	______________
110.	hyster/o-	______	______________
111.	-ia	______	______________
112.	-iasis	______	______________

		Word Part	Definition
113.	iatr/o-	______	______________
114.	-ic	______	______________
115.	-ician	______	______________
116.	-ics	______	______________
117.	-in	______	______________
118.	incis/o-	______	______________
119.	induct/o-	______	______________
120.	-ine	______	______________
121.	inflammat/o-	______	______________
122.	infra-	______	______________
123.	inject/o-	______	______________
124.	insemin/o-	______	______________
125.	intern/o-	______	______________
126.	intra-	______	______________
127.	involut/o-	______	______________
128.	-ion	______	______________
129.	isch/o-	______	______________
130.	-ist	______	______________
131.	-itis	______	______________
132.	-ity	______	______________
133.	-ive	______	______________
134.	-ization	______	______________
135.	labi/o-	______	______________
136.	lact/i-	______	______________
137.	lact/o-	______	______________
138.	lapar/o-	______	______________
139.	later/o-	______	______________
140.	lei/o-	______	______________
141.	leuk/o-	______	______________
142.	ligat/o-	______	______________
143.	lith/o-	______	______________
144.	lob/o-	______	______________
145.	log/o-	______	______________
146.	-logy	______	______________
147.	ly/o-	______	______________
148.	mal-	______	______________
149.	malign/o-	______	______________
150.	mamm/a-	______	______________
151.	mamm/o-	______	______________
152.	manu/o-	______	______________
153.	mast/o-	______	______________
154.	melan/o-	______	______________

		Word Part	Definition			Word Part	Definition
155.	men/o-	______	________________	196.	perine/o-	______	________________
156.	menstru/o-	______	________________	197.	-pexy	______	________________
157.	-ment	______	________________	198.	phor/o-	______	________________
158.	metri/o-	______	________________	199.	phot/o-	______	________________
159.	metr/o-	______	________________	200.	phylact/o-	______	________________
160.	-metry	______	________________	201.	physic/o-	______	________________
161.	mult/i-	______	________________	202.	placent/o-	______	________________
162.	my/o-	______	________________	203.	plasm/o-	______	________________
163.	-nate	______	________________	204.	plas/o-	______	________________
164.	nat/o-	______	________________	205.	-plasty	______	________________
165.	ne/o-	______	________________	206.	-pnea	______	________________
166.	nuch/o-	______	________________	207.	pne/o-	______	________________
167.	null/i-	______	________________	208.	poly-	______	________________
168.	obstetr/o-	______	________________	209.	post-	______	________________
169.	-ol	______	________________	210.	pre-	______	________________
170.	olig/o-	______	________________	211.	pregn/o-	______	________________
171.	-oma	______	________________	212.	prim/i-	______	________________
172.	om/o-	______	________________	213.	pro-	______	________________
173.	o/o-	______	________________	214.	-probe	______	________________
174.	oophor/o-	______	________________	215.	product/o-	______	________________
175.	-opsy	______	________________	216.	pub/o-	______	________________
176.	-or	______	________________	217.	py/o-	______	________________
177.	-ory	______	________________	218.	radic/o-	______	________________
178.	-osis	______	________________	219.	re-	______	________________
179.	-ous	______	________________	220.	recept/o-	______	________________
180.	ovari/o-	______	________________	221.	rect/o-	______	________________
181.	ov/i-	______	________________	222.	reduct/o-	______	________________
182.	ovul/o-	______	________________	223.	retro-	______	________________
183.	ox/y-	______	________________	224.	-rrhage	______	________________
184.	pareun/o-	______	________________	225.	rrhag/o-	______	________________
185.	pariet/o-	______	________________	226.	-rrhaphy	______	________________
186.	par/o-	______	________________	227.	-rrhea	______	________________
187.	-partum	______	________________	228.	salping/o-	______	________________
188.	parturit/o-	______	________________	229.	-salpinx	______	________________
189.	-pause	______	________________	230.	sarc/o-	______	________________
180.	paus/o-	______	________________	231.	-scope	______	________________
191.	ped/o-	______	________________	232.	-scopy	______	________________
192.	pelv/i-	______	________________	233.	secret/o-	______	________________
193.	pelv/o-	______	________________	234.	-some	______	________________
194.	pendul/o-	______	________________	235.	son/o-	______	________________
195.	peri-	______	________________	236.	spir/o-	______	________________

		Word Part	Definition			Word Part	Definition
237.	-stalsis	______	______________	249.	trop/o-	______	______________
238.	stere/o-	______	______________	250.	tub/o-	______	______________
239.	surg/o-	______	______________	251.	-ule	______	______________
240.	suspens/o-	______	______________	252.	ultra-	______	______________
241.	tact/o-	______	______________	253.	umbilic/o-	______	______________
242.	therapeut/o-	______	______________	254.	urethr/o-	______	______________
243.	-therapy	______	______________	255.	uter/o-	______	______________
244.	-tic	______	______________	256.	vagin/o-	______	______________
245.	toc/o-	______	______________	257.	–verse	______	______________
246.	-tomy	______	______________	258.	vers/o-	______	______________
247.	tox/o-	______	______________	259.	vulv/o-	______	______________
248.	trans-	______	______________	260.	xer/o-	______	______________

Symptoms, Signs, and Diseases

Matching Exercise

Match each numbered word or phrase to its description.

1.	breasts	____ System to describe stages of breast development
2.	nipples	____ Gynecologic exam that uses both hands
3.	dorsal lithotomy	____ Can be pendulous
4.	breast skin	____ Instrument that pushes apart the vaginal walls
5.	Tanner stage	____ Axillary ones are enlarged from breast cancer
6.	lymph nodes	____ Standard gynecologic examination position
7.	uterus	____ Can be inverted or retracted
8.	vaginal speculum	____ Peau d' orange dimpling associated with cancer
9.	bimanual	____ When prolapsed, its cervix can be seen at the vaginal introitus

Circle Exercise

Circle the correct word from the choices given.

1. Galactorrhea is a disease that affects the (**breasts, perineum, vagina**).
2. (**Amenorrhea, Dysmenorrhea, Menometrorrhagia**) is the complete absence of monthly menstrual periods.
3. (**Cervical, Endometrial, Ovarian**) cancer is the most difficult to detect and is often widespread before symptoms become severe.
4. Dyspareunia and dysmenorrhea are symptoms of (**endometriosis, menopause, pregnancy**).
5. A yeast infection in the vagina is known as (**anovulation, candidiasis, hydrosalpinx**).
6. (**Menometrorrhagia, Metrorrhagia, Myometritis**) is an inflammation or infection in the muscular wall of the uterus.
7. An ectopic pregnancy can result in (**eclampsia, hemosalpinx, involution**).
8. Mastitis is a postpartum inflammation of the (**breast, perineum, uterus**).
9. (**Gestational diabetes mellitus, Prolapsed cord, Salpingitis**) cuts off the supply of oxygen to the fetus.
10. Yellowish discoloration of the skin in the neonate is known as (**acrocyanosis, apnea, jaundice**).
11. Pain during sexual intercourse is known as (**abortion, dyspareunia, eclampsia**).

Matching Exercise

Match each numbered word or phrase to its description.

1.	candidiasis	_____	Yeast infection of the vagina
2.	endometriosis	_____	Discharge of milk from the breast without pregnancy
3.	galactorrhea	_____	Climacteric
4.	leiomyomata	_____	Prolapse of the uterus
5.	menopause	_____	Many smooth muscle tumors of the uterus
6.	oligomenorrhea	_____	Pus in the fallopian tube
7.	pyosalpinx	_____	Scanty menstrual flow
8.	uterine descensus	_____	"Chocolate cysts" in the ovary

Word-Building Exercise

Use the combining forms, prefixes, and suffixes given here to build medical words that match the definitions given. Write the word that you build on the blank line. Some word parts may be used more than once. The first one has been done for you.

Word Parts

a- (away from, without)
-al (pertaining to)
an- (without, not)
-ation (a process; being or having)
-cele (hernia)
cyst/o- (bladder; fluid-filled sac; semisolid cyst)
dys- (painful, difficult, abnormal)
ectop/o- (outside of a place)
fibr/o- (fiber)
flex/o- (bending)
-ia (condition, state, thing)
-ic (pertaining to)
-ion (action; condition)
-itis (inflammation of)
lei/o- (smooth)
leuk/o- (white)
men/o- (month)
my/o- (muscle)
-oma (tumor, mass)
ovul/o- (ovum, egg)
paus/o- (cessation)
peri- (around)
plas/o- (growth, formation)
poly- (many, much)
pre- (before; in front of)
retro- (behind, backward)
-rrhea (flow, discharge)
vagin/o- (vagina)

1. Painful menstruation (*dys- + men/o- + -rrhea*) *dysmenorrhea*
2. Pertaining to symptoms that occur around the onset of menopause ______________________
3. Pertaining to having many cysts in the ovary ______________________
4. Having (the ovaries) not release an ovum ______________________
5. Tumor of the smooth muscle (of the wall of the uterus) ______________________
6. Condition (of the uterus) in which it is bent backwards ______________________
7. White discharge (from the vagina) ______________________
8. Hernia of the bladder (into the vagina) ______________________
9. Tumor of fibrous cyst (in the breast) ______________________
10. Without the flow of menstruation ______________________
11. Condition of abnormal growth or formation (of cells) ______________________
12. Inflammation of the vagina ______________________
13. Pertaining to (a pregnancy) that is outside of its normal place ______________________

Laboratory, Radiology, Surgery, and Drugs

True or False

Indicate whether each statement is true or false by writing T or F on the line.

1. ____ The presence of the BRCA1 gene greatly increases the risk of developing fibrocystic disease of the breast.
2. ____ A fine-needle aspiration biopsy uses a small needle to inject drugs into a cancerous tumor.
3. ____ Dysplasia is an abnormality of the cell that always means it is malignant.
4. ____ The estrogen receptor assay predicts whether estrogen-blocking drugs will be successful in treating a patient's breast cancer.
5. ____ Bacterial or viral infections of the vagina can cause abnormal Pap smear results.
6. ____ A cold knife conization is a type of cryosurgery.
7. ____ A lumpectomy is a more extensive procedure than a mastectomy.
8. ____ A hysteropexy is also known as a uterine suspension.
9. ____ Hormone replacement therapy treats the vaginal dryness and hot flashes associated with menopause.
10. ____ Hysterosalpingography can show blockage in the fallopian tubes.

Matching Exercise

Match each numbered word or phrase to its description.

1. incisional biopsy	_____ Used to hold the cervix in a fixed position during an examination
2. colposcope	_____ Low-power microscope used to examine the cervix
3. Pap smear	_____ X-ray image of the breast
4. cryoprobe	_____ Only part of the tumor is excised
5. mammogram	_____ Instrument used to freeze cervical lesions
6. ultrasound	_____ Ring instrument with a sharp edge for scraping
7. curet	_____ Uses sound waves to produce an image
8. tenaculum	_____ Drug used to stop premature labor
9. laparoscope	_____ Exfoliative cytology
10. tocolytic	_____ Fiberoptic endoscope

Multiple Choice

Circle the choice that best answers the question.

1. Surgical procedure used to suture a weakness in the vaginal wall.
   a. cystocele c. conization
   b. cryosurgery d. colporrhaphy
2. A hysterectomy can be performed ________________________.
   a. through the vagina c. laparoscopically
   b. through the abdominal wall d. all of the above.
3. A breast lift is another name for a/an ________________________.
   a. augmentation mammoplasty c. reduction mammoplasty
   b. mastopexy d. mastectomy
4. Drugs used to treat dysmenorrhea include ________________________.
   a. NSAID drugs c. antiviral drugs
   b. antibiotic drugs d. HRT

Abbreviations

Matching Exercise

Match each abbreviation to its definition.

1.	ASC-US	_____ Due date
2.	BSE	_____ Untreated, this can cause adhesions, scarring, and infertility
3.	Bx	_____ Uses a loop with electrical current running through it to cut away tissue
4.	CIS	_____ Uterus and bilateral fallopian tubes and ovaries are surgically removed
5.	EDC	_____ Includes physical symptoms of PMS plus mood disorder
6.	FSH	_____ Surgical flap to reconstruct breast after mastectomy
7.	HRT	_____ Abbreviation for biopsy
8.	LEEP	_____ Drug therapy to treat the symptoms of menopause
9.	OCP	_____ Drug to prevent pregnancy
10.	PID	_____ Cancer still confined to one location
11.	PMDD	_____ Hormone that makes the follicles produce a mature ovum
12.	TAH-BSO	_____ Abnormal Pap smear finding
13.	TRAM	_____ Having a vaginal birth after a prior cesarean section
14.	VBAC	_____ Important way to detect breast cancer

Applied Skills

Plural Noun and Adjective Spelling

Fill in the blanks with the correct word form. Be sure to check your spelling. The first one has been done for you.

	Singular Noun	Plural Noun	Adjective
1.	areola	*areolae*	*areolar*
2.	amnion		______
3.	breast	______	______
4.	cervix		______
5.	fetus	______	______
6.	fundus		______
7.	gonad	______	______
8.	ovary	______	______
9.	ovum	______	
10.	perineum		______
11.	placenta		______
12.	umbilicus		______
13.	uterus		______
14.	vagina		______

English and Medical Word Equivalents

For each English word, write its equivalent medical word.

	English Word	Medical Word
1.	breasts	______
2.	afterbirth	______
3.	baby	______
4.	bag of waters	______
5.	false labor	
6.	getting your tubes tied	______
7.	soft spot	______
8.	womb	______
9.	morning sickness	______

Analysis of a Medical Report

This exercise contains a History and Physical Examination done in the neonatal intensive care unit. Read the report and answer the questions.

HISTORY AND PHYSICAL EXAMINATION

PATIENT:	KAISER, Baby Boy
MEDICAL RECORD NUMBER:	03-7843
DATE OF BIRTH:	November 19, 20xx
DATE OF ADMISSION TO NICU:	November 19, 20xx

HISTORY
This is a 3360 g, full-term white male infant, who was transferred from the delivery room to the NICU after birth because of respiratory distress. The infant was born to a 34-year-old mother with an EDB of 11/22/xx, and he had an EGA of 40 weeks.

MATERNAL HISTORY
The mother was G2, TPAL 0-0-1-0 with a SAB 2 years ago. The mother had prenatal care beginning in the first trimester of this pregnancy. She took prenatal vitamins. She denied the use of alcohol, smoking, or drugs. A sonogram on 10/10/xx showed a single fetus in breech presentation at 35 weeks' gestation.

LABOR AND DELIVERY HISTORY
The membranes ruptured spontaneously 14 hours prior to the onset of labor. The mother had a temperature of 103.2 degrees prior to delivery and was started on an antibiotic drug. A version of the breech was performed. Labor was induced and lasted 8 hours.

The baby was born via normal spontaneous vaginal delivery. Apgars were 8 and 8 at 1 and 5 minutes respectively. There was no evidence of meconium aspiration on visualization of the vocal cords. The infant was tachypneic despite suctioning and the administration of blow-by oxygen and was brought to the neonatal intensive care unit.

PHYSICAL EXAMINATION
Heart rate 200 beats/minute, respiratory rate 70/minute, temperature 101.2, weight 3360 g, length 54 cm, head circumference 33.5 cm. General: Full-term, AGA male. Alert, active, responsive. Head: Molding present. Fontanels soft. Palate intact. Eyes: Pupils equal and reactive to light. Chest symmetrical. Now pink in room air with only mild tachypnea and mild sternal retractions. Breath sounds equal bilaterally. Clavicles intact. Abdomen: Bowel sounds present. No hepatosplenomegaly. There is a 3-vessel umbilical cord. Genitalia normal. Anus patent. Neurologic: Strong cry, strong suck, normal muscle tone.

IMPRESSION
Term male infant, estimated gestational age of 38.5 weeks, appropriate for gestational age. Rule out pneumonia.

PLAN
Admit to the neonatal intensive care unit. Vital signs q.1h. until stable.
Cardiorespiratory monitor. Intravenous fluids of dextrose 10% in water at 80 cc/kg/day.
Hold oral feedings for now. Vitamin K 1 mg IM. Chest x-ray to rule out pneumonia.

Bonita C. Grant, M.D.

Bonita C. Grant, M.D.

BCG: cgm
D: 11/19/xx
T: 11/19/xx

WORD ANALYSIS QUESTIONS

1. Give the definitions of these abbreviations.
   a. AGA ______________________________
   b. EDB ______________________________
   c. EGA ______________________________
   d. NICU ______________________________
   e. SAB ______________________________
2. A sonogram showed the fetus at 35 weeks' gestation. If you wanted to use the adjective form of *gestation,* you would say, "The fetus had a ______________ age of 35 weeks."
3. Divide *gestational* into its three word parts and define each word part.

Word Part	**Definition**
______	______________
______	______________
______	______________

4. Divide *amniotic* into its two word parts and define each word part.

Word Part	**Definition**
______	______________
______	______________

5. Divide *prenatal* into its three word parts and define each word part.

Word Part	**Definition**
______	______________
______	______________
______	______________

6. What is the abbreviation for the medical phrase *normal spontaneous vaginal delivery*? ______________

FACT FINDING QUESTIONS

1. The sonogram (ultrasound) done on 10/10/xx showed what fetal presentation? ______________
2. What procedure was performed to correct this presentation? Circle the correct answer.

   Apgar **repeat sonogram** **version** **vaginal delivery**
3. What does the mother's TPAL score of 0-0-1-0 mean? ______________
4. What abnormality of the head was noted on the physical examination? ______________
5. The newborn's estimated gestational age was 38.5 weeks. Is this a term newborn? **Yes** **No**
6. Where are the fontanels located? ______________

CRITICAL THINKING QUESTIONS

1. Circle the route by which vitamin K was given to the newborn.

   orally **topically in the eyes** **intramuscularly**
2. Rupture of the membranes many hours prior to delivery can cause infection in the newborn. What information is given in the record that tells you that the newborn did develop an infection? ______________
3. Circle the correct answer. Meconium-stained amniotic fluid means that the newborn experienced (**apnea, fetal distress, premature birth**).

Pronunciation Checklist

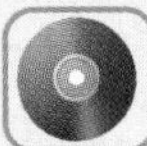

Read each word and its pronunciation. Practice pronouncing each word. Verify your pronunciation by listening to the Pronunciation List on the CD-ROM. Check the box next to the word after you master its pronunciation.

- ❑ abortion (ah-BOR-shun)
- ❑ abruptio placentae (ab-RUP-shee-oh plah-SEN-tee)
- ❑ acrocyanosis (AK-roh-SY-ah-NOH-sis)
- ❑ adenocarcinoma (AD-eh-noh-KAR-sih-NOH-mah)
- ❑ adnexa (ad-NEK-sah)
- ❑ adnexal (ad-NEK-sal)
- ❑ alpha fetoprotein (AL-fah FEE-toh-PROH-teen)
- ❑ amenorrhea (AH-meh-noh-REE-ah)
- ❑ amniocentesis (AM-nee-oh-sen-TEE-sis)
- ❑ amnion (AM-nee-on)
- ❑ amniotic fluid (AM-nee-AWT-ik FLOO-id)
- ❑ amniotomy (AM-nee-AWT-oh-mee)
- ❑ androgen (AN-droh-jen)
- ❑ anovulation (AN-awv-yoo-LAY-shun)
- ❑ anteflexion (AN-tee-FLEK-shun)
- ❑ antepartum (AN-tee-PAR-tum)
- ❑ antibiotic drug (AN-tee-by-AWT-ik DRUHG) (AN-tih-by-AWT-ik)
- ❑ antibody (AN-tee-BAWD-ee) (AN-tih-BAWD-ee)
- ❑ apnea (AP-nee-ah)
- ❑ apneic (AP-nee-ik)
- ❑ areola (ah-REE-oh-lah)
- ❑ areolae (ah-REE-oh-lee)
- ❑ areolar (ah-REE-oh-lar)
- ❑ aspiration (AS-pih-RAY-shun)
- ❑ assay (AS-say)
- ❑ augmentation mammaplasty (AWG-men-TAY-shun MAM-ah-plas-tee)
- ❑ Bartholin's glands (BAR-thoh-linz GLANZ)
- ❑ bilateral (by-LAT-er-al)
- ❑ bimanual examination (by-MAN-yoo-al eg-ZAM-ih-NAY-shun)
- ❑ biophysical profile (BY-oh-FIZ-ih-kal PRO-file)
- ❑ biopsy (BY-awp-see)
- ❑ biparietal diameter (BY-pah-RY-eh-tal dy-AM-eh-ter)
- ❑ Braxton Hicks contraction (BRAK-ston HIKS con-TRAK-shun)
- ❑ breast (BREST)
- ❑ breech (BREECH)
- ❑ cancerous (KAN-ser-us)
- ❑ candidiasis (KAN-dih-DY-ah-sis)
- ❑ carcinoma (KAR-sih-NOH-mah)
- ❑ carcinoma in situ (KAR-sih-NOH-mah IN SY-too)
- ❑ cephalic presentation (seh-FAL-ik PREE-sen-TAY-shun)
- ❑ cephalopelvic disproportion (SEF-ah-loh-PEL-vik DIS-proh-POR-shun)
- ❑ cerclage (sir-CLAWJ)
- ❑ cervical (SER-vih-kal)
- ❑ cervical canal (SER-vih-kal kah-NAL)
- ❑ cervical os (SER-vih-kal AWS)
- ❑ cervix (SER-viks)
- ❑ cesarean section (seh-ZAY-ree-an SEK-shun)
- ❑ chemotherapy drug (KEE-moh-THAIR-ah-pee DRUHG)
- ❑ chorion (KOH-ree-on)
- ❑ chorionic (KOH-ree-ON-ik)
- ❑ chorionic villus sampling (KOH-ree-ON-ik VIL-us SAM-pling)
- ❑ chromosome (KROH-moh-sohm)
- ❑ cilia (SIL-ee-ah)
- ❑ climacteric (kly-MAK-ter-ik)
- ❑ clitoris (KLIT-oh-ris)
- ❑ colostrum (koh-LAWS-trum)
- ❑ colporrhaphy (kol-POR-ah-fee)
- ❑ conception (con-SEP-shun)
- ❑ congenital (con-JEN-ih-tal)
- ❑ conization (KOH-nih-ZAY-shun)
- ❑ contraception (CON-trah-SEP-shun)
- ❑ corpus (KOR-pus)
- ❑ corpus luteum (KOR-pus LOO-tee-um)
- ❑ crowning (KROWN-ing)
- ❑ cryoprobe (KRY-oh-prohb)
- ❑ cryosurgery (KRY-oh-SER-jer-ee)
- ❑ culdoscopy (kul-DAWS-koh-pee)
- ❑ curettage (kyoo-reh-TAHZH)
- ❑ curet (kyoo-RET)
- ❑ cystocele (SIS-toh-seel)
- ❑ cytology (sy-TAWL-oh-jee)
- ❑ descensus (dee-SEN-sus)
- ❑ dilation (dy-LAY-shun)
- ❑ dissection (dih-SEK-shun)
- ❑ dorsal lithotomy (DOR-sal lih-THAWT-oh-mee)
- ❑ dysfunctional uterine bleeding (dis-FUNK-shun-al YOO-ter-in BLEED-ing)
- ❑ dysmenorrhea (DIS-men-oh-REE-ah)
- ❑ dyspareunia (DIS-pah-ROO-nee-ah)
- ❑ dysplasia (dis-PLAY-zee-ah)
- ❑ dysplastic (dis-PLAS-tik)
- ❑ dystocia (dis-TOH-see-ah)
- ❑ eclampsia (ee-KLAMP-see-ah)
- ❑ ectocervical (EK-toh-SER-vih-kal)
- ❑ ectopic pregnancy (ek-TOP-ik PREG-nan-see)
- ❑ effacement (eh-FAYS-ment)
- ❑ embolization (EM-bol-ih-ZAY-shun)
- ❑ embryo (EM-bree-oh)
- ❑ embryonic (EM-bree-ON-ik)
- ❑ endocervical (EN-doh-SER-vih-kal)
- ❑ endometrial (EN-doh-MEE-tree-al)
- ❑ endometrial ablation (EN-doh-MEE-tree-al ab-LAY-shun)
- ❑ endometriosis (EN-doh-MEE-tree-OH-sis)
- ❑ endometrium (EN-doh-MEE-tree-um)
- ❑ endoscope (EN-doh-skohp)
- ❑ epidural anesthesia (EP-ih-DYOO-ral AN-es-THEE-zee-ah)
- ❑ episiotomy (eh-PIS-ee-AWT-oh-mee)
- ❑ estradiol (ES-trah-DY-awl)
- ❑ excisional biopsy (ek-SIZH-un-al BY-awp-see)
- ❑ exfoliative cytology (eks-FOH-lee-ah-tiv sy-TAWL-oh-jee)
- ❑ fallopian tube (fah-LOH-pee-an TOOB)
- ❑ fertilization (FER-til-ih-ZAY-shun)
- ❑ fetal (FEE-tal)
- ❑ fetus (FEE-tus)
- ❑ fibrocystic disease (FY-broh-SIS-tik dih-ZEEZ)
- ❑ fimbriae (FIM-bree-ee)
- ❑ follicle (FAWL-ih-kl)
- ❑ follicle-stimulating hormone (FAWL-ih-kl STIM-yoo-lay-ting HOR-mohn)
- ❑ fontanel (FAWN-tah-NEL)
- ❑ fornix (FOR-niks)
- ❑ fraternal twins (frah-TER-nal TWINZ)
- ❑ fundal (FUN-dal)
- ❑ fundus (FUN-dus)
- ❑ galactorrhea (gah-LAK-toh-REE-ah)
- ❑ gamete (GAM-eet)
- ❑ gene (JEEN)
- ❑ genetic (jeh-NET-ik)
- ❑ genital (JEN-ih-tal)
- ❑ genitalia (JEN-ih-TAY-lee-ah)

- ❑ gestation (jes-TAY-shun)
- ❑ gestational diabetes mellitus (jes-TAY-shun-al DY-ah-BEE-teez MEL-ih-tus)
- ❑ gonad (GOH-nad)
- ❑ gonadotropin (GOH-nah-doh-TROH-pin)
- ❑ gravida (GRAV-ih-dah)
- ❑ gynecologic (GY-neh-koh-LAW-jik)
- ❑ gynecologist (GY-neh-KAWL-oh-jist)
- ❑ gynecology (GY-neh-KAWL-oh-jee)
- ❑ hemosalpinx (HEE-moh-SAL-pinks)
- ❑ human papillomavirus (HYOO-man PAP-ih-LOH-mah-VY-rus)
- ❑ hydatidiform mole (HY-dah-TID-ih-form MOHL)
- ❑ hydrosalpinx (HY-droh-SAL-pinx)
- ❑ hymen (HY-men)
- ❑ hyperbilirubinemia (HY-per-BIL-ih-ROO-bih-NEE-mee-ah)
- ❑ hyperemesis gravidarum (HY-per-EM-eh-sis GRAV-ih-DAIR-um)
- ❑ hysterectomy (HIS-ter-EK-toh-mee)
- ❑ hysteropexy (HIS-ter-oh-pek-see)
- ❑ hysterosalpingogram (HIS-ter-oh-sal-PING-goh-gram)
- ❑ hysterosalpingography (HIS-ter-oh-SAL-ping-GAWG-rah-fee)
- ❑ incisional biopsy (in-SIZH-un-al BY-awp-see)
- ❑ incompetent cervix (in-COM-peh-tent SER-viks)
- ❑ induction (in-DUK-shun)
- ❑ inframammary (IN-frah-MAM-ah-ree)
- ❑ infundibulum (IN-fun-DIB-yoo-lum)
- ❑ insemination (in-SEM-ih-NAY-shun)
- ❑ intracytoplasmic sperm injection (IN-trah-SY-toh-PLAS-mik SPERM in-JEK-shun)
- ❑ intrafallopian transfer (IN-trah-fah-LOH-pee-an TRANS-fer)
- ❑ intrauterine cavity (IN-trah-YOO-ter-in) (IN-trah-YOO-ter-ine) (KAV-ih-tee)
- ❑ introitus (in-TROH-ih-tus)
- ❑ *in vitro* fertilization (IN VEE-troh FER-til-ih-ZAY-shun)
- ❑ involution (IN-voh-LOO-shun)
- ❑ involutional melancholy (IN-voh-LOO-shun-al MEL-an-KOH-lee-ah)
- ❑ ischemic phase (is-KEE-mik FAYZ)
- ❑ jaundice (JAWN-dis)
- ❑ labial (LAY-bee-al)
- ❑ labia majora (LAY-bee-ah mah-JOR-ah)
- ❑ labia minora (LAY-bee-ah my-NOR-ah)
- ❑ lactation (lak-TAY-shun)
- ❑ lactiferous duct (lak-TIF-er-us DUHKT)
- ❑ lactiferous lobule (lak-TIF-er-us LAWB-yool)
- ❑ laparoscope (LAP-ah-roh-skohp)
- ❑ laparoscopy (LAP-ah-RAWS-koh-pee)
- ❑ lecithin (LES-ih-thin)
- ❑ leiomyoma (LIE-oh-my-OH-mah)
- ❑ leiomyomata (LIE-oh-my-OH-mah-tah)
- ❑ leiomyosarcoma (LIE-oh-MY-oh-sar-KOH-mah)
- ❑ leukorrhea (LOO-koh-REE-ah)
- ❑ ligament (LIG-ah-ment)
- ❑ lochia (LOH-kee-ah)
- ❑ lumen (LOO-men)
- ❑ lumpectomy (lum-PEK-toh-mee)
- ❑ luteinizing hormone (LOO-tee-ih-ny-zing HOR-mohn)
- ❑ malignancy (mah-LIG-nan-see)
- ❑ malpresentation (MAL-pree-sen-TAY-shun)
- ❑ mammaplasty (MAM-ah-plas-tee)
- ❑ mammary glands (MAM-ah-ree GLANZ)
- ❑ mammogram (MAM-oh-gram)
- ❑ mammography (mah-MAWG-rah-fee)
- ❑ mammoplasty (MAM-oh-plas-tee)
- ❑ mastectomy (mas-TEK-toh-mee)
- ❑ mastitis (mas-TY-tis)
- ❑ mastopexy (MAS-toh-pek-see)
- ❑ meconium (meh-KOH-nee-um)
- ❑ meconium aspiration (meh-KOH-nee-um AS-pih-RAY-shun)
- ❑ meiosis (my-OH-sis)
- ❑ menarche (meh-NAR-kee)
- ❑ menometrorrhagia (MEN-oh-MEE-troh-RAY-jee-ah)
- ❑ menopausal (MEN-oh-PAW-zal)
- ❑ menopause (MEN-oh-pawz)
- ❑ menorrhagia (MEN-oh-RAY-jee-ah)
- ❑ menses (MEN-seez)
- ❑ menstrual (MEN-stroo-al)
- ❑ menstruate (MEN-stroo-ate)
- ❑ menstruation (MEN-stroo-AA-shun)
- ❑ metrorrhagia (MEE-troh-RAY-jee-ah)
- ❑ mitosis (my-TOH-sis)
- ❑ mons pubis (MAWNZ PYOO-bis)
- ❑ multigravida (MUL-tih-GRAV-ih-dah)
- ❑ multiparous (mul-TIP-ah-rus)
- ❑ myomectomy (MY-oh-MEK-toh-mee)
- ❑ myometrial (MY-oh-MEE-tree-al)
- ❑ myometritis (MY-oh-mee-TRY-tis)
- ❑ myometrium (MY-oh-MEE-tree-um)
- ❑ Nägele's rule (NAY-gelz ROOL)
- ❑ neonatal (NEE-oh-NAY-tal)
- ❑ neonate (NEE-oh-nayt)
- ❑ neonatologist (NEE-oh-nay-TAWL-oh-jist)
- ❑ neonatology (NEE-oh-nay-TAWL-oh-jee)
- ❑ nipple (NIP-l)
- ❑ nuchal cord (NOO-kal CORD)
- ❑ nulligravida (NUL-ih-GRAV-ih-dah)
- ❑ nurse midwife (NURS MID-wyfe)
- ❑ obstetrician (AWB-steh-TRISH-an)
- ❑ obstetrics (awb-STET-riks)
- ❑ oligohydramnios (OL-ih-goh-hy-DRAM-nee-ohs)
- ❑ oligomenorrhea (OL-ih-goh-MEN-oh-REE-ah)
- ❑ oocyte (OH-oh-site)
- ❑ oogenesis (oh-oh-JEN-eh-sis)
- ❑ oophorectomy (OH-of-or-EK-toh-mee)
- ❑ ova (OH-vah)
- ❑ ovarian (oh-VAIR-ee-an)
- ❑ ovary (OH-vah-ree)
- ❑ oviduct (OH-vih-dukt)
- ❑ ovulation (AWV-yoo-LAY-shun)
- ❑ ovum (OH-vum)
- ❑ oxytocin (AWK-see-TOH-sin)
- ❑ para (PAIR-ah)
- ❑ parturition (PAR-tyoo-RIH-shun)
- ❑ peau d' orange (poh-deh-RAHNJ)
- ❑ pediatrician (PEE-dee-ah-TRISH-an)
- ❑ pediatrics (PEE-dee-AT-riks)
- ❑ pelvic cavity (PEL-vik KAV-ih-tee)
- ❑ pelvic inflammatory disease (PEL-vik in-FLAM-ah-tor-ee dih-ZEEZ)
- ❑ pelvimetry (pel-VIM-ih-tree)
- ❑ pendulous breast (PEN-dyoo-lus BREST)
- ❑ perimenopausal (PAIR-ee-MEN-oh-PAW-zal)
- ❑ perineal (PAIR-ih-NEE-al)
- ❑ perineum (PAIR-ih-NEE-um)
- ❑ peristalsis (PAIR-ih-STAL-sis)
- ❑ phototherapy (FOH-toh-THAIR-ah-pee)
- ❑ pica (PY-kah) (PEE-kah)
- ❑ placenta (plah-SEN-tah)
- ❑ placenta previa (plah-SEN-tah PREE-vee-ah)
- ❑ placental (plah-SEN-tal)
- ❑ polycystic disease (PAWL-ee-SIS-tik dih-ZEEZ)
- ❑ polyhydramnios (PAWL-ee-hy-DRAM-nee-ohs)
- ❑ postnatal (post-NAY-tal)
- ❑ postpartum (post-PAR-tum)
- ❑ postpartum depression (post-PAR-tum dee-PRESH-un)
- ❑ postpartum hemorrhage (post-PAR-tum HEM-oh-rij)

- ❑ preeclampsia (PREE-ee-KLAMP-see-ah)
- ❑ pregnant (PREG-nant)
- ❑ premenstrual dysphoric disorder (pree-MEN-stroo-al dis-FOR-ik dis-OR-der)
- ❑ premenstrual syndrome (pree-MEN-stroo-al SIN-drohm)
- ❑ prenatal (pree-NAY-tal)
- ❑ primigravida (PRY-mih-GRAV-ih-dah)
- ❑ progesterone (proh-JES-ter-ohn)
- ❑ prolapse (PROH-laps)
- ❑ proliferative phase (proh-LIF-er-ah-tiv FAYZ)
- ❑ prophylactic (PROH-fih-LAK-tik)
- ❑ prostaglandin (PRAWS-tah-GLAN-din)
- ❑ prosthesis (praws-THEE-sis)
- ❑ pubic (PYOO-bik)
- ❑ pyometritis (PY-oh-mee-TRY-tis)
- ❑ pyosalpinx (PY-oh-SAL-pinks)
- ❑ radical mastectomy (RAD-ih-kal mas-TEK-toh-mee)
- ❑ receptor (ree-SEP-tor)
- ❑ reconstructive breast surgery (REE-con-STRUK-tiv BREST SER-jer-ee)
- ❑ reduction mammaplasty (ree-DUK-shun MAM-ah-plas-tee)
- ❑ reproductive system (REE-proh-DUK-tiv SIS-tem)
- ❑ retroflexion (RET-roh-FLEK-shun)
- ❑ retroversion (RET-roh-VER-shun)
- ❑ salpingectomy (SAL-pin-JEK-toh-mee)
- ❑ salpingitis (SAL-pin-JY-tis)
- ❑ salpingo-oophorectomy (sal-PING-goh-OH-of-or-EK-toh-mee)
- ❑ secretory phase (SEE-kreh-toh-ree FAYZ)
- ❑ Skene's glands (SKEENZ GLANZ)
- ❑ sonogram (SAWN-oh-gram)
- ❑ speculum (SPEK-yoo-lum)
- ❑ sphingomyelin (SFING-goh-MY-eh-lin)
- ❑ stereotactic biopsy (STAIR-ee-oh-TAK-tik BY-awp-see)
- ❑ surfactant (ser-FAK-tant)
- ❑ tampon (TAM-pawn)
- ❑ tenaculum (teh-NAK-yoo-lum)
- ❑ therapeutic abortion (THAIR-ah-PYOO-tik ah-BOR-shun)
- ❑ tocolytic drug (TOH-koh-LIT-ik DRUHG)
- ❑ transvaginal ultrasound (trans-VAJ-ih-nal UL-trah-sound)
- ❑ transverse rectus abdominis muscle (trans-VERS REK-tus ab-DAWM-ih-nis MUS-el)
- ❑ trimester (TRY-mes-ter) (try-MES-ter)
- ❑ tubal anastomosis (TOO-bal ah-NAS-toh-MOH-sis)
- ❑ tubal ligation (TOO-bal ly-GAY-shun)
- ❑ tubal pregnancy (TOO-bal PREG-nan-see)
- ❑ ultrasonography (UL-trah-soh-NAWG-rah-fee)
- ❑ ultrasound (UL-trah-sound)
- ❑ umbilical (um-BIL-ih-kal)
- ❑ umbilicus (um-BIL-ih-kus) (UM-bih-LIE-kus)
- ❑ urethral glands (yoo-REE-thral GLANZ)
- ❑ uterine (YOO-ter-in) (YOO-ter-ine)
- ❑ uterine inertia (YOO-ter-in) (YOO-ter-ine) (in-ER-shee-ah)
- ❑ uterine suspension (YOO-ter-in) (YOO-ter-ine sus-PEN-shun)
- ❑ uterus (YOO-ter-us)
- ❑ vagina (vah-JY-nah)
- ❑ vaginal (VAJ-ih-nal)
- ❑ vaginitis (VAJ-ih-NY-tis)
- ❑ vaginosis (VAJ-ih-NOH-sis)
- ❑ vernix caseosa (VER-niks KAY-see-OH-sah)
- ❑ version (VER-zhun)
- ❑ vertex presentation (VER-teks PREE-sen-TAY-shun)
- ❑ vulva (VUL-vah)
- ❑ vulvar (VUL-var)
- ❑ xeromammogram (ZEER-oh-MAM-oh-gram)
- ❑ xeromammography (ZEER-oh-mah-MAWG-rah-fee)
- ❑ zygote (ZY-goht)

Experience Multimedia

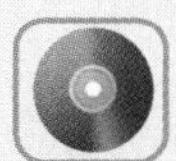

CD-ROM Learning Activities Checklist

Check off the box as you complete each learning activity.

❑ **CD-ROM Learning Activity 13.1:** ***ANATOMY WORD PARTS FLASHCARDS***
Use flashcards to help you memorize word parts. Make your own flashcards or print out prepared flashcards. Also see the electronic flashcard game. Time: 20 minutes.

❑ **CD-ROM Learning Activity 13.2:** ***MEDICINE IN ACTION***
Watch a video clip of a cesarean section. Time: 20 minutes.

❑ **CD-ROM Learning Activity 13.3:** ***DISEASE AND OTHER WORD PARTS FLASHCARDS***
A continuation of the flashcard learning activity. Time: 20 minutes.

❑ **CD-ROM Learning Activity 13.4:** ***MEMORY AIDS***
Use memory aids to help you memorize medical words and meanings. Time: 5 minutes.

❑ **CD-ROM Learning Activity 13.5:** ***MEDICAL LANGUAGE SPOKEN HERE***
Listen to actual medical reports and spell the missing medical words. Time: 20 minutes.

❑ **CD-ROM Learning Activity 13.6:** ***SPELLING CHALLENGE***
Listen to a pronounced medical word and then spell it. Time: 5 minutes.

❑ **CD-ROM Learning Activity 13.7:** ***MEDICAL LANGUAGE PRONUNCIATION***
Listen to a pronounced medical word and then practice pronouncing it. Time: 30 minutes.

❑ **CD-ROM Learning Activity 13.8:** ***EDUCATIONAL FUN AND GAMES***
Enjoy these fun activities while reinforcing your knowledge. Time: 15 minutes.

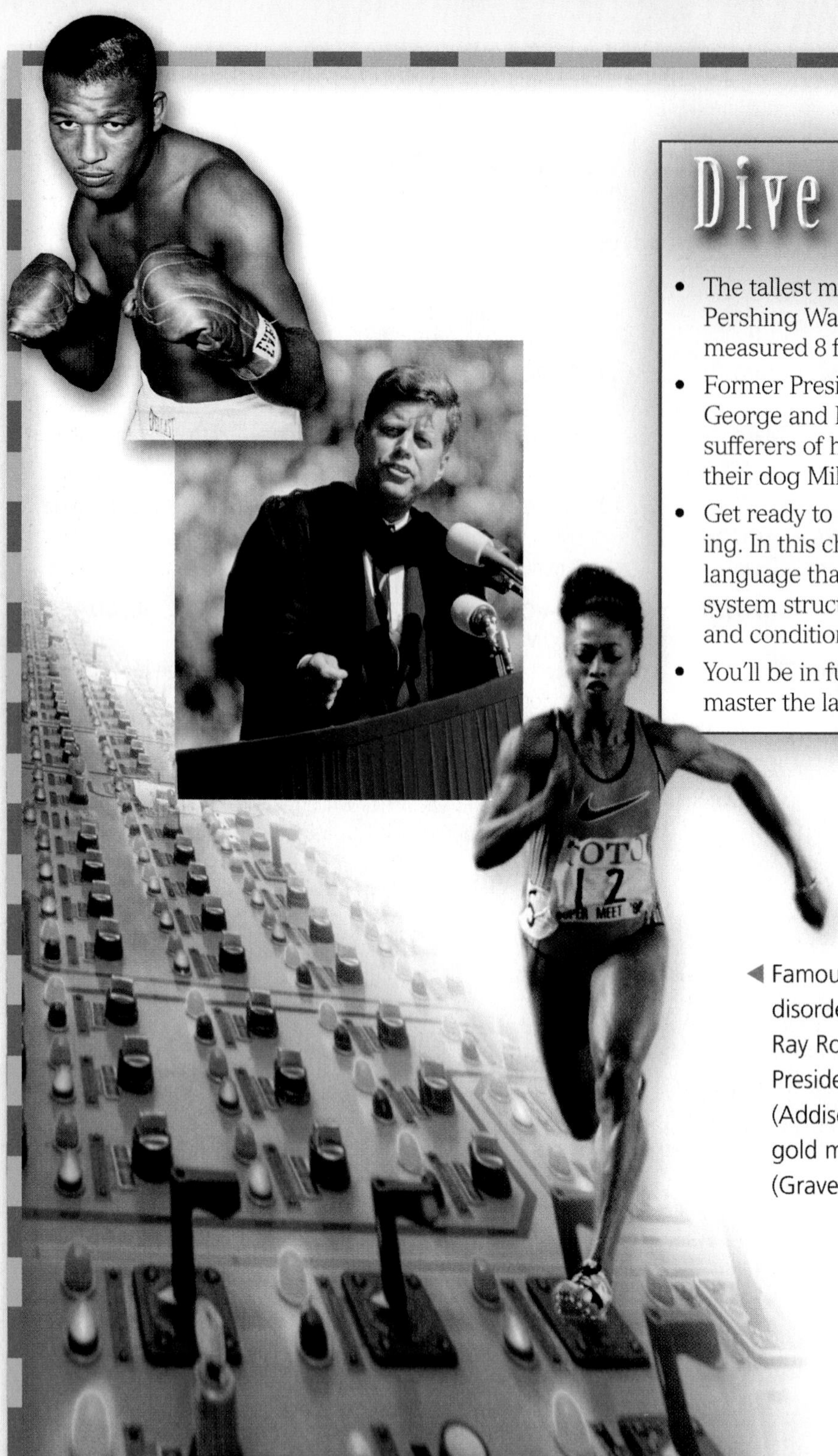

Dive In!

- The tallest man on record was Robert Pershing Wadlow of Illinois, who measured 8 feet, 11.1 inches.
- Former President and First Lady George and Barbara Bush are both sufferers of hyperthyroidism. Even their dog Millie had thyroid problems.
- Get ready to regulate your understanding. In this chapter we'll explore the language that describes the endocrine system structures, functions, diseases, and conditions.
- You'll be in full control once you master the language of endocrinology!

◀ Famous sufferers of endocrine disorders: boxing legend Sugar Ray Robinson (diabetes mellitus); President John F. Kennedy (Addison's disease); Olympic gold medalist Gail Devers (Graves' disease).

Medicine Through HISTORY

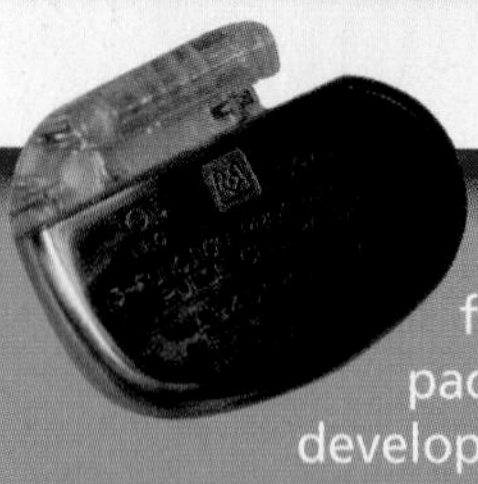

1952
The first cardiac pacemaker is developed

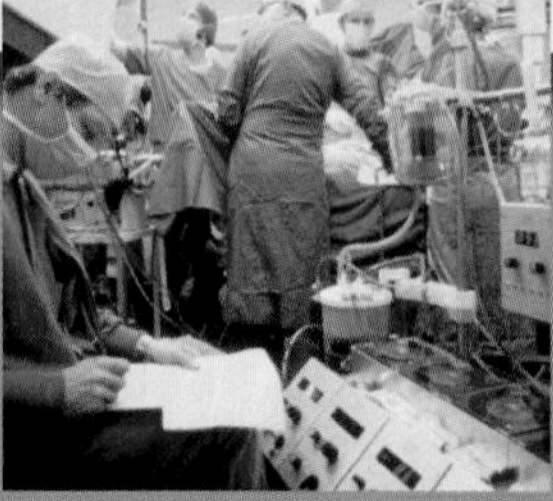

1953
The heart-lung machine for use during open heart surgery is invented by Dr. John Gibbon

1955 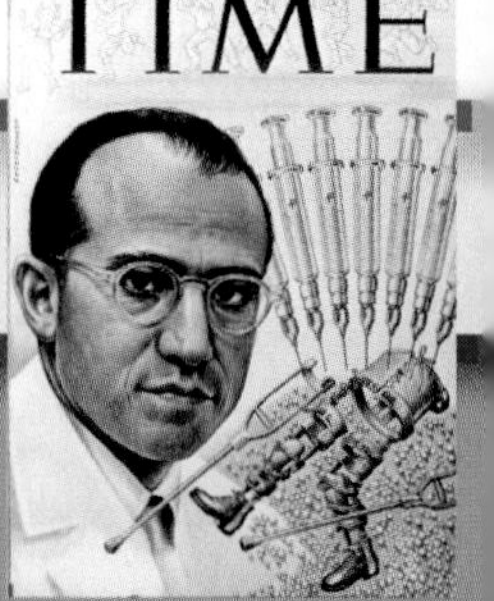
The first polio vaccine (a solution of dead virus) is developed by Dr. Jonas Salk. The oral polio vaccine that uses live, weakened virus is developed by Dr. Albert Sabin in 1961

CHAPTER 14 Endocrinology

Endocrine System

Endocrinology (EN-doh-krin-AWL-oh-jee) is the medical specialty that studies the anatomy and physiology of the endocrine system and uses diagnostic tests, medical and surgical procedures, and drugs to treat endocrine system diseases.

◀ The endocrine system contains organs and glands that secrete hormones to regulate various body functions.

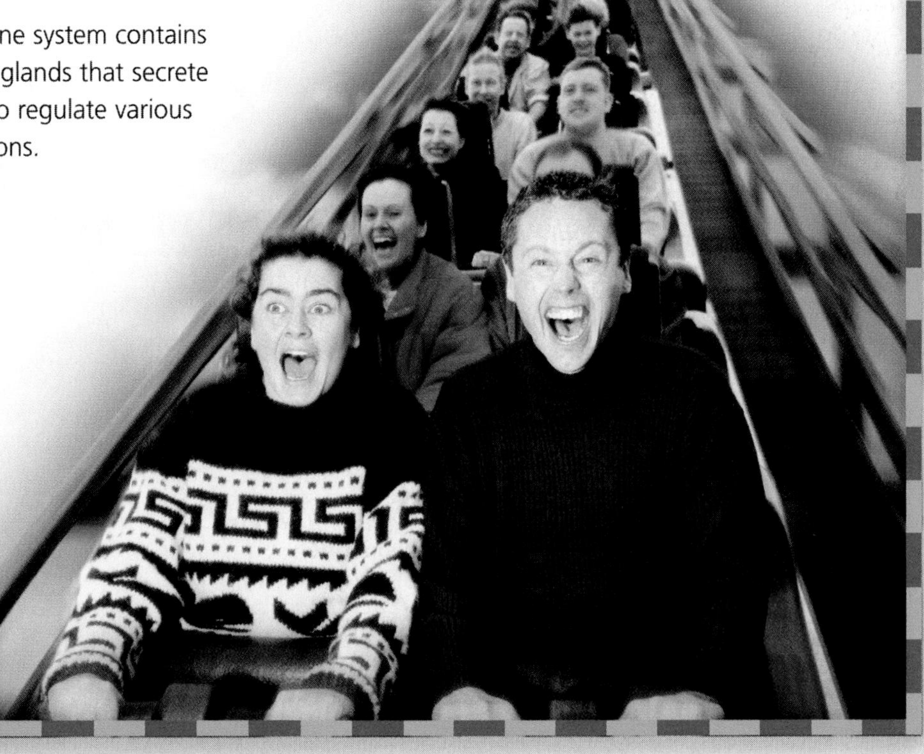

▶ A roller coaster of hormones are being secreted in the bodies of these riders as they experience fear, stress, joy, and excitement.

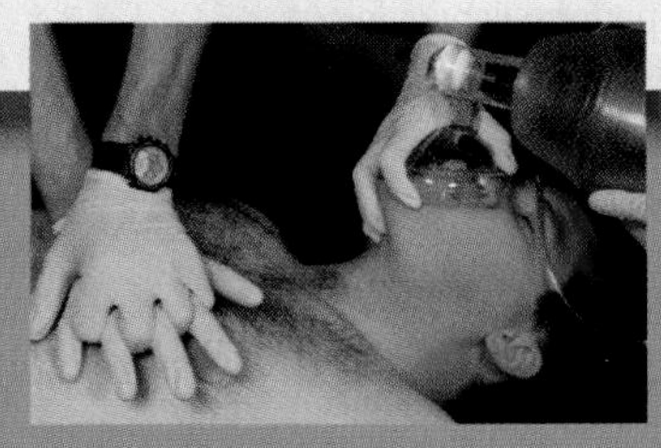

1957

The development of cardiopulmonary resuscitation (CPR) techniques begins with the creation of the ABCs (airway, breathing, circulation)

1959

Patients with Down syndrome and mental retardation are found to have an abnormal number of chromosomes

Measure Your Progress: Learning Objectives

After you study this chapter, you should be able to

1. Identify the anatomical structures of the endocrine system by correctly labeling them on anatomical illustrations.
2. Describe the actions of hormones released by endocrine glands.
3. Build endocrine words from combining forms, prefixes, and suffixes.
4. Describe common endocrine diseases.
5. Describe common endocrine diagnostic laboratory and radiology tests.
6. Describe common endocrine medical and surgical procedures and drug categories.
7. Define common endocrine abbreviations.
8. Correctly spell and pronounce endocrine words.
9. Apply your skills by analyzing an endocrinology report.
10. Test your knowledge of endocrinology by completing review exercises at the end of the chapter and learning activities on the CD-ROM.

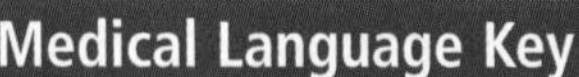

Medical Language Key

To unlock the meaning of a medical word, first define each word part. Then put the word part definitions in order, beginning with the suffix, followed by the first word part, then the other word parts in order.

	Word Part	Word Part Definition
SUFFIX	-logy	*the study of*
PREFIX	endo-	*innermost, within*
COMBINING FORM	crin/o-	*secrete*

Endocrinology: *The study of the organs and glands within the body that secrete hormones.*

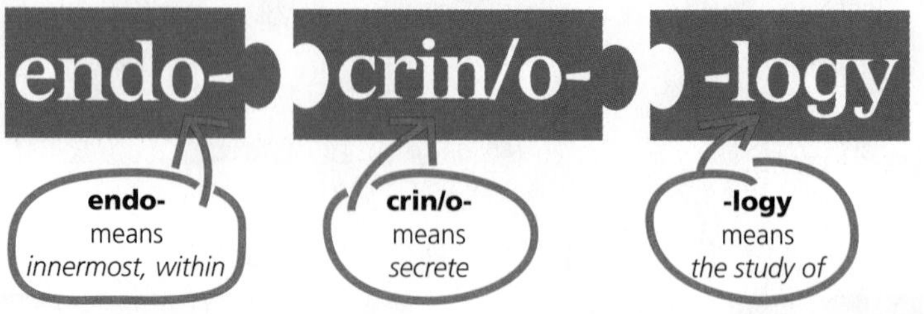

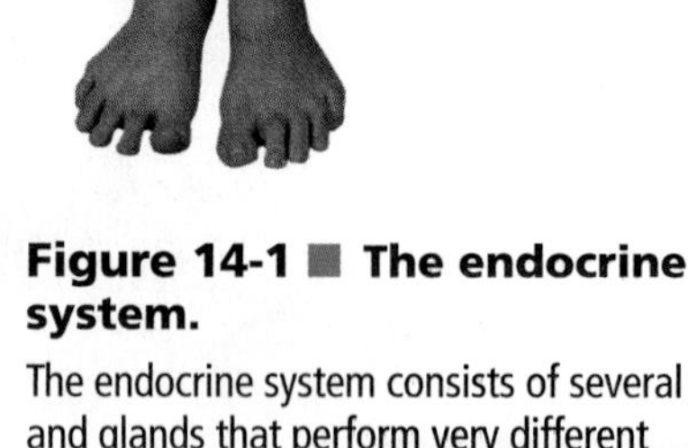

Figure 14-1 ■ The endocrine system.

The endocrine system consists of several organs and glands that perform very different functions. They are related to each other because they all secrete hormones into the blood.

www.prenhall.com/turley

For interactive flashcards, real-life video clips, games, exercises, and audio pronunciations please explore the companion CD-ROM in the back of the book. Click on the companion website for bonus chapters, additional resources, and links to on-line learning.

Anatomy and Physiology

The **endocrine system** is different from other body systems in that its organs and **glands** are in different parts of the body and are not physically connected to each other (see Figure 14-1 ■). The endocrine system includes the hypothalamus, pituitary gland, pineal body, thyroid gland, parathyroid glands, thymus, pancreas, adrenal glands, ovaries, and testes. Some of these organs and glands are influenced by the secretions of the pituitary gland, but this is not true of all of them. However, they are all alike in these ways:

1. They release substances known as **hormones.**
2. They release their hormones directly into the blood and not through ducts.
3. Their hormones regulate specific body functions.

The function of the endocrine system is to keep the body in **homeostasis.** This is a state of equilibrium in which the internal environment of the body is kept in a balanced and steady state so that all of the body systems can function optimally. Homeostasis involves regulation of body fluids, acid-base balance, temperature, metabolism, and other factors.

Word Alert

SOUND-ALIKE WORDS

endocrine (adjective) descriptive word for glands and organs that release hormones directly into the blood

Example: The thyroid gland is one of the glands of the endocrine system.

exocrine (adjective) descriptive word for glands that release substances through ducts and not directly into the blood

Example: The sebaceous glands are exocrine glands that are overactive in the adolescent years.

---

endocrine (EN-doh-krin) (EN-doh-krine)
endo- *innermost, within*
-crine *a thing that secretes*
Every medical word must contain a combining form. The suffix of *endocrine* contains the combining form *crin/o-*.

Add words to make a correct and complete definition of *endocrine: A thing [organ or gland] that secretes [hormones] within [the body].*

system (SIS-tem)
System is derived from a Greek word meaning *combination of parts to make an organized whole.*

gland (GLAND)
Gland is derived from a Latin word meaning *acorn.* Some glands are the size of acorns, but others are not.

glandular (GLAN-dyoo-lar)
glandul/o- *gland*
-ar *pertaining to*

hormone (HOR-mohn)
Hormone is derived from a Greek word meaning *to set in motion.*

hormonal (hor-MOH-nal)
hormon/o- *hormone*
-al *pertaining to*

homeostasis (HOH-mee-oh-STAY-sis)
home/o- *same*
-stasis *condition of standing still; staying in one place*

Anatomy of the Endocrine System

Hypothalamus

The **hypothalamus** is located in the brain just below the thalamus. It forms the floor of the third ventricle and the stalk that connects to the pituitary gland (see Figure 14-2 ■). The hypothalamus functions as part of both the nervous system and the endocrine system. Its function as part of the nervous system was discussed in Neurology (Chapter 10). As part of the endocrine system, the hypothalamus secretes releasing and inhibiting substances that stimulate or inhibit the secretion of hormones produced by the anterior pituitary gland. The hypothalamus also produces two hormones (antidiuretic hormone [ADH] and oxytocin) that are stored in the posterior pituitary gland. These hormones are released when the hypothalamus sends nerve impulses to the posterior pituitary gland.

hypothalamus (HY-poh-THAL-ah-mus)

hypothalamic (HY-poh-thah-LAM-ik)
hypo- *below; deficient*
thalam/o- *thalamus*
-ic *pertaining to*

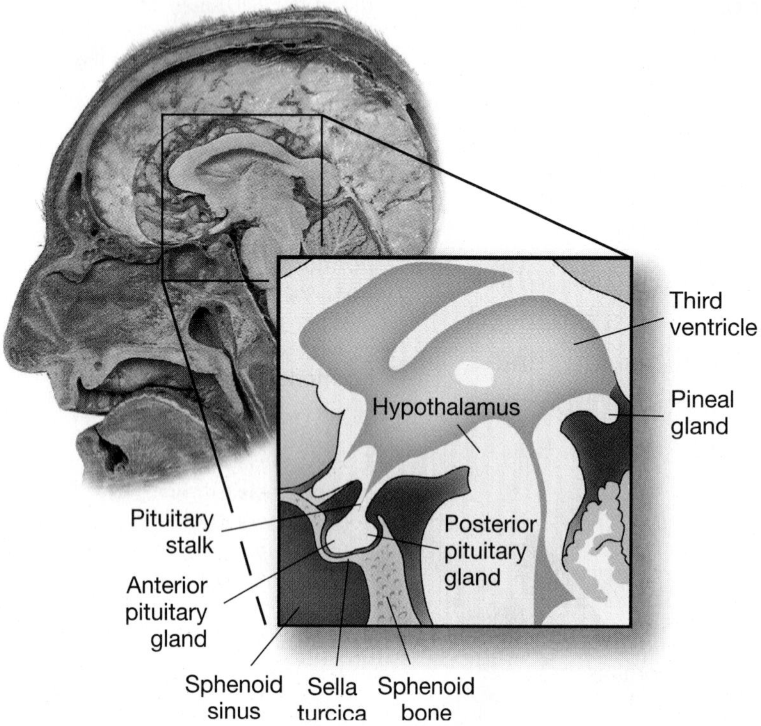

Figure 14-2 ■ Endocrine glands in the cranial cavity.

The hypothalamus forms the floor of the third ventricle and the stalk of tissue that goes to the pituitary gland. The pituitary gland is about the size of a pea and weighs only a fraction of an ounce. Even so, the pituitary gland is known as the master gland of the body. The pineal gland is located posterior to the hypothalamus.

Pituitary Gland

The **pituitary gland** is located in the brain just posterior to the sphenoid sinus (see Figure 14-2). It is a very small, teardrop-shaped gland at the end of a thin stalk of tissue that is an extension from the hypothalamus. The pituitary gland sits in a tiny bony cup (the **sella turcica**) in the sphenoid bone of the cranium. The pituitary gland, or hypophysis, is known as the master gland of the body. It is actually composed of two different glands that function independently of each other: the **anterior pituitary gland** (or **adenohypophysis**) and the **posterior pituitary gland (neurohypophysis)**.

Anterior Pituitary Gland The anterior pituitary gland produces and secretes seven hormones (see Figure 14-3 ■).

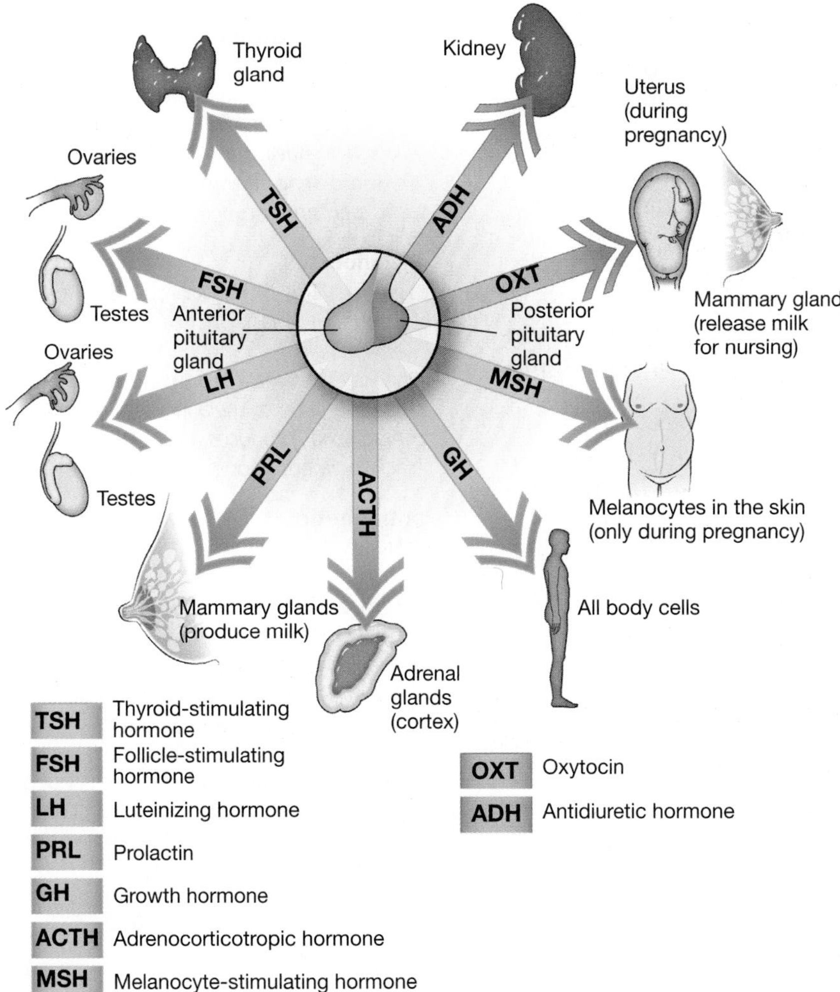

Figure 14-3 ■ Hormones of the anterior and posterior pituitary gland.

The anterior pituitary gland produces and secretes seven different hormones. The posterior pituitary gland releases two hormones that are actually produced by the hypothalamus.

pituitary (pih-TOO-eh-TAIR-ee)
pituit/o- *pituitary gland*
-ary *pertaining to*
Pituitary is derived from a Latin word meaning *mucous secretions from the nose.* The Romans thought that nasal mucus came from the pituitary gland. So *pituitary* originally meant *pertaining to mucous secretions from the nose.*

sella turcica (SEL-ah TUR-sih-kah)
Sella turcica is a Latin phrase meaning *saddle of a Turk* because this bony cup resembles the high pommel and deep seat characteristic of ancient Turkish saddles.

anterior (an-TEER-ee-or)
anter/o- *before; front part*
-ior *pertaining to*

adenohypophysis (AD-eh-noh-hy-PAWF-ih-sis)
aden/o- *gland*
hypo- *below; deficient*
-physis *state of growing*
Adenohypophysis refers to the anterior pituitary gland that produces and secretes hormones like a true gland.

posterior (pohs-TEER-ee-or)
poster/o- *back part*
-ior *pertaining to*

neurohypophysis (NYOOR-oh-hy-PAWF-ih-sis)
neur/o- *nerve*
hypo- *below; deficient*
-physis *state of growing*
Neurohypophysis refers to the posterior pituitary gland that is below the hypothalamus. It does not make or secrete its own hormones but releases hormones produced by the hypothalamus when signaled to do so by nerves from the hypothalamus.

1. **Thyroid-stimulating hormone (TSH).** Stimulates the thyroid gland to secrete thyroid hormones T_3 and T_4.
2. **Follicle-stimulating hormone (FSH).** In females, this hormone stimulates the ovaries to develop follicles, produce mature ova, and secrete estradiol. In males, it stimulates the seminiferous tubules of the testes to produce sperm.
3. **Luteinizing hormone (LH).** In females, this hormone triggers ovulation (rupture of the follicle to release the mature egg). It stimulates the corpus luteum (ruptured ovarian follicle) to secrete estradiol and progesterone. In males, it stimulates the interstitial cells of the testes to secrete testosterone.
4. **Prolactin.** Stimulates the development of the milk glands of the breasts during puberty and the production of milk during pregnancy.
5. **Adrenocorticotropic hormone (ACTH).** Stimulates the cortex of the adrenal gland to secrete the hormones aldosterone, cortisol and androgens.
6. **Growth hormone (GH).** Stimulates cell growth and protein synthesis in all body cells. Increases height and weight during puberty.
7. **Melanocyte-stimulating hormone (MSH).** This hormone does not have any significant function and is not normally produced in adults. In pregnant women, however, it is produced and it stimulates melanocytes in the skin to produce pigmentation of the face and abdomen, as discussed in Dermatology (Chapter 7).

Posterior Pituitary Gland The posterior pituitary gland releases two hormones that are produced in the hypothalamus (see Figure 14-3).

1. **Antidiuretic hormone (ADH).** ADH causes sodium and water to be reabsorbed from the tubules of the kidneys back into the blood. This decreases urine output and increases blood volume and blood pressure.
2. **Oxytocin.** Oxytocin stimulates the pregnant uterus to contract and begin labor. It also causes the breasts to release milk for nursing ("the let-down reflex") when the newborn baby cries or sucks.

thyroid (THY-royd)

stimulate (STIM-yoo-layt)
stimul/o- *exciting, strengthening*
-ate *composed of; pertaining to*

follicle (FAWL-ih-kl)

luteinizing (LOO-tee-ih-NY-zing)
Luteinizing hormone derives its name from the corpus luteum of the ovary.

prolactin (proh-LAK-tin)
pro- *before*
lact/o- *milk*
-in *a substance*
Add words to make a correct and complete definition of *prolactin: a substance [that must be released] before milk [can be produced].*

adrenocorticotropic
(ah-DREE-noh-KOR-tih-koh-TROHP-ik)
adren/o- *adrenal gland*
cortic/o- *cortex (outer region)*
trop/o- *having an affinity for; stimulating; turning*
-ic *pertaining to*

melanocyte
(meh-LAN-oh-site) (MEL-ah-noh-site)
melan/o- *black*
-cyte *cell*
Add words to make a correct and complete definition of *melanocyte: A cell [in the skin that produces a dark brown or] black [pigment known as melanin].*

antidiuretic (AN-tee-DY-yoo-RET-ik)
(AN-tih-DY-yoo-RET-ik)
anti- *against*
dia- *complete; completely through*
oure/o- *urine*
-tic *pertaining to*
The *a* in *dia-* and the *o* in *oure/o-* are dropped when the word is formed. A diuretic drug increases urine production. Antidiuretic hormone (ADH) has the opposite effect. It decreases urine production.

oxytocin (AWK-see-TOH-sin)
ox/y- *oxygen; quick*
toc/o- *labor and childbirth*
-in *a substance*

Did You Know?

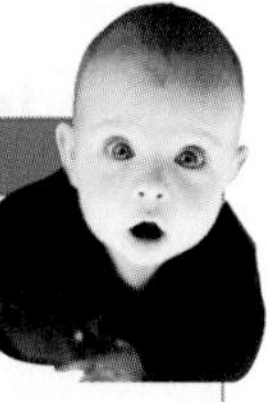

Follicle-stimulating hormone (FSH) and luteinizing hormone (LH) stimulate the male and female sex glands (gonads). Together, FSH and LH are known as **gonadotropins.**

gonadotropin
(GOH-nah-doh-TROH-pin)
gonad/o- *gonads (ovaries and testes)*
trop/o- *having an affinity for; stimulating; turning*
-in *a substance*

Pineal Body

The **pineal body** is located posterior to the hypothalamus (see Figure 14-2). It is a smooth, fingertip-shaped tissue that secretes the hormone **melatonin.** It maintains the body's internal clock and the 24-hour wake-sleep cycle (the **circadian rhythm**) and regulates the onset and duration of sleep.

pineal (PIN-ee-al)
Pineal is derived from a Latin word meaning *pine cone.* The pineal body was thought to resemble that shape.

melatonin (MEL-ah-TOHN-in)

circadian rhythm (ser-KAY-dee-an RITH-um)
Circadian is a combination of the prefix *circa-* (about), part of the Latin word *diem* (one day) and the *suffix -an* (pertaining to).

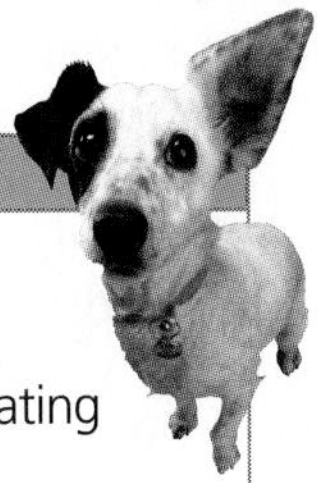

Word Alert

SOUND-ALIKE MEDICAL WORDS

melanin (noun) Dark brown or black pigment produced by melanocytes in the skin. Melanocyte-stimulating hormone (MSH) and sunlight stimulate the melanocytes to form melanin.

Example: Sunshine increases the level of melanin in the skin, causing it to tan.

melatonin (noun) Hormone secreted by the pineal gland. Associated with wake-sleep cycles. Increased levels occur during winter.

Example: Daylight and sunshine decrease melatonin levels in the brain, helping us to be awake during the daytime.

Thyroid Gland

The **thyroid gland** is an irregularly shaped gland that has two **lobes** connected by a thin bridge of tissue known as the **isthmus.** The thyroid gland is located in the neck on either side of and across the surface of the trachea (see Figure 14-4■). The thyroid gland secretes three hormones.

thyroid (THY-royd)
thyr/o- *shield-shaped structure (thyroid gland)*
-oid *resembling*

lobe (LOHB)

isthmus (IS-mus)
Isthmus is derived from a Greek word meaning *a neck of land between two larger land masses.*

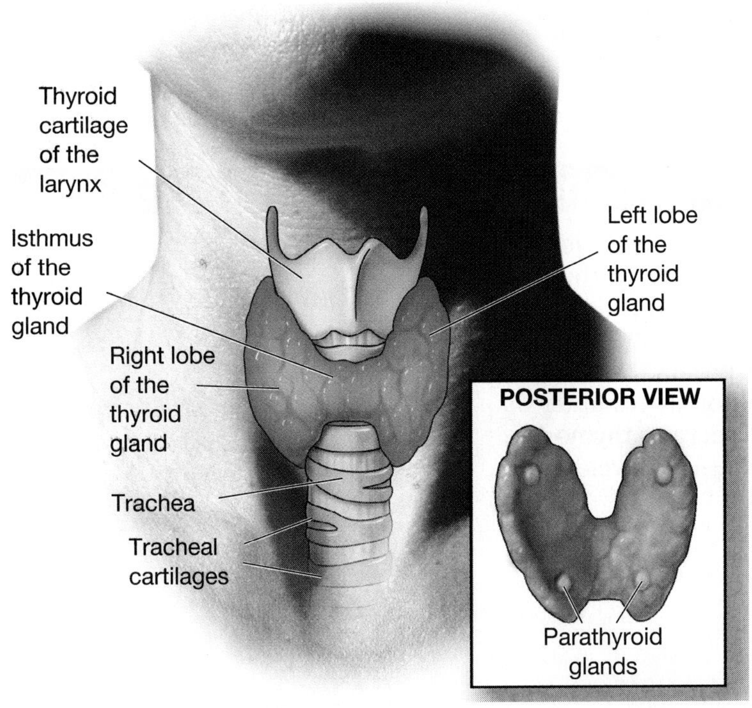

Figure 14-4 ■ Thyroid gland and parathyroid glands.

An anterior view of the thyroid gland, showing its two lobes connected by the isthmus, a bridge of tissue. The thyroid cartilage mirrors the shield-like shape of the thyroid gland. However, the thyroid cartilage actually forms the wall of the larynx and is not part of the thyroid gland or the endocrine system. The parathyroid glands are located on the posterior surface of the thyroid gland.

1. **T_3 or triiodothyronine** increases the rate of cellular metabolism. Production of T_3 is dependent on adequate amounts of iodine in the diet.
2. **T_4 or thyroxine** is produced and then most of it is changed into T_3 by the liver.
3. **Calcitonin** regulates the amount of calcium in the blood. If the calcium level is too high, calcitonin moves calcium from the blood and deposits it in the bones. Calcitonin has an opposite action from that of parathyroid hormone from the parathyroid glands.

The thyroid gland secretes T_3 and T_4 when stimulated by TSH from the anterior pituitary gland. The thyroid gland secretes calcitonin in response to the calcium level in the blood. When the thyroid gland is functioning properly, producing neither too much nor too little of these hormones, this steady state is known as **euthyroidism.**

triiodothyronine
(try-EYE-oh-doh-THY-roh-neen)
tri- *three*
iod/o- *iodine*
thyr/o- *shield-shaped structure (thyroid gland)*
-nine *pertaining to a single chemical substance*
Each molecule of T_3 contains three iodine atoms.

thyroxine (thy-RAWK-seen)
(thy-RAWK-sin)
Thyroxine is a combination of *thyr/o-* (shield-shaped structure [thyroid gland]), *ox/y-* (oxygen), and the letters *in* from the word *indole* (a chemical compound).

calcitonin (KAL-sih-TOH-nin)
calc/i- *calcium*
ton/o- *pressure, tone*
-in *a substance*

euthyroidism (yoo-THY-royd-izm)
eu- *normal, good*
thyroid/o- *thyroid gland*
-ism *process; disease from a specific cause*

Parathyroid Glands

The four tiny **parathyroid glands** are located on the posterior side of the thyroid gland, two on each lobe (see Figure 14-4). The parathyroid glands secrete **parathyroid hormone,** which regulates the amount of calcium in the blood. If the calcium level is too low, parathyroid hormone moves calcium from the bones to the blood. Parathyroid hormone has an opposite action from that of calcitonin secreted by the thyroid gland.

parathyroid (PAIR-ah-THY-royd)
para- *beside, apart from; two parts of a pair; abnormal*
thyr/o- *shield-shaped structure (thyroid gland)*
-oid *resembling*
Some word parts have more than one definition. The best definition of *parathyroid* is *resembling two parts of a pair beside the thyroid gland.*

Thymus Gland

The **thymus gland** is a small, grainy gland located in the thoracic cavity posterior to the sternum. During childhood and puberty, the thymus gland is large, but it shrinks to a much smaller size during adulthood. The thymus gland functions as part of both the body's immune response and the endocrine system. Its function as part of the immune response was discussed in Hematology and Immunology (Chapter 6). As part of the endocrine system, the thymus gland secretes **thymosins,** which cause immature T lymphocytes in the thymus to develop and mature.

thymus (THY-mus)

thymic (THY-mik)
thym/o- *thymus; rage*
-ic *pertaining to*

thymosin (thy-MOH-sin)
Thymosin is a combination of the original Greek spelling *thymos* (thymus) and the suffix *-in* (a substance).

Pancreas

The **pancreas** is an elongated, triangular, somewhat lumpy gland that is located posterior to the stomach. The head of the pancreas is tucked into a loop of the duodenum, the body of the pancreas lies horizontally, and the tail of the pancreas tapers to a point (see Figure 14-5 ■). The pancreas functions as part of both the digestive system and the endocrine system. Its function as part of the digestive system was discussed in Gastroenterology (Chapter 3). As part of the endocrine system, the pancreas secretes three hormones directly into the blood from the **islets of Langerhans.**

1. **Glucagon** is secreted by **alpha cells** in the islets of Langerhans. When blood glucose levels are low, this hormone breaks down **glycogen** (a form of glucose stored in the liver and skeletal muscles) to form **glucose.**
2. **Insulin** is secreted by **beta cells** in the islets of Langerhans. The pancreas secretes insulin in response to a high blood glucose level. Insulin transports glucose to the cell, links with an insulin receptor on the cell membrane, and transports glucose inside the cell where it is metabolized.
3. **Somatostatin** is secreted by **delta cells** in the islets of Langerhans. This hormone inhibits the release of growth hormone (from the anterior pituitary gland), glucagon, and insulin.

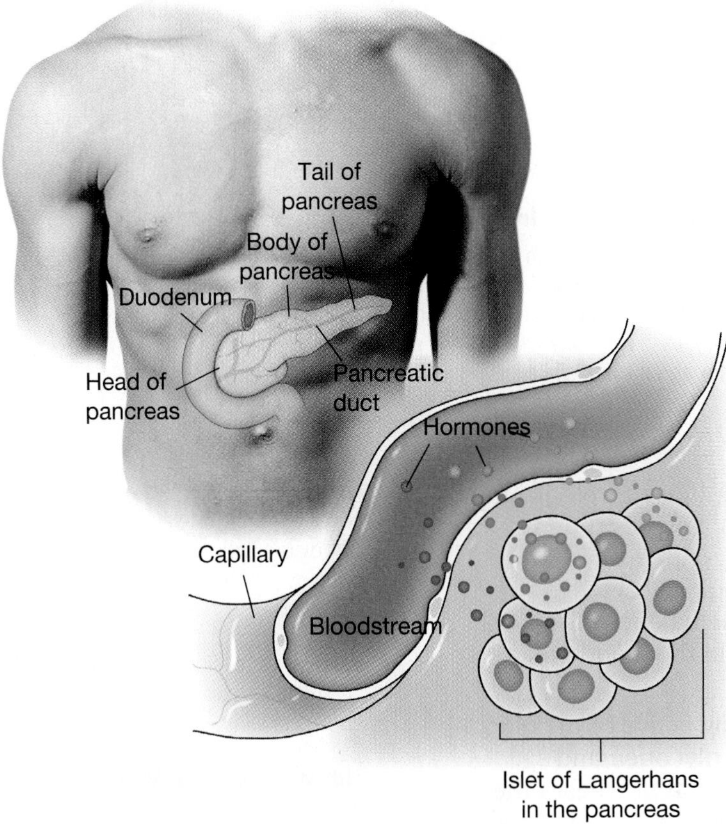

Figure 14-5 ■ Pancreas.

The pancreas is composed of small groups (or islands) of cells known as the islets of Langerhans. These are scattered throughout the pancreas. Each islet is located next to a capillary so that the secreted hormones (glucagon, insulin, and somatostatin) can move directly into the blood.

pancreas (PAN-kree-as)
Pancreas is derived from a Greek word meaning *sweetbread.* The pancreas of large animals was considered a culinary delicacy.

pancreatic (PAN-kree-AT-ik)
pancreat/o- *pancreas*
-ic *pertaining to*

islets of Langerhans
(EYE-lets of LAHNG-er-hanz)
Islets are small islands of cells. The islets of Langerhans were named by Paul Langerhans (1847–1888), a German anatomist. This is an example of an eponym: a person from whom something takes its name.

Alpha, beta, and *delta* are the first, second, and fourth letters of the Greek alphabet. *Gamma,* the third letter of the Greek alphabet, was not used to name structures because it is out of alphabetical order with respect to the English alphabet.

glucagon (GLOO-kah-gawn)
gluc/o- *glucose (sugar)*
ag/o- *to lead to*
-on *substance; structure*
Glucagon is a substance that can be broken down to produce glucose.

glycogen (GLY-koh-jen)
glyc/o- *glucose (sugar)*
-gen *that which produces*

glucose (GLOO-kohs)
gluc/o- *glucose (sugar)*
-ose *full of*

insulin (IN-soo-lin)
insul/o- *island*
-in *a substance*
Insulin is secreted by little "islands of cells," the islets of Langerhans.

somatostatin (SOH-mah-toh-STAT-in)
somat/o- *body*
stat/o- *standing still; staying in one place*
-in *a substance*
Add words to make a correct and complete definition of *somatostatin: A substance [that makes the] body [to be] standing still [without growth].* Somatostatin inhibits the hormone that causes growth in the body.

Adrenal Glands

The two **adrenal glands** are slightly folded mounds that are draped over the superior ends of each of the two kidneys (see Figure 14-6 ■). Each adrenal gland is divided into an outer layer and inner area. The outer layer (cortex) and the inner area (medulla) function as two different endocrine glands, each producing its own set of hormones.

adrenal (ah-DREE-nal)
ad- *toward*
ren/o- *kidney*
-al *pertaining to*

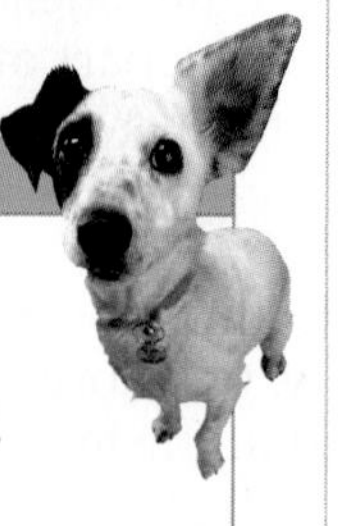

Word Alert

SOUND-ALIKE WORDS

aden/o- (combining form) a gland
Example: An adenoma is a benign tumor of a gland.

adren/o- (combining form) adrenal gland
Example: Each adrenal gland sits on top of a kidney.

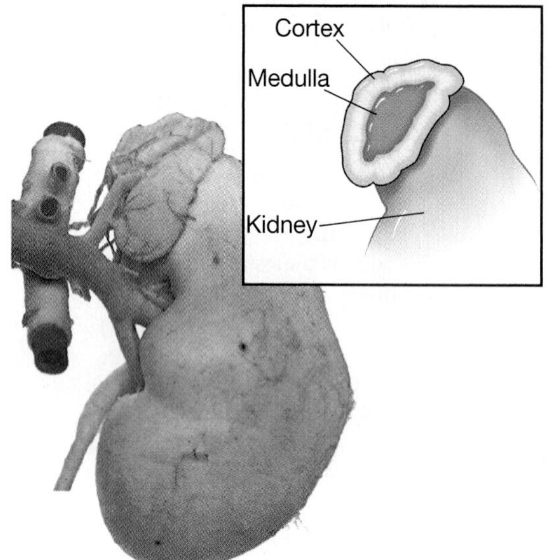

Figure 14-6 ■ Adrenal gland.
The adrenal glands are in very close proximity to the kidneys, but the adrenal glands are part of the endocrine system while the kidneys belong to the urinary system. Each adrenal is draped over the top of a kidney like a soft, thick cap. The two parts of the adrenal gland, the cortex and the medulla, function as two separate endocrine glands.

Adrenal Cortex The **adrenal cortex** secretes these three groups of hormones: mineralocorticoids, glucocorticoids, and androgens.

1. **Aldosterone.** The most abundant and biologically active of the **mineralocorticoid** hormones. It regulates the balance of minerals (electrolytes), keeping sodium (and water) in the blood while excreting potassium in the urine.
2. **Cortisol.** The most abundant and biologically active of the **glucocorticoid** hormones. It breaks down stored glycogen and increases the amount of glucose in the blood. It decreases the formation of proteins and new tissue, and it exerts a strong anti-inflammatory effect.
3. **Androgens.** Androgens are male hormones. The adrenal gland secretes some androgens. (It does not secrete the most biologically active androgen, testosterone.)

cortex (KOR-teks)
cortices (KOR-tih-seez)
Cortex is a Latin singular noun meaning *outer covering or bark.* Form the plural by changing *-ex* to *-ices.*

cortical (KOR-tih-kal)
cortic/o- *cortex (outer region)*
-al *pertaining to*

aldosterone (al-DAWS-ter-ohn)

mineralocorticoid (MIN-er-AL-oh-KOR-tih-koyd)
mineral/o- *mineral; electrolyte*
cortic/o- *cortex (outer region)*
-oid *resembling*

The adrenal cortex secretes aldosterone when the blood pressure is low. The adrenal cortex secretes all three hormones when stimulated by ACTH from the anterior pituitary gland.

Adrenal Medulla The **adrenal medulla** secretes the hormones **epinephrine** and **norepinephrine** into the blood when it is stimulated by nerves of the sympathetic or parasympathetic nervous system, as discussed in Neurology (Chapter 10).

Connections

Neurology (Chapter 10). Epinephrine is a neurotransmitter for the sympathetic nervous system. When a person experiences danger or anger, epinephrine prepares the body to either fight or run away from the danger. This is the "fight or flight" response. Epinephrine increases the heart rate, constricts the smooth muscle of the blood vessels to raise the blood pressure, increases the respiratory rate, and dilates the bronchi to increase air flow to the lungs.

cortisol (KOR-tih-sawl)
Cortisol is a combination of *cortisone* (the chemical precursor of cortisol) and the suffix *-ol* (chemical substance).

glucocorticoid (GLOO-koh-KOR-tih-koyd)
gluc/o- *glucose (sugar)*
cortic/o- *cortex (outer region)*
-oid *resembling*

androgen (AN-droh-jen)
andr/o- *male*
-gen *that which produces*

medulla (meh-DUL-ah) (meh-DYOOL-ah)
medullae (meh-DUL-ee) (meh-DYOOL-ee)
Medulla is a Latin singular feminine noun meaning *middle.* Form the plural by changing *-a* to *-ae.*

medullary (MED-yoo-LAIR-ee)
medull/o- *medulla (inner region)*
-ary *pertaining to*

epinephrine (EP-ih-NEF-rin)

norepinephrine (NOR-ep-ih-NEF-rin)
The prefix *nor-* refers to a specific chemical modification to a chemical structure.

Ovaries

The **ovaries** are small, oval-shaped glands located in the pelvic cavity. The ovaries function as part of both the female reproductive system and the endocrine system. Their function as part of the female reproductive system was discussed in Gynecology and Obstetrics (Chapter 13). As part of the endocrine system, the follicles of the ovary produce and secrete **estradiol** when stimulated by FSH from the anterior pituitary gland. Estradiol is the most abundant and most biologically active of the female hormones. The corpus luteum (ruptured ovarian follicle) produces and secretes estradiol and **progesterone** when stimulated by LH from the anterior pituitary gland. The cells around the follicle produce and secrete androgens when stimulated by LH from the anterior pituitary gland.

ovary (OH-vah-ree)
Ovary is derived from a Latin word meaning *egg.*

ovarian (oh-VAIR-ee-an)
ovari/o- *ovary*
-an *pertaining to*

estradiol (ES-trah-DY-awl)
estr/a- *female*
di- *two*
-ol *chemical substance*
A molecule of estradiol contains two atoms of oxygen.

progesterone (proh-JES-ter-ohn)
Progesterone is a combination of the prefix *pro-* (before), the combining form *gest/o-* (from conception to birth), the letters *er* from *sterol* (a category of chemicals), and the suffix- *one* (a chemical substance).

Testes

The **testes** or **testicles** are egg-shaped glands located outside the body in the scrotum, a pouch of skin behind the penis. The testes function as part of both the male genitourinary system and the endocrine system. Their function as part of the male genitourinary system was discussed in Male Reproductive Medicine (Chapter 12). As part of the endocrine system, the seminiferous tubules of the testes produce sperm when stimulated by FSH from the anterior pituitary gland. Interstitial cells of the testes secrete testosterone when stimulated by LH from the anterior pituitary gland. **Testosterone** is the most abundant and biologically active of all the androgens (male hormones).

testis (TES-tis)
testes (TES-teez)
Testis is a Latin singular noun. Form the plural by changing *-is* to *-es*.

testicle (TES-tih-kl)
testicles (TES-tih-kls)
Testicle is a combination of *testis* and the suffix *-cle* (small thing).

testicular (tes-TIK-yoo-lar)
testicul/o- *testis; testicle*
-ar *pertaining to*

testosterone (tes-TAWS-teh-rohn)

Physiology of Hormone Response and Feedback

While the nervous system uses neurotransmitters as chemical messengers that travel the distance between two neurons, the endocrine system uses hormones as chemical messengers. Hormones are secreted into the blood and travel throughout the body. Some neurotransmitters (epinephrine, norepinephrine, and dopamine) are also hormones because they are secreted by a gland and travel in the blood. As they travel in the blood, hormones seek out specific target organs whose **receptors** they can bind with. A hormone is like a key that can unlock one or more receptors on a target organ and produce an effect. Other keys (other hormones), however, cannot unlock those receptors.

A unique feature of the endocrine system is the "chain reaction" sequence of hormones: A hormone released by one organ or gland can stimulate another organ or gland to release its hormones that then bind to receptors on a target organ.

The action of hormones can involve **stimulation** or **inhibition.** Some hormones, like the releasing hormones of the hypothalamus, stimulate a gland or organ to release its hormones. Other hormones, like the inhibiting hormone of the hypothalamus, keep a gland or organ from releasing its hormones.

receptor (ree-SEP-ter)
recept/o- *receive*
-or *person or thing that produces or does*

stimulation (STIM-yoo-LAY-shun)
stimul/o- *exciting, strengthening*
-ation *a process; being or having*

inhibition (IN-hih-BISH-un)
inhibit/o- *block; hold back*
-ion *action; condition*

Some hormones, like T_3 and T_4, work in conjunction with one another to accomplish the same result. This is known as **synergism.** Other hormones, like calcitonin and parathyroid hormone, exert opposite effects. This is known as **antagonism** (see Figure 14-7 ■).

The endocrine system maintains body homeostasis through the use of hormones and a negative feedback mechanism. For example, after the anterior pituitary gland secretes thyroid-stimulating hormone, it then monitors the blood to see if it can detect normal levels of the two thyroid hormones. If these hormones are not present (negative feedback), the anterior pituitary will secrete more thyroid-stimulating hormone to stimulate the thyroid.

synergism (SIN-er-jizm)
syn- *together*
erg/o- *activity; work*
-ism *process; disease from a specific cause*

antagonism (an-TAG-on-izm)
antagon/o- *oppose or work against*
-ism *process; disease from a specific cause*

	ACTION	HORMONE	SOURCE
BODY METABOLISM	↑ Increased metabolism	T_3 and T_4	Thyroid
BLOOD GLUCOSE	↑ Increased blood glucose (stored glycogen converted to glucose)	Cortisol	Adrenal cortex
	↑ Increased blood glucose	Epinephrine	Adrenal medulla
	↑ Increased blood glucose	Glucagon	Pancreas
	↓ Decreased blood glucose (glucose metabolized by cells or stored as glycogen)	Insulin	Pancreas
BLOOD CALCIUM	↑ Increased blood calcium	Parathyroid hormone	Parathyroid
	↓ Decreased blood calcium	Calcitonin	Thyroid
BLOOD SODIUM	↑ Increased blood sodium (more sodium reabsorbed from kidney tubules)	Aldosterone	Adrenal cortex

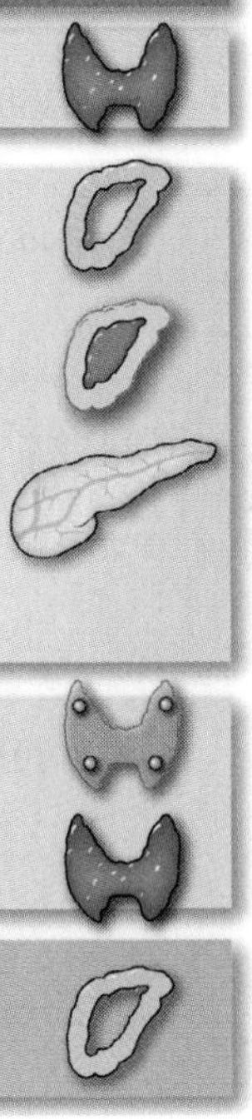

Figure 14-7 ■ Effects of hormones.
Hormones from the various endocrine glands affect body metabolism, blood glucose, blood calcium, and blood sodium in complementary or opposite ways.

Vocabulary Review

Anatomy and Physiology

Now that you have studied the anatomy and physiology of the endocrine system, take time to review those new words and descriptions. Memorize the combining forms and their definitions before going on to the next section.

Word or Phrase	Combining Form and Definition	Description
adrenal cortex	adren/o- *adrenal gland*	Outermost part of the adrenal gland. It produces and secretes three groups of hormones: mineralocorticoids (aldosterone), glucocorticoids (cortisol), and some androgens (male hormones).
adrenal glands	adren/o- *adrenal gland*	Endocrine glands on top of the kidneys. Each adrenal gland contains two parts: the cortex and the medulla. Both parts secrete hormones.
adrenal medulla	adren/o- *adrenal gland*	Innermost part of the adrenal gland. It produces and secretes the hormones epinephrine and norepinephrine.
adrenocortico-tropic hormone (ACTH)	adren/o- *adrenal gland* cortic/o- *cortex (outer region)* trop/o- *having an affinity for; stimulating; turning*	Hormone secreted by the anterior pituitary gland. It stimulates the adrenal cortex to secrete all three of its hormones.
aldosterone		Most abundant and biologically active of the mineralocorticoid hormones secreted by the adrenal cortex. It regulates the balance of electrolytes, keeping sodium (and water) in the blood while excreting potassium in the urine.
androgens	andr/o- *male*	Category that includes naturally occurring male hormones like testosterone from the testes, other androgens from the adrenal cortex, as well as manufactured male hormones used in drugs
antagonism	antagon/o- *oppose or work against*	Process in which two hormones exert opposite effects
anterior pituitary gland	anter/o- *before; front part* pituit/o- *pituitary gland* aden/o- *gland*	Part of the pituitary gland that secretes thyroid-stimulating hormone (TSH), follicle-stimulating hormone (FSH), luteinizing hormone (LH), prolactin, adrenocorticotropic hormone (ACTH), growth hormone (GH), and melanocyte-stimulating hormone (MSH). Also known as the **adenohypophysis.**
antidiuretic hormone (ADH)		Hormone produced by the hypothalamus but stored in and released by the posterior pituitary gland. It stimulates the kidneys to move water back into the blood to increase the volume of the blood.
calcitonin	calc/i- *calcium*	Hormone secreted by the thyroid gland. Along with parathyroid hormone, it regulates the amount of calcium in the blood. If the calcium level is too high, calcitonin moves calcium from the blood and deposits it in the bones.
cortisol		Most abundant and biologically active of the glucocorticoid hormones secreted by the adrenal cortex. It increases the level of glucose in the blood, decreases the formation of proteins and new tissues, and has an anti-inflammatory effect. The adrenal cortex secretes cortisol when stimulated by ACTH from the anterior pituitary gland.

Word or Phrase	Combining Form and Definition	Description
endocrine system	crin/o- *secrete*	Body system that includes organs and glands that secrete hormones into the blood.
epinephrine		Hormone secreted by the adrenal medulla in response to stimulation by nerves of the sympathetic nervous system.
estradiol	estr/a- *female*	Female hormone that is the most abundant and biologically active of all the estrogens. Estradiol is produced and secreted by the follicles and corpus luteum of the ovary when stimulated by FSH from the anterior pituitary gland.
euthyroidism	thyroid/o- *thyroid gland*	State of normal functioning of the hormones of the thyroid gland
follicle-stimulating hormone (FSH)	stimul/o- *exciting, strengthening*	Hormone secreted by the anterior pituitary gland. In females, it stimulates the ovary to develop follicles. It stimulates the follicles to secrete estradiol. In males, it stimulates the seminiferous tubules of the testes to produce sperm.
gland	glandul/o- *gland*	One of the structures of the endocrine system that secretes hormones directly into the blood
glucagon	gluc/o- *glucose (sugar)*	Hormone secreted by alpha cells in the islets of Langerhans in the pancreas. It breaks down glycogen to form glucose.
glucocorticoids	gluc/o- *glucose (sugar)* cortic/o- *cortex (outer region)*	Group of hormones secreted by the adrenal cortex. See *cortisol.*
glucose	gluc/o- *glucose (sugar)*	A simple sugar found in foods and also the sugar in the blood. It is produced when the hormone glucagon breaks down glycogen.
glycogen	glyc/o- *glucose (sugar)*	The form that glucose (sugar) takes when it is stored in the liver and skeletal muscles
gonadotropins	gonad/o- *gonads (ovaries and testes)* trop/o- *having an affinity for; stimulating; turning*	Category of hormones that stimulate the male and female gonads. Includes follicle-stimulating hormone (FSH) and luteinizing hormone (LH).
growth hormone (GH)		Hormone secreted by the anterior pituitary gland. It stimulates all the tissues of the body to grow.
homeostasis	home/o- *same*	State of equilibrium of the internal environment of the body, including fluid balance, acid-base balance, temperature, metabolism, and so forth, to keep all the body systems functioning optimally
hormone	hormon/o- *hormone*	Chemical messenger of the endocrine system that is secreted by a gland or organ and travels through the blood
hypothalamus	thalam/o- *thalamus*	Endocrine gland located in the brain just below the thalamus. It produces (but does not secrete) antidiuretic hormone (ADH) and oxytocin.
inhibition	inhibit/o- *block; hold back*	Action of a hormone to prevent an organ or gland from secreting its hormones
insulin	insul/o- *island*	Hormone secreted by the beta cells of the islets of Langerhans in the pancreas. It transports glucose to the cells.

Word or Phrase	Combining Form and Definition	Description
luteinizing hormone (LH)		Hormone secreted by the anterior pituitary gland. In females, it triggers ovulation. It stimulates the corpus luteum to secrete estradiol and progesterone. In males, it stimulates the interstitial cells of the testes to secrete testosterone.
melanocyte-stimulating hormone (MSH)	melan/o- *black*	Hormone secreted by the anterior pituitary gland. It stimulates melanocytes in the skin to produce the pigment melanin during. pregnancy.
melatonin		Hormone secreted by the pineal body. It maintains the 24-hour wake-sleep cycle known as the **circadian rhythm.**
mineralocorticoids	mineral/o- *mineral; electrolyte* cortic/o- *cortex (outer region)*	Group of hormones secreted by the adrenal cortex. See *aldosterone.*
norepinephrine		Hormone secreted by the adrenal medulla in response to stimulation by nerves of the parasympathetic nervous system.
ovaries	ovari/o- *ovary*	Endocrine glands near the uterus. FSH from the anterior pituitary gland stimulates the ovary to develop follicles and stimulates the follicles to secrete estradiol. LH from the anterior pituitary gland stimulates the cells around the follicle to secrete androgens. LH triggers ovulation and stimulates the corpus luteum to secrete estradiol and progesterone.
oxytocin	ox/y- *oxygen; quick* toc/o- *labor and childbirth*	Hormone produced by the hypothalamus but stored in and released by the posterior pituitary gland. It stimulates the uterus to contract during labor and releases milk for nursing ("the let-down reflex" from the breasts).
pancreas	pancreat/o- *pancreas*	Endocrine gland posterior to the stomach that contains the islets of Langerhans (alpha, beta, and delta cells) that produce and secrete the hormones glucagon, insulin, and somatostatin.
parathyroid glands	thyr/o- *shield-shaped structure (thyroid gland)*	Four endocrine glands on the posterior lobes of the thyroid gland. They produce and secrete parathyroid hormone.
parathyroid hormone	thyr/o- *shield-shaped structure (thyroid gland)*	Hormone secreted by the parathyroid glands. Along with calcitonin from the thyroid gland, it regulates the amount of calcium in the blood. If the calcium level is too low, parathyroid hormone moves calcium from the bones to the blood.
pineal gland		Endocrine gland in the brain that lies posterior to the pituitary gland. It secretes the hormone melatonin, which controls the body's circadian rhythm.
pituitary gland	pituit/o- *pituitary gland*	Endocrine gland in the brain that is connected by a stalk of tissue to the hypothalamus. It sits in the bony sella turcica of the sphenoid bone. Also known as the hypophysis. It is known as the master gland of the body. It consists of the anterior pituitary gland and the posterior pituitary gland.
posterior pituitary gland	poster/o- *back part* pituit/o- *pituitary gland* neur/o- *nerve*	Part of the pituitary gland that stores and releases antidiuretic hormone (ADH) and oxytocin produced by the hypothalamus. Also known as the **neurohypophysis.**

Word or Phrase	Combining Form and Definition	Description
progesterone	gest/o- *from conception to birth*	Female hormone produced and secreted by the corpus luteum of the ovary when stimulated by LH from the anterior pituitary gland
prolactin	lact/o- *milk*	Hormone secreted by the anterior pituitary gland. It stimulates lactiferous glands of the breasts to develop during puberty and to produce milk during pregnancy.
receptor	recept/o- *receive*	Structure on the cell membrane of a target organ or gland where a hormone binds
somatostatin	somat/o- *body* stat/o- *standing still; staying in one place*	Hormone secreted by the delta cells of the islets of Langerhans in the pancreas. It inhibits the release of growth hormone, glucagon, and insulin.
stimulation	stimul/o- *exciting, strengthening*	Action of a hormone to cause an organ or gland to release its hormones
synergism	erg/o- *work*	Process in which two hormones work together to accomplish the same result
T_3	iod/o- *iodine* thyr/o- *shield-shaped structure (thyroid gland)*	Hormone secreted by the thyroid gland. It increases the rate of cellular metabolism. Also known as **triiodothyronine.**
T_4	thyr/o- *shield-shaped structure (thyroid gland)*	Hormone secreted by the thyroid gland. Most of it is changed into T_3 by the liver. Also known as **thyroxine.**
testes	test/o- *testis* testicul/o- *testes; testicle*	Endocrine glands on either side of the scrotum. Also known as **testicles.** FSH from the anterior pituitary gland stimulates their seminiferous tubules to produce sperm. LH from the anterior pituitary gland stimulates their interstitial cells to produce and secrete testosterone.
testosterone	test/o- *testis*	Male hormone that is the most abundant and most biologically active of the androgens. Testosterone is produced and secreted by the interstitial cells of the testes when stimulated by LH from the anterior pituitary gland.
thymus	thym/o- *thymus gland*	Endocrine gland posterior to the sternum that produces and secretes the group of hormones known as **thymosins.** They cause immature T lymphocytes in the thymus to mature.
thyroid gland	thyr/o- *shield-shaped structure (thyroid gland)*	Endocrine gland in the neck that produces and secretes the hormones T_3, T_4, and calcitonin. Its two lobes and narrow connecting bridge (isthmus) give it a shieldlike shape.
thyroid-stimulating hormone (TSH)	thyr/o- *shield-shaped structure (thyroid gland)* stimul/o- *exciting, strengthening*	Hormone secreted by the anterior pituitary gland that stimulates the thyroid to secrete T_3 and T_4

Labeling Exercise

A. *Match each anatomy word or phrase to its numbered structure in Figure 14-8 ■. Write that word or phrase on the blank line next to the number. Use the Answer Key at the end of the book to check your answers.*

adrenal gland	pancreas	pituitary gland	thymus
hypothalamus	parathyroid glands	testis	thyroid gland
ovary	pineal body		

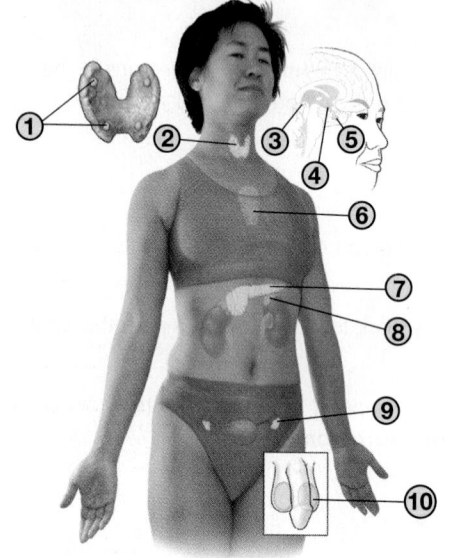

1. ____________________
2. ____________________
3. ____________________
4. ____________________
5. ____________________
6. ____________________
7. ____________________
8. ____________________
9. ____________________
10. ____________________

Figure 14-8 ■

B. *Match each anatomy word or phrase to its numbered structure in Figure 14-9 ■. Write that word or phrase on the blank line next to its number.*

isthmus of thyroid gland	parathyroid glands	thyroid cartilage	tracheal cartilage
left lobe of the thyroid gland	right lobe of the thyroid gland	trachea	

1. ____________________
2. ____________________
3. ____________________
4. ____________________
5. ____________________
6. ____________________
7. ____________________

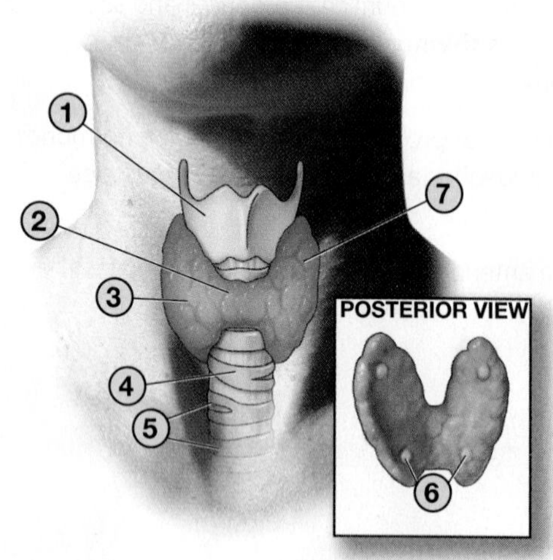

Figure 14-9 ■

Building Medical Words

Combining Forms

Here are the endocrine combining forms you have learned so far. Next to each combining form, write its meaning. Use the Answer Key at the end of the book to check your answers. The first one has been done for you.

	Combining Form	Medical Meaning		Combining Form	Medical Meaning
1.	ovari/o-	ovary	23.	medull/o-	______
2.	aden/o-	______	24.	melan/o-	______
3.	adren/o-	______	25.	mineral/o-	______
4.	ag/o-	______	26.	neur/o-	______
5.	andr/o-	______	27.	ox/y-	______
6.	antagan/o-	______	28.	pancreat/o-	______
7.	anter/o-	______	29.	pituit/o-	______
8.	calc/i-	______	30.	poster/o-	______
9.	cortic/o-	______	31.	recept/o-	______
10.	crin/o-	______	32.	ren/o-	______
11.	erg/o-	______	33.	somat/o-	______
12.	estr/a-	______	34.	stat/o-	______
13.	glandul/o-	______	35.	stimul/o-	______
14.	gluc/o-	______	36.	testicul/o-	______
15.	glyc/o-	______	37.	thalam/o-	______
16.	gonad/o-	______	38.	thym/o-	______
17.	home/o-	______	39.	thyr/o-	______
18.	hormon/o-	______	40.	thyroid/o-	______
19.	inhibit/o-	______	41.	toc/o-	______
20.	insul/o-	______	42.	ton/o-	______
21.	iod/o-	______	43.	trop/o-	______
22.	lact/o-	______			

Combining Forms and Suffixes

Read the definition hint for the medical word you are to build. Look at the combining form that is given. Write the correct suffix on the blank line. Then write the medical word. (Remember: You may need to remove the combining vowel. Always remove the hyphens and slash.) Use the Answer Key at the end of the book to check your answers. The first one has been done for you.

SUFFIX LIST

-al (pertaining to)	-ary (pertaining to)	-ic (pertaining to)
-an (pertaining to	-ation (a process; being or having)	-oid (resembling)
-ar (pertaining to)	-gen (that which produces)	-stasis (condition of standing still)

	Definition Hint	Combining Form	Suffix	Write the Medical Word
1.	Pertaining to the thymus	thym/o-	-ic	thymic
2.	Pertaining to substances from endocrine glands	hormon/o-	________	________
3.	Substance that produces male characteristics	andr/o-	________	________
4.	Pertaining to the medulla	medull/o-	________	________
5.	Pertaining to the ovaries	ovari/o-	________	________
6.	Condition of staying the same	home/o-	________	________
7.	Process of exciting	stimul/o-	________	________
8.	Resembling a shield-shaped structure	thyr/o-	________	________
9.	Pertaining to the pancreas	pancreat/o-	________	________
10.	Pertaining to the testicle	testicul/o-	________	________

Combining Forms and Prefixes

Read the definition hint for the medical word you are to build. Look at the medical word or word part that is given. It already contains a combining form and a suffix. Write the correct prefix on the blank line. Then write the medical word. (Remember: You may need to remove the combining vowel. Always remove the hyphens and slash.) Use the Answer Key at the end of the book to check your answers. The first one has been done for you.

PREFIX LIST

eu- (normal, good)	para- (beside; apart from; two parts of a pair; abnormal)	pro- (before)
hypo- (below; deficient)		syn- (together)

	Definition Hint	Prefix	Medical Word or Word Part	Write the Medical Word
1.	Pertaining to something that grows below	hypo-	physial	hypophysial
2.	Process of normal thyroid	________	thyroidism	________
3.	Pertaining to two parts of a pair beside the thyroid gland	________	thyroid	________
4.	Pertaining to a gland below the thalamus	________	thalamic	________
5.	Substance (hormone) that acts before milk comes in	________	lactin	________
6.	Process of working together	________	ergism	________

Symptoms, Signs, and Diseases

Anterior Pituitary Gland: All Hormones

Word or Phase	Word Part and Definition	Description
hyperpituitarism	**hyperpituitarism** (HY-per-pih-TOO-ih-tah-rizm) **hyper-** *above; more than normal* **pituitar/o-** *pituitary gland* **-ism** *process; disease from a specific cause* **hypersecretion** (HY-per-seh-KREE-shun) **hyper-** *above; more than normal* **secret/o-** *produce; secrete* **-ion** *action; condition* **adenoma** (AD-eh-NOH-mah) **aden/o-** *gland* **-oma** *tumor, mass* **adenomata** (AD-eh-NOH-mah-tah) *Adenoma* is a Greek noun. Form the plural by changing *-oma* to *-omata.*	**Hypersecretion** of one or all of the hormones from the anterior pituitary gland. Caused by a benign tumor (**adenoma**) in the pituitary gland. Treatment: Surgery to remove the tumor.
hypopituitarism	**hypopituitarism** (HY-poh-pih-TOO-ih-tah-rizm) **hypo-** *below; deficient* **pituitar/o-** *pituitary gland* **-ism** *process; disease from a specific cause* **hyposecretion** (HY-poh-seh-KREE-shun) **hypo-** *below; deficient* **secret/o-** *produce; secrete* **-ion** *action; condition* **panhypopituitarism** (pan-HY-poh-pih-TOO-eh-tah-rizm) **pan-** *all* **hypo-** *below; deficient* **pituitar/o-** *pituitary gland* **-ism** *process; disease from a specific cause*	**Hyposecretion** of one or all of the hormones of the anterior pituitary gland. Caused by injury or a defect in the pituitary gland itself. **Panhypopituitarism** is a condition in which there is hyposecretion of all of the hormones of the anterior pituitary gland. Treatment: Drug therapy to replace those hormones.

Anterior Pituitary Gland: Prolactin

Word or Phase	Word Part and Definition	Description
galactorrhea	**galactorrhea** (gah-LAK-toh-REE-ah) **galact/o-** *milk* **-rrhea** *flow, discharge*	Hypersecretion of prolactin. This causes secretion of milk from the breasts, even though the patient is not pregnant. Also causes cessation of menstrual cycles by inhibiting secretion of FSH and LH. Treatment: Drug to suppress the production of prolactin. Surgery to remove the adenoma from the anterior pituitary gland.
failure of lactation	**lactation** (lak-TAY-shun) **lact/o-** *milk* **-ation** *a process; being or having*	Hyposecretion of prolactin. This causes lack of development of lactiferous glands in the breasts during puberty and inability of the breasts to produce sufficient milk for breastfeeding after the baby is born. Treatment: None.

Anterior Pituitary Gland: Growth Hormone

Word or Phase	Word Part and Definition	Description
gigantism	**gigantism** (jy-GAN-tizm) (JY-gan-tizm) **gigant/o-** *giant* **-ism** *process; disease from a specific cause*	Hypersecretion of growth hormone during childhood and puberty. Causes all the bones and tissues to grow continuously. Treatment: Drug to suppress the production of growth hormone. Radiation therapy. Surgery to remove the adenoma from the anterior pituitary gland.
acromegaly	**acromegaly** (AK-roh-MEG-ah-lee) **acr/o-** *extremity; highest point* **-megaly** *enlargement*	Hypersecretion of growth hormone during adulthood. Because the growth plates at the ends of the long bones are already fused, the patient cannot grow taller. Growth hormone causes the facial features to become wider and enlarged and the jaw enlarges. The hands and feet become wider (see Figure 14-10■). Treatment: Drug to suppress the production of growth hormone. Radiation therapy. Surgery to remove the adenoma from the anterior pituitary gland.

Did You Know?

The tallest man who ever lived suffered from gigantism. His name was Robert Wadlow. He was born in 1918 in Illinois and was of average weight and length at birth. By the time he was 18 years old, he was 8′11″ and weighed 491 pounds. He wore size 37AA shoes that were over 18″ in length. He died in 1940, at the age of 22.

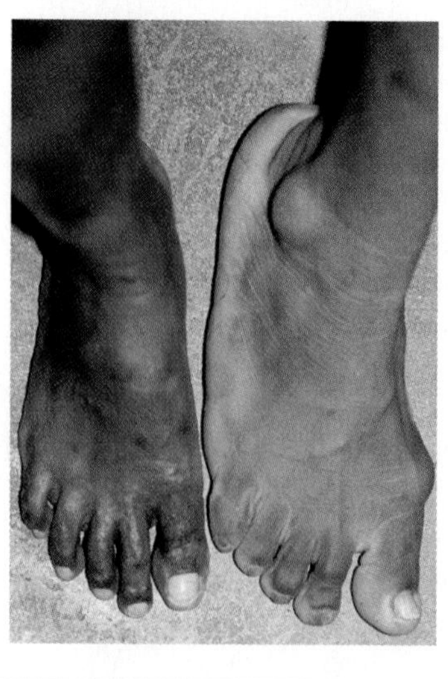

Figure 14-10 ■ Acromegaly. Increased levels of growth hormone in adulthood cause the face and extremities to widen rather than grow longer. The foot on the left is normal. The foot on the right shows acromegaly with enlargement and widening.

Word or Phase	Word Part and Definition	Description
dwarfism	**dwarfism** (DWORF-izm) *Dwarfism* is a combination of the word *dwarf* and the suffix *-ism* (process; disease from a specific cause).	Hyposecretion of growth hormone during childhood and puberty. Causes a lack of growth and short stature but with normal body proportions. Treatment: Growth hormone drug. Note: Dwarfism has many other causes. One common cause, achondroplasia, is a genetic mutation in which cartilage does not convert to bone. This results in a dwarf with small extremities but a normal sized trunk. Short stature in an otherwise normal person can also be caused by severe malnutrition, very short parents (heredity), or severe kidney or heart disease.
Posterior Pituitary Gland: Antidiuretic Hormone (ADH)		
syndrome of inappropriate ADH (SIADH)		Hypersecretion of antidiuretic hormone (ADH). ADH moves water from the renal tubules back into the blood. Too much ADH causes fluid and electrolyte imbalance. Treatment: Restriction of water intake. Surgery to remove the adenoma from the posterior pituitary gland.
diabetes insipidus (DI)	**diabetes** (DY-ah-BEE-teez) *Diabetes* is a Greek word meaning *a siphon.* **insipidus** (in-SIP-ih-dus) *Insipidus* is a Latin word meaning *lacking a distinctive taste.* Patients with diabetes insipidus have tasteless, dilute urine, like water. **polyuria** (PAWL-ee-YOO-ree-ah) **poly-** *many, much* **ur/o-** *urine; urinary system* **-ia** *condition, state, thing* **polydipsia** (PAWL-ee-DIP-see-ah) **poly-** *many, much* **dips/o-** *thirst* **-ia** *condition, state, thing*	Hyposecretion of antidiuretic hormone (ADH). Causes excessive amounts of water to be excreted in the urine (**polyuria**). Other symptoms include weakness, thirst (due to water loss and dehydration), and increased intake of fluids (**polydipsia**). Treatment: Antidiuretic hormone drug.
Posterior Pituitary Gland: Oxytocin		
		There is no specific disease associated with hypersecretion of oxytocin.
postpartum hemorrhage	**postpartum** (post-PAR-tum) **post-** *after, behind* **-partum** *childbirth* **hemorrhage** (HEM-oh-rij) **hem/o-** *blood* **-rrhage** *excessive flow or discharge*	Hyposecretion of oxytocin. This causes continual bleeding from the uterus at the site where the placenta separates at birth. Treatment: Oxytocin drug.

Word or Phase	Word Part and Definition	Description
uterine inertia	**uterine** (YOO-ter-in) (YOO-ter-ine) **uter/o-** *uterus* **-ine** *pertaining to* **inertia** (in-ER-shah) (in-ER-shee-ah) *Inertia* is a Latin word meaning *inactivity or laziness.*	Hyposecretion of oxytocin. Causes weak or uncoordinated contractions of the pregnant uterus during labor. Treatment: Oxytocin drug.
Pineal Gland: Melatonin		
seasonal affective disorder (SAD)	**affective** (ah-FEK-tiv) **affect/o-** *state of mind; mood; to have an influence on* **-ive** *pertaining to*	Hypersecretion of melatonin. Melatonin is normally produced during the dark hours of each day. During the winter months when the nights are longer and there are fewer hours of bright sunlight, melatonin and melatonin-stimulating hormone (MSH) levels are increased. This can trigger seasonal affective disorder, a mood disorder characterized by depression, weight gain, and an increased desire for food and sleep. Treatment: Exposing the skin to sunlight or light from a light box for several hours each day.
		There is no specific disease associated with hyposecretion of melatonin.
Thyroid Gland: T_3 and T_4 Thyroid Hormones		
goiter	**goiter** (GOY-ter) *Goiter* is derived from a French word for *throat.* **thyromegaly** (THY-roh-MEG-ah-lee) **thyr/o-** *shield-shaped structure (thyroid gland)* **-megaly** *enlargement* **iodine** (EYE-oh-dine) (EYE-oh-deen) **nontoxic** (non-TAWK-sik) **non-** *not* **tox/o-** *poison* **-ic** *pertaining to* **endemic** (en-DEM-ik) **en-** *in, within, inward* **dem/o-** *people; population* **-ic** *pertaining to* **adenoma** (AD-eh-NOH-mah) **aden/o-** *gland* **-oma** *tumor, mass*	Chronic and progressive enlargement of the thyroid gland (see Figure 14-11■). Mild-to-moderate thyroid gland enlargement is known as **thyromegaly**. The physician can feel enlargement on physical examination (see Figure 14-12■) even before it becomes visible. Causes of goiter and thyromegaly include the following: 1. A lack of **iodine** in the soil and the diet. This causes the thyroid gland to enlarge to be able to capture more iodine. This is known as a **simple goiter,** a **nontoxic goiter,** or an **endemic goiter** (because it occurs in people who live in a geographic area where the soil is poor in iodine). 2. An **adenoma** or **nodule** growing in the thyroid gland. This enlarges that part of the gland. This is known as an **adenomatous goiter** or a **nodular goiter.** If there are many nodules, this is known as a **multinodular goiter.** 3. An autoimmune disease such as Hashimoto's thyroiditis or Graves' disease. Treatment: Addition of iodine to the diet. Surgical removal of adenoma or nodule. **Figure 14-11 ■ Goiter.** A goiter can be a mild, subtle swelling in the neck, or it can enlarge enough to cause difficulty swallowing and breathing.

Word or Phase	Word Part and Definition	Description
goiter (*continued*)	**adenomatous** (AD-eh-NOH-mah-tus) aden/o- *gland* -oma *tumor, mass* -tous *pertaining to* **nodule** (NAWD-yool) nod/o- *node (knob of tissue)* -ule *small thing* **nodular** (NAWD-yoo-lar) nod/o- *node (knob of tissue)* -ular *pertaining to something small thing* **multinodular** (MUL-tee-NAWD-yoo-lar) mult/i- *many* nod/o- *node (knob of tissue)* -ular *pertaining to something small*	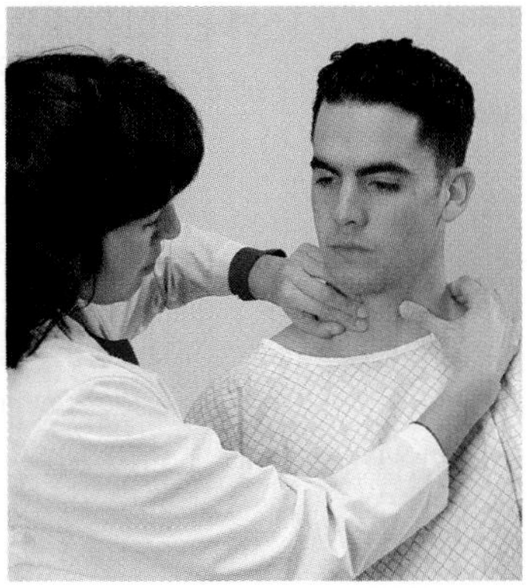 **Figure 14-12 ■ Physical examination of the thyroid gland.** The anterior location of the thyroid gland means that even mild enlargement can be detected. This physician is palpating the edges of the patient's thyroid gland to determine its size.
Graves' disease	**Graves' disease** (GRAYVZ) Named by Robert Graves (1796–1853), an Irish physician. **toxic** (TAWK-sik) tox/o- *poison* -ic *pertaining to* **exophthalmos** (EK-sawf-THAL-mohs) *Exophthalmos* is a combination of the prefix *ex-* (away from, out) and the Greek word *ophthalmos* (eye).	The most common form of hyperthyroidism. This is an autoimmune disease in which the body produces antibodies that stimulate TSH receptors on the thyroid gland, increasing the production of thyroid hormones. The entire thyroid gland is enlarged (**diffuse toxic goiter**), and there is **exophthalmos** in which the eyes bulge and appear to stare because of the large amount of white sclerae that is visible around the pupils) (see Figure 14-13■). Treatment: Drug that suppresses the production of T_3 and T_4 or surgical removal of the thyroid gland (thyroidectomy). 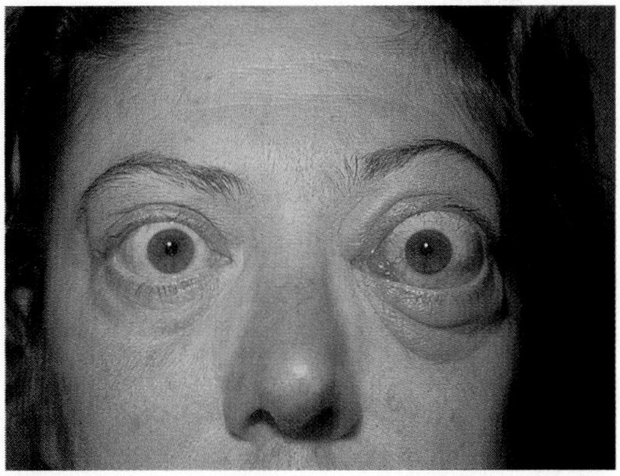 **Figure 14-13 ■ Exophthalmos.** Exophthalmos is a well-known symptom of hyperthyroidism. Edema in the tissues behind the eyeballs causes them to protrude forward to an abnormal degree.

Word or Phase	Word Part and Definition	Description
hyperthyroidism	**hyperthyroidism** (HY-per-THY-royd-izm) **hyper-** *above; more than normal* **thyroid/o-** *thyroid gland* **-ism** *process; disease from a specific cause* **thyrotoxicosis** (THY-roh-TAWK-sih-KOH-sis) **thyr/o-** *shield-shaped structure (thyroid gland)* **toxic/o-** *poison, toxin* **-osis** *condition; abnormal condition; process* Add words to make a correct and complete definition of *thyrotoxicosis: An abnormal condition [in which hypersecretion of the] thyroid gland [acts as a] poison or toxin [to the body].*	Hypersecretion of T_3 and T_4 thyroid hormones. Caused by an adenoma or a nodule in the thyroid gland. (It can also be caused by hypersecretion of TSH from an adenoma in the anterior pituitary gland.) There is thyroid enlargement that can be felt on palpation of the neck. The eyes are dry and irritated with slow eyelid closing (known as lid lag). There are tremors of the hands, tachycardia, palpitations, restlessness, nervousness, diarrhea, insomnia, fatigue, and generalized weight loss. Hyperthyroidism is also known as **thyrotoxicosis** because of the toxic effect of high levels of thyroid hormones. The sudden onset of severe hyperthyroidism is known as a **thyroid storm.** Treatment: Drug that suppresses the production of T_3 and T_4 or surgical removal of the thyroid gland (thyroidectomy).
hypothyroidism	**hypothyroidism** (HY-poh-THY-royd-izm) **hypo-** *below; deficient* **thyroid/o-** *thyroid gland* **-ism** *process; disease from a specific cause* **myxedema** (MIK-seh-DEE-mah) **myx/o-** *mucus-like substance* **-edema** *swelling* In myxedema, a mucus-like thick substance deposited in the subcutaneous and connective tissues causes edema. **congenital** (con-JEN-ih-tal) **congenit/o-** *present at birth* **-al** *pertaining to* **cretinism** (KREE-tin-izm) *Cretinism* is a combination of the word *cretin* and the suffix *-ism* (process; disease from a specific cause). *Crétin* is a French word meaning *mentally deficient person.*	Hyposecretion of T_3 and T_4 thyroid hormones. Caused by thyroiditis or by drugs prescribed to treat hyperthyroidism. (It can also be caused by hyposecretion of TSH from the anterior pituitary gland.) Mild hypothyroidism in adults is characterized by fatigue, decreased body temperature, dry hair and skin, constipation, and weight gain. Severe hypothyroidism in adults is characterized by **myxedema** with swelling of the subcutaneous and connective tissues in various parts of the body, tingling in the hands and feet because of nerve compression, an enlarged heart, bradycardia, an enlarged tongue, slow speech, and mental impairment. **Congenital** hypothyroidism is a deficiency of thyroid hormone production in an infant; if untreated, this causes mental retardation (**cretinism**). Treatment: T_3 and T_4 thyroid hormone drug. **Connections** **Dietetics.** The ancient Chinese used seaweed to treat thyroid enlargement; it was effective because seaweed contains iodine. There have been few cases of endemic goiter in the United States since the introduction of iodized table salt in 1924.
thyroid carcinoma	**carcinoma** (KAR-sih-NOH-mah) **carcin/o-** *cancer* **-oma** *tumor, mass*	Malignant tumor of the thyroid gland. There is hoarseness, neck pain, and enlargement of the lymph nodes. Treatment: Radioactive iodine to destroy thyroid cells or thyroidectomy.

Word or Phase	Word Part and Definition	Description
thyroid nodule	**nodule** (NAWD-yool) **nod/o-** *node (knob of tissue)* **-ule** *small thing*	One or many small tumors that arise from the thyroid gland itself. It is usually benign, but can sometimes be cancerous. Treatment: Thyroidectomy if many nodules.
thyroiditis	**thyroiditis** (THY-roy-DY-tis) **thyroid/o-** *thyroid gland* **-itis** *inflammation of* **Hashimoto** (HAH-shee-MOH-toh) Named by Hakaru Hashimoto (1881–1934), a Japanese surgeon.	Chronic inflammation and progressive destruction of the thyroid gland. The most common form is **Hashimoto's thyroiditis,** an autoimmune disorder in which the body forms antibodies against its own thyroid gland. The thyroid becomes inflamed and enlarged (goiter). Over time, the patient develops hypothyroidism as thyroid tissue is destroyed and replaced by fibrous tissue. Treatment: T_3 and T_4 thyroid hormone drug.
	Parathyroid Glands: Parathyroid Hormone	
hyperpara-thyroidism	**hyperparathyroidism** (HY-per-PAIR-ah-THY-royd-izm) **hyper-** *above; more than normal* **para-** *beside, apart from; two parts of a pair; abnormal* **thyroid/o-** *thyroid gland* **-ism** *process; disease from a specific cause* **hypercalcemia** (HY-per-kal-SEE-mee-ah) **hyper-** *above; more than normal* **calc/o-** *calcium* **-emia** *condition of the blood; substance in the blood*	Hypersecretion of parathyroid hormone. Caused by an adenoma in the parathyroid glands. The calcium level in the blood becomes very high (**hypercalcemia**) as the bones lose calcium and become demineralized and prone to fracture. Excess calcium in the blood is excreted in the urine, and this can form kidney stones. Treatment: Surgery to remove the parathyroid glands.
hypopara-thyroidism	**hypoparathyroidism** (HY-poh-PAIR-ah-THY-royd-izm) **hypo-** *below; deficient* **para-** *beside, apart from; two parts of a pair; abnormal* **thyroid/o-** *thyroid gland* **-ism** *process; disease from a specific cause* **hypocalcemia** (HY-poh-kal-SEE-mee-ah) **hypo-** *below; deficient* **calc/o-** *calcium* **-emia** *condition of the blood; substance in the blood*	Hyposecretion of parathyroid hormone. Caused by accidental removal of the parathyroid glands during a thyroidectomy. The calcium level in the blood becomes very low (**hypocalcemia**), causing irritability of the nerves and skeletal muscle cramps or sustained muscle spasm (tetany). Treatment: Parathyroid hormone drug.

Pancreas: Insulin

Word or Phase	Word Part and Definition	Description
hyperinsulinism	**hyperinsulinism** (HY-per-IN-soo-lin-izm) **hyper-** *above; more than normal* **insulin/o-** *insulin* **-ism** *process; disease from a specific cause* **resistance** (ree-ZIS-tans) **resist/o-** *withstand the effect of* **-ance** *state of*	Hypersecretion of insulin. Caused by a tumor in the pancreas or by **insulin resistance syndrome (IRS),** in which receptors on body cells show resistance and do not allow insulin to bring glucose into the cell to be metabolized. The pancreas secretes large amounts of insulin to over come the resistance. When the pancreas can no longer secrete large amounts of insulin, the patient develops type 2 diabetes mellitus. Treatment: Surgery to remove the tumor. Oral antidiabetic drugs to treat type 2 diabetes mellitus. 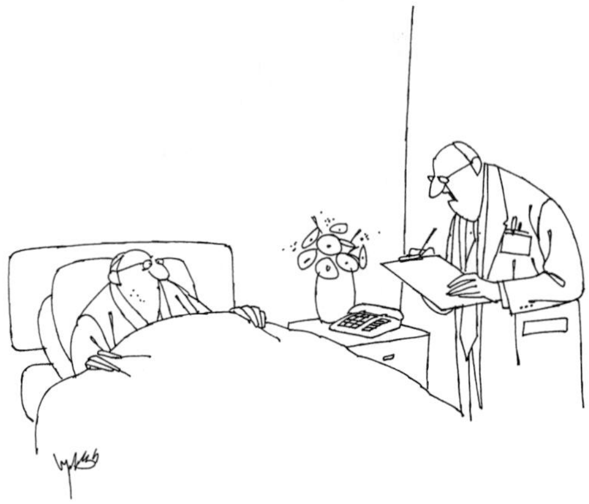 "Your chart says you have IRS . . . It's either a problem with insulin resistance syndrome or the Internal Revenue Service."
diabetes mellitus (DM)	**diabetes** (DY-ah-BEE-teez) *Diabetes* is a Greek word meaning *a siphon.* **mellitus** (MEL-ih-tus) *Mellitus* means *honeyed* because of the large amounts of glucose present in the urine. In ancient times, when physicians tasted the urine of diabetics, they found that it tasted sweet. **hyperglycemia** (HY-per-gly-SEE-mee-ah) **hyper-** *above; more than normal* **glyc/o-** *glucose (sugar)* **-emia** *condition of the blood; substance in the blood* **diabetic** (DY-ah-BET-ik) **diabet/o-** *diabetes* **-ic** *pertaining to*	Hyposecretion of insulin. There is an elevated level of glucose in the blood (**hyperglycemia**). A person who has diabetes is said to be a **diabetic.** Excess glucose in the blood is excreted in the urine (**glycosuria**). If blood glucose levels remain high, there is increased urine production (**polyuria**) and the patient drinks often (**polydipsia**). The patient also feels hungry and eats often (**polyphagia**) because the glucose in the blood cannot enter the cells without insulin. A brittle diabetic is one who is being treated for diabetes but has difficulty controlling blood glucose levels, with frequent swings from hyperglycemia to hypoglycemia. **Type 1 diabetes mellitus** is caused by destruction of the beta cells of the islets of Langerhans in the pancreas. The pancreas secretes little or no insulin. Type 1 diabetes mellitus is an autoimmune response that may be triggered by a viral infection or an inherited genetic predisposition. Type 1 diabetes mellitus begins in childhood or adolescence (see Table 14-1). Treatment: Daily injections of insulin, diet management, weight control, exercise. *(continued)*

Word or Phase	Word Part and Definition	Description
diabetes mellitus *(continued)*	**glycosuria** (GLY-koh-SYOO-ree-ah) glycos/o- *glucose (sugar)* ur/o- *urine; urinary system* -ia *condition, state, thing* **polyuria** (PAWL-ee-YOO-ree-ah) poly- *many, much* ur/o- *urine; urinary system* -ia *condition, state, thing* **polydipsia** (PAWL-ee-DIP-see-ah) poly- *many, much* dips/o- *thirst* -ia *condition, state, thing* **polyphagia** (PAWL-ee-FAY-jee-ah) poly- *many, much* phag/o- *eating, swallowing* -ia *condition, state, thing* **gestational** (jes-TAY-shun-al) gestat/o- *from conception to birth* -ation *a process; being or having* -al *pertaining to*	**Type 2 diabetes mellitus** is caused by decreased function of the beta cells and decreased amounts of insulin coupled with a decreased number of insulin receptors on the cell membranes. Type 2 diabetes mellitus begins in middle age with a gradual onset. Risk factors include obesity and a family history of diabetes. Treatment: Diet management, weight control, exercise. Oral antidiabetic drugs are often needed. Occasionally, insulin injections are needed. "Sugar diabetes" is a layperson's phrase that refers to diabetes mellitus type 1 or type 2. **Gestational diabetes mellitus** occurs only during pregnancy and resolves once the pregnancy is delivered; however, many patients develop type 2 diabetes later in life.

Word Alert

SOUND-ALIKE WORDS

diabetes insipidus — Caused by hyposecretion of antidiuretic hormone (ADH) from the posterior pituitary gland.

diabetes mellitus — Caused by hyposecretion of insulin by the pancreas

A Closer Look

Excessive urination (polyuria) is a symptom of both diabetes insipidus and diabetes mellitus, but for different reasons. In diabetes insipidus, a lack of ADH causes excessive production of urine. In diabetes mellitus, excess glucose is excreted in the urine, pulling water with it because of osmotic pressure.

Table 14-1 Diabetes Mellitus

Type	Type 1	Type 2
Former Names	Insulin-dependent diabetes mellitus (IDDM)	Non–insulin-dependent diabetes mellitus (NIDDM)
	Juvenile-onset diabetes mellitus	Adult-onset diabetes mellitus
Onset	Childhood, young adulthood	Middle age
Contributing Factors	Viral trigger, heredity	Obesity, heredity
Treatment	Insulin, diet management, weight control, exercise	Oral antidiabetic drugs, sometimes insulin, diet management, weight control, exercise

Word or Phase	Word Part and Definition	Description
diabetic ketoacidosis	**ketoacidosis** (KEE-toh-AS-ih-DOH-sis) ket/o- *ketones* acid/o- *acid (low pH)* -osis *condition; abnormal condition; process* **ketones** (KEE-tohnz)	Excessive amounts of **ketones** in the blood. When there is no insulin to metabolize glucose, the body turns to other sources of energy like fat or protein. Body fat contains the most calories per gram, but body fat does not metabolize cleanly and leaves ketones, an acidic byproduct. The patient's breath has a unique "fruity" or "nail polish" odor from the high levels of glucose and ketones in the blood. Large amounts of ketones lower the pH of the blood to the point that chemical reactions in the body cannot occur and the patient becomes unconscious (diabetic coma). Treatment: Insulin and glucose drugs.
hypoglycemia	**hypoglycemia** (HY-poh-gly-SEE-mee-ah) hypo- *below; deficient* glyc/o- *glucose (sugar)* -emia *condition of the blood; substance in the blood*	Low levels of glucose in the blood. Caused by diabetics who take an antidiabetic pill or inject insulin but then miss a meal. (It can also occur in nondiabetic patients who are dieting or fasting.) There is headache, dizziness, sweating, shakiness, and tunnel vision. If left untreated, hypoglycemia can progress to insulin shock and then coma as the blood glucose level becomes too low to support brain activity. Treatment: Glucose in food or as a drug.

A Closer Look

Diabetic complications include diseases of various organs of the body because of the effects of diabetes mellitus.

neuropathy (nyoo-RAWP-ah-thee)
neur/o- *nerve*
-pathy *disease, suffering*

nephropathy (neh-FRAWP-ah-thee)
nephr/o- *kidney; nephron*
-pathy *disease, suffering*

retinopathy (RET-ih-NAWP-ah-thee)
retin/o- *retina (of the eye)*
-pathy *disease, suffering*

1. **Diabetic neuropathy.** Decreased or abnormal sensation in the extremities because of nerve damage due to demyelinization of the nerves.
2. **Diabetic nephropathy.** Degenerative changes, fibrosis, and scarring in the nephrons of the kidneys because of the local effects of biochemical imbalances.
3. **Diabetic retinopathy.** Degenerative changes of the retina of the eye because of the local effects of biochemical imbalances. There is formation of new, abnormally fragile blood vessels that produce frequent hemorrhages.
4. Atherosclerosis. Fatty deposits and plaque formation with hardening of the arteries is accelerated in diabetes mellitus because of abnormalities in fat metabolism.
5. Impotence. Nerve damage and atherosclerosis of the arteries to the penis result in difficulty having an erection.

Connections

Podiatry. Diabetic patients are at high risk for developing gangrene of the feet. They are advised to see a podiatrist or physician to have their toenails trimmed. Poor eyesight (from age and diabetic retinopathy) coupled with decreased sensation in the lower extremities (diabetic neuropathy) makes it easy for diabetic patients to cut themselves when trimming their toenails. Small cuts do not heal because of poor blood flow from atherosclerosis and may progress to gangrene of the foot.

Adrenal Cortex: Aldosterone

Word or Phase	Word Part and Definition	Description
hyperaldosteronism	**hyperaldosteronism** (HY-per-al-DAWS-ter-ohn-izm) *Hyperaldosteronism* is a combination of the prefix *hyper-* (above; more than normal), *aldosterone* (with the -e deleted) and the suffix *-ism* (process; disease from a specific cause).	Hypersecretion of aldosterone. Caused by an adenoma in the adrenal cortex. (It can also be caused by hypersecretion of ACTH from an adenoma in the anterior pituitary gland.) Excess aldosterone (1) holds large amounts of sodium in the blood (this causes hypertension) and (2) sends large amounts of potassium to be excreted in the urine (this causes electrolyte imbalance and weakness). Treatment: Surgery to remove the adenoma from the adrenal cortex or anterior pituitary gland.
hypoaldosteronism	**hypoaldosteronism** (HY-poh-al-DAWS-ter-ohn-izm)	Hyposecretion of aldosterone. Rare condition caused by an inherited genetic abnormality of the adrenal cortex. Treatment: Aldosterone drug.

Adrenal Cortex: Cortisol

Word or Phase	Word Part and Definition	Description
Cushing's syndrome	**Cushing** (KOOSH-ing) Named by Harvey Cushing (1869–1939), an American surgeon. **syndrome** (SIN-drohm) **syn-** *together* **-drome** *a running* A syndrome is many different symptoms and signs that make up one disease.	Hypersecretion of cortisol. Caused by an adenoma in the adrenal cortex. (When it is caused by hypersecretion of ACTH from an adenoma in the anterior pituitary gland, this is known as Cushing's disease.) It can also occur in a patient who takes corticosteroid drugs on a long-term basis because of an autoimmune disease. Cushing's syndrome is characterized by many different symptoms. Excess cortisol breaks down too much glycogen and causes elevated levels of glucose in the blood. This results in weight gain, with deposits of fat in the face (moon face) (see Figure 14-14■), upper back (buffalo hump), and abdomen. There is also a wasted appearance in the muscles of the extremities and weakness because of the lack of protein synthesis. Hypersecretion of ACTH from the pituitary gland causes the adrenal cortex to produce excess androgens, and this produces dark facial hair and amenorrhea in women. Treatment: Surgery to remove the adenoma from the adrenal cortex or anterior pituitary gland. 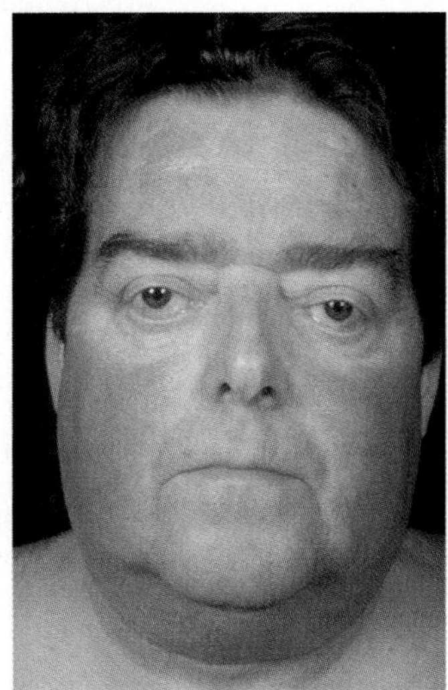 **Figure 14-14 ■ Cushing's syndrome.** This patient shows the characteristic signs of Cushing's syndrome. There is deposition of fat in the cheeks with a moon face appearance. At the same time there is break down of protein in the connective tissues of the skin. The skin becomes thin, allowing blood vessels to show through and give the cheeks a reddened appearance.

Word or Phase	Word Part and Definition	Description
Addison's disease	**Addison** (AD-ih-son) Named by Thomas Addison (1793–1860), an English physician.	Hyposecretion of cortisol. This is an autoimmune disease in which the body produces antibodies that destroy the adrenal cortex. (It can also be caused by hyposecretion of ACTH from the anterior pituitary gland.) There are low levels of blood glucose, fatigue, weight loss, and decreased ability to tolerate stress, disease, or surgery. Patients have an unusual bronzed color to the skin, even in areas not exposed to the sun. Treatment: Corticosteroid drugs.
Adrenal Cortex: Androgens		
adrenogenital syndrome	**adrenogenital** (ah-DREE-noh-JEN-ih-tal) **adren/o-** *adrenal gland* **genit/o-** *genitalia* **-al** *pertaining to* **virilism** (VIR-ih-lizm) **viril/o-** *masculine* **-ism** *process; disease from a specific cause* **hirsutism** (HER-soo-tizm) **hirsut/o-** *hairy* **-ism** *process; disease from a specific cause*	Hypersecretion of androgens. Caused by an adenoma in the adrenal gland. In girls, it causes the clitorus and labia to enlarge and resemble a penis and scrotum. In boys, it causes precocious puberty. In adult females, it causes **virilism** with masculine facial features and body build, **hirsutism** (excessive, dark hair on the forearms and face), and amenorrhea). Treatment: Surgery to remove the adenoma from the adrenal cortex.
		There is no specific disease associated with hyposecretion of androgens.
Adrenal Medulla: Epinephrine and Norepinephrine		
pheochromocytoma	**pheochromocytoma** (FEE-oh-KROH-moh-sy-TOH-mah) **phe/o-** *gray* **chrom/o-** *color* **cyt/o-** *cell* **-oma** *tumor, mass* Add words to make a correct and complete definition of *pheochromocytoma: tumor [with a] gray color to the cells [when viewed under the microscope].*	Hypersecretion of epinephrine and norepinephrine. Caused by an adenoma in the adrenal medulla. There are headaches and severe hypertension that can cause a stroke. Treatment: Surgery to remove the adenoma from the adrenal medulla.
		There is no specific disease associated with hyposecretion of epinephrine and norepinephrine.

Ovaries: Estradiol and Progesterone

Word or Phase	Word Part and Definition	Description
precocious puberty	**precocious** (prih-KOH-shus) *Precocious* is an English word meaning *pertaining to premature development.* **puberty** (PYOO-ber-tee) *Puberty* is derived from a Latin word meaning *grown up.*	Hypersecretion of estradiol. Caused by an adenoma in the ovary. (It can also be caused by hypersecretion of FSH and LH from an adenoma in the anterior pituitary gland.) There is premature development of the breasts, menstruation, and ovulation in a child. Treatment: Surgery to remove the adenoma.
infertility		Imbalance or lack of estradiol or progesterone. (It can also be caused by a lack of FSH and LH from the anterior pituitary gland.) There is a lack of ovulation, abnormal menstruation, or history of miscarriage. Treatment: Hormone drugs.
menopause	**menopause** (MEN-oh-pawz) **men/o-** *month* **-pause** *cessation*	Hyposecretion of estradiol. Caused by the aging process in which the ovaries secrete progressively less estradiol. There is vaginal dryness, thinning of the hair, and lack of sex drive. As the hypothalamus senses low estradiol levels, it stimulates the anterior pituitary gland to secrete FSH and LH to stimulate the ovary. This causes hot flashes. Treatment: Hormone replacement therapy.

Testes: Testosterone

Word or Phase	Word Part and Definition	Description
precocious puberty		Hypersecretion of testosterone. Caused by an adenoma in the testis. (It can also be caused by hypersecretion of FSH and LH from an adenoma in the anterior pituitary gland.) There is premature development of a beard, deepening of the voice, and sperm production in a child. Treatment: Surgery to remove the adenoma.
gynecomastia	**gynecomastia** (GY-neh-koh-MAS-tee-ah) **gynec/o-** *female, woman* **mast/o-** *breast; mastoid process* **-ia** *condition, state, thing*	Enlargement of the male breasts. In the male, androgens secreted by the adrenal cortex and testosterone secreted by the testes are converted to estradiol. Any change in the adrenal cortex or the testes decreases the total amount of androgens/testosterone and increases the relative amount of estradiol, creating an imbalance of androgens and estradiol. Caused by puberty, aging, surgical removal of the testes, or estrogen drug treatment for prostate cancer. Treatment: Androgen drug. Plastic surgery to decrease breast size.
infertility	**infertility** (IN-fer-TIL-ih-tee) **in-** *in; without; not* **fertil/o-** *able to conceive a child* **-ity** *state; condition*	Hyposecretion of testosterone. Caused by failure of one or both of the testes to descend into the scrotum before birth. Also caused by surgical removal of a testis because of cancer. (It can also be caused by an imbalance or lack of FSH and LH from the anterior pituitary gland.) Causes lack of sperm production. Treatment: Surgery to bring the testes into the scrotum. Androgen drug.

Diagnostic Procedures

Blood Tests

Word or Phase	Word Part and Definition	Description
antithyroglobulin antibodies	**antithyroglobulin** (AN-tee-THY-roh-GLAWB-yoo-lin) **anti-** *against* **thyr/o-** *shield-shaped structure (thyroid gland)* **globul/o-** *shaped like a globe* **-in** *a substance* **antibody** (AN-tee-BAWD-ee) (AN-tih-BAWD-ee) **anti-** *against* **-body** *a structure or thing*	Blood test that detects antibodies against thyroglobulin (precursor hormone to T_3 and T_4) in the thyroid gland. A positive test result indicates Hashimoto's thyroiditis.
calcium	**calcium** (KAL-see-um)	Blood test that measures the level of calcium. Used to evaluate the function of the parathyroid gland.
cortisol level	**cortisol** (KOR-tih-sawl) **hydroxycorticosteroids** (hy-DRAWK-see-KOR-tih-koh-STAIR-oydz)	Blood test that measures the level of cortisol. Used to evaluate the function of the adrenal cortex and the anterior pituitary gland. A metabolite of cortisol, **17-hydroxycorticosteroids,** can also be measured in the urine to indirectly measure the level of cortisol.
fasting blood sugar (FBS)		Blood test that measures the level of glucose after the patient has fasted (not eaten) for at least 12 hours. Used to evaluate the function of the pancreas.
FSH assay and LH assay	**assay** (AS-say) *Assay* is derived from an Old French word meaning *to weigh.*	Blood test that measures the levels of follicle-stimulating hormone (FSH) and luteinizing hormone (LH). Used to evaluate the function of the anterior pituitary gland and the ovaries and testes.
glucose self-testing	**glucose** (GLOO-kohs) **gluc/o-** *glucose (sugar)* **-ose** *full of*	Self-test blood test that measures the level of glucose. Diabetic patients test their own blood sugar level one or more times each day (see Figure 14-15■).

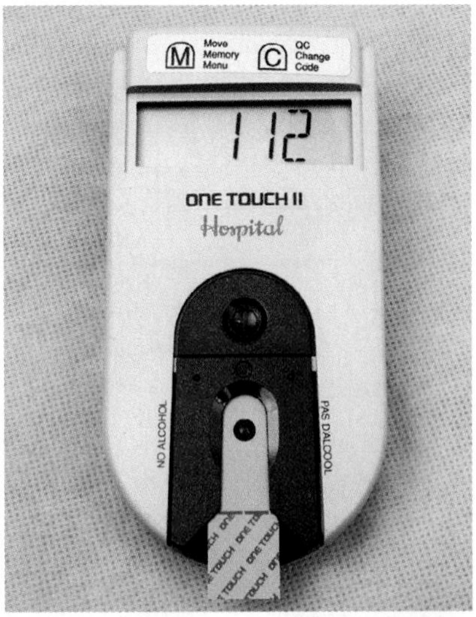

Figure 14-15 ■ Blood glucose monitor.

The patient pricks the fingertip and the drop of blood is placed on a test strip. It is inserted into the blood glucose monitor and the monitor displays the numerical value of the patient's blood glucose level.

Word or Phase	Word Part and Definition	Description
glucose tolerance test (GTT)	**Glucola** (gloo-KOH-lah) **dextrose** (DEKS-trohs) **dextr/o-** *right; sugar* **-ose** *full of* Dextrose is a molecule of glucose that bends to the right any light rays that pass through it. It is the form in which glucose is given intravenously.	Blood and urine tests that measure the level of glucose. Used to evaluate the function of the pancreas. After the patient has fasted for 12 hours, blood and urine specimens are obtained. Then the patient drinks glucose (in a sugary drink known as **Glucola**) or is given **dextrose** intravenously. Blood and urine specimens are obtained every hour for four hours. Normally, the blood glucose returns to normal within one to two hours. High blood and urine levels of glucose indicate diabetes mellitus. Also known as an **oral glucose tolerance test (OGTT).**
growth hormone		Blood test that measures the level of growth hormone (GH). Used to evaluate the function of the anterior pituitary gland.
hemoglobin A_{1C} (HbA_{1C})	**hemoglobin A_{1C}** (HEE-moh-gloh-bin AA-one-see) **glycohemoglobin** (GLY-koh-HEE-moh-gloh-bin) **glycosylated** (gly-KOH-sih-lay-ted)	Blood test that measures the A_{1C} fraction of hemoglobin in red blood cells. Hemoglobin A_{1C} binds with glucose. Because red blood cells only live about 12 weeks, the hemoglobin A_{1C} result indicates the average level of blood glucose during the previous 12 weeks. Used to monitor how well diabetic patients are controlling blood sugar with diet and drugs. Also known as **glycohemoglobin** or **glycosylated hemoglobin.**
testosterone		Blood test that measures the levels of total testosterone and free testosterone from the testes. Used to evaluate the function of the testes and the anterior pituitary gland.
thyroid function tests (TFTs)		Blood test that measures the levels of T_3, T_4, and TSH. Used to evaluate the function of the thyroid gland and the anterior pituitary gland. The test uses radioimmunoassay (RIA) technique in which antibodies labeled with radioactive isotopes combine with the hormone and the amount of radioactivity is measured. Another value, the free thyroxine index (FTI) or T_7, can be calculated from this.
Urine Tests		
ADH stimulation test		Urine test that measures the concentration of urine. Used to evaluate the function of the posterior pituitary gland. Water is withheld for 12 hours and a urine specimen is obtained. Then ADH is given (as the drug vasopressin), the patient drinks water, and another urine specimen is obtained. In a patient with diabetes insipidus, the second urine specimen will be more concentrated because of the ADH (vasopressin). Also known as the **water deprivation test.**
estradiol		Urine test that measures the level of estradiol. Used to evaluate the function of the ovaries and the anterior pituitary gland.
vanillylmandelic acid (VMA)	**vanillylmandelic acid** (VAN-ih-lil-man-DEL-ik AS-id)	A 24-hour urine test that measures the levels of epinephrine and norepinephrine. Used to evaluate the function of the adrenal medulla. Vanillylmandelic acid (VMA), a byproduct of these hormones, is measured.
urine dipstick		Urine test that measures glucose, ketones, and other substances in the urine. Rapid screening test used to evaluate diabetic patients.

Radiology Tests

Word or Phase	Word Part and Definition	Description
radioactive iodine uptake (RAIU) and thyroid scan	**radioactive** (RAY-dee-oh-AK-tiv) radi/o- *radius (forearm bone); x-ray; radiation* act/o- *active* -ive *pertaining to* **iodine** (EYE-oh-dine) (EYE-oh-deen)	Nuclear medicine procedure that combines a radioactive iodine uptake procedure and a thyroid scan. The radioactive iodine uptake demonstrates how well the thyroid gland is able to absorb iodine from the blood. The thyroid scan shows the size and shape of the thyroid gland. Two radioactive tracers are given, orally and intravenously. A normal scan will show uniform distribution of radioactive tracer throughout the thyroid gland. An adenoma appears as a bright ("hot") spot because of its increased uptake of radioactive iodine compared to the rest of the gland. A darker area (a "cold" spot) can either be a cyst or a cancerous tumor of the thyroid gland (neither of which take up iodine) (see Figure 14-16■). **Figure 14-16 ■ Thyroid scan.** This patient's thyroid scan shows a large, dark area in the inferior portion of one lobe. This is a "cold" spot, an area of decreased uptake of radioactive tracer. A "cold" spot can be a cyst or a cancerous tumor.

Medical and Surgical Procedures

Medical Procedures

Word or Phase	Word Part and Definition	Description
ADA diet		Special physician-prescribed diet for diabetic patients that follows the guidelines of the American Diabetes Association (ADA). The amounts of carbohydrate and fat are limited. The physician orders the upper limit for total daily number of calories for a diabetic patient in the hospital. Example: 1200-calorie ADA diet. Rather than using the ADA diet, diabetic patients can just count calories. A dietitian or diabetes educator helps the patient plan a menu that fits lifestyle and food preferences.

Surgical Procedures

Word or Phase	Word Part and Definition	Description
adrenalectomy	**adrenalectomy** (ah-DREE-nal-EK-toh-mee) adrenal/o- *adrenal gland* -ectomy *surgical excision*	Surgical procedure to remove the adrenal gland because of an adenoma or cancerous tumor.

Word or Phase	Word Part and Definition	Description
fine-needle biopsy	**biopsy** (BY-awp-see) **bi/o-** *life; living organisms; living tissue* **-opsy** *the process of viewing*	Surgical procedure that uses a fine needle to take a small sample of tissue from a thyroid nodule seen on a thyroid scan. The tissue is sent to the laboratory to determine if it is benign or malignant.
parathyroidectomy	**parathyroidectomy** (PAIR-ah-THY-roy-DEK-toh-mee) **para-** *beside, apart from; two parts of a pair; abnormal* **thyroid/o-** *thyroid gland* **-ectomy** *surgical excision*	Surgical procedure to remove one or more of the parathyroid glands to control hyperparathyoidism. Also, a parathyroidectomy can occur accidentally when the thyroid gland is surgically removed.
thymectomy	**thymectomy** (thy-MEK-toh-mee) **thym/o-** *thymus; rage* **-ectomy** *surgical excision*	Surgical procedure to remove the thymus in patients with myasthenia gravis.
thyroidectomy	**thyroidectomy** (THY-roy-DEK-toh-mee) **thyroid/o-** *thyroid gland* **-ectomy** *surgical excision* **lobectomy** (loh-BEK-toh-mee) **lob/o-** *lobe of an organ* **-ectomy** *surgical excision*	Surgical procedure to remove the thyroid gland. All of the thyroid gland or just one part (one lobe) can be removed (**subtotal thyroidectomy** or **thyroid lobectomy**).
transsphenoidal hypophysectomy	**transsphenoidal** (TRANS-sfee-NOY-dal) **trans-** *across, through* **sphenoid/o-** *sphenoid bone or sinus* **-al** *pertaining to* **hypophysectomy** (HY-pawf-ih-SEK-toh-mee) **hypophys/o-** *pituitary gland* **-ectomy** *surgical excision*	Surgical procedure to remove an adenoma from the pituitary gland (hypophysis). The pituitary gland is difficult to visualize through an incision in the cranium, so the incision is made through the sphenoid sinus.

Drug Categories

Several different categories of drugs are used to treat the symptoms, signs, and diseases of the endocrine system. The most common drugs in each category are listed.

Category	Word Part and Definition	Description	Example
antidiabetic drugs	**antidiabetic** (AN-tee-DY-ah-BET-ik) **anti-** *against* **diabet/o-** *diabetes* **-ic** *pertaining to*	Treat type 2 diabetes mellitus by stimulating the pancreas to produce more insulin. These drugs are given orally. They are not insulin and they are not used to treat patients with type 1 diabetes mellitus.	DiaBeta, Diabinese, Glucotrol
antithyroid drugs	**antithyroid** (AN-tee-THY-royd) (AN-tih-THY-royd)	Treat hyperthyroidism by inhibiting the production of T_3 and T_4.	Tapazole

Category	Word Part and Definition	Description	Example
corticosteroid drugs	**corticosteroid** (KOR-tih-koh-STAIR-oyd) corticl/o- *cortex (outer region)* -steroid *steroid*	Mimic the action of hormones from the adrenal cortex. Used to suppress inflammation. Used to treat Addison's disease.	cortisone, Decadron, hydrocortisone (cortisol) Florinef for Addison's disease.
growth hormone drugs		Provide growth hormone.	Humatrope, Protropin
insulin	**insulin** (IN-soo-lin)	Treats type 1 diabetes mellitus. Can be used for type 2 diabetes mellitus that cannot be controlled with oral antidiabetic drugs. Insulin must be injected from one to several times each day to control the blood sugar (see Figure 14-17■). Insulin is classified according to how quickly it acts (which depends on the size of the insulin crystal) and how many hours its therapeutic action continues (see Figure 14-18■).	rapid-acting insulins (regular, Humalog, Humulin R, Novolin R, NovoLog), intermediate-acting insulins (NPH, Humulin N, Novolin N), long-acting insulins (ultralente, Humulin U)

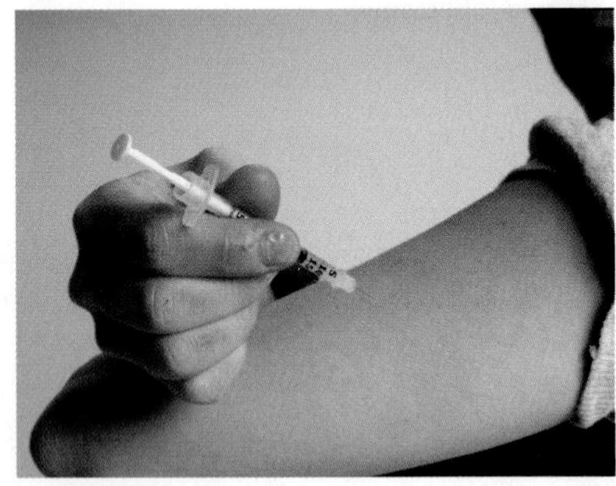

Figure 14-17 ■ Insulin injection.

Insulin is a liquid drug that must be injected subcutaneously into the fat layer beneath the skin. The needle is inserted at an angle so that it does not go into the muscle layer. The back of the arms, abdomen, and many other sites can be used for insulin injections. A new site must be selected for each injection.

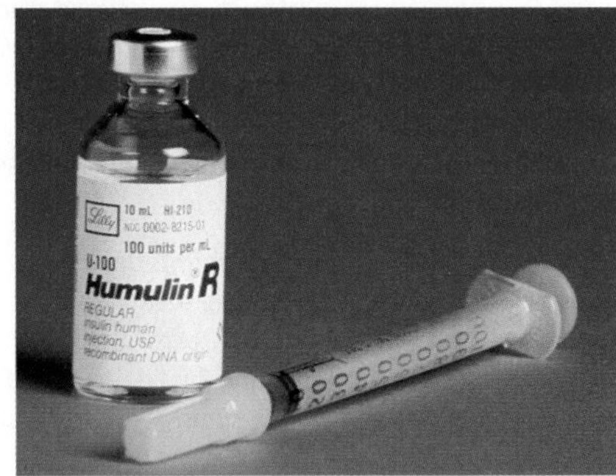

Figure 14-18 ■ Humulin R insulin.

This insulin is a rapid-acting insulin. The *R* stands for *regular*. Humulin is a trade name for insulin that is manufactured by using recombinant DNA technology. In the past insulin was produced from ground-up animal pancreas.

Category	Word Part and Definition	Description	Example
radioactive sodium iodide 131 (I-131)		Treats hyperthyroidism. Given orally. It is taken up by the thyroid gland and emits low-level beta and gamma radiation that destroys thyroid cells. It has a short half-life and is excreted in the urine, limiting the number of cells that are destroyed. Some functioning thyroid gland tissue can remain.	
thyroid supplement drugs		Treat a lack of thyroid hormones and hypothyroidism.	Cytomel, Synthroid, Thyrolar

Abbreviations

ACTH	adrenocorticotropic hormone
ADA	American Diabetes Association or American Dietetic Association
ADH	antidiuretic hormone
Ca, Ca^{++}	calcium
CDE	certified diabetes educator
DI	diabetes insipidus
DKA	diabetic ketoacidosis
DM	diabetes mellitus
FBS	fasting blood sugar
FSH	follicle-stimulating hormone
FTI	free thyroxine index
GH	growth hormone
GTT	glucose tolerance test
HbA_{1C}	hemoglobin A_{1C}
IDDM	insulin-dependent diabetes mellitus
IRS	insulin resistance syndrome
K, K^+	potassium
LH	luteinizing hormone
MSH	melanocyte-stimulating hormone
Na, Na^+	sodium
NIDDM	non–insulin-dependent diabetes mellitus
NPH	neutral protamine Hagedorn (type of insulin)
OGTT	oral glucose tolerance test
RAIU	radioactive iodine uptake
RIA	radioimmunoassay
SAD	seasonal affective disorder
SIADH	syndrome of inappropriate ADH
T_3	triiodothyronine
T_4	thyroxine
T_7	free thyroxine index (FTI)
TFTs	thyroid function tests
TSH	thyroid-stimulating hormone
VMA	vanillylmandelic acid

Word Alert

ABBREVIATIONS

Abbreviations are commonly used in all types of medical documentation; however, they can mean different things to different people and their meaning can be misinterpreted. Always verify the meaning of an abbreviation.

ADA stands for *American Diabetes Association,* but it can also stand for *American Dietetic Association.*

Ca stands for *calcium,* but it can also stand for *cancer.*

GTT stands for *glucose tolerance test,* but *gtt.* stands for *drops.*

NPH stands for *neutral protamine Hagedorn* (insulin), but it can also stand for *normal pressure hydrocephalus.*

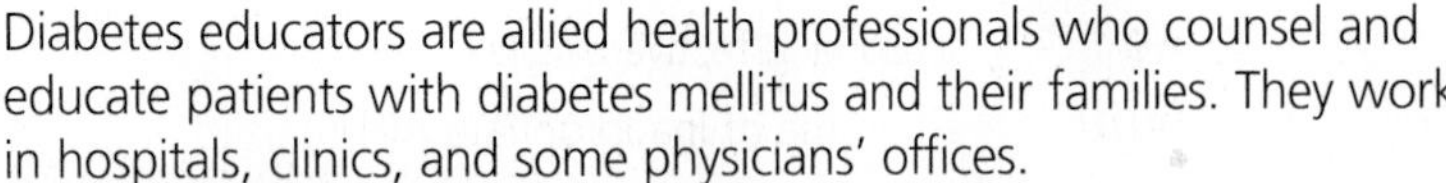

Career Focus

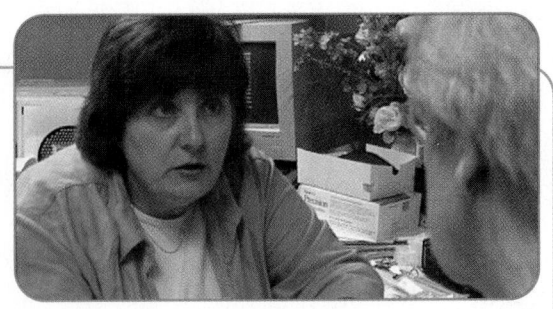

Meet Maureen, a diabetes educator.

"I worked in a large city hospital which had a very large diabetic population, and that's how I got interested in the disease. On a typical day we see patients who have had diabetes anywhere from just a few weeks to years. Diabetic education has really changed a lot, because we're really trying to empower the patient. The person lives with diabetes every day, so they should have the tools to take care of their diabetes. The more information they have, the better choices that they're going to make. What we try and do is teach them how—about their food, how to monitor their blood sugar, what their medications are and how to take them properly and consistently and what do they do if their blood sugars are either too high or too low."

Diabetes educators are allied health professionals who counsel and educate patients with diabetes mellitus and their families. They work in hospitals, clinics, and some physicians' offices.

Endocrinologists are physicians who practice in the specialty of endocrinology. They diagnose and treat patients with diseases of the endocrine system. Some endocrinologists who specialize and become **diabetologists** only treat patients with diabetes mellitus. Physicians can take additional training and become board certified in the subspecialties of reproductive endocrinology or pediatric endocrinology. Surgery on the endocrine system is performed by a general surgeon or a neurosurgeon. Cancerous tumors of the endocrine system are treated medically by an oncologist or surgically by a general surgeon or neurosurgeon.

endocrinologist
(EN-doh-krih-NAWL-oh-jist)
endo- *innermost, within*
crin/o- *secrete*
log/o- *the study of*
-ist *one who specializes in*

diabetologist (DY-ah-beh-TAWL-oh-jist)
diabet/o- *diabetes*
log/o- *the study of*
-ist *one who specializes in*

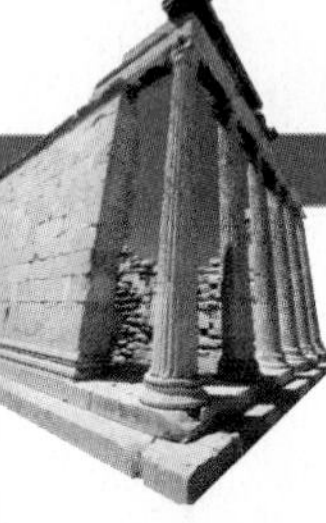

It's Greek to Me!

Did you notice that some endocrine system words have two different combining forms? Combining forms from both Greek and Latin languages remain a part of medical language today.

English Word	Greek	Latin	Examples of Medical Words
male, masculine	andr/o-	viril/o-	androgens, virilism
milk	galact/o-	lact/o-	galactorrhea, lactation
pituitary gland	hypophys/o-	pituit/o-	adenohypophysis, pituitary

CHAPTER REVIEW EXERCISES

Review all the material in this chapter by completing the review exercises in this section. Use the Answer Key at the end of the book to check your answers.

Anatomy and Physiology

Location Exercise

Identify the area of the body where each of these endocrine structures is located. The first one has been done for you.

Endocrine Gland or Organ	Location
1. hypothalamus	in the brain below the third ventricle
2. pituitary gland	______
3. pineal gland	______
4. thyroid gland	______
5. parathyroid glands	______
6. thymus	______
7. pancreas	______
8. adrenal glands	______
9. ovaries	______
10. testes	______

Unscramble and Match

Unscramble the letters to spell a hormone. Write its correct spelling on the blank line, then match the hormone with the gland or organ that secretes it. Note: Some glands or organs will have more than one hormone. The first one has been done for you.

1. nnsuiil	insulin	____	anterior pituitary gland
2. daltsoerone	______	____	posterior pituitary gland
3. HST	______	____	pineal gland
4. cooxtoyin	______	____	thyroid gland
5. HACT	______	1	pancreas
6. nacggoul	______	____	adrenal cortex
7. HDA	______	____	adrenal medulla
8. ephpiinener	______	____	testes
9. tttesosroeen	______	____	ovaries
10. tlcainrop	______		
11. tolmeanin	______		
12. dloiaerst	______		
13. yxhtroienr	______		

Circle Exercise

Circle the correct word from the choices given.

1. The (**pineal gland, pancreas, testis**) secretes the male hormone testosterone.
2. The (**ovary, pituitary, thymus**) secretes estradiol and is responsible for sexual characteristics in the female.
3. The (**ovaries, parathyroid glands, testes**) are four small glands located on the thyroid gland.
4. The (**adrenal gland, pancreas, pituitary gland**) contains two areas called the cortex and the medulla.
5. The (**adrenal gland, pituitary gland, thymus**) shrinks in size in adults.

Medical Language Word Parts

Name that Word Part

Identify each of the word parts given here by writing the correct letter (P, C, or S) on the line beside it. Then write the definition of the word part on the blank line. The first one has been done for you.

Prefix = P **Combining Form = C** **Suffix = S**

		Word Part	Definition
1.	-al	S	pertaining to
2.	acid/o-		
3.	acr/o-		
4.	act/o-		
5.	aden/o-		
6.	ad-		
7.	adrenal/o-		
8.	adren/o-		
9.	affect/o-		
10.	ag/o-		
11.	-an		
12.	-ance		
13.	andr/o-		
14.	antagon/o-		
15.	anter/o-		
16.	anti-		
17.	-ar		
18.	-ary		
19.	-ate		
20.	-ation		
21.	bi/o-		
22.	-body		
23.	calc/i-		
24.	calc/o-		
25.	carcin/o-		
26.	chrom/o-		
27.	congenit/o-		
28.	cortic/o-		
29.	-crine		
30.	crin/o-		
31.	-cyte		
32.	cyt/o-		
33.	dem/o-		
34.	dextr/o-		
35.	di-		
36.	dia-		
37.	diabet/o-		
38.	dips/o-		
39.	-drome		
40.	-ectomy		
41.	-edema		
42.	-emia		
43.	en-		
44.	endo-		
45.	erg/o-		
46.	estr/a-		
47.	eu-		
48.	fertil/o-		
49.	galact/o-		
50.	-gen		
51.	genit/o-		
52.	gestat/o-		
53.	gest/o-		
54.	gigant/o-		
55.	globul/o-		
56.	gluc/o-		
57.	glyc/o-		
58.	glycos/o-		
59.	gonad/o-		
60.	gynec/o-		
61.	hirsut/o-		
62.	home/o-		
63.	hormon/o-		
64.	hyper-		
65.	hypo-		
66.	hypophys/o-		
67.	-ia		
68.	-ial		
69.	-ic		
70.	in-		

	Word Part	Definition			Word Part	Definition
71.	-in	______	__________________	111.	ovari/o-	______	__________________
72.	-ine	______	__________________	112.	ox/y-	______	__________________
73.	inhibit/o-	______	__________________	113.	pan-	______	__________________
74.	insulin/o-	______	__________________	114.	pancreat/o-	______	__________________
75.	insul/o-	______	__________________	115.	para-	______	__________________
76.	iod/o-	______	__________________	116.	-pathy	______	__________________
77.	-ion	______	__________________	117.	-pause	______	__________________
78.	-ior	______	__________________	118.	phag/o-	______	__________________
79.	-ism	______	__________________	119.	phe/o-	______	__________________
80.	-ist	______	__________________	120.	-physis	______	__________________
81.	-itis	______	__________________	121.	pituitar/o-	______	__________________
82.	-ity	______	__________________	122.	pituit/o-	______	__________________
83.	-ive	______	__________________	123.	poly-	______	__________________
84.	ket/o-	______	__________________	124.	poster/o-	______	__________________
85.	lact/o-	______	__________________	125.	pro-	______	__________________
86.	lob/o-	______	__________________	126.	radi/o-	______	__________________
87.	log/o-	______	__________________	127.	recept/o-	______	__________________
88.	-logy	______	__________________	128.	ren/o-	______	__________________
89.	mast/o-	______	__________________	129.	resist/o-	______	__________________
90.	medull/o-	______	__________________	130.	retin/o-	______	__________________
91.	-megaly	______	__________________	131.	-rrhea	______	__________________
92.	melan/o-	______	__________________	132.	secret/o-	______	__________________
93.	men/o-	______	__________________	133.	somat/o-	______	__________________
94.	mineral/o-	______	__________________	134.	sphenoid/o-	______	__________________
95.	mult/i-	______	__________________	135.	-stasis	______	__________________
96.	myx/o-	______	__________________	136.	stat/o-	______	__________________
97.	nephr/o-	______	__________________	137.	-steroid	______	__________________
98.	neur/o-	______	__________________	138.	stimul/o-	______	__________________
99.	-nine	______	__________________	139.	syn-	______	__________________
100.	nod/o-	______	__________________	140.	testicul/o-	______	__________________
101.	non-	______	__________________	141.	thalam/o-	______	__________________
102.	-oid	______	__________________	142.	thym/o-	______	__________________
103.	-ol	______	__________________	143.	thyr/o-	______	__________________
104.	-oma	______	__________________	144.	thyroid/o-	______	__________________
105.	-on	______	__________________	145.	-tic	______	__________________
106.	-opsy	______	__________________	146.	toc/o-	______	__________________
107.	-or	______	__________________	147.	ton/o-	______	__________________
108.	-ose	______	__________________	148.	-tous	______	__________________
109.	-osis	______	__________________	149.	toxic/o-	______	__________________
110.	oure/o-	______	__________________	150.	tox/o-	______	__________________

		Word Part	Definition			Word Part	Definition
151.	trans-	______	______________	155.	-ule	______	______________
152.	tri-	______	______________	156.	ur/o-	______	______________
153.	trop/o-	______	______________	157.	uter/o-	______	______________
154.	-ular	______	______________	158.	viril/o-	______	______________

Symptoms, Signs, and Diseases

Matching Exercise

Match each numbered word or phrase to its description.

1.	thyromegaly	____ Bulging, staring eyes
2.	diabetes insipidus	____ Excessive thirst
3.	myxedema	____ Not enough ADH
4.	exophthalmos	____ Hyposecretion of estradiol
5.	galactorrhea	____ Too little oxytocin
6.	gigantism	____ Severe hypothyroidism in an adult
7.	menopause	____ Milk secretion from breasts of nonpregnant female
8.	polydipsia	____ Enlargement of the thyroid gland
9.	uterine inertia	____ Hypersecretion of growth hormone during childhood

True or False

Indicate whether each statement is true or false by writing T or F on the line.

1. ____ A goiter is also known as thyromegaly.
2. ____ Diabetes insipidus is also known as sugar diabetes.
3. ____ Addison's disease is also known as thyrotoxicosis.
4. ____ Cretinism in a child is caused by a lack of the same hormone as dwarfism in an child.
5. ____ Gestational diabetes only occurs in men.
6. ____ Moon face and buffalo hump are characteristics of Cushing's syndrome.
7. ____ Gynecomastia is the overproduction of milk by the breasts during pregnancy.

Divide and Conquer

Separate these endocrine words into their component parts (prefix, combining form, and suffix). Note: Some words do not contain all three word parts. The first one has been done for you.

Medical Word	Prefix	Combining Form	Suffix
1. biopsy	______	bi/o-	-opsy
2. hyperthyroidism	______	______	______
3. polydipsia	______	______	______
4. thyroidectomy	______	______	______
5. thyroiditis	______	______	______
6. adenoma	______	______	______
7. glycosuria	______	______	______
8. endocrinology	______	______	______

Word-Building Exercise

Use the combining forms, prefixes, and suffixes here to build medical words that match the definitions given. Write the word that you build on the blank line. Some word parts may be used more than once. The first one has been done for you.

Word Parts

acr/o- (extremity; highest point)
aden/o- (gland)
dips/o- (thirst)
-emia (condition of the blood; substance in the blood)
galact/o- (milk)
glyc/o- (glucose)
gynec/o- (female, woman)
hyper- (above; more than normal)
-ia (condition, state, thing)
-ism (process; disease from a specific cause)
mast/o- (breast; mastoid process)
-megaly (enlargement)
-oma (tumor, mass)
para- (beside, apart from; two parts of a pair; abnormal)
poly- (many, much)
-rrhea (flow, discharge)
thyr/o- (shield-shaped structure [thyroid gland])
thyroid/o- (thyroid gland)
-tous (pertaining to)
ur/o- (urine; urinary system)

1. Condition with excessive secretion of parathyroid hormone (You think *hyper-* + *para-* + *thyroid/o-* + *-ism*).
   You write hyperparathyroidism
2. Excessive production of urine __________
3. Flow of milk from the breasts of a nonpregnant woman __________
4. Enlargement of the face, hands, and feet __________
5. Tumor of a gland __________
6. Enlarged thyroid gland __________
7. Elevated levels of sugar in the blood __________
8. Condition of great thirst __________
9. Enlargement of the breasts in a man __________
10. Pertaining to a tumor of a gland __________

Laboratory, Radiology, Surgery, and Drugs

Circle Exercise

Circle the correct word from the choices given.

1. Which disease is associated with the adrenal cortex? (**diabetes, thyroiditis, virilism**)
2. A cold or hot nodule might be seen on a/an (**ACTH stimulation test, fasting blood sugar, thyroid scan**).
3. A large volume of urine could indicate (**diabetes insipidus, precocious puberty, thyroid storm**).
4. HbA_{1C} is also known as (**antithyroglobulin antibodies, FSH, glycosylated hemoglobin**).
5. A person taking Synthroid would have had the (**adrenal gland, ovary, thyroid gland**) surgically removed.
6. All of the following are laboratory tests for diabetes EXCEPT (**calcium, fasting blood sugar, GTT**).
7. Thyroid function tests include all of the following EXCEPT (**estradiol, T_4, TSH**).

Matching Exercise

Match each numbered word or phrase to its description.

1.	antidiabetic drugs	_____ Surgical treatment for myasthenia gravis
2.	corticosteroid drugs	_____ Removes just part of the thyroid gland
3.	insulin	_____ Used to treat patients with type 2 diabetes mellitus
4.	lobectomy	_____ Patients with Addison's disease must take these
5.	radioactive I-131	_____ This drug is given by subcutaneous injection
6.	thymectomy	_____ Emits gamma radiation that destroys the thyroid

Laboratory Test Exercise

Review this form for ordering laboratory tests. Find each of the following tests related to endocrinology and put a check in the box next to it.

electrolyte panel	potassium	T_3, total
glucose, fasting	prolactin	T_4, total
glucose tolerance test (GGT)	sodium	TSH

PANELS AND PROFILES			TESTS		
968T		Lipid Panel	19687W		Bilirubin (Direct)
315F		Electrolyte Panel	265F		HBsAg
10256F		Hepatic Function Panel	51870R		HB Core Antibody
10165F		Basic Metabolic Panel	1012F		Cardio CRP
10231A		Comprehensive Metabolic Panel	23242E		GGT
10306F		Hepatitis Panel, Acute	28852E		Protein, Total
182Aaa		Obstetric Panel	141A		CBC Hemogram
18T		Chem-Screen Panel (Basic)	21105R		hCG, Qualitative, Serum
554T		Chem-Screen Panel (Basic with HDL)	10321A		ANA
7971A		Chem-Screen Panel (Basic with HDL, TIBC)	80185		Cardio CRP with Lipid Profile
TESTS			26F		PT with INR
56713E		Lead, Blood	232Aaa		UA, Dipstick
2782A		Antibody Screen	42A		CBC with Diff
3556F		Iron, TIBC	20867W		HDL Cholesterol
20933E		Cholesterol	31732E		PTT
3084111E		Uric Acid	34F		UA, Dipstick and Microscopic
53348W		Rubella Antibody	20396R		CEA
27771E		Phosphate	45443E		Hematocrit
2111600E		Creatinine	28571E		PSA, Total
29868W		Testosterone, Total	66902E		WBC count
9704F		Creatinine Clearance	20750E		Chloride
19752E		Bilirubin (Total)	7187W		Hemoglobin
30536Rrr		T3, Total	4259T		HIV-1 Antibody
687T		Protein Electrophoresis	45484R		Hemoglobin A1c
3563444R		Digoxin	67868R		Alk Phosphatase
15214R		Glucose, 2-Hour Postprandial	24984R		Iron
30502E		T3, Uptake	28512E		Sodium
7773E		Platelet Count	17426R		ALT
39685R		Dilantin (phenytoin)	MICROBIOLOGY		
30494R		Triglycerides	112680E		Group A Beta Strep Culture, Throat
26013E		Magnesium	5827W		Group B Beta Strep Culture, Genitals
15586R		Glucose, Fasting	49932E		Chlamydia, Endocervix/Urethra
30237W		T4, Free	6007W		Culture, Blood
28233E		Potassium	2692E		Culture, Genitals
19208W		AST	2649T		Culture, HSV
30163E		TSH	612A		Culture, Sputum
22764R		Ferritin	6262E		Culture, Throat
20008W		Calcium	6304R		Culture, Urine
54726F		Occult Blood, Stool	50286R		Gonococcus, Endocervix/Urethra
51839W		HAV Antibody, Total	6643E		Gram Stain
430A		Blood Group and Rh Type	STOOL PATHOGENS		
28399W		Progesterone	10045F		Culture, Stool
30262E		T4, Total	4475F		Culture, Campylobacter
20289W		Carbon Dioxide	10018T		Culture, Salmonella
1156F		RPR	86140A		E. coli Toxins
30940E		Urea Nitrogen	1099T		Ova and Parasites
17417W		Albumin	VENIPUNCTURE		
28423E		Prolactin	63180		Venipuncture

Abbreviations

Abbreviation Exercise

Give the abbreviation for the following definitions.

1. Type 1 diabetes mellitus __________
2. A group of tests that pertain to thyroid gland function __________
3. Blood test that measures glucose level after not eating __________
4. Diabetes with burning of fat and acidic blood __________
5. Organization for diabetes education and information __________
6. Measures the average blood sugar over several months __________
7. Depression related to low levels of light __________
8. Certified instructor who teaches about diabetic diets __________
9. Syndrome in which receptors resist the effect of insulin __________
10. Triiodothyronine __________

Applied Skills

Plural Noun and Adjective Spelling

Fill in the blanks with the correct word form. Be sure to check your spelling. The first one has been done for you.

Singular Noun	Plural Noun	Adjective
1. hypophysis		hypophysial
2. adenoma	______	______
	______	
3. cortex	______	______
4. gland	______	______
5. hormone	______	______

Singular Noun	Plural Noun	Adjective
6. hypothalamus		______
7. medulla	______	______
8. ovary	______	______
9. pancreas		______
10. testis	______	______
11. thymus		______

Analysis of a Medical Report

This exercise contains a physician's office chart note in the SOAP note format. Read the report and answer the questions.

CHART NOTE

S: This is a 54-year-old male who presents with fatigue. He also has headaches. Because of a history of some visual field deficits during his headaches, his ophthalmologist ordered an MRI of the brain. I reviewed the films and did not see anything but the expected postsurgical changes of the brain. Lab tests show that he does have some residual function of the pituitary gland, so his endocrinologist only placed him on testosterone patches and thyroid hormone replacement (Synthroid). He also has a history of depression, which could explain the fatigue and headache, or they could be due to low thyroid hormone replacement levels.

O: HEENT: Normal. Lungs: Clear to auscultation. Cardiovascular: Regular rate and rhythm, without murmurs, rubs, or gallops. Abdomen: Nondistended, nontender. Extremities: No edema.

A:

1. Fatigue. Possibly hypothyroidism. Will check T_3, T_4, and TSH levels.
2. Headache, possibly within the context of depression. He is on a rather low dose of an antidepressant drug at this time.
3. Hypopituitarism.

P:

1. Will obtain an FSH, LH, free and total testosterone, and baseline ACTH.
2. Follow up in 1 week.

Edward Allen Selcher, M.D.

Edward Allen Selcher, M.D.

EAS:blg
D: 11/19/xx
T: 11/19/xx

WORD ANALYSIS QUESTIONS

1. Divide *endocrinologist* into its four word parts and define each word part.

Word Part	Definition
______	______
______	______
______	______
______	______

2. Divide *hypopituitarism* into its three word parts and define each word part.

Word Part	Definition
______	______
______	______
______	______

3. What is the abbreviation for *thyroid-stimulating hormone*? ______

FACT FINDING QUESTIONS

1. Besides the physician who dictated this report, what two physician specialists have also recently seen the patient?

    ____

    ____

2. What two hormones does the patient already take as drugs for hormone replacement therapy?

    ____

    ____

3. What do the abbreviations *ACTH, FSH,* and *LH* stand for?

    ADH: ______________________________

    FSH: ______________________________

    LH: ______________________________

4. The patient is taking Synthroid for his (**headaches, hypothyroidism, lungs**). Circle the correct answer.

CRITICAL THINKING QUESTIONS

1. The patient's fatigue, headache, and visual field defect could be signs of a recurring tumor in the brain. What test has already been done to look for a tumor?

    ____

2. The patient's MRI of the brain showed postsurgical changes, meaning changes that are present because of a surgery that was done. Which endocrine gland was operated on in the past?

    ____

3. Which of the patient's drugs correlates with doing the lab tests for T_3, T_4, and TSH?

    ____

4. In a physician's office chart note format, what do the initials *S, O, A,* and *P* stand for? (*Hint:* See the section on the health record in Chapter 1).

    S: ______________________________

    O: ______________________________

    A: ______________________________

    P: ______________________________

Pronunciation Checklist

Read each word and its pronunciation. Practice pronouncing each word. Verify your pronunciation by listening to the Pronunciation List on the CD-ROM. Check the box next to the word after you master its pronunciation.

- ❑ acromegaly (AK-roh-MEG-ah-lee)
- ❑ Addison's disease (AD-ih-sonz dih-ZEEZ)
- ❑ adenohypophysis (AD-eh-noh-hy-PAWF-ih-sis)
- ❑ adenoma (AD-eh-NOH-mah)
- ❑ adenomata (AD-eh-NOH-mah-tah)
- ❑ adenomatous (AD-eh-NOH-mah-tus)
- ❑ adrenal (ah-DREE-nal)
- ❑ adrenalectomy (ah-DREE-nal-EK-toh-mee)
- ❑ adrenocorticotropic (ah-DREE-noh-KOR-tih-koh-TROHP-ik)
- ❑ adrenogenital syndrome (ah-DREE-noh-JEN-ih-tal SIN-drohm)
- ❑ aldosterone (al-DAWS-ter-ohn)
- ❑ androgens (AN-droh-jens)
- ❑ antagonism (an-TAG-on-izm)
- ❑ anterior (an-TEER-ee-or)
- ❑ antidiabetic drug (AN-tee-DY-ah-BET-ik DRUHG)
- ❑ antidiuretic hormone (AN-tee-DY-yoo-RET-ik HOR-mohn)
- ❑ antithyroglobulin antibody (AN-tee-THY-roh-GLAWB-yoo-lin AN-tee-BAWD-ee) (AN-tih-BAWD-ee)
- ❑ antithyroid drug (AN-tee-THY-royd DRUHG)
- ❑ biopsy (BY-awp-see)
- ❑ calcitonin (KAL-sih-TOH-nin)
- ❑ calcium (KAL-see-um)
- ❑ carcinoma (KAR-sih-NOH-mah)
- ❑ circadian rhythm (ser-KAY-dee-an RITH-um)
- ❑ congenital (con-JEN-ih-tal)
- ❑ cortex (KOR-teks)
- ❑ cortical (KOR-tih-kal)
- ❑ cortices (KOR-tih-seez)
- ❑ corticosteroid drug (KOR-tih-koh-STAIR-oyd DRUHG)
- ❑ cortisol (KOR-tih-sawl)
- ❑ cretinism (KREE-tin-izm)
- ❑ Cushing's disease (KOOSH-ingz dih-ZEEZ)
- ❑ Cushing's syndrome (KOOSH-ingz SIN-drohm)
- ❑ diabetes educator (DY-ah-BEE-teez ED-jyoo-kay-ter)
- ❑ diabetes insipidus (DY-ah-BEE-teez in-SIP-ih-dus)
- ❑ diabetes mellitus (DY-ah-BEE-teez MEL-ih-tus)
- ❑ diabetic (DY-ah-BET-ik)
- ❑ diabetic ketoacidosis (DY-ah-BET-ik KEE-toh-AS-ih-DOH-sis)
- ❑ diabetic nephropathy (DY-ah-BET-ik neh-FRAWP-ah-thee)
- ❑ diabetic neuropathy (DY-ah-BET-ik nyoo-RAWP-ah-thee)
- ❑ diabetic retinopathy (DY-ah-BET-ik RET-ih-NAWP-ah-thee)
- ❑ diabetologist (DY-ah-beh-TAWL-oh-jist)
- ❑ dwarfism (DWORF-izm)
- ❑ endemic goiter (en-DEM-ik GOY-ter)
- ❑ endocrine system (EN-doh-krin SIS-tem) (EN-doh-krine)
- ❑ endocrinologist (EN-doh-krih-NAWL-oh-jist)
- ❑ endocrinology (EN-doh-krih-NAWL-oh-jee)
- ❑ epinephrine (EP-ih-NEF-rin)
- ❑ estradiol (ES-trah-DY-awl)
- ❑ euthyroidism (yoo-THY-royd-izm)
- ❑ exophthalmos (EK-sawf-THAL-mohs)
- ❑ follicle (FAWL-ih-kl)
- ❑ galactorrhea (gah-LAK-toh-REE-ah)
- ❑ gestational diabetes (jes-TAY-shun-al DY-ah-BEE-teez)
- ❑ gigantism (jy-GAN-tizm) (JY-gan-tizm)
- ❑ gland (GLAND)
- ❑ glandular (GLAN-dyoo-lar)
- ❑ glucagon (GLOO-kah-gawn)
- ❑ glucocorticoid (GLOO-koh-KOR-tih-koyd)
- ❑ glycogen (GLY-koh-jen)
- ❑ glycohemoglobin (GLY-koh-HEE-moh-gloh-bin)
- ❑ glucose (GLOO-kohs)
- ❑ glycosuria (GLY-koh-SYOO-ree-ah)
- ❑ glycosylated hemoglobin (gly-KOH-sih-lay-ted HEE-moh-gloh-bin)
- ❑ goiter (GOY-ter)
- ❑ gonadotropin (GOH-nah-doh-TROH-pin)
- ❑ Graves' disease (GRAYVZ dih-ZEEZ)
- ❑ gynecomastia (GY-neh-koh-MAS-tee-ah)
- ❑ Hashimoto's thyroiditis (HAH-shee-MOH-tohz THY-roy-DY-tis)
- ❑ hemoglobin A_{1c} (HEE-moh-gloh-bihn AA-one-see)
- ❑ hirsutism (HER-soo-tizm)
- ❑ homeostasis (HOH-mee-oh-STAY-sis)
- ❑ hormonal (hor-MOH-nal)
- ❑ hormone (HOR-mohn)
- ❑ hydroxycorticosteroids (hy-DRAWK-see-KOR-tih-koh-STAIR-oydz)
- ❑ hyperaldosteronism (HY-per-al-DAWS-ter-ohn-izm)
- ❑ hypercalcemia (HY-per-kal-SEE-mee-ah)
- ❑ hyperglycemia (HY-per-gly-SEE-mee-ah)
- ❑ hyperinsulinism (HY-per-IN-soo-lin-izm)
- ❑ hyperparathyroidism (HY-per-PAIR-ah-THY-royd-izm)
- ❑ hyperpituitarism (HY-per-pih-TOO-ih-tah-rizm)
- ❑ hypersecretion (HY-per-seh-KREE-shun)
- ❑ hyperthyroidism (HY-per-THY-royd-izm)
- ❑ hypoaldosteronism (HY-poh-al-DAWS-ter-ohn-izm)
- ❑ hypocalcemia (HY-poh-kal-SEE-mee-ah)
- ❑ hypoglycemia (HY-poh-gly-SEE-mee-ah)
- ❑ hypoparathyroidism (HY-poh-PAIR-ah-THY-royd-izm)
- ❑ hypophysial (HY-poh-FIZ-ee-al)
- ❑ hypophysis (hy-PAWF-ih-sis)
- ❑ hypopituitarism (HY-poh-pih-TOO-ih-tah-rizm)
- ❑ hyposecretion (HY-poh-seh-KREE-shun)
- ❑ hypothalamic (HY-poh-thah-LAM-ik)
- ❑ hypothalamus (HY-poh-THAL-ah-mus)
- ❑ hypothyroidism (HY-poh-THY-royd-izm)
- ❑ infertility (IN-fer-TIL-ih-tee)
- ❑ inhibition (IN-hih-BISH-un)
- ❑ insulin (IN-soo-lin)
- ❑ insulin resistance syndrome (IN-soo-lin ree-ZIS-tans SIN-drohm)
- ❑ iodine (EYE-oh-dine) (EYE-oh-deen)
- ❑ islets of Langerhans (EYE-lets of LAHNG-er-hanz)
- ❑ isthmus (IS-mus)
- ❑ ketones (KEE-tohnz)
- ❑ lactatation (lak-TAY-shun)
- ❑ lobe (LOHB)
- ❑ lobectomy (loh-BEK-toh-mee)
- ❑ luteinizing (LOO-tee-in-NY-zing)
- ❑ medulla (meh-DUL-ah) (meh-DYOOL-ah)
- ❑ medullae (meh-DUL-ee) (meh-DYOOL-ee)
- ❑ medullary (MED-yoo-LAIR-ee)
- ❑ melanocyte (meh-LAN-oh-site) (MEL-ah-noh-site)

- ❑ melatonin (MEL-ah-TOHN-in)
- ❑ menopause (MEN-oh-pawz)
- ❑ micronodular goiter (MY-kroh-NAWD-yoo-lar GOY-ter)
- ❑ mineralocorticoid (MIN-er-al-oh-KOR-tih-koyd)
- ❑ multinodular goiter (MUL-tee-NAWD-yoo-lar GOY-ter)
- ❑ myxedema (MIK-seh-DEE-mah)
- ❑ neurohypophysis (NYOOR-oh-hy-PAWF-ih-sis)
- ❑ nodular (NAWD-yoo-lar)
- ❑ nodule (NAWD-yool)
- ❑ nontoxic goiter (non-TAWK-sik GOY-ter)
- ❑ norepinephrine (NOR-ep-ih-NEF-rin)
- ❑ ovarian (oh-VAIR-ee-an)
- ❑ ovary (OH-vah-ree)
- ❑ oxytocin (AWK-see-TOH-sin)
- ❑ pancreas (PAN-kree-as)
- ❑ pancreatic (PAN-kree-AT-ik)
- ❑ panhypopituitarism (pan-HY-poh-pih-TOO-eh-tah-rizm)
- ❑ parathyroid (PAIR-ah-THY-royd)
- ❑ parathyroidectomy (PAIR-ah-THY-roy-DEK-toh-mee)
- ❑ pheochromocytoma (FEE-oh-KROH-moh-sy-TOH-mah)
- ❑ pineal (PIN-ee-al)
- ❑ pituitary (pih-TOO-eh-TAIR-ee)
- ❑ polydipsia (PAWL-ee-DIP-see-ah)
- ❑ polyphagia (PAWL-ee-FAY-jee-ah)
- ❑ polyuria (PAWL-ee-YOO-ree-ah)
- ❑ posterior (pohs-TEER-ee-or)
- ❑ precocious puberty (prih-KOH-shus PYOO-ber-tee)
- ❑ progesterone (proh-JES-ter-ohn)
- ❑ prolactin (proh-LAK-tin)
- ❑ radioactive iodine (RAY-dee-oh-AK-tiv EYE-oh-dine) (EYE-oh-deen)
- ❑ receptor (ree-SEP-tor)
- ❑ seasonal affective disorder (SEE-son-al ah-FEK-tiv dis-OR-der)
- ❑ sella turcica (SEL-ah TUR-sih-kah)
- ❑ somatostatin (SOH-mah-toh-STAT-in)
- ❑ stimulate (STIM-yoo-layt)
- ❑ stimulation (STIM-yoo-LAY-shun)
- ❑ synergism (SIN-er-jizm)
- ❑ testes (TES-teez)
- ❑ testicle (TES-tih-kl)
- ❑ testicular (tes-TIK-yoo-lar)
- ❑ testis (TES-tis)
- ❑ testosterone (tes-TAWS-teh-rohn)
- ❑ tetany (TET-ah-nee)
- ❑ thymectomy (thy-MEK-toh-mee)
- ❑ thymic (THY-mik)
- ❑ thymosin (thy-MOH-sin)
- ❑ thymus (THY-mus)
- ❑ thyroid (THY-royd)
- ❑ thyroidectomy (THY-roy-DEK-toh-mee)
- ❑ thyroiditis (THY-roy-DY-tis)
- ❑ thyromegaly (THY-roh-MEG-ah-lee)
- ❑ thyrotoxicosis (THY-roh-TAWK-sih-KOH-sis)
- ❑ thyroxine (thy-RAWK-seen) (thy-RAWK-sin)
- ❑ toxic goiter (TAWK-sik GOY-ter)
- ❑ transsphenoidal hypophysectomy (TRANS-sfee-NOY-dal HY-pawf-ih-SEK-toh-mee)
- ❑ triiodothyronine (try-EYE-oh-doh-THY-roh-neen)
- ❑ uterine inertia (YOO-ter-in) (YOO-ter-ine) (in-ER-shah) (in-ER-shee-ah)
- ❑ vanillylmandelic acid (VAN-ih-lil-man-DEL-ik AS-id)
- ❑ virilism (VIR-ih-lizm)

Experience Multimedia

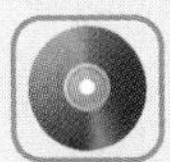

CD-ROM Learning Activities Checklist

Check off the box as you complete each learning activity.

❑ **CD-ROM Learning Activity 14.1: *ANATOMY WORD PARTS FLASHCARDS***
Use flashcards to help you memorize word parts. Make your own flashcards or print out prepared flashcards. Also see the electronic flashcard game. Time: 20 minutes.

❑ **CD-ROM Learning Activity 14.2: *MEDICINE IN ACTION***
Learn about the drug insulin and watch a video clip of how it is given. Time: 5 minutes.

❑ **CD-ROM Learning Activity 14.3: *DISEASE AND OTHER WORD PARTS FLASHCARDS***
A continuation of the flashcard learning activity. Time: 20 minutes.

❑ **CD-ROM Learning Activity 14.4: *MEMORY AIDS***
Use memory aids to help you memorize medical words and meanings. Time: 5 minutes.

❑ **CD-ROM Learning Activity 14.5: *MEDICAL LANGUAGE SPOKEN HERE***
Listen to actual medical reports and spell the missing medical words. Time: 20 minutes.

❑ **CD-ROM Learning Activity 14.6: *SPELLING CHALLENGE***
Listen to a pronounced medical word and then spell it. Time: 5 minutes.

❑ **CD-ROM Learning Activity 14.7: *MEDICAL LANGUAGE PRONUNCIATION***
Listen to a pronounced medical word and then practice pronouncing it. Time: 30 minutes.

❑ **CD-ROM Learning Activity 14.8: *EDUCATIONAL FUN AND GAMES***
Enjoy these fun activities while reinforcing your knowledge. Time: 15 minutes.

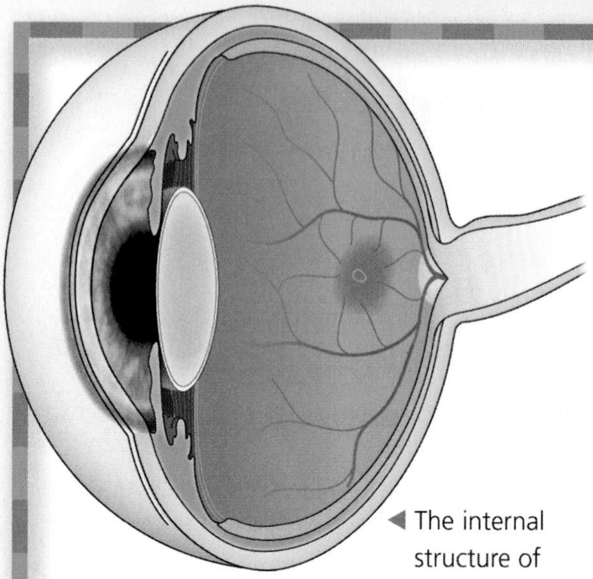

◀ The internal structure of the eye.

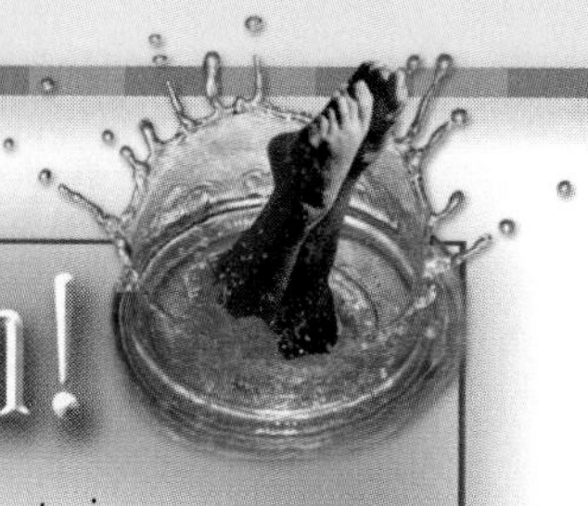

Dive In!

- Women blink nearly twice as much as men.
- After his retirement, Crayola's most senior crayon maker Emerson Moser revealed that he was actually colorblind.
- Leonardo DiVinci devised the first concept for the contact lens.
- Set your sights on becoming a star pupil. In this chapter we'll explore the language that describes the eye structures, functions, diseases, and conditions.
- You'll be seeing clearly once you master the language of opthalmology!

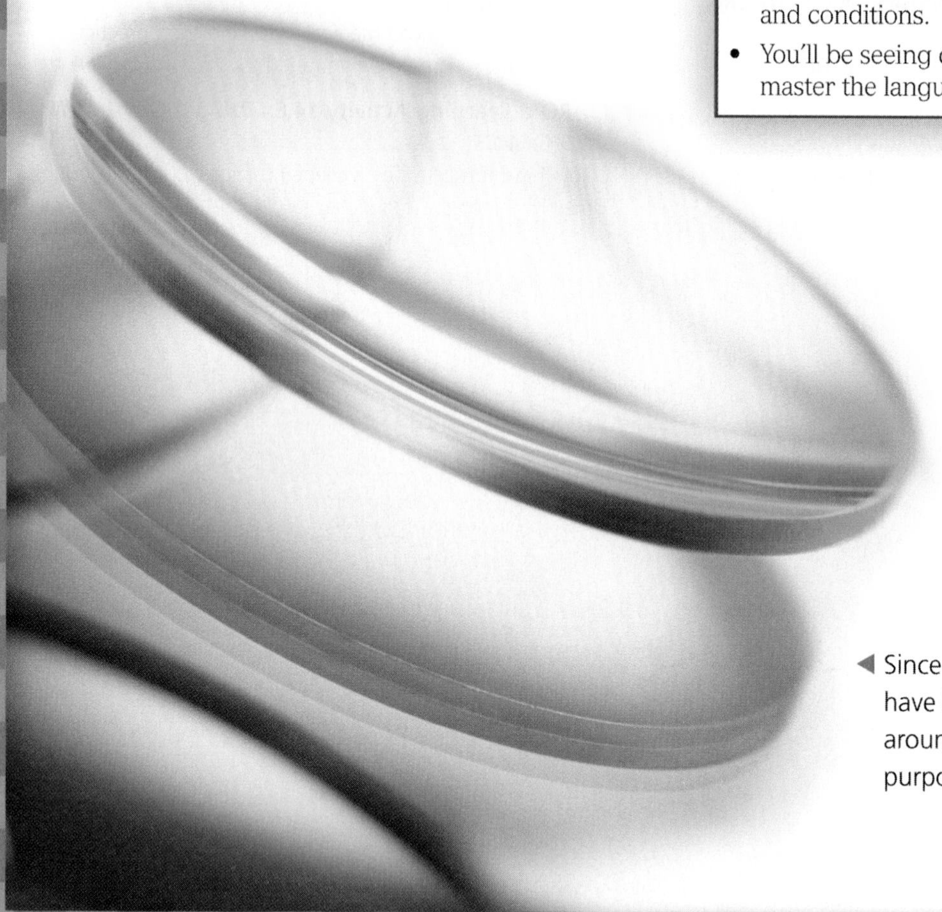

◀ Since the 1940s contact lenses have been used by millions around the world for corrective purposes.

Medicine Through HISTORY

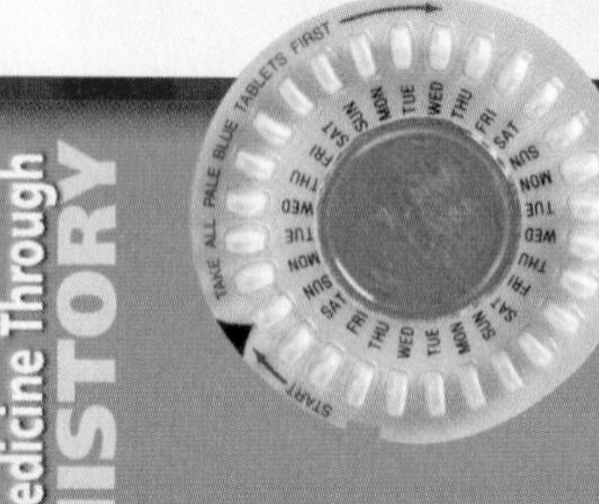

1960

The first oral contraceptive pill is introduced

1961

The first breast silicone implant surgery is performed

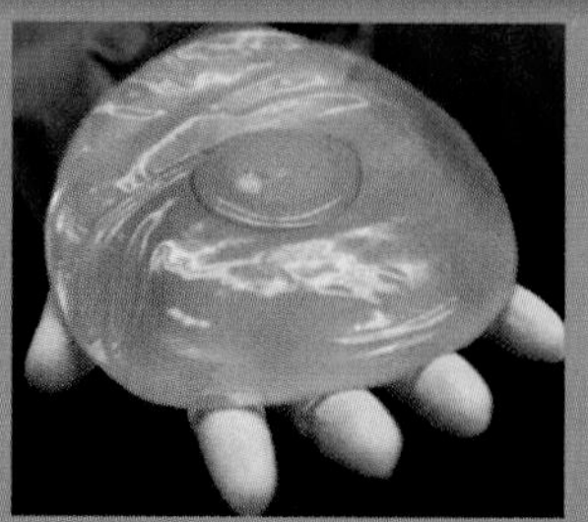

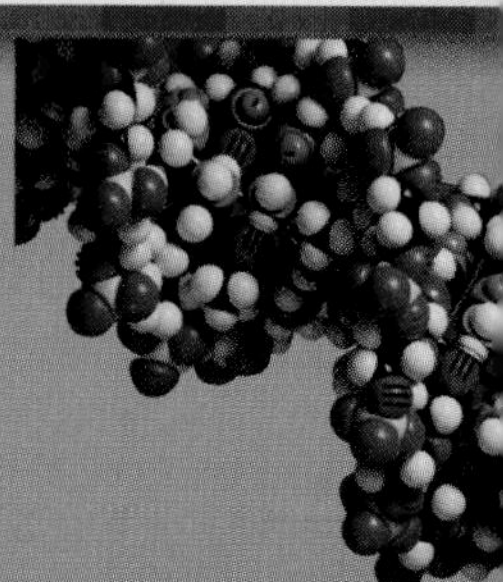

CHAPTER 15

Ophthalmology

Eye

Ophthalmology (OFF-thal-MAWL-oh-jee) is the medical specialty that studies the anatomy and physiology of the eye and uses diagnostic tests, medical and surgical procedures, and drugs to treat eye diseases.

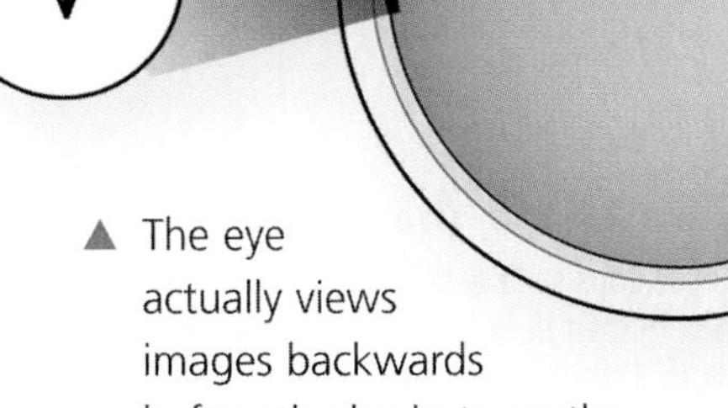

▲ The eye actually views images backwards before the brain turns the image right side up.

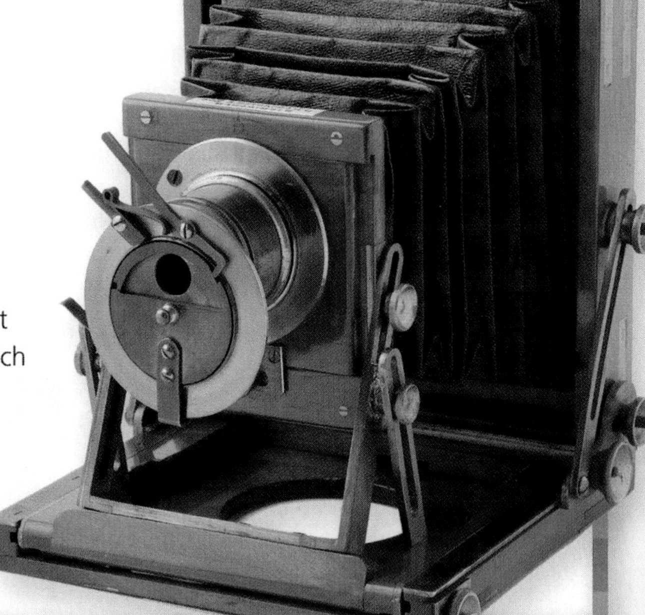

▶ Cameras process light to create images, much like the human eye.

1962

Watson and Crick receive the Nobel Prize for identifying the double-helix structure of DNA in the nucleus of a cell

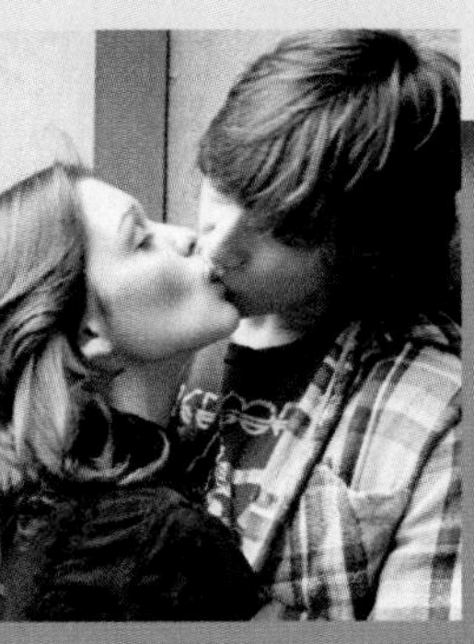

1964

Epstein-Barr virus is discovered to be the cause of "kissing disease" (infectious mononucleosis)

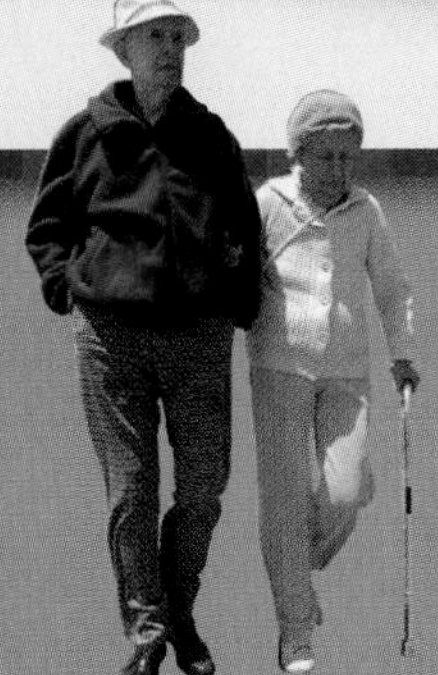

1965

Medicare and Medicaid begin to provide medical coverage for the elderly and the poor

Measure Your Progress: Learning Objectives

After you study this chapter, you should be able to

1. Identify the anatomical structures of the eye by correctly labeling them on anatomical illustrations.
2. Describe the process of vision.
3. Build medical words from combining forms, prefixes, and suffixes.
4. Describe common eye diseases.
5. Describe common eye diagnostic laboratory and radiology tests.
6. Describe common eye medical and surgical procedures and drug categories.
7. Define common eye abbreviations.
8. Correctly spell and pronounce eye words.
9. Apply your skills by analyzing an ophthalmology report.
10. Test your knowledge of ophthalmology by completing review exercises at the end of the chapter and learning activities on the CD-ROM.

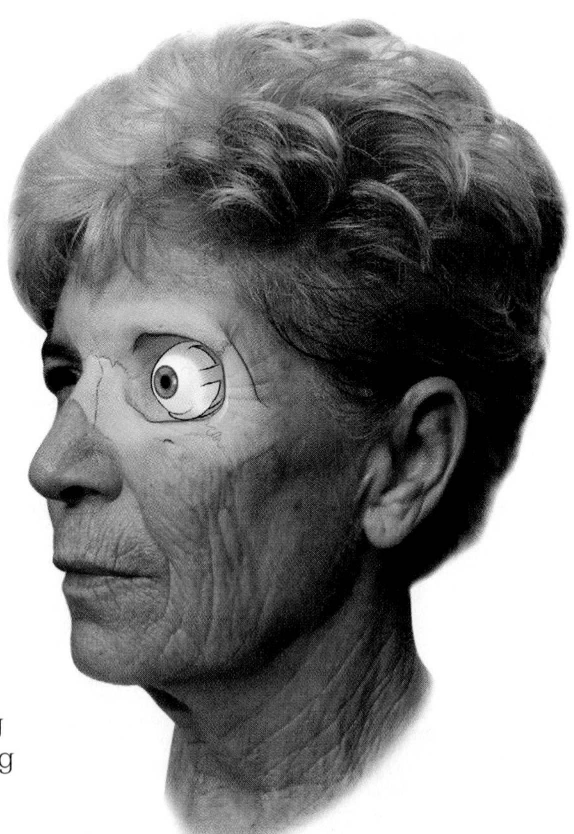

Figure 15-1 ■ The eye.

The eyes consist of two identical but individual organs that sit in hollow areas in the anterior cranium. The eyes are complex structures, and they also connect to the visual cortex in the brain to provide the special sense of sight.

Medical Language Key

To unlock the meaning of a medical word, first define each word part. Then put the word part definitions in order, beginning with the suffix, followed by the first word part.

	Word Part	Word Part Definition
SUFFIX	-logy	*the study of*
COMBINING FORM	ophthalm/o-	*eye*

Ophthalmology: ***The study of the eye.***

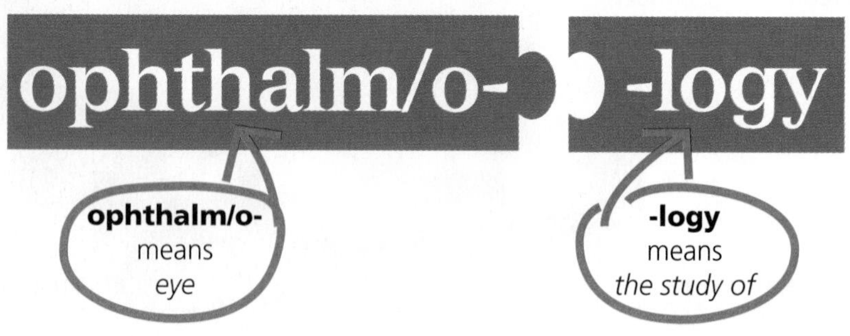

ophthalm/o-
-logy
ophthalm/o- means eye
-logy means the study of

www.prenhall.com/turley

For interactive flashcards, real-life video clips, games, exercises, and audio pronunciations please explore the companion CD-ROM in the back of the book. Click on the companion website for bonus chapters, additional resources, and links to on-line learning.

Anatomy and Physiology

The eyes make up a body system that consists of two identical main organs and many associated structures (see Figure 15-1 ■). Each eyeball or **optic globe** is located within the **orbit,** a bony **socket** in the anterior cranium. The orbit surrounds all but the anterior surface of the eye. The walls of the orbit are made up of several different cranial and facial bones. The orbit does not have a continuous bony posterior wall. There are several openings in its posterior wall where the optic nerve (cranial nerve II), as well as arteries and veins, come through to reach the eye. Within the orbit is a layer of fat that cushions and protects the eyeball on all sides. The function of the eyes is to provide visual information that can be interpreted by the visual cortex in the brain to become the sense of sight.

optic (AWP-tik)
opt/o- *eye; vision*
-ic *pertaining to*

orbit (OR-bit)
Orbit is derived from a Latin word meaning *round circuit.*

orbital (OR-bih-tal)
orbit/o- *orbit (eye socket)*
-al *pertaining to*

socket (SAW-kit)
Socket is derived from a Latin word meaning *sock and shoe.* The eye and the bony orbit fit together like a sock in a shoe.

Anatomy of the Eye

Eyelid and Conjunctiva

The upper and lower eyelids protect the delicate tissues of the eye. They blink to continually refresh a layer of tears to keep the surface of the eye moist. They also prevent foreign substances from entering the eye. At the edges of the eyelids are **sebaceous (meibomian) glands** that secrete oil. The oil acts as a barrier to keep tears in the eye. The red, triangular tissue at the medial corner where the eyelids meet is the **caruncle.**

The eyelashes form a protective barrier that extends outward from the eye to catch foreign substances before they come in contact with the eye.

The **conjunctiva** is a delicate, transparent mucous membrane that covers the insides of the eyelids and continues across the anterior surface of the eye. The conjunctiva produces watery, clear mucus that allows the eyelids to slide easily across the surface of the eye with each blink. This mucus also helps trap particles that enter the eye.

sebaceous (seh-BAY-shus)
sebace/o- *sebum (oil)*
-ous *pertaining to*

meibomian (my-BOH-mee-an)
Meibomian glands were named by Heinrich Meibom (1638–1700), a German anatomist. This is an example of an eponym: a person from whom something takes its name.

caruncle (KAR-ung-kl)
Caruncle is a Latin word meaning *small, fleshy mass.*

conjunctiva (CON-junk-TY-vah) (con-JUNK-tih-vah)
conjunctivae (CON-junk-TY-vee) (con-JUNK-tih-vee)

conjunctival (CON-junk-TY-val) (con-JUNK-tih-val)
conjunctiv/o- *conjunctiva*
-al *pertaining to*

Sclera and Cornea

The **sclera** is a tough, fibrous connective tissue that forms a continuous outer layer around the eyeball. This tissue is white and opaque, and on the anterior surface of the eye it is known as the white of the eye (see Figure 15-2 ■). The sclera protects the internal structures of the eye and maintains the shape of the eye. The sclera is the site of attachment for all of the muscles that move the eye.

Across the anterior part of the eye, the sclera changes into a transparent layer known as the **cornea** (see Figure 15-4). The transitional area where this occurs is known as the **limbus** (see Figure 15-2). The cornea allows light to enter the eye. It also bends or refracts the light rays. The cornea itself contains no blood vessels, not even capillaries. It receives oxygen and nutrients from tears that flow across its surface and from aqueous humor that flows in the anterior chamber beneath it. The cornea does have nerves, however, and is the most sensitive area on the anterior surface of the eye.

sclera (SKLEER-ah)
sclerae (SKLEER-ee)
Sclera is a Latin word meaning *hard.*

scleral (SKLEER-al)
scler/o- *hard; sclera (white of the eye)*
-al *pertaining to*

cornea (KOR-nee-ah)
corneae (KOR-nee-ee)
Cornea is derived from a Latin word meaning *horny sheath.*

corneal (KOR-nee-al)
corne/o- *cornea*
-al *pertaining to*

limbus (LIM-bus)
Limbus is a Latin word meaning *border.*

limbic (LIM-bik)
limb/o- *edge, border*
-ic *pertaining to*

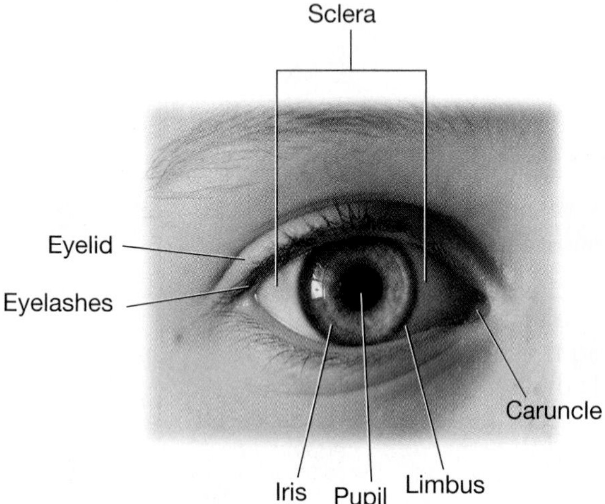

Figure 15-2 ■ The anterior surface of the eye and associated structures. The anterior surface is the only part of the eye that is visible on the surface of the body.

Iris and Pupil

The iris and pupil lie directly posterior to the cornea and can be clearly seen through the cornea. The **iris** is a circular tissue whose color is genetically determined. At the center of the iris is the **pupil,** a round opening that allows light rays to enter the eye (see Figure 15-2). The pupil itself appears black because very little light is reflected from the back of the eye. However, if you take a picture with flash photography, the intense light is reflected from the back of the eye, and the photograph shows an eye with a red pupil.

iris (EYE-ris)
irides (IHR-ih-deez)
Iris is a Greek word meaning *rainbow of colors.*

iridal (IHR-ih-dal) (EYE-rih-dal)
irid/o- *iris (colored part of the eye)*
-al *pertaining to*

pupil (PYOO-pil)
Pupil is derived from a Latin word meaning *little girl or doll,* because you can see a tiny reflection of yourself when you look closely at someone else's pupil.

pupillary (PYOO-pih-lair-ee)
pupill/o- *pupil of the eye*
-ary *pertaining to*

In bright light, muscles in the iris contract, constricting (reducing the size of) the pupil. This process, known as **miosis,** keeps too much light from entering the eye. In dim light, muscles in the iris relax, dilating (enlarging the size of) the pupil. This process, known as **mydriasis,** allows more light to enter the eye.

miosis (my-OH-sis)
mi/o- *lessening*
-osis *condition; abnormal condition; process*
Some word parts have more than one definition. The best definition of *miosis* is a *process of lessening [the size of the pupil].*

mydriasis (mih-DRY-eh-sis)
mydr/o- *widening*
-iasis *state of; process of*

Connections

Genetics. Eye color is a genetically determined trait. Chromosome 15 contains genes for brown/blue and brown/brown eye colors. Chromosome 19 has a gene for blue/green eye colors. Each parent contributes combinations of these genes to their baby.

At birth, all babies' eyes appear slate gray to blue in color because of the lack of the brown pigment melanin in the iris. Exposure to light triggers the production of melanin by melanocytes in the iris. Babies who inherit a brown/brown or brown/blue gene have a large number of melanocytes in their iris, and they develop dark brown or light brown eyes. Babies who inherit a blue/blue or a blue/green gene have no melanocytes in the iris.

Lacrimal Gland

The **lacrimal gland** is located near the superior-lateral aspect of the eye, just under the edge of the bony orbit (see Figure 15-3 ■). The lacrimal gland continuously produces and releases tears through the **lacrimal ducts** to moisten the eye. Large amounts of tears are produced when the eye is irritated or invaded by a foreign substance and during times of emotional distress. Tears also contain an antibacterial enzyme to prevent bacterial infections. At the medial aspects of the upper and lower eyelids, two tiny openings drain excess tears from the eye. The tears flow through small canals into the **lacrimal sac** and finally into the **nasolacrimal duct** that carries tears to the inside of the nose. That is why when your eyes water, your nose also runs!

lacrimal (LAK-rih-mal)
lacrim/o- *tears*
-al *pertaining to*

duct (DUHKT)
Duct is derived from a Latin word meaning *to lead.*

sac (SAK)
Sac is derived from a Latin word meaning *a bag.*

nasolacrimal (NAY-soh-LAK-rih-mal)
nas/o- *nose*
lacrim/o- *tears*
-al *pertaining to*

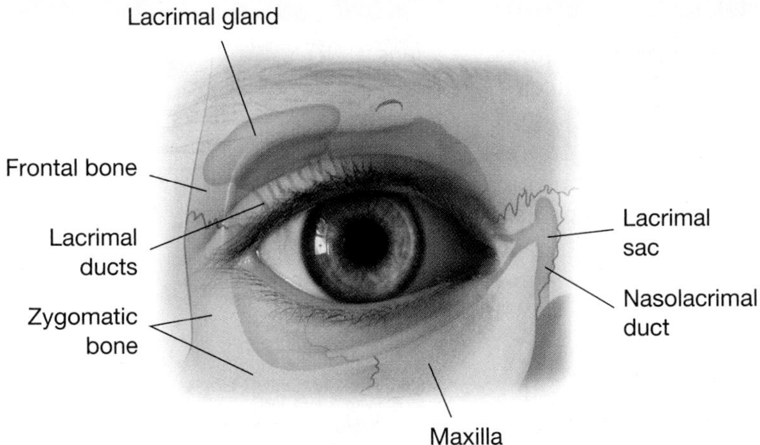

Figure 15-3 ■ Lacrimal glands.
The lacrimal glands release tears that lubricate the anterior surface of the eye. Excess tears leave the eye through small openings and eventually drain into the nose.

Choroid and Ciliary Body

The **choroid** is a spongy membrane of blood vessels that is part of the internal structure of the eye (see Figure 15-4■). It begins at the outer edges of the iris. It cannot be seen on the anterior surface of the eye because (unlike the iris) it lies beneath the opaque sclera. The blood vessels of the choroid supply blood to the entire eyeball.

The **ciliary body** is an extension of the choroid that lies posterior to the iris (see Figure 15-4). It contains thin ligaments that suspend the lens in place behind the iris. The ciliary body also contains tiny muscles that attach to the lens and change the shape of the lens to focus light rays coming through the pupil. The ciliary body also produces aqueous humor.

The **uvea** or **uveal tract** is a collective word for the structures of the iris, choroid, and ciliary body.

choroid (KOH-royd)
Choroid is derived from a Greek word meaning *like a membrane.*

choroidal (koh-ROY-dal)
choroid/o- *choroid (middle layer around the eye)*
-al *pertaining to*

ciliary (SIL-ee-air-ee)
cili/o- *hairlike structure*
-ary *pertaining to*

uvea (YOO-vee-ah)
Uvea is derived from a Latin word meaning *a grape.* The eyeball resembled a grape and the structures of the uvea were like the skin of the grape.

uveal (YOO-vee-al)
uve/o- *uvea of the eye*
-al *pertaining to*

tract (TRAKT)
Tract is derived from a Latin word meaning *path or track.*

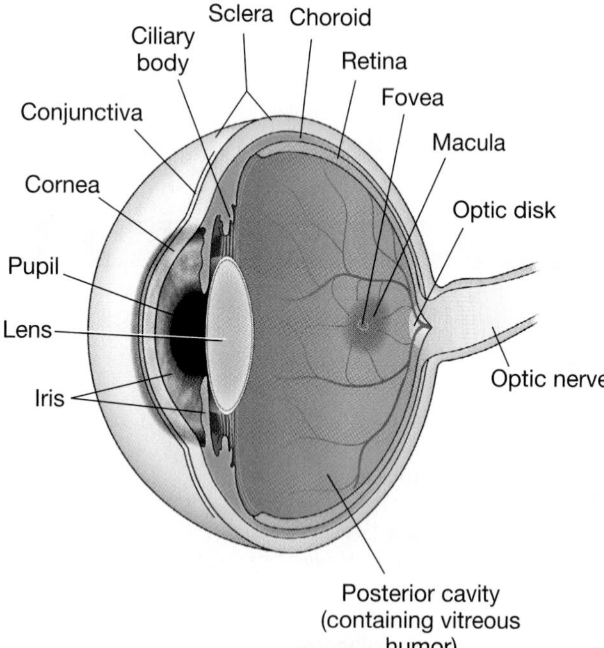

Figure 15-4 ■ Internal structures of the eye.
The iris and the pupil are visible through the clear cornea. The three layers of the sclera, choroid, and retina surround the posterior portion of the eye. The ciliary body is the anterior extension of the choroid. The retina lines the wall of the posterior cavity of the eye and contains the macula (area of sharpest vision) and the optic disk (area where the optic nerve enters).

Lens

The **lens** is a clear, hard disk that is made of transparent protein molecules arranged in a crystalline fashion (see Figure 15-4). The muscles and ligaments of the ciliary body pull on the lens and change its shape so that light rays coming into the pupil are bent and focused onto the retina. The lens becomes more concave for near vision or thinner for far vision. The lens is enclosed in a clear membrane, the **lens capsule.**

lens (LENZ)
lenses (LEN-sez)
Lens is a Latin word meaning *lentil.* The two curved sides of a lentil seed resemble a lens, and the lentil plant itself is named *Lens culinaris.*

lenticular (len-TIK-yoo-lar)
lenticul/o- *lens*
-ar *pertaining to*

capsule (KAP-sool)
Capsule is derived from a Latin word meaning *little box.*

capsular (KAP-soo-lar)
capsul/o- *capsule (enveloping structure)*
-ar *pertaining to*

Anterior and Posterior Chambers

The **anterior chamber** is a small area between the cornea and the iris (see Figure 15-5 ■). The **posterior chamber** is a narrow space posterior to the iris. The iris forms a dividing wall between the anterior and posterior chambers of the anterior eye. The only opening in this wall is the pupil. The anterior and posterior chambers are filled with aqueous humor.

Aqueous humor is a clear, watery fluid that is continuously produced by the ciliary body. Aqueous humor carries nutrients and oxygen to the cornea and lens. Aqueous humor flows from the ciliary body, through the posterior chamber, through the pupil, and into the anterior chamber. It then passes through the **trabecular meshwork,** an area of interlacing fibers located in the angle where the edges of the iris and cornea meet. It drains through a small opening in the sclera (canal of Schlemm), and then it is absorbed into veins and taken away by the blood. The rate of production of aqueous humor normally equals the rate of drainage.

anterior (an-TEER-ee-or)
anter/o- *before; front part*
-ior *pertaining to*

posterior (pohs-TEER-ee-or)
poster/o- *back part*
-ior *pertaining to*

aqueous humor
(AA-kwee-us HYOO-mor)
aque/o- *watery substance*
-ous *pertaining to*
Humor is derived from a Latin word meaning *liquid.*

trabecular (trah-BEK-yoo-lar)
trabecul/o- *trabecula (mesh)*
-ar *pertaining to*
Trabecula is a Latin word meaning *a little beam.*

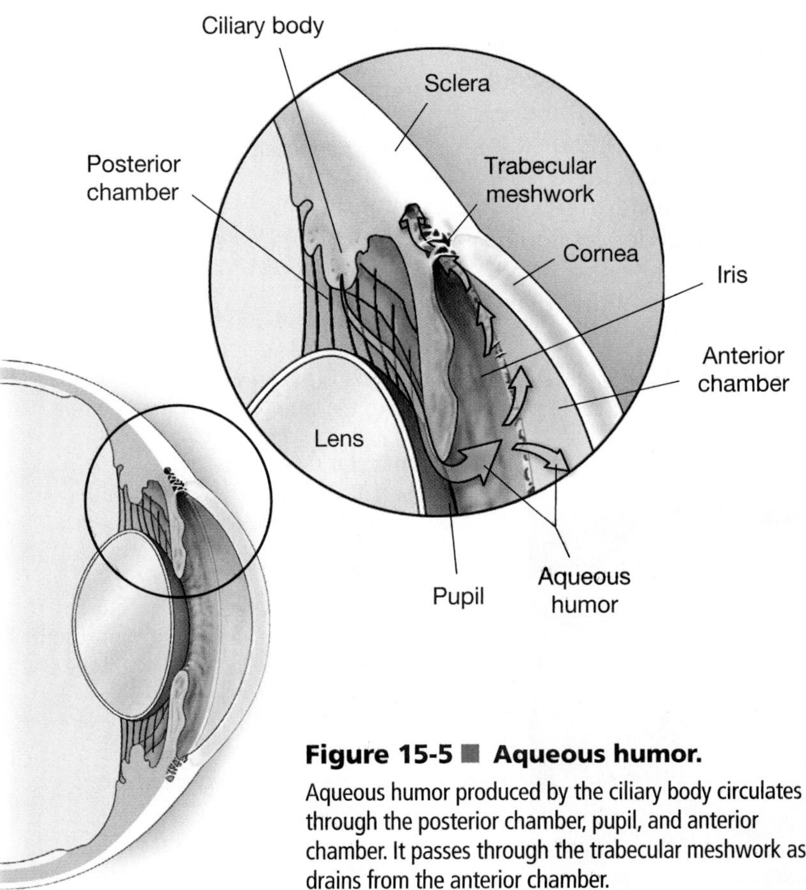

Figure 15-5 ■ Aqueous humor.

Aqueous humor produced by the ciliary body circulates through the posterior chamber, pupil, and anterior chamber. It passes through the trabecular meshwork as it drains from the anterior chamber.

Posterior Cavity

The **posterior cavity** is the largest area in the eye. It lies between the lens and the back of the eye (see Figure 15-4). It is filled with **vitreous humor,** a clear, gel-like substance that gives shape to the eye.

cavity (KAV-ih-tee)
cav/o- *hollow space*
-ity *state; condition*

vitreous humor (VIT-ree-us HYOO-mor)
vitre/o- *vitreous humor; transparent substance*
-ous *pertaining to*
Vitreous is derived from a Latin word meaning *glass.* Although the vitreous is clear like glass, it is not hard like glass.

Retina

The **retina** is a thin layer of tissue that lines the walls of the posterior cavity (see Figure 15-4). The choroid layer lies beneath the retina and provides blood to the retina.

There are several distinctive landmarks on the retina (see Figures 15-4 and 15-6■). The **optic disk** is a bright, yellow-white circle with sharp edges on the side of the retina closest to the nose. The **optic nerve** (cranial nerve II) enters the eye at the optic disk. The retinal arteries also originate from the optic disk and spread across the eye, and the retinal veins leave the eye at the optic disk. The optic disk is not stimulated by light or color and does not produce any visual images. It is known as the blind spot. The **macula** is a dark yellow-orange area lateral to the optic disk. The **fovea** is a small depression in the center of the macula. The fovea lies directly opposite the pupil. Light rays entering the pupil fall on the macula, specifically the fovea, which is the area of greatest visual acuity. **Fundus** is a general word for the retina, whose curved sides and posterior wall form part of a sphere-shaped structure.

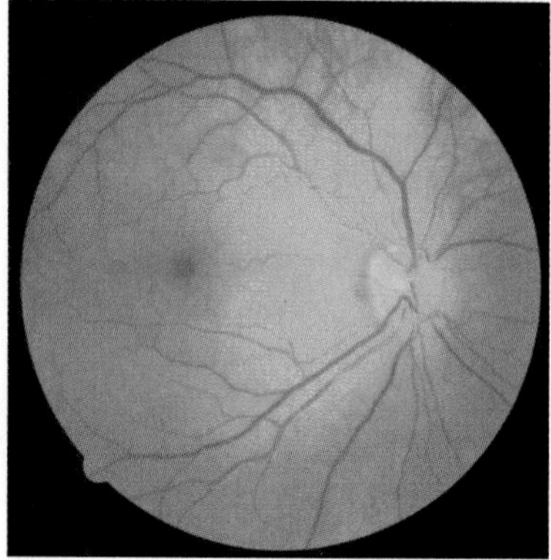

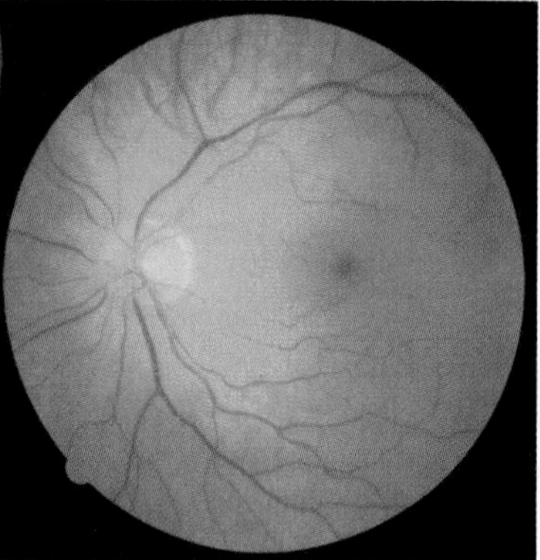

Figure 15-6 ■ The retina.

Dilation of the pupil permits visualization of the retina. The structures of the optic disk, macula, and retinal blood vessels can be clearly seen. Note that the size and shape of these structures are not identical in both eyes of the same patient.

retina (RET-ih-nah)
retinae (RET-ih-nee)
Retina is derived from a word meaning *netlike coat. Retina* is a Latin singular feminine noun. Form the plural by changing *-a* to *-ae.*

retinal (RET-ih-nal)
retin/o- *retina*
-al *pertaining to*

optic (AWP-tik)
opt/o- *eye; vision*
-ic *pertaining to*

macula (MAK-yoo-lah)
maculae (MAK-yoo-lee)
Macula is a Latin singular feminine noun. Form the plural by changing *-a* to *-ae.*

macular (MAK-yoo-lar)
macul/o- *small area or spot*
-ar *pertaining to*

fovea (FOH-vee-ah)
foveae (FOH-vee-ee)
Fovea is a Latin singular feminine noun meaning *pit or depression.* Form the plural by changing *-a* to *-ae.*

foveal (FOH-vee-al)
fove/o- *small, depressed area*
-al *pertaining to*

fundus (FUN-dus)
fundi (FUN-die)
Fundus is a Latin singular masculine noun meaning *part farthest from the opening.* The fundus is the part of the eye that is farthest away from the pupil. Form the plural by changing *-us* to *-i.*

fundal (FUN-dal)
fund/o- *fundus (part farthest from the opening)*
-al *pertaining to*

Word Alert

SOUND-ALIKE WORDS

macula (noun) Dark, orange-yellow area with indistinct margins located on the retina.

Example: The macula showed degenerative changes.

macule (noun) Small, flat, pigmented spot on the skin.

Example: Sun exposure increases the number of macules (freckles) on the skin.

macular (adjective) Descriptive word that pertains to the macula of the eye and a macule on the skin.

Examples: The patient has macular degeneration of the eye.
The patient has a macular-papular rash on the skin.

Extraocular Muscles

The **extraocular muscles** control the movements of the eye. They are attached to the sclera by tendons. Four of these muscles are straight muscles and have the word **rectus** (straight) in their names. The other two muscles wrap around the eye in a slanted manner and have the word **oblique** (slanted) in their names (see Figure 15-7 ■). The extraocular muscles and the muscles that move the eyelids are controlled by nerve impulses from cranial nerves III through VI that originate in the brain.

Extraocular Muscles

- **Superior rectus muscle:** Turns the eye superiorly
- **Inferior rectus muscle:** Turns the eye inferiorly
- **Medial rectus muscle:** Turns the eye medially (toward the midline)
- **Lateral rectus muscle:** Turns the eye laterally (away from the midline)
- **Superior oblique muscle:** Turns the eye inferiorly plus medially
- **Inferior oblique muscle:** Turns the eye superiorly plus laterally

extraocular (EKS-trah-AWK-yoo-lar)
extra- *outside of*
ocul/o- *eye*
-ar *pertaining to*

rectus (REK-tus)
Rectus is a Latin word meaning *straight.*

oblique (ob-LEEK)
Oblique is derived from a Latin word meaning *lateral or slanting.*

superior (soo-PEER-ee-or)
super/o- *above*
-ior *pertaining to*

inferior (in-FEER-ee-or)
infer/o- *below*
-ior *pertaining to*

medial (MEE-dee-al)
medi/o- *middle*
-al *pertaining to*

lateral (LAT-er-al)
later/o- *side*
-al *pertaining to*

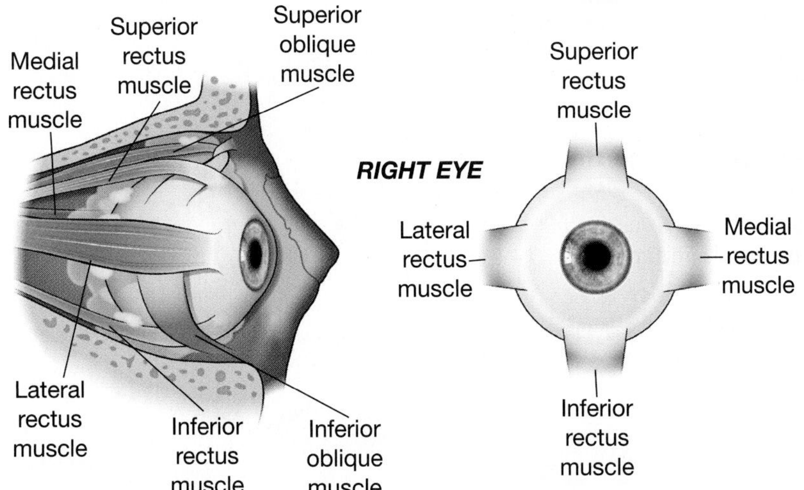

Figure 15-7 ■ Extraocular muscles.

The eye can move in all directions because of the six different extraocular muscles attached to the sclera.

Physiology of Vision

Light rays from an object pass through the cornea, which bends the rays to begin to focus them. The light rays then enter the pupil and pass through the lens. Muscles in the ciliary body contract or relax ligaments attached to the lens to focus the light rays. Light rays from objects directly in the line of vision fall on the macula (specifically the fovea), and these objects produce the clearest, sharpest image. Other parts of the retina pick up light rays from other objects in the visual field.

The retina contains special light-sensitive cells known as rods and cones. **Rods** are sensitive to all levels of light but not to color. Rods function in daytime and nighttime vision. It only takes one photon (light particle) to activate a rod, so rods can detect objects in very low light, but they only produce a somewhat grainy black-and-white image of that object. There are no rods in the macula of the retina.

rod (RAWD)
Rods are so-named because one end of each cell is shaped like a cylindrical rod.

Cones are sensitive only to color. There are three types of cones: those that respond to red light, those that respond to green light, and those that respond to blue light. The cones are concentrated in the macula. It takes many photons to activate a cone, which is why it is difficult to see colors in dim light. Cones produce a sharp color image that is superimposed on the black-and-white image created by the rods.

cone (kohn)
Cones are so-named because the end of each cell is shaped like an ice cream cone.

At this point, because of the way in which the light rays have been bent, the image of the object is actually upside down and facing in the opposite direction when it touches the retina (see Figure 15-8■).

Rods and cones everywhere in the retina respond to the light rays and relay an image to the optic nerve. The image is then converted to nerve impulses that are transmitted to the optic nerve.

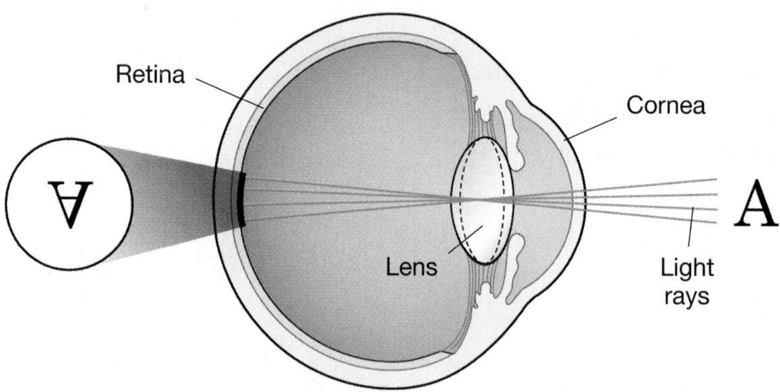

Figure 15-8 ■ Light rays coming from an object to the retina.

The cornea and lens focus light rays from an object onto the retina. An object directly in the line of vision produces an image on the macula. This image is sharp and clear, but upside down and backward.

The optic nerve (cranial nerve II) from each eye travels to the **optic chiasm,** a crossing point in the brain. There, parts of the optic nerve from the right eye cross over and join the left optic nerve. Also parts of the optic nerve from the left eye cross over and joint the right optic nerve. This merges a section of the visual field of one eye with that of the other eye and creates three-dimensional, **stereoscopic vision** with a perception of depth or distance.

From there, both optic nerves travel to the **thalamus** in the brain. The thalamus is a relay station that sends sensory nerve impulses to the right or left **visual cortex** (see Figure 15-9 ■). Each visual cortex is spread across the surface of the occipital lobe of one hemisphere of the cerebrum. The visual cortices merge the images from both eyes to create a single, three-dimensional image. The visual cortex turns the image right side up and faces it in its original direction so that it matches the object that was seen.

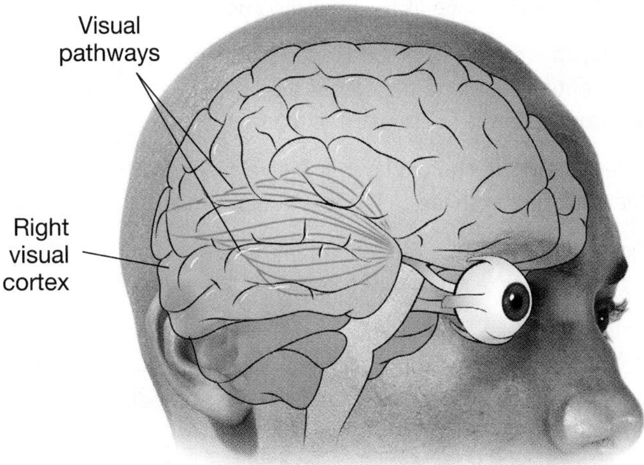

Figure 15-9 ■ Visual cortex of the brain.

Images of an object travel as nerve impulses through cranial nerve II (optic nerve) to the optic chiasm, to the thalamus, and then to the visual cortex where they are interpreted. There are two visual cortices, in the right and left occipital lobes.

chiasm (KY-azm)
Chiasm is derived from a Greek word meaning *two crossing lines.*

stereoscopic (STAIR-ee-oh-SKAWP-ik)
stere/o- *three dimensions*
scop/o- *examine with an instrument*
-ic *pertaining to*
In this case, the "instrument" is the eye itself.

vision (VIZH-un)
vis/o- *sight; vision*
-ion *action; condition*

thalamus (THAL-ah-mus)

visual (VIZH-yoo-al)
vis/o- *sight; vision*
-ual *pertaining to*

cortex (KOR-teks)
Cortex is a Latin word meaning *bark.* The visual cortex covers the surface of the occipital lobe like bark covers a tree.

Vocabulary Review

Anatomy and Physiology

Now that you have studied the anatomy and physiology of the eye, take time to review those new words and descriptions. Memorize the combining forms and their definitions before going on to the next section.

Word or Phrase	Combining Form and Definition	Description
anterior chamber	anter/o- *before; front part*	Small area between the cornea and the surface of the iris. Aqueous humor circulates through it.
aqueous humor	aque/o- *watery substance*	Clear, watery fluid produced by the ciliary body. It circulates through the posterior and anterior chambers and takes nutrients and oxygen to the cornea and lens.
caruncle		Red, triangular tissue at the medial corner of the eye
choroid	choroid/o- *choroid (middle layer around the eye)*	Spongy membrane of blood vessels that begins at the iris and continues around the eye. In the posterior cavity, it is the middle layer between the sclera and the retina.
ciliary body	cili/o- *hairlike structure*	Extension of the choroid layer. It lies posterior to the iris. It has muscles that change the shape of the lens. It also produces aqueous humor.
cones		Light-sensitive cells in the retina that detect colored light. There are three types of cones, each of which responds to either red, green, or blue light.
conjunctiva	conjunctiv/o- *conjunctiva*	Delicate, transparent mucous membrane that covers the inside of the eyelids and the anterior surface of the eye. It produces clear, watery mucus.
cornea	corne/o- *cornea*	Transparent layer over the anterior part of the eye. It is a continuation of the white sclera.
extraocular muscles	ocul/o- *eye*	Six muscles that control the movements of the eye in all directions. They include the superior rectus, inferior rectus, medial rectus, lateral rectus, superior oblique, and inferior oblique muscles.
fovea	fove/o- *small, depressed area*	Small depression in the center of the macula. This area of greatest visual acuity lies directly opposite the pupil.
fundus	fund/o- *fundus (part farthest from the opening)*	General word for the retina and its structures
iris	irid/o- *iris (colored part of the eye)*	Colored ring of tissue whose muscles contract or relax to change the size of the pupil in its center
lacrimal gland	lacrim/o- *tears*	Gland located near the superior-lateral aspect of the eye. It produces and releases tears through the **lacrimal ducts.**
lacrimal sac	lacrim/o- *tears*	Small structure that collects tears as they drain from the medial aspect of the eye. It empties into the nasolacrimal duct.
lens	lenticul/o- *lens*	Clear, hard disk in the internal eye. The muscles of the ciliary body change the lens shape to focus light rays on the retina.
lens capsule	capsul/o- *capsule (enveloping structure)*	Clear membrane that envelopes the lens

Word or Phrase	Combining Form and Definition	Description
limbus	limb/o- *edge, border*	Border between the transparent edge of the cornea and the white, fibrous sclera
macula	macul/o- *small area or spot*	Dark yellow-orange area with indistinct edges in the retina. It contains the fovea.
miosis	mi/o- *lessening*	Contraction of the iris muscle to decrease the size of the pupil and limit the amount of light entering the eye
mydriasis	mydr/o- *widening*	Relaxation of the iris muscle to increase the size of the pupil and increase the amount of light entering the eye
nasolacrimal duct	nas/o- *nose* lacrim/o- *tears*	Tube that carries tears from the lacrimal sac to the inside of the nose
optic chiasm	opt/o- *eye; vision*	Crossroads in the brain where parts of the right and left optic nerves cross and join the other optic nerve
optic disk	opt/o- *eye; vision*	Bright yellow-white circle on the retina where the optic nerve and retinal arteries enter the posterior cavity. It cannot perceive visual images and is known as the blind spot.
optic globe	opt/o- *eye; vision*	The eyeball
optic nerve	opt/o- *eye; vision*	Cranial nerve II. A sensory nerve that carries nerve impulses of visual images from the rods and cones of the retina to the visual cortex in the brain.
orbit	orbit/o- *orbit (eye socket)*	Bony socket in the cranium that surrounds all but the anterior part of the eyeball
posterior cavity	poster/o- *back part* cav/o- *hollow space*	Large space in the posterior aspect of the eye. It contains vitreous humor.
posterior chamber	poster/o- *back part*	Thin space behind the iris. Aqueous humor circulates through it.
pupil	pupill/o- *pupil of the eye*	Dark, round, central opening in the iris that allows light rays to enter the internal eye
retina	retin/o- *retina*	Membrane lining the posterior cavity. It contains rods and cones. Landmarks on the retina include the optic disk and the macula.
rods		Light-sensitive cells in the retina. They detect black and white and function in daytime and nighttime vision.
sclera	scler/o- *hard; sclera (white of the eye)*	White, tough, fibrous connective tissue that forms the outer layer around most of the eye. Also known as the white of the eye.
sebaceous glands	sebace/o- *sebum (oil)*	Oil glands at the edges of the eyelids. Also called **meibomian glands.**
stereoscopic vision	stere/o- *three dimensions* scop/o- *examine with an instrument*	Three-dimensional vision with depth perception

Word or Phrase	Combining Form and Definition	Description
thalamus		Relay station in the brain that receives sensory nerve impulses from the optic nerves and sends them to the visual centers in the occipital lobes of the brain
trabecular meshwork	trabecul/o- *trabecula (mesh)*	Area of interlacing fibers through which the aqueous humor is filtered. It is located in the anterior chamber in the angle where the edges of the iris and the cornea meet.
uveal tract	uve/o- *uvea of the eye*	Collective word for the iris, choroid, and ciliary body. Also known as the **uvea.**
visual cortex	vis/o- *sight; vision*	Areas in the right and left occipital lobes of the brain. They merge images from both eyes to create a single image that is right side up and in its original direction, matching the original object that was seen.
vitreous humor	vitre/o- *transparent substance*	Clear, gel-like substance that fills the posterior cavity of the eye

Labeling Exercise

A. *Match each anatomy word or phrase to its numbered structure in Figure 15-10 ■. Write that word or phrase on the blank line next to its number. Use the Answer Key at the end of the book to check your answers.*

caruncle	lacrimal gland and ducts	limbus	pupil
iris	lacrimal sac	nasolacrimal duct	sclera

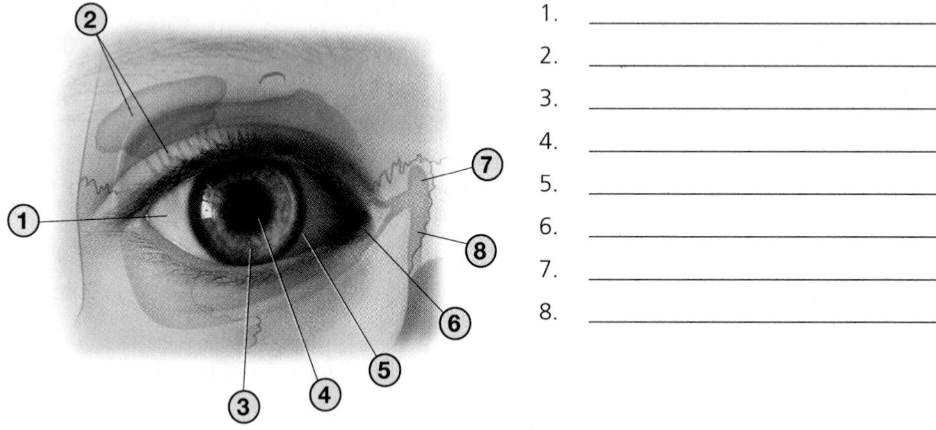

1. ____________________
2. ____________________
3. ____________________
4. ____________________
5. ____________________
6. ____________________
7. ____________________
8. ____________________

Figure 15-10 ■

B. *Match each anatomy word or phrase to its numbered structure in Figure 15-11 ■.*

choroid	fovea	optic disk	pupil
ciliary body	iris	optic nerve	retina
conjunctivae	lens	posterior cavity	sclera
cornea	macula		

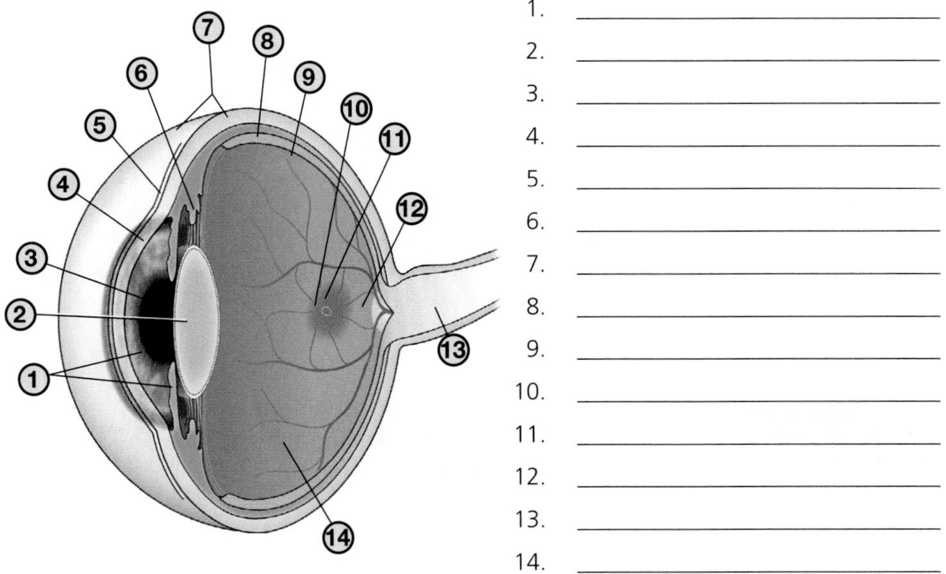

1. ______________
2. ______________
3. ______________
4. ______________
5. ______________
6. ______________
7. ______________
8. ______________
9. ______________
10. ______________
11. ______________
12. ______________
13. ______________
14. ______________

Figure 15-11 ■

Building Medical Words

Combining Forms

Here are the combining forms you have learned so far. Next to each combining form, write its meaning. Use the Answer Key at the end of the book to check your answers. The first one has been done for you.

Combining Form	Medical Meaning	Combining Form	Medical Meaning
1. anter/o-	before; front part	14. later/o-	
2. aque/o-		15. lenticul/o-	
3. capsul/o-		16. limb/o-	
4. cav/o-		17. macul/o-	
5. choroid/o-		18. medi/o-	
6. cili/o-		19. mi/o-	
7. conjunctiv/o-		20. mydr/o-	
8. corne/o-		21. nas/o-	
9. fove/o-		22. ocul/o-	
10. fund/o-		23. ophthalm/o-	
11. infer/o-		24. opt/o-	
12. irid/o-		25. orbit/o-	
13. lacrim/o-		26. poster/o-	

Combining Form	Medical Meaning
27. pupill/o-	______
28. retin/o-	______
29. scler/o-	______
30. scop/o-	______
31. sebace/o-	______
32. stere/o-	______
33. super/o-	______
34. trabecul/o-	______
35. uve/o-	______
36. vis/o-	______
37. vitre/o-	______

Combining Forms and Suffixes

Read the definition hint for the medical word you are to build. Look at the combining form that is given. Write the correct suffix on the blank line. Then write the medical word. (Remember: You may need to remove the combining vowel. Always remove the hyphens and slash.) Use the Answer Key at the end of the book to check your answers. The first one has been done for you.

SUFFIX LIST

-al (pertaining to)	-ic (pertaining to)	-ity (state; condition)
-ar (pertaining to)	-ion (condition; action)	-ous (pertaining to)
-ary (pertaining to)	-ior (pertaining to)	-ual (pertaining to)
-iasis (state of; process of)		

Definition Hint	Combining Form	Suffix	Write the Medical Word
1. Pertaining to the cornea	corne/o-	-al	*corneal*
2. Pertaining to the retina	retin/o-	______	______
3. Pertaining to the back part	poster/o-	______	______
4. Pertaining to the pupil	pupill/o-	______	______
5. Pertaining to the white of the eye	scler/o-	______	______
6. Process of the pupil dilating or widening	mydr/o-	______	______
7. Pertaining to sight or vision	opt/o-	______	______
8. Pertaining to the eye socket	orbit/o-	______	______
9. Pertaining to the lens	lenticul/o-	______	______
10. Pertaining to a watery substance	aque/o-	______	______
11. State of being a hollow space	cav/o-	______	______
12. Condition of having sight	vis/o-	______	______
13. Pertaining to sight and vision	vis/o-	______	______

Symptoms, Signs, and Diseases

Eyelid

Word or Phrase	Word Part and Definition	Description
blepharitis	**blepharitis** (BLEF-ah-RY-tis) **blephar/o-** *eyelid* **-itis** *inflammation of*	Inflammation or infection of the eyelid with redness, crusts, and scales at the bases of the eyelashes. Acute blepharitis is caused by allergy or infection. Chronic blepharitis is caused by acne rosacea, seborrheic dermatitis, or an infection from microscopic mites that live in the sebaceous glands and eyelash follicles. Treatment: Antibiotic or steroid ophthalmic ointment.
blepharoptosis	**blepharoptosis** (BLEF-ah-rawp-TOH-sis) (BLEF-ah-RAWP-toh-sis) **blephar/o-** *eyelid* **-ptosis** *state of prolapse or drooping; falling*	Drooping of the upper eyelid from excessive fat or sagging of the tissues due to age. Can also be from a disease that affects the muscles or nerves (for example, myasthenia gravis or stroke). Treatment: Blepharoplasty.
ectropion	**ectropion** (ek-TROH-pee-on) **ec-** *out, outward* **trop/o-** *having an affinity for; stimulating; turning* **-ion** *action; condition* Some word parts have more than one definition: The best definition of *ectropion* is *a condition of outward turning [of the eyelid].*	Weakening of connective tissue in the lower eyelid in older patients. The lower eyelid turns outward (see Figure 15-12 ■), exposing the conjunctiva and causing dryness and chronic conjunctivitis. Treatment: Lubricating eye drops or surgical correction. **Figure 15-12 ■ An ectropion.** The exposed conjunctiva becomes inflamed and tears spill out, leaving the surface of the eye dry and irritated.
entropion	**entropion** (en-TROH-pee-on) **en-** *in, within, inward* **trop/o-** *having an affinity for; stimulating; turning* **-ion** *action; condition*	Weakening of the muscle in the lower eyelid in older patients. The lower eyelid turns inward, causing the eyelashes to touch the eye, which results in chronic conjunctivitis and pain. Treatment: Lubricating eye drops or surgical correction.
hordeolum	**hordeolum** (hor-DEE-oh-lum) *Hordeolum* is derived from a Latin word meaning *barley* because a hordeolum can look like a white grain of barley. **chalazion** (kah-LAY-zee-on) *Chalazion* is a Greek word meaning *small lump.*	Red, painful swelling or pimple containing pus near the edge of the eyelid. Caused by a bacterial infection (staphylococcus) in a sebaceous (meibomian) gland. Also known as a stye. Sometimes, the hordeolum becomes a **chalazion,** a small, firm, painless lump. Treatment: Antibiotic drug for a hordeolum. Warm compresses or surgical excision for a chalazion.

Lacrimal Gland

Word or Phrase	Word Part and Definition	Description
dacryocystitis	**dacryocystitis** (DAK-ree-oh-sis-TY-tis) **dacry/o-** *lacrimal sac; tears* **cyst/o-** *bladder; fluid-filled sac; semisolid cyst* **-itis** *inflammation of*	Infection of the lacrimal sac by the bacterium that causes skin, nose, and ear infections. The lacrimal sac is tender and contains pus. Treatment: Oral antibiotic drug.
xerophthalmia	**xerophthalmia** (ZEER-off-THAL-mee-ah) **xer/o-** *dry* **ophthalm/o-** *eye* **-ia** *condition, state, thing*	Insufficient production of tears with eye irritation. Associated with the aging process or an ectropion. Can also be caused by certain medications. Also known as dry eyes syndrome. Treatment: Artificial tears eye drops. Surgery: Insertion of silicone plugs into the tear ducts to keep tears in the eye.

Sclera, Cornea, and Conjunctiva

Word or Phrase	Word Part and Definition	Description
conjunctivitis	**conjunctivitis** (con-JUNK-tih-VY-tis) **conjunctiv/o-** *conjunctiva* **-itis** *inflammation of*	Inflamed, reddened, and swollen conjunctivae with dilated blood vessels on the sclerae. Caused by a foreign substance in the eye, a chemical splashed in the eye, allergens or pollution in the air, chlorinated water in swimming pools, mechanical irritation from eyelashes (entropion), or dryness due to a lack of tears. Also caused by a bacterial or viral infection. Acute contagious bacterial conjunctivitis with mucus discharge is known as pinkeye. Treatment: Corticosteroid eye drops for inflammation. Antibiotic eye drops or oral antibiotic drug for infection. **Connections** **Neonatology.** When a woman with the sexually transmitted disease gonorrhea gives birth, the eyes of the newborn may become infected from the birth canal. A gonorrheal infection of the eye causes conjunctivitis and can cause blindness. By state law, all newborns are given antibiotic eye drops after birth to prevent blindness caused by gonorrhea. Chlamydia, another organism that causes a sexually transmitted disease of the genital tract, can also cause conjunctivitis in the newborn.
corneal abrasion	**abrasion** (ah-BRAY-shun) **abras/o-** *scrape off* **-ion** *action; condition* **ulcer** (UL-ser) *Ulcer* is a Latin word meaning *a sore.* **ulcerative** (UL-ser-ah-tiv) **ulcerat/o-** *ulcer* **-ive** *pertaining to* **keratitis** (KER-ah-TY-tis) **kerat/o-** *cornea* **-itis** *inflammation of*	Loss of the superficial layers of the cornea due to trauma or repetitive irritation, like a foreign particle under a contact lens. Chronic bacterial infection in an abrasion causes a **corneal ulcer** with sloughing off of necrotic tissue. Also known as **ulcerative keratitis.** Treatment: Corticosteroid drugs for inflammation; antibiotic drugs for infection. Surgery: Corneal transplant.

Word or Phrase	Word Part and Definition	Description
exophthalmos	**exophthalmos** (EKS-off-THAL-mohs) *Exophthalmos* is a combination of the prefix *ex-* and the Greek word *ophthalmos* (eye).	Pronounced outward bulging of the anterior surface of the eye with a startled, staring expression. If just one eye is affected, it often has a tumor behind it. If both eyes are affected, the patient usually has hyperthyroidism (see Figure 14-13).
scleral icterus	**icterus** (IK-ter-us) *Icterus* is a Greek word meaning *jaundice.* **icteric** (ik-TER-ik) icter/o- *jaundice* -ic *pertaining to* **jaundice** (JAWN-dis) *Jaundice* is derived from a French word meaning *yellow.* **anicteric** (AN-ik-TER-ik) an- *without, not* icter/o- *jaundice* -ic *pertaining to*	Yellow coloration of the conjunctivae which makes the sclerae also appear yellow. Caused by **jaundice** due to liver disease (see Figure 15-13 ■). In a patient without jaundice, the sclerae are said to be **anicteric**. **Figure 15-13 ■ Scleral icterus.** This patient's eye shows a yellow discoloration due to high levels of bilirubin that his diseased liver is unable to conjugate.
Iris, Pupil, and Anterior Chamber		
anisocoria	**anisocoria** (an-EYE-soh-KOH-ree-ah) anis/o- *unequal* cor/o- *pupil* -ia *condition, state, thing*	Unequal sizes of the pupils. Caused by glaucoma, head trauma, stroke, or a tumor that damages the cranial nerve that causes the iris to dilate and constrict. Treatment: Correct the underlying cause.
glaucoma	**glaucoma** (glaw-KOH-mah) *Glaucoma* is a combination of *glauc/o-* (silver gray or green) and the suffix *-oma* (tumor, mass). Its meaning actually describes a cataract because these two diseases were thought to be the same until the early 1700s. **intraocular** (IN-trah-AWK-yoo-lar) intra- *within* ocul/o- *eye* -ar *pertaining to*	Increased **intraocular pressure (IOP)** because aqueous humor cannot circulate freely. In open-angle glaucoma, the angle where the edges of the iris and cornea touch is normal and open, but the trabecular meshwork is blocked. Open-angle glaucoma is painless but destroys peripheral vision, leaving the patient with tunnel vision. In closed-angle glaucoma, the angle is too small and blocks the aqueous humor. Closed-angle glaucoma causes severe pain, blurred vision, and photophobia. Glaucoma can progress to blindness. Treatment: Eye drops to lower the intraocular pressure. Surgery: Laser trabeculoplasty.

Word or Phrase	Word Part and Definition	Description
hyphema	**hyphema** (hy-FEE-mah) *Hyphema* is derived from a Greek word meaning *condition of blood throughout.*	Blood in the anterior chamber. Caused by trauma or increased intraocular pressure. Treatment: Corticosteroid eye drops or oral drugs.
photophobia	**photophobia** (FOH-toh-FOH-bee-ah) **phot/o-** *light* **phob/o-** *fear or avoidance* **-ia** *condition, state, thing*	Abnormal sensitivity to bright light. Can be associated with inflammation and external or internal diseases of the eye or increased intracranial pressure. Treatment: Correct the underlying cause.
uveitis	**uveitis** (YOO-vee-EYE-tis) **uve/o-** *uvea of the eye* **-itis** *inflammation of* **iritis** (eye-RY-tis) **ir/o-** *iris (colored part of the eye)* **-itis** *inflammation of* **choroiditis** (KOH-roy-DY-tis) **choroid/o-** *choroid (middle layer around the eye)* **-itis** *inflammation of*	Inflammation or infection of the uveal tract. Can be caused by infection in the eye or another part of the body, allergy, trauma, or autoimmune disorders. **Iritis** affects the iris. **Choroiditis** affects the choroid membrane. Treatment: Correct the underlying cause.
Lens		
aphakia	**aphakia** (ah-FAY-kee-ah) **a-** *away from, without* **phak/o-** *lens of the eye* **-ia** *condition, state, thing* **aphakic** (ah-FAY-kik) **a-** *away from, without* **phak/o-** *lens of the eye* **-ic** *pertaining to*	Condition in which the lens of the eye has been surgically removed. In most patients, an artificial intraocular lens is put into the eye during the cataract surgery. Some cataract patients are not good candidates for an artificial intraocular lens. Their cataract is removed, but they wear special cataract eyeglasses, and they remain **aphakic.**
cataract	**cataract** (KAT-ah-rakt) *Cataract* is derived from a Greek word meaning *a waterfall.* Looking through a cataract can be like looking through a waterfall or a piece of waxed paper.	Clouding of the lens (see Figure 15-14■). Protein molecules in the lens begin to clump together. Caused by aging, sun exposure, eye trauma, smoking, and some medications. Vision becomes dull and blurry with faded colors and a yellowish tint around lights. Congenital cataracts are present at birth. Treatment: Cataract surgery.

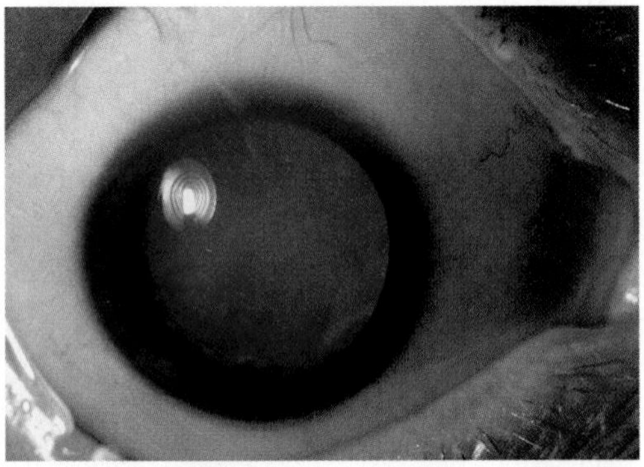

Figure 15-14 ■ Cataract.

As a cataract develops, the lens gradually becomes cloudy and opaque. The vision is blurry and colors are faded and yellowed.

Word or Phrase	Word Part and Definition	Description
presbyopia	**presbyopia** (PREZ-bee-OH-pee-ah) **presby/o-** *old age* **-opia** *condition of vision*	Loss of flexibility of the lens with blurry near vision and loss of accommodation. Caused by aging. Treatment: Corrective eyeglasses.
Posterior Cavity and Retina		
color blindness		Genetic condition in which the cones, particularly green or red ones, are absent or do not contain enough visual pigment to respond to the light from colored objects. Treatment: None.
diabetic retinopathy	**diabetic** (DY-ah-BET-ik) **diabet/o-** *diabetes* **-ic** *pertaining to* **retinopathy** (RET-ih-NAWP-ah-thee) **retin/o-** *retina* **-pathy** *disease, suffering*	Chronic, progressive condition in which new, fragile retinal blood vessels are formed in patients with uncontrolled diabetes mellitus. These contain microaneurysms that leak, forming exudates (dried fluid deposits) on the retina. They also rupture easily, causing intraocular hemorrhage. Treatment: Management of diabetes mellitus. Surgery with laser photocoagulation.
floaters and flashers		Floaters are clumps, dots, or strings of collagen molecules that form in the vitreous humor because of aging. Flashers are brief bursts of bright light that occur when the vitreous humor pulls on the retina. Treatment: None.
macular degeneration	**macular** (MAK-yoo-lar) **macul/o-** *small area or spot* **-ar** *pertaining to* **degeneration** (DEE-jen-er-AA-shun) **de-** *reversal of; without* **gener/o-** *production; creation* **-ation** *a process; being or having*	Chronic, progressive loss of central vision as the macula degenerates. In older patients, this is known as age-related macular degeneration (ARMD). In dry macular degeneration (the most common type), the macula deteriorates with age. In wet macular degeneration, abnormal blood vessels grow under the macula. They are fragile and leak, causing the macula to lift away from the retina. Treatment: Laser therapy to destroy abnormal blood vessels.
night blindness		Marked decrease in visual acuity at night or in dim light. This occurs with aging or when the diet does not contain enough vitamin A. Treatment: Dietary supplement, if needed.
papilledema	**papilledema** (PAP-il-ah-DEE-mah) **papill/o-** *elevated structure* **-edema** *swelling*	Inflammation and edema of the optic disk. Caused by increased intracranial pressure from a brain tumor or head trauma. Also known as a choked disk. Treatment: Correct the underlying cause.
retinal detachment	**detachment** (dee-TACH-ment) *Detachment* is a combination of *detach* (to separate) and the suffix *-ment* (action; state).	Separation of the retina from the choroid layer beneath it. This can be caused by head trauma. It can occur gradually during aging as the vitreous humor changes from a gel to a watery consistency that flows into tears in the retina and separates the two layers. In diabetic patients, hemorrhage of the fragile retinal blood vessels can separate the layers. Treatment: Retinopexy with cryotherapy or laser photocoagulation.
retinitis pigmentosa (RP)	**retinitis pigmentosa** (RET-ih-NY-tis PIG-men-TOH-sah) **retin/o-** *retina* **-itis** *inflammation of*	Inherited abnormality linked to 70 different genes. The retina has abnormal deposits of pigmentation behind the rods and cones, causing loss of color vision or night vision and loss of central or peripheral vision. It can progress to blindness. Treatment: None.

Word or Phrase	Word Part and Definition	Description
retinoblastoma	**retinoblastoma** (RET-ih-noh-blas-TOH-mah) **retin/o-** *retina* **blast/o-** *immature; embryonic* **-oma** *tumor, mass*	Cancerous tumor of the retina in children, arising from abnormal embryonic retinal cells. Treatment: Chemotherapy, radiation therapy, and surgical excision.
retinopathy of prematurity	**retinopathy** (RET-ih-NAWP-ah-thee) **retin/o-** *retina* **-pathy** *disease, suffering* **prematurity** (PREE-mah-TYOOR-ih-tee) **pre-** *before; in front of* **matur/o-** *mature* **-ity** *state; condition* **retrolental** (REH-troh-LEN-tal) **retro-** *behind, backward* **lent/o-** *lens of the eye* **-al** *pertaining to* **fibroplasia** (FY-broh-PLAY-zee-ah) **fibr/o-** *fiber* **plas/o-** *growth, formation* **-ia** *condition, state, thing*	Retinal tissue is replaced with fibrous tissue because of therapy using high levels of oxygen in premature babies with immature lungs. Also known as **retrolental fibroplasia.** Treatment: Laser photocoagulation.
Extraocular Muscles		
nystagmus	**nystagmus** (nis-TAG-mus) *Nystagmus* is derived from a Greek word meaning *nodding.*	Involuntary rhythmic motions of the eye, particularly when looking to the side. Each back-and-forth motion is known as a "beat." Nystagmus can be caused by multiple sclerosis or Meniere's disease. Treatment: Correct the underlying cause.
strabismus	**strabismus** (strah-BIZ-mus) *Strabismus* is derived from a Greek word meaning *squinting.* **esotropia** (ES-oh-TROH-pee-ah) **es/o-** *inward* **trop/o-** *having an affinity for; stimulating; turning* **-ia** *condition, state, thing* **exotropia** (EKS-oh-TROH-pee-ah) **ex/o-** *away from, external, outward* **trop/o-** *having an affinity for; stimulating; turning* **-ia** *condition, state, thing*	Deviation of one or both eyes medially or laterally. Medial deviation is known as **esotropia** or cross-eye (see Figure 15-15 ■). Lateral deviation is known as **exotropia** or wall-eye. Treatment: Surgery repositioning of the extraocular muscles. This is done during early childhood. **Figure 15-15 ■ Esotropia.** In this type of strabismus, one or both eyes deviate medially toward the nose. Surgical correction is necessary for the patient to develop normal vision.

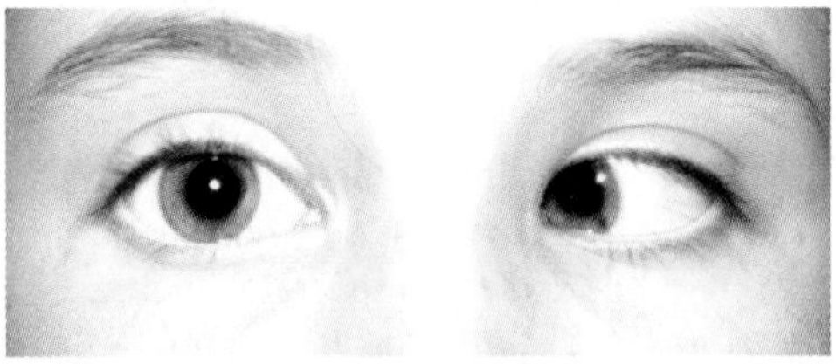

Refractive Disorders of the Eyes

Word or Phrase	Word Part and Definition	Description
astigmatism	**astigmatism** (ah-STIG-mah-tizm) **a-** *away from, without* **stigmat/o-** *point, mark* **-ism** *process; disease from a specific cause*	Surface of the cornea is curved more steeply on one side of the eye than on the other, so there is no single point of focus. The patient's vision is blurry both near and at a distance. Treatment: Corrective lenses or surgery.
hyperopia	**hyperopia** (HY-per-OH-pee-ah) **hyper-** *above; more than normal* **-opia** *condition of vision* Add words to make a correct and complete definition of *hyperopia: vision [that is sharp at] more than normal [distance].*	Farsightedness. Light rays from a far object focus correctly on the retina, creating a sharp image. However, light rays from a near object come into focus posterior to the retina, creating a blurred image (see Figure 15-16■). 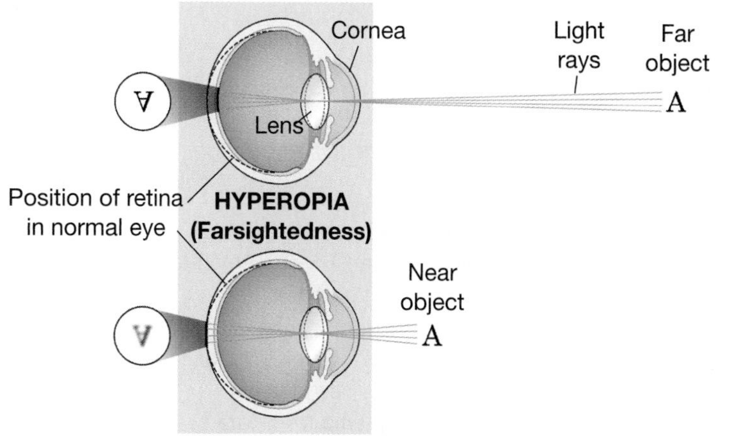 **Figure 15-16 ■ Hyperopia.** There is an abnormally short distance between the cornea and the retina. The patient can clearly see things that are at a distance (farsightedness), but near vision is blurry.
myopia	**myopia** (my-OH-pee-ah) **myop/o-** *near* **-opia** *condition of vision* *Myopia* is derived from the Greek word *myein* (*to shut*) and *-opia* (*condition of vision*). Patients with myopia often half-close their eyelids to improve their vision.	Nearsightedness. Light rays from a near object focus correctly on the retina, creating a sharp image. However, light rays from a far object come into focus anterior to the retina, creating a blurred image (see Figure 15-17■). 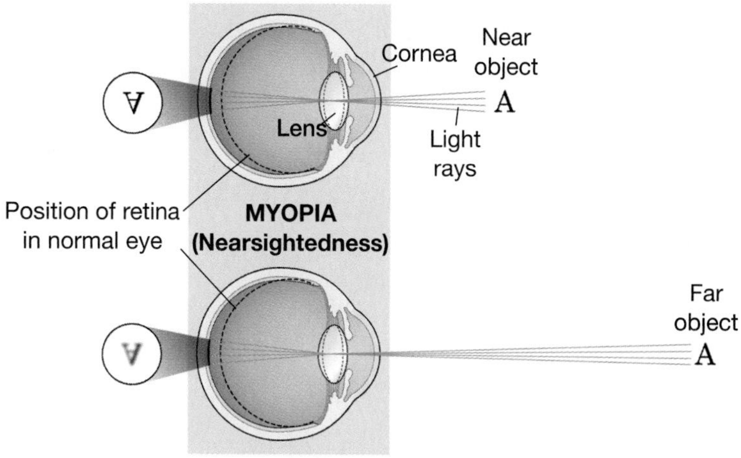 **Figure 15-17 ■ Myopia.** There is an abnormally long distance between the cornea and the retina. The patient can clearly see things that are close by, but far vision is blurry.

Conditions of the Brain and Visual Cortex

Word or Phrase	Word Part and Definition	Description
amblyopia	**amblyopia** (AM-blee-OH-pee-ah) **ambly/o-** *dimness* **-opia** *condition of vision* Add words to make a correct and complete definition of *amblyopia: vision [suppression] and dimness [in one eye].*	To prevent double vision, the brain ignores the visual image from an eye with strabismus (the most common cause) or an eye in which the vision is unfocused or cloudy. Also known as lazy eye. Amblyopia may continue even after the strabismus or other defect is surgically corrected. Treatment: The normal eye is patched until the brain accepts the visual image from the other eye.
blindness		Condition of complete or partial loss of vision. Patients whose best visual acuity is 20/200 even with corrective lenses are legally blind. Caused by trauma, eye diseases, or defects in the structure of the eye, optic nerve, or visual cortex in the brain. Treatment: Correct the underlying cause.
diplopia	**diplopia** (dih-PLOH-pee-ah) **dipl/o-** *double* **-opia** *condition of vision*	Two visual fields are seen rather than one fused image. Can be caused by ambylopia, by tumors or trauma that increase the intracranial pressure, or by multiple sclerosis that affects nerve conduction to the visual cortex in the brain. Treatment: Correct the underlying cause.
scotoma	**scotoma** (skoh-TOH-mah) **scotomata** (skoh-TOH-mah-tah) **scot/o-** *darkness* **-oma** *tumor, mass* *Scotoma* is a Greek singular noun. Form the plural by changing *-oma* to *-omata.* Although a scotoma is not a tumor or mass, its effect is as if a mass was blocking the vision. **hemianopia** (HEM-ee-ah-NOH-pee-ah) **hemi-** *one half* **an-** *without, not* **-opia** *condition of vision*	Temporary or permanent visual field defect in one or both eyes. These vary in size and can be patchy or solid, stationary or moving. This is caused by glaucoma, diabetic retinopathy, or macular degeneration when various parts of the retina or optic nerve branches are destroyed. Also, a hemorrhage (stroke), tumor, or trauma on one side of the brain can cause a scotoma in the opposite visual field. **Hemianopia** is loss of one half of the visual field (right or left, top or bottom). Prior to a migraine headache, a patient may see a scintillating scotoma, a moving line of brilliantly flashing bars of light. Also known as hemianopsia. Treatment: Correct the underlying cause.

Diagnostic Procedures

Eye Tests

Word or Phrase	Word Part and Definition	Description
color blindness testing		Diagnostic procedure to determine the degree of red or green color blindness. Each successive color plate requires a higher discrimination of color perception. Color plates with numbers are used to test adults (see Figure 15-18 ■), while color plates with circles, squares, or animals are used to test children. 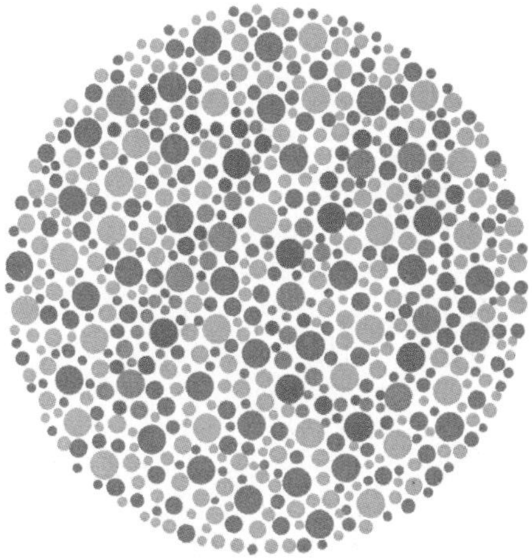 **Figure 15-18 ■ The Ishihara color plate for testing color blindness.** A patient with green color blindness would not be able to distinguish the *70* printed in green.
fluorescein angiography	**fluorescein** (floo-RES-een) **angiography** (AN-jee-AWG-rah-fee) **angi/o-** *blood vessel; lymphatic vessel* **-graphy** *process of recording* **angiogram** (AN-jee-oh-gram) **angi/o-** *blood vessel; lymphatic vessel* **-gram** *a record or picture*	Diagnostic procedure in which fluorescein, an orange fluorescent dye, is injected intravenously. The dye travels to the retinal artery in the eye. It glows fluorescent green on flash photography of the retina. The photographic image is known as an **angiogram.** It reveals retinal microaneurysms, leaking, and hemorrhages common in diabetic patients.

Word or Phrase	Word Part and Definition	Description
fluorescein staining	**fluorescein** (floo-RES-een)	Diagnostic procedure in which fluorescein, an orange fluorescent dye, is applied topically to the cornea and used to detect corneal abrasions and ulcers. As a blue light is used to examine the eye, corneal abrasions and ulcers appear as fluorescent green.
gonioscopy	**gonioscopy** (GOH-nee-AWS-koh-pee) **goni/o-** *angle* **-scopy** *process of using an instrument to examine*	Diagnostic procedure for glaucoma. It uses a slit lamp with a special lens that illuminates the trabecular meshwork.
slit-lamp examination		Diagnostic procedure to look for abnormalities of the cornea, anterior chamber, iris, or lens. The slit lamp combines a low-power microscope (biomicroscope) for magnification with a high-intensity light beam whose width can be adjusted down to a slit (see Figure 15-19 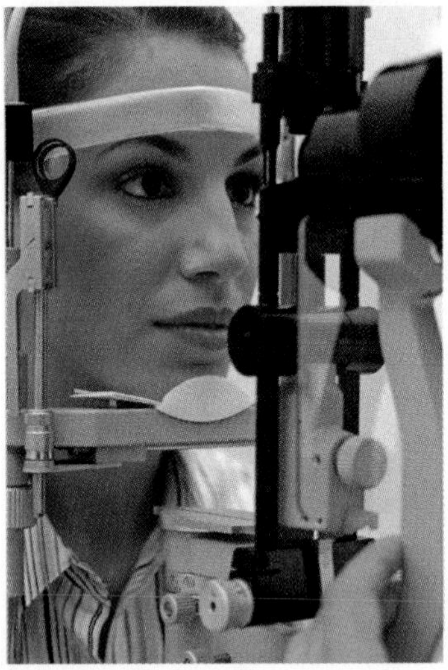 ■). **Figure 15-19 ■ Slit lamp examination.** The patient's chin and forehead are in a fixed position as the slit lamp moves around to magnify, illuminate, and view the eye from different angles.
tonometry	**tonometry** (toh-NAWM-eh-tree) **ton/o-** *pressure, tone* **-metry** *process of measuring* **tonometer** (toh-NAWM-eh-ter) **ton/o-** *pressure, tone* **-meter** *instrument used to measure*	Diagnostic procedure for increased intraocular pressure and glaucoma. The small, flat disk of the **tonometer** is pressed against the cornea to record the intraocular pressure. Alternatively, air-puff tonometry emits a short burst of air and measures the pressure of the air rebounding from the cornea without touching the patient's eye.

Word or Phrase	Word Part and Definition	Description
visual acuity testing	**visual** (VIZH-yoo-al) **vis/o-** *sight; vision* **-ual** *pertaining to* **acuity** (ah-KYOO-ih-tee) **acu/o-** *needle; sharpness* **-ity** *state; condition*	Diagnostic procedure for near and distance vision. Each eye is tested separately. A card with typed sentences of decreasing print size is held at a preset distance of 16 inches to test the near vision. The Snellen chart is used to test distance vision. Each line on the card or the chart corresponds to a visual acuity rating. Normal visual acuity is 20/20. The numerator stands for 20 feet, the standard distance between the chart and the patient. The denominator stands for the distance at which a person with normal vision could see that line on the chart. The Tumbling E chart has capital *E*s facing in various directions, and the patient indicates which way the legs of the *E* are pointing. Children or patients who are illiterate are tested with charts that use pictures. For a patient with severe vision problems, visual acuity can be recorded as either count fingers or light perception.
Radiologic Tests		
ultrasonography	**ultrasonography** (UL-trah-soh-NAWG-rah-fee) **ultra-** *beyond; higher* **son/o-** *sound* **-graphy** *process of recording* **sonogram** (SAWN-oh-gram) **son/o-** *sound* **-gram** *a record or picture*	Radiologic procedure that uses high-frequency sound waves to create an image of the eye. A-scan ultrasound measures the eye prior to intraocular lens insertion. B-scan creates a two-dimensional image of the inside of the eye to show tumors or hemorrhages. The ultrasound image is known as a **sonogram.**

Medical and Surgical Procedures

Medical Procedures

Word or Phrase	Word Part and Definition	Description
accommodation	**accommodation** (ah-KAWM-oh-DAY-shun) **accommod/o-** *to adapt* **-ation** *a process; being or having*	Medical procedure to test the ability of the ciliary muscles and ligaments to contract and flex the lens as demonstrated on near and distance visual acuity tests.
convergence	**convergence** (con-VER-jens) **converg/o-** *coming together* **-ence** *state of*	Medical procedure to test the ability of both eyes to turn medially. The physician holds up an index finger and moves it progressively closer to the patient's nose to test the function of the medial rectus muscles. The maximum convergence is called the near point.

Word or Phrase	Word Part and Definition	Description
dilated funduscopy	**funduscopy** (fun-DUHS-koh-pee) **fundu/o-** *fundus (part farthest from the opening)* **-scopy** *process of using an instrument to examine* **funduscopic** (FUN-duh-SKAWP-ik) **fundu/o-** *fundus (part farthest from the opening)* **scop/o-** *examine with an instrument* **-ic** *pertaining to* **mydriatic** (MIH-dree-AT-ik) **mydr/o-** *widening* **-iatic** *pertaining to a state or process* **cycloplegia** (SY-kloh-PLEE-jee-ah) **cycl/o-** *ciliary body of the eye; cycle* **pleg/o-** *paralysis* **-ia** *condition, state, thing* **ophthalmoscope** (off-THAL-moh-skohp) **ophthalm/o-** *eye* **-scope** *instrument used to examine*	Medical procedure to examine the posterior cavity. **Mydriatic** eye drops are used to dilate the pupil (a process known as **cycloplegia**). An **ophthalmoscope,** a handheld instrument with a light and changeable lenses of different strengths, is used to examine the retina from all angles. The physician dials in the correct lens that produces a sharp image while compensating for both his visual defects and those of the patient. Alternatively, the patient can be placed in a darkened room to dilate the pupils. A strobe light creates a sudden flash to illuminate the retina while a Polaroid® picture is taken. This method is able to show about 30% of the retina. Any abnormalities of the retina must be further examined with a dilated funduscopic exam.
eye patching		Medical procedure in which the eye is covered with a soft bandage and a hard outer shield after eye trauma or eye surgery. Also, a normal eye can be patched to treat amblyopia.
gaze testing	**conjugate** (CON-joo-gayt) **conjug/o-** *joined together* **-ate** *composed of; pertaining to* **dysconjugate** (dis-CON-joo-gayt) **dys-** *painful, difficult, abnormal* **conjug/o-** *joined together* **-ate** *composed of; pertaining to* Some word parts have more than one definition. The best definition of *dysconjugate* is *pertaining to abnormally joined together [eye movements]*.	Medical procedure to test the extraocular muscles. The patient follows the physician's finger from side to side and up and down. **Conjugate gaze** is when both eyes move together as a unit. This is documented in the patient's record as EOMI (extraocular movements intact). **Dysconjugate gaze** is when the eyes do not move together.

Word or Phrase	Word Part and Definition	Description
peripheral vision	**peripheral** (peh-RIF-eh-ral) peripher/o- *outer aspects* -al *pertaining to*	Medical procedure to test the visual acuity at the edges of the visual field. The patient looks straight ahead while the physician moves an object from behind the patient's head toward the edge of the visual field (from the top, bottom, and both sides). The patient indicates when the object is first seen. Alternatively, a computer projects dots onto a screen with a grid and the patient indicates when a dot is seen.
phorometry	**phorometry** (foh-RAWM-eh-tree) phor/o- *range* -metry *process of measuring* **phorometer** (foh-RAWM-eh-ter) phor/o- *range* -meter *instrument used to measure*	Medical procedure to select the strength of lens that corrects the patient's refractive error and gives 20/20 vision. The specifications of that lens are written as a prescription that is duplicated in eyeglasses or contact lenses. A **phorometer** (see Figure 15-20 ■) holds lenses of successive strengths that are dialed into place as the patient looks through the lens at a Snellen chart. Each eye is tested separately. 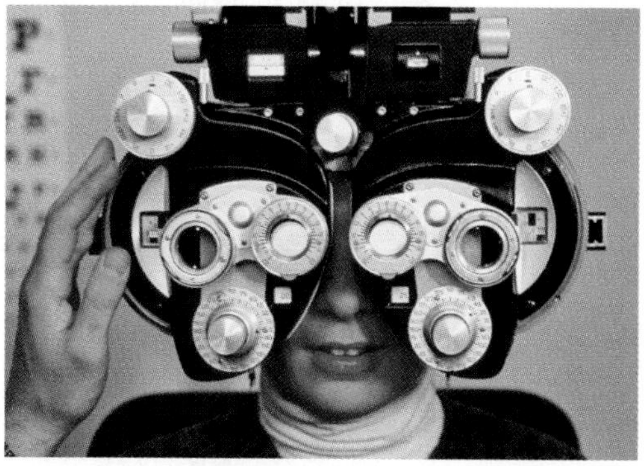 **Figure 15-20 ■ Phorometer.** This instrument helps the ophthalmologist select the most accurate corrective lens for the patient.
pupillary response		Medical procedure to test that the pupils constrict briskly and equally in response to a bright light (see Figure 15-21 ■). This is documented in the patient's record as *PERRL* (pupils equal, round, and reactive to light). 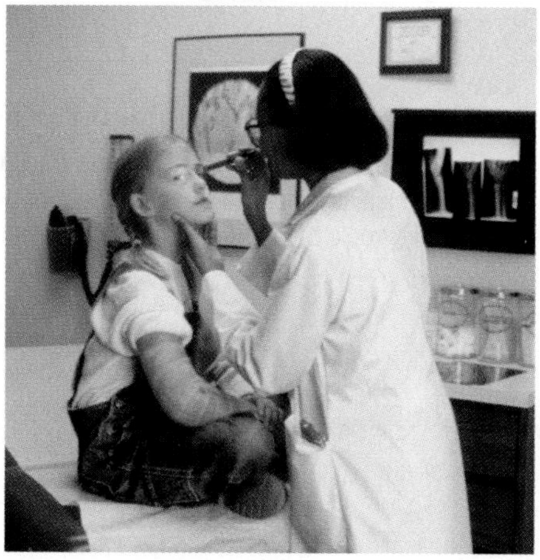 **Figure 15-21 ■ Pupillary response.** This physician is using a penlight to check the response of the pupils. This girl suffered a broken arm and a mild concussion. A sluggish or unequal pupillary response to light could indicate bleeding or edema in the brain.

A Closer Look

A prescription for corrective eyeglasses includes a number of different measurements (see Figure 15-22 ■).

Sphere. Numbers indicate prism diopters (PD), a unit of measurement for the refractive power of a lens. The higher the number, the more powerful the lens. A plus sign (+) in front of the number means a convex lens is needed. A convex lens (thicker in the center than at the edges) is used to correct farsightedness. A minus sign (−) in front of the number means a concave lens is needed. A concave lens (thinner in the center and thicker at the edges) is used to correct nearsightedness.

Cylinder. The extent of astigmatism of the cornea is also measured in diopters. The number given is the difference between the most curved and least curved areas on the central part of the cornea.

Axis. The most curved to least curved areas of the cornea can be oriented in any direction. The axis is given as the number of degrees (from 1 to 180) of deviation from a horizontal line (0 degrees).

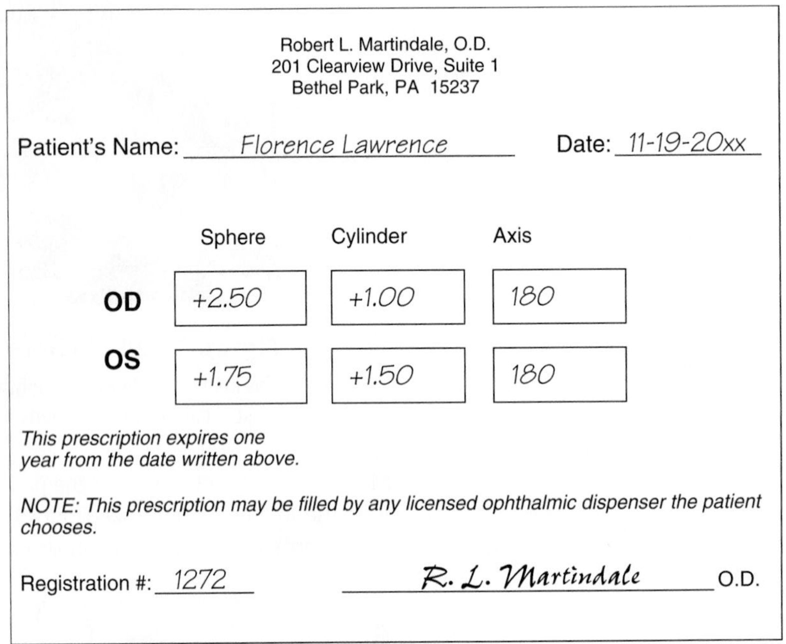

Robert L. Martindale, O.D.
201 Clearview Drive, Suite 1
Bethel Park, PA 15237

Patient's Name: *Florence Lawrence* Date: *11-19-20xx*

	Sphere	Cylinder	Axis
OD	+2.50	+1.00	180
OS	+1.75	+1.50	180

This prescription expires one year from the date written above.

NOTE: This prescription may be filled by any licensed ophthalmic dispenser the patient chooses.

Registration #: 1272 *R. L. Martindale* O.D.

Figure 15-22 ■ Eyeglasses prescription.

This patient has moderate hyperopia (farsightedness). The plus sign (+) indicates that a convex lens is needed to correct the refractive error, with the right eye (OD) being slightly worse than the left eye (OS).

Surgical Procedures

Word or Phrase	Word Part and Definition	Description
blepharoplasty	**blepharoplasty** (BLEF-ah-roh-PLAS-tee) **blephar/o-** *eyelid* **-plasty** *process of reshaping by surgery*	Plastic surgery procedure to the eyelids to remove fat and sagging skin. Often done in conjunction with a face-lift.
capsulotomy	**capsulotomy** (KAP-soo-LAWT-oh-mee) **capsul/o-** *capsule (enveloping structure)* **-tomy** *process of cutting or making an incision*	Surgical procedure that is only done after a cataract extraction when the remaining posterior lens capsule becomes cloudy or wrinkled. A YAG laser is used to make an opening in the capsule to restore normal vision.
cataract extraction	**extracapsular** (EKS-trah-KAP-soo-lar) **extra-** *outside of* **capsul/o-** *capsule (enveloping structure)* **-ar** *pertaining to* **extraction** (ek-STRAK-shun) **ex-** *out, away from* **tract/o-** *pulling* **-ion** *action; condition* **phacoemulsification** (FAY-koh-ee-MUL-sih-fih-KAY-shun) **phac/o-** *lens of the eye* **emulsific/o-** *particles suspended in a solution* **-ation** *a process; being or having* **intracapsular** (IN-trah-KAP-soo-lar) **intra-** *within* **capsul/o-** *capsule (enveloping structure)* **-ar** *pertaining to*	Surgical procedure to remove a lens affected by a cataract. Preoperatively, a laser is used to measure the length of the eye and the curvature of the cornea so that a customized IOL can be created that corrects the patient's vision. In **extracapsular cataract extraction (ECCE),** an incision is made in the sclera to remove the lens but the posterior lens capsule is left in place. In **phacoemulsification,** a small, self-sealing (stitchless) incision is made in the cornea. An ultrasonic probe is inserted and sound waves are used to break up the lens. The pieces are removed with irrigation and aspiration. In both operations, the central part of the lens is removed and replaced with an artificial intraocular lens (IOL) implant. The implant folds to pass through the incision and then unfolds. **Intracapsular cataract extraction (ICCE)** in which the entire lens and lens capsule are removed is performed less often.
corneal transplantation	**transplantation** (TRANS-plan-TAY-shun) **transplant/o-** *move something to another place* **-ation** *a process; being or having*	Surgical procedure to replace a damaged or diseased cornea. The cornea is removed with a trephine (a round cookie-cutter instrument with a sharp edge). Then a donor cornea is sutured in place with zig-zag sutures. Donor corneas are obtained from people who have died of illness or accident and willed their organs to others.
enucleation	**enucleation** (EE-noo-klee-AA-shun) **enucle/o-** *to remove the kernel or nucleus* **-ation** *a process; being or having*	Surgical procedure to remove the eye from the orbit because of trauma or tumor.

Word or Phrase	Word Part and Definition	Description
hyperopia surgery	**conductive** (con-DUK-tiv) **conduct/o-** *carrying, conveying* **-ive** *pertaining to* **keratoplasty** (KER-ah-toh-PLAS-tee) **kerat/o-** *cornea* **-plasty** *process of reshaping by surgery* **laser** (LAY-zer) *Laser* is an acronym for the words *light amplification by stimulated emission of radiation.* **thermal** (THER-mal) **therm/o-** *heat* **-al** *pertaining to*	Surgical procedure to correct farsightedness. Uses heat to shrink tissues around the edge of the cornea to produce a greater curvature in the cornea that corrects the refractive error. **Conductive keratoplasty (CK)** uses radiowaves delivered by a probe as thin as a hair in spots around the edge of the cornea. **Laser thermal keratoplasty (LTK)** uses a laser to simultaneously place spots in two concentric circles around the cornea.
laser photocoagulation	**laser** (LAY-zer) **photocoagulation** (FOH-toh-koh-AG-yoo-LAY-shun) **phot/o-** *light* **coagul/o-** *clotting* **-ation** *a process; being or having* **vitrectomy** (vih-TREK-toh-mee) **vitre/o-** *vitreous humor; transparent substance* **-ectomy** *surgical excision*	Surgical procedure to seal leaking or hemorrhaging retinal blood vessels or reattach a detached retina. Light from the laser creates heat that coagulates the tissues (see Figure 15-23 ■). If there is blood in the vitreous humor, the light from the laser cannot reach the retina, and a **vitrectomy** must be done first to remove the vitreous humor and replace it with a synthetic substitute. 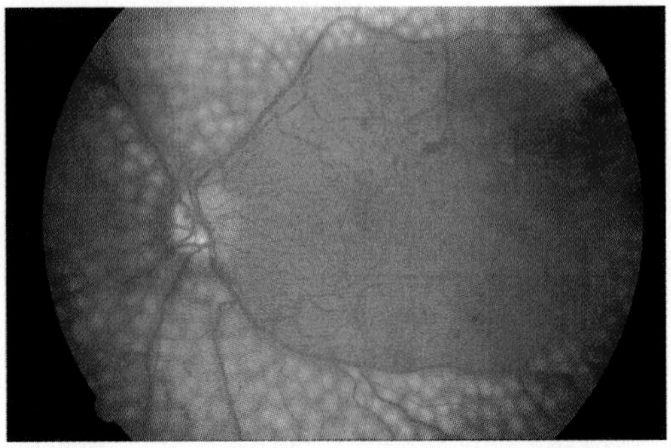 **Figure 15-23 ■ Laser photocoagulation.** This procedure is used to treat the leaking or hemorrhaging blood vessels associated with diabetic retinopathy. Here, the laser has been used in multiple spots to coagulate the tissues around the optic disk.

Word or Phrase	Word Part and Definition	Description
myopia surgery	**laser** (LAY-zer) **in situ** (in SY-too) *In situ* is a Latin phrase meaning *at that site and not extending into other sites.* **keratomileusis** (KER-ah-toh-my-LOO-sis) **kerat/o-** *cornea* **-mileusis** *process of carving* **microkeratome** (MY-kroh-KER-ah-tohm) **micr/o-** *small* **kerat/o-** *cornea* **-tome** *instrument used to cut; an area with distinct edges* **photorefractive** (FOH-toh-ree-FRAK-tiv) **phot/o-** *light* **refract/o-** *bend or deflect* **-ive** *pertaining to* **keratectomy** (KER-ah-TEK-toh-mee) **kerat/o-** *cornea* **-ectomy** *surgical excision*	Surgical procedure to correct nearsightedness. A three-dimensional corneal map is created preoperatively and programmed into the laser. In **laser-assisted *in situ* keratomileusis (LASIK),** a **microkeratome** creates a very thin flap on the surface of the cornea. The flap is peeled back, and an excimer laser (a cold laser that cuts tissue without heating it) is used to reshape the underlying cornea. The surface flap is then positioned back in place. In **photorefractive keratectomy (PRK),** the excimer laser reshapes the curvature of the cornea without the creation of a corneal surface flap.
retinopexy	**retinopexy** (RET-ih-noh-PEK-see) **retin/o-** *retina* **-pexy** *process of surgically fixing in place* **cryotherapy** (KRY-oh-THAIR-ah-pee) **cry/o-** *cold* **-therapy** *treatment*	Surgical procedure to reattach a detached retina. **Cryotherapy** is used to freeze the tissue and fix all three layers (sclera, choroid, retina) together. Alternatively, laser photocoagulation can be done to heat spots on the retina to coagulate and seal them to the layers beneath.
strabismus surgery	**resection** (ree-SEK-shun) **resect/o-** *to cut out and remove* **-ion** *action; condition* **recession** (ree-SESH-un) **recess/o-** *to move back* **-ion** *action; condition*	Surgical procedure to correct esotropia or exotropia. In a **resection,** the extraocular muscle on one side is shortened and in a **recession,** the extraocular muscle on the other side is lengthened and reattached.

Word or Phrase	Word Part and Definition	Description
trabeculoplasty	**trabeculoplasty** (trah-BEK-yoo-loh-PLAS-tee) **trabecul/o-** *trabecula (mesh)* **-plasty** *process of reshaping by surgery*	Surgical procedure to treat open-angle glaucoma. An argon laser is used to create small holes in half of the trabecular meshwork to increase the flow of aqueous humor. The procedure is usually effective for five years, at which time another trabeculoplasty can be performed on the untreated half of the trabecular meshwork.

Drug Categories

Several different categories of drugs are used to treat the symptoms, signs, and diseases of the eye. The most common drugs in each category are listed. Note: All drugs used topically in the eye are specially formulated from a solution that is physiologically similar to the fluids of the eye so as not to damage the delicate tissues of the eye.

Category	Word Part and Definition	Description	Examples
antibiotic drugs	**antibiotic** (AN-tee-by-AWT-ik) (AN-tih-by-AWT-ik) **anti-** *against* **bi/o-** *life; living organisms; living tissue* **-tic** *pertaining to*	Treat bacterial infections of the eye. Antibiotics are not effective against viral infections of the eye.	Genoptic, Ocuflox
antiviral drugs	**antiviral** (AN-tee-VY-ral) (AN-tih-VY-ral) **anti-** *against* **vir/o-** *virus* **-al** *pertaining to*	Treat viral infections of the eye, specifically herpes simplex virus.	Viroptic
chemotherapy drugs	**chemotherapy** (KEE-moh-THAIR-ah-pee) **chem/o-** *chemical, drug* **-therapy** *treatment*	Kill rapidly dividing cancer cells in the eye.	carboplatin, Cytoxan, vincristine
corticosteroid drugs	**corticosteroid** (KOR-tih-koh-STAIR-oyd) **cortic/o-** *cortex (outer region)* **-steroid** *steroid*	Treat inflammation of the eye.	Flarex, Inflamase Forte, Maxidex
drugs for glaucoma		Act by decreasing the amount of aqueous humor or by constricting the pupil to open up the angle between the iris and the cornea.	Azopt, Betoptic, Ocupress, pilocarpine
mydriatic drugs	**mydriatic** (MIH-dree-AT-ik) **mydr/o-** *widening* **-iatic** *pertaining to a state or process*	Dilate the pupil and prepare the eye for an internal examination.	atropine, Mydriacyl

Abbreviations

ARMD	age-related macular degeneration
CK	conductive keratoplasty
ECCE	extracapsular cataract extraction
EOM	extraocular movements
EOMI	extraocular muscles intact
HEENT	head, eyes, ears, nose, and throat
ICCE	intracapsular cataract extraction
IOL	intraocular lens
IOP	intraocular pressure
LASIK	laser-assisted *in situ* keratomileusis
LTK	laser thermal keratoplasty
OD, O.D.	right eye (oculus dexter)
O.D.	Doctor of Optometry
OS, O.S.	left eye (oculus sinister)
OU, O.U.	both eyes (oculus uterque)
PD	prism diopter
PERRL	pupils equal, round, and reactive to light
PERRLA	pupils equal, round, reactive to light and accommodation
PRK	photorefractive keratectomy
ROP	retinopathy of prematurity
RP	retinitis pigmentosa
VF	visual field

Word Alert

MEDICAL ABBREVIATIONS

Abbreviations are commonly used in all types of medical documents; however, they can mean different things to different people and their meaning can be misinterpreted. Always verify the meaning of an abbreviation.

O.D. stands for *right eye* or *Doctor of Optometry,* but it also stands for *overdose.*

LASIK stands for *laser assisted* in situ *keratomileusis,* but it can be mistaken for *Lasix,* the trade name of a diuretic drug.

Career Focus

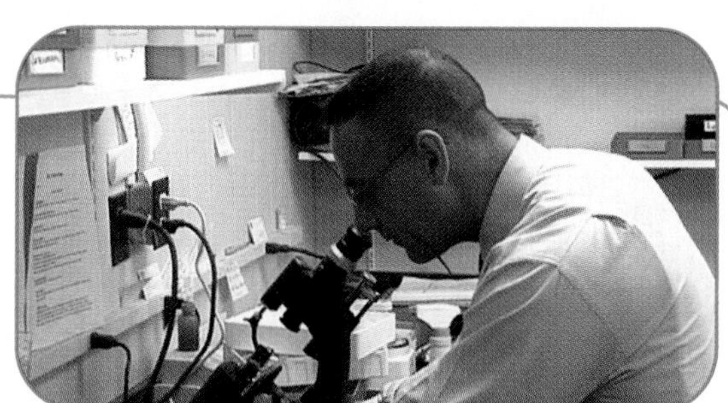

Meet Paul, an optician.

"I pick up where the ophthalmologist or optometrist leaves off, by looking at the prescription and suggesting to the patient the selection of frame styles or lens styles. Either we have the lenses here in stock, or we'll order them from a servicing lab that actually manufactures the lens. We use a lensometer to read the prescription of the lens, and we have to make sure we place the optical center of the lens in front of the patient's pupil. This is a fairly busy practice. From 8:00 A.M. to closing, patients come in to purchase new eyewear or have their old eyewear repaired. I've been dealing with the public all my life. When you dispense a pair of glasses to someone and it puts a new light on everything, it's gratifying; it really is."

Opticians are allied health professionals who use automated equipment to cut, grind, and finish lenses to exact specifications based on a written prescription from an optometrist or ophthalmologist. They also prepare contact lenses and instruct the patient in their care and handling. Opticians work in optical stores or in the office of an optometrist or ophthalmologist.

Optometrists are doctors of **optometry** (O.D.) who have graduated from a school of optometry. They diagnose and treat patients with vision problems and diseases of the eyes. They write prescriptions for eyeglasses and contact lenses. They can administer and prescribe ophthalmic drugs. Optometrists do not perform eye surgery.

Ophthalmologists are physicians (M.D.) who practice in the medical specialty of ophthalmology. They do all of the things an optometrist does, but they are also able to perform surgery on the eye. Cancerous tumors of the eye are treated medically by an oncologist or surgically by an opthalmologist.

optician (op-TISH-un)
opt/o- *eye; vision*
-ician *a skilled professional or expert*

optometrist (op-TAWM-eh-trist)
opt/o- *eye; vision*
metr/o- *measurement*
-ist *one who specializes in*

optometry (op-TAWM-eh-tree)
opt/o- *eye; vision*
-metry *process of measuring*

ophthalmologist (OFF-thal-MAWL-oh-jist)
ophthalm/o- *eye*
log/o- *the study of*
-ist *one who specializes in*

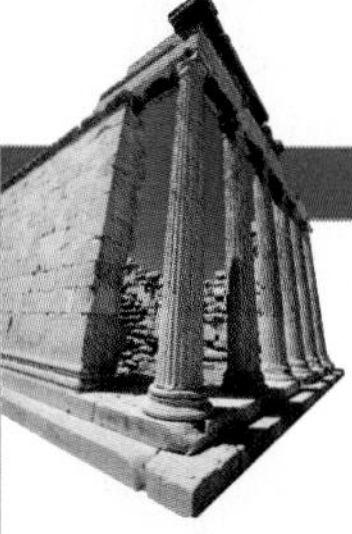

It's Greek to Me!

Did you notice that some eye words have two different combining forms? Combining forms from both Greek and Latin languages remain a part of medical language today.

English Word	Greek	Latin	Examples of Medical Words
eye	ophthalm/o-	ocul/o-	ophthalmology, ocular
lens	phac/o-, phak/o-	lenticul/o-, lent/o-	phacoemulsification, aphakia, lenticular, retrolental
pupil	cor/o-	pupill/o-	anisocoria, pupillary
sight, vision	opt/o-	vis/o-	optic, visual

Chapter Review Exercises

Review all the material in this chapter by completing the review exercises in this section. Use the Answer Key at the end of the book to check your answers.

Anatomy and Physiology

Matching Exercise

Match each numbered word or phrase to its description.

1.	ciliary body	____ Turns the eyeball upwards
2.	conjunctiva	____ Center of the macula
3.	fovea	____ Support the lens
4.	limbus	____ Includes iris, choroid, and ciliary body
5.	mydriasis	____ Enlarging of the size of the pupil
6.	optic chiasm	____ The bony socket that holds the eyeball
7.	orbit	____ Filters aqueous humor
8.	superior rectus muscle	____ Edge of the cornea where it joins the sclera
9.	suspensory ligaments	____ Where the brain processes visual images
10.	trabecular meshwork	____ Produces aqueous humor
11.	uveal tract	____ Mucous membrane on underside of eyelid
12.	visual cortex	____ Where the optic nerves cross

Circle Exercise

Circle the correct word from the choices given.

1. The (**iris, limbus, orbit**) is the colored, circular structure around the pupil.
2. The red, triangular tissue at the medial corner of the eye is the (**caruncle, lacrimal gland, trabecular meshwork**).
3. The (**cornea, iris, sclera**) is the tough, fibrous, white outer covering of the eye.
4. The blind spot on the retina corresponds to the (**fundus, macula, optic disk**).
5. Color vision comes from cells known as (**cones, rods, visual cortices**).
6. Cranial nerve (**II, III, IV, V**) is the optic nerve for vision.

True or False

Indicate whether each statement is true or false by writing T or F on the line.

1. ____ The nasolacrimal duct carries vitreous humor.
2. ____ The sclera is the clear part of the cornea.
3. ____ Eye color is a genetically determined trait.
4. ____ Muscles in the pupil make it dilate or constrict.
5. ____ At birth, all babies' eyes appear gray-blue.
6. ____ Vitreous humor is a clear, watery fluid.
7. ____ Stereoscopic vision is three dimensional.

Sequencing Exercise

Beginning where light enters the eye, use the list of words and phrases to help you sequence the structures of the eye in the correct order.

aqueous humor	cornea	light rays from an object	pupil
conjunctiva	fovea	optic nerve	vitreous humor

1. Light rays from object → 2. ______ → 3. ______ →
4. ______ → 5. ______ → 6. ______ →
7. ______ → 8. ______

Medical Language Word Parts

Name that Word Part

Identify each of the word parts given here by writing in the correct letter (P, C, or S) on the line beside it. Then write the definition of the word part on the blank line. The first one has been done for you.

Prefix = P **Combining Form = C** **Suffix = S**

	Word Part	Definition		Word Part	Definition
1. -al	S	pertaining to	25. coagul/o-		
2. a-			26. conduct/o-		
3. abras/o-			27. conjug/o-		
4. accommod/o-			28. conjunctiv/o-		
5. acu/o-			29. converg/o-		
6. ambly/o-			30. corne/o-		
7. an-			31. cor/o-		
8. angi/o-			32. cortic/o-		
9. anis/o-			33. cry/o-		
10. anter/o-			34. cycl/o-		
11. anti-			35. cyst/o-		
12. aque/o-			36. dacry/o-		
13. -ar			37. de-		
14. -ary			38. diabet/o-		
15. -ate			39. dipl/o-		
16. -ation			40. dys-		
17. bi/o-			41. ec-		
18. blast/o-			42. -ectomy		
19. blephar/o-			43. -edema		
20. capsul/o-			44. emulsific/o-		
21. cav/o-			45. en-		
22. chem/o-			46. -ence		
23. choroid/o-			47. enucle/o-		
24. cili/o-			48. es/o-		

	Word Part	Definition
49. ex-	_____	_______________
50. ex/o-	_____	_______________
51. extra-	_____	_______________
52. fibr/o-	_____	_______________
53. fove/o-	_____	_______________
54. fund/o-	_____	_______________
55. fundu/o-	_____	_______________
56. gener/o-	_____	_______________
57. goni/o-	_____	_______________
58. -gram	_____	_______________
59. -graphy	_____	_______________
60. hemi-	_____	_______________
61. hyper-	_____	_______________
62. -ia	_____	_______________
63. -iasis	_____	_______________
64. -iatic	_____	_______________
65. -ic	_____	_______________
66. -ician	_____	_______________
67. icter/o-	_____	_______________
68. infer/o-	_____	_______________
69. intra-	_____	_______________
70. -ion	_____	_______________
71. -ior	_____	_______________
72. irid/o-	_____	_______________
73. ir/o-	_____	_______________
74. -ism	_____	_______________
75. -ist	_____	_______________
76. -itis	_____	_______________
77. -ity	_____	_______________
78. -ive	_____	_______________
79. kerat/o-	_____	_______________
80. lacrim/o-	_____	_______________
81. later/o-	_____	_______________
82. lenticul/o-	_____	_______________
83. lent/o-	_____	_______________
84. limb/o-	_____	_______________
85. log/o-	_____	_______________
86. -logy	_____	_______________
87. macul/o-	_____	_______________
88. matur/o-	_____	_______________
89. medi/o-	_____	_______________
90. -meter	_____	_______________

	Word Part	Definition
91. metr/o-	_____	_______________
92. -metry	_____	_______________
93. micr/o-	_____	_______________
94. -mileusis	_____	_______________
95. mi/o-	_____	_______________
96. mydr/o-	_____	_______________
97. nas/o-	_____	_______________
98. ocul/o-	_____	_______________
99. -oma	_____	_______________
100. ophthalm/o-	_____	_______________
101. -opia	_____	_______________
102. opt/o-	_____	_______________
103. orbit/o-	_____	_______________
104. -osis	_____	_______________
105. -ous	_____	_______________
106. papill/o-	_____	_______________
107. -pathy	_____	_______________
108. peripher/o-	_____	_______________
109. -pexy	_____	_______________
110. phac/o-	_____	_______________
111. phak/o-	_____	_______________
112. phob/o-	_____	_______________
113. phor/o-	_____	_______________
114. phot/o-	_____	_______________
115. plas/o-	_____	_______________
116. -plasty	_____	_______________
117. pleg/o-	_____	_______________
118. poster/o-	_____	_______________
119. pre-	_____	_______________
120. presby/o-	_____	_______________
121. -ptosis	_____	_______________
122. pupill/o-	_____	_______________
123. recess/o-	_____	_______________
124. refract/o-	_____	_______________
125. resect/o-	_____	_______________
126. retin/o-	_____	_______________
127. retro-	_____	_______________
128. scler/o-	_____	_______________
129. -scope	_____	_______________
130. scop/o-	_____	_______________
131. -scopy	_____	_______________
132. scot/o-	_____	_______________

	Word Part	Definition		Word Part	Definition
133. sebace/o-	______	______	145. trabecul/o-	______	______
134. son/o-	______	______	146. tract/o-	______	______
135. stere/o-	______	______	147. transplant/o-	______	______
136. -steroid	______	______	148. trop/o-	______	______
137. stigmat/o-	______	______	149. -ual	______	______
138. super/o-	______	______	150. ulcerat/o-	______	______
139. -therapy	______	______	151. ultra-	______	______
140. therm/o-	______	______	152. uve/o-	______	______
141. -tic	______	______	153. vir/o-	______	______
142. -tome	______	______	154. vis/o-	______	______
143. -tomy	______	______	155. vitre/o-	______	______
144. ton/o-	______	______	156. xer/o-	______	______

Word-Building Exercise

Use the combining forms, prefixes, and suffixes given here to build medical words that match the definitions given. Write the word that you build on the blank line. Some word parts may be used more than once. The first one has been done for you.

Word Parts

blephar/o- (eyelid)	-ia (condition, state, thing)	ophthalm/o- (eye)	presby/o- (old age)
conjunctiv/o- (conjunctiva)	ir/o- (iris)	phob/o- (fear or avoidance)	-ptosis (state of prolapse or drooping; falling)
dipl/o- (double)	-itis (inflammation of)	phot/o- (light)	xer/o- (dry)
hyper- (above; more than normal)	-logy (the study of)	-plasty (process of reshaping by surgery)	
	-opia (condition of vision)		

1. Inflammation of the conjunctiva (You think *conjunctiv/o-* + *-itis*). You write conjunctivitis
2. Farsightedness ______
3. Inflammation of the eyelid ______
4. Sensitivity of the eyes to light ______
5. Changes in the vision in older patients ______
6. Study of the eye ______
7. Double vision ______
8. Dry eye syndrome ______
9. Inflammation of the iris ______
10. Drooping of the eyelid ______
11. Plastic surgery for eyelids ______

Symptoms, Signs, and Diseases

Circle Exercise

Circle the correct word from the choices given.

1. Involuntary beats of the eye when looking to the side is called (**diplopia, nystagmus, strabismus**).
2. A patient with exophthalmos often has (**blindness, glaucoma, hyperthyroidism**).
3. Increased intraocular pressure is caused by (**conjunctivitis, glaucoma, presbyopia**).
4. Clumps of vitreous humor cause (**color blindness, floaters, strabismus**).
5. Farsightedness is (**astigmatism, hyperopia, myopia**).

Matching Exercise

Match each numbered word or phrase to its description.

1.	anisocoria	_____ Malignant eye tumor in children
2.	blepharitis	_____ Also known as a stye
3.	cataract	_____ A type of strabismus
4.	entropion	_____ Caused by mites in the eyelash follicles
5.	exotropia	_____ Blurry, opaque lens
6.	glaucoma	_____ Lower eyelid turns in
7.	hordeolum	_____ Visual field defect
8.	macular degeneration	_____ Loss of peripheral vision
9.	pinkeye	_____ Unequal pupils
10.	retinoblastoma	_____ Acute contagious bacterial conjunctivitis
11.	scotoma	_____ Loss of central vision

Laboratory, Radiology, Surgery, and Drugs

True or False

Indicate whether each statement is true or false by writing T or F on the line.

1. ____ Gonioscopy is used to visualize the trabecular meshwork.
2. ____ Diopters are drugs that dilate the pupil.
3. ____ A blepharoplasty removes fat and sagging skin from the eyelid.
4. ____ LASIK and PRK are used to surgically correct nearsightedness.
5. ____ Corticosteroid drugs are used to dilate the pupil before an eye exam.

Matching Exercise

Match each numbered word or phrase to its description.

1.	convergence	_____ What can be seen at the edge of the visual field
2.	penlight	_____ Used to do a funduscopic examination
3.	conjugate gaze	_____ Lens can change shape to focus
4.	peripheral vision	_____ Eyes move together as a unit
5.	accommodation	_____ Used to check the pupil response
6.	ophthalmoscope	_____ Both eyes focus on the near point
7.	angiogram	_____ Test for glaucoma
8.	Ishihara	_____ Laser seals leaking retinal blood vessels
9.	phacoemulsification	_____ Used to treat a detached retina
10.	phorometer	_____ Holds lenses of successive strengths
11.	photocoagulation	_____ Fluorescein outlines the retinal blood vessels
12.	retinopexy	_____ Color blindness test
13.	Snellen	_____ Surgical procedure to treat glaucoma
14.	tonometry	_____ Visual acuity test
15.	trabeculoplasty	_____ Part of cataract surgery

Abbreviations

Matching Exercise

Match each numbered abbreviation to its definition.

1.	IOL	_____ Eye movements are intact
2.	IOP	_____ Premature babies get this eye disease
3.	LASIK	_____ Placed within the eye after cataract surgery
4.	O.S.	_____ Pupils react normally
5.	OU	_____ Surgery for nearsightedness
6.	ROP	_____ Glaucoma causes this
7.	EOMI	_____ Left eye
8.	PERRL	_____ Both eyes

Applied Skills

Plural Noun and Adjective Spelling

Fill in the blanks with the correct word form. Be sure to check your spelling. The first one has been done for you.

Singular Noun	Plural Noun	Adjective	Singular Noun	Plural Noun	Adjective
1. sclera	sclerae	scleral	5. cornea	____________	____________
2. iris	____________	____________	6. retina	____________	____________
3. pupil	____________	____________	7. macula	____________	____________
4. conjunctiva	____________	____________	8. fundus	____________	____________

Analysis of a Medical Report

This exercise contains a Consultation Report from a specialist physician. Read the report and answer the questions.

CONSULTATION REPORT

PATIENT NAME: BROWN, Rubeetha

PATIENT NUMBER: 04-7223

DATE OF CONSULTATION: November 19, 20xx

HISTORY OF PRESENT ILLNESS

This 54-year-old, African American female comes in today as a referral from her primary care physician. She is complaining of bloodshot eyes, headaches, large floaters in her visual field, and blurred vision at close range.

PAST HISTORY

She has had myopia since childhood (onset at age 12). She was diagnosed by a neurologist as having migraines with an aura of scintillating scotomas followed by a temporary visual field defect of hemianopia "like a gray curtain" coming down. She denies a history of hyperthyroidism, although she has been tested for this on several occasions. She denies hypertension, heart disease, or diabetes. She has some mild osteoarthritis, particularly in her right knee. Past surgeries include a tonsillectomy and an appendectomy in the remote past.

SOCIAL HISTORY

She is married and has 2 children, both living away from home. She works in the member services department of an HMO and does paperwork and computer work all day.

PHYSICAL EXAMINATION

The conjunctivae are injected, and the sclerae are anicteric. There is a soft, movable mass in the margin of the right upper eyelid. The patient states that this was from a trauma and has remained unchanged for many years. This is not a chalazion, just scar tissue. There is a moderate amount of crusted exudate on the eyelids. There is mild exophthalmos bilaterally. PERRL. Extraocular movements intact. Dilating drops were instilled in each eye, and funduscopy was performed. There is evidence of a developing cataract in the right eye. The retinas bilaterally were normal. There was no suggestion of macular degeneration, and the cup-to-disk ratio was normal. There were no microaneurysms or hemorrhages. There were small clumps of vitreous humor visible in the posterior cavity.

VISUAL TESTING

Distance vision without glasses was 20/200 in both eyes. Peripheral vision was normal. Depth perception was normal. Tonometry showed normal intraocular pressures in both eyes.

DIAGNOSES

1. Eye strain and new-onset presbyopia.
2. Severe myopia. Wears corrective lenses for distance vision.
3. Stage I cataract, O.D.
4. Blepharitis.
5. Vitreous floaters. The patient was advised that although these are annoying and appear large, they are actually small and benign and are the result of the aging process.

PLAN

1. The patient has been given a prescription for new eyeglasses. These will be bifocal lenses to correct her myopia and her new-onset presbyopia.
2. The patient was asked to gently cleanse the eyelids and apply bacitracin ophthalmic ointment b.i.d.
3. The patient has been advised of her increased risk of developing glaucoma given her age and race and was advised to have an annual eye examination with tonometry. Follow up in 1 year to evaluate the status of her cataract and do a glaucoma check.

Lauren J. Spiner, M.D.

Lauren J. Spiner, M.D.

LJS: jtr

D: 11/19/xx

T: 11/19/xx

WORD ANALYSIS QUESTIONS

1. A funduscopy was performed. If you wanted to use the adjective form of funduscopy, you would say, "The patient had a ______________________ examination performed."
2. Divide *intraocular* into its three word parts and define each word part.

Word Part	Definition
________	________________________
________	________________________
________	________________________

3. Divide *anicteric* into its three word parts and define each word part.

Word Part	Definition
________	________________________
________	________________________
________	________________________

FACT FINDING QUESTIONS

1. What part of the eye does a funduscopy examine? ______________________
2. What eye condition has the patient had since childhood? ______________________
3. What two visual symptoms does the patient have before the onset of a migraine? ______________________
4. The normal tonometry results ruled out what disease? ______________________
5. The mass on the patient's eyelid is a chalazion. **True** **False**
6. What is the meaning of PERRL? ______________________
7. What abbreviation tells you that the patient's cataract was in the right eye? ______________________

CRITICAL THINKING QUESTIONS

1. The physical finding of crusted exudates on the eyelids corresponds to which diagnosis?______________________
2. Examination of which part of the eye tells you that the patient does not have liver disease?______________________
3. Why have physicians in the past tested the patient for hyperthyroidism? ______________________

Pronunciation Checklist

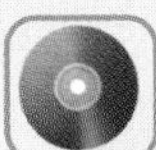

Read each word and its pronunciation. Practice pronouncing each word. Verify your pronunciation by listening to the Pronunciation List on the CD-ROM. Check the box next to the word after you master its pronunciation.

- ❑ accommodation (ah-KAWM-oh-DAY-shun)
- ❑ amblyopia (AM-blee-OH-pee-ah)
- ❑ anicteric sclerae (AN-ik-TER-ik SKLEER-ee)
- ❑ anisocoria (an-EYE-soh-KOH-ree-ah)
- ❑ anterior chamber (an-TEER-ee-or CHAYM-ber)
- ❑ antibiotic drug (AN-tee-by-AWT-ik DRUHG) (AN-tih-by-AWT-ik)
- ❑ antiviral drug (AN-tee-VY-ral DRUHG)
- ❑ aphakia (ah-FAY-kee-ah)
- ❑ aphakic (ah-FAY-kik)
- ❑ aqueous humor (AA-kwee-us HYOO-mor)
- ❑ astigmatism (ah-STIG-mah-tizm)
- ❑ blepharitis (BLEF-ah-RY-tis)
- ❑ blepharoplasty (BLEF-ah-roh-PLAS-tee)
- ❑ blepharoptosis (BLEF-ah-rawp-TOH-sis)
- ❑ capsular (KAP-soo-lar)
- ❑ capsule (KAP-sool)
- ❑ capsulotomy (KAP-soo-LAWT-oh-mee)
- ❑ caruncle (KAR-ung-kl)
- ❑ cataract (KAT-ah-rakt)
- ❑ chalazion (kah-LAY-zee-on)
- ❑ chemotherapy drug (KEE-moh-THAIR-ah-pee DRUHG)
- ❑ choroid (KOH-royd)
- ❑ choroidal (koh-ROY-dal)
- ❑ choroiditis (KOH-roy-DY-tis)
- ❑ ciliary body (SIL-ee-air-ee BAW-dee)
- ❑ conductive keratoplasty (con-DUK-tiv KER-ah-toh-PLAS-tee)
- ❑ conjugate gaze (CON-joo-gayt GAYZ)
- ❑ conjunctiva (CON-junk-TY-vah) (con-JUNK-tih-vah)
- ❑ conjunctivae (CON-junk-TY-vee) (con-JUNK-tih-vee)
- ❑ conjunctival (CON-junk-TY-val) (con-JUNK-tih-val)
- ❑ conjunctivitis (con-JUNK-tih-VY-tis)
- ❑ convergence (con-VER-jens)
- ❑ cornea (KOR-nee-ah)
- ❑ corneae (KOR-nee-ee)
- ❑ corneal (KOR-nee-al)
- ❑ corneal abrasion (KOR-nee-al ah-BRAY-shun)
- ❑ corneal transplantation (KOR-nee-al TRANS-plan-TAY-shun)
- ❑ corneal ulcer (KOR-nee-al UL-ser)
- ❑ corticosteroid drug (KOR-tih-koh-STAIR-oyd DRUHG)
- ❑ cryotherapy (KRY-oh-THAIR-ah-pee)
- ❑ cycloplegia (SY-kloh-PLEE-jee-ah)
- ❑ dacryocystitis (DAK-ree-oh-sis-TY-tis)
- ❑ diabetic retinopathy (DY-ah-BET-ik RET-ih-NAWP-ah-thee)
- ❑ diplopia (dih-PLOH-pee-ah)
- ❑ dysconjugate gaze (dis-CON-joo-gayt GAYZ)
- ❑ ectropion (ek-TROH-pee-on)
- ❑ entropion (en-TROH-pee-on)
- ❑ enucleation (EE-noo-klee-AA-shun)
- ❑ esotropia (ES-oh-TROH-pee-ah)
- ❑ exophthalmos (EKS-off-THAL-mohs)
- ❑ exotropia (EKS-oh-TROH-pee-ah)
- ❑ extracapsular cataract extraction (EKS-trah-KAP-soo-lar KAT-ah-rakt ek-STRAK-shun)
- ❑ extraocular muscle (EKS-trah-AWK-yoo-lar MUS-el)
- ❑ fluorescein angiogram (floo-RES-een AN-jee-oh-gram)
- ❑ fluorescein angiography (floo-RES-een AN-jee-AWG-rah-fee)
- ❑ fovea (FOH-vee-ah)
- ❑ foveae (FOH-vee-ee)
- ❑ foveal (FOH-vee-al)
- ❑ fundal (FUN-dal)
- ❑ fundi (FUN-die)
- ❑ fundus (FUN-dus)
- ❑ funduscopic (FUN-duh-SKAWP-ik)
- ❑ funduscopy (fun-DUHS-koh-pee)
- ❑ glaucoma (glaw-KOH-mah)
- ❑ gonioscopy (GOH-nee-AWS-koh-pee)
- ❑ hemianopia (HEM-ee-ah-NOH-pee-ah)
- ❑ hordeolum (hor-DEE-oh-lum)
- ❑ hyperopia (HY-per-OH-pee-ah)
- ❑ hyphema (hy-FEE-mah)
- ❑ inferior oblique muscle (in-FEER-ee-or awb-LEEK MUS-el)
- ❑ inferior rectus muscle (in-FEER-ee-or REK-tus MUS-el)
- ❑ *in situ* keratomileusis (in SY-too KER-ah-toh-my-LOO-sis)
- ❑ intracapsular cataract extraction (IN-trah-KAP-soo-lar KAT-ah-rakt ek-STRAK-shun)
- ❑ intraocular (IN-trah-AWK-yoo-lar)
- ❑ iridal (IHR-ih-dal) (EYE-rih-dal)
- ❑ irides (IHR-ih-deez)
- ❑ iris (EYE-ris)
- ❑ iritis (eye-RY-tis)
- ❑ jaundice (JAWN-dis)
- ❑ keratitis (KER-ah-TY-tis)
- ❑ lacrimal duct (LAK-rih-mal DUHKT)
- ❑ lacrimal gland (LAK-rih-mal GLAND)
- ❑ lacrimal sac (LAK-rih-mal SAK)
- ❑ laser photocoagulation (LAY-zer FOH-toh-koh-AG-yoo-LAY-shun)
- ❑ laser thermal keratoplasty (LAY-zer THER-mal KER-ah-toh-PLAS-tee)
- ❑ lateral rectus muscle (LAT-er-al REK-tus MUS-el)
- ❑ lens (LENZ)
- ❑ lens capsule (LENZ KAP-sool)
- ❑ lenses (LEN-sez)
- ❑ lenticular (len-TIK-yoo-lar)
- ❑ limbic (LIM-bik)
- ❑ limbus (LIM-bus)
- ❑ macula (MAK-yoo-lah)
- ❑ maculae (MAK-yoo-lee)
- ❑ macular (MAK-yoo-lar)
- ❑ macular degeneraton (MAK-yoo-lar DEE-jen-er-AA-shun)
- ❑ medial rectus muscle (MEE-dee-al REK-tus MUS-el)
- ❑ meibomian gland (my-BOH-mee-an GLAND)
- ❑ microkeratome (MY-kroh-KER-ah-tohm)
- ❑ miosis (my-OH-sis)
- ❑ mydriasis (mih-DRY-eh-sis)
- ❑ mydriatic drug (MIH-dree-AT-ik DRUHG)
- ❑ myopia (my-OH-pee-ah)
- ❑ nasolacrimal duct (NAY-soh-LAK-rih-mal DUHKT)
- ❑ nystagmus (nis-TAG-mus)
- ❑ ocular (AWK-yoo-lar)
- ❑ ophthalmologist (OFF-thal-MAWL-oh-jist)
- ❑ ophthalmology (OFF-thal-MAWL-oh-jee)
- ❑ ophthalmoscope (off-THAL-moh-skohp)
- ❑ optic chiasm (AWP-tik KY-azm)
- ❑ optic disk (AWP-tik DISK)
- ❑ optic globe (AWP-tik GLOHB)
- ❑ optician (op-TISH-un)

- ❑ optic nerve (AWP-tik NERV)
- ❑ optometrist (op-TAWM-eh-trist)
- ❑ optometry (op-TAWM-eh-tree)
- ❑ orbit (OR-bit)
- ❑ papilledema (PAP-il-ah-DEE-mah)
- ❑ peripheral vision (peh-RIF-eh-ral VIZH-un)
- ❑ phacoemulsification (FAY-koh-ee-MUL-sih-fih-KAY-shun)
- ❑ phorometer (foh-RAWM-eh-ter)
- ❑ phorometry (foh-RAWM-eh-tree)
- ❑ photophobia (FOH-toh-FOH-bee-ah)
- ❑ photorefractive keratectomy (FOH-toh-ree-FRAK-tiv KER-ah-TEK-toh-mee)
- ❑ posterior cavity (pohs-TEER-ee-or KAV-ih-tee)
- ❑ posterior chamber (pohs-TEER-ee-or CHAYM-ber)
- ❑ presbyopia (PREZ-bee-OH-pee-ah)
- ❑ pupil (PYOO-pil)
- ❑ pupillary (PYOO-pih-lair-ee)
- ❑ recession (ree-SESH-un)
- ❑ resection (ree-SEK-shun)
- ❑ retina (RET-ih-nah)
- ❑ retinae (RET-ih-nee)
- ❑ retinal (RET-ih-nal)
- ❑ retinal detachment (RET-ih-nal dee-TACH-ment)
- ❑ retinitis pigmentosa (RET-ih-NY-tis PIG-men-TOH-sah)
- ❑ retinoblastoma (RET-ih-noh-blas-TOH-mah)
- ❑ retinopathy of prematurity (RET-ih-NAWP-ah-thee of PREE-mah-TYOOR-ih-tee)
- ❑ retinopexy (RET-ih-noh-PEK-see)
- ❑ retrolental fibroplasia (REH-troh-LEN-tal FY-broh-PLAY-see-ah)
- ❑ sclera (SKLEER-ah)
- ❑ sclerae (SKLEER-ee)
- ❑ scleral (SKLEER-al)
- ❑ scleral icterus (SKLEER-al IK-ter-us)
- ❑ scotoma (skoh-TOH-mah)
- ❑ scotomata (skoh-TOH-mah-tah)
- ❑ sebaceous gland (seh-BAY-shus GLAND)
- ❑ socket (SAW-kit)
- ❑ sonogram (SAWN-oh-gram)
- ❑ stereoscopic vision (STAIR-ee-oh-SKAWP-ik VIZH-un)
- ❑ strabismus (strah-BIZ-mus)
- ❑ superior oblique muscle (soo-PEER-ee-or awb-LEEK MUS-el)
- ❑ superior rectus muscle (soo-PEER-ee-or REK-tus MUS-el)
- ❑ thalamus (THAL-ah-mus)
- ❑ tonometer (toh-NAWM-eh-ter)
- ❑ tonometry (toh-NAWM-eh-tree)
- ❑ trabecular meshwork (trah-BEK-yoo-lar MESH-wurk)
- ❑ trabeculoplasty (trah-BEK-yoo-loh-PLAS-tee)
- ❑ ulcerative keratitis (UL-ser-ah-tiv KER-ah-TY-tis)
- ❑ ultrasonography (UL-trah-soh-NAWG-rah-fee)
- ❑ uvea (YOO-vee-ah)
- ❑ uveal tract (YOO-vee-al TRAKT)
- ❑ uveitis (YOO-vee-EYE-tis)
- ❑ visual acuity (VIZH-yoo-al ah-KYOO-ih-tee)
- ❑ visual cortex (VIZH-yoo-al KOR-teks)
- ❑ visual field (VIZH-yoo-al FEELD)
- ❑ vitrectomy (vih-TREK-toh-mee)
- ❑ vitreous humor (VIT-ree-us HYOO-mor)
- ❑ xerophthalmia (ZEER-off-THAL-mee-ah)

Experience Multimedia

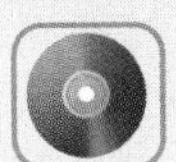

CD-ROM Learning Activities Checklist

Check off the box as you complete each learning activity.

❑ **CD-ROM Learning Activity 15.1: *ANATOMY WORD PARTS FLASHCARDS***
Use flashcards to help you memorize word parts. Make your own flashcards or print out prepared flashcards. Also see the electronic flashcard game. Time: 20 minutes.

❑ **CD-ROM Learning Activity 15.2: *MEDICINE IN ACTION***
Watch a video clip about macular degeneration. Time: 5 minutes.

❑ **CD-ROM Learning Activity 15.3: *DISEASE AND OTHER WORD PARTS FLASHCARDS***
A continuation of the flashcard learning activity. Time: 20 minutes.

❑ **CD-ROM Learning Activity 15.4: *MEMORY AIDS***
Use memory aids to help you memorize medical words and meanings. Time: 5 minutes.

❑ **CD-ROM Learning Activity 15.5: *MEDICAL LANGUAGE SPOKEN HERE***
Listen to actual medical reports and spell the missing medical words. Time: 20 minutes.

❑ **CD-ROM Learning Activity 15.6: *SPELLING CHALLENGE***
Listen to a pronounced medical word and then spell it. Time: 5 minutes.

❑ **CD-ROM Learning Activity 15.7: *MEDICAL LANGUAGE PRONUNCIATION***
Listen to a pronounced medical word and then practice pronouncing it. Time: 30 minutes.

❑ **CD-ROM Learning Activity 15.8: *EDUCATIONAL FUN AND GAMES***
Enjoy these fun activities while reinforcing your knowledge. Time: 15 minutes.

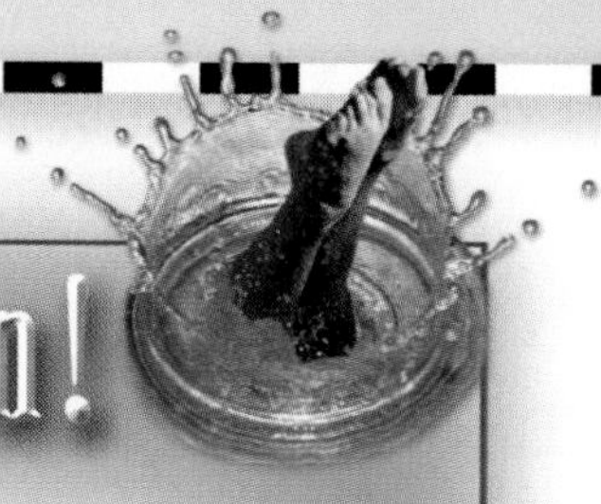

Dive In!

- While our eyes remain the same size from birth, our ears and nose never stop growing.
- Humans can tell the difference between about 10,000 odors.
- This may be tough to swallow, but listen carefully. In this chapter we'll explore the language that describes the structures, functions, diseases, and conditions of the ears, nose, and throat.
- You'll sniff out the truth once you master the language of otolaryngology!

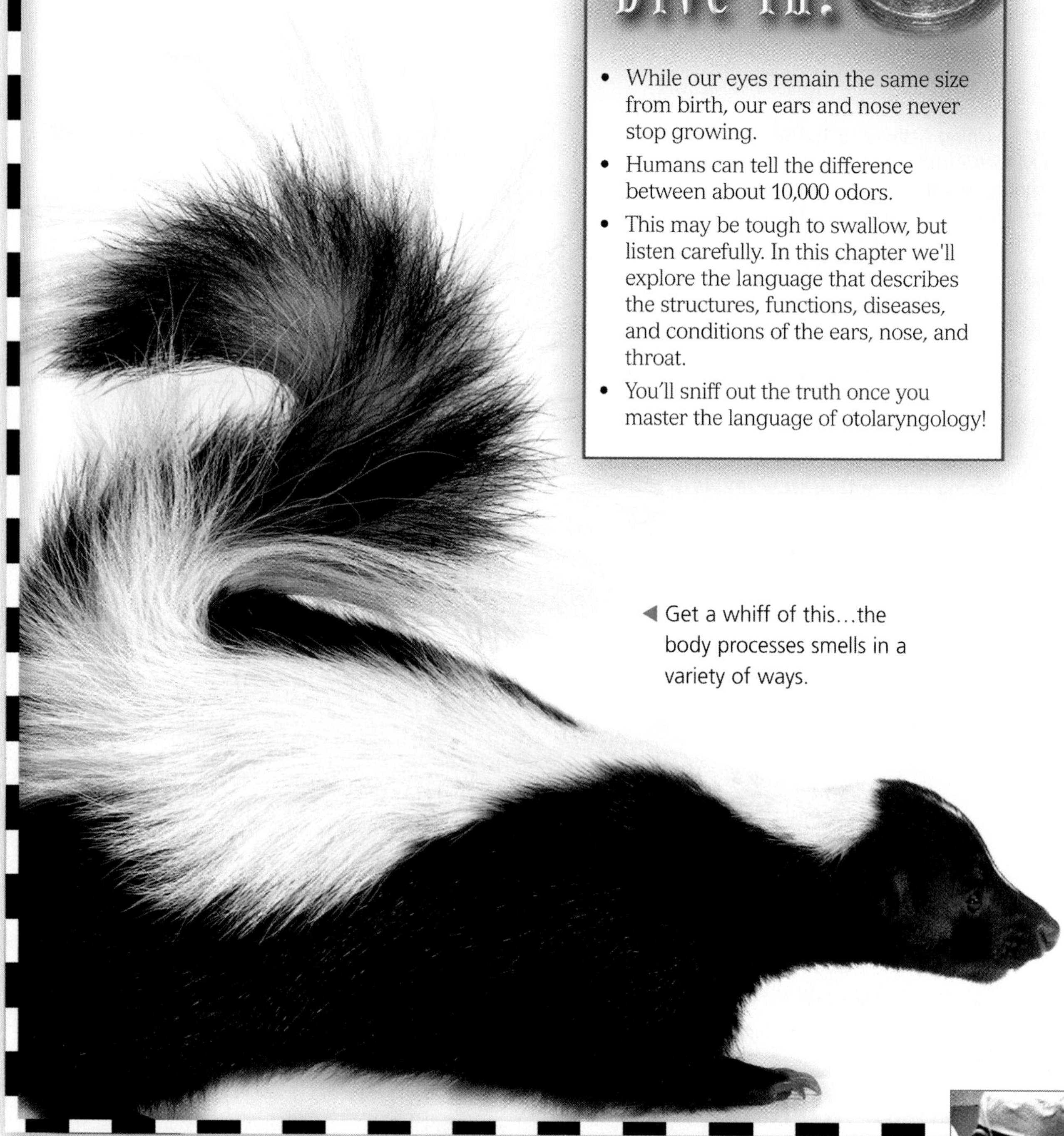

◀ Get a whiff of this…the body processes smells in a variety of ways.

Medicine Through HISTORY

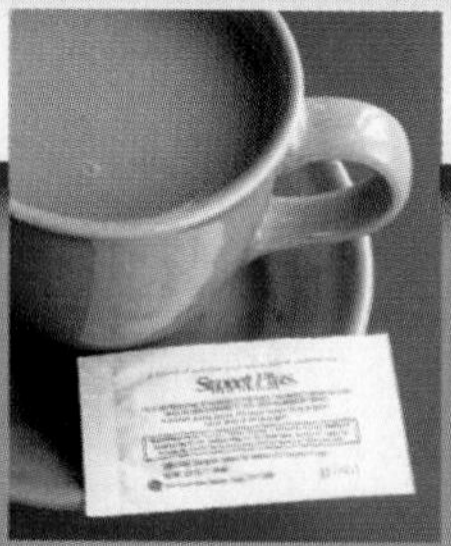

1965

Aspartame, the first artificial sweetener, is developed

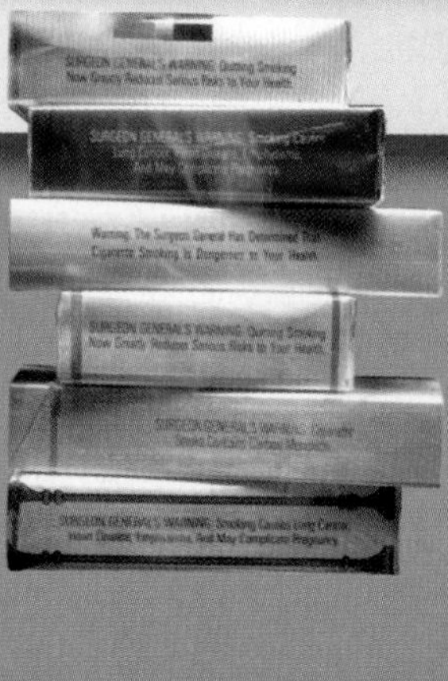

1965

Congress requires a warning label on cigarette packages to say that smoking is hazardous to your health

1967

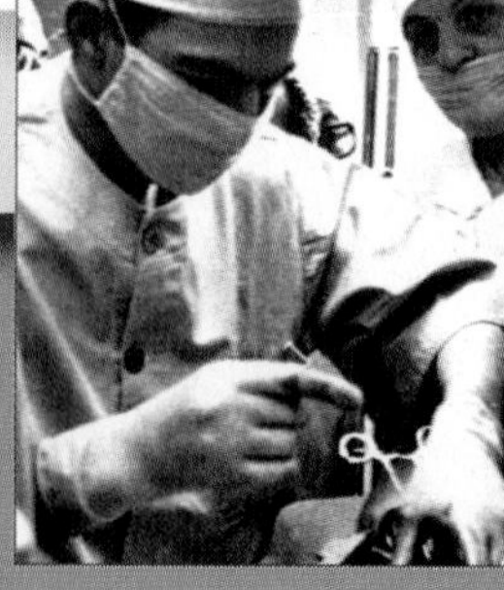

Dr. Christiaan Barnard performs the first heart transplant operation

CHAPTER 16

Otolaryngology

Ears, Nose, and Throat

Otolaryngology (OH-toh-LAIR-ing-GAWL-oh-jee) is the medical specialty that studies the anatomy and physiology of the ears, nose, mouth, and throat (ENT) and uses diagnostic tests, medical and surgical procedures, and drugs to treat ENT diseases.

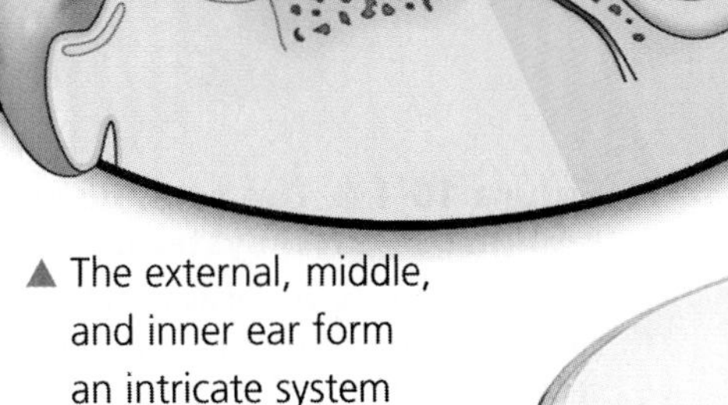

▲ The external, middle, and inner ear form an intricate system to process hearing and enable balance.

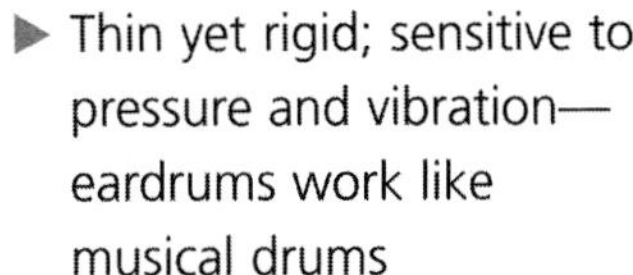

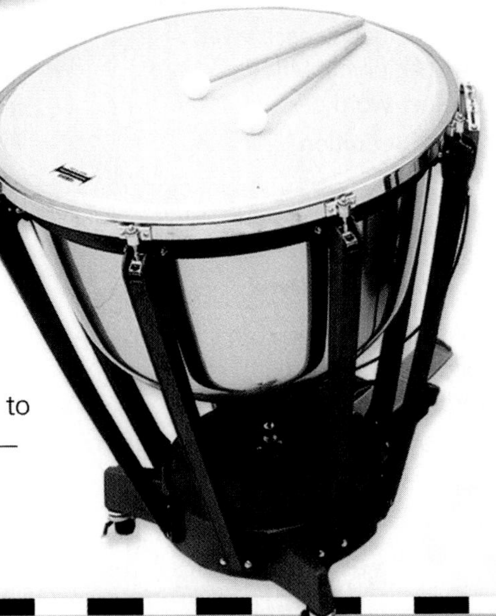

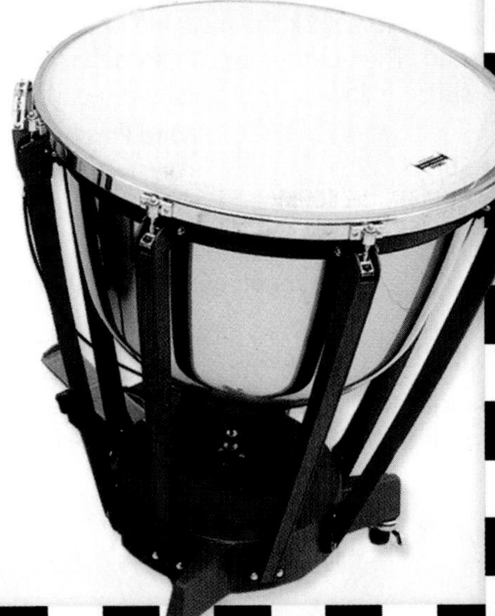

▶ Thin yet rigid; sensitive to pressure and vibration—eardrums work like musical drums

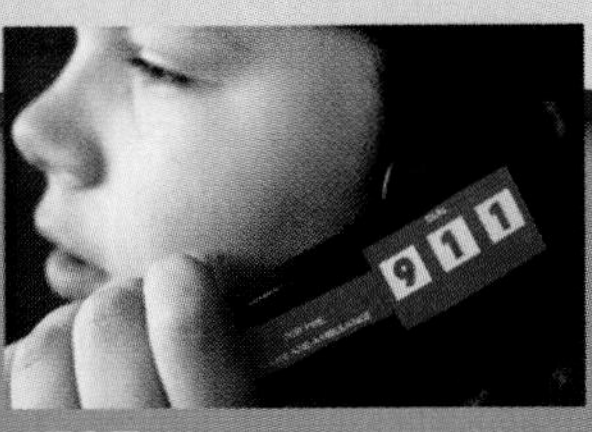

1968

AT&T announces a new national emergency telephone number: 911

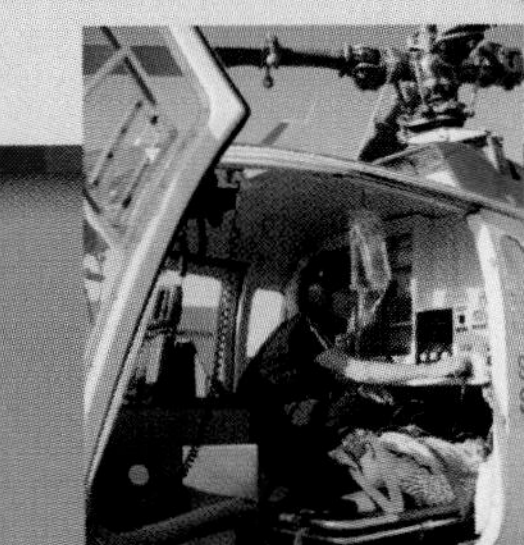

1969

The first Shock Trauma Unit is established at the University of Maryland

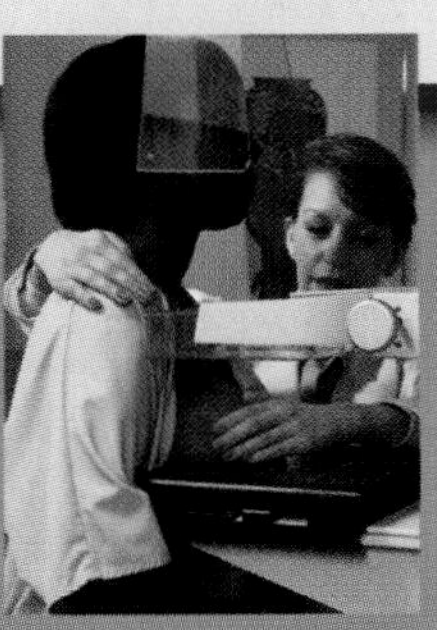

1969

The first mammography of the breast is performed

Measure Your Progress: Learning Objectives

After you study this chapter, you should be able to

1. Identify the anatomical structures of the ears, nose, and throat (ENT) system by correctly labeling them on anatomical illustrations.
2. Describe the process of hearing.
3. Build ENT words from combining forms, prefixes, and suffixes.
4. Describe common ENT diseases.
5. Describe common ENT diagnostic laboratory and radiology tests.
6. Describe common ENT medical and surgical procedures and drug categories.
7. Define common ENT abbreviations.
8. Correctly spell and pronounce ENT words.
9. Apply your skills by analyzing an otolaryngology report.
10. Test your knowledge of otolaryngology by completing review exercises at the end of the chapter and learning activities on the CD-ROM.

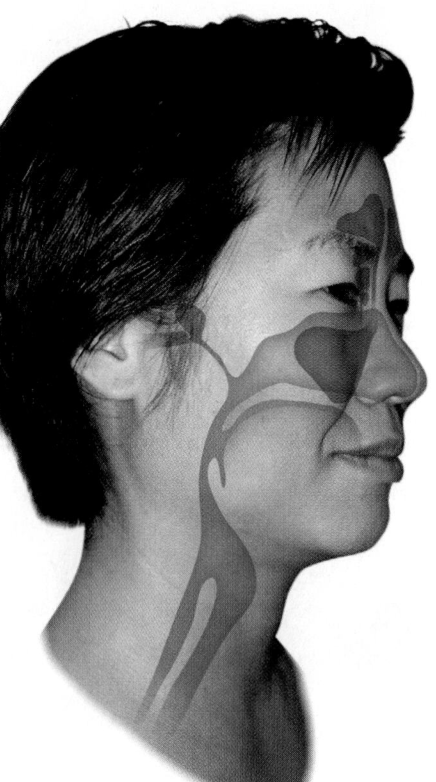

Figure 16-1 ■ The ears, nose, and throat (ENT) system.

The ENT system consists of many different structures in the head and neck. Note how each of these individual structures is interrelated and connected to one another.

Medical Language Key

To unlock the meaning of a medical word, first define each word part. Then put the word part definitions in order, beginning with the suffix, followed by the first word part, then the other word parts in order.

	Word Part	Word Part Definition
SUFFIX	-logy	*the study of*
COMBINING FORM	ot/o-	*ear*
COMBINING FORM	laryng/o-	*larynx (voice box)*

Otolaryngology: ***The study of the ears, [nose], and larynx.***

Although the word *otolaryngology* does not contain combining forms for the nose, mouth, throat, or neck, it is understood that these structures are included in this medical specialty. The word *otorhinolaryngology* does include the combining form *rhin/o-* for nose.

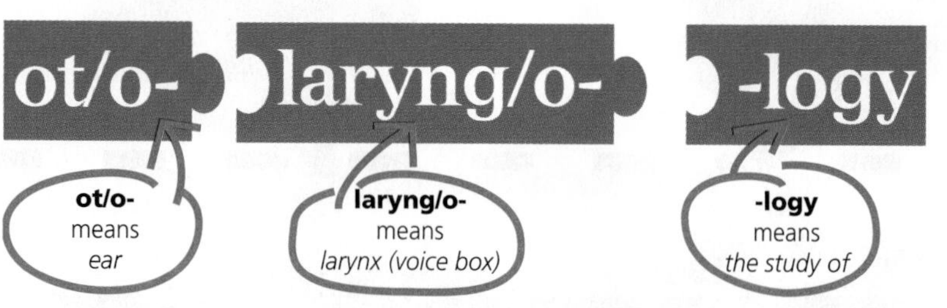
ot/o-
laryng/o-
-logy
ot/o- means ear
laryng/o- means larynx (voice box)
-logy means the study of

www.prenhall.com/turley

For interactive flashcards, real-life video clips, games, exercises, and audio pronunciations please explore the companion CD-ROM in the back of the book. Click on the companion website for bonus chapters, additional resources, and links to on-line learning.

Anatomy and Physiology

The **ears, nose, and throat (ENT) system** is a compact body system that is contained entirely in the head and neck (see Figure 16-1■). The head contains the external and internal structures of the ears, nose, and mouth, and the internal structures of the sinuses. The neck contains the internal structures of the pharynx and larynx. The ENT system has several functions. It shares some structures with the gastrointestinal system and the respiratory system and serves as a passageway for food and air. The ENT system also contains lymphoid tissue that functions as part of the immune response. The body's senses of hearing and smell are also part of the ENT system. The structures of the ENT system (along with the respiratory system) are used to generate sounds that, when formed by the mouth, tongue, and lips, become speech.

Anatomy of the ENT System

External Ear

The external ear is known as the **auricle** or **pinna** (see Figure 16-2■). The **helix** is the outer rim of tissue and cartilage that forms a *C* and ends at the ear lobe. The **external auditory meatus** is the opening that leads into the **external auditory canal (EAC).** The **tragus** is the triangular cartilage anterior to the meatus. The canal has glands that secrete

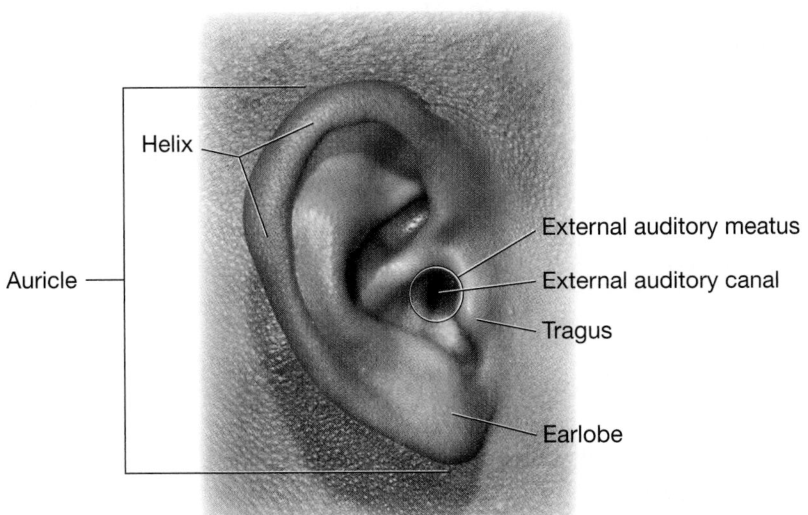

Figure 16-2 ■ External ear.

The external ear is composed of several types and shapes of tissue and cartilage. The external ear also includes the external auditory canal that travels into the temporal bone of the cranium.

auricle (AW-rih-kl)
aur/i- *ear*
-cle *small thing*

auricular (aw-RIK-yoo-lar)
auricul/o- *ear*
-ar *pertaining to*

pinna (PIN-ah)
pinnae (PIN-ee)
Pinna is a Latin singular feminine noun meaning *wing or fin.* Form the plural by changing *-a* to *-ae.*

helix (HEE-liks)
Helix is a Greek word meaning *coil.*

external (eks-TER-nal)
extern/o- *outside*
-al *pertaining to*

auditory (AW-dih-toh-ree)
audit/o- *the sense of hearing*
-ory *having the function of*

meatus (mee-AA-tus)
meati (mee-AA-tie)
Meatus is derived from a Latin singular masculine noun meaning *a passage.* Form the plural by changing *-us* to *-i.*

cerumen, a waxy, sticky substance that traps dirt and has an antibiotic action against microorganisms that enter the canal. At the end of the canal is the **tympanic membrane (TM)** or eardrum, a thin dividing wall between the external ear and the middle ear (see Figure 16-3 ■). Muscles of the neck attach to the mastoid process. The **mastoid process,** a bony projection of the temporal bone, lies just behind the external ear. The mastoid process is not solid bone; it contains tiny cavities filled with air.

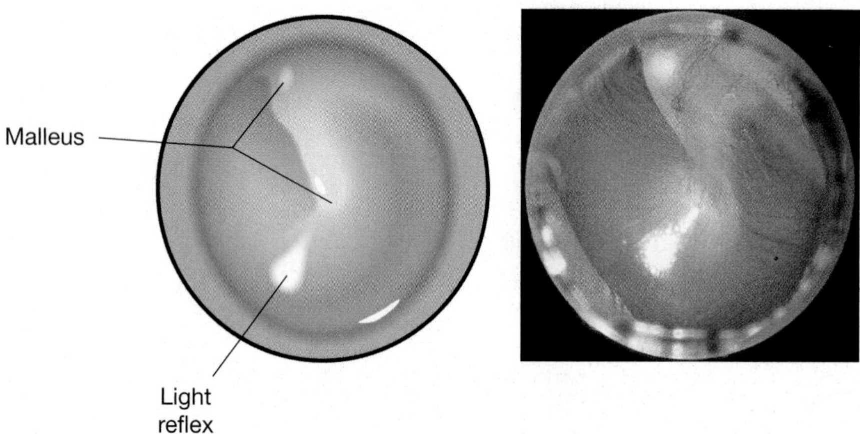

Figure 16-3 ■ Tympanic membrane.

The tympanic membrane has a gray, pearly color and is so thin that the malleus can be seen behind it. A shiny, reflective strip (reflected light from the otoscope) is seen that is known as the light reflex. This is a characteristic of a normal tympanic membrane.

canal (kah-NAL)
Canal is derived from a Latin word meaning *channel.*

tragus (TRAY-gus)
tragi (TRAY-jeye)
Tragus is a Latin singular masculine noun meaning *goat.* In old age, coarse hairs on the tragus resemble the beard of a goat! Form the plural by changing *-us* to *-i.*

cerumen (seh-ROO-men)
Cerumen is derived from a Latin word meaning *wax.*

tympanic (tim-PAN-ik)
tympan/o- *tympanic membrane (eardrum)*
-ic *pertaining to*

mastoid (MASS-toyd)
mast/o- *breast; mastoid process*
-oid *resembling*
The mastoid process is not made of breast tissue, but it was thought to resemble the rounded shape of a breast by the ancient Greeks. *Process* is derived from a Latin word meaning *a projection.*

Middle Ear

The middle ear is a hollow area inside the temporal bone of the skull (see Figure 16-4 ■). It contains three tiny bones: the **malleus, incus,** and **stapes,** collectively known as the **ossicles.** The ossicles are connected to each other by tiny ligaments to form the **ossicular chain.** The first bone, the malleus, is shaped like a hammer. It is connected to the tympanic

Word Alert

SOUND-ALIKE MEDICAL WORDS

malleus (noun) first bone of the middle ear
Example: An infection in the middle ear caused scar tissue around the malleus and affected the patient's hearing.

malleolus (noun) bony projection on each side of the leg near the ankle
Example: The lateral malleolus is a bony projection that arises from the distal fibula.

malleus (MAL-ee-us)
mallei (MAL-ee-eye)
Malleus is a Latin singular masculine noun meaning *a hammer.* Form the plural by changing *-us* to *-i.*

mallear (MAL-ee-ar)
malle/o- *malleus (hammer-shaped bone)*
-ar *pertaining to*

incus (ING-kus)
incudes (in-KYOO-deez)
Incus is a Latin word meaning *anvil.*

incudal (IN-kyoo-dal)
incud/o- *incus (anvil-shaped bone)*
-al *pertaining to*

stapes (STAY-peez)
stapedes (STAY-pee-deez)
Stapes is a Latin word meaning *stirrup.*

membrane. Because the tympanic membrane is nearly transparent, the malleus can be seen through it. The second bone, the incus, is shaped like an anvil. The last ossicle, the stirrup-shaped stapes, fits into a tiny opening in the temporal bone known as the **oval window.** The **round window,** another opening in the temporal bone, is covered by a membrane. The middle ear is connected to the upper throat by the **eustachian tube.** The eustachian tube allows air pressure in the middle ear to equalize with air pressure in the mouth and outside of the body.

stapedial (stay-PEE-dee-al)
staped/o- *stapes (stirrup-shaped bone)*
-ial *pertaining to*

ossicle (AWS-ih-kl)
Ossicle is derived from a Latin word meaning *little bone.*

ossicular (aw-SIK-yoo-lar)
ossicul/o- *ossicle (little bone)*
-ar *pertaining to*

eustachian (yoo-STAY-shun)
The eustachian tube was named by Bartolommeo Eustachio (1524–1574), an Italian anatomist. This is an example of an eponym: a person from whom something takes it name.

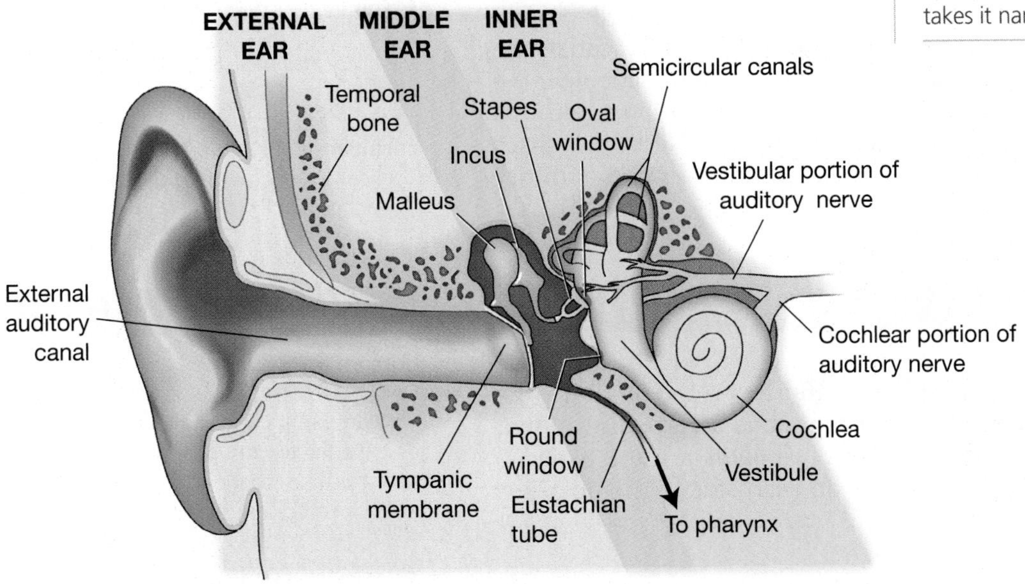

Figure 16-4 ■ Structures of the middle ear and inner ear.

Notice the shapes of the malleus, incus, and stapes. Do they look like a hammer, anvil, and stirrup to you? The structures of the inner ear send information about balance and hearing to the brain via the branches of the auditory nerve.

Inner Ear

A wall of temporal bone divides the middle ear from the inner ear, with only the openings of the round window and oval window to connect the two cavities. The inner ear contains three tiny, fluid-filled structures: the vestibule, the semicircular canals, and the cochlea (see Figure 16-4). The **vestibule,** the first structure of the inner ear, is in contact with both the oval and round windows to the middle ear. One end of the vestibule divides to form the three **semicircular canals,** each of which is oriented in a different plane: horizontally, vertically, and obliquely. When you tilt your head forward, backwards, or to the side, the semicircular canals relay the position of your head, and this information is interpreted by the brain to help you keep your balance. Nerve impulses from the semicircular canals travel along the vestibular branch of the auditory nerve (cranial nerve VIII) to the brain. The other end of the vestibule coils on itself to form the snail-shell–shaped **cochlea.** When sound waves enter your external auditory canal, the vibrations are transmitted through the middle ear to the cochlea, the cochlea relays the frequency and intensity of the vibrations, and this information is interpreted by the brain as sounds. Nerve impulses from the cochlea travel along the cochlear branch of the auditory nerve (cranial nerve VIII) to the brain.

vestibule (VES-tih-byool)
Vestibule is derived from a Latin word meaning *small entrance chamber.*

vestibular (ves-TIB-yoo-lar)
vestibul/o- *vestibule (entrance)*
-ar *pertaining to*

semicircular (SEM-ee-SIR-kyoo-lar)
semi- *half, partly*
circul/o- *circle*
-ar *pertaining to*

cochlea (KOHK-lee-ah)
cochleae (KOHK-lee-ee)
Cochlea is a Latin singular feminine noun meaning *snail shell.* Form the plural by changing *-a* to *-ae.*

cochlear (KOHK-lee-ar)
cochle/o- *cochlea (of the inner ear)*
-ar *pertaining to*

External Nose

The external nose is supported by the nasal bone, which forms the bridge and **dorsum** of the nose (see Figure 16-5■). At the nasal tip, the bone is replaced by cartilage. The **nasal septum** is a vertical wall that divides the nose into right and left sides. The **nares** are the external openings or nostrils. The flared cartilage on each side of the nostril is the nasal **ala.**

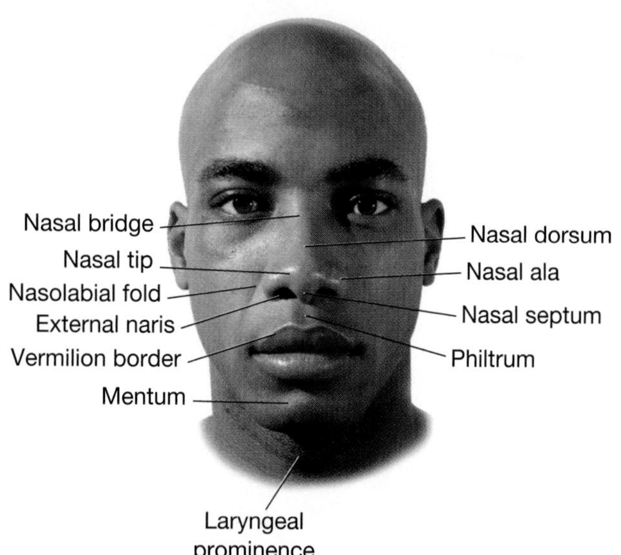

Figure 16-5 ■ External nose, mouth, and neck.

The external nose is supported by the nasal bone, which transitions to cartilage at the tip of the nose. The tissues of the mouth and chin are supported by the maxilla and mandible. The laryngeal prominence is composed of cartilage.

dorsum (DOR-sum)
Dorsum usually means the back or posterior part, but it can also be used to describe the top or uppermost part of certain structures, as the dorsum or top of the nose or foot or the dorsal fin on a shark.

dorsal (DOR-sal)
dors/o- *back; dorsum; uppermost part*
-al *pertaining to*

nasal (NAY-zal)
nas/o- *nose*
-al *pertaining to*
Nasal is the adjective form for *nose.*

septum (SEP-tum)
Septum is derived from a Latin word meaning *a partition.*

septal (SEP-tal)
sept/o- *septum (dividing wall)*
-al *pertaining to*

naris (NAY-ris)
nares (NAY-reez)
Naris is a Latin word meaning *nostril.*

ala (AA-lah)
alae (AA-lee)
Ala is a Latin singular feminine noun meaning *wing.* Form the plural by changing *-a* to *-ae.*

Nasal Cavity

The **nasal cavity** inside the nose is formed by the ethmoid bone (on its roof and sides) and by the maxilla as the hard palate (see Figure 16-6■). The nasal septum, the dividing wall between the two nostrils, is made of cartilage but becomes bone as it merges with the ethmoid bone in the posterior nasal cavity. Along the walls of the nasal cavity are a series of three long, bony projections, known as the **superior, middle, and inferior turbinates** or **nasal conchae.** These jut out into the nasal cavity to divide and slow down inhaled air so that it can pick up warmth and moisture. The nasal cavity is lined with **nasal mucosa,** a mucous membrane that continuously produces **mucus.**

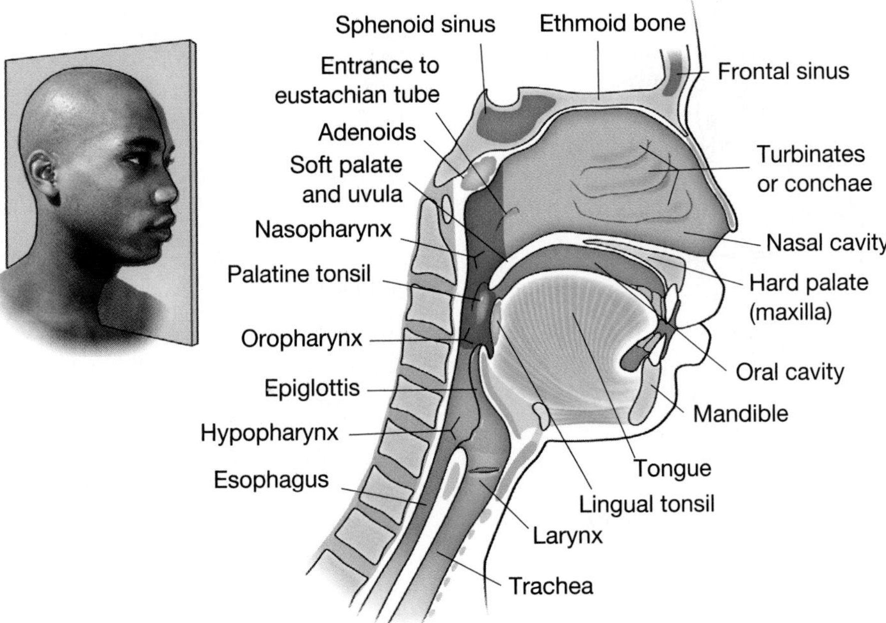

Figure 16-6 ■ Structures of the internal nose, mouth, and throat.

This midsagittal cut section of the head and neck reveals the turbinates of the nasal cavity, the structures of the oral cavity, the tonsils and adenoids, and the three parts of the pharynx (nasopharynx, oropharynx, and hypopharynx). Note how anatomically close the pharynx is to the bones of the spinal column.

nasal (NAY-zal)
nas/o- *nose*
-al *pertaining to*
Nasal is the adjective form for *nose.*

cavity (KAV-ih-tee)
cav/o- *hollow space*
-ity *state; condition*

superior (soo-PEER-ee-or)
super/o- *above*
-ior *pertaining to*

inferior (in-FEER-ee-or)
infer/o- *below*
-ior *pertaining to*

turbinate (TER-bih-nayt)
turbin/o- *scroll-like structure; turbinate*
-ate *composed of; pertaining to*
Turbinate is derived from a Latin word meaning *something that spins like a top.* Each turbinate bone is rolled within itself, like a turban or a scroll.

concha (CON-kah)
conchae (CON-kee)
Concha is a Latin word meaning *a shell.*

mucosa (myoo-KOH-sah)
Mucosa is a Latin word meaning *mucus.*

mucosal (myoo-KOH-sal)
mucos/o- *mucous membrane*
-al *pertaining to*

mucus (MYOO-kus)

Sinuses

A **sinus** is a hollow cavity within a cranial or facial bone (see Figures 16-6 and 16-7 ■). There are four pairs of sinuses, each located in the bone for which they are named. The **frontal sinuses** are in the frontal bone, just above each eyebrow. The **maxillary sinuses,** the largest of the sinuses, are in the maxilla on either side of the nose. The **ethmoid sinuses,** groups of small air cells, are located in the ethmoid bone, between the nose and the eyes. The **sphenoid sinuses** are located in the sphenoid bone, posterior to the eye and deep inside the skull in front of the pituitary gland of the brain. All of the sinuses are lined with mucosa. As a group, these are also known as the **paranasal sinuses.**

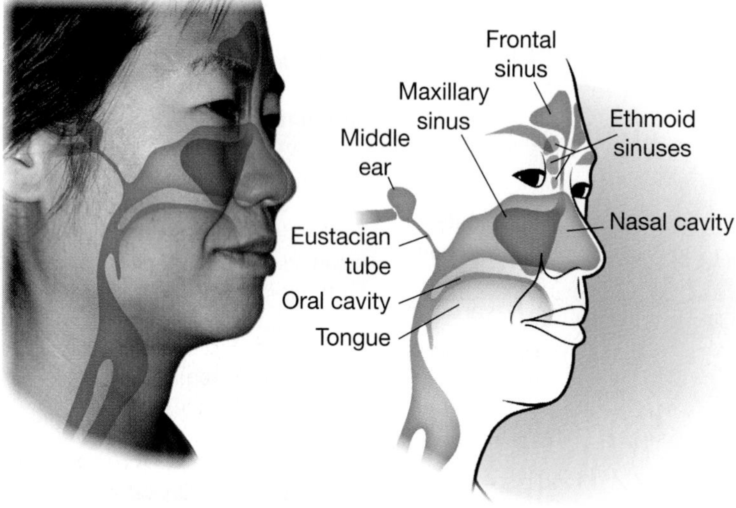

Figure 16-7 ■ Sinuses.
The sinuses are hollow cavities lined with mucosa within the frontal, maxillary, ethmoid, and sphenoid bones of the cranium and face.

sinus (SY-nus)
Sinus is a Latin word meaning *hollow cavity.* The Latin plural is also *sinus*. An English plural can be formed by adding *-es* (sinuses).

frontal (FRUN-tal)
front/o- *front*
-al *pertaining to*

maxillary (MAK-sih-lair-ee)
maxill/o- *maxilla (upper jaw)*
-ary *pertaining to*

ethmoid (ETH-moyd)
ethm/o- *sieve*
-oid *resembling*
The ethmoid bone is very porous with many small, hollow spaces that resemble a sieve.

sphenoid (SFEE-noyd)
sphen/o- *wedge shape*
-oid *resembling*

paranasal (PAIR-ah-NAY-zal)
para- *beside, apart from; two parts of a pair; abnormal*
nas/o- *nose*
-al *pertaining to*
Some word parts have more than one definition. The best definition of *paranasal* is *pertaining to beside the nose.*

External Mouth and Chin

The tissues of the lips, part of the cheeks, and the chin are supported by the maxilla (upper jawbone) and mandible (lower jawbone) (see Figure 16-5). The **nasolabial fold** is the oblique skin crease in the cheek, going from the edge of the nose to the corner of the mouth. The **philtrum** is a vertical groove in the skin of the upper lip. The **vermilion border** is the pink-red border around the lips. The mandible or lower jawbone supports the tissues of the lower lip and chin. The chin is also known as the **mentum.**

nasolabial (NAY-zoh-LAY-bee-al)
nas/o- *nose*
labi/o- *lip; labium*
-al *pertaining to*

philtrum (FIL-trum)
Philtrum is derived from a Greek word meaning *love potion or charm.*

vermilion (ver-MIL-yon)
Vermilion is an English word meaning *bright red.*

mentum (MEN-tum)
Mentum is a Latin word meaning *chin.*

mental (MEN-tal)
ment/o- *mind; chin*
-al *pertaining to*
Some word parts have more than one definition. The best definition of *mental* (in otolaryngology) is *pertaining to the chin.*

Oral Cavity

The **oral cavity** or mouth contains the tongue, hard palate, soft palate and uvula, teeth, and salivary glands. The oral cavity is lined with the **oral mucosa,** which is known as **buccal mucosa** in the cheek area. The hard **palate** or roof of the mouth divides the oral cavity from the nasal cavity (see Figure 16-6). The hard palate is made up of three different bones: the maxilla, then the palatine bone, and the vomer bone as the most posterior section. The posterior hard palate transitions to the tissue of the soft palate and the **uvula,** the fleshy hanging part of the soft palate. The mandible forms the floor of the mouth, and the base of the **tongue** is attached to it. **Submental lymph nodes** underneath the chin contain lymphocytes and macrophages that attack bacteria and viruses that enter the body through the oral cavity. Each end of the mandible is attached to the temporal bone of the cranium at the moveable **temporomandibular joint (TMJ).** The salivary glands were discussed in Gastroenterology (Chapter 3).

oral (OR-al)
or/o- *mouth*
-al *pertaining to*
Oral is the adjective form for *mouth.*

buccal (BUHK-al)
bucc/o- *cheek*
-al *pertaining to*

palate (PAL-at)

palatal (PAL-ah-tal)
palat/o- *palate*
-al *pertaining to*

glossal (GLAWS-al)
gloss/o- *tongue*
-al *pertaining to*
Glossal and *lingual* are the adjective forms for *tongue.*

uvula (YOO-vyoo-lah)
Uvula is derived from a Latin word that means *little grape.*

submental (sub-MEN-tal)
sub- *below; underneath; less than*
ment/o- *mind; chin*
-al *pertaining to*
Some word parts have more than one definition. The best definition of *submental* is *pertaining to underneath the chin.*

temporomandibular (TEM-poh-roh-man-DIB-yoo-lar)
tempor/o- *temple (side of the head)*
mandibul/o- *mandible (lower jaw)*
-ar *pertaining to*

Pharynx

The **pharynx** or throat is divided into three areas: the nasopharynx, the oropharynx, and the hypopharynx (see Figure 16-6). As the nasal cavity continues posteriorly, it becomes the **nasopharynx** or uppermost portion of the throat. The openings at the ends of the eustachian tubes are in the nasopharynx. The roof and walls of the nasopharynx contain the pharyngeal tonsil, a collection of lymphoid tissue commonly known as the **adenoids.** As the nasopharynx continues inferiorly, it

pharynx (FAIR-ingks)
Pharynx is a Greek word meaning *throat.*

pharyngeal (fah-RIN-jee-al)
pharyng/o- *pharynx (throat)*
-eal *pertaining to*

nasopharynx (NAY-zoh-FAIR-ingks)
nas/o- *nose*
-pharynx *pharynx (throat)*

nasopharyngeal (NAY-zoh-fah-RIN-jee-al)
nas/o- *nose*
pharyng/o- *pharynx (throat)*
-eal *pertaining to*

adenoids (AD-eh-noydz)
aden/o- *gland*
-oid *resembling*

becomes the **oropharynx** or middle portion of the throat. The oropharynx begins at the level of the soft palate and ends at the epiglottis. The oropharynx contains the **palatine tonsils,** areas of lymphoid tissue on either side of the throat where the soft palate arches downward (see Figure 16-8■). The **hypopharynx** begins at the base of the tongue and ends at the entrances to the esophagus and larynx. The hypopharynx contains the **lingual tonsils,** located on either side of the base of the tongue. The tonsils and adenoids are part of the lymphatic system, and they function in the immune response. They contain lymphocytes and macrophages that attack bacteria and viruses in the tissues around the oral cavity.

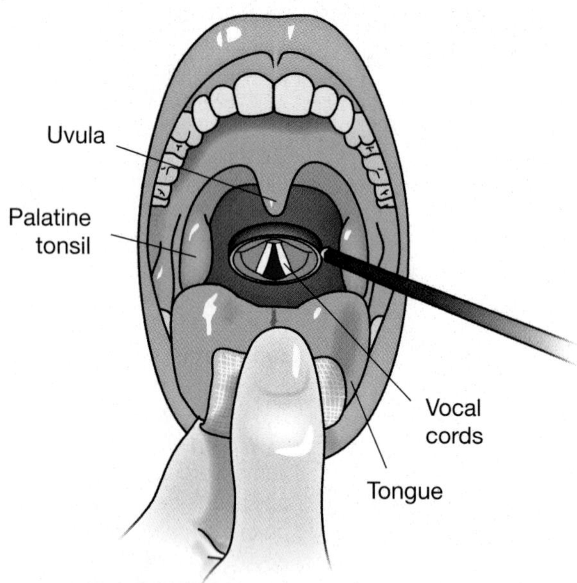

Figure 16-8 ■ Pharynx.

By holding the tongue with a piece of gauze and pulling it forward, the pharynx can be examined. The palatine tonsils can be seen on either side of the oropharynx. A laryngeal mirror placed in the oropharynx can be used to visualize the vocal cords in the larynx. The image of the vocal cords as reflected in the mirror is upside down as compared to the actual position of the vocal cords. The laryngeal mirror can be turned to face upward to examine the nasopharynx.

oropharynx (OR-oh-FAIR-ingks)
or/o- *mouth*
-pharynx *pharynx (throat)*

oropharyngeal (OR-oh-fah-RIN-jee-al)
or/o- *mouth*
pharyng/o- *pharynx (throat)*
-eal *pertaining to*

palatine (PAL-ah-teen)
palat/o- *palate*
-ine *pertaining to*
Palatine and *palatal* are both adjective forms for *palate*.

tonsil (TAWN-sil)
Tonsil is derived from a Latin word that means *a little oar or a stake.*

tonsillar (TAWN-sih-lar)
tonsill/o- *tonsil*
-ar *pertaining to*

hypopharynx (HY-poh-FAIR-ingks)
hypo- *below; deficient*
-pharynx *pharynx (throat)*

hypopharyngeal (HY-poh-fah-RIN-jee-al)
hypo- *below; deficient*
pharyng/o- *pharynx (throat)*
-eal *pertaining to*

lingual (LING-gwal)
lingu/o- *tongue*
-al *pertaining to*

Larynx

At its inferior end, the pharynx divides into two parts: the larynx that leads to the trachea and the esophagus that leads to the stomach. The **larynx** or voice box is a short, triangular structure. The larynx is surrounded by two thick rings of cartilage that can be clearly seen at the front of the neck as the **laryngeal prominence** (Adam's apple) (see Figure 16-5). At the superior end of the larynx just below the base of the tongue is the **epiglottis,** a lidlike structure (see Figure 16-6). During swallowing, the larynx moves superiorly and closes against the epiglottis to keep food from entering the lungs. In the middle of the larynx is the **glottis,** a V-shaped structure of mucous membranes, ligaments, and the **vocal cords** (see Figure 16-8). The larynx remains open during breathing, speaking, or singing to allow air to pass over the vocal cords.

A man has a large larynx and long vocal cords that vibrate at a slow frequency and produce a voice with a low pitch. A woman has shorter vocal cords and a voice with a higher pitch. Muscles in the larynx relax or tighten the vocal cords to lower or raise the pitch. The volume of air from the lungs affects how loud or soft the voice is. The sound waves also resonate in the sinuses, adding fullness to the voice in speech or singing.

During speech, the vocal cords close partially or entirely. Exhaled air from the lungs causes the vocal cords to vibrate. The surface layer of each vocal cord is looser than the layers beneath it, and this layer vibrates in a wavelike fashion at a frequency of up to 100 times per second. These vibrations produce sound waves. These sound waves travel through the vocal cords and past the soft palate, tongue, and lips, all of which shape the sound waves into the words as we speak.

larynx (LAIR-ingks)

laryngeal (lah-RIN-jee-al)
laryng/o- *larynx (voice box)*
-eal *pertaining to*

epiglottis (EP-ih-GLAWT-is)
epi- *upon, above*
glott/o- *glottis (of the larynx)*
-ic *pertaining to*

glottis (GLAWT-is)
Glottis is a Greek word meaning *opening of the larynx.*

vocal (VOH-kal)
voc/o- *voice*
-al *pertaining to*

Physiology of the Sense of Hearing

The external ear captures sound waves. They travel down the external auditory canal to the tympanic membrane (see Figure 16-9 ■). There, the sound waves are converted to mechanical motion as they cause the tympanic membrane to move inward and outward. As it moves, the tympanic membrane moves the malleus, then the incus, and then the stapes. The stapes transmits this mechanical motion to the oval window. This causes inner ear fluid on the other side of the oval window to begin to vibrate. The vibration is transmitted throughout the length of the cochlea. Within the cochlea, tiny hairs detect different frequencies of sound, sending nerve impulses through the cochlear branch of the **auditory nerve** (cranial nerve VIII) to the **auditory cortex** in each temporal lobe of the brain. The location in the cochlea of the stimulated hairs correlates to the frequency of the sound. How many of the hairs were stimulated correlates to the loudness of the sound.

When the vibration has traveled through the cochlea, it comes back to the vestibule where it causes the round window to bulge. The round window acts as a safety valve in the otherwise rigid bony walls around the inner ear.

auditory (AW-dih-toh-ree)
audit/o- *the sense of hearing*
-ory *having the function of*

cortex (KOR-teks)
Cortex is a Latin word meaning *bark.* The auditory cortex covers part of the surface of the temporal lobe like bark covers a tree.

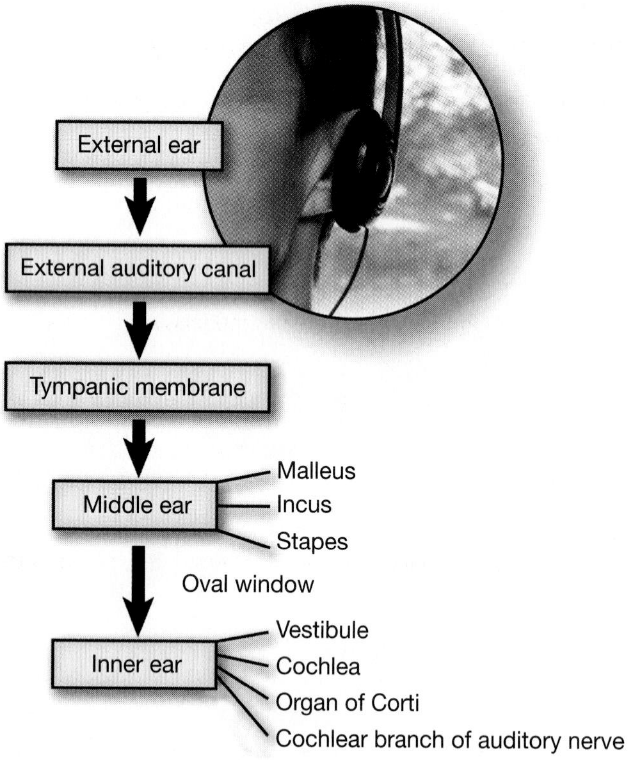

Figure 16-9 ■ The sense of hearing.
Sounds travel as sound waves through the external and middle ear. Then they travel as nerve impulses through the inner ear to the cochlear branch of the auditory nerve (cranial nerve VIII).

Vocabulary Review

Anatomy and Physiology

Now that you have studied the anatomy and physiology of the ENT system, take time to review those new words and descriptions. Memorize the combining forms and their definitions before going on to the next section.

Ears

Word or Phrase	Combining Form and Definition	Description
auditory cortex	audit/o- *the sense of hearing*	Area of the temporal lobe of the brain where nerve impulses from the auditory nerve are interpreted for the sense of hearing.
auditory nerve	audit/o- *the sense of hearing*	Cranial nerve VIII that conducts nerve impulses from the semicircular canals and the cochlea to the brain to maintain balance and for the sense of hearing
auricle	aur/i- *ear*	The visible external ear. Also known as the pinna.
cerumen		Sticky wax that traps dirt in the external auditory canal.
cochlea	cochle/o- *cochlea*	Structure of the inner ear associated with the sense of hearing. It relays information to the brain via the cochlear branch of the auditory nerve.
eustachian tube		Tube that connects the middle ear to the nasopharynx and equalizes the air pressure in the middle ear
external auditory meatus	extern/o- *outside* audit/o- *the sense of hearing*	Opening at the entrance to the external auditory canal
external auditory canal	audit/o- *the sense of hearing*	Passageway from the external ear to the middle ear. It contains glands that secrete cerumen.
helix		Rim of tissue and cartilage that forms the *C* shape of the external ear
incus	incud/o- *incus (anvil-shaped bone)*	Second bone of the middle ear. It is attached to the malleus on one end and the stapes on the other end. Also known as the anvil.
malleus	malle/o- *malleus (hammer-shaped bone)*	First bone of the middle ear. It is attached to the tympanic membrane on one end and to the incus on the other end. Also known as the hammer.
mastoid process	mast/o- *breast; mastoid process*	Bony projection of the temporal bone behind the ear where the neck muscles attach. It resembles the shape of a breast although it is bone, not breast tissue.
ossicles	ossicul/o- *ossicle (little bone)*	The three tiny bones of the middle ear: malleus, incus, and stapes. Also known as the ossicular chain.
oval window		Opening in the temporal bone between the middle ear and the vestibule of the inner ear. The opening is covered by the end of the stapes.
round window		Opening in the temporal bone between the middle ear and the vestibule of the inner ear. The opening is covered with a membrane.
semicircular canals	circul/o- *circle*	Three separate but intertwined canals in the inner ear that are oriented in different planes (horizontally, vertically, obliquely). They help the body keep its balance. They relay information to the brain via the vestibular branch of the auditory nerve.

Word or Phrase	Combining Form and Definition	Description
stapes	**staped/o-** *stapes (stirrup-shaped bone)*	Third bone of the middle ear. It is attached to the incus on one end and the oval window on the other end. Also known as the stirrup.
tragus		Triangular cartilage anterior to the external auditory meatus
tympanic membrane	**tympan/o-** *tympanic membrane (eardrum)*	Membrane that divides the external ear from the middle ear. Also known as the eardrum.
vestibule	**vestibul/o-** *vestibule (entrance)*	First structure of the inner ear. Tubular structure filled with fluid that contacts the oval window and round window. The ends of the vestibule become the semicircular canals and the cochlea.
		Nose
ala		Flared cartilage on each side of the nostril
mucosa	**mucos/o-** *mucous membrane*	Mucous membrane lining the nasal cavity that warms and moisturizes the incoming air. It also produces **mucus** to trap foreign particles.
naris		One nostril, the opening into the nasal cavity
nasal cavity	**nas/o-** *nose* **cav/o-** *hollow space*	Hollow area inside the nose that is formed by the ethmoid and maxillary bones. It is lined with mucosa.
nasal dorsum	**dors/o-** *back; dorsum; uppermost part*	Uppermost surface of the external nose. It is supported by the nasal bone.
nasal septum	**sept/o-** *septum (dividing wall)*	Wall of cartilage and bone that divides the right and left nostrils from each other
turbinates	**turbin/o-** *scroll-like structure; turbinate* **super/o-** *above* **infer/o-** *below*	Three long projections (superior, middle, inferior) of the ethmoid bone that jut into the nasal cavity. They break up and give moisture to air as it enters the nose. Also known as the **nasal conchae.**
		Sinuses
ethmoid sinuses	**ethm/o-** *sieve*	Groups of small air cells in the ethmoid bone between the nose and the eye
frontal sinuses	**front/o-** *front*	Pair of sinuses above each eyebrow in the frontal bone of the skull
maxillary sinuses	**maxill/o-** *maxilla (upper jaw)*	Largest of the sinuses. Pair of sinuses on either side of the nose in the maxillary bone (upper jaw)
sinus		Hollow cavity within a bone of the cranium. The **paranasal sinuses** include all of the sinuses.
sphenoid sinuses	**sphen/o-** *wedge shape*	Sinuses in the sphenoid bone posterior to the nasal cavity and next to the pituitary gland of the brain

Mouth

Word or Phrase	Combining Form and Definition	Description
buccal mucosa	bucc/o- *cheek*	Mucosa specifically in the cheek area of the oral cavity
hard palate	palat/o- *palate*	Bone that divides the nasal cavity from the oral cavity. It includes the maxilla, palatine, and vomer bones. Also known as the roof of the mouth.
mentum	ment/o- *mind; chin*	The chin. The most anterior part of the lower jaw bone or mandible.
nasolabial fold	nas/o- *nose* labi/o- *lip; labrum*	Skin crease in the cheek from the nose to the corner of the mouth
oral cavity	or/o- *mouth* mucos/o- *mucous membrane*	Hollow area inside of the mouth that contains the tongue, teeth, hard and soft palates, uvula, and salivary glands. It is lined with **oral mucosa.**
philtrum		Area with vertical grooves in the skin of the upper lip.
soft palate	palat/o- *palate*	Soft tissue extension of the hard palate at the back of the throat. It ends with the **uvula.**
submental lymph nodes	ment/o- *mind; chin*	Lymph nodes underneath the chin
temporo-mandibular joint	tempor/o- *temple (side of the head)*	Moveable joint where ligaments attach each end of the mandible to the temporal bone of the cranium
tongue	gloss/o- *tongue* lingu/o- *tongue*	Large muscle in the oral cavity that is attached to the mandible
vermillion border		Edge of pink-red around the lips

Pharynx and Larynx

Word or Phrase	Combining Form and Definition	Description
adenoids	aden/o- *gland*	Lymphoid tissue in the superior part of the nasopharynx. Also known as the pharyngeal tonsils.
epiglottis	glott/o- *glottis (of the larynx)*	Lidlike structure that covers the top of the larynx during swallowing
glottis	glott/o- *glottis (of the larynx)*	V-shaped structure of mucous membranes and vocal cords within the larynx
hypopharynx	pharyng/o- *pharynx (throat)*	Most posterior portion of the throat from the base of the tongue to the entrances to the esophagus and trachea
larynx	laryng/o- *larynx (voice box)*	Triangular structure in the anterior neck (visible as the laryngeal prominence or Adam's apple) that contains the vocal cords
lingual tonsils	lingu/o- *tongue* tonsill/o- *tonsil*	Lymphoid tissue located on both sides of the base of the tongue in the hypopharynx

Word or Phrase	Combining Form and Definition	Descriptions
nasopharynx	nas/o- *nose* pharyng/o- *pharynx (throat)*	Uppermost portion of the throat where the posterior nares unite. The nasopharynx contains the openings for the eustachian tubes and the adenoids.
oropharynx	or/o- *mouth* pharyng/o- *pharynx (throat)*	Middle portion of the throat just behind the the oral cavity. It begins at the level of the soft palate and ends at the epiglottis. It contains the palatine tonsils.
palatine tonsils	palat/o- *palate* tonsill/o- *tonsil*	Lymphoid tissue on either side of the throat where the soft palate arches downward in the oropharynx
pharynx	pharyng/o- *pharynx (throat)*	The throat. It is composed of the nasopharynx, oropharynx, and hypopharynx.
vocal cords	voc/o- *voice*	Connective tissue bands in the larynx that vibrate and produce sounds for speaking and singing

Labeling Exercise

A. *Match each anatomy word or phrase to its numbered structure in Figure 16-10■. Write that word or phrase on the blank line next to its number. Use the Answer Key at the end of the book to check your answers.*

cochlea	incus	round window	tympanic membrane
cochlear branch of auditory nerve	malleus	semicircular canals	vestibular branch of auditory nerve
eustachian tube	oval window	stapes	vestibule
external auditory canal	pharynx	temporal bone	

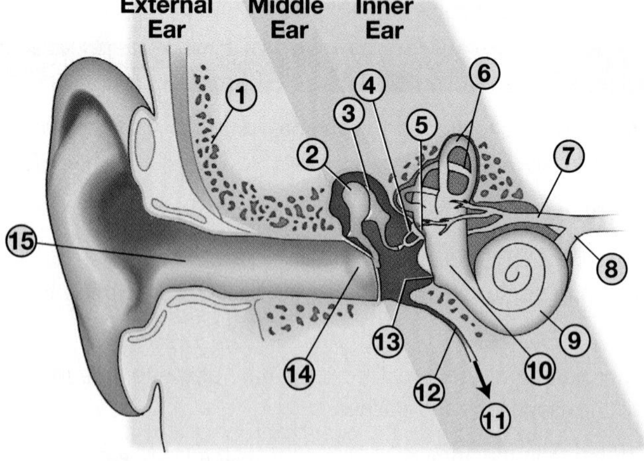

Figure 16-10 ■

1. ______________
2. ______________
3. ______________
4. ______________
5. ______________
6. ______________
7. ______________
8. ______________
9. ______________
10. ______________
11. ______________
12. ______________
13. ______________
14. ______________
15. ______________

B. *Match each anatomy word or phrase to its numbered structure in Figure 16-11 ■.*

adenoids	hypopharynx	nasopharynx	soft palate and uvula
entrance to eustachian tube	larynx	oral cavity	sphenoid sinus
epiglottis	lingual tonsil	oropharynx	tongue
frontal sinus	mandible	palatine tonsil	turbinates or conchae
hard palate	nasal cavity		

Figure 16-11 ■

1. ______________________
2. ______________________
3. ______________________
4. ______________________
5. ______________________
6. ______________________
7. ______________________
8. ______________________
9. ______________________
10. ______________________
11. ______________________
12. ______________________
13. ______________________
14. ______________________
15. ______________________
16. ______________________
17. ______________________
18. ______________________

Building Medical Words

Combining Forms

Here are the combining forms you have learned so far. Next to each combining form, write its meaning. Use the Answer Key at the end of the book to check your answers. The first one has been done for you.

Combining Form	Medical Meaning	Combining Form	Medical Meaning
1. aden/o-	gland	9. ethm/o-	
2. audit/o-		10. extern/o-	
3. aur/i-		11. front/o-	
4. auricul/o-		12. gloss/o-	
5. bucc/o-		13. glott/o-	
6. cav/o-		14. incud/o-	
7. cochle/o-		15. infer/o-	
8. dors/o-		16. labi/o-	

17. laryng/o- ________________
18. lingu/o- ________________
19. malle/o- ________________
20. mandibul/o- ________________
21. mast/o- ________________
22. maxill/o- ________________
23. ment/o- ________________
24. mucos/o- ________________
25. nas/o- ________________
26. or/o- ________________
27. ossicul/o- ________________
28. palat/o- ________________
29. pharyng/o- ________________
30. sept/o- ________________
31. sphen/o- ________________
32. staped/o- ________________
33. super/o- ________________
34. tempor/o- ________________
35. tonsill/o- ________________
36. turbin/o- ________________
37. tympan/o- ________________
38. vestibul/o- ________________
39. voc/o- ________________

Combining Forms and Suffixes

Read the definition hint for the medical word you are to build. Look at the combining form that is given. Write the correct suffix on the blank line. Then write the medical word. (Remember: You may need to remove the combining vowel. Always remove the hyphens and slash.) Use the Answer Key at the end of the book to check your answers. The first one has been done for you.

SUFFIX LIST

-al (pertaining to)	-cle (small thing)	-ine (pertaining to)
-ar (pertaining to)	-eal (pertaining to)	-oid resembling)
-ate (composed of; pertaining to)	-ial (pertaining to)	-ory (having the function of)
	-ic (pertaining to)	

Definition Hint	Combining Form	Suffix	Write the Medical Word
1. Pertaining to the pinna	aur/i-	-cle	*auricle*
2. Pertaining to the nose	nas/o-	______	________________
3. Having the function of the sense of hearing	audit/o-	______	________________
4. Pertaining to the eardrum	tympan/o-	______	________________
5. Pertaining to the septum	sept/o-	______	________________
6. Composed of a structure like a scroll	turbin/o-	______	________________
7. Pertaining to a tonsil	tonsill/o-	______	________________
8. Pertaining to the cheek	bucc/o-	______	________________
9. Pertaining to the stapes	staped/o-	______	________________
10. Resembling a sievelike bone	ethm/o-	______	________________
11. Pertaining to the pharynx	pharyng/o-	______	________________
12. Pertaining to the tongue	gloss/o-	______	________________
13. Pertaining to tonsils near the palate	palat/o-	______	________________

Symptoms, Signs, and Diseases

Ears

Word or Phrase	Word Part and Definition	Description
acoustic neuroma	**acoustic** (ah-KOOS-tik) acous/o- *hearing, sound* -tic *pertaining to* **neuroma** (nyoo-ROH-mah) neur/o- *nerve* -oma *tumor, mass* **benign** (bee-NINE) *Benign* is derived from a Latin word meaning *kind, not cancerous.*	**Benign** tumor of the nerve cells of the auditory nerve. Depending on its location in the ear, it can cause symptoms of pain, dizziness, or hearing loss. Treatment: Surgical excision.
cerumen impaction	**impaction** (im-PAK-shun) impact/o- *wedged in* -ion *action; condition*	Cerumen (earwax), epithelial cells, and hair form a mass that occludes the external auditory canal. Occurs most commonly in the elderly because of dryness of the skin, thick cerumen, and growth of hair in the external auditory canal. Treatment: Removal with forceps (see Figure 16-12 ■).

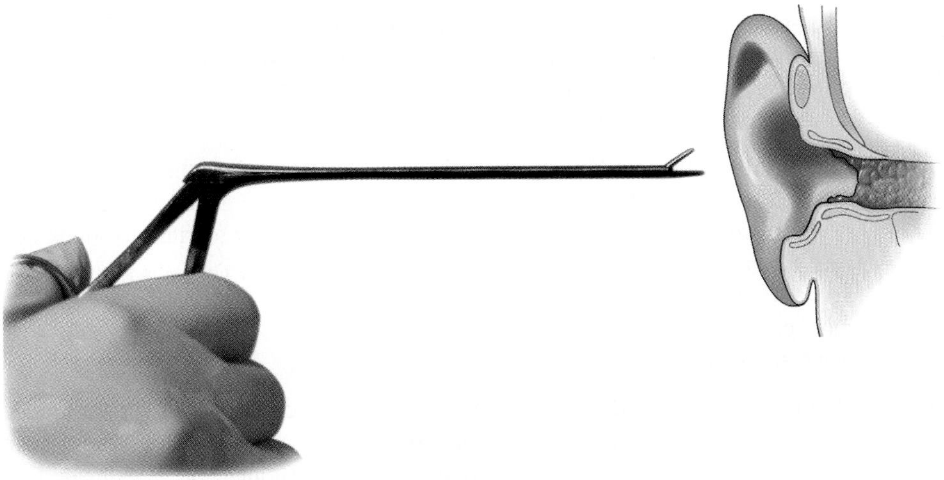

Figure 16-12 ■ Cerumen impaction.

Alligator forceps are used to enter the external auditory canal and remove impacted cerumen or foreign bodies. Alligator forceps are so-named because the shape resembles the long nose and open, biting jaws of an alligator.

Word or Phrase	Word Part and Definition	Description
cholesteatoma	**cholesteatoma** (koh-LES-tee-ah-TOH-mah) *Cholesteatoma* is a combination of the word *cholesterol,* the Greek word *stear* (animal fat), and the suffix *-oma* (tumor, mass).	Benign, slow-growing mass in the middle ear, composed of cholesterol deposits and epithelial cells. It can eventually destroy the bones of the middle ear and extend into the mastoid air cells. The underlying cause is chronic otitis media. Treatment: Surgical excision.

Word or Phrase	Word Part and Definition	Description
hearing loss	**conductive** (con-DUK-tiv) conduct/o- *carrying, conveying* -ive *pertaining to* **sensorineural** (SEN-soh-ree-NYOOR-al) sensor/i- *sensory* neur/o- *nerve* -al *pertaining to* **presbyacusis** (PREZ-bee-ah-KOO-sis) presby/o- *old age* -acusis *hearing* **anacusis** (AN-ah-KOO-sis) an- *without, not* -acusis *hearing*	Progressive, permanent decline in the ability to hear sounds in one or both ears. A foreign body or infection in the external auditory canal, perforation of the tympanic membrane, fluid behind the tympanic membrane, or degeneration of the ossicles of the middle ear keep sound waves from reaching the inner ear. This is known as **conductive hearing loss.** Otosclerosis, disease of the cochlea, damage to the inner ear from excessive noise, or aging prevent generation of nerve impulses to the auditory nerve. This is known as **sensorineural hearing loss.** A combination of both conductive and sensorineural hearing loss is called **mixed hearing loss. Low-frequency hearing loss** is the inability to hear low-pitched tones. **High-frequency hearing loss** is the inability to hear high-pitched tones. Patients with a hearing loss are said to be hearing impaired or hard of hearing. **Presbyacusis** is bilateral hearing loss due to aging. Total deafness is known as **anacusis.** Deaf-mutism is deafness coupled with the inability to speak. Treatment: Correct the underlying cause. Hearing aid; in some cases a cochlear implant may be done. **Did You Know?** Tone deafness is not a type of hearing loss. It is the inability to identify musical notes and sing in tune with them.
hemotympanum	**hemotympanum** (HEE-moh-TIM-pah-num) *Hemotympanum* is a combination of *hem/o-* (blood) and the Latin word *tympanum* (eardrum).	Blood in the middle ear space behind the tympanic membrane. It can be caused by infection or trauma (head trauma, a slap to the ear, or a nearby explosion). Treatment: None usually needed.
labyrinthitis	**labyrinthitis** (LAB-ih-rin-THY-tis) labyrinth/o- *labyrinth (in the inner ear)* -itis *inflammation of* The labyrinth includes all the inner ear structures. A labyrinth is a mazelike passageway.	Bacterial or viral infection of the semicircular canals of the inner ear, causing severe vertigo. Treatment: Antibiotic drug for a bacterial infection. Viruses are not sensitive to antibiotic drugs.
Ménière's disease	**Ménière's** (MEN-eh-AIRZ) Ménière's disease was named by Prosper Ménière (1799–1862), a French physician.	Edema of the semicircular canals with destruction of the cochlea, causing hearing loss, tinnitus, and vertigo. It can be triggered by head trauma or middle ear infections. Treatment: Correct the underlying cause.
motion sickness	**dysequilibrium** (DIS-ee-kwih-LIB-ree-um) *Dysequilibrium* is a combination of the prefix *dys-* (painful, difficult, abnormal) and the word *equilibrium* (evenly balanced).	**Dysequilibrium** with headache, dizziness, nausea, and vomiting caused by riding in a car, boat, or airplane. Treatment: Drug to treat motion sickness.

Word or Phrase	Word Part and Definition	Description
otitis externa	**otitis externa** (oh-TY-tis eks-TER-nah) **ot/o-** *ear* **-itis** *inflammation of* *Externa* is a Latin word meaning *external.* **otalgia** (oh-TAL-jee-ah) **ot/o-** *ear* **alg/o-** *pain* **-ia** *condition, state, thing*	Bacterial infection of the external auditory canal. There is throbbing earache pain (**otalgia**) with a swollen, red canal and serous or purulent drainage. Caused by a foreign body in the ear or the patient scratching or probing inside the ear. Also seen in swimmers whose ear canals are rubbed by ear plugs or softened by exposure to water. Also known as swimmer's ear. Treatment: Correct the underlying cause. Topical or oral antibiotic drug.
otitis media	**otitis media** (oh-TY-tis MEE-dee-ah) *Media* is a Latin word meaning *middle.* **myringitis** (MIR-in-JY-tis) **myring/o-** *tympanic membrane (eardrum)* **-itis** *inflammation of* **effusion** (ee-FYOO-shun) **effus/o-** *a pouring out* **-ion** *action; condition* **serous** (SEER-us) **ser/o-** *serum of the blood; serumlike fluid* **-ous** *pertaining to* **suppurative** (SUP-yoor-ah-tiv) **suppur/o-** *pus formation* **-ative** *pertaining to* **mastoiditis** (MAS-toy-DY-tis) **mastoid/o-** *mastoid process* **-itis** *inflammation of*	Acute or chronic bacterial infection of the middle ear. Symptoms include **myringitis** (redness and inflammation of the tympanic membrane), otalgia, a feeling of pressure, and bulging of the tympanic membrane (see Figure 16-13 ■). There can be an **effusion** (a collection of fluid behind the tympanic membrane that creates an air-fluid level). This fluid can be **serous** (clear) or **suppurative** (with pus). In children, the effusion can be so thick that it is called glue ear. Otitis media is common in young children because the short eustachian tube is in a nearly horizontal position that allows bacteria to enter from the nasopharynx. If left untreated, the tympanic membrane can rupture or the bones of the middle ear can degenerate, resulting in permanent hearing loss. The mastoid bone can become infected (**mastoiditis**). Treatment: Antibiotic drug. Surgery to insert tubes to drain the middle ear.

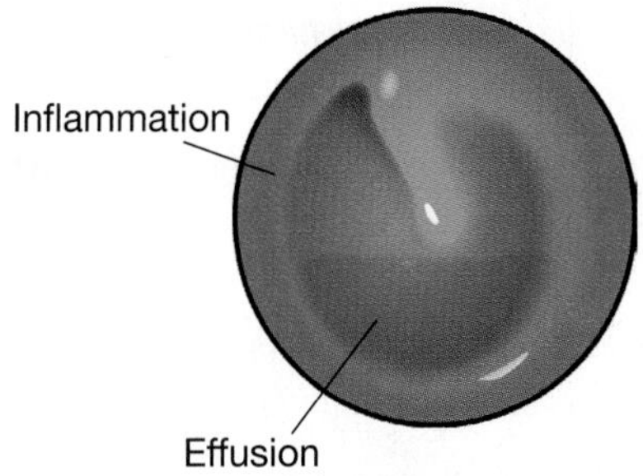

Figure 16-13 ■ Myringitis.

The tympanic membrane is red and inflamed or it may appear injected with streaks of red. There is dullness with no light reflex. There is a loss of normal landmarks (visibility of malleus) with bulging into the external auditory canal. An effusion in the middle ear can create an air-fluid level that can be seen through the tympanic membrane.

Word Alert

SOUND-ALIKE MEDICAL WORDS

mastoiditis (noun) infection of the air cells of the bone of the mastoid process

Example: The middle ear infection progressed to become mastoiditis.

mastitis (noun) infection of the mammary glands of the breast

Example: Mastitis can develop in nursing mothers.

Word or Phrase	Word Part and Definition	Description
otorrhea	**otorrhea** (OH-toh-REE-ah) **ot/o-** *ear* **-rrhea** *flow, discharge*	Drainage of serous fluid or pus from the ear. It can be caused by otitis externa or otitis media (with a ruptured tympanic membrane). It can also be caused by a fracture of the temporal bone of the cranium with leakage of cerebrospinal fluid. Treatment: Correct the underlying cause.
otosclerosis	**otosclerosis** (OH-toh-skleh-ROH-sis) **ot/o-** *ear* **scler/o-** *hard; sclera (white of the eye)* **-osis** *condition; abnormal condition; process*	Abnormal formation of bone in the inner ear, particularly between the stapes and the oval window. The stapes becomes immoveable, causing conductive hearing loss. Certain families have a genetic predisposition to develop otosclerosis. Treatment: Hearing aid, stapedectomy.
ruptured tympanic membrane		Tear in the tympanic membrane due to excessive pressure or infection. In pilots and deep sea divers, unequal air pressure in the middle ear compared to the surrounding air or water pressure can rupture the tympanic membrane. Treatment: Tympanoplasty.
tinnitus	**tinnitus** (TIN-ih-tus) (tih-NY-tus) *Tinnitus* is a Latin word meaning *a jingling or clinking sound.*	Sounds (buzzing, ringing, hissing, or roaring) that are heard constantly or intermittently in one or both ears, even in a quiet environment. It is caused by exposure to excess noise and associated with hearing loss. It can also be related to overuse of aspirin. Treatment: Soft background noise like the hum of a fan or the use of a device that generates "white noise" can mask tinnitus and allow the patient to sleep.
vertigo	**vertigo** (VER-tih-goh) *Vertigo* is a Latin word meaning *dizziness or turning.*	Sensation of being off balance when the body is not moving. Caused by upper respiratory infection, middle or inner ear infection, head trauma, degenerative changes of the semicircular canals, or Ménière's disease. Treatment: Correct the underlying cause.
Nose and Sinuses		
allergic rhinitis	**allergic** (ah-LER-jik) **allerg/o-** *allergy* **-ic** *pertaining to* **rhinitis** (ry-NY-tis) **rhin/o-** *nose* **-itis** *inflammation of* **rhinorrhea** (RY-noh-REE-ah) **rhin/o-** *nose* **-rrhea** *flow, discharge* **hypertrophy** (hy-PER-troh-fee) **hyper-** *above; more than normal* **-trophy** *process of development* **postnasal** (post-NAY-zal) **post-** *after, behind* **nas/o-** *nose* **-al** *pertaining to*	Allergic symptoms in the nose. In response to an inhaled antigen (pollen, dust, animal dander, mold), the immune response releases histamine. This produces nasal stuffiness, sneezing, **rhinorrhea** (clear mucus discharge from the nose), hypertrophy of the turbinates with red, edematous, and boggy mucous membranes, and **postnasal drip (PND)**. When this occurs in spring or fall and coincides with the blooming of certain trees and plants (grasses, maple trees, roses, goldenrod), it is known as seasonal allergy or hay fever. Treatment: Antihistamine drugs, decongestant drugs, corticosteroid drugs.

Word or Phrase	Word Part and Definition	Description
anosmia	**anosmia** (an-AWZ-mee-ah) **an-** *without, not* **osm/o-** *the sense of smell* **-ia** *condition, state, thing*	Loss of the sense of smell. Most often caused by head trauma.
epistaxis	**epistaxis** (EP-ih-STAK-sis) *Epistaxis* is derived from a Greek word meaning *blood falling from the nose.*	Sudden, sometimes severe, bleeding from the nose. Due to irritation or dryness of the nasal mucosa and the rupture of a small artery just beneath the mucous membrane. It can also be caused by trauma to the nose. Also known as a nosebleed. Treatment: Topical cautery with heat or chemicals to stop the bleeding.
polyp	**polyp** (PAWL-ip) *Polyp* is derived from a Latin word meaning *many feet.* The base (foot) of a polyp can have many different shapes, from wide and round to a thin stalk.	Benign growth from the mucous membrane of the nose or sinuses. A single polyp may grow large enough to limit the flow of air, or there may be several polyps. Treatment: Polypectomy.
rhinophyma	**rhinophyma** (RY-noh-FY-mah) **rhin/o-** *nose* **-phyma** *tumor, growth*	Redness and hypertrophy of the nose with small-to-large, irregular lumps in the skin. It is caused by an increased number of sebaceous glands and acne rosacea. Treatment: Topical drugs for acne rosacea.
septal deviation		Lateral displacement of the nasal septum, significantly narrowing one of the nasal airways. This can be a congenital condition or it can be caused by trauma to the nose. Treatment: Septoplasty.
sinusitis	**sinusitis** (SY-nyoo-SY-tis) **sinus/o-** *sinus* **-itis** *inflammation of* **pansinusitis** (PAN-sy-nyoo-SY-tis) **pan-** *all* **sinus/o-** *sinus* **-itis** *inflammation of*	Acute or chronic bacterial infection in one or all of the sinus cavities. Symptoms include headache, pain in the face over the sinus, postnasal drainage, fatigue, and fever. **Pansinusitis** involves all the sinuses or all the sinuses on one side of the face. Treatment: Antibiotic drug. Sinus surgery.
upper respiratory infection (URI)		Bacterial or viral infection of the nose that can spread to the throat and ears. The nose is a part of the respiratory system as well as the ENT system. Also known as a common cold or head cold. Treatment: Antibiotic drug for a bacterial infection.
Mouth, Throat, and Neck		
cancer of the mouth and neck	**malignant** (mah-LIG-nant) **malign/o-** *intentionally causing harm; cancer* **-ant** *pertaining to* **carcinoma** (KAR-sih-NOH-mah) **carcin/o-** *cancer* **-oma** *tumor, mass*	**Malignant** tumor (**carcinoma**) from squamous epithelial cells in the oral cavity (lips, tongue, gums, cheeks), throat, or larynx. Smoking and using smokeless tobacco can cause oral cancer and cancer of the larynx. Treatment: Surgical excision.

Word or Phrase	Word Part and Definition	Description
cervical lymphadenopathy	**cervical** (SER-vih-kal) **cervic/o-** *neck; cervix* **-al** *pertaining to* **lymphadenopathy** (lim-FAD-eh-NAWP-eh-thee) **lymph/o-** *lymph; lymphatic system* **aden/o-** *gland* **-pathy** *disease, suffering*	Enlargement of the lymph nodes in the neck. Caused by infection, cancer, or the spread of a cancerous tumor from another site. Treatment: Correct the underlying cause.
cleft lip and palate	**cleft** (KLEFT) **unilateral** (YOO-nih-LAT-eh-ral) **uni-** *single, not paired* **later/o-** *side* **-al** *pertaining to* **bilateral** (by-LAT-eh-ral) **bi-** *two* **later/o-** *side* **-al** *pertaining to*	Congenital deformity in which the maxilla fails to join before birth. The resulting cleft in the bone and skin can be **unilateral** or **bilateral** (see Figure 16-14 ■). The cleft can also extend into the soft palate. Treatment: Surgical correction. **Figure 16-14 ■ Cleft lip.** This infant has a bilateral cleft lip and palate and has difficulty feeding from the breast or bottle because milk flows into the nasal cavity where it could be inhaled into the lungs. Note the feeding tube inserted in the right nostril and taped to the cheek.
cold sores	**herpes simplex** (HER-peez SIM-pleks)	Recurring, painful clusters of blisters, erupting on the lips or nose, and caused by infection with **herpes simplex virus** type 1. After the initial infection, the virus remains dormant in the skin until triggers of stress, sunlight, illness, or menstruation cause it to erupt again. Also known as fever blisters. Treatment: Topical antiviral drug. (Note: Herpes simplex type 2 causes genital herpes, a sexually transmitted disease.)
glossitis	**glossitis** (glaw-SY-tis) **gloss/o-** *tongue* **-itis** *inflammation of*	Inflammation of the tongue. Caused by irritation from a food, infection, or vitamin B deficiency. Treatment: Correct the underlying cause.
laryngitis	**laryngitis** (LAIR-in-JY-tis) **laryng/o-** *larynx (voice box)* **-itis** *inflammation of*	Hoarseness or complete loss of the voice, difficulty swallowing, and cough due to swelling and inflammation of the larynx. Caused by a bacterial or viral infection. Treatment: Antibiotic drug for a bacterial infection.
leukoplakia	**leukoplakia** (LOO-koh-PLAY-kee-ah) **leuk/o-** *white* **plak/o-** *plaque* **-ia** *condition, state, thing*	Benign, thickened, white patch on the mucous membrane of the mouth. It is caused by tobacco use; it can become cancerous. Also caused by Epstein-Barr virus infection in AIDS patients. Treatment: Correct the underlying cause.

Word or Phrase	Word Part and Definition	Description
pharyngitis	**pharyngitis** (FAIR-in-JY-tis) pharyng/o- *pharynx (throat)* -itis *inflammation of* **streptococcus** (STREP-toh-KAWK-uhs) strept/o- *curved* -coccus *spherical bacterium* Streptococci are individual spherical bacteria that join together to form curved chains.	Bacterial or viral infection of the throat. When the bacteria group A beta-hemolytic **streptococcus** causes the infection, it is known as **strep throat.** It is important to diagnose strep throat and treat it with an antibiotic drug so that it does not cause the complication of rheumatic heart disease. Treatment: Antibiotic drug.
temporomandibular joint (TMJ) syndrome	**temporomandibular** (TEM-poh-roh-man-DIB-yoo-lar) tempor/o- *temple (side of the head)* mandibul/o- *mandible (lower jaw)* -ar *pertaining to* **syndrome** (SIN-drohm) syn- *together* -drome *a running* A syndrome is a group of different symptoms and signs that are all related to one disease.	Dysfunction of the temporomandibular joint with clicking, pain, muscle spasm, and difficulty opening the jaw. Caused by chewing on only one side of the mouth, clenching or grinding the teeth (often during sleep), or misalignment of the teeth. Treatment: Dental bite guard worn at night, correction of misaligned teeth.
thrush	***Candida albicans*** (KAN-dih-dah AL-bih-kanz) **candidiasis** (KAN-dih-DY-ah-sis)	Oral infection caused by the yeastlike fungus *Candida albicans.* It coats the tongue and oral mucosa (see Figure 16-15 ■). Thrush is common in infants, but is also seen in the mouths of immunocompromised patients with AIDS because their immune response cannot control its growth. Also seen after a course of antibiotic drugs kills bacteria in the mouth, allowing overgrowth of *Candida albicans.* Also known as **oral candidiasis.** Treatment: Oral antiyeast drug. 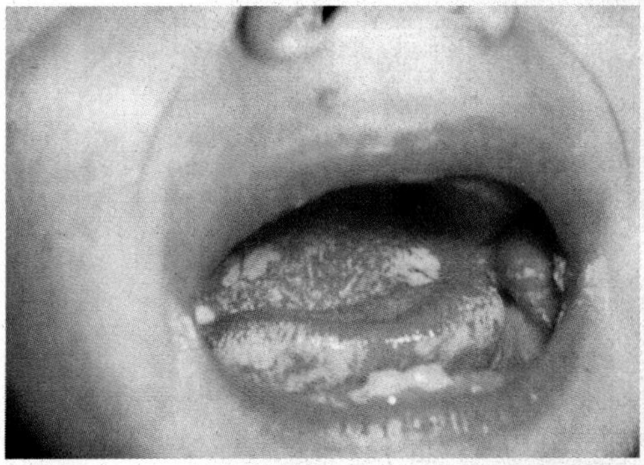 **Figure 16-15 ■ Thrush.** The warm, moist environment of the mouth is the perfect growth medium for *Candida albicans.* It forms a thick white coating that resembles curdled milk, but cannot be wiped away.

<table>
<tr><th>Word or Phrase</th><th>Word Part and Definition</th><th>Description</th></tr>
<tr><td>tonsillitis</td><td>tonsillitis (TAWN-sih-LY-tis)
tonsill/o- tonsil
-itis inflammation of</td><td>Acute or chronic bacterial infection of the pharynx and palatine tonsils (see Figure 16-16 ■), with sore throat, difficulty swallowing, and mouth breathing and snoring. The tonsils hypertrophy and the tonsillar crypts contain pus and debris. The adenoids may also hypertrophy and block the eustachian tubes. Treatment: Antibiotic drug, tonsillectomy.

Figure 16-16 ■ Tonsillitis.
This patient has an acute inflammation and hypertrophy of the palatine tonsils on either side of the oropharynx. The uvula and posterior oropharynx are also inflamed.

Word Alert
MEDICAL WORD SPELLING
tonsil — the lymph tissue in the throat — spelled with one l
tonsillitis — an inflammation or infection of the tonsils — spelled with two l's
tonsillectomy — surgical excision of the tonsils — spelled with two l's</td></tr>
<tr><td>vocal cord nodule or polyp</td><td>nodule (NAWD-yool)
Nodule is derived from a Latin word meaning small knot or node.

polyp (PAWL-ip)</td><td>Benign growth on the surface of the vocal cord. A nodule is a small fibrous growth. A polyp is a larger, soft, benign growth that contains blood vessels. Caused by strain from constant talking or singing or chronic irritation from smoking or allergies. There is hoarseness and change in the quality of the voice. Treatment: Voice rest, surgical excision.</td></tr>
</table>

Diagnostic Procedures

Hearing Tests

Word or Phrase	Word Part and Definition	Description
audiometry	**audiometry** (AW-dee-AWM-eh-tree) audi/o- *the sense of hearing* -metry *process of measuring* **audiometer** (AW-dee-AWM-eh-ter) audi/o- *the sense of hearing* -meter *instrument used to measure* **hertz** (HERTS) *Hertz* was named by Heinrich Hertz (1857–1894), a German physicist. **decibel** (DES-ih-bel) *Decibel* is a combination of *deci-* (one tenth) and *bel* (a unit for the power of sound that was named by Alexander Graham Bell). **audiogram** (AW-dee-oh-gram) audi/o- *the sense of hearing* -gram *a record or picture*	Hearing test that measures hearing acuity and documents hearing loss. The patient puts on headphones that are connected to an **audiometer** that produces a series of pure tones, each at a different frequency (pitch) and varying in intensity (loudness). The frequency of a tone is measured in **hertz (Hz).** The intensity of a tone is measured in **decibels (dB).** The patient presses a button to signal when the sound is heard. The result, which is printed on graph paper, is known as an **audiogram.** In **speech audiometry,** the patient hears spoken words and sentences. If he or she can repeat 50% of the words correctly, then this is the threshold of hearing ability for speech sounds. Both pure tone audiometry and speech audiometry are used to determine whether a patient needs a hearing aid.
brainstem auditory evoked response (BAER)		Analyzes the brain's response to sounds. The patient listens as an audiometer produces a series of clicks. Electroencephalography (EEG) is performed at the same time. A lesion or tumor in the auditory cortex of the brain or on the auditory nerve will produce an abnormal BAER. Also known as an **auditory brainstem response (ABR).**

Word or Phrase	Word Part and Definition	Description
Rinne and Weber hearing tests	**Rinne** (RIN-eh) The Rinne test was named by Friederich Rinne (1819–1868), a German physician. **Weber** (VAH-ber) The Weber test was named by Ernst Weber (1795–1898), a German physiologist.	The Rinne tuning fork test evaluates bone conduction versus air conduction of sound in one ear at a time (see Figure 16-17 ■). A vibrating tuning fork is placed against the mastoid process behind the ear to test bone conduction of sound. Then it is placed next to (but not touching) the same ear. If the sound is louder when the tuning fork is next to the ear, then hearing in that ear is normal and the test is said to be positive (because air conduction normally is greater than bone conduction). If the sound is louder when the tuning fork touches the mastoid process, then the patient has a conductive hearing loss. The Weber tuning fork test evaluates bone conduction of sound in both ears at the same time. The vibrating tuning fork is placed against the center of the forehead or on the top of the head. The sound should be heard equally in both ears. 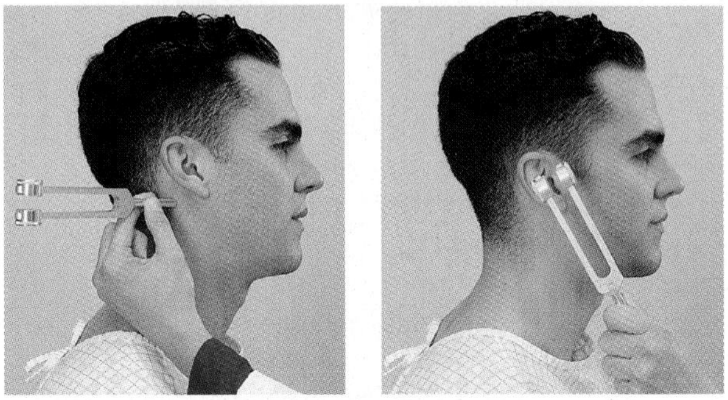 **Figure 16-17 ■ Rinne test.** This hearing test uses a vibrating tuning fork to compare bone conduction of sound to air conduction of sound for the same ear.
tympanometry	**tympanometry** (TIM-pah-NAWM-eh-tree) **tympan/o-** *tympanic membrane (eardrum)* **-metry** *process of measuring* **impedance** (im-PEE-dans) **tympanogram** (tim-PAN-oh-gram) **tympan/o-** *tympanic membrane (eardrum)* **-gram** *a record or picture*	Hearing test that measures the ability of the tympanic membrane and the bones of the middle ear to move back and forth. Air pressure (rather than sound vibration) is applied to the external auditory canal. If infection or disease has fixed the middle ear bones, then the tympanic membrane will move very little. This resistance to movement is called **impedance.** The result, which is printed on graph paper, is called a **tympanogram.** **Did You Know?** The ear can hear sounds with a frequency as low as 20 Hz or as high as 20,000 Hz. In contrast, a dog can hear from 20 Hz to 45,000 Hz, and a porpoise can hear from 75 Hz to 150,000 Hz. A tuning fork of 256 Hz is used to test the hearing. This frequency corresponds to middle C on the piano.

Laboratory and Radiologic Tests

Word or Phrase	Word Part and Definition	Description
culture and sensitivity (C&S)	**culture** (KUL-chur) **sensitivity** (SEN-sih-TIV-ih-tee) sensitiv/o- *affected by, sensitive to* -ity *state; condition*	Laboratory test that puts a swab of material from the nose, tonsils, or throat (see Figure 16-18 ■) onto culture medium in a Petri dish to identify the cause of an infection. Microorganisms grow into colonies, and the specific disease-causing microorganism is identified and tested to determine its sensitivity to various antibiotic drugs. **Figure 16-18 ■ Throat swab.** This child is having a swab taken of the oropharynx. The material on the swab will be sent to the laboratory for a culture and sensitivity test.
rapid strep test		Test kit for strep throat. It detects beta-hemolytic group A streptococcus, which causes a purplish pink line to appear. Unlike a standard culture and sensitivity test, the result of a rapid strep test is available within the hour so that the physician can immediately prescribe an antibiotic drug.
sinus series		Plain x-rays are taken from various angles to show all of the sinuses and confirm or rule out a diagnosis of sinusitis. Sinusitis shows as cloudy, opacified sinuses with thickened mucous membranes. Sometimes an air-fluid level can be seen within the sinus.

Medical and Surgical Procedures

Medical Procedures

Word or Phrase	Word Part and Definition	Description
nose, sinus, mouth, and throat examinations	**speculum** (SPEK-yoo-lum) *Speculum* is a Latin word meaning *instrument used to look.*	A nasal **speculum** is used to widen the nostril, and a penlight is used to light the nasal cavity. The frontal and maxillary sinuses are examined for tenderness by pressing with the fingertips on the forehead and cheekbones. A tongue depressor, penlight, and a laryngeal mirror are used to examine the mouth and throat. 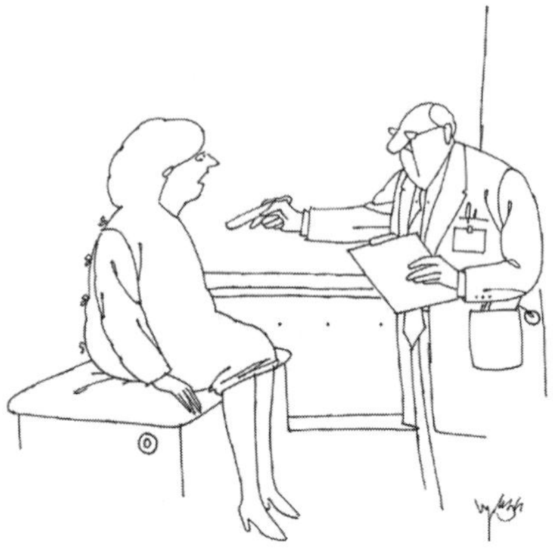 That's all you want me to say, . . . Ah?
otoscopy	**otoscopy** (oh-TAWS-koh-pee) **ot/o-** *ear* **-scopy** *process of using an instrument to examine*	Medical procedure to examine the external auditory canals and tympanic membranes (see Figure 16-19 ■). The physician gently pulls the helix back and up to straighten the external auditory canal and better visualize the tympanic membrane. In infants younger than 3, the helix is 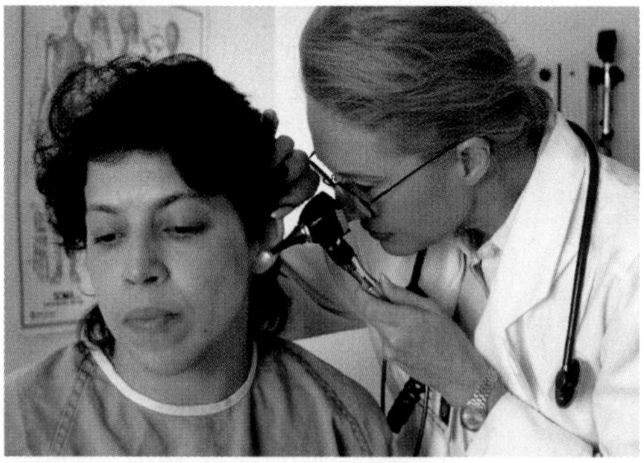 **Figure 16-19 ■ Otoscopy.** The physician is using a otoscope to examine this patient's left internal auditory canal and tympanic membrane. Before each use, a disposable black plastic tip or speculum is fitted over the part of the otoscope that enters the patient's ear.

Word or Phrase	Word Part and Definition	Description
otoscopy (*continued*)	**otoscope** (OH-toh-skohp) ot/o- *ear* -scope *instrument used to examine*	pulled back and down. The **otoscope** provides light and magnification. When pressed against the external auditory meatus, the otoscope forms an air-tight seal. To assess the mobility of the tympanic membrane, some otoscopes have a rubber bulb that is squeezed to force air into the external auditory canal. A normal tympanic membrane moves in and out in response to this procedure.
Romberg's sign	**Romberg** (RAWM-berg) Named by Moritz Romberg (1795–1873), a German physician.	Medical procedure to assess equilibrium. The patient stands with the feet together and the eyes closed. Swaying or falling to one side indicates a loss of balance and inner ear dysfunction.
Surgical Procedures		
cheiloplasty	**cheiloplasty** (KY-loh-PLAS-tee) cheil/o- *lip* -plasty *process of reshaping by surgery*	Surgical procedure to repair the lip, usually because of a laceration.
cochlear implant		Surgical procedure to implant a small, battery-powered implant beneath the skin behind the ear. Wires are placed from the implant through the round window and into the cochlea of the inner ear. When the implant "hears" a sound, it sends an electrical impulse to stimulate the cochlear nerve.
endoscopic sinus surgery	**endoscopic** (EN-doh-SKAWP-ik) endo- *innermost, within* scop/o- *examine with an instrument* -ic *pertaining to* **endoscope** (EN-doh-skohp) endo- *innermost, within* -scope *instrument used to examine* **endoscopy** (en-DAWS-koh-pee) endo- *innermost, within* -scopy *process of using an instrument to examine*	Surgical procedure that uses an **endoscope** (a flexible, fiberoptic scope with a magnifying lens and a light source) to examine the nose, sinuses, or throat. **Endoscopy** is used to remove tissue and fluid or perform a biopsy.
mastoidectomy	**mastoidectomy** (MASS-toy-DEK-toh-mee) mastoid/o- *mastoid process* -ectomy *surgical excision*	Surgical procedure to remove part of the mastoid process of the temporal bone because of infection.

Word or Phrase	Word Part and Definition	Description
myringotomy	**myringotomy** (MEER-ing-GAWT-oh-mee) **myring/o-** *tympanic membrane (eardrum)* **-tomy** *process of cutting or making an incision* **myringotome** (mih-RING-goh-tohm) **myring/o-** *tympanic membrane (eardrum)* **-tome** *instrument used to cut; an area with distinct edges* **tympanostomy** (TIM-pan-AWS-toh-mee) **tympan/o-** *tympanic membrane (eardrum)* **-stomy** *surgically created opening*	Surgical procedure that uses a **myringotome** to make an incision in the tympanic membrane to drain fluid from the middle ear. For chronic middle ear infections, a ventilating tube can also be inserted through the incision to form a permanent opening into the middle ear (see Figure 16-20■). That procedure is known as a **tympanostomy.** 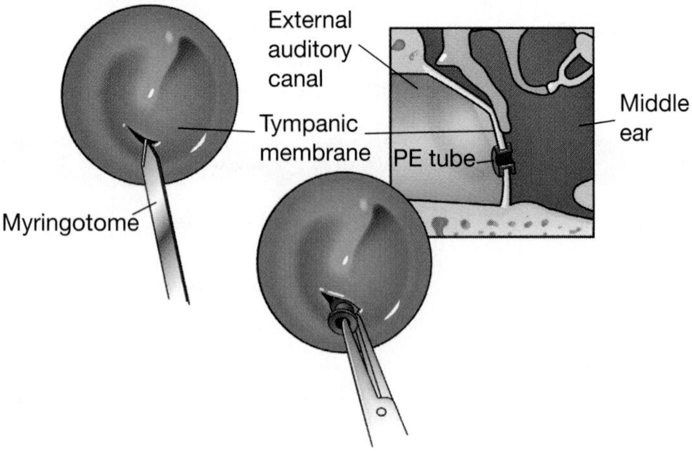 External auditory canal / Tympanic membrane / Middle ear / PE tube / Myringotome **Figure 16-20 ■ Myringotomy and tympanostomy.** A myringotome is used to make an incision in the tympanic membrane. Then a small ventilating tube (tympanostomy tube) is inserted through the incision. This is also known as a PE tube because it is made of polyethylene.
polypectomy	**polypectomy** (PAWL-ih-PEK-toh-mee) **polyp/o-** *polyp* **-ectomy** *surgical excision*	Surgical procedure to remove polyps from the nasal cavity, sinuses, or vocal cords.
otoplasty	**otoplasty** (OH-toh-PLAS-tee) **ot/o-** *ear* **-plasty** *process of reshaping by surgery*	Surgical procedure that uses plastic surgery to correct deformities of the external ear. When it corrects protruding ears, it is known as an ear pinning.
radical neck dissection	**radical** (RAD-ih-kal) **radic/o-** *all parts including the root* **-al** *pertaining to* **dissection** (dy-SEK-shun) **dissect/o-** *to cut apart* **-ion** *action; condition* **glossectomy** (glaw-SEK-toh-mee) **gloss/o-** *tongue* **-ectomy** *surgical excision* **laryngectomy** (LAIR-in-JEK-toh-mee) **laryng/o-** *larynx (voice box)* **-ectomy** *surgical excision*	Surgical procedure to treat extensive cancer of the mouth and neck. Parts of the jaw bone, tongue (partial **glossectomy**), lymph nodes, and muscles of the neck may be removed. The larynx can also be removed (**laryngectomy**).

Word or Phrase	Word Part and Definition	Description
rhinoplasty	**rhinoplasty** (RY-noh-PLAS-tee) **rhin/o-** *nose* **-plasty** *process of reshaping by surgery*	Surgical procedure that uses plastic surgery to change the size or shape of the nose.
stapedectomy	**stapedectomy** (STAY-pee-DEK-toh-mee) **staped/o-** *stapes (stirrup-shaped bone)* **-ectomy** *surgical excision*	Surgical procedure for otosclerosis to remove the diseased part of the stapes and replace it with a prosthetic device.
tonsillectomy and adenoidectomy (T&A)	**tonsillectomy** (TAWN-sih-LEK-toh-mee) **tonsill/o-** *tonsil* **-ectomy** *surgical excision* **adenoidectomy** (AD-eh-noy-DEK-toh-mee) **aden/o-** *gland* **-oid** *resembling* **–ectomy** *surgical excision*	Surgical procedure to remove the tonsils and adenoids in patients with chronic tonsillitis and hypertrophy of the tonsils and adenoids.
tympanoplasty	**tympanoplasty** (TIM-pah-noh-PLAS-tee) (TIM-pah-noh-PLAS-tee) **tympan/o-** *tympanic membrane (eardrum)* **-plasty** *process of reshaping by surgery*	Surgical procedure to reconstruct a ruptured tympanic membrane.

Drug Categories

Several different categories of drugs are used to treat the symptoms, signs, and diseases of the ENT system. The most common drugs in each category are listed.

Category	Word Part and Definition	Description	Examples
antibiotic drugs	**antibiotic** (AN-tee-by-AWT-ik) (AN-tih-by-AWT-ik) **anti-** *against* **bi/o-** *life; living organisms; living tissue* **-tic** *pertaining to*	Treat bacterial infections of the ears, nose, sinuses, or throat. Antibiotic drugs are not effective against viral infections.	amoxicillin, Bactrim, Septra
antihistamine drugs	**antihistamine** (AN-tee-HIS-tah-meen) *Antihistamine* is a combination of the prefix *anti-* (against) and the word *histamine*.	Block the effect of histamine released during an allergic reaction. Histamine causes symptoms of runny, itchy nose and swollen mucous membranes.	Allegra, Benadryl, Claritin, Zyrtec

Category	Word Part and Definition	Description	Examples
antitussive drugs	**antitussive** (AN-tee-TUS-iv) anti- *against* tuss/o- *cough* -ive *pertaining to*	Suppress the cough center in the brain. Some of these drugs contain a narcotic.	dextromethorphan, Hycodan, Robitussin
antiyeast drugs	**antiyeast** (AN-tee-YEEST) *Antiyeast* is a combination of the prefix *anti-* (against) and the word *yeast.*	Treat yeast infections (oral candidiasis, thrush) of the mouth caused by *Candida albicans.* Solution is swished and swallowed.	nystatin, Mycostatin
chemotherapy drugs	**chemotherapy** (KEE-moh-THAIR-ah-pee) chem/o- *chemical, drug* -therapy *treatment*	Kill rapidly dividing cancer cells in the ears, nose, or throat.	bleomycin, methotrexate, Taxol
corticosteroid drugs	**corticosteroid** (KOR-tih-koh-STAIR-oyd) cortic/o- *cortex (outer region)* -steroid *steroid*	Treat inflammation of the ears, nose, or mouth. Topical nose drops, ear drops, or oral drug.	Beconase, Flonase, Rhinocort
decongestant drugs	**decongestant** (DEE-con-JES-tant) de- *reversal of; without* congest/o- *accumulation of fluid* -ant *pertaining to*	Constrict blood vessels and decrease swelling of the mucous membranes of the nose and sinuses due to colds and allergies. Topical nasal sprays or oral drugs.	Afrin, Dristan, Drixoral, Sudafed
drugs used to treat vertigo and motion sickness		Decrease the sensitivity of the inner ear to motion and keep nerve impulses from the inner ear from reaching the vomiting center in the brain.	Antivert, Dramamine, Transderm-Scop

Connections

ototoxicity
(OH-toh-tawk-SIS-ih-tee)
ot/o- *ear*
toxic/o- *poison, toxin*
-ity *state; condition*

Pharmacology. Aminoglycoside antibiotic drugs are known to damage the cochlea. This drug effect is known as **ototoxicity.** Patients taking aminoglycosides need to have audiograms done periodically to monitor their hearing.

Abbreviations

ABR	auditory brainstem response
AD, A.D.	auris dextra (right ear)
AS, A.S.	auris sinister (left ear)
AU, A.U.	auris uterque (both ears)
BAER	brainstem auditory evoked response
BOM	bilateral otitis media
C&S	culture and sensitivity
dB, db	decibel
EAC	external auditory canal
ENT	ears, nose, and throat
HEENT	head, eyes, ears, nose, and throat
Hz	hertz
PE	polyethylene (tube)
PND	postnasal drip (or drainage)
SOM	serous otitis media
T&A	tonsillectomy and adenoidectomy
TM	tympanic membrane
TMJ	temporomandibular joint
URI	upper respiratory infection

Word Alert

MEDICAL ABBREVIATIONS

Abbreviations are commonly used in all types of medical documents; however, they can mean different things to different people and their meaning can be misinterpreted. Always verify the meaning of an abbreviation.

C&S stands for *culture and sensitivity,* but the sound-alike abbreviation *CNS* stands for *central nervous system.*

PND stands for *postnasal drip,* but it can also stand for *paroxysmal nocturnal dyspnea.*

TM stands for *tympanic membrane,* but *TMJ* stands for *temporomandibular joint.*

Career Focus

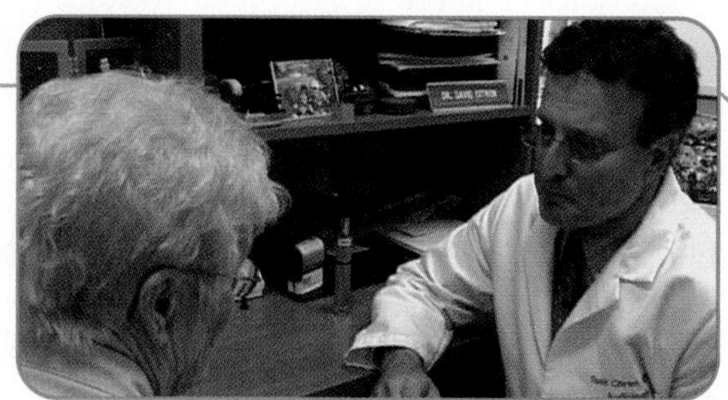

Meet David, an audiologist.

"Audiology is very exciting, not just because of all the changes in technology that have occurred, but also the fact that the profession is growing. One very large change is in the area of newborn hearing screening. Now we can screen babies right at birth. There are technologically advanced hearing aids. All of them are programmable by computer; we can individualize each person's hearing profile by programming the hearing aid to meet their specific needs. We tend to see a lot of people who have balance problems because one area of audiology deals with assessing and treating dizziness and vertigo. All audiologists need to have a doctoral degree and the reason for that is because of all the things we do—our scope of practice has grown so much."

Audiologists are allied health professionals who perform hearing tests, diagnose hearing loss, and determine how patients can best use their remaining hearing. They also make and fit hearing aids. Audiologists work in schools, hospitals, physicians' offices, and their own private offices.

Otolaryngologists or **otorhinolaryngologists** are physicians who practice in the medical specialty of otolaryngology. They diagnose and treat patients with diseases of the ears, nose, or throat. They are also known as ENT specialists. When otolaryngologists perform surgery, they are known as head and neck surgeons or **oral and maxillofacial surgeons.** Physicians can take additional training and become board certified in the subspecialties of pediatric otolaryngology, plastic surgery of the head and neck, or allergy and immunology. Malignancies of the ears, nose, and throat are treated medically by an oncologist or surgically by a head and neck surgeon or oral surgeon.

audiologist (AW-dee-AWL-oh-jist)
audi/o- *the sense of hearing*
log/o- *the study of*
-ist *one who specializes in*

otolaryngologist (OH-toh-LAIR-ing-GAWL-oh-jist)
ot/o- *ear*
laryng/o- *larynx (voice box)*
log/o- *the study of*
-ist *one who specializes in*

otorhinolaryngologist (OH-toh-RY-noh-LAIR-ing-GAWL-oh-jist)
ot/o- *ear*
rhin/o- *nose*
laryng/o- *larynx (voice box)*
log/o- *the study of*
-ist *one who specializes in*

maxillofacial (MAK-sil-oh-FAY-shal)
maxill/o- *maxilla (upper jaw)*
faci/o- *face*
-al *pertaining to*

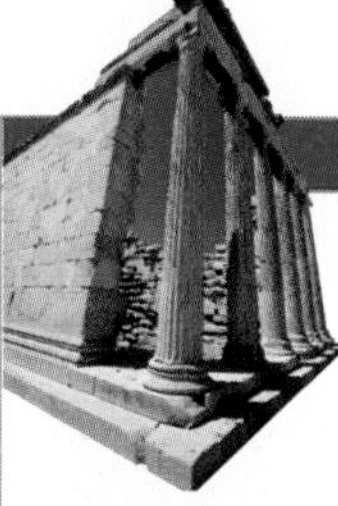

It's Greek to Me!

Did you notice that some ENT words have two different combining forms? Combining forms from both Greek and Latin languages remain a part of medical language today.

English Word	Greek	Latin	Examples of Medical Words
ear	ot/o-	aur/i-	otic, auricle
eardrum	tympan/o-	myring/o-	tympanic membrane, myringotomy
hearing	acous/o-	aud/i-, audit/o-	acoustic neuroma, audiogram, auditory canal
lip	cheil/o-	labi/o-	cheiloplasty, nasolabial
nose	rhin/o-	nas/o-	rhinoplasty, nasal
tongue	gloss/o-	lingu/o-	glossectomy, lingual

CHAPTER REVIEW EXERCISES

Review all of the material in this chapter by completing the review exercises in this section. Use the Answer Key at the end of the book to check your answers.

Anatomy and Physiology

Matching Exercise

Match each numbered word or phrase to its location. Note: Some locations have more than one correct answer.

1.	adenoids	_____ External ear
2.	alae	_____ Middle ear
3.	cochlea	_____ Inner ear
4.	conchae	_____ External nose
5.	helix	_____ Nasal cavity
6.	incus	_____ External mouth
7.	malleus	_____ Pharynx
8.	nares	
9.	nasal septum	
10.	nasopharynx	
11.	ossicles	
12.	philtrum	
13.	pinna	
14.	semicircular canals	
15.	stapes	
16.	tonsils	
17.	tragus	
18.	turbinates	
19.	vermilion border	
20.	vestibule	

True or False

Indicate whether each statement is true or false by writing T or F on the line.

1. ____ The semicircular canals help the body keep its balance.
2. ____ The eustachian tube connects the nasal cavity to the inner ear.
3. ____ The sinuses in the cheek on either side of the nose are the maxillary sinuses.
4. ____ The chin is also known as the mentum.
5. ____ The lingual tonsils are located on either side of the base of the tongue.
6. ____ The pinna is another name for the tragus.
7. ____ The ossicular chain is located in the semicircular canals of the inner ear.
8. ____ The tympanic membrane divides the external auditory canal from the middle ear.

Sequencing Exercise

Beginning where the sound enters the external ear, use the list of anatomical structures given here to help you sequence the structures of the ear in their correct order.

auditory cortex of the brain	external auditory canal	tympanic membrane	incus
malleus	stapes	vestibule	
cochlea	auditory nerve	oval window	

1. External auditory canal → 2. ______ → 3. ______ →
4. ______ → 5. ______ → 6. ______ →
7. ______ → 8. ______ → 9. ______ →
10. ______

Medical Language Word Parts

Name that Word Part

Identify each of the word parts given here by writing in the correct letter (P, C, or S) on the line beside it. Then write the definition of the word part on the blank line. The first one has been done for you.

Prefix = P **Combining Form = C** **Suffix = S**

	Word Part	Definition		Word Part	Definition
1. -al	S	pertaining to	26. -cle		
2. acous/o-			27. -coccus		
3. -acusis			28. cochle/o-		
4. aden/o-			29. conduct/o-		
5. alg/o-			30. congest/o-		
6. allerg/o-			31. cortic/o-		
7. an-			32. de-		
8. -ant			33. dissect/o-		
9. anti-			34. dors/o-		
10. -ar			35. -drome		
11. -ary			36. -eal		
12. -ate			37. -ectomy		
13. -ative			38. effus/o-		
14. audi/o-			39. endo-		
15. audit/o-			40. epi-		
16. aur/i-			41. ethm/o-		
17. auricul/o-			42. extern/o-		
18. bi-			43. faci/o-		
19. bi/o-			44. front/o-		
20. bucc/o-			45. gloss/o-		
21. carcin/o-			46. glott/o-		
22. cav/o-			47. -gram		
23. cervic/o-			48. hyper-		
24. cheil/o-			49. hypo-		
25. chem/o-			50. -ia		

		Word Part	Definition
51.	-ial	______	______________
52.	-ic	______	______________
53.	impact/o-	______	______________
54.	incud/o-	______	______________
55.	-ine	______	______________
56.	-ion	______	______________
57.	-ist	______	______________
58.	-itis	______	______________
59.	-ity	______	______________
60.	-ive	______	______________
61.	labi/o-	______	______________
62.	labyrinth/o-	______	______________
63.	laryng/o-	______	______________
64.	later/o-	______	______________
65.	leuk/o-	______	______________
66.	lingu/o-	______	______________
67.	log/o-	______	______________
68.	-logy	______	______________
69.	lymph/o-	______	______________
70.	malign/o-	______	______________
71.	malle/o-	______	______________
72.	mandibul/o-	______	______________
73.	mast/o-	______	______________
74.	mastoid/o-	______	______________
75.	maxill/o-	______	______________
76.	ment/o-	______	______________
77.	-meter	______	______________
78.	-metry	______	______________
79.	mucos/o-	______	______________
80.	myring/o-	______	______________
81.	nas/o-	______	______________
82.	neur/o-	______	______________
83.	-oid	______	______________
84.	-oma	______	______________
85.	or/o-	______	______________
86.	-ory	______	______________
87.	osm/o-	______	______________
88.	-ous	______	______________
89.	-osis	______	______________
90.	ossicul/o-	______	______________
91.	ot/o-	______	______________
92.	palat/o-	______	______________
93.	pan-	______	______________
94.	para-	______	______________

		Word Part	Definition
95.	-pathy	______	______________
96.	pharyng/o-	______	______________
97.	-pharynx	______	______________
98.	-phyma	______	______________
99.	plak/o-	______	______________
100.	-plasty	______	______________
101.	polyp/o-	______	______________
102.	post-	______	______________
103.	presby/o-	______	______________
104.	radicul/o-	______	______________
105.	rhin/o-	______	______________
106.	-rrhea	______	______________
107.	scler/o-	______	______________
108.	-scope	______	______________
109.	scop/o-	______	______________
110.	-scopy	______	______________
111.	sensitiv/o-	______	______________
112.	sensor/i-	______	______________
113.	sept/o-	______	______________
114.	ser/o-	______	______________
115.	sinus/o-	______	______________
116.	sphen/o-	______	______________
117.	staped/o-	______	______________
118.	-steroid	______	______________
119.	-stomy	______	______________
120.	strept/o-	______	______________
121.	sub-	______	______________
122.	suppur/o-	______	______________
123.	syn-	______	______________
124.	tempor/o-	______	______________
125.	-therapy	______	______________
126.	-tic	______	______________
127.	-tome	______	______________
128.	-tomy	______	______________
129.	tonsill/o-	______	______________
130.	toxic/o-	______	______________
131.	-trophy	______	______________
132.	turbin/o-	______	______________
133.	tuss/o-	______	______________
134.	tympan/o-	______	______________
135.	uni-	______	______________
136.	vestibul/o-	______	______________
137.	voc/o-	______	______________

Word-Building Exercise

Use the combining forms, prefixes, and suffixes given here to build medical words that match the definitions given. Write the word that you build on the blank line. Some word parts may be used more than once. The first one has been done for you.

Word Parts		
-acusis (hearing)	-metry (process of measuring)	-rrhea (flow, drainage)
an- (without, not)	myring/o- (tympanic membrane)	-scope (instrument used to examine)
audit/o- (hearing)	-ory (pertaining to)	sinus/o- (sinus)
endo- (innermost, within)	ot/o- (ear)	-tomy (process of cutting or making an incision)
-itis (inflammation of)	presby/o- (old age)	tympan/o- (tympanic membrane)

1. Pertaining to hearing (You think *audit/o-* + *-ory*). You write auditory
2. Incision into the eardrum ____________
3. Instrument used to examine within (the sinuses) ____________
4. Decreased hearing in old age ____________
5. Inflammation or infection of the ear ____________
6. Total deafness without hearing ____________
7. Drainage flowing from the ear ____________
8. Inflammation or infection of the sinus ____________
9. Process of measuring the movement of the tympanic membrane ____________
10. Instrument used to examine the ear ____________

Symptoms, Signs, and Diseases

True or False

Indicate whether each statement is true or false by writing T or F on the line.

1. ____ Misalignment of the mandible can cause a vocal cord nodule.
2. ____ Hemotympanum can be caused by pressure, trauma, or otitis media.
3. ____ Sensorineural hearing loss is caused by a problem in the inner ear.
4. ____ Untreated middle ear infections can progress to otitis externa.
5. ____ The landmarks are distinctive features of the nasopharynx.
6. ____ The palatine tonsils are also called the adenoids.
7. ____ A benign growth of the mucous membranes of the nose is known as epistaxis.
8. ____ Rhinorrhea is serous drainage from the middle ear.
9. ____ Buzzing or ringing sounds in the ear are known as tinnitus.

Matching Exercise

Match each numbered word or phrase to its description.

1.	anosmia	_____ Loss of sense of smell
2.	cold sores	_____ Ringing or buzzing in the ears
3.	epistaxis	_____ Mouth infection with *Candida albicans*
4.	hemotympanum	_____ Fluid that contains pus
5.	otitis externa	_____ Blood in the middle ear behind the eardrum
6.	otosclerosis	_____ Bleeding from the nose
7.	suppurative	_____ Swimmer's ear
8.	thrush	_____ Caused by herpes simplex virus type 1
9.	tinnitus	_____ Dizziness
10.	vertigo	_____ Abnormal bone forms at stapes and oval window

Laboratory, Radiology, Surgery, and Drugs

Matching Exercise

Match each numbered word or phrase to its description.

1.	antihistamine	_____ Uses a vibrating tuning fork
2.	antitussive	_____ Drug used to suppress coughing
3.	audiometry	_____ Procedure to view the sinuses
4.	cheiloplasty	_____ Plastic surgery on the nose
5.	cochlear implant	_____ Grows microorganism on a culture medium
6.	culture	_____ View the ear with a lighted instrument
7.	endoscopy	_____ Drug used to treat allergies
8.	otoscopy	_____ Test that measures the hearing
9.	rhinoplasty	_____ Placed in the inner ear to correct total deafness
10.	Rinne test	_____ Plastic surgery to repair the lip

Abbreviations

Matching Exercise

Match each numbered abbreviation to its definition.

1.	AD	_____ Tonsillectomy and adenoidectomy
2.	BOM	_____ Temporomandibular joint
3.	C&S	_____ Postnasal drip
4.	ENT	_____ Bilateral otitis media
5.	PND	_____ Ears, nose, and throat
6.	T&A	_____ Right ear
7.	TMJ	_____ Culture and sensitivity

Applied Skills

English and Medical Word Equivalents

For each English word, write its equivalent medical word. The first one has been done for you.

English Word	Medical Word
1. ear canal	*external auditory canal*
2. eardrum	____________
3. earwax	____________
4. hammer-shaped bone	____________
5. anvil-shaped bone	____________
6. stirrup-shaped bone	____________
7. nostril	____________
8. throat	____________
9. voice box, Adam's apple	____________
10. seasonal allergies	____________
11. common cold	____________
12. total deafness	____________
13. nosebleed	____________
14. earache	____________
15. sore throat	____________
16. ringing in the ears	____________

Dictionary Challenge

On the job, you will often encounter new medical words. Practice your medical dictionary skills by looking up the medical word in bold. Write the definition on the line provided.

OFFICE CHART NOTE (EXCERPT)

DIAGNOSIS: **Rhinitis medicamentosa,** secondary to chronic Afrin use. The patient will take prednisone 20 mg every day for 5 days to decrease the inflammation. She will return in 3 weeks for a full evaluation of her allergies.

rhinitis medicamentosa: ______________________________

Analysis of a Medical Report

This report is a physician office chart note. Read the report and answer the questions that follow.

OFFICE NOTE

PATIENT NAME: ARQUETTE, Geanne

RECORD NUMBER: 144-26-9842

DATE OF VISIT: November 19, 20xx

S: This 22-year-old mother of 2 children developed a slight fever, a sore throat, and a head cold that developed over a few days after both children had similar symptoms. She states that both children are in day care and many children at the day care center have been ill. A few days later, she also had the acute onset of severe pain and pressure over her right cheekbone and right forehead, but this subsided somewhat more recently. She continued to go to work but, within the last few days, has been experiencing increasingly severe fatigue, is slightly dizzy at times, and has some pain in her ears.

O: On physical examination today, she has only a slightly increased temperature. She denies pain on palpation of her forehead and cheekbone areas on either side. However, in both ears the TMs are red and bulging outward.

A:

1. Bilateral acute otitis media.
2. Previously acute but now subacute sinusitis.

P: Amoxicillin 500 mg PO b.i.d. × 10 days. She is to call if she has any exacerbation of her symptoms.

Irene S. Klinitski, M.D.

Irene S. Klinitski, M.D.

ISK: mtt
D: 11/19/xx
T: 11/19/xx

WORD ANALYSIS QUESTIONS

1. Divide *sinusitis* into its two word parts and define each word part.

Word Part **Definition**

__________ ____________________

__________ ____________________

2. Divide *bilateral* into its three word parts and define each word part.

Word Part **Definition**

__________ ____________________

__________ ____________________

__________ ____________________

3. What does the abbreviation *TMs* stand for? ____________________

FACT FINDING QUESTIONS

1. Which of the patient's symptoms began with an acute onset? ____________________
2. What technique was used to do the physical examination of the sinuses? ____________________
3. What disease is now subacute? ____________________
4. What drug was prescribed for the patient? ____________________

CRITICAL THINKING QUESTIONS

1. Which of the four headings in this report gives the physician's diagnosis? ____________________
2. Which sinuses are located beneath the forehead and cheekbones? ____________________
3. In Diagnosis #1, what abbreviation could be used instead of saying *both ears* or *bilateral?* ____________________
4. Describe what symptoms or signs would be considered an exacerbation that might lead the patient to call the office, as instructed. ____________________

Pronunciation Checklist

Read each word and its pronunciation. Practice pronouncing each word. Verify your pronunciation by listening to the Pronunciation List on the CD-ROM. Check the box next to the word after you master its pronunciation.

- ❑ acoustic neuroma (ah-KOOS-tik nyoo-ROH-mah)
- ❑ adenoidectomy (AD-eh-noy-DEK-toh-mee)
- ❑ adenoids (AD-eh-noydz)
- ❑ ala (AA-lah)
- ❑ alae (AA-lee)
- ❑ allergic rhinitis (ah-LER-jik ry-NY-tis)
- ❑ anacusis (AN-ah-KOO-sis)
- ❑ anosmia (an-AWZ-mee-ah)
- ❑ antibiotic drug (AN-tee-by-AWT-ik DRUHG) (AN-tih-by-AWT-ik)
- ❑ antihistamine drug (AN-tee-HIS-tah-meen DRUHG)
- ❑ antitussive drug (AN-tee-TUS-iv DRUHG)
- ❑ antiyeast drug (AN-tee-YEEST DRUHG)
- ❑ audiogram (AW-dee-oh-gram)
- ❑ audiologist (AW-dee-AWL-oh-jist)
- ❑ audiometer (AW-dee-AWM-eh-ter)
- ❑ audiometry (AW-dee-AWM-eh-tree)
- ❑ auditory (AW-dih-toh-ree)
- ❑ auricle (AW-rih-kl)
- ❑ auricular (aw-RIK-yoo-lar)
- ❑ benign (bee-NINE)
- ❑ bilateral (by-LAT-eh-ral)
- ❑ buccal mucosa (BUHK-al myoo-KOH-sah)
- ❑ *Candida albicans* (KAN-dih-dah AL-bih-kanz)
- ❑ candidiasis (KAN-dih-DY-ah-sis)
- ❑ carcinoma (KAR-sih-NOH-mah)
- ❑ cerumen (seh-ROO-men)
- ❑ cerumen impaction (seh-ROO-men im-PAK-shun)
- ❑ cervical lymphadenopathy (SER-vih-kal lim-FAD-eh-NAWP-eh-thee)
- ❑ cheiloplasty (KY-loh-PLAS-tee)
- ❑ chemotherapy drug (KEE-moh-THAIR-ah-pee DRUHG)
- ❑ cholesteatoma (koh-LES-tee-ah-TOH-mah)
- ❑ cochlea (KOHK-lee-ah)
- ❑ cochleae (KOHK-lee-ee)
- ❑ concha (CON-kah)
- ❑ conductive (con-DUK-tiv)
- ❑ corticosteroid drug (KOR-tih-koh-STAIR-oyd DRUHG)
- ❑ culture and sensitivity (KUL-chur and SEN-sih-TIV-ih-tee)
- ❑ decibel (DES-ih-bel)
- ❑ decongestant drug (DEE-con-JES-tant DRUHG)
- ❑ dorsal (DOR-sal)
- ❑ dorsum (DOR-sum)
- ❑ dysequilibrium (DIS-ee-kwih-LIB-ree-um)
- ❑ effusion (ee-FYOO-shun)
- ❑ endoscope (EN-doh-skohp)
- ❑ endoscopic (EN-doh-SKAWP-ik)
- ❑ endoscopy (en-DAWS-koh-pee)
- ❑ epiglottis (EP-ih-GLAWT-is)
- ❑ epistaxis (EP-ih-STAK-sis)
- ❑ ethmoid sinus (ETH-moyd SY-nus)
- ❑ eustachian (yoo-STAY-shun)
- ❑ external auditory canal (eks-TER-nal AW-dih-toh-ree kah-NAL)
- ❑ external auditory meatus (eks-TER-nal AW-dih-toh-ree mee-AA-tus)
- ❑ frontal sinus (FRUN-tal SY-nus)
- ❑ glossal (GLAWS-al)
- ❑ glossectomy (glaw-SEK-toh-mee)
- ❑ glossitis (glaw-SY-tis)
- ❑ glottis (GLAWT-is)
- ❑ helix (HEE-liks)
- ❑ hemotympanum (HEE-moh-TIM-pah-num)
- ❑ herpes simplex virus (HER-peez SIM-pleks VY-rus)
- ❑ hertz (HERTS)
- ❑ hypopharyngeal (HY-poh-fah-RIN-jee-al)
- ❑ hypopharynx (HY-poh-FAIR-ingks)
- ❑ impedance (im-PEE-dans)
- ❑ incudal (IN-kyoo-dal)
- ❑ incudes (in-KYOO-deez)
- ❑ incus (ING-kus)
- ❑ labyrinthitis (LAB-ih-rin-THY-tis)
- ❑ laryngeal (lah-RIN-jee-al)
- ❑ laryngectomy (LAIR-in-JEK-toh-mee)
- ❑ laryngitis (LAIR-in-JY-tis)
- ❑ larynx (LAIR-ingks)
- ❑ leukoplakia (LOO-koh-PLAY-kee-ah)
- ❑ lingual (LING-gwal)
- ❑ lingual tonsil (LING-gwal TAWN-sil)
- ❑ malignant (mah-LIG-nant)
- ❑ mallear (MAL-ee-ar)
- ❑ mallei (MAL-ee-eye)
- ❑ malleus (MAL-ee-us)
- ❑ mastoid (MASS-toyd)
- ❑ mastoidectomy (MASS-toy-DEK-toh-mee)
- ❑ mastoiditis (MASS-toy-DY-tis)
- ❑ maxillary sinus (MAK-sih-lair-ee SY-nus)
- ❑ maxillofacial surgeon (MAK-sil-oh-FAY-shal SER-jun)
- ❑ meati (mee-AA-tie)
- ❑ meatus (mee-AA-tus)
- ❑ Ménière's disease (MEN-eh-AIRZ dih-ZEEZ)
- ❑ mental (MEN-tal)
- ❑ mentum (MEN-tum)
- ❑ mucosa (myoo-KOH-sah)
- ❑ mucosal (myoo-KOH-al)
- ❑ mucosal hypertrophy (myoo-KOH-sal hy-PER-troh-fee)
- ❑ mucus (MYOO-kus)
- ❑ myringitis (MIR-in-JY-tis)
- ❑ myringotome (mih-RING-goh-tohm)
- ❑ myringotomy (MEER-ing-GAWT-oh-mee)
- ❑ nares (NAY-reez)
- ❑ naris (NAY-ris)
- ❑ nasal (NAY-zal)
- ❑ nasal cavity (NAY-zal KAV-ih-tee)
- ❑ nasolabial (NAY-zoh-LAY-bee-al)
- ❑ nasopharyngeal (NAY-zoh-fah-RIN-jee-al)
- ❑ nasopharynx (NAY-zoh-FAIR-ingks)
- ❑ nodule (NAWD-yool)
- ❑ oral cavity (OR-al KAV-ih-tee)
- ❑ oral mucosa (OR-al myoo-KOH-sah)
- ❑ oropharyngeal (OR-oh-fah-RIN-jee-al)
- ❑ oropharynx (OR-oh-FAIR-ingks)
- ❑ ossicle (AWS-ih-kl)
- ❑ ossicular (aw-SIK-yoo-lar)
- ❑ otalgia (oh-TAL-jee-ah)
- ❑ otitis externa (oh-TY-tis eks-TER-nah)
- ❑ otitis media (oh-TY-tis MEE-dee-ah)
- ❑ otolaryngologist (OH-toh-LAIR-ing-GAWL-oh-jist)
- ❑ otolaryngology (OH-toh-LAIR-ing-GAWL-oh-jee)
- ❑ otorhinolaryngologist (OH-toh-RY-noh-LAIR-ing-GAWL-oh-jist)
- ❑ otoplasty (OH-toh-PLAS-tee)
- ❑ otorrhea (OH-toh-REE-ah)
- ❑ otosclerosis (OH-toh-skleh-ROH-sis)
- ❑ otoscope (OH-toh-skohp)
- ❑ otoscopy (oh-TAWS-koh-pee)
- ❑ palatal (PAL-ah-tal)
- ❑ palate (PAL-at)

- ❑ palatine tonsil (PAL-ah-teen TAWN-sil)
- ❑ pansinusitis (PAN-sy-nyoo-SY-tis)
- ❑ paranasal sinus (PAIR-ah-NAY-zal SY-nus)
- ❑ pharyngeal (fah-RIN-jee-al)
- ❑ pharyngitis (FAIR-in-JY-tis)
- ❑ pharynx (FAIR-ingks)
- ❑ philtrum (FIL-trum)
- ❑ pinna (PIN-ah)
- ❑ pinnae (PIN-ee)
- ❑ polyp (PAWL-ip)
- ❑ polypectomy (PAWL-ih-PEK-toh-mee)
- ❑ postnasal (post-NAY-zal)
- ❑ presbyacusis (PREZ-bee-ah-KOO-sis)
- ❑ radical neck dissection (RAD-ih-kal NEK dy-SEK-shun)
- ❑ rhinophyma (RY-noh-FY-mah)
- ❑ rhinoplasty (RY-noh-PLAS-tee)
- ❑ rhinorrhea (RY-noh-REE-ah)
- ❑ Rinne test (RIN-eh TEST)
- ❑ Romberg's sign (RAWM-bergz sine)
- ❑ sensorineural (SEN-soh-ree-NYOOR-al)
- ❑ septal (SEP-tal)
- ❑ septum (SEP-tum)
- ❑ serous (SEER-us)
- ❑ sinus (SY-nus)
- ❑ sinusitis (SY-nyoo-SY-tis)
- ❑ speculum (SPEK-yoo-lum)
- ❑ sphenoid sinus (SFEE-noyd SY-nus)
- ❑ stapedectomy (STAY-pee-DEK-toh-mee)
- ❑ stapedes (STAY-pee-deez)
- ❑ stapedial (stay-PEE-dee-al)
- ❑ stapes (STAY-peez)
- ❑ streptococcus (STREP-toh-KAWK-uhs)
- ❑ submandibular (SUB-man-DIB-yoo-lar)
- ❑ submental (sub-MEN-tal)
- ❑ suppurative (SUP-yoor-ah-tiv)
- ❑ temporomandibular joint (TEM-poh-roh-man-DIB-yoo-lar JOYNT)
- ❑ temporomandibular joint syndrome (TEM-poh-roh-man-DIB-yoo-lar JOYNT SIN-drohm)
- ❑ tinnitus (TIN-ih-tus) (tih-NY-tus)
- ❑ tonsil (TAWN-sil)
- ❑ tonsillar (TAWN-sih-lar)
- ❑ tonsillectomy (TAWN-sih-LEK-toh-mee)
- ❑ tonsillitis (TAWN-sih-LY-tis)
- ❑ tragi (TRAY-jeye)
- ❑ tragus (TRAY-gus)
- ❑ turbinate (TER-bih-nayt)
- ❑ tympanic membrane (tim-PAN-ik MEM-brayn)
- ❑ tympanogram (tim-PAN-oh-gram)
- ❑ tympanometry (TIM-pah-NAWM-eh-tree)
- ❑ tympanoplasty (TIM-pah-noh-PLAS-tee) (TIM-pah-noh-PLAS-tee)
- ❑ tympanostomy (TIM-pan-AWS-toh-mee)
- ❑ unilateral (YOO-nih-LAT-eh-ral)
- ❑ vermilion (ver-MIL-yon)
- ❑ vertigo (VER-tih-goh)
- ❑ vestibular (ves-TIB-yoo-lar)
- ❑ vestibule (VES-tih-byool)
- ❑ vocal cord (VOH-kal KORD)
- ❑ Weber test (VAH-ber TEST)

Experience Multimedia

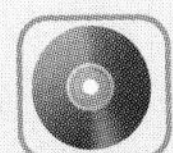

CD-ROM Learning Activities Checklist

Check off the box as you complete each learning activity.

❑ **CD-ROM Learning Activity 16.1: *ANATOMY WORD PARTS FLASHCARDS***
Use flashcards to help you memorize word parts. Make your own flashcards or print out prepared flashcards. Also see the electronic flashcard game. Time: 20 minutes.

❑ **CD-ROM Learning Activity 16.2: *MEDICINE IN ACTION***
Watch an animation clip about the middle ear. Time: 5 minutes.

❑ **CD-ROM Learning Activity 16.3: *DISEASE AND OTHER WORD PARTS FLASHCARDS***
A continuation of the flashcard learning activity. Time: 20 minutes.

❑ **CD-ROM Learning Activity 16.4: *MEMORY AIDS***
Use memory aids to help you memorize medical words and meanings. Time: 5 minutes.

❑ **CD-ROM Learning Activity 16.5: *MEDICAL LANGUAGE SPOKEN HERE***
Listen to actual medical reports and spell the missing medical words. Time: 20 minutes.

❑ **CD-ROM Learning Activity 16.6: *SPELLING CHALLENGE***
Listen to a pronounced medical word and then spell it. Time: 5 minutes.

❑ **CD-ROM Learning Activity 16.7: *MEDICAL LANGUAGE PRONUNCIATION***
Listen to a pronounced medical word and then practice pronouncing it. Time: 30 minutes.

❑ **CD-ROM Learning Activity 16.8: *EDUCATIONAL FUN AND GAMES***
Enjoy these fun activities while reinforcing your knowledge. Time: 15 minutes.

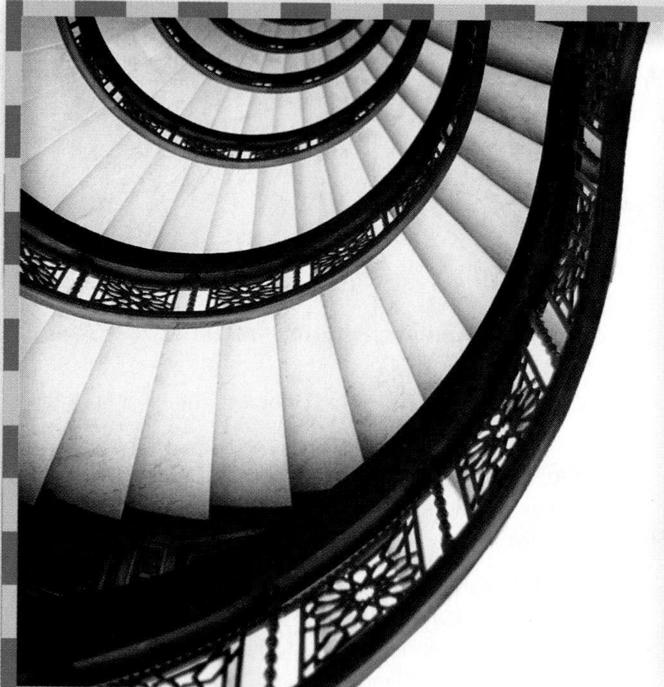

Dive In!

- On average people fear spiders more than they do death.
- A few of the famous people who have had depressive mood disorders: Ludwig von Beethoven, Abraham Lincoln, Marilyn Monroe, John Lennon, Kurt Cobain
- Don't panic. It's time to get in the mood. In this chapter we'll explore the language that describes the structures, functions, diseases, and conditions that pertain to psychiatry.
- You'll be on your best behavior once you master the language of the mind!

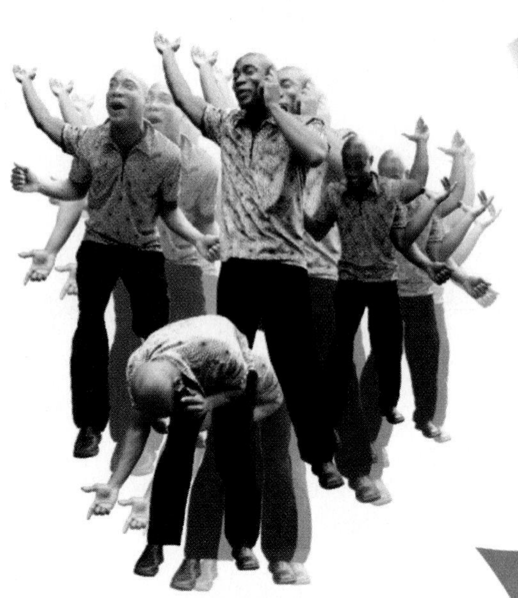

Mania

Depression

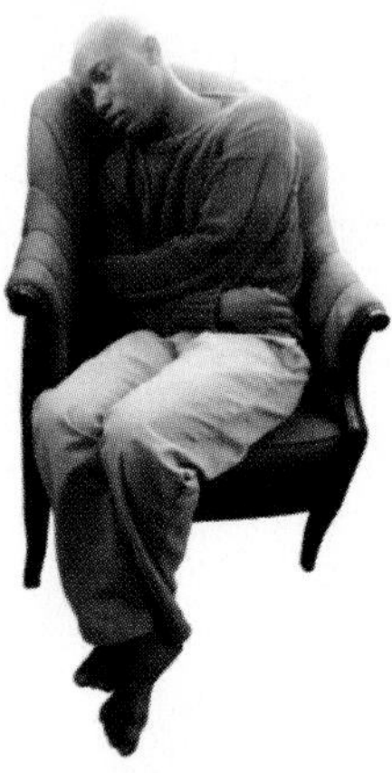

Bipolar disorder is characterized by chronic mood swings between the extremes of depression and mania.

Medicine Through HISTORY

1969

The antianxiety drug Valium becomes the number one prescription drug in the United States with 30 million tablets manufactured each day

1971

The computerized axial tomography (CAT) scan, a radiologic procedure that takes pictures of the body in slices, is introduced

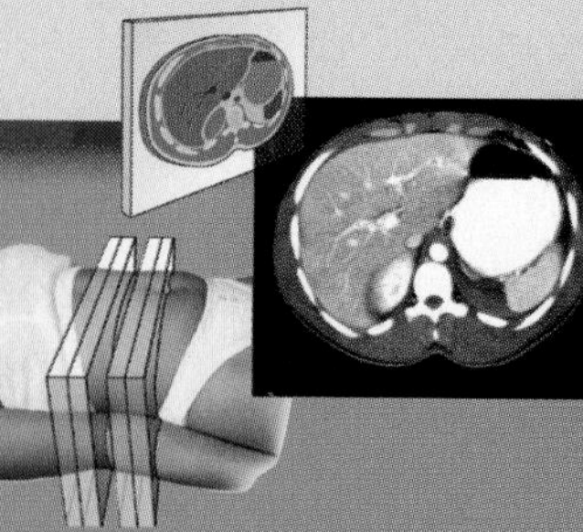

CHAPTER 17 Psychiatry

Psychiatry (sy-KY-ah-tree) is the medical specialty that studies the anatomy and physiology of the brain and the functioning of the mind and uses diagnostic tests, medical and psychiatric procedures, and drugs to treat psychiatric diseases.

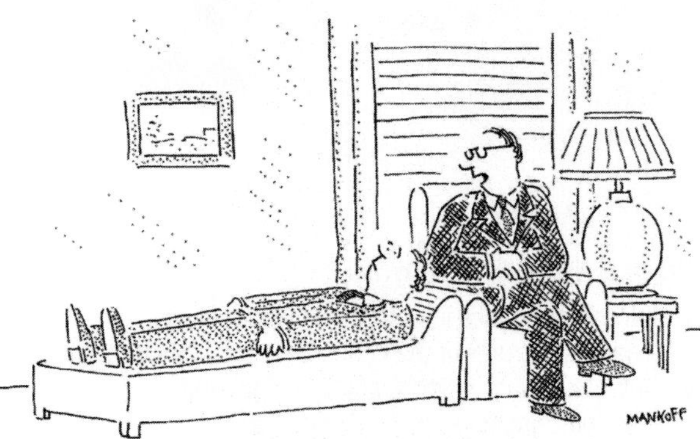

"Wow! You need professional help."

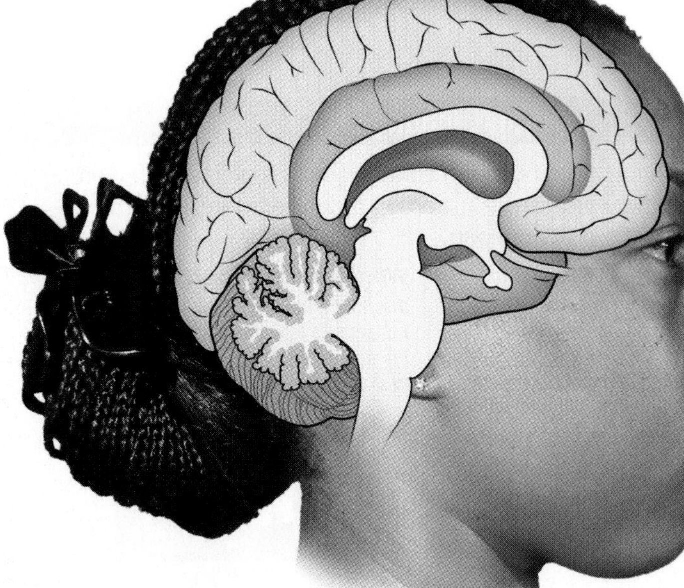

▶ The limbic system processes memories and controls emotion, mood, motivation, and behavior.

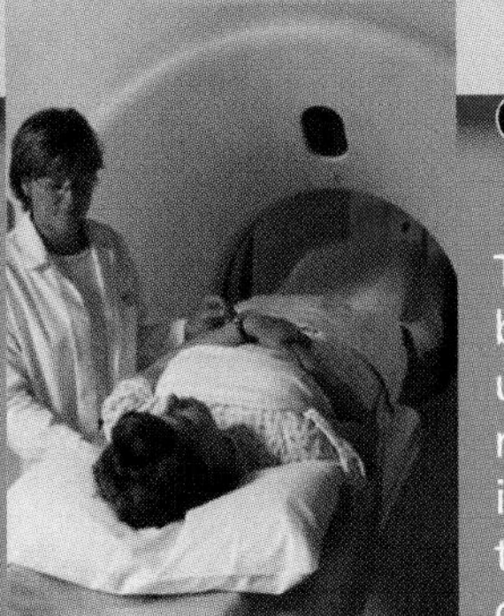

1977

The first whole-body scanner using magnetic resonance imaging (MRI) technology is constructed

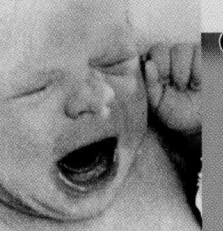

1978

Louise Brown becomes the first baby to be conceived by in vitro fertilization techniques. She was nicknamed the "test tube baby"

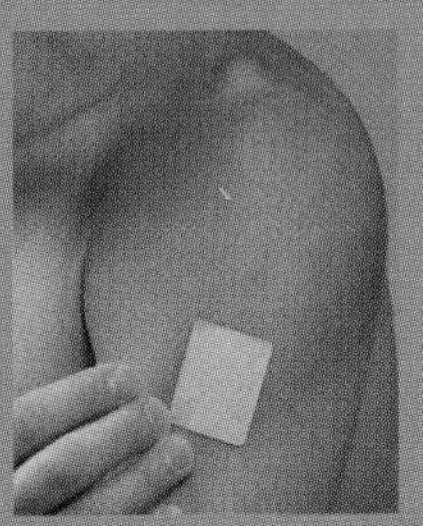

1981

Ciba-Geigy introduces the first transdermal patch drug delivery system

Measure Your Progress: Learning Objectives

After you study this chapter, you should be able to

1. Identify the anatomical structures of the brain that are related to psychiatry.
2. Describe the process of an emotional response.
3. Build psychiatric words from combining forms, prefixes, and suffixes.
4. Describe common psychiatric diseases.
5. Describe common psychiatric diagnostic tests.
6. Identify common psychiatric procedures and drug categories.
7. Define common psychiatric abbreviations.
8. Correctly spell and pronounce psychiatric words.
9. Test your knowledge of psychiatry by completing review exercises at the end of the chapter and learning activities on the CD-ROM.

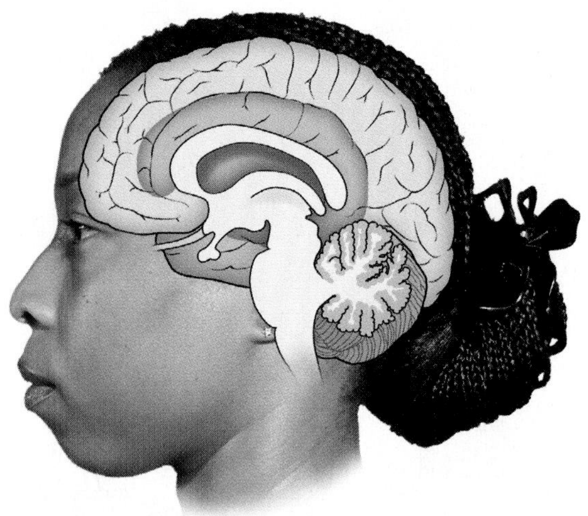

Figure 17-1 ■ The mind.

The mind is a complex interaction between specific anatomical structures of the brain, the mental functions of reasoning, learning, memory, and conscious and subconscious emotions, drives, and desires.

Medical Language Key

To unlock the meaning of a medical word, first define each word part. Then put the word part definitions in order, beginning with the suffix, followed by the first word part.

	Word Part	Word Part Definition
SUFFIX	-iatry	*medical treatment*
COMBINING FORM	psych/o-	*mind*

Psychiatry: ***The medical treatment of the mind.***

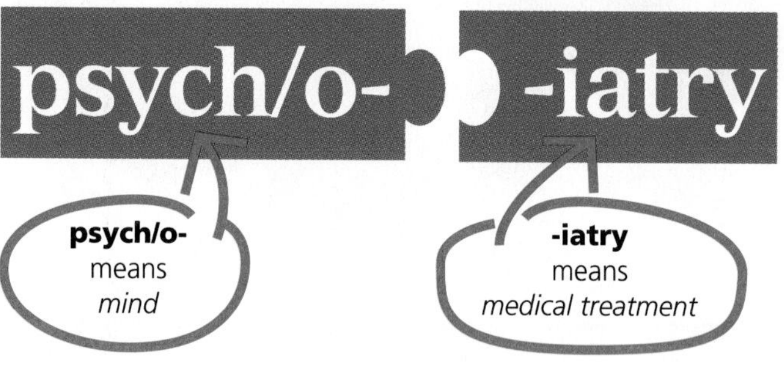

www.prenhall.com/turley

For interactive flashcards, real-life video clips, games, exercises, and audio pronunciations please explore the companion CD-ROM in the back of the book. Click on the companion website for bonus chapters, additional resources, and links to on-line learning.

Anatomy and Physiology

The anatomical structures that pertain to psychiatry are located in the brain (see Figure 17-1■). In addition, psychiatry is concerned with physical symptoms and signs as well as behaviors that are produced by thoughts and emotions (for example, rapid heart rate and agitation during anger, crying with depression, hyperventilation and chest pains with anxiety, and so forth).

Anatomy Related to Psychiatry

Limbic Lobe and Limbic System

The **limbic lobe** is an area of the brain that is located around the medial edges of the two cerebral hemispheres (just superior to the corpus callosum that joins the hemispheres). It includes small areas from each of the lobes of the brain plus a longer extension into the temporal lobe. The limbic lobe is also known as the **cingulate gyrus** because it is in the form of a curved, encircling layer.

The **limbic system** consists of the limbic lobe, thalamus, hypothalamus, and several other smaller structures in the brain (see Figure 17-2■). The limbic system links the unconscious mind to the conscious mind. The limbic system processes memories and controls emotion, mood, memory, motivation, and behavior.

limbic (LIM-bik)
limb/o- *edge, border*
-ic *pertaining to*

cingulate (SIN-gyoo-layt)
Cingulum is a Latin word meaning *a girdle that surrounds.*

gyrus (JY-rus)
Gyrus is a Latin word meaning *curved structure.*

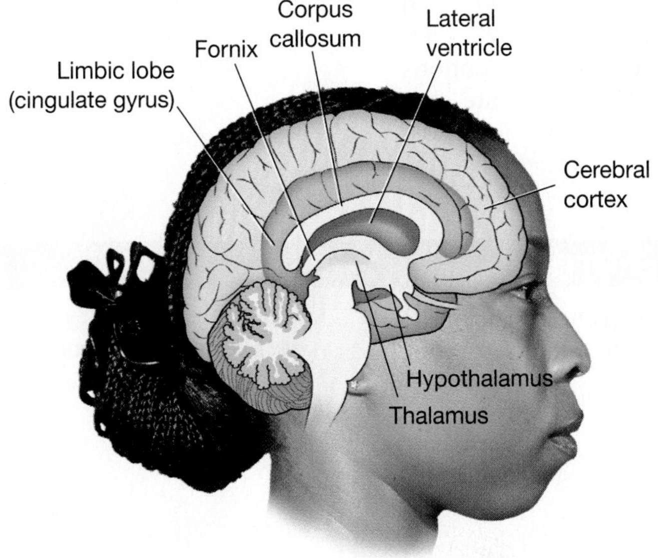

Figure 17-2 ■ Limbic lobe.

This midsagittal section of the brain shows the limbic lobe and some of the structures of the limbic system. The hippocampus and amygdaloid body in each temporal lobe are not visible on this view.

Thalamus

The **thalamus** acts as a relay station, receiving nerve impulses from the five senses (sight, hearing, touch, taste, smell) and relaying them to the sensory and motor areas of the cerebral cortex.

thalamus (THAL-ah-mus)

Hypothalamus

The **hypothalamus,** located below the thalamus, forms the floor of the third ventricle. The hypothalamus controls emotions of pleasure, excitement, fear, anger, sexual arousal, and bodily responses to these emotions. The hypothalamus also contains the feeding center and satiety center. The hypothalamus regulates the sex drive and sexual behavior. (This behavior is also regulated by the male and female sex hormones and by conscious thought processes from the cerebral cortex.)

During times of fear or anger, the hypothalamus sends nerve impulses to the sympathetic nervous system to increase the heart rate and respiratory rate as part of the "fight or flight" response to danger.

hypothalamus (HY-poh-THAL-ah-mus)

Hippocampus

The **hippocampus** is an elongated structure with a head and a tail that is located in each temporal lobe. The hippocampus controls long-term memory and facilitates comparison between present and past emotions and experiences. The tail of the hippocampus connects to the hypothalamus.

hippocampus (HIP-oh-KAM-pus)
Hippocampus is a Latin word meaning *seahorse.* The structure of the hippocampus was thought to resemble the head and tail of a seahorse.

Amygdaloid Bodies

The **amygdaloid body** is an almond-shaped area of grey, unmyelinated nerve tissue located in each temporal lobe. The amygdaloid bodies are involved in interpreting facial expressions and new social situations and identifying which situations are dangerous. They integrate sensory information, thoughts, and long-term memories and are most active with the emotions of fear, anger, and rage.

amygdaloid (ah-MIG-dah-loyd)
amygdal/o- *almond shape*
-oid *resembling*

Fornix

The **fornix** is a tract of myelinated nerves along the arched floor of the lateral ventricles. It connects the hippocampus in each temporal lobe to the thalamus and each amygdaloid body.

fornix (FOR-niks)
Fornix is a Latin word meaning *arch.*

Physiology of Emotion and Behavior

A current thought, sensory input from one of the five senses, a recalled memory, or a combination of all three can trigger an emotion. An **emotion** is an intense state of feelings. An intense emotion connected with a particular situation causes that situation to imprint deeply in long-term memory. That situation, when later called to mind, brings with it those same intense emotions.

The presence of an emotion in the thoughts produces an outward display on the face (the person's **affect**) (see Figure 17-3■), changes in behavior, and physical symptoms and signs in the body. A person's emotional state of mind may reflect many emotions at the same time (fear, guilt, and anger), but the prevailing, predominant emotion is known as the person's **mood.**

Emotions are normal forms of expression, but extremely intense, long-lasting, inappropriate, or absent emotions are signs of mental illness. Injury to the brain or changes in the levels of various neurotransmitters in the brain can produce abnormal emotions and behaviors.

The frontal lobe is the site of reasoning, judgment, planning, organizing, personality, creativity, and recent memories of all of those things. The frontal lobe exerts conscious control over alertness, concentration, and emotions. The frontal lobe also analyzes situations, predicts future events, and weighs the benefits or consequences of actions taken. Injury to the frontal lobe can produce these psychiatric symptoms: flat affect, disinterest, inability to concentrate, inappropriate laughing or crying, inappropriate social or sexual behavior, indifference to the consequences of behavior and actions, inability to plan or modify behavior, inability to abide by or create rules to govern behavior, inability to keep commitments, impulsiveness, and absence of goal-directed behavior.

Injury to the hypothalamus can cause overeating and obesity, disinterest in eating, or sleep abnormalities of insomnia or excessive sleepiness.

Hyperstimulation of the amygdaloid bodies can cause violent, aggressive behavior. Injury to or degeneration of the amygdaloid bodies can cause a loss of the emotions of anger and fear. The patient may recognize a person's face but cannot say if that person is a friend or an enemy. The patient is also unaware of dangerous situations.

Injury to or degeneration of either hippocampus can cause the loss of all long-term memory. A patient with Alzheimer's disease with degeneration of those areas may be unable to recognize his/her own face in the mirror.

Neurotransmitters are chemicals that relay messages from one neuron to the next. Neurotransmitters play an important role in emotion and behavior. Increased, decreased, or unbalanced levels of neurotransmitters can cause abnormal emotions and behaviors.

1. **Epinephrine.** Neurotransmitter for the sympathetic nervous system. It is released when a person experiences fear or anger in order to prepare the body for "fight or flight." Increased levels of epinephrine cause anxiety, social phobia, performance phobia, and panic attacks.
2. **Norepinephrine.** Neurotransmitter for the parasympathetic nervous system. It controls the day-to-day function of the involun-

emotion (ee-MOH-shun)
emot/o- *moving, stirring up*
-ion *action; condition*

affect (AF-fekt)
Affect is derived from a Latin word meaning *state of mind.*

affective (af-FEK-tiv)
affect/o- *state of mind; mood; to have an influence on*
-ive *pertaining to*

mood (MOOD)

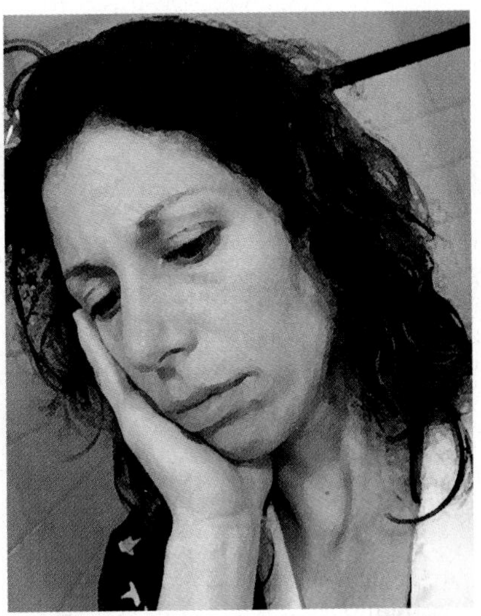

Figure 17-3 ■ Mood.
This woman's affect or facial expression reflects sadness and depression. Emotions are inward thoughts that produce an outward display in the body through the facial affect, body position, and behavior.

neurotransmitter (NYOOR-oh-trans-MIT-er)
neur/o- *nerve*
trans- *across, through*
mitt/o- *to send*
-er *person or thing that produces or does*

epinephrine (EP-ih-NEF-rin)

norepinephrine (NOR-ep-ih-NEF-rin)

tary processes in the body. Increased levels cause aggression, infatuation, and mania. Decreased levels cause depression.

3. **Dopamine.** Neurotransmitter in the brain. Increased levels are caused by cocaine, narcotics, and alcohol and produce the euphoria and excitement ("high") experienced by addicts. Increased levels are also associated with infatuation. Increased levels of dopamine in the limbic system coupled with decreased levels of dopamine in the frontal lobe cause paranoia. Decreased levels cause schizophrenia and depression.

dopamine (DOHP-ah-meen)

4. **Serotonin.** Neurotransmitter in the brain and spinal cord. Decreased levels of serotonin cause depression. Decreased levels of serotonin coupled with increased levels of norepinephrine cause violent behavior.

serotonin (SER-oh-TOH-nin)

5. **GABA.** Neurotransmitter in the brain. Decreased levels cause anxiety. GABA stands for gamma-amino butyric acid.

Vocabulary Review

Anatomy and Physiology

Now that you have studied the anatomy and physiology that pertains to psychiatry, take time to review those new words and descriptions. Memorize the combining forms and their definitions before going on to the next section.

Word or Phrase	Combining Form and Definition	Description
affect	**affect/o-** *state of mind; mood; to have an influence on*	Outward display on the face of the inward emotions and thoughts
amygdaloid body	**amygdal/o-** *almond shape*	Almond-shaped area within each temporal lobe. It interprets facial expressions and new social situations to identify danger. It integrates with long-term memory and is particularly active in the emotions of fear, anger, and rage.
dopamine		Neurotransmitter in the brain
emotion	**emot/o-** *moving, stirring up*	Intense state of feelings
epinephrine		Neurotransmitter of the sympathetic nervous system. It prepares the body for "fight or flight."
fornix		Tract of nerves that joins all the parts of the limbic system
GABA		Neurotransmitter in the brain
hippocampus		Irregular, curved area within each temporal lobe that controls long-term memory and compares past and present emotions and experiences
hypothalamus		Controls emotions (pleasure, excitement, fear, anger, sexual arousal) and bodily responses to emotions. Regulates the sex drive. Contains the feeding and satiety centers. Functions as part of the "fight or flight" response of the sympathetic nervous system.
limbic lobe	**limb/o-** *edge, border*	Curved, encircling area of the brain that includes the medial edges of the two cerebral hemispheres and extends into the temporal lobes. Also known as the **cingulate gyrus.**

Word or Phrase	Combining Form and Definition	Description
limbic system	limb/o- *edge, border*	Related structures in the brain that control emotion, mood, memory, motivation, and behavior and link the conscious to the unconscious mind. The limbic system consists of the thalamus, hypothalamus, hippocampus, amygdaloid bodies, and fornix.
mood		Prevailing, predominant emotion affecting a person's state of mind
neurotransmitter	neur/o- *nerve* mitt/o- *to send*	Chemicals that relay messages from one neuron to another
norepinephrine		Neurotransmitter of the parasympathetic nervous system. It controls the daily involuntary processes of the body.
serotonin		Neurotransmitter in the brain and spinal cord
thalamus		Relay station that receives nerve impulses from the senses and relays them to the sensory and motor areas of the cerebral cortex

Building Medical Words

Combining Forms

Here are the combining forms you have learned so far. Next to each combining form, write its meaning. Use the Answer Key at the end of the book to check your answers. The first one has been done for you.

Combining Form	Medical Meaning	Combining Form	Medical Meaning
1. amygdal/o-	almond shape	4. limb/o-	______
2. affect/o-	______	5. neur/o-	______
3. emot/o-	______	6. mitt/o-	______

Combining Forms and Suffixes

Read the definition hint for the medical word you are to build. Look at the combining form that is given. Write the correct suffix on the blank line. Then write the medical word. (Remember: You may need to remove the combining vowel. Always remove the hyphens and slash.) Use the Answer Key at the end of the book to check your answers. The first one has been done for you.

SUFFIX LIST			
-ic (pertaining to)	-ion (action; condition)	-ive (pertaining to)	-oid (resembling)

Definition Hint	Combining Form	Suffix	Write the Medical Word
1. Resembling an almond in shape	amygdal/o-	-oid	amygdaloid
2. Pertaining to the edge or border	limb/o-	______	______
3. Condition or action of stirring up	emot/o-	______	______
4. Pertaining to state of mind or mood	affect/o-	______	______

Symptoms, Signs, and Mental Disorders

Anxiety Disorders

Anxiety disorders are characterized by the predominant emotion of anxiety, with uneasiness, uncertainty, dread, worry, apprehension, or fear. Bodily symptoms and signs include inability to think clearly, dizziness, dry mouth, chest tightness, palpitations, upset stomach, diarrhea, fine tremor, sweaty palms, inability to relax, heightened startle reflex, fatigue, and irritability. Anxiety itself is an appropriate response to danger, but anxiety disorders are not associated with a specific dangerous situation, person, or thing. Treatment: Antianxiety drugs, antidepressant drugs, psychotherapy, group therapy.

Word or Phrase	Word Part and Definition	Description
generalized anxiety disorder	**anxiety** (ang-ZY-eh-tee) **anxi/o-** *fear, worry* **-ety** *condition, state*	Dwelling on issues that involve "What if . . ." and predicting or fearing that the worst thing will happen to self, family, or friends.
obsessive-compulsive disorder	**obsession** (awb-SESH-un) **obsess/o-** *besieged by thoughts* **-ion** *action; condition* **obsessive** (awb-SES-iv) **obsess/o-** *besieged by thoughts* **-ive** *pertaining to* **compulsion** (com-PAWL-shun) **compuls/o-** *drive or compel* **-ion** *action; condition* **compulsive** (com-PAWL-siv) **compuls/o-** *drive or compel* **-ive** *pertaining to*	Constant, persistent, uncontrollable thoughts (obsessions) that occupy the mind, cause anxiety, and compel the patient to perform excessive, repetitive, meaningless activities (compulsions) for fear of what might happen if these are not done. These activities include washing and cleaning; checking work again and again; checking doors and locks; ordering, labeling, and arranging belongings in a particular sequence; hoarding useless collections of things with an inability to discard things; and repetitive thinking, counting, praying, or making mental lists. These activities consume a significant portion of each day.
panic disorder	**panic** (PAN-ik) *Panic* is derived from *Pan* (the mythical Greek god who could cause sudden fear) and the suffix *-ic* (pertaining to).	Sudden attacks of severe, overwhelming anxiety without an identifiable cause. Patients often feel that they are choking or dying of a heart attack.
phobia	**phobia** (FOH-bee-ah) **phob/o-** *fear* **-ia** *condition, state, thing* **phobic** (FOH-bik) **phob/o-** *fear* **-ic** *pertaining to*	Intense, unreasonable fear of a specific thing or situation or even the thought of it (see Table 17-1 and Figure 17-4■). Phobias occur when the unconscious mind avoids a real, ongoing conflict by projecting the anxiety onto an unrelated situation or object. Avoidance of the phobia can severely restrict the normal activities of daily life. **Did You Know?** Fear of the number 13 is known as *triskaidekaphobia.* (The Greek word for 13 is *triskaideka.*) Not all phobias are associated with fears or mental disorders. Photophobia is the avoidance of light, a common occurrence in patients with migraine headaches.

Table 17-1 Common Phobias

Phobia	Description	Word Part and Definition
acrophobia	Fear of heights	**acrophobia** (AK-roh-FOH-bee-ah) **acr/o-** *extremity; highest point* **phob/o-** *fear* **-ia** *condition, state, thing*
agoraphobia	Fear of crowds or public places	**agoraphobia** (AG-or-ah-FOH-bee-ah) **agor/a-** *open areas or space* **phob/o-** *fear* **-ia** *condition, state, thing*
arachnophobia	Fear of spiders	**arachnophobia** (ah-RAK-noh-FOH-bee-ah) **arachn/o-** *spider, spider web* **phob/o-** *fear* **-ia** *condition, state, thing*
claustrophobia	Fear of closed-in spaces	**claustrophobia** (KLAW-stroh-FOH-bee-ah) **claustr/o-** *enclosed space* **phob/o-** *fear* **-ia** *condition, state, thing*
microphobia	Fear of germs	**microphobia** (MY-kroh-FOH-bee-ah) **micr/o-** *small* **phob/o-** *fear* **-ia** *condition, state, thing*
ophidiophobia	Fear of snakes	**ophidiophobia** (oh-FID-ee-oh-FOH-bee-ah) **ophidi/o-** *snake* **phob/o-** *fear* **-ia** *condition, state, thing*
social phobia	Fear of being embarrassed or humiliated in front of others or in a public place or fear of being the center of attention	**social** (SOH-shal) **soci/o-** *human beings; community* **-al** *pertaining to*
thanatophobia	Fear of death	**thanatophobia** (THAN-ah-toh-FOH-bee-ah) **thanat/o-** *death* **phob/o-** *fear* **-ia** *condition, state, thing*
xenophobia	Fear of strangers	**xenophobia** (ZEN-oh-FOH-bee-ah) **xen/o-** *foreign* **phob/o-** *fear* **-ia** *condition, state, thing*

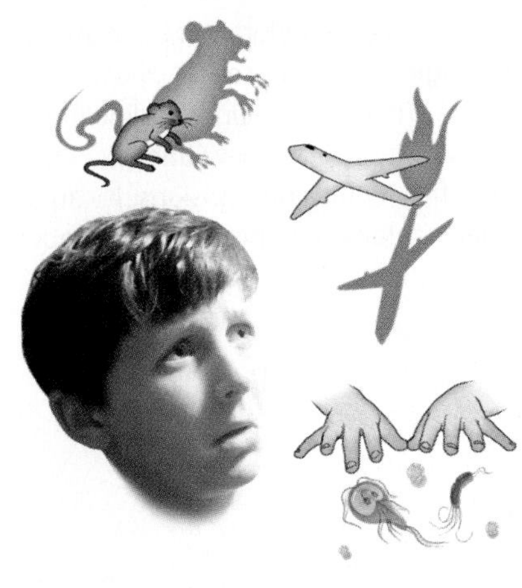

Figure 17-4 ■ Phobia.
Phobias are intense, exaggerated fears of a specific thing or situation.

Word or Phrase	Word Part and Definition	Description
posttraumatic stress disorder (PTSD)	**posttraumatic** (POST-trah-MAT-ik) **post-** *after, behind* **traumat/o-** *injury* **-ic** *pertaining to*	Continuing, disabling reaction to an excessively traumatic situation or event, such as a war, terrorist attack, torture, rape, kidnapping, natural disaster (earthquake, flood), explosion, or fire. The patient feels helpless, has a numbed emotional response with disinterest in people and current events, and relives the trauma of the event over and over. Other symptoms include chronic anxiety, insomnia, irritability, and occasional violent outbursts. Previously known as combat fatigue.

Cognitive Disorders

Cognitive disorders are characterized by a temporary or permanent impairment of thinking and memory. Treatment: Supportive care, drugs to slow memory loss or improve cognitive function, or psychotherapy.

Word or Phrase	Word Part and Definition	Description
amnesia	**amnesia** (am-NEE-zee-ah) **amnes/o-** *forgetfulness* **-ia** *condition, state, thing* **amnestic** (am-NES-tik) **amnes/o-** *forgetfulness* **-tic** *pertaining to* **retrograde** (RET-roh-grayd) **retro-** *behind, backward* **-grade** *going* **anterograde** (AN-ter-oh-grayd) **anter/o-** *before; front part* **-grade** *going* **global** (GLOH-bal) **glob/o-** *shaped like a globe; comprehensive* **-al** *pertaining to*	Partial or total loss of long-term memory due to trauma or disease of the hippocampus. The patient is said to be **amnestic.** In **retrograde amnesia,** no events before the onset of the amnesia can be recalled. In **anterograde amnesia,** no events after the onset of the amnesia can be recalled. In **global amnesia,** all memories are lost.
delirium	**delirium** (deh-LEER-ee-um) (dee-LEER-ee-um) *Delirium* is a Latin word meaning *off the track.* **delirium tremens** (dee-LEER-ee-um TREM-enz)	Acute confusion, disorientation, and agitation due to toxic levels of body chemicals, drugs, or alcohol in the blood that affect the brain. **Delirium tremens (DT)** is caused by withdrawal symptoms from alcoholic intoxication and includes restlessness, tremors of the hands, hallucinations, sweating, and increased heart rate.
dementia	**dementia** (dee-MEN-shee-ah) **de-** *reversal of; without* **ment/o-** *mind; chin* **-ia** *condition, state, thing* **cognitive** (KAWG-nih-tiv) **cognit/o-** *thinking* **-ive** *pertaining to*	Gradual but progressive deterioration of **cognitive function** due to old age or a neurologic disease process. Alzheimer's is the most common type of dementia. There is a gradual decline in mental abilities, with forgetfulness, inability to learn new things, inability to perform daily activities, and difficulty making decisions. It can also include personality changes, anxiety, irritability, poor judgment, impulsiveness, hostility, combativeness, depression, and delusions.

Childhood Disorders

Childhood disorders include any behavioral abnormality having to do with feeding, eating, elimination, learning, or motor skills—all major developmental areas of childhood. Treatment: Drugs for ADHD, psychotherapy, group therapy, family therapy.

Word or Phrase	Word Part and Definition	Description
attention-deficit hyperactivity disorder (ADHD)		Distractability, short attention span, inability to follow directions, restlessness, hyperactivity, emotional lability, and impulsiveness. It may be caused by mild brain damage at birth, genetic factors, or other abnormalities. It is five times more common in boys than in girls. Most children outgrow the symptoms by late childhood. Previously known as minimal brain dysfunction and attention deficit disorder.
autism	**autism** (AW-tizm) aut/o- *self* -ism *process; disease from a specific cause* **echolalia** (EK-oh-LAY-lee-ah) ech/o- *echo (sound wave)* -lalia *condition of speech*	Inability to communicate or form significant relationships with others, and a lack of interest in doing so. Patients may be of normal intelligence or may be mentally retarded. Speech may not develop or may be abnormal with **echolalia** (automatically repeating what someone else has said). Patients avoid physical contact and eye contact, but are fascinated by certain objects. There are ritualistic, repetitive behaviors.
encopresis	**encopresis** (EN-koh-PREE-sis) en- *in, within, inward* copr/o- *feces, stool* -esis *condition of*	Repeated passage of stool into the clothing in a child older than age 5 who does not have gastrointestinal illness or disability.
oppositional defiant disorder	**oppositional** (AWP-ih-ZISH-un-al) oppos/o- *forceful resistance* -ition *condition of having* -al *pertaining to*	Persistent, aggressive behavior (fighting, arguing, provoking, annoying), defiance of and refusal to obey rules, disrespect for authority figures, with anger, stubbornness, and touchiness. **Conduct disorder** is a more severe form in which patients physically and sexually assault others, destroy property, steal, set fires, or run away from home.
reactive attachment disorder	**reactive** (ree-AK-tiv) react/o- *reverse movement* -ive *pertaining to*	Inability to emotionally bond and form intimate relationships with others because of severe abuse or neglect of the patient's basic needs before age 2 when trust is established. There is a lack of trust, watchful wariness, poor eye contact, lack of empathy, inability to show genuine affection, and a lack of a conscience. The patient is difficult to comfort and resists physical contact like being held or cuddled, but sometimes exhibits inappropriate friendliness to strangers.
Tourette's syndrome	**Tourette** (TOOR-et) Tourette's syndrome was named by Georges Gilles de la Tourette (1857–1904), a French physician. This is an example of an eponym: a person from whom something takes its name. **coprolalia** (KAWP-roh-LAY-lee-ah) copr/o- *feces, stool* -lalia *condition of speech*	Frequent, spontaneous, involuntary movement tics (eye blinking, throat clearing, arm thrusting) and vocal tics (grunts, barks), or comments that are socially inappropriate, vulgar, obscene [**coprolalia**], or racist). The patient can only temporarily suppress these tics. There may also be echolalia, obsessive-compulsive disorder, and hyperactivity.

Eating Disorders

Eating disorders are characterized by abnormal eating patterns, distorted body image, fear, guilt, and depression. The majority of patients are young women. Treatment: Antidepressant drugs, psychotherapy, family therapy.

Word or Phrase	Word Part and Definition	Description
anorexia nervosa	**anorexia nervosa** (AN-oh-REK-see-ah ner-VOH-sah) **an-** *without, not* **orex/o-** *appetite* **-ia** *condition, state, thing* Remember, anorexia is a simple loss of appetite due to illness. It is not a psychiatric disorder.	Extreme, chronic fear of being fat and an obsession with becoming thinner. The patient is driven to decrease food intake to the point of starvation (see Figure 17-5 ■). Patients deny being too thin. They deny abnormal eating habits and try to keep these a secret from family and friends by making excuses for not eating and wearing clothes that conceal their extreme weight loss. **Figure 17-5 ■ Anorexia nervosa.** This patient has long-standing anorexia nervosa. All of the subcutaneous fat on the body is gone because of chronic decreased food intake to the point of starvation. This patient would still deny being too thin and would, in fact, appear to herself as being fat if she looked in a mirror.
bulimia	**bulimia** (byool-LIM-ee-ah) *Bulimia* is a combination of two Greek words meaning *ox* and *hunger* plus the suffix *-ia* (condition, state, thing).	Patients gorge themselves on excessive amounts of food (binge eating) and then, for fear of gaining weight, they rid (purge) themselves of food by using laxatives or by self-induced vomiting. Long-term vomiting wears away tooth enamel and can cause inflammation and ulcers in the esophagus.

Dissociative Disorders

Dissociative disorders are characterized by a breakdown between the conscious mind and the person's identity, personality, and memory. This breakdown is precipitated by a traumatic event or by continuing trauma endured at an early age. Treatment: Psychotherapy.

Word or Phrase	Word Part and Definition	Description
depersonalization	**depersonalization** (dee-PER-son-al-ih-ZAY-shun) *Depersonalization* is a combination of the prefix *de-* (reversal of, without), the word *personal,* and the suffix *-ization* (the process of making, creating, or inserting). **dissociative** (dih-SOH-see-ah-tiv) **dis-** *away from* **soci/o-** *human beings; community* **-ative** *pertaining to*	Loss of connection (**dissociative** process) between personal thoughts and a sense of self and the environment. Patients feel as if they are in a dream or watching a movie of themselves, and things feel unreal and strange.

Word or Phrase	Word Part and Definition	Description
fugue	**fugue** (FYOOG) *Fugue* is a Latin word meaning *flight.*	Impulsive flight from one's life and familiar surroundings after a traumatic event. The patient begins a new life in a new location and functions normally but is unable to remember anything of the past.
identity disorder		Loss of connection between the normally integrated functions of conscious thought, perception of the environment, identity, and memory. This is done in an effort to repress traumatic memories. Two or more distinct personalities are present, each with its own identity (made up of some facets of the original personality) and history. Each personality is capable of independent thoughts and actions and may be unaware of the other personalities. Previously known as multiple personality disorder or split personality.

Factitious Disorders

Factitious disorders are characterized by physical and/or psychological symptoms that are consciously made up (fabricated) by the patient, which the patient knows are not real. Patients pretend to be sick (often with symptoms that are difficult to evaluate) or even make themselves sick because of a desire to be cared for. They are intelligent and knowledgeable about medicine, but they are experienced, expert liars who often fool several physicians.

Word or Phrase	Word Part and Definition	Description
malingering	**malingering** (mah-LING-ger-ing) *Malingering* is derived from a French word meaning *weak.* **factitious** (fak-TISH-us) **factiti/o-** *artificial, contrived* **-ous** *pertaining to*	Exhibiting **factitious** medical or psychiatric symptoms in order to get a tangible reward, like narcotic drugs or disability payments. Patients are aware that they are lying and know exactly what they want to achieve from their deceptions.
Munchausen syndrome	**Munchausen** (moon-CHOW-zen) This syndrome was named for a German nobleman, Baron Karl Munchausen, who was a well-known liar.	Exhibiting factitious medical or psychiatric symptoms. Patients are aware that they are lying, but are unaware that their motivation is the desire for assistance, attention, compassion, pity, and being excused from the normal expectations of life. Patients are not concerned about the cost of multiple tests, treatments, or surgeries and, in fact, desire to have them.
Munchausen by proxy	**proxy** (PRAWK-see) *Proxy* is an English word meaning *a person who is authorized to act in place of another person.*	Patient creates illness in another person, usually a child. This is a form of child abuse in which the parent, usually the mother, makes up a medical history, induces physical symptoms with drugs, or contaminates laboratory tests. The patient vicariously lives the role of being sick while simultaneously enjoying attention as the sacrificing, loving caregiver.

Somatoform Disorders

Somatoform disorders are characterized by excessive physical complaints that are dramatic but do not fit any medical disease. Diagnostic tests are negative. There is pain in various places in the body with anxiety. Patients have poor insight into their problem and may have experienced trauma prior to the onset of symptoms. Treatment: Psychotherapy, antianxiety drugs. *Somatoform* (soh-MAT-oh-form) is a combination of *somat/o-* (body) and *-form* (having the form of).

Word or Phrase	Word Part and Definition	Description
body dysmorphic disorder	**dysmorphic** (dis-MOR-fik) **dys-** *painful, difficult, abnormal* **morph/o-** *shape* **-ic** *pertaining to*	Overconcern with minor defects in the appearance of the body, particularly the face, with the demand for frequent plastic surgery.

Word or Phrase	Word Part and Definition	Description
conversion disorder	**conversion** (con-VER-shun) **con-** *with* **vers/o-** *to travel; to turn* **-ion** *action; condition* **somatoform** (soh-MAT-oh-form) **somat/o-** *body* **-form** *having the form of* **repression** (ree-PRESH-un) **repress/o-** *press back* **-ion** *action; condition*	**Somatoform** (neurologic, sensory, or motor) deficits that occur without any physical basis. There may be sudden blindness, deafness, paralysis, or the inability to speak. There is **repression** of overwhelming anxiety or internal conflict which then undergoes a conversion to physical symptoms.
hypochondriasis	**hypochondriasis** (HY-poh-con-DRY-ah-sis) **hypo-** *below; deficient* **chondr/o-** *cartilage* **-iasis** *state of; process of* *Hypochondrium* is a Greek word for the areas of the abdomen below the cartilage of the ribs. These areas contain the liver and spleen, which the ancient Greeks thought contained humors that caused moods.	Preoccupation with and misinterpretation of minor bodily sensations with the fear that these indicate disease. Patients are convinced they have a serious illness and make frequent trips to the doctor despite medical evidence and reassurance to the contrary. The patient is known as a hypochondriac.

Sexual and Gender Identity Disorders

Sexual and gender identity disorders are characterized by abnormalities in accepting one's own sexual gender or focusing sexual attention on an object or a person other than a consenting adult. Gender identity is the sexual designation that a person correctly or incorrectly assigns to himself or herself based on physical and psychological characteristics as well as parental and societal expectations. Treatment: Psychotherapy.

Word or Phrase	Word Part and Definition	Description
exhibitionism	**exhibitionism** (EK-sih-BISH-un-izm) **exhibit/o-** *showing* **-ion** *action; condition* **-ism** *process; disease from a specific cause*	Obtaining power, control, and sexual arousal by exposing the genital area in public areas to strangers. The patient is known as an exhibitionist.
fetishism	**fetishism** (FET-ish-izm) *Fetishism* is a combination of the Latin word *fetish* (charm) and the suffix *-ism* (process; disease from a specific cause).	Obtaining sexual arousal from objects rather than a person. Patients devote a great deal of time to obtaining and using the object, which, for men, often includes women's clothing.
masochism	**masochism** (MAS-oh-kizm) *Masochism* was named for Leopold von Sacher-Masoch (1836–1895), an Austrian novelist who wrote about a man (himself) with these characteristics.	Obtaining sexual arousal through abuse, pain, humiliation, or bondage deliberately caused by another person. The patient is known as a masochist.

Word or Phrase	Word Part and Definition	Description
pedophilia	**pedophilia** (PEE-doh-FIL-ee-ah) **ped/o-** *child* **phil/o-** *attraction to, fondness for* **-ia** *condition, state, thing* **pedophile** (PEE-doh-file) **ped/o-** *child* **-phile** *person who is attracted to or fond of*	Obtaining power, control, and sexual arousal through contact or sexual acts with preadolescent children. The patient is known as a pedophile.
rape	**rape** (RAYP) **rapist** (RAY-pist) **rap/o-** *to seize and drag away* **-ist** *one who specializes in*	Obtaining power, control, and sexual arousal through forced sexual intercourse with a nonconsenting adult. Statutory rape is sexual intercourse with a minor (defined by most states as a person under the age of 18). The patient is known as a rapist. **Incest** is rape of a child by a parent or relative.
sadism	**sadism** (SAY-dizm) (SAD-izm) *Sadism* is named for Count Marquis de Sade (1740–1814), a French novelist who had these characteristics and wrote about them.	Obtaining power, control, and sexual arousal by deliberately causing abuse, pain, humiliation, or bondage to another person. The patient is known as a sadist.
transsexualism	**transsexualism** (tranz-SEK-shoo-ah-lizm) **trans-** *across, through* **sex/o-** *sex* **-ual** *pertaining to* **-ism** *process; disease from a specific cause*	Person's belief that he or she has been assigned (by anatomy, parents, or society) the wrong gender identity. The patient desires to change his or her outward appearance to the opposite sex in order to match what is already felt in the mind as being the true personal identity. Treatment may include a sex change operation.
transvestism	**transvestism** (trans-VES-tizm) **trans-** *across, through* **vest/o-** *to dress* **-ism** *process; disease from a specific cause*	Obtaining sexual arousal by wearing clothes belonging to the opposite sex or posing as someone of the opposite sex. The patient is known as a transvestite.
voyeurism	**voyeurism** (VOY-yer-izm) *Voyeurism* is a combination of a French word meaning *to see* and the suffix *-ism* (process; disease from a specific cause).	Obtaining power, control, and sexual arousal by secretively viewing other people who are naked or having sexual relations. The elements of risk and danger as well as knowingly violating another's privacy are part of the experience. The patient is known as a voyeur.

Impulse Control Disorders

Impulse control disorders are characterized by strong, persistent thoughts that occupy the mind and cause tension as the patient decides whether or not to act on them. When the act is performed, the patient feels relief or even pleasure. Treatment: Psychotherapy, counseling with anger management, family therapy.

Word or Phrase	Word Part and Definition	Description
intermittent explosive disorder	**homicidal** (HOHM-ih-SY-dal) hom/i- *man* cid/o- *killing* -al *pertaining to* **ideation** (EYE-dee-AA-shun) *Ideation* is a combination of *idea* and the suffix *-ation* (a process; being or having).	Sudden, explosively violent, unprovoked attacks of rage that are out of proportion to the stress experienced. Patients always place the blame on other people or circumstances for making them angry. Involves assault, battery, and is often associated with domestic violence. During a psychiatric interview, this patient is asked if he has any **homicidal ideation** about actually killing someone.
kleptomania	**kleptomania** (KLEP-toh-MAY-nee-ah) klept/o- *to steal* -mania *condition of frenzy*	Overwhelming impulse to steal things that have little or no value. These things are not stolen out of anger or revenge, and the patient sometimes even secretively returns them. Unlike shoplifting, the patient does not steal in order to obtain something without paying for it. The patient is known as a kleptomaniac.
pathological gambling	**pathological** (PATH-oh-LAWJ-ih-kal) path/o- *disease, suffering* log/o- *the study of* -ical *pertaining to*	Constant gambling that interferes with normal life and work activities and creates severe financial problems. Patients lie about how much money they have lost and often place bigger bets to win back lost money.
pyromania	**pyromania** (PY-roh-MAY-nee-ah) pyr/o- *fire; burning* -mania *condition of frenzy*	Deliberately setting fires for the pleasure of watching the fire and the people sent to fight the fire. Fires are not set to take revenge, conceal a crime, or collect insurance money. The patient is known as a pyromaniac.
trichotillomania	**trichotillomania** (TRIK-oh-TIL-oh-MAY-nee-ah) trich/o- *hair* till/o- *to pull out* -mania *condition of frenzy*	Repetitive pulling out of hair from the head.

Substance-Related Disorders

Substance-related disorders are characterized by the frequent or constant use and abuse of drugs or chemicals to achieve a desired physical or emotional effect (a "high," sedation, or hallucinations). The drugs may be prescription drugs, tobacco, alcohol, or illegal street drugs. After a brief period of use, patients experience **dependence** (need for the substance in order to prevent withdrawal symptoms). Later, patients exhibit **tolerance** (decreasing effect even with increasing amounts of the substance). Much of the patient's life may center on drug-seeking behavior. Patients are aware of the serious medical conditions related to the use of the substance, but they choose to ignore this and continue to use the substance. **Addiction** is a state of complete physical and psychological dependence on a substance. Treatment: Psychotherapy, group therapy, family therapy, support groups, aversion therapy, medical support for withdrawal symptoms.

The following substances and drugs are related to this disorder.

- Alcohol (beer, wine, liquor, ETOH, rubbing alcohol, wood alcohol)
- Amphetamines (central nervous system stimulant drugs; diet pills, speed)
- Cannabis (marijuana, hashish)
- Cocaine
- **Hallucinogens** (LSD, PCP)
- Inhalants (fumes from paint, paint thinner, cleaning fluid, lighter fluid, liquid glue, correction fluid, felt-tipped markers, or gasoline; aerosol propellant from spray cans)
- Nicotine (cigarettes, cigars, chewing tobacco)
- Opioids (narcotic drugs like morphine, codeine, Demerol, OxyContin; heroin)
- Sedatives and antianxiety drugs (barbiturates, sleeping pills, Valium)

dependence (dee-PEN-dens)
depend/o- *to hang onto*
-ence *state of*

tolerance (TAWL-er-ans)
toler/o- *to become accustomed to*
-ance *state of*

addiction (ah-DIK-shun)
addict/o- *surrender to; be controlled by*
-ion *action; condition*

hallucinogen (hah-LOO-sih-noh-jen)
hallucin/o- *imagined perception*
-gen *that which produces*

Affective or Mood Disorders

Mood disorders are characterized by the chronic, persistent presence (longer than six months) of depression or mood swings alternating in cycles between depression and mania. Normal feelings of sadness that diminish over time are considered appropriate and not categorized as a mood disorder. Mood disorders are also known as **affective disorders** because the effect of the mood can be seen in the patient's affect. Treatment: Psychotherapy, antidepressant drugs, drugs for mania.

Word or Phrase	Word Part and Definition	Description
bipolar disorder	**bipolar** (by-POH-lar) **bi-** *two* **pol/o-** *pole* **-ar** *pertaining to* **mania** (MAY-nee-ah) *Mania* is a Greek word meaning *frenzy.* **euphoria** (yoo-FOR-ee-ah) **eu-** *normal, good* **phor/o-** *range* **-ia** *condition, state, thing* **manic** (MAN-ik) *Manic* is derived from a Greek word meaning *affected by frenzy.*	Chronic mood swings between **mania** and depression (see Figure 17-6■). Patients with mania are hyperactive with limitless energy and extreme happiness (**euphoria**). They have feelings of power and mastery, need little sleep, and are intensely interested in and talk about one thing after another (flight of ideas), making and then quickly discarding plans. Gradually, their thoughts get out of control, and they are unable to concentrate and show increasingly poor judgment and recklessness. After an episode of mania, the patient swings abruptly into severe depression. Also known as **manic-depressive disorder.**

(continued)

Word or Phrase	Word Part and Definition	Description
	depressive (dee-PRES-iv) **depress/o-** *press down* **-ive** *pertaining to*	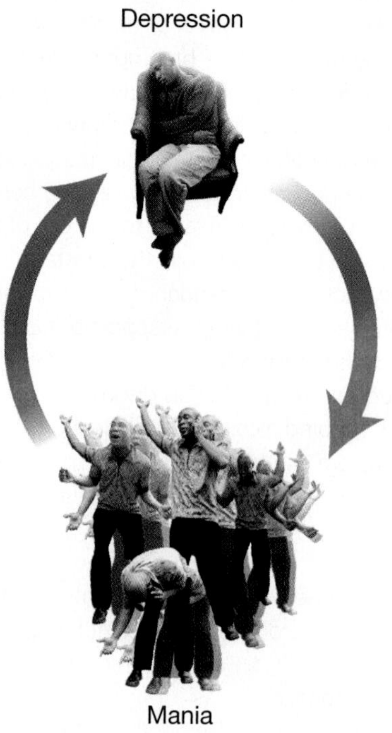 Depression Mania **Figure 17-6 ■ Bipolar disorder.** Depression and mania are characterized by emotions and behaviors that are at opposite poles or ends from each other.
cyclothymia	**cyclothymia** (SY-kloh-THY-mee-ah) **cycl/o-** *cycle; circle* **thym/o-** *thymus; rage* **-ia** *condition, state, thing*	Chronic, mild bipolar disorder. In between mood swings, the patient is free from symptoms and signs for several months.
dysthymia	**dysthymia** (dis-THY-mee-ah) **dys-** *painful, difficult, abnormal* **thym/o-** *thymus; rage* **-ia** *condition, state, thing*	Chronic, mild-to-moderate depression.
major depression	**depression** (dee-PRESH-un) **depress/o-** *press down* **-ion** *action; condition* **apathy** (AP-ah-thee) **a-** *away from, without* **-pathy** *disease, suffering* **anhedonia** (AN-hee-DOH-nee-ah) **an-** *without, not* **hedon/o-** *pleasure* **-ia** *condition, state, thing* **suicidal** (SOO-ih-SY-dal) **su/i-** *self* **cid/o-** *killing* **-al** *pertaining to*	Chronic, severe symptoms of depression with **apathy** (indifference), hopelessness, helplessness, worthlessness, crying, insomnia, lack of pleasure in any activity (**anhedonia**), increased or decreased appetite, inability to make decisions or concentrate, fatigue, and slowed movements. During the psychiatric interview, a depressed patient is asked if he has **suicidal ideation** or suicide attempts. **Did You Know?** Depression was previously known as *melancholia.* This word was derived from *melan/o-* (black) and *chol/e-* (bile, gall) and meant *black bile* because the ancient Greeks thought that the body contained four "humors" (blood, yellow bile, black bile, and phlegm) that caused different moods.

Word or Phrase	Word Part and Definition	Description
premenstrual dysphoric disorder (PMDD)	**premenstrual** (pree-MEN-stroo-al) **pre-** *before, in front of* **menstru/o-** *monthly discharge of blood* **-al** *pertaining to* **dysphoric** (dis-FOR-ik) **dys-** *painful, difficult, abnormal* **phor/o-** *to bear, to carry* **-ic** *pertaining to*	Occurs before the onset of the menstrual cycle and combines the symptoms of premenstrual syndrome (PMS) (breast, joint, and muscle pains) with depression, anxiety, tearfulness, difficulty concentrating, and sleep and eating disturbances.
seasonal affective disorder (SAD)	**affective** (ah-FEK-tiv) **affect/o-** *state of mind; mood; to have an infuence on* **-ive** *pertaining to*	Caused by hypersecretion of melatonin from the pineal gland in the brain. Melatonin is normally produced during the dark hours of each day. More dark hours and less sunshine during winter months increase the production of melatonin, and this causes symptoms of depression, weight gain, and altered sleeping habits. Treatment: Exposure to sunlight or the use of a light box for several hours each day.

Psychosis

Psychoses are characterized by a loss of touch with reality and a disintegration of the thought processes. There is a change in affect and behavior, with inability to communicate effectively or maintain life activities. Schizophrenia is the most common form of psychosis. Treatment: Antipsychotic drugs, psychotherapy. *Psychosis* (sy-KOH-sis) is a combination of *psych/o-* (mind) and *-osis* (condition; abnormal condition; process).

Word or Phrase	Word Part and Definition	Description
delusional disorder	**delusional** (dee-LOO-zhun-al) **delus/o-** *false belief* **-ion** *action; condition* **-al** *pertaining to* **delusion** (dee-LOO-zhun) **delus/o-** *false belief* **-ion** *action; condition* *Delusion* is derived from a Latin word meaning *to deceive.* **paranoia** (PAIR-ah-NOY-ah) *Paranoia* is derived from a Greek word meaning *condition of thinking abnormal thoughts.*	Continued false beliefs (delusions) concerning events of everyday life. These beliefs are fixed and unchanging despite the efforts of others to persuade or evidence showing otherwise. Common delusions: other people or even strangers are in love with you, your husband or wife is unfaithful, other people are trying to hurt or kill you (delusions of persecution, also known as **paranoia**), or you have the powers of a god or are a famous person (delusions of grandeur).

Word or Phrase	Word Part and Definition	Description
schizophrenia	**schizophrenia** (SKIZ-oh-FREE-nee-ah) (SKIT-soh-FREE-nee-ah) **schiz/o-** *split* **phren/o-** *mind; diaphragm* **-ia** *condition, state, thing* Some word parts have more than one definition. The best definition of *schizophrenia* is *condition of a split mind.* **schizophrenic** (SKIZ-oh-FREN-ik) (SKIT-soh-FREN-ik) **schiz/o-** *split* **phren/o-** *mind; diaphragm* **-ic** *pertaining to* **hallucination** (hah-LOO-sih-NAY-shun) **hallucin/o-** *imagined perception* **-ation** *a process; being or having* **neologism** (nee-AWL-oh-jizm) **ne/o-** *new* **log/o-** *word; the study of* **-ism** *process; disease from a specific cause* **catatonia** (KAT-ah-TOH-nee-ah) **cata-** *down* **ton/o-** *pressure, tone* **-ia** *condition, state, thing* **catatonic** (KAT-ah-TAWN-ik) **cata-** *down* **ton/o-** *pressure, tone* **-ic** *pertaining to* **catalepsy** (KAT-ah-LEP-see) **cata-** *down* **-lepsy** *seizure* **hebephrenia** (HEE-bah-FREE-nee-ah) (HEB-ee-FREE-nee-ah) **hebe/o-** *youth* **phren/o-** *diaphragm; mind* **-ia** *condition, state, thing*	Chronic loss of touch with reality in most or all aspects of life with bizarre behavior and breakdown of thought processes. Patients have **hallucinations** (false impressions of vision, smell, sound, taste, or touch). The most common is an auditory hallucination of a voice telling them to do certain things. Patients have delusions of persecution and delusions that others are controlling their thoughts or that they can use their thoughts to control events. Some patients' thoughts are so chaotic that their spoken words are completely meaningless, and they may use **neologisms.** Patients' emotions and affect are inappropriate and do not correspond to what they are saying. Some patients are rigid and in a stupor (**catatonia**) or their extremities stay fixed in whatever position they are placed (**catalepsy**), while others show childish, silly behavior (**hebephrenia**). Many patients have their first episode as young adults following a stressful event. Others develop symptoms more slowly over time. **Did You Know?** *Insanity* is derived from two Latin words meaning *not sound.* Literature has long depicted an insane person as a lunatic who is influenced by the phases of the moon, with the most severe symptoms during a full moon. *Lunatic* is derived from the Latin word *lun/o-* (moon).

Personality Disorders

Personality disorders are characterized by a disturbance in one or more aspects of the personality (which is the combination of thoughts, beliefs, emotions, and behaviors that are unique to each person). Patients with personality disorders experience difficulty in interpersonal relationships (marriage, work, social). They are unable to adapt their rigid views, they fail to meet the needs of others, and they have a tendency to blame others for their own failures. Treatment: Psychotherapy, group therapy, family therapy.

Word or Phrase	Word Part and Definition	Description
antisocial personality	**antisocial** (AN-tee-SOH-shal) anti- *against* soci/o- *human beings; community* -al *pertaining to* **personality** (PER-son-AL-ih-tee) person/o- *person* -al *pertaining to* -ity *state; condition*	Disregard for written and unwritten rules and standards of conduct (laws, morals, ethics) of society. Patients lie, steal, and manipulate, showing no empathy for others or guilt or remorse for their actions. There is also fighting, failure to attend school (truancy), vandalism, sexual promiscuity, excessive drinking, the use of illegal drugs, and criminal acts. Previously known as sociopaths or psychopaths.
avoidant personality		Avoidance of social contact because of excessive shyness and extreme fear and sensitivity to criticism or rejection.
borderline personality		Inability to sustain a stable relationship. Patients fear abandonment and panic when they are alone, rushing into intense, but self-destructive relationships. They tend to see things in black and white—all good or all bad with no middle ground. They are hypersensitive with strong emotions that can easily change. They have poor tolerance to stress and often overreact.
dependent personality	**dependent** (dee-PEN-dent) depend/o- *to hang onto* -ent *pertaining to*	Expects and wants to be told what to do and what to think. Patients are passive, have difficulty making decisions, and want others to take care of them and the details of their life.
narcissistic personality	**narcissism** (NAWR-sih-sizm) *Narcissism* is derived from the Greek myth of Narcissos, a young man who shunned the love of others because he was in love with his own reflection in the water. **histrionic** (HIS-tree-AW-nik) *Histrionic* is derived from a Latin word meaning *an actor.*	Exaggerated sense of self worth and importance. Patients feel superior to others and believe they are entitled to be the center of attention and to receive compliments, admiration, and affection. They are angry, demanding, and manipulative if others receive more than they do. Their demand to be noticed can be emotional, dramatic, and done for its effect (**histrionic**).
obsessive-compulsive personality		Inflexible and perfectionistic. Patients feel that everything must be accounted for and in its place, nothing can be left to chance, and they are unwilling to compromise. Patients feel that there is always one best way to do everything and they expect others to act accordingly. Patients keep lists and schedules and are concerned about productivity, but may be so consumed by minor details that they sometimes cannot get the job done. These patients do not actually have obsessive-compulsive disorder (which was discussed previously).

Diagnostic Procedures

Blood and Urine Tests

Word or Phrase	Word Part and Definition	Description
drug level		Blood test to determine the level of an antipsychotic drug in patients who are noncompliant with their medication schedule.
urine test for drugs		Urine test to detect illegal drugs.

Radiologic Procedures

Word or Phrase	Word Part and Definition	Description
CT scan or MRI scan		Radiologic procedure used to document loss of brain tissue or structural abnormalities of the brain that might contribute to a psychiatric illness.
PET scan		Radiologic procedure that shows areas of abnormal metabolism in the brain related to dementia and Alzheimer's disease.

Psychiatric Procedures and Tests

Word or Phrase	Word Part and Definition	Description
Beck Depression Inventory (BDI)		Assesses the degree of depression. Screening tool that is filled out by the patient. Each item offers four answers that show progressively more depressed emotions: I do not feel sad (0 points), I feel sad (1 point), I am sad all the time (2 points), I am so sad I can't stand it (3 points). The patient selects the statement that most closely matches his/her feelings.
Holmes Social Readjustment Rating Scale	**stressor** (STRES-or) **stress/o-** *disturbing stimulus* **-or** *person or thing that produces or does*	Assigns point values to various **stressors** (negative and positive life events) to measure the total amount of stress in a patient's life. Death of spouse (100 points), divorce (73 points), death of family member (63 points), personal illness (53 points), marriage (50 points), retirement (45 points), pregnancy (40 points), change in finances (38 points), change in jobs (36 points), change in schools (25 points), vacation (13 points), Christmas (12 points).
intelligence testing		Intelligence tests are administered if the patient is suspected of having any degree of mental impairment or retardation.

Word or Phrase	Word Part and Definition	Description
psychiatric diagnosis	**psychiatric** (SY-kee-AT-rik) psych/o- *mind* iatr/o- *physician; medical treatment* -ic *pertaining to*	Stated in a specific way that involves five axes or aspects, as required by the American Psychiatric Association's publication *Diagnostic and Statistical Manual of Mental Disorders,* fourth edition (DSM-IV) (see Table 17-2).

Table 17-2 Psychiatric Diagnosis Format

Axis I	Any psychiatric disorders (except personality disorders and mental retardation).
Axis II	Personality disorders and mental retardation.
Axis III	Medical symptoms, signs, and diseases. (Physical examination, neurological examination, and mental status examination are performed.)
Axis IV	Psychosocial and Environmental Problems. (Problems with marriage, family, neighbors, community, school, work, housing, finances, health care, police, or the courts)
Axis V	Global Assessment of Functioning (GAF). The GAF Scale ranges from 1 to 100 points. A person who is able to manage life's problems, functions in all areas of life, and exhibits no symptoms or signs of mental disorder scores between 91 and 100. Patients with moderate psychiatric disorders or moderate difficulty functioning in social, work, and school situations score between 51 and 60. Patients in constant, severe danger of hurting themselves or others score less than 10 points.

Word or Phrase	Word Part and Definition	Description
psychiatric interview		Provides the first insights into the patient's mental illness. Done in a psychiatrist's office or clinic or during admission to an acute care hospital or psychiatric hospital. The patient (or other person if the patient is unable to answer) is asked why he came for care, who brought him for care, what stressors are going on in his life, and about any previous psychiatric illness. The interviewer notes the patient's general appearance and behavior and listens to the patient's answers to analyze speech, content of thoughts, abstract reasoning, insight, and judgment.
Rorschach test	**Rorschach** (ROHR-shahk) Rorschach test was named by Hermann Rorschach (1884–1922), a Swiss psychiatrist.	Uses cards with abstract shapes on them. Patients are asked to describe what the shape of the inkblot represents to them. Also known as the inkblot test.
Thematic Apperception Test (TAT)	**apperception** (AP-er-SEP-shun) appercept/o- *fully perceived* -ion *action; condition*	Assesses personality, emotions, attitudes, motivation, and conflicts. The patient is shown 31 different pictures of social or interpersonal situations. The patient describes what is happening in the picture or what the theme of the picture is.

Psychiatric Therapies

Word or Phrase	Word Part and Definition	Description
art therapy	**therapy** (THAIR-ah-pee) **therapeutic** (THAIR-ah-PYOO-tik) therapeut/o- *treatment* -ic *pertaining to*	Drawing or creating other types of art while talking about it with an art therapist. Art therapy relieves stress, allows patients to express their thoughts and emotions safely, and helps them gain insight into their problems. Art therapy helps small children express something they saw or something that was done to them that they cannot describe in words.
aversion therapy	**aversion** (ah-VUHR-shun) a- *away from, without* vers/o- *to travel; to turn* -ion *action; condition*	The patient thinks about a desired, but destructive, behavior and this is coupled with a mild electrical shock or noxious smells like ammonia. This is a form of conditioning that creates an aversion to doing that behavior. Used to treat drug and cigarette addiction and sexual identity issues.
cognitive-behavioral therapy (CBT)	**cognitive** (KAWG-nih-tiv) cognit/o- *thinking* -ive *pertaining to* **behavioral** (bee-HAYV-yer-al) behav/o- *activity or manner of acting* -ior *pertaining to* -al *pertaining to*	Therapy based on the premise that beliefs and attitudes (not people or events) cause undesirable or destructive emotions, and thought patterns and behaviors are learned and can be unlearned. Patients are taught to use guided imagery and self-counseling to produce desirable emotions and behavior. Used to treat anxiety, panic attacks, phobias, depression, eating disorders, and other behaviors.
detoxication	**detoxication** (dee-TAWKS-ih-KAY-shun) de- *reversal of; without* toxic/o- *poison, toxin* -ation *a process; being or having*	Observation of an alcohol-addicted patient undergoing withdrawal. Drugs are given, as needed, to minimize withdrawal symptoms and prevent seizures. Also known as detoxification.
electroconvulsive therapy (ECT)	**electroconvulsive** (ee-LEK-troh-con-VUL-siv) electr/o- *electricity* convuls/o- *seizure* -ive *pertaining to*	Uses an electrical current and electrodes on the head to produce seizures (convulsions). Patients are given sedative and muscle relaxant drugs to make them unconscious and relaxed. The seizure lasts about one minute and the patient awakens within one hour. Used to treat severe depression and schizophrenia. ECT relieves symptoms more quickly than antidepressant drugs (that can take up to a month to become effective). Also known as electroshock therapy.
family therapy		Involves the entire family, not just the patient. The focus is on relationships and conflicts between family members. What family members say to each other, how they say it, and how they act toward each other can be dysfunctional. The family often labels one family member (the patient) as the troublemaker, while others can do no wrong. Unless corrected, these fixed roles inhibit changing and adopting more appropriate behaviors.

Word or Phrase	Word Part and Definition	Description
group therapy		Provides simultaneous therapy to several patients who have a similar mental illness like anxiety, depression, or being a victim of sexual abuse (see Figure 17-7 ■). Group members share experiences and insights and provide feedback and emotional support to each other. **Figure 17-7 ■ Group therapy.** This psychologist is conducting a group therapy session. Group members support or challenge each other while gaining insight into their own problems.
hypnosis	**hypnosis** (hip-NOH-sis) **hypn/o-** *sleep* **-osis** *condition; abnormal condition; process*	Places the patient in a sleeplike trance (patient is still able to remember who they are and what is happening). The therapist makes suggestions that are incorporated in the patient's subconscious mind and later acted upon consciously to some degree. Used to treat anxiety and phobias and to help patients stop smoking or lose weight. Also known as hypnotherapy.
play therapy		Uses toys and other objects (often dolls) to help young children express emotions and reenact traumatic or abusive events (on a small scale they can control). Used to treat social withdrawal, anxiety, depression, aggression, and ADHD.
psychoanalysis	**psychoanalysis** (SY-koh-ah-NAL-ih-sis) **psych/o-** *mind* **analy/o-** *to separate* **-osis** *condition; abnormal condition; process*	Based on the ideas of conscious and subconscious as developed by Sigmund Freud to analyze a patient's thoughts and behavior. It includes intepretation of dreams and hypnosis.
psychotherapy	**psychotherapy** (SY-koh-THAIR-ah-pee) **psych/o-** *mind* **-therapy** *treatment*	Any therapy (except drug therapy and electroconvulsive therapy) that uses verbal or nonverbal communication between a patient or a group of patients and a psychologist or psychiatrist to treat a mental disorder.

Word or Phrase	Word Part and Definition	Description
systematic desensitization	**desensitization** (dee-SEN-sih-tih-ZAY-shun) **de-** *reversal of, without* **sensit/o-** *affected by, sensitive to* **-ization** *process of making, creating, or inserting*	Technique in which patients imagine about 10 different scenarios involving a specific phobia (for example, fear of spiders). Each scenario is associated with progressively greater anxiety. The patient practices relaxation techniques before and after visualizing the first scenario. When the first scenario no longer causes anxiety, patients move on to the second, and so forth until they are no longer sensitive to that phobia.
therapeutic milieu	**milieu** (meel-YOO) *Milieu* is a French word meaning *middle place.*	Stable, structured, and safe emotional and physical environment that provides ongoing therapy of various types for a psychiatric patient.

Drug Categories

Several different categories of drugs are used to treat the symptoms and signs of mental disorders. The most common drugs in each category are listed.

Category	Word Part and Definition	Description	Examples
antianxiety drugs	**antianxiety** (AN-tee-ang-ZY-eh-tee) **anti-** *against* **anxi/o-** *fear, worry* **-ety** *condition, state* **anxiolytic** (ANG-zee-oh-LIT-ik) **anxi/o-** *fear, worry* **ly/o-** *break down, separate, dissolve* **-tic** *pertaining to* **tranquilizer** (TRANG-kwih-ly-zer) **tranquil/o-** *calm* **-izer** *thing that affects in a particular way*	Treat anxiety and neurosis. Also known as anxiolytic drugs and minor tranquilizers.	Effexor, Librium, Tranxene, Valium
antidepressant drugs	**antidepressant** (AN-tee-dee-PRES-ant) **anti-** *against* **depress/o-** *press down* **-ant** *pertaining to*	Treat depression by prolonging the action of norepinephrine or serotonin. Classes include tricyclic, tetracyclic, and monoamine oxidase (MAO) inhibitor drugs. Another class, selective serotonin reuptake inhibitors (SSRI), only acts on serotonin.	Paxil, Zoloft

Did You Know?

Valium is derived from the Latin word *valere,* which means *to be healthy.* The wild European plant valerian has been known since the time of Hippocrates to calm the nerves.

Category	Word Part and Definition	Description	Examples
antipsychotic drugs	**antipsychotic** (AN-tee-sy-KAWT-ik) **anti-** *against* **psych/o-** *mind* **-tic** *pertaining to*	Treat psychosis, paranoia, and schizophrenia by blocking dopamine receptors in the limbic system. Also known as neuroleptics and major tranquilizers.	Haldol, Prozac, Risperdal, Thorazine, Zyprexa

Connections

tardive (TAR-dive)
tard/o- *late, slow*
-ive *pertaining to*

dyskinesia (DIS-kih-NEE-zee-ah)
dys- *painful, difficult, abnormal*
kines/o- *movement*
-ia *condition, state, thing*

Pharmacology. Many schizophrenic patients are noncompliant with taking their antipsychotic medication because of a severe side effect known as **tardive dyskinesia** that develops as a late complication of treatment. It causes involuntary, repetitive movements of the face (grimacing, lip smacking, eye blinking, tongue movements) and can also include movements of the arms and legs.

Category	Word Part and Definition	Description	Examples
drugs for alcoholism		Inhibit an enzyme that metabolizes the breakdown products of alcohol. Patients on this drug who drink alcohol experience headache, dizziness, nausea, and even arrhythmias. This unpleasant reaction is a detriment to drinking alcohol.	Antabuse
drugs for mania		Inhibits the action of excessive norepinephrine while increasing the sensitivity of serotonin receptors.	lithium (Lithobid)

Abbreviations

ADD	attention deficit disorder
ADHD	attention deficit hyperactivity disorder
BDI	Beck Depression Inventory
CBT	cognitive behavioral therapy
CNS	central nervous system
DT	delirium tremens
ECT	electroconvulsive therapy
ETOH	alcohol (liquor)
LSD	lysergic acid diethylamide (a street drug)
MAO	monoamine oxidase (inhibitor drug)
OCD	obsessive-compulsive disorder
OD	overdose
PCP	phencyclidine (angel dust, a street drug)
PMDD	premenstrual dysphoric disorder
PTSD	posttraumatic stress disorder
Psy	psychiatry, psychology
Psych	psychiatry, psychology
SAD	seasonal affective disorder
SSRI	selective serotonin reuptake inhibitor
TAT	Thematic Apperception Test

Career Focus

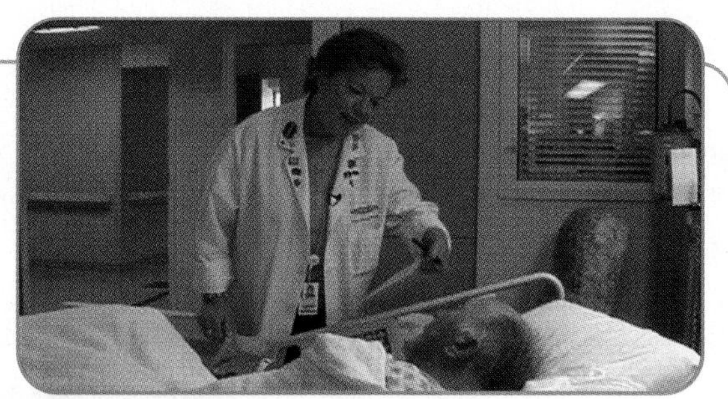

Meet Patricia, a social worker.

"There are all kinds of jobs you can do when you're a social worker. You can work in nursing homes. You can work in rehab centers. You can work on your own and do private counseling with people who've just gotten a terminal diagnosis. You can work with children. You can work in schools. One of the reasons why I love it is because you never know what you're going to be doing in a day. I'm assigned to a pulmonologist. Each day we go over his case list, and we prioritize who needs to be seen first, who needs home care, who needs nursing home placement, who needs help with prescriptions, who needs somebody to just go in and talk to them. I see my role as helping patients who are in an unfamiliar environment. It's not the best time of their lives. I use medical terminology all day long, especially when calling in the clinical information to the insurance companies."

Social workers are allied health professionals who obtain medical, housing, financial, or other community services and support for patients or clients. Social workers work in the department of human services in government offices, clinics, nursing homes, hospitals, and in psychiatric hospitals.

Psychologists are mental health practitioners who have a doctoral degree (Ph.D.) in **psychology.** They work in psychiatric hospitals, outpatient clinics, and school systems. They administer psychological and intelligence tests and act as therapists for various types of counseling and psychotherapy sessions (family, group, marriage). They are not physicians and cannot prescribe drug therapy.

Psychiatrists are physicians who practice in the mental health specialty of psychiatry. They diagnose and treat patients with mental illness. Physicians can take additional training and become board certified in the subspecialties of child and adolescent psychiatry, geriatric psychiatry, psychosomatic medicine, addiction psychiatry, or forensic psychiatry.

social (SOH-shal)
soci/o- *human beings; community*
-al *pertaining to*

psychologist (sy-KAWL-oh-jist)
psych/o- *mind*
log/o- *the study of*
-ist *one who specializes in*

psychology (sy-KAWL-oh-jee)
psych/o- *mind*
-logy *the study of*

psychiatrist (sy-KY-ah-trist)
psych/o- *mind*
iatr/o- *physician; medical treatment*
-ist *one who specializes in*

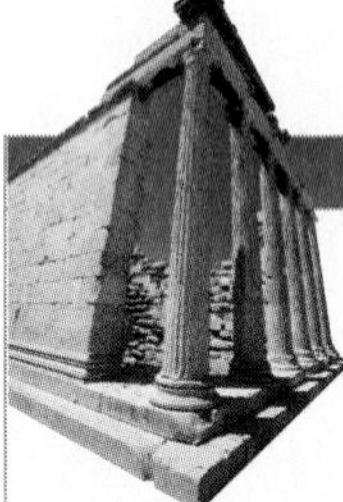

It's Greek to Me!

Did you notice that some psychiatric words have two different combining forms? Combining forms from both Greek and Latin languages remain a part of medical language today.

English Word	Greek	Latin	Examples of Medical Words
mind	phren/o-	ment/o-	schizophrenia, mental, dementia
	psych/o-		psychotherapy
self	aut/o-	su/i-	autism, suicide

CHAPTER REVIEW EXERCISES

Review all the material in this chapter by completing the review exercises in this section. Use the Answer Key at the end of the book to check your answers.

Anatomy and Physiology

Matching Exercise

Match each numbered word or phrase to its description. Some structures may have more than one correct description.

1. amygdaloid bodies
2. fornix
3. hippocampus
4. hypothalamus
5. thalamus

_____ Tract of nerves that joins all parts of the limbic system
_____ Contains the satiety and feeding centers
_____ Almond-shaped structures
_____ Relay station that sends sensory impulses to the brain
_____ Interprets facial expressions and new social situations
_____ Forms the floor of the third ventricle
_____ Sends nerve signals for "fight or flight"
_____ Located in both of the temporal lobes
_____ Located along the floor of the lateral ventricles
_____ Looks like a seahorse
_____ Particularly active in the emotions of fear, anger, and rage

True or False

Indicate whether each statement is true or false by writing T or F on the line.

1. ____ The hippocampus is the entire anatomical system of the brain that deals with emotions.
2. ____ The limbic lobe is also known as the cingulate gyrus.
3. ____ The hippocampus is involved in short-term and long-term memory.
4. ____ An emotion is an intense state of feeling.
5. ____ The outward expression on a person's face of the inward emotions is known as the mood.
6. ____ Neurotransmitters are chemicals that relay messages from one neuron to the next.
7. ____ Injury to the frontal lobe can produce a flat affect and inability to concentrate.

Matching Exercise

Match each numbered word or phrase to its description. Some neurotransmitters may be used more than once.

1. dopamine
2. epinephrine
3. GABA
4. norepinephrine
5. serotonin

_____ Decreased levels associated with depression
_____ Decreased levels associated with anxiety
_____ Increased levels associated with panic attacks, phobias
_____ Decreased levels associated with schizophrenia
_____ "Fight or flight" of the sympathetic nervous system
_____ Increased levels associated with infatuation

Medical Language Word Parts

Name That Word Part

Identify each of the word parts given here by writing in the correct letter (P, C, or S) on the line beside it. Then write the definition of the word part on the blank line. The first one has been done for you.

Prefix = P **Combining Form = C** **Suffix = S**

		Word Part	Definition			Word Part	Definition
1.	-al	S	pertaining to	35.	delus/o-	______	______
2.	a-	______	______	36.	depend/o-	______	______
3.	acr/o-	______	______	37.	depress/o-	______	______
4.	addict/o-	______	______	38.	dis-	______	______
5.	affect/o-	______	______	39.	dys-	______	______
6.	agor/a-	______	______	40.	ech/o-	______	______
7.	amygdal/o-	______	______	41.	electr/o-	______	______
8.	amnes/o-	______	______	42.	emot/o-	______	______
9.	an-	______	______	43.	en-	______	______
10.	analy/o-	______	______	44.	-ence	______	______
11.	-ance	______	______	45.	-ent	______	______
12.	-ant	______	______	46.	-er	______	______
13.	anter/o-	______	______	47.	-esis	______	______
14.	anti-	______	______	48.	eu-	______	______
15.	anxi/o-	______	______	49.	-ety	______	______
16.	appercept/o-	______	______	50.	exhibit/o-	______	______
17.	-ar	______	______	51.	factiti/o-	______	______
18.	arachn/o-	______	______	52.	-form	______	______
19.	-ation	______	______	53.	-gen	______	______
20.	-ative	______	______	54.	glob/o-	______	______
21.	aut/o-	______	______	55.	-grade	______	______
22.	behav/o-	______	______	56.	hallucin/o-	______	______
23.	bi-	______	______	57.	hebe/o-	______	______
24.	cata-	______	______	58.	hedon/o-	______	______
25.	chondr/o-	______	______	59.	hom/i-	______	______
26.	cid/o-	______	______	50.	hypn/o-	______	______
27.	claustr/o-	______	______	61.	hypo-	______	______
28.	cognit/o-	______	______	62.	-ia	______	______
29.	compuls/o-	______	______	63.	-iasis	______	______
30.	con-	______	______	64.	iatr/o-	______	______
31.	convuls/o-	______	______	65.	-iatry	______	______
32.	copr/o-	______	______	66.	-ic	______	______
33.	cycl/o-	______	______	67.	-ical	______	______
34.	de-	______	______	68.	-ion	______	______

	Word Part	Definition		Word Part	Definition
69. -ior	______	______________	107. phob/o-	______	______________
70. -ism	______	______________	108. phor/o-	______	______________
71. -ist	______	______________	109. phren/o-	______	______________
72. -ition	______	______________	110. pol/o-	______	______________
73. -ity	______	______________	111. post-	______	______________
74. -ive	______	______________	112. pre-	______	______________
75. -ization	______	______________	113. psych/o-	______	______________
76. -izer	______	______________	114. pyr/o-	______	______________
77. kines/o	______	______________	115. rap/o-	______	______________
78. klept/o-	______	______________	116. react/o-	______	______________
79. -lalia	______	______________	117. repress/o-	______	______________
80. -lepsy	______	______________	118. retro-	______	______________
81. limb/o-	______	______________	119. sex/o-	______	______________
82. log/o-	______	______________	120. schiz/o-	______	______________
83. -logy	______	______________	121. sensit/o-	______	______________
84. ly/o-	______	______________	122. soci/o-	______	______________
85. -mania	______	______________	123. somat/o-	______	______________
86. menstru/o-	______	______________	124. stress/o-	______	______________
87. ment/o-	______	______________	125. su/i-	______	______________
88. micr/o-	______	______________	126. tard/o-	______	______________
89. mitt/o-	______	______________	127. thanat/o-	______	______________
90. morph/o-	______	______________	128. therapeut/o-	______	______________
91. ne/o-	______	______________	129. -therapy	______	______________
92. neur/o-	______	______________	130. thym/o-	______	______________
93. obsess/o-	______	______________	131. -tic	______	______________
94. -oid	______	______________	132. till/o-	______	______________
95. ophidi/o-	______	______________	133. toler/o-	______	______________
96. oppos/o-	______	______________	134. ton/o-	______	______________
97. -or	______	______________	135. toxic/o-	______	______________
98. orex/o-	______	______________	136. tranquil/o-	______	______________
99. -osis	______	______________	137. trans-	______	______________
100. -ous	______	______________	138. traumat/o-	______	______________
101. path/o-	______	______________	139. trich/o-	______	______________
102. -pathy	______	______________	140. -ual	______	______________
103. ped/o-	______	______________	141. vers/o-	______	______________
104. person/o-	______	______________	142. vest/o-	______	______________
105. -phile	______	______________	143. xen/o-	______	______________
106. phil/o-	______	______________			

Word-Building Exercise

Use the combining forms, prefixes, and suffixes given here to build medical words that match the definitions given. Write the word that you build on the blank line. Some word parts may be used more than once. The first one has been done for you.

Word Parts			
acr/o- (extremity; highest point)	de- (reversal of, without)	-ion (action; condition)	-mania (frenzy)
-al (pertaining to)	emot/o- (moving, stirring)	-ive (pertaining to)	ment/o- (mind; chin)
cognit/o- (thinking)	-ia (condition, state, thing)	klept/o- (to steal)	phob/o- (fear)
compuls/o- (drive or compel)			

1. Pertaining to the mind (You think *ment/o-* + *-al*). You write mental ____________
2. Condition (of thoughts) that drive or compel ____________
3. State of being afraid of heights ____________
4. Pertaining to thinking ____________
5. Frenzy to steal things ____________
6. Condition of moving or stirring (the feelings) ____________
7. Condition of being without the mind ____________

Symptoms, Signs, and Mental Disorders

Circle Exercise

Circle the correct word from the choices given.

1. (**Delirium, Panic, Rage**) is a sudden attack of overwhelming anxiety.
2. (**Avoidance, Bulimia, Delusion**) is bingeing on food and then vomiting.
3. (**Delirium, Delirium tremens, Schizophrenia**) is part of the symptoms of withdrawal from alcohol intoxication.
4. Retrograde amnesia causes the patient to forget events that happened (**after, before, during**) a traumatic event.
5. Autistic children can show (**echolalia, encopresis, euphoria**) in their speech.
6. Affective disorders are also known as (**depression, emotions, mood disorders**).
7. Hopelessness, helplessness, and worthlessness are symptoms of (**apathy, depression, withdrawal**).
8. Manic-depressive disorder is also known as (**bipolar disorder, intermittent explosive disorder, sadism**).
9. Making another person sick so that you can get attention is a sign of (**autism, Munchausen by proxy, psychosis**).
10. Doing something for its emotional and dramatic effect is being (**autistic, histrionic, obsessive**).

Matching Exercise

Match each numbered word or phrase to its description.

1.	addiction	_____ Constantly worried about "What if . . ."
2.	anhedonia	_____ Feels superior to others and deserving of attention
3.	conversion disorder	_____ Physical and psychological dependence on a substance
4.	dysthymia	_____ Performs excessive, repetitive, meaningless activities
5.	fugue	_____ Forgetting one's old life and beginning a new life elsewhere
6.	generalized anxiety disorder	_____ Sudden, severe, overwhelming anxiety
7.	identity disorder	_____ Most common psychosis
8.	kleptomania	_____ Stealing things of no value
9.	malingering	_____ Mild, chronic depression
10.	narcissism	_____ Lack of pleasure in any activity
11.	obsessive-compulsive disorder	_____ Sudden blindness or paralysis because of repressed internal conflict
12.	panic attack	_____ Multiple personality disorder
13.	schizophrenia	_____ Pretending to be in pain in order to get narcotic drugs
14.	sociopath	_____ Dressing as someone of the opposite sex
15.	transvestism	_____ Antisocial personality prone to violence and criminal acts

True or False

Indicate whether each statement is true or false by writing T or F on the line.

1. ____ Mental disorder is the same thing as a mental illness.
2. ____ Tardive dyskinesia is characterized by eye blinking, arm thrusting, grunts, and vulgar or socially inappropriate comments.
3. ____ Anorexia is the brief name for anorexia nervosa.
4. ____ A hypochondriac fears minor body sensations indicate a disease.
5. ____ Childish, silly behavior in schizophrenic patients is known as autism.
6. ____ Obsessive-compulsive disorder is the mildest form of obsessive-compulsive personality.
7. ____ Neologisms are made-up words whose meanings are known only to the patient.
8. ____ A fetish is an object used to produce sexual arousal.

Divide and Conquer

Separate these words into their component parts (prefix, combining form, suffix). Note: Some words do not contain all three word parts. The first one has been done for you.

Medical Word	Prefix	Combining Form	Suffix
1. anorexia	*an-*	*orex/o-*	*-ia*
2. anxiety	______	______	______
3. autism	______	______	______
4. bipolar	______	______	______
5. dementia	______	______	______
6. dysmorphic	______	______	______
7. hallucination	______	______	______
8. hypochondriasis	______	______	______
9. mental	______	______	______
10. microphobia	______	______	______
11. neologism	______	______	______
12. pedophile	______	______	______
13. phobic	______	______	______
14. posttraumatic	______	______	______

Matching Exercise

Match each numbered word or phrase to its description.

1. acrophobia	_____ Fear of closed-in spaces
2. agoraphobia	_____ Fear of strangers
3. arachnophobia	_____ Fear of germs
4. claustrophobia	_____ Fear of death
5. microphobia	_____ Fear of spiders
6. ophidiophobia	_____ Fear of crowds or public places
7. thanatophobia	_____ Fear of heights
8. xenophobia	_____ Fear of snakes

Diagnostic Procedures, Therapies, and Drugs

True or False

Indicate whether each statement is true or false by writing T or F on the line.

1. ____ The Rorschach test is another name for the inkblot test.
2. ____ MAO and SSRI are types of drugs used to treat alcoholism.
3. ____ A PET scan looks at abnormal metabolism in the brain of a patient with dementia.
4. ____ Even positive life events are associated with levels of stress.
5. ____ The *Diagnostic and Statistical Manual of Mental Disorders* is published by the American Medical Association.
6. ____ An axis is a way of expressing the severity of a patient's depression.
7. ____ Detoxication is an appropriate therapy for a patient with psychosis.
8. ____ A dysfunctional family often labels one family member as the troublemaker.
9. ____ Hypnosis is also known as hypnotherapy.
10. ____ The mania of bipolar disorder is treated with the drug lithium.
11. ____ Tardive dyskinesia can be a severe side effect of antipsychotic drugs.

Matching Exercise

Match each numbered word or phrase to its description.

1. aversion therapy	______ Stable, structured, safe environment for therapy
2. cognitive-behavioral therapy	______ All family members receive therapy
3. family therapy	______ Thoughts can be changed
4. group therapy	______ Uses toys and dolls to reenact trauma
5. play therapy	______ Members support each other in therapy
6. psychoanalysis	______ Uses noxious substances like ammonia
7. therapeutic milieu	______ Based on the work of Freud

Abbreviations

Matching Exercise

Match the abbreviation to its definition.

1.	ADHD	_____ Illegal, hallucinogenic drug
2.	BDI	_____ Alcohol
3.	ECT	_____ Administration of electricity to cause convulsions
4.	ETOH	_____ Characterized by distractability and hyperactivity
5.	LSD	_____ Occurs during the winter months
6.	MAO	_____ Type of antidepressant drug
7.	OCD	_____ Mood disorder during premenstrual time
8.	PMDD	_____ Characterized by meaningless rituals
9.	PTSD	_____ Happens after war, terrorist attacks, or kidnapping
10.	SAD	_____ Test to assess the extent of depression

Applied Skills

Proofreading and Spelling Exercise

Read the following paragraph and identify any misspelled medical words. Write the correct spelling of the word on the blank line.

Pyschiatry is the study of the mind, as is psychology. Our inner emotions are expressed as our outward effect. The neurotransmitters dopamin and seratonin are associated with depression. Mild depression is known as disthymia. Suiside attempts are not uncommon in depressed patients, but homocidal ideation is usually expressed by patients who are schizofrenic or have an antisocial personalty. Psychotic patients have strong feelings of paranoya and suspect others are trying to kill them. Patients who always need to be the center of attention are narcistic. Narcotics are drugs and inhalants are substances of abuse and adiction. A theraputic milyoo is a safe, secure environment for therapy.

1. ____________________
2. ____________________
3. ____________________
4. ____________________
5. ____________________
6. ____________________
7. ____________________
8. ____________________
9. ____________________
10. ____________________
11. ____________________
12. ____________________
13. ____________________
14. ____________________

Analysis of a Medical Report

This exercise contains a letter from a psychiatrist to the patient's primary care physician. Read the report and answer the questions.

Joseph Gildron, M.D.
Centennial Medical Building, Suite 201
2859 Bonnie Brae Road
Ebensberg, PA 15890

Re: HARDISH, Janine

Dear Dr. Gildron:

Thank you for referring your patient, Mrs. Janine Hardish, to me for psychiatric evaluation.

The patient is a 39-year-old, divorced Caucasian female. She lives in a single-family dwelling with her 2 children. In the past, she has worked part-time as a nurses' aide, but is not currently working because of feeling weak, dizzy, and tired. She states that she also feels depressed and hopeless. She claims that she has crying episodes every other day and difficulty sleeping at night.

She presents as a well-groomed lady whose clothes are neat, clean, and in good condition. Her hair is combed and her nails are clean and well-manicured. Her affect is moderately bright, and she is alert and oriented to time, person, and place. She is able to answer questions easily, logically, and with a moderate amount of detail. Her thought content is well-organized without evidence of flight of ideas or loose associations. Her fund of knowledge appears to be adequate. She is able to count backwards from 100 and to do serial 7s. Her memory for recent and remote events is intact. She was able to name the last 5 presidents. She is able to think of 18 words that begin with the letter "f" in 45 seconds (an above-normal result). However, she states that she feels that her memory is impaired.

She denies delusions or hallucinations. She denies feelings of being persecuted or plotted against. She denies suicidal or homicidal ideation.

She has little contact with her ex-husband. She is experiencing some difficulty with her finances at this time; her husband does send child support payments, but she is not currently working. Her oldest son is experiencing difficulties in his schoolwork and recently was pulled over by the police and given a ticket for driving over the speed limit.

She has been taking Elavil 2 mg P.O. at bedtime, as prescribed by you; however, she has also obtained a prescription for another tricyclic antidepressant from another physician and is taking this as well as Ambien for sleep.

It is my opinion that this patient is able to care for her own personal needs, is mentally intact, and has little difficulty relating to others.

DIAGNOSIS

Axis I Factitious disorder, not otherwise specified.

Axis II None.

Axis III Normal mental status and psychiatric evaluation. A complete physical and neurologic examination was not performed. No known documented physical illness.

Axis IV Moderate degree of psychosocial stressors.

Axis V GAF score is not computed because of factitious disorder.

Thank you for your referral of this patient.

Sincerely,

Daniel P. Bentley, M.D.

Daniel P. Bentley, M.D.

DPB:jbt
D: 11/19/20xx
T: 11/19/20xx

WORD ANALYSIS QUESTIONS

1. Divide *psychosocial* into its three word parts and define each word part.

   Word Part **Definition**

   ________ ____________________

   ________ ____________________

   ________ ____________________

2. Divide *factitious* into its two word parts and define each word part.

   Word Part **Definition**

   ________ ____________________

   ________ ____________________

3. Divide *homicidal* into its three word parts and define each word part.

   Word Part **Definition**

   ________ ____________________

   ________ ____________________

   ________ ____________________

4. A patient who has entertained ideas of suicide is said to be ____________ (adjective form).

FACT FINDING QUESTIONS

1. Define *factitious disorder.* ____________________
2. Name 3 psychosocial stressors that the patient is currently experiencing.

   a. ____________________

   b. ____________________

   c. ____________________

3. What evidence of drug-seeking behavior is mentioned in this report? ____________________

CRITICAL THINKING QUESTIONS

1. Flight of ideas is associated with which of these diseases? **bipolar disorder** **gender identity issues** **suicide**
2. How are delusions different from hallucinations? ____________________
3. Feelings of being persecuted or plotted against can be labeled as what mental illness? ____________________

Pronunciation Checklist

Read each word and its pronunciation. Practice pronouncing each word. Verify your pronunciation by listening to the Pronunciation List on the CD-ROM. Check the box next to the word after you master its pronunciation.

- ❑ acrophobia (AK-roh-FOH-bee-ah)
- ❑ addiction (ah-DIK-shun)
- ❑ affect (AF-fekt)
- ❑ affective (ah-FEK-tiv)
- ❑ agoraphobia (AG-or-ah-FOH-bee-ah)
- ❑ amnesia (am-NEE-zee-ah)
- ❑ amnestic (am-NES-tik)
- ❑ amygdaloid (ah-MIG-dah-loyd)
- ❑ anhedonia (AN-hee-DOH-nee-ah)
- ❑ anorexia nervosa (AN-oh-REK-see-ah ner-VOH-sah)
- ❑ anterograde amnesia (AN-ter-oh-grayd am-NEE-zee-ah)
- ❑ antianxiety drug (AN-tee-ang-ZY-eh-tee DRUHG)
- ❑ antidepressant drug (AN-tee-dee-PRES-ant DRUHG)
- ❑ antipsychotic drug (AN-tee-sy-KAWT-ik DRUHG)
- ❑ antisocial personality (AN-tee-SOH-shal PER-son-AL-ih-tee)
- ❑ anxiety (ang-ZY-eh-tee)
- ❑ apathy (AP-ah-thee)
- ❑ arachnophobia (ah-RAK-noh-FOH-bee-ah)
- ❑ autism (AW-tizm)
- ❑ aversion therapy (ah-VUHR-shun THAIR-ah-pee)
- ❑ behavioral (bee-HAYV-yer-al)
- ❑ bipolar disorder (by-POH-lar dis-OR-der)
- ❑ bulimia (byool-LIM-ee-ah)
- ❑ catalepsy (KAT-ah-LEP-see)
- ❑ catatonia (KAT-ah-TOH-nee-ah)
- ❑ catatonic (KAT-ah-TAWN-ik)
- ❑ cingulate gyrus (SIN-gyoo-layt JY-rus)
- ❑ claustrophobia (KLAW-stroh-FOH-bee-ah)
- ❑ cognitive (KAWG-nih-tiv)
- ❑ compulsion (com-PAWL-shun)
- ❑ compulsive (com-PAWL-siv)
- ❑ conversion (con-VER-shun)
- ❑ coprolalia (KAWP-roh-LAY-lee-ah)
- ❑ cyclothymia (SY-kloh-THY-mee-ah)
- ❑ delirium (deh-LEER-ee-um) (dee-LEER-ee-um)
- ❑ delirium tremens (dee-LEER-ee-um TREM-enz)
- ❑ delusion (dee-LOO-zhun)
- ❑ delusional (dee-LOO-zhun-al)
- ❑ dementia (dee-MEN-shee-ah)
- ❑ dependence (dee-PEN-dens)
- ❑ dependent personality (dee-PEN-dent PER-son-AL-ih-tee)
- ❑ depersonalization (dee-PER-son-al-ih-ZAY-shun)
- ❑ depression (dee-PRESH-un)
- ❑ depressive (dee-PRES-iv)
- ❑ desensitization therapy (dee-SEN-sih-tih-ZAY-shun THAIR-ah-pee)
- ❑ detoxification (dee-TAWK-sih-fih-KAY-shun)
- ❑ dissociative disorder (dih-SOH-see-ah-tiv dis-OR-der)
- ❑ dopamine (DOHP-ah-meen)
- ❑ dysmorphic (dis-MOR-fik)
- ❑ dysthymia (dis-THY-mee-ah)
- ❑ echolalia (EK-oh-LAY-lee-ah)
- ❑ electroconvulsive therapy (ee-LEK-troh-con-VUL-siv THAIR-ah-pee)
- ❑ emotion (ee-MOH-shun)
- ❑ encopresis (EN-koh-PREE-sis)
- ❑ epinephrine (EP-ih-NEF-rin)
- ❑ euphoria (yoo-FOR-ee-ah)
- ❑ exhibitionism (EK-sih-BISH-un-izm)
- ❑ factitious disorder (fak-TISH-us dis-OR-der)
- ❑ fetishism (FET-ish-izm)
- ❑ fornix (FOR-niks)
- ❑ fugue (FYOOG)
- ❑ global amnesia (GLOH-bal am-NEE-zee-ah)
- ❑ hallucination (hah-LOO-sih-NAY-shun)
- ❑ hallucinogen (hah-LOO-sin-oh-jen)
- ❑ hebephrenia (HEE-bah-FREE-nee-ah) (HEB-ee-FREE-nee-ah)
- ❑ hippocampus (HIP-oh-KAM-pus)
- ❑ histronic personality (HIH-stree-AW-nik PER-son-AL-ih-tee)
- ❑ homicidal ideation (HOHM-ih-SY-dal EYE-dee-AA-shun)
- ❑ hypochondriasis (HY-poh-con-DRY-ah-sis)
- ❑ hypnosis (hip-NOH-sis)
- ❑ hypothalamus (HY-poh-THAL-ah-mus)
- ❑ kleptomania (KLEP-toh-MAY-nee-ah)
- ❑ limbic lobe (LIM-bik LOHB)
- ❑ limbic system (LIM-bik SIS-tem)
- ❑ malingering (mah-LING-ger-ing)
- ❑ mania (MAY-nee-ah)
- ❑ manic (MAN-ik)
- ❑ masochism (MAS-oh-kizm)
- ❑ microphobia (MY-kroh-FOH-bee-ah)
- ❑ milieu (meel-YOO)
- ❑ Munchausen (moon-CHOW-zen)
- ❑ Munchausen by proxy (moon-CHOW-zen by PRAWK-see)
- ❑ narcissism (NAWR-sih-sizm)
- ❑ narcissistic personality (NAWR-sih-SIS-tik PER-son-AL-ih-tee)
- ❑ neologism (nee-AWL-oh-jizm)
- ❑ neurotransmitter (NYOOR-oh-TRANS-mit-er)
- ❑ norepinephrine (NOR-ep-ih-NEF-rin)
- ❑ obsession (awb-SESH-un)
- ❑ obsessive-compulsive disorder (awb-SES-iv com-PAWL-siv dis-OR-der)
- ❑ ophidiophobia (oh-FID-ee-oh-FOH-bee-ah)
- ❑ oppositional defiant disorder (AWP-ih-SIH-shun-al dee-FY-ant dis-OR-der)
- ❑ panic (PAN-ik)
- ❑ paranoia (PAIR-ah-NOY-ah)
- ❑ pathological (PATH-oh-LAWJ-ih-kal)
- ❑ pedophile (PEE-doh-file)
- ❑ pedophilia (PEE-doh-FIL-ee-ah)
- ❑ personality (PER-son-AL-ih-tee)
- ❑ phobia (FOH-bee-ah)
- ❑ phobic (FOH-bik)
- ❑ posttraumatic stress disorder (POST-trah-MAT-ik STRES dis-OR-der)
- ❑ premenstrual dysphoric syndrome (pree-MEN-stroo-al dis-FOR-ik SIN-drohm)
- ❑ psychiatric (SY-kee-AT-rik)
- ❑ psychiatrist (sy-KY-ah-trist)
- ❑ psychiatry (sy-KY-ah-tree)
- ❑ psychoanalysis (SY-koh-ah-NAL-ih-sis)
- ❑ psychologist (sy-KAWL-oh-jist)
- ❑ psychology (sy-KAWL-oh-jee)
- ❑ psychosis (sy-KOH-sis)
- ❑ psychotherapy (SY-koh-THAIR-ah-pee)
- ❑ pyromania (PY-roh-MAY-nee-ah)
- ❑ rape (RAYP)
- ❑ rapist (RAY-pist)
- ❑ reactive attachment disorder (ree-AK-tiv ah-TACH-ment dis-OR-der)

- ❑ repression (ree-PRESH-un)
- ❑ retrograde amnesia (RET-roh-grayd am-NEE-zee-ah)
- ❑ Rorschach test (ROHR-shahk TEST)
- ❑ sadism (SAY-dizm) (SAD-izm)
- ❑ schizophrenia (SKIZ-oh-FREE-nee-ah) (SKIT-soh-FREE-nee-ah)
- ❑ schizophrenic (SKIZ-oh-FREN-ik) (SKIT-soh-FREN-ik)
- ❑ serotonin (SER-oh-TOH-nin)
- ❑ social phobia (SOH-shal FOH-bee-ah)
- ❑ social worker (SOH-shal WER-ker)
- ❑ somatoform (soh-MAT-oh-form)
- ❑ suicidal ideation (SOO-ih-SY-dal EYE-dee-AA-shun)
- ❑ thalamus (THAL-ah-mus)
- ❑ thanatophobia (THAN-ah-toh-FOH-bee-ah)
- ❑ Thematic Apperception Test (thee-MAT-ik AP-er-SEP-shun TEST)
- ❑ therapeutic milieu (THAIR-ah-PYOO-tik meel-YOO)
- ❑ therapy (THAIR-ah-pee)
- ❑ tolerance (TAWL-er-ans)
- ❑ Tourette's syndrome (TOOR-etz SIN-drohm)
- ❑ transsexualism (tranz-SEK-shoo-ah-lizm)
- ❑ transvestism (trans-VES-tizm)
- ❑ trichotillomania (TRIK-oh-TIL-oh-MAY-nee-ah)
- ❑ voyeurism (VOY-yer-izm)
- ❑ xenophobia (ZEN-oh-FOH-bee-ah)

Experience Multimedia

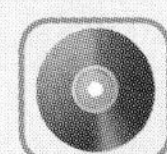

CD-ROM Learning Activities Checklist

Check off the box as you complete each learning activity.

- ❑ **CD-ROM Learning Activity 17.1: *ANATOMY WORD PARTS FLASHCARDS***
  Use flashcards to help you memorize word parts. Make your own flashcards or print out prepared flashcards.
  Time: 20 minutes.
- ❑ **CD-ROM Learning Activity 17.2: *MEDICINE IN ACTION***
  Watch a video clip about an autistic patient. Time: 5 minutes.
- ❑ **CD-ROM Learning Activity 17.3: *DISEASE AND OTHER WORD PARTS FLASHCARDS***
  A continuation of the flashcard learning activity. Time: 20 minutes.
- ❑ **CD-ROM Learning Activity 17.4: *MEMORY AIDS***
  Use memory aids to help you memorize medical words and meanings. Time: 5 minutes.
- ❑ **CD-ROM Learning Activity 17.5: *MEDICAL LANGUAGE SPOKEN HERE***
  Listen to actual medical reports and spell the missing medical words. Time: 10 minutes.
- ❑ **CD-ROM Learning Activity 17.6: *SPELLING CHALLENGE***
  Listen to a pronounced medical word and then spell it. Time: 5 minutes.
- ❑ **CD-ROM Learning Activity 17.7: *MEDICAL LANGUAGE PRONUNCIATION***
  Listen to a pronounced medical word and then practice pronouncing it. Time: 30 minutes.
- ❑ **CD-ROM Learning Activity 17.8: *EDUCATIONAL FUN AND GAMES***
  Enjoy these fun activities while reinforcing your knowledge. Time: 15 minutes.

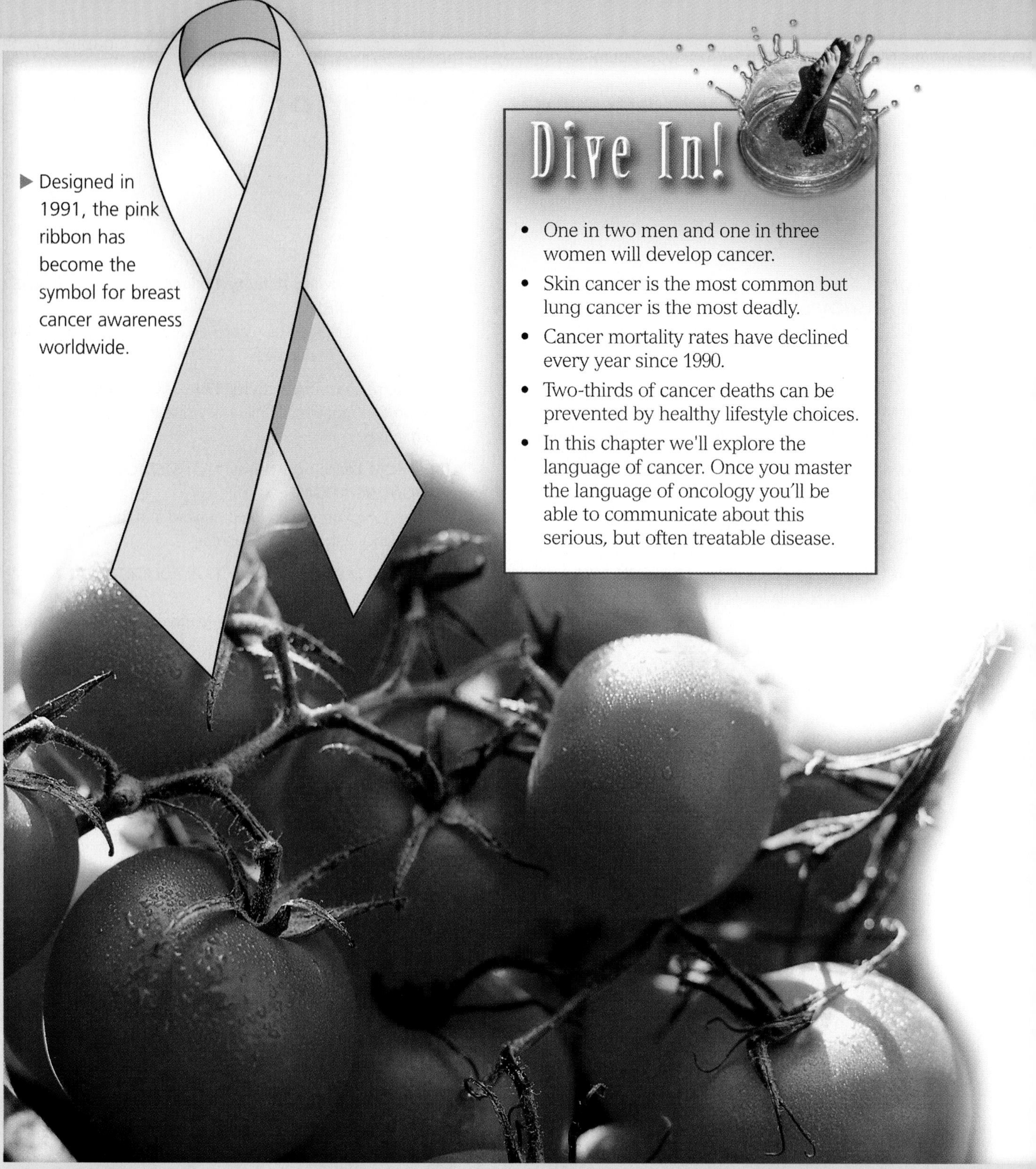

Designed in 1991, the pink ribbon has become the symbol for breast cancer awareness worldwide.

Dive In!

- One in two men and one in three women will develop cancer.
- Skin cancer is the most common but lung cancer is the most deadly.
- Cancer mortality rates have declined every year since 1990.
- Two-thirds of cancer deaths can be prevented by healthy lifestyle choices.
- In this chapter we'll explore the language of cancer. Once you master the language of oncology you'll be able to communicate about this serious, but often treatable disease.

Medicine Through HISTORY

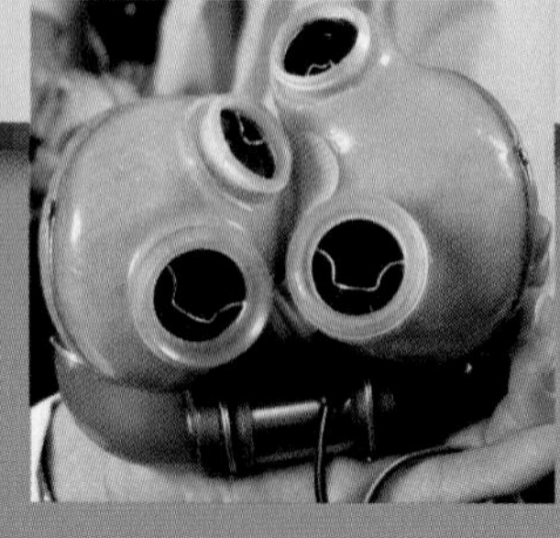

1982

Barney Clark is the first person to receive an implanted artificial heart, the Jarvik-7 created by Dr. Robert Jarvik

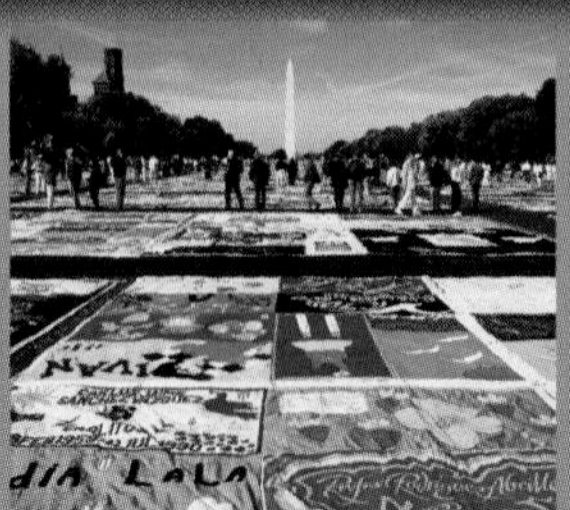

1982

The phrase acquired immunodeficiency syndrome (AIDS) is first used

1984

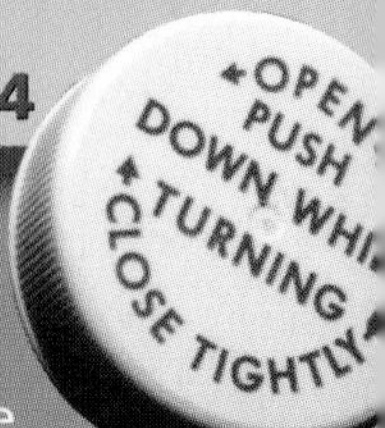

OPEN PUSH DOWN WHI TURNING CLOSE TIGHTLY

The child-proof safety cap fo medicine bottles is invented

CHAPTER 18 Oncology

▼ Cells are marvels of engineering, but change in their structure or function can result in cancer.

Oncology (ong-KAWL-oh-jee) is the medical specialty that studies the anatomy and physiology of a cancer cell and uses diagnostic tests, medical and surgical procedures, and drugs to treat cancerous diseases.

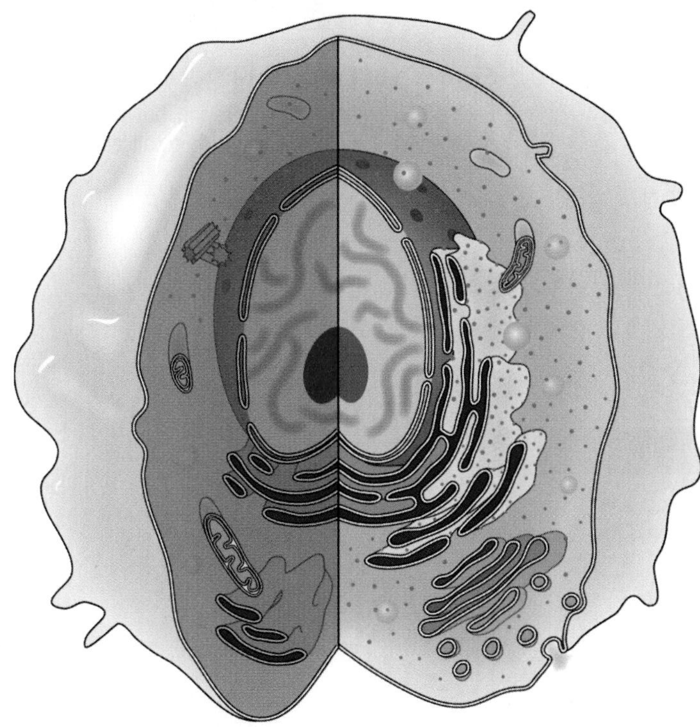

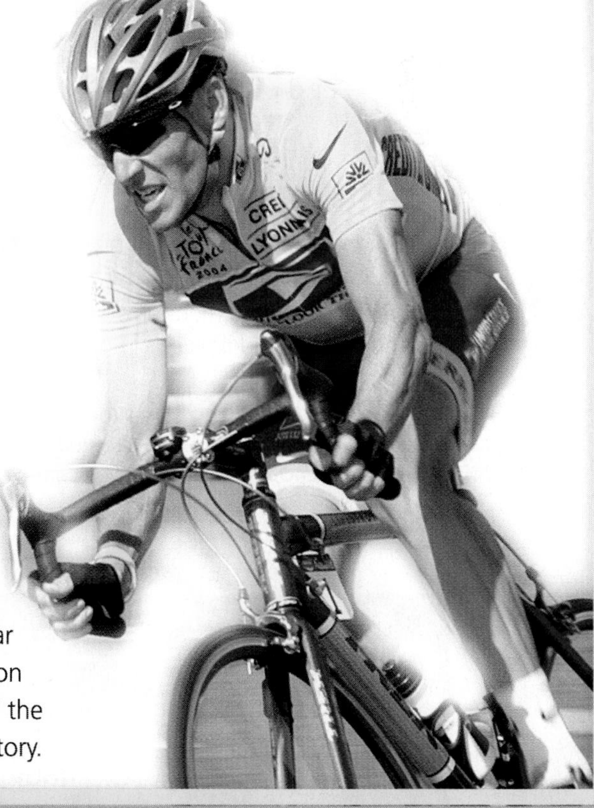

◀ Pass the ketchup! Lycopene is an antioxidant found in tomatoes that may help reduce the risk of prostate cancer.

▶ Lance Armstrong overcame testicular cancer and went on to become one of the best cyclists in history.

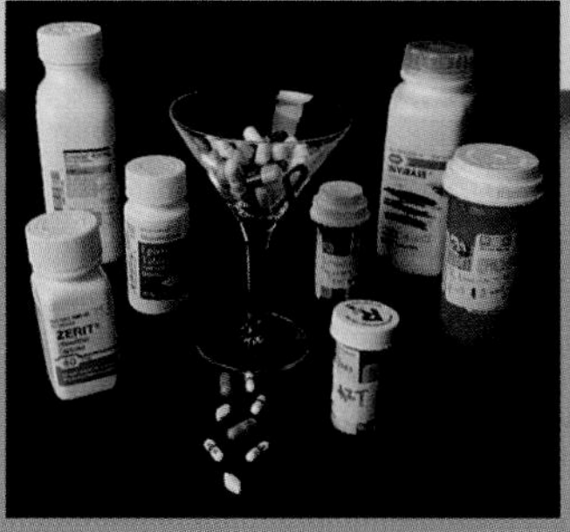

1984

AZT (Retrovir) is introduced as part of the drug "cocktail" to treat AIDS

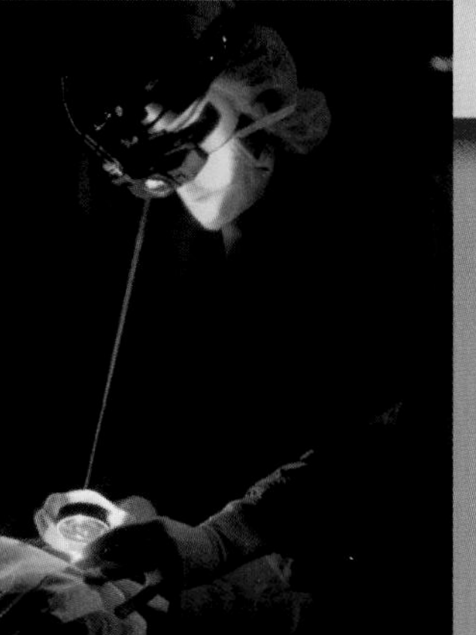

1988

Cataract surgery using a laser is first performed by Dr. Patricia Bath. She is also the first African American female physician to receive a patent for a medical device.

Measure Your Progress: Learning Objectives

After you study this chapter, you should be able to

1. Identify the anatomical structures of a cell by correctly labeling them on an anatomical illustration.
2. List six characteristics of cancerous cells and tumors.
3. Describe the process by which normal cells become cancerous cells.
4. Build oncologic words from combining forms, prefixes, and suffixes.
5. Describe common oncologic diseases.
6. Describe common oncologic diagnostic laboratory and radiology tests.
7. Describe common oncologic medical and surgical procedures and drug categories.
8. Define common oncologic abbreviations.
9. Apply your skills by analyzing an oncology report.
10. Test your knowledge of oncology by completing review exercises at the end of the chapter and learning activities on the CD-ROM.

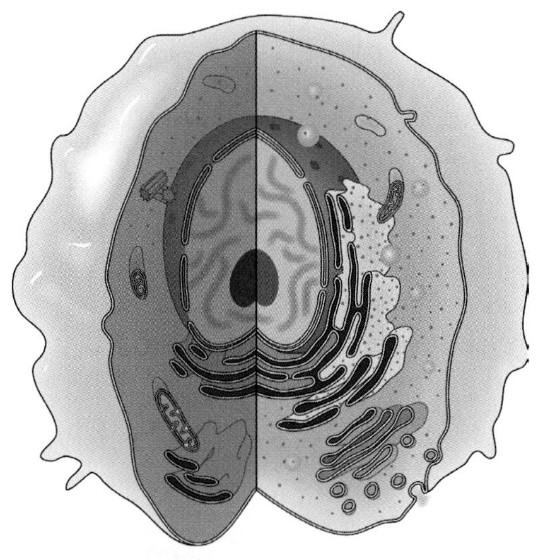

Figure 18-1 ■ A cell.

Each cell is a marvel of engineering, but a change in its structure or function can result in cancer.

Medical Language Key

To unlock the meaning of a medical word, first define each word part. Then put the word part definitions in order, beginning with the suffix, followed by the first word part.

	Word Part	Word Part Definition
SUFFIX	-logy	*the study of*
COMBINING FORM	onc/o-	*tumor, mass*

Oncology: *The study of [cancerous] tumors and masses.*

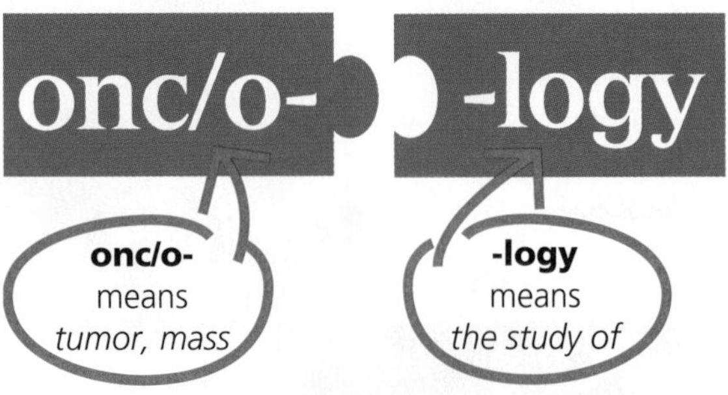

www.prenhall.com/turley

For interactive flashcards, real-life video clips, games, exercises, and audio pronunciations please explore the companion CD-ROM in the back of the book. Click on the companion website for bonus chapters, additional resources, and links to on-line learning.

Anatomy and Physiology

Unlike the other medical specialties you have already studied, the medical specialty of oncology is not based on a particular body system. Oncology encompasses all of the body systems because cancer can occur anywhere in the body.

Cancer arises from various types of cells and tissues that often lend their names to the cancer. Cancer begins as a single normal cell (see Figure 18-1 ■) that becomes an abnormal cell, and so we will begin our study of oncology by studying the structure and function of a normal cell.

cancer (KAN-ser)
Cancer is a Latin word meaning *a crab.* Cancer reaches out and eats away at nearby tissues much like the pincers on a crab reach out to nearby objects.

cancerous (KAN-ser-us)
cancer/o- *cancer*
-ous *pertaining to*

Anatomy Related to Oncology

Cells

A **cell** is the smallest independently functioning structure in the body that can reproduce itself by division. Cells come in many shapes and sizes, but all cells contain certain basic structures (see Figure 18-2 ■). The **cell membrane** around the cell is a permeable barrier that protects and supports the **intracellular contents.** It allows water and nutrients to enter the cell and cellular waste products to leave the cell. It also contains ion pumps that actively bring electrolytes (sodium, potassium, and so forth) in and out of the cell. The **cytoplasm** is a gel-like substance that fills the cell.

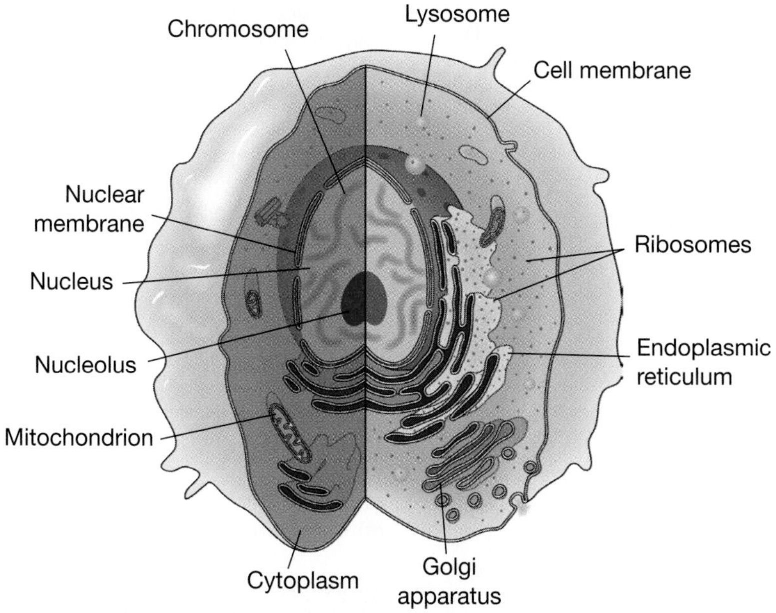

Figure 18-2 ■ The structures of a cell.

A cell consists of many different structures, each of which plays a unique role in securing nutrients, producing energy, building proteins, fighting invading pathogens, or overseeing cellular division and other cellular activities.

cell (SEL)
Cell is derived from a Latin word meaning *a storeroom or chamber.*

cellular (SEL-yoo-lar)
cellul/o- *cell*
-ar *pertaining to*

intracellular (IN-trah-SEL-yoo-lar)
intra- *within*
cellul/o- *cell*
-ar *pertaining to*

cytoplasm (SY-toh-plazm)
cyt/o- *cell*
-plasm *growth; formed substance*

The cytoplasm contains a variety of dissolved substances as well as several different embedded structures that are collectively known as **organelles.**

- **Chromosomes.** Paired structures within the nucleus. Each cell nucleus contains 23 pairs of chromosomes for a total of 46 chromosomes. In each pair of chromosomes, one of the chromosomes was inherited from the mother and the other was inherited from the father. A single chromosome is made of one long DNA (**deoxyribonucleic acid**) molecule. The DNA molecule consists of repeating pairs of amino acids sequenced along two strands to form a double helix. A **gene** is one segment of a DNA molecule that contains enough amino acid pairs to furnish the information needed to produce one protein molecule. In a cell that is not dividing, each long DNA molecule is loosely coiled, giving the nucleus a woven, grainy appearance under the microscope. As the cell prepares to divide, each DNA molecule coils tightly, making the chromosomes visible as rodlike structures in the nucleus.
- **Endoplasmic reticulum.** Network of channels throughout the cytoplasm that transports materials within the cell. Also the site of protein, fat, and glycogen synthesis.
- **Golgi apparatus.** Curved, stacked membranes that process and store proteins (hormones or enzymes) that will be released by the cell. It also makes lysosomes and the digestive enzymes in them.
- **Lysosomes.** Small sacs that contain powerful digestive enzymes to destroy a bacterium or virus that invades the cell. When a cell dies, the lysosomes disintegrate and release their enzymes within the cell, and the cell is slowly destroyed.
- **Messenger RNA.** Messenger RNA (**ribonucleic acid**) duplicates the information contained in a gene and carries that information to the ribosome where it is used to assemble amino acids to produce a protein molecule.
- **Mitochondria.** Large, individual, capsule-shaped structures with sectioned chambers that produce and store ATP, a high-energy molecule obtained from the metabolism of glucose. As needed, the mitochondria convert ATP to ADP to release energy for cellular activities.

organelle (OR-gah-NEL) (OR-gah-nel)
organ/o- *organ*
-elle *little thing*

chromosome (KROH-moh-sohm)
chrom/o- *color*
-some *a body*
Add words to make a correct and complete definition of *chromosome: a body [that takes on] color [when stained].*

chromosomal (KROH-moh-SOH-mal)
chrom/o- *color*
som/o- *a body*
-al *pertaining to*

deoxyribonucleic acid
(dee-AWK-see-RY-boh-noo-KLEE-ik AS-id)

gene (JEEN)
Gene is derived from a Greek word meaning *to produce.*

genetic (jeh-NET-ik)
gene/o- *gene*
-tic *pertaining to*

endoplasmic (EN-doh-PLAS-mik)
endo- *innermost, within*
plasm/o- *plasma; formed substance*
-ic *pertaining to*

reticulum (reh-TIK-yoo-lum)
Reticulum is a Latin word meaning *a little net.*

Golgi (GOHL-jee)
The Golgi apparatus was named by Camillo Golgi (1843–1926), an Italian neurologist. This is an example of an eponym: a person from whom something takes its name.

lysosome (LY-soh-sohm)
lys/o- *break down or dissolve*
-some *a body*
Add words to make a correct and complete definition of *lysosome: a body [that contains enzymes that] break down or dissolve [a bacterium or virus].*

ribonucleic acid
(RY-boh-nyoo-KLEE-ik AS-id)

mitochondrion (MY-toh-CON-dree-on)
mitochondria (MY-toh-CON-dree-ah)

mitochondrial (MY-toh-CON-dree-al)
mit/o- *threadlike structure*
chondri/o- *little granule*
-al *pertaining to*
Mitochondria vary in shape from a thread to a rod to a sphere.

- **Nucleus.** Large, round, centralized body that is surrounded by a nuclear membrane. Through the action of DNA, it controls all of the activities that take place within the cell, such as the production of cellular proteins and the production of enzymes to control metabolism in the cell. The **nucleolus** is a round, central region within the nucleus. It produces RNA and ribosomes.
- **Ribosomes.** Granular structures located throughout the cytoplasm and on the endoplasmic reticulum. Ribosomes contain RNA and proteins and are the site of protein synthesis.

nucleus (NYOO-klee-us)
nuclei (NYOO-klee-eye)
Nucleus is a Latin singular masculine noun meaning *kernal.* Form the plural by changing *-us* to *-i.*

nuclear (NYOO-klee-ar)
nucle/o- *nucleus*
-ar *pertaining to*

nucleolus (nyoo-KLEE-oh-lus)
nucleoli (nyoo-KLEE-oh-lie)
Nucleolus is a Latin singular masculine noun meaning *little nucleus.* Form the plural by changing *-us* to *-i.*

nucleolar (nyoo-KLEE-oh-lar)
nucleol/o- *nucleolus*
-ar *pertaining to*

ribosome (RY-boh-sohm)
rib/o- *ribonucleic acid*
-some *a body*

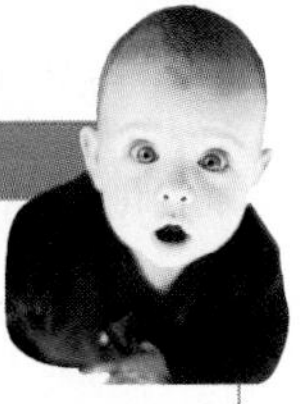

Did You Know?

Most body cells contain one central nucleus. However, mature erythrocytes (red blood cells) do not contain any nucleus, and each skeletal muscle cell contains several nuclei.

Physiology of Cellular Division and Cancer

Mitosis is the process by which a cell divides. Mitosis begins in the nucleus as each chromosome makes an exact copy of itself. (The double helix of its DNA molecule splits down its length and rebuilds to form another double helix.) All of the chromosomes and their identical copies align themselves along threadlike filaments in the nucleus and then separate to opposite sides of the nucleus. Then the entire nucleus and cytoplasm split, forming two cells that are identical to the original cell.

Normal body cells divide in an orderly fashion and in response to a particular need. During puberty, growth hormone causes the cells of the body to divide as a child grows. During times of blood loss, the hormone erythropoietin stimulates stem cells in the bone marrow to divide and produce more mature erythrocytes (red blood cells). In an adult who is healthy and no longer growing, the **mitotic rate** is controlled by cells. The rate of mitosis is different for different types of cells. Skin cells have a high rate of mitosis because they are constantly being shed from the surface of the body. In contrast, muscle cells divide less frequently. **Supressor genes,** a group of genes in the DNA of each cell, inhibit mitosis and keep each cell from dividing excessively.

mitosis (my-TOH-sis)
mit/o- *threadlike structure*
-osis *condition; abnormal condition; process*
Add words to make a correct and complete definition of *mitosis: a condition [of cell division during which the chromosomes align along] threadlike structures [in the nucleus].*

mitotic (my-TAWT-ik)
mit/o- *threadlike structure*
-tic *pertaining to*

suppressor (soo-PRES-or)
suppress/o- *press down*
-or *person or thing that produces or does*

A Closer Look

The p53 gene is the most important suppressor gene. It is located on chromosome 17 in every cell. It is inactive until DNA in the cell's nucleus is damaged. The p53 gene recognizes the DNA damage and activates proteins to repair the damage. While the DNA is being repaired, the p53 gene inhibits mitosis to decrease the chance of producing more defective cells. Because of their role in preventing the formation of cancer cells, suppressor genes are also known as tumor suppressor genes. If the DNA cannot be repaired, the p53 gene directs the cell to shut down. This is known as **apoptosis** or programmed cell death.

apoptosis (AP-awp-TOH-sis)
apo- *away from*
-ptosis *state of prolapse or drooping; falling*
Apoptosis is the falling away of a cell from life to death.

Damage to the DNA molecule of a chromosome consists of **genetic mutations** that delete genes, reverse their normal order, or break off segments of genes and insert them into other chromosomes (a process known as **translocation**).

Damage to DNA can be caused by a number of different factors: carcinogens, pathogens, or heredity. Most of these factors do not immediately cause cancer. It is only after prolonged exposure that the cellular DNA is damaged beyond repair.

mutation (myoo-TAY-shun)
mutat/o- *to change*
-ion *action; condition*

translocation (TRANS-loh-KAY-shun)
trans- *across, through*
locat/o- *a place*
-ion *action; condition*

Factors that Contribute to the Development of Cancer (see Figure 18-3 ■)

1. **Carcinogens** (environmental substances)

   radiation (sunlight, x-rays, radiation therapy, nuclear weapons)

   chemicals (insecticides, dyes)

   fumes (industrial pollution, radon gas from the soil, cigarette tar and smoke, automobile exhaust)

   foreign particles that cause chronic irritation (asbestos)

   some chemotherapy drugs

   some hormone drugs

2. **Pathogens** (bacteria and viruses)

   Chronic irritation and inflammation from a bacterial or viral infection can eventually damage DNA.

   The human papillomavirus causes genital warts and chronic inflammation that can lead to cervical cancer in women.

   Oncogenes are mutated genes within viral RNA. When the virus enters and infects a normal cell, its oncogene becomes incorporated into the normal cell's DNA, changing it into a cancerous cell.

carcinogen (KAR-SIN-oh-jen)
carcin/o- *cancer*
-gen *that which produces*

pathogen (PATH-oh-jen)
path/o- *disease, suffering*
-gen *that which produces*

oncogene (AWNG-koh-jeen)
onc/o- *tumor, mass*
-gene *gene*

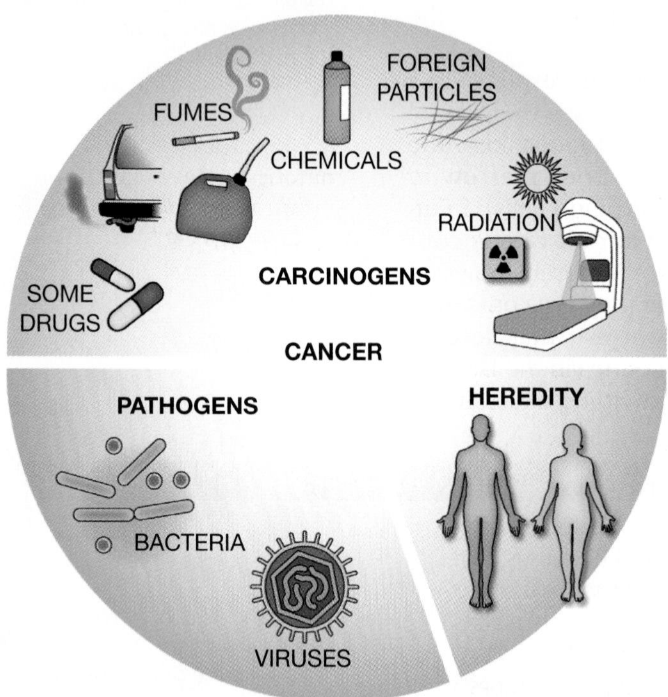

Figure 18-3 ■ Causes of cancer.
Cancer is caused by carcinogens in the environment, pathogens (bacteria and viruses), and oncogenes (genes within a virus).

Human immunodeficiency virus (HIV) weakens the immune response until the body is unable to destroy newly formed cancerous cells.

3. **Heredity.** Some persons inherit damaged DNA or an oncogene from one of their parents.

heredity (heh-RED-ih-tee)
hered/o- *genetic inheritance*
-ity *state; condition*

If the DNA in a chromosome is damaged, and the damaged area includes the p53 gene, then the cell loses the mechanism with which to repair itself. The damage remains, and the damaged cell cannot stop itself from dividing and producing more damaged cells. More than one half of all cancer cells show damage to the p53 gene. However, even if the p53 gene is not functioning, the body has other means of detecting and destroying cancerous cells.

1. Specialized lymphocytes known as NK cells (natural killer cells) detect, engulf, and destroy a cancerous cell.
2. If NK cells do not destroy a cancerous cell, the lymphatic system takes it up as it collects tissue fluid to make lymph. The lymph carries the cancerous cell to a lymph node where it is filtered out of the lymph. In the lymph node, macrophages phagocytize and destroy the cancerous cell.
3. Lymph nodes release **tumor necrosis factor,** a substance that causes a cancer cell to become necrotic and die.

tumor (TOO-mor)
Tumor is a Latin word meaning *a swelling.*

necrosis (neh-KROH-sis)
necr/o- *death*
-osis *condition; abnormal condition; process*

Cancerous cells that are not destroyed by any of these means go on to grow and form cancerous tumors.

Characteristics of Cancerous Cells and Tumors

1. Cancerous cells are not part of and do not contribute to the normal structure and function of the body. Once a single cancerous cell has been produced, it stops functioning as a normal cell and takes on the characteristics of a cancerous cell.
2. Cancerous cells lack differentiation and cannot perform the specialized functions of normal cells.

A Closer Look

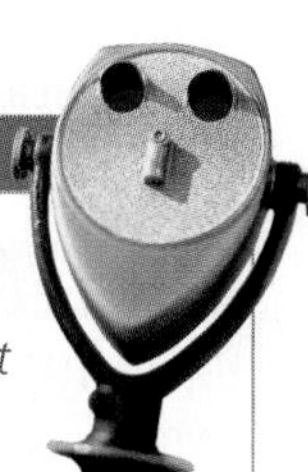

A human being begins as a single cell that immediately begins to divide. By the end of the first week of life, the individual cells begin to differentiate, migrating to various parts of the body and changing into specialized cells that produce specific tissues (like muscle or bone) with different shapes and functions. This process is known as **cellular differentiation.** Cancer cells arise from a particular type of tissue (like muscle or bone), but then lose this differentiation and revert back to an immature, embryonal, **undifferentiated** appearance.

differentiation (DIF-er-EN-shee-AA-shun)
differentiat/o- *being distinct or specialized*
-ion *action; condition*

undifferentiated (un-DIF-er-EN-shee-aa-ted)
un- *not*
differentiat/o- *being distinct or specialized*
-ed *pertaining to*

3. Cancerous cells are of varying sizes and are not arranged in an orderly fashion (stacked on top of each other or all oriented in the same direction) like normal cells.
4. Cancerous cells divide more rapidly than normal cells. Cancerous tumors grow more quickly than normal tissue.

5. The growth of cancerous cells cannot be easily controlled by the body.
6. Cancerous cells form a tumor that is irregular in shape and is not **encapsulated** like a benign tumor.
7. A cancerous tumor releases a substance that causes blood vessels in the surrounding tissues to grow into the tumor to provide it with nutrients. This process is known as **angiogenesis.** The tumor grows rapidly but often has a central core of tissue that is necrotic because the blood supply was inadequate.
8. Cancerous tumors are **invasive.** They penetrate (infiltrate) normal tissues around them, hindering tissue function and destroying normal cells.
9. Cancerous cells break off and move through the blood vessels and lymphatic vessels to other sites in the body. This process is known as **metastasis.** The cancerous cells are said to **metastasize** and are characterized as being **metastatic** (see Figure 18-4 ■).

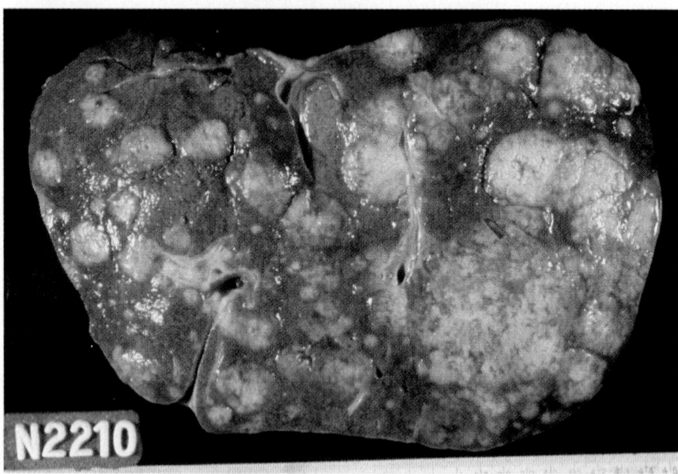

Figure 18-4 ■ Metastases.
This liver was removed from a patient who died of cancer. It shows multiple areas of metatasis of cancer from a primary site elsewhere in the body.

Did You Know?

In his 1974 text, *An Introduction to Drugs,* Michael C. Gerald wrote: "Cancerous cells are the anarchists of the body, for they know no law, pay no regard for the commonwealth, serve no useful function, and cause disharmony and death in their surrounds."

encapsulated (en-KAP-soo-lay-ted)
en- *in, within, inward*
capsul/o- *capsule (enveloping structure)*
-ated *pertaining to a condition; composed of*

angiogenesis (AN-jee-oh-JEN-eh-sis)
angi/o- *blood vessel; lymphatic vessel*
gen/o- *arising from; produced by*
-esis *condition*

invasive (in-VAY-siv)
invas/o- *to go into*
-ive *pertaining to*

metastasis (meh-TAS-tah-sis)
metastases (meh-TAS-tah-seez)
meta- *after, subsequent to; transition; change*
-stasis *condition of standing still; staying in one place*
Add words to make a correct and complete definition of *metastasis: Condition of [a cell that is normally] staying in one place [undergoing] change [and moving to other parts of the body].*

metastasize (meh-TAS-tah-size)
meta- *after, subsequent to; transition; change*
stas/o- *standing still; staying in one place*
-ize *affecting in a particular way*

metastatic (MET-ah-STAT-ik)
meta- *after, subsequent to; transition; change*
stat/o- *standing still; staying in one place*
-ic *pertaining to*

Vocabulary Review

Now that you have studied the anatomy and physiology of normal cells and cancerous cells, take time to review those new words and descriptions. Memorize the combining forms and their definitions before going on to the next section.

Word or Phrase	Combining Form and Definition	Description
angiogenesis	angi/o- *blood vessel; lymphatic vessel* gen/o- *arising from; produced by*	Process by which a cancerous tumor causes blood vessels in the surrounding tissues to grow into the tumor and provide it with nutrients
apoptosis		Programmed cell death in which the p53 gene directs the cell to shut down when its DNA is too damaged to be repaired
cell	cellul/o- *cell*	Smallest, independently functioning structure in the body that can reproduce itself by division
cell membrane		Permeable barrier that surrounds a cell and holds in the cytoplasm. It allows water and nutrients to enter and waste products to leave the cell.
carcinogen	carcin/o- *cancer*	Environmental substance that can contribute to the development of cancer
chromosome	chrom/o- *color*	Paired, rodlike structures within the nucleus. Each cell contains 46 chromosomes (23 pairs).
cytoplasm	cyt/o- *cell*	Gel-like intracellular substance. Organelles are embedded in it.
differentiation	differentiat/o- *being distinct or specialized*	Process by which embryonic cells assume different shapes and function in different parts of the body
DNA		Deoxyribonucleic acid. Sequenced pairs of amino acids that form a double helix chain within a chromosome. One segment of DNA makes up a gene.
encapsulated	capsul/o- *capsule (enveloping structure)*	Having a capsule or enveloping structure around it. Benign tumors have a capsule; cancerous tumors do not.
endoplasmic reticulum	plasm/o- *plasma; formed substance*	Organelle that consists of a network of channels that transport materials within the cell. Also the site of protein, fat, and glycogen synthesis.
gene		An area on a chromosome that contains all the DNA information needed to produce one type of protein molecule
genetic mutation	gene/o- *gene* mutat/o- *to change*	Damage to the DNA molecule that deletes genes, reverses the normal order of genes, or breaks off gene segments from one chromosome and inserts them in another chromosome
Gogli apparatus		Organelle that consists of curved, stacked membranes that process and store intracellular hormones and enzymes. Also makes lysosomes and their digestive enzymes.
heredity	hered/o- *genetic inheritance*	Genetic inheritance passed on from the DNA of the father and mother to the child. Genetic mutations that cause cancer can be inherited.
intracellular	cellul/o- *cell*	Within a cell

Word or Phrase	Combining Form and Definition	Description
invasive	invas/o- *to go into*	Characteristic of cancerous tumors. They penetrate and destroy the normal cells around them, compromising tissue functions.
lysosome	lys/o- *break down or dissolve*	Organelle that consists of a small sac with digestive enzymes in it. It destroys pathogens that invade the cell.
messenger RNA		RNA that duplicates DNA information in the nucleus and carries that information to the ribosome.
metastasis	stat/o- *standing still; staying in one place*	Process by which cancerous cells break off from a tumor and move through the blood vessels or lymphatic vessels to other sites in the body
mitochondrium	mit/o- *threadlike structure*	Organelle that produces and stores ATP and then converts it to ADP to release energy for cellular activities
mitosis	mit/o- *threadlike structure*	Process of cellular division. The chromosomes duplicate and then migrate to either end of the cell as the cell divides to become two. The rate of cellular division is known as the **mitotic rate.**
nucleolus	nucleol/o- *nucleolus*	Round, central region within the nucleus. It makes RNA and ribosomes.
nucleus	nucle/o- *nucleus*	Large, round, centralized intracellular body that contains chromosomes and their DNA. It controls all of the cell's activities. It is surrounded by a nuclear membrane.
oncogene	onc/o- *tumor, mass*	Damaged and mutated genes that cause a cell to become cancerous. A virus can carry an oncogene in its RNA. Then when it enters a normal cell, the oncogene becomes incorporated into the cell's DNA and changes it into a cancerous cell.
organelle	organ/o- *organ*	Small structures in the cytoplasm that have various specialized functions. Organelles include mitochondria, ribosomes, the endoplasmic reticulum, the Golgi apparatus, and lysosomes.
pathogen	path/o- *disease, suffering*	Microorganism (bacterium, virus, and so forth) that causes infection
ribosome	rib/o- *ribonucleic acid*	Granular organelle located throughout the cytoplasm and on the endoplasmic reticulum. Ribosomes contain RNA and proteins and are the site of protein synthesis.
RNA		Ribonucleic acid created in the nucleolus and stored in ribosomes
suppressor genes	suppress/o- *press down*	Group of genes in the DNA of each cell that inhibits mitosis. The p53 gene is the most important suppressor gene.
translocation	locat/o- *a place*	Damage to the DNA that breaks off a gene segment from one chromosome and puts it into another chromosome
tumor necrosis factor	necr/o- *death*	Substance released from lymph nodes that kills cancerous cells
undifferentiated	differentiat/o- *being distinct or specialized*	Cells that are immature and embryonal in appearance and behavior

Labeling Exercise

Match each anatomy word or phrase to its numbered structure in Figure 18-5■. Write that word or phrase on the blank line next to its number. Use the Answer Key at the end of the book to check your answers.

cell membrane	endoplasmic reticulum	mitochondrian	nucleus
chromosome	Golgi apparatus	nuclear membrane	ribosomes
cytoplasm	lysosome	nucleolus	

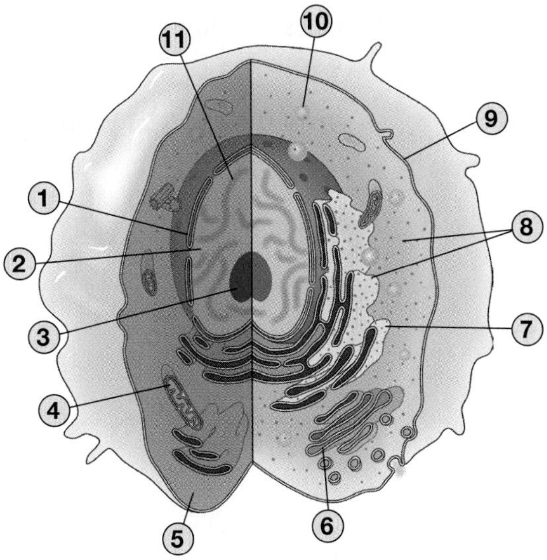

1. ______________
2. ______________
3. ______________
4. ______________
5. ______________
6. ______________
7. ______________
8. ______________
9. ______________
10. ______________
11. ______________

Figure 18-5 ■

Building Medical Words

Combining Forms

Here are the combining forms you have learned so far. Next to each combining form, write its meaning. Use the Answer Key at the end of the book to check your answers. The first one has been done for you.

	Combining Form	Medical Meaning		Combining Form	Medical Meaning
1.	differentiat/o-	being distinct or specialized	15.	lys/o-	
2.	angi/o-		16.	mit/o-	
3.	cancer/o-		17.	mutat/o-	
4.	capsul/o-		18.	necr/o-	
5.	carcin/o-		19.	nucle/o-	
6.	cellul/o-		20.	nucleol/o-	
7.	chondri/o-		21.	onc/o-	
8.	chrom/o-		22.	organ/o-	
9.	cyt/o-		23.	plasm/o-	
10.	gene/o-		24.	rib/o-	
11.	gen/o-		25.	som/o-	
12.	hered/o-		26.	stas/o-	
13.	invas/o-		27.	stat/o-	
14.	locat/o-		28.	suppress/o-	

Combining Forms and Suffixes

Read the definition hint for the medical word you are to build. Look at the combining form that is given. Write the correct suffix on the blank line. Then write the medical word. (Remember: You may need to remove the combining vowel. Always remove the hyphens and slash.) Use the Answer Key at the end of the book to check your answers. The first one has been done for you.

SUFFIX LIST		
-ar (pertaining to)	-ion (action; condition)	-ous (pertaining to)
-elle (little thing)	-ity (state; condition)	-plasm (growth; formed structure)
-gen (that which produces)	-ive (pertaining to)	-some (a body)
-gene (gene)	-osis (condition; abnormal condition; process)	-tic (pertaining to)

	Definition Hint	Combining Form	Suffix	Write the Medical Word
1.	A body of ribonucleic acid	rib/o-	-some	ribosome
2.	Pertaining to cancer	cancer/o-	________	________
3.	Condition of death	necr/o-	________	________
4.	Pertaining to go into	invas/o-	________	________
5.	Pertaining to genes	gene/o-	________	________
6.	Formed substance that makes up a cell	cyt/o-	________	________
7.	Little organ	organ/o-	________	________
8.	Pertaining to a cell	cellul/o-	________	________
9.	A body that (contains an enzyme that) breaks down things	lys/o-	________	________
10.	That which produces cancer	carcin/o-	________	________
11.	Gene that causes a tumor or mass	onc/o-	________	________
12.	State of genetic inheritance	hered/o-	________	________
13.	Pertaining to the nucleus	nucle/o-	________	________
14.	A body that has a color (when stained)	chrom/o-	________	________
15.	Action that involves a change	mutat/o-	________	________

Symptoms, Signs, and Types of Cancer

General

Word or Phrase	Word Part and Definition	Description
anaplasia	**anaplasia** (AN-ah-PLAY-zee-ah) (AN-ah-PLAY-zha) ana- *apart from; excessive* plas/o- *growth, formation* -ia *condition, state, thing*	Condition in which normal cells that are mature and differentiated become cancerous cells that are undifferentiated in appearance and behavior
cancer	**cancer** (KAN-ser) **cancerous** (KAN-ser-us)	General word for any type of **cancerous** cell or tumor. There are four broad categories of cancer: carcinoma, sarcoma, leukemia, and embryonal cell carcinoma. Cancer is treated with chemotherapy, radiation therapy, surgery, or a combination of these, depending on the type and extent of the cancer.
carcinoid tumor	**carcinoid** (KAR-sih-noyd) carcin/o- *cancer* -oid *resembling*	Slow-growing cancerous tumor that seldom metastasizes. It does not exhibit all of the characteristics of cancer. It occurs mainly in the digestive tract. **Carcinoid syndrome** is a set of symptoms caused by the release of the hormone serotonin from a carcinoid tumor.
carcinomatosis	**carcinomatosis** (KAR-sih-NOH-mah-TOH-sis) *Carcinomatosis* is a combination of *carcinomata* (the plural form of carcinoma) and the suffix *-osis* (condition; abnormal condition; process).	General word for a condition in which cancerous tumors are present in multiple sites in the body
dysplasia	**dysplasia** (dis-PLAY-zee-ah) (dis-PLAY-zha) dys- *painful, difficult, abnormal* plas/o- *growth, formation* -ia *condition, state, thing* **dysplastic** (dis-PLAS-tik) dys- *painful, difficult, abnormal* plas/o- *growth, formation* -tic *pertaining to* Some word parts have more than one definition. The best definition of *dysplastic* is *pertaining to abnormal growth or formation [of cells].*	Condition of atypical cells that are abnormal in size, shape, or organization, but have not yet become cancerous. These cells are said to be **dysplastic.** Dysplasia is the result of chronic irritation and inflammation.
lymphadenopathy	**lymphadenopathy** (LIM-fad-eh-NAWP-ah-thee) lymph/o- *lymph; lymphatic system* aden/o- *gland* -pathy *disease, suffering*	Enlarged lymph nodes. The lymph nodes trap cancerous cells that break away from the site of the original tumor. The lymph node itself then becomes a site of cancer. Chains of lymph nodes in the neck, axillae, and groin regions are common sites of lymphadenopathy.

Word or Phrase	Word Part and Definition	Description
neoplasm	**neoplasm** (NEE-oh-plazm) **ne/o-** *new* **-plasm** *growth; formed substance* **neoplasia** (NEE-oh-PLAY-zee-ah) **ne/o-** *new* **plas/o-** *growth, formation* **-ia** *condition, state, thing* **tumor** (TOO-mor) *Tumor* is a Latin word meaning *a swelling.* **malignant** (mah-LIG-nant) **malign/o-** *intentionally causing harm; cancer* **-ant** *pertaining to* **benign** (bee-NINE) *Benign* is derived from a Latin word meaning *kind, not cancerous.*	General word for any growing tissue that is not part of normal body structure or function. Neoplasms are also known as **tumors. Neoplasia** is the process by which a neoplasm develops. Neoplasms are either **malignant** or **benign.** Malignant neoplasms are known as cancer.
relapse	**relapse** (REE-laps) *Relapse* is derived from a Latin word meaning *to slide back.*	Return of the symptoms or signs of cancer after a period of improvement or even remission
remission	**remission** (ree-MISH-un) **remiss/o-** *send back* **-ion** *action; condition*	Period of time during which there are no symptoms or signs of cancer. A remission occurs after the successful treatment of cancer.
site of the tumor	**in situ** (in SY-too) *In situ* is a Latin phrase meaning *in the site of origin.*	Area where the cancerous cell first formed and grew into a cancerous tumor is known as the **primary site.** When the tumor is still contained in that area it is said to be **in situ.** When the tumor spreads or metastasizes via the blood or lymphatic system to a distant part of the body, that area is known as the **secondary site.** There is always just one primary site, but there may be several secondary sites.

Did You Know?

Screening examinations are extremely important in the early detection of cancer. Self-examination of the breasts and testes is performed by the patient. Other examinations, such as mammography and colonoscopy, should be performed at regular intervals by healthcare professionals.

WARNING SIGNS OF SOME COMMON TYPES OF CANCER

The American Cancer Society promotes the use of the acronym CAUTION as a memory aid to help healthcare professionals and others remember the ways in which early cancer can present.

- **C** Change in bowel or bladder habits
- **A** A sore that does not heal
- **U** Unusual bleeding or discharge
- **T** Thickening or lump
- **I** Indigestion or trouble swallowing
- **O** Obvious changes in a wart or mole
- **N** Nagging cough or hoarseness

Carcinomas

Word or Phrase	Word Part and Definition	Description
adenocarcinoma	**adenocarcinoma** (AD-eh-noh-KAR-sih-NOH-mah) aden/o- *gland* carcin/o- *cancer* -oma *tumor, mass* **ductal** (DUK-tal) duct/o- *bring or move; a duct* -al *pertaining to*	Cancer of the epithelial cells that line the ducts of the lactiferous glands of the breast (see Figure 18-6 ■). Adenocarcinoma can also occur in the ducts of the gallbladder, pancreas, prostate gland, or salivary gland. Also known as **ductal cell carcinoma.** **Figure 18-6 ■ Breast cancer.** A pink ribbon is the symbol for the fight against adenocarcinoma of the breast (breast cancer). **Did You Know?** Advanced adenocarcinoma of the breast can cause dimpling of the skin of the breast when the tumor pulls on the fine supporting tissues around the milk ducts. This condition, known by the French phrase *peau d' orange* (peel of the orange), appears very much like the irregular, dimpled surface of an orange.
carcinoma	**carcinoma** (KAR-sih-NOH-mah) carcin/o- *cancer* -oma *tumor, mass*	Cancer of epithelial cells in the skin and mucous membranes of organs. Carcinomas grow more slowly that sarcomas, but they occur more frequently. Carcinomas usually metastasize via the lymphatic system.
basal cell carcinoma	**basal** (BAY-sal) bas/o- *base of a structure* -al *pertaining to*	Cancer of the deepest layer (base layer) of the epidermis of the skin (see Figure 18-7■) **Figure 18-7 ■ Basal cell carcinoma.** This basal cell carcinoma of the skin shows a characteristic asymmetrical shape with a central ulcerated area. There is crusting from oozing tissue fluid and periodic bleeding that formed a scab.

Word or Phrase	Word Part and Definition	Description
bronchogenic carcinoma	**bronchogenic** (BRONG-koh-JEN-ik) **bronch/o-** *bronchus* **gen/o-** *arising from; produced by* **-ic** *pertaining to*	Cancer of the mucous membranes lining the bronchi of the lungs
cholangio-carcinoma	**cholangiocarcinoma** (koh-LAN-jee-oh-KAR-sih-NOH-mah) **cholangi/o-** *bile duct* **carcin/o-** *cancer* **-oma** *tumor, mass*	Cancer of the epithelial cells lining the ducts of the gallbladder. This is a type of adenocarcinoma.
endometrial carcinoma	**endometrial** (EN-doh-MEE-tree-al) **endo-** *innermost, within* **metri/o-** *uterus (womb)* **-al** *pertaining to*	Cancer of the endometrium that lines the intrauterine cavity of the uterus
hepatocellular carcinoma	**hepatocellular** (HEP-ah-to-SEL-yoo-lar) **hepat/o-** *liver* **cellul/o-** *cell* **-ar** *pertaining to* **hepatoma** (HEP-ah-TOH-mah) **hepat/o-** *liver* **-oma** *tumor, mass*	Cancer of the liver cells. Also known as a **hepatoma.**
small cell carcinoma		Cancer of the epithelial cells of the lungs. The cells are small and round or oval (in contrast to large cell carcinoma, a less common type of lung cancer which has larger cells). Also known as oat cell carcinoma.
squamous cell carcinoma	**squamous** (SKWAY-mus) **squam/o-** *scalelike cell* **-ous** *pertaining to*	Cancer of the squamous cells (top layer) of epidermis of the skin
transitional cell carcinoma	**transitional** (trans-ZISH-un-al) **transit/o-** *changing over from one thing to another* **-ion** *action; condition* **-al** *pertaining to*	Cancer of the epithelial cells lining the urinary tract. Transitional cells are unique in that their shape transitions (changes) each time the ureters or bladder become filled with urine.
malignant melanoma	**melanoma** (MEL-ah-NOH-mah) **melan/o-** *black* **-oma** *tumor, mass*	Cancer of melanocytes (pigment cells) of the skin (see Figure 7-20)

Sarcomas

Word or Phrase	Word Part and Definition	Description
angiosarcoma	**angiosarcoma** (AN-jee-oh-sar-KOH-mah) **angi/o-** *blood vessel; lymphatic vessel* **sarc/o-** *connective tissue* **-oma** *tumor, mass*	Cancer of a blood vessel or lymphatic vessel
astrocytoma	**astrocytoma** (AS-troh-sy-TOH-mah) **astr/o-** *starlike structure* **cyt/o-** *cell* **-oma** *tumor, mass* The many branching parts of an astrocyte give it a starlike appearance.	Cancer of an astrocyte (branching cell that supports neurons) in the cerebrum of the brain
chondrosarcoma	**chondrosarcoma** (CON-droh-sar-KOH-mah) **chondr/o-** *cartilage* **sarc/o-** *connective tissue* **-oma** *tumor, mass*	Cancer of the cartilage
Ewing's sarcoma	**Ewing** (YOO-ing) Ewing's sarcoma was named by James Ewing (1866–1943), an American pathologist.	Cancer of the growth area (epiphysial plate) at the end of a bone, usually of an arm or leg
fibrosarcoma	**fibrosarcoma** (FY-broh-sar-KOH-mah) **fibr/o-** *fiber* **sarc/o-** *connective tissue* **-oma** *tumor, mass*	Cancer of a tendon, ligament, aponeurosis, or scar tissue
glioblastoma multiforme	**glioblastoma multiforme** (GLY-oh-blas-TOH-mah mul-tee-FOR-may) **gli/o-** *substance that holds things together* **blast/o-** *immature; embryonic* **-oma** *tumor, mass*	Cancer of an immature astrocyte (branching cell that supports neurons) in the cerebrum of the brain

Word or Phrase	Word Part and Definition	Description
Kaposi's sarcoma	**Kaposi** (KAH-poh-see) Kaposi's sarcoma was named by Moritz Kaposi Khan (1837–1902), an Australian dermatologist.	Cancer of the skin and subcutaneous tissue (see Figure 18-8■) 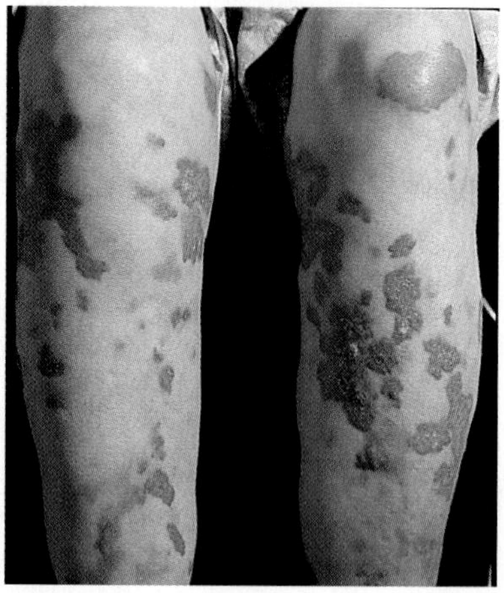 **Figure 18-8 ■ Kaposi's sarcoma.** This previously rare cancer is now commonly seen in AIDS patients because of their impaired immune response. The cancer involves the skin, subcutaneous tissue, and internal organs.
leiomyosarcoma	**leiomyosarcoma** (LIE-oh-MY-oh-sar-KOH-mah) **lei/o-** *smooth* **my/o-** *muscle* **sarc/o-** *connective tissue* **-oma** *tumor, mass*	Cancer of a smooth (involuntary) muscle tumor in the uterus, digestive tract, bladder, or prostate gland
liposarcoma	**liposarcoma** (LY-poh-sar-KOH-mah) **lip/o-** *lipid (fat)* **sarc/o-** *connective tissue* **-oma** *tumor, mass*	Cancer of the fatty tissue
myosarcoma	**myosarcoma** (MY-oh-sar-KOH-mah) **my/o-** *muscle* **sarc/o-** *connective tissue* **-oma** *tumor, mass*	Cancer of a muscle
neurofibrosarcoma	**neurofibrosarcoma** (NYOOR-oh-FY-broh-sar-KOH-mah) **neur/o-** *nerve* **fibr/o-** *fiber* **sarc/o-** *connective tissue* **-oma** *tumor, mass*	Cancer of Schwann cells around a cranial nerve or peripheral nerve
oligodendroglioma	**oligodendroglioma** (OHL-ih-goh-DEN-droh-glee-OH-mah) **olig/o-** *scanty* **dendr/o-** *branching structure* **gli/o-** *substance that holds things together* **-oma** *tumor, mass*	Cancer of an oligodendroglia, a myelin-forming cell in the brain or spinal cord. It has only a few branching structures coming from the cell.

Word or Phrase	Word Part and Definition	Description
osteosarcoma	**osteosarcoma** (AWS-tee-oh-sar-KOH-mah) oste/o- *bone* sarc/o- *connective tissue* -oma *tumor, mass* **osteogenic** (AWS-tee-oh-JEN-ik) oste/o- *bone* gen/o- *arising from; produced by* -ic *pertaining to*	Cancer of a bone (see Figure 18-9■). Also known as **osteogenic sarcoma.** **Figure 18-9 ■ Osteosarcoma.** This 11-year-old girl had an osteosarcoma of the distal end of the femur. The tumor infiltrated through the bone into the soft tissues around the bone.
rhabdomyo-sarcoma	**rhabdomyosarcoma** (RAB-doh-MY-oh-sar-KOH-mah) rhabd/o- *rod shaped* my/o- *muscle* sarc/o- *connective tissue* -oma *tumor, mass* The immature muscle cells in this tumor are shaped like a rod.	Cancer of a skeletal (voluntary) muscle in the arms or legs
sarcoma	**sarcoma** (sar-KOH-mah) sarc/o- *connective tissue* -oma *tumor, mass*	Cancer of connective tissues (cartilage, bone, tendon, ligament, aponeurosis, fascia, fat, subcutaneous tissue), muscles, or nerves. Sarcomas grow rapidly and most often show anaplasia of their cells. Sarcomas usually metastasize via the circulatory system.
Cancers of the Blood and Lymphatic System		
leukemia	**leukemia** (loo-KEE-mee-ah) leuk/o- *white* -emia *condition of the blood; substance in the blood* **myelogenous** (MY-eh-LAWJ-eh-nus) myel/o- *bone marrow; spinal cord; myelin* gen/o- *arising from; produced by* -ous *pertaining to* **lymphocytic** (LIM-foh-SIT-ik) lymph/o- *lymph; lymphatic system* cyt/o- *cell* -ic *pertaining to*	Cancer of leukocytes (white blood cells), including lymphoblasts that mature into lymphocytes, as well as myeloblasts and myelocytes that mature into neutrophils, eosinophils, or basophils). Leukemia is named according to the type of leukocyte that is the most prevalent and whether the onset of symptoms is acute or chronic. Types of leukemia include acute **myelogenous leukemia** (AML), chronic myelogenous leukemia (CML), acute **lymphocytic leukemia** (ALL), and chronic lymphocytic leukemia (CLL).

Word or Phrase	Word Part and Definition	Description
lymphoma	**lymphoma** (lim-FOH-mah) **lymph/o-** *lymph; lymphatic system* **-oma** *tumor, mass* **Hodgkin** (HAWJ-kin) Hodgkin's lymphoma was named by Thomas Hodgkin, (1798–1866), an English physician.	Cancer of a lymph node, lymphoid tissue, or T or B lymphocytes. There are two types of lymphomas. **Hodgkin's lymphoma,** the most common type, shows characteristic Reed-Sternberg cells (large, atypical lymphocytes) on biopsy. **Non-Hodgkin's lymphoma,** a group of more than 20 different lymphomas, does not have Reed-Sternberg cells. A lymphoma that originates in a lymph node should not be confused with metastasis to a lymph node from a primary tumor located elsewhere in the body.
multiple myeloma	**myeloma** (MY-eh-LOH-mah) **myel/o-** *bone marrow; spinal cord; myelin* **-oma** *tumor, mass* Some word parts have more than one definition. The best definition of *myeloma* is *a tumor of the bone marrow.*	Cancer of the bone marrow. It contains clumps of malignant plasma cells. Normal plasma cells are B lymphocytes that produce antibodies (immunoglobulins) when activated by a pathogen. Malignant plasma cells produce abnormal antibodies known as Bence Jones protein. The patient's immune response is abnormal because of decreased levels of normal plasma cells and antibodies.
	Embryonal Cell Cancer	
choriocarcinoma	**choriocarcinoma** (KOH-ree-oh-KAR-sih-NOH-mah) **chori/o-** *chorion (fetal membrane)* **carcin/o-** *cancer* **-oma** *tumor, mass*	Cancer that develops during pregnancy. It involves the chorion, the membrane that surrounds the developing embryo and will later become the placenta.
dysgerminoma	**dysgerminoma** (DIS-jer-mih-NOH-mah) **dys-** *painful, difficult, abnormal* **germin/o-** *embryonic tissue* **-oma** *tumor, mass*	Cancer of an immature oocyte in the ovary that occurs in young adulthood in females. It is a type of germ cell tumor.
embryonal cell cancer	**embryonal** (EM-bree-oh-nal) **embryon/o-** *embryo; immature form* **-al** *pertaining to*	Cancer of an embryonal cell that does not mature and differentiate like a normal cell. First becomes apparent during childhood or adolescence.
germ cell tumor		Cancer of a germ cell or embryonal cell (oocyte or spermatoblast) in the ovary or testis. Also known as germinoma.
hepatoblastoma	**hepatoblastoma** (HEP-ah-toh-blas-TOH-mah) **hepat/o-** *liver* **blast/o-** *immature; embryonic* **-oma** *tumor, mass*	Cancer of an embryonal cell in the liver that occurs in young children
neuroblastoma	**neuroblastoma** (NYOOR-oh-blas-TOH-mah) **neur/o-** *nerve* **blast/o-** *immature; embryonic* **-oma** *tumor, mass*	Cancer of an embryonal nerve cell in the autonomic nervous system. This cancer occurs in young children.

Word or Phrase	Word Part and Definition	Description
retinoblastoma	**retinoblastoma** (RET-ih-noh-blas-TOH-mah) **retin/o-** *retina* **blast/o-** *immature; embryonic* **-oma** *tumor, mass*	Cancer of an embryonal cell in the retina. This cancer occurs in young children.
seminoma	**seminoma** (SEM-ih-NOH-mah) **semin/o-** *spermatozoon; semen* **-oma** *tumor, mass* Add words to make a correct and complete definition of *seminoma: tumor or mass [of the testes that produces] spermatozoon.*	Cancer of an immature spermatoblast in the testis that occurs in young adulthood in males. It is a type of germ cell tumor.
teratoma	**teratoma** (TER-ah-TOH-mah) **terat/o-** *bizarre form* **-oma** *tumor, mass* *Terat/o-* is derived from a Greek word meaning *monster.*	Cancer of the ovary or testis that contains cells from other parts of the body. In the ovary, a teratoma can be malignant but usually is in the form of a benign dermoid cyst that contains hair and sometimes even teeth. However, a teratoma in the testis is almost always malignant.
Wilms' tumor (nephroblastoma)	**Wilms' tumor** (WILMZ TOO-mor) **nephroblastoma** (NEF-roh-blas-TOH-mah) **nephr/o-** *kidney; nephron* **blast/o-** *immature; embryonic* **-oma** *tumor, mass*	Cancer of an embryonal cell of the kidney that occurs in young children.

Diagnostic Procedures

Cytology Tests

Word or Phrase	Word Part and Definition	Description
bone marrow aspiration	**aspiration** (AS-pih-RAY-shun) **aspir/o-** *to breathe in; to suck in* **-ation** *a process; being or having*	Cytology test to diagnose leukemia or lymphoma and monitor its progression. Bone marrow is taken from the posterior iliac crest to examine all the stages of cell development (stem cell to mature cell) under the microscope.
exfoliative cytology	**exfoliative** (eks-FOH-lee-ah-tiv) *Exfoliative* is derived from a Latin word meaning *falling off of leaves.* **cytology** (sy-TAWL-oh-jee) **cyt/o-** *cell* **-logy** *the study of*	Cytology test that uses cells in secretions or scraped or washed from the body. The sample is examined under the microscope to look for abnormal or cancerous cells. Examples: Pap smear of the cervix, bronchial or gastric washings, sputum collection.

Word or Phrase	Word Part and Definition	Description
frozen section		Cytology test that involves freezing a tissue specimen obtained from a biopsy. Thin slices of the specimen are stained and examined under the microscope. This procedure is done in the laboratory during surgery so that the surgeon knows immediately whether the tissue is cancerous or not. Freezing the tissue distorts some of the architecture, and so a permanent section is also done using a paraffin-like substance to make the tissue firm.
Her2/neu		Cytology test that detects a gene that affects the prognosis and treatment options for breast cancer, ovarian cancer, and bladder cancer. A tumor that is Her2/neu positive is an aggressive tumor that is resistant to hormone therapy and some chemotherapy drugs.
karyotype	**karyotype** (KAIR-ee-oh-type) **kary/o-** *nucleus* **-type** *particular kind of; a model of*	Cytology test used to examine the chromosomes under the microscope. A photograph of the karyotype (see Figure 18-10 ■) is studied to look for chromosomal deletions or translocations. A translocation of chromosome 9 to chromosome 22, the *Philadelphia chromosome,* is diagnostic of chronic myelogenous leukemia. A translocation between chromosomes 11 and 22 causes Ewing's sarcoma. 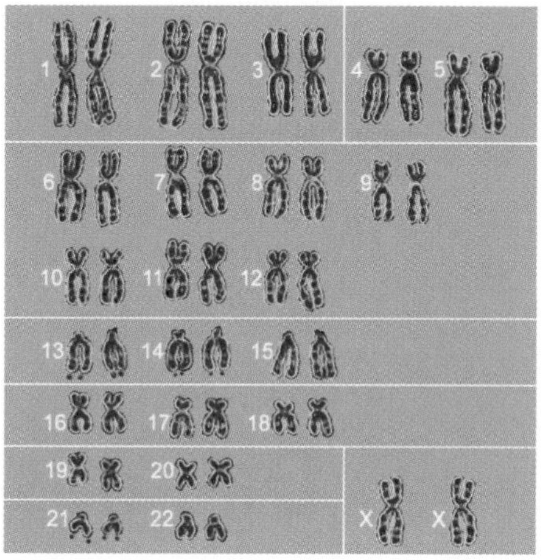 **Figure 18-10 ■ A normal karyotype.** There are 23 pairs of chromosomes. Pairs 1–22 are shown here with pair 23 (the sex chromosomes) in the bottom right-hand corner. Two X sex chromosomes make this patient a female.
receptor assays	**receptor** (ree-SEP-tor) **recept/o-** *receive* **-or** *person or thing that produces or does* **assay** (AS-say) *Assay* is derived from a French word meaning *to weigh.*	Cytology test that measures the number of **estrogen receptors (ER)** or **progesterone receptors (PR)** in the cell to determine the prognosis and treatment options for breast cancer. A tumor with increased numbers of ER or PR receptors (ER-positive or PR-positive) is dependent on those hormones and is most sensitive to treatment with male hormone therapy that creates the opposite hormonal environment.

Blood Tests

Word or Phrase	Word Part and Definition	Description
alpha fetoprotein (AFP)	**alpha fetoprotein** (AL-fah FEE-toh-PRO-teen)	Blood test that detects a protein normally present in a fetus but not in adults. Elevated levels of AFP are seen with cancer of the liver, testes, and ovaries. The higher the level, the more advanced the cancer. AFP can also be elevated in noncancerous conditions like cirrhosis and hepatitis.
blood smear		Blood test done manually to examine the characteristics of erythrocytes and leukocytes under the microscope when an abnormal automated complete blood count (CBC) suggests leukemia.
BRCA1 or BRCA2 gene		Blood test for the BRCA1 or BRCA2 gene, genetic mutations that significantly increase the risk of breast cancer. The BRCA1 gene also increases the risk of ovarian cancer. This test is performed when there is a strong family history of breast or ovarian cancer. BRCA stands for **br**east **ca**ncer.
carcinoembryonic antigen (CEA)	**carcinoembryonic** (KAR-sih-noh-EM-bree-AW-nik) **carcin/o-** *cancer* **embryon/o-** *embryo; immature form* **-ic** *pertaining to* **antigen** (AN-tih-jen) *Antigen* is a combination of the word *antibody* with *-body* deleted and the suffix *-gen* (that which produces).	Blood test that detects a protein normally present in an embryo but not in adults. Elevated levels of CEA are seen with several different cancers; the higher the level, the more advanced the cancer is. CEA can also be elevated in patients with noncancerous diseases of the colon or liver and in patients who smoke.
human chorionic gonadotropin (HCG)	**chorionic** (KOH-ree-ON-ik) **chorion/o-** *chorion (fetal membrane)* **-ic** *pertaining to* **gonadotropin** (GOH-nad-oh-TROH-pin) **gonad/o-** *gonads (ovaries and testes)* **trop/o-** *having an affinity for; stimulating; turning* **-in** *a substance*	Blood test that detects a hormone normally present during pregnancy but not at other times. Elevated levels of HCG are seen with cancer of the testes and choriocarcinoma. HCG can also be elevated in patients with noncancerous diseases like cirrhosis, duodenal ulcer, and inflammatory bowel disease.
prostate-specific antigen (PSA)		Blood test that measures a protein from the prostate gland. Elevated levels of PSA are seen in cancer of the prostate gland. The higher the level, the more advanced the cancer. Both free PSA and total PSA levels can be measured.
tumor markers		Blood test that detects antigens on the surface of cancer cells. Tumor markers are used to evaluate the extent of the cancer and the effectiveness of the treatment being given. They include CA 15-3 (breast cancer), CA 19-9 (cancer of the pancreas and bile ducts), CA 27.29 (cancer of the breast), and CA 125 (cancer of the ovary). AFP, CEA, and HCG are also classified as tumor markers.

Urine Tests

Word or Phrase	Word Part and Definition	Description
urinalysis (UA)	**urinalysis** (YOO-rih-NAL-ih-sis) *Urinalysis* is a combination of the combining form *urin/o-* (urine; urinary system) plus a shortened form of *analysis.*	Urine test that detects chemical compounds in the urine that are indicative of various types of cancers. These compounds include Bence Jones protein (multiple myeloma), vanillylmandelic acid (VMA) (neuroblastoma), and 5-HIAA (carcinoid syndrome).

Radiology and Nuclear Medicine Procedures

Word or Phrase	Word Part and Definition	Description
computed axial tomography (CAT, CT)	**tomography** (toh-MAWG-rah-fee) **tom/o-** *a cut, slice, or layer* **-graphy** *process of recording*	Radiologic procedure that uses x-rays to create many individual, closely spaced images (slices). The computer can combine these into a three-dimensional image to precisely locate a tumor or metatases. Radiopaque contrast dye can also be injected to provide more detail.
lymphangiography	**lymphangiography** (lim-FAN-jee-AWG-rah-fee) **lymph/o-** *lymph; lymphatic system* **angi/o-** *blood vessel; lymphatic vessel* **-graphy** *process of recording* **lymphangiogram** (lim-FAN-jee-oh-gram) **lymph/o-** *lymph; lymphatic system* **angi/o-** *blood vessel; lymphatic vessel* **-gram** *a record or picture*	Radiologic procedure in which a radiopaque contrast dye is injected into a lymphatic vessel. X-rays are taken as the dye travels through the lymphatic vessels to demonstrate enlarged lymph nodes, lymphomas, and areas of blocked lymph drainage. The x-ray image is known as a **lymphangiogram.**
magnetic resonance imaging (MRI)	**magnetic** (mag-NET-ik) **magnet/o-** *magnet* **-ic** *pertaining to*	Radiologic procedure that uses a magnetic field and radiowaves to align protons in the body and cause them to emit signals. Magnetic resonance imaging is a tomography that creates many individual "slice" images that the computer combines into a three-dimensional image to precisely locate a tumor or metastases. Radiopaque contrast dye can also be injected to provide more detail. An MRI scan does not use x-rays so the patient is not exposed to any radiation.
mammography	**mammography** (mah-MAWG-rah-fee) **mamm/o-** *breast* **-graphy** *process of recording* **mammogram** (MAM-oh-gram) **mamm/o-** *breast* **-gram** *a picture or record*	Radiologic procedure that uses x-rays to produce an image of the breast to detect tumors. The breast is compressed between two flat surfaces to decrease its thickness and increase the quality of the image. The x-ray image is known as a **mammogram** (see Figure 18-11■). **Figure 18-11 ■ Mammogram.** This patient has a cancerous tumor of the breast, seen as a dense white mass in the center of the breast. Note its characteristic irregular edge with infiltration into the surrounding breast tissue. The normal dense supporting fibers and lactiferous ducts are visible as white streaks throughout the breast. The fatty tissues of the breast appear dark gray.

Word or Phrase	Word Part and Definition	Description
scintigraphy	**scintigraphy** (sin-TIG-rah-fee) **scint/i-** *point of light* **-graphy** *process of recording* The combining form *scint/i-* is derived from a Latin word meaning *a spark.* **scintigram** (SIN-tih-gram) **scint/i-** *point of light* **-gram** *a record or picture*	Nuclear medicine procedure that uses a radioactive tracer that collects in particular organs or tissues. A gamma camera scans and counts the radioactivity (gamma rays) and creates an image known as a **scintigram.** Areas of increased uptake are abnormal and can be infection, cancer, or metatases.
ultrasonography	**ultrasonography** (UL-trah-soh-NAWG-rah-fee) **ultra-** *beyond, higher* **son/o-** *sound* **-graphy** *process of recording* **ultrasound** (UHL-trah-sound) *Ultrasound* is a combination of the prefix *ultra-* (beyond; higher) and the word *sound.* Ultrasound uses ultra high-frequency sound waves to produce an image. **sonography** (soh-NAWG-rah-fee) **son/o-** *sound* **-graphy** *process of recording* **sonogram** (SAWN-oh-gram) **son/o-** *sound* **-gram** *a record or picture*	Radiologic procedure that uses ultra high-frequency sound waves to produce an image. Used to differentiate benign, fluid-filled tumors (cysts) from solid tumors that need to be biopsied. Used to evaluate the breasts, abdominal organs, pelvic organs, and testes. Also known as **sonography** and the ultrasound image is known as a **sonogram.**

Medical, Surgical, and Radiation Therapy Procedures

Medical Procedures

Word or Phrase	Word Part and Definition	Description
bone marrow transplantation (BMT)	**transplantation** (TRANS-plan-TAY-shun) **transplant/o-** *move something to another place* **-ation** *a process; being or having*	Medical treatment for patients with leukemia and lymphoma. Red bone marrow is harvested from the posterior iliac crest of a matched donor. The patient is treated with high-dose chemotherapy drugs or radiation to destroy all cancerous cells (this also destroys all the red marrow cells). The donor bone marrow is administered through a central intravenous line, travels through the blood, and implants in the bones. In two to four weeks, the donor marrow begins to produce normal blood cells. In **stem cell transplantation,** stem cells (rather than marrow) from the patient or a matched donor are collected by apheresis of the peripheral blood. Matched stem cells from umbilical cord blood can also be given.

Word or Phrase	Word Part and Definition	Description
cryosurgery	**cryosurgery** (KRY-oh-SER-jer-ee) **cry/o-** *cold* **surg/o-** *operative procedure* **-ery** *process of*	Medical procedure in which liquid nitrogen is sprayed or painted onto a small malignant lesion. The liquid nitrogen freezes and destroys the tissue.
electrosurgery	**electrosurgery** (ee-LEK-troh-SER-jer-ee) **electr/o-** *electricity* **surg/o-** *operative procedure* **-ery** *process of* **fulguration** (FUL-guh-RAY-shun) **fulgur/o-** *spark of electricity* **-ation** *a process; being or having* **electrodesiccation** (ee-LEK-troh-DES-ih-KAY-shun) **electr/o-** *electricity* **desicc/o-** *to dry up* **-ation** *a process; being or having*	Medical procedure that uses electrical current to remove small cancerous tumors on the skin. The electrical current passes through an electrode and evaporates the intracellular contents of the cancerous cell. In **fulguration,** the electrode is held away from the skin and transmits the electrical current as a spark to the skin surface. In **electrodesiccation,** the electrode is touched to or inserted into the cancerous tumor.
grading		Medical procedure that classifies cancer by how well differentiated the cells appear under the microscope. Normal cells appear well differentiated and characteristic of that tissue type. Poorly differentiated or undifferentiated cells lack evidence of specialization and appear immature and embryonic. The greater the number of undifferentiated cells, the poorer the prognosis.
insertion of devices to administer chemotherapy drugs	**intravenous** (IN-trah-VEE-nus) **intra-** *within* **ven/o-** *vein* **-ous** *pertaining to* **peripheral** (peh-RIF-eh-ral) **peripher/o-** *outer aspects* **-al** *pertaining to* *Peripheral* has the opposite meaning of *central.* **intrathecal** (IN-trah-THEE-kal) **intra-** *within* **thec/o-** *sheath or layers of membranes* **-al** *pertaining to* *Intrathecal* refers to the layer of membranes around the spinal cord. **catheter** (KATH-eh-ter) *Catheter* is derived from a Greek word meaning *to send down.*	Medical procedure to insert an **intravenous line,** a PICC line, or an intrathecal catheter. A **peripherally inserted central catheter** (PICC) is inserted into the arm and threaded into the superior vena cava. Chemotherapy drugs administered through this catheter circulate through the blood. An **intrathecal catheter** is inserted after a lumbar puncture is performed. Chemotherapy drugs administered through this catheter circulate through the cerebrospinal fluid. **Intravesical chemotherapy** is administered through a catheter inserted into the bladder. The chemotherapy drug is held in the bladder for several hours and then removed. This procedure is done weekly for several weeks.

Word or Phrase	Word Part and Definition	Description
insertion of devices to administer chemotherapy drugs *(continued)*	**intravesical** (IN-trah-VES-ih-kal) **intra-** *within* **vesic/o-** *bladder; fluid-filled sac* **-al** *pertaining to*	
staging		Medical (or surgical) procedure that classifies cancer by how far it has spread in the body. The TNM staging system is used to describe the size of the tumor and whether the tumor has spread to lymph nodes and other sites (see Table 18-1).

Table 18-1 Classification Systems for Cancer

TNM System	
T	Size of the primary tumor (T1 through T4)
N	Number of regional lymph nodes affected (N1 through N4)
M	Presence or absence of metastases to other sites in the body (M0 or M1)
Other Systems	
Bethesda System	Cervical cancer
CIN Classification	Cervical cancer
Clark Level	Malignant melanoma
Dukes Classification	Cancer of the colon or rectum
FIGO Staging	Ovarian cancer
Gleason Score	Adenocarcinoma of the prostate
Jewett Classification	Bladder carcinoma

Surgical Procedures

Word or Phrase	Word Part and Definition	Description
biopsy (Bx)	**biopsy** (BY-awp-see) **bi/o-** *life; living organisms; living tissue* **-opsy** *process of viewing*	Surgical procedure to remove tissue from a suspected cancerous tumor.
core needle biopsy		A large-gauge needle is inserted into the tumor to obtain several long cores of tissue.
excisional biopsy	**excisional** (ek-SIZH-un-al) **excis/o-** *to cut out* **-ion** *action; condition* **-al** *pertaining to*	An incision is made to expose the suspected cancer, and the entire tumor is removed along with a surrounding margin of normal tissue.
fine-needle aspiration	**aspiration** (AS-pih-RAY-shun) **aspir/o-** *to breathe in; to suck in* **-ation** *a process; being or having*	A very fine needle is inserted into the tumor, and the fluid or tissue inside the tumor is aspirated into the attached syringe by pulling back on its plunger.

Word or Phrase	Word Part and Definition	Description
incisional biopsy	**incisional** (in-SIZH-un-al) **incis/o-** *to cut into* **-ion** *action; condition* **-al** *pertaining to*	An incision is made to expose the suspected cancer, and part (but not all) of the tumor is removed.
punch biopsy		Special forceps are used to grasp part of the tumor. As the forceps closes, it punches out a small, cylindrical tissue specimen. Multiple punch biopsies can be taken at one time.
sentinel node biopsy	**sentinel** (SEN-tih-nal) *Sentinel* is an English word that means *something that stands guard.*	The sentinel lymph node, the first lymph node that receives drainage from the site of the primary tumor, is removed.
stereotactic biopsy	**stereotactic** (STAIR-ee-oh-TAK-tik) **stere/o-** *three dimensions* **tact/o-** *touch* **-ic** *pertaining to*	Uses a CT scan to pinpoint the location of the mass in three dimensions and guide the biopsy needle.
vacuum-assisted biopsy		A probe with a cutting device is inserted through the skin and rotated around to take multiple specimens. The specimens are then suctioned out.
debulking	**debulk** (dee-BULK) *Debulk* is a combination of the prefix *de-* (reversal of; without) and the word *bulk.*	Surgical procedure to excise part of a bulky, unresectable tumor. This is done to reduce the size of the tumor and make the patient more comfortable or to leave a smaller tumor that can be treated with chemotherapy or radiation therapy.
en bloc resection	**en bloc** (en BLAWK) *En bloc* is a French phrase meaning *as a whole.* **resection** (ree-SEK-shun) **resect/o-** *to cut out and remove* **-ion** *action; condition*	A surgical procedure to excise the tumor and surrounding structures, which are taken as one block of tissue.
endoscopy	**endoscopy** (en-DAWS-koh-pee) **endo-** *innermost, within* **-scopy** *process of using an instrument to examine* Every medical word must contain a combining form. The suffix of *endoscopy* contains the combining form *scop/o-.*	Surgical procedure that uses a fiberoptic endoscope to examine a body cavity for signs of abnormal tissues or tumors. Grasping and cutting instruments are inserted through the endoscope to perform biopsies.
excision of a tumor	**excision** (ek-SIZH-un) **excis/o-** *to cut out* **-ion** *action; condition*	Surgical procedure to remove all or part of a cancerous tumor. In a wide excision, the tumor plus a wide margin of normal tissue around it is excised.
exenteration	**exenteration** (eks-EN-ter-AA-shun) **ex-** *out, away from* **enter/o-** *intestine* **-ation** *a process; being or having*	Surgical procedure to excise the tumor as well as all the nearby organs. Used to treat widely metastatic cancer in the abdominopelvic cavity.

Word or Phrase	Word Part and Definition	Description
exploratory laparotomy	**exploratory** (eks-PLOR-ah-TOHR-ee) **explorat/o-** *to search out* **-ory** *having the function of* **laparotomy** (LAP-ah-ROT-ah-mee) **lapar/o-** *abdomen* **-tomy** *process of cutting or making an incision*	Surgical procedure that uses an abdominal incision to widely open the abdominopelvic cavity so that it can be explored.
insertion of devices to administer chemotherapy drugs	**venous** (VEE-nus) **ven/o-** *vein* **-ous** *pertaining to* **intra-arterial** (IN-trah-ar-TEE-ree-al) **intra-** *within* **arteri/o-** *artery* **-al** *pertaining to* **intraperitoneal** (IN-trah-PAIR-ih-toh-NEE-al) **intra-** *within* **peritone/o-** *peritoneum* **-al** *pertaining to* **implantable** (im-PLANT-ah-bl) **implant/o-** *placed within* **-able** *able to be* **port** (PORT)	Surgical procedure to insert a central venous catheter, an intra-arterial catheter, an intraperitoneal catheter, or an implantable port to administer liquid chemotherapy drugs (see Figure 18-12 ■), or an implantable wafer to slowly release a chemotherapy drug. A **central venous catheter** (Broviac, Hickman, or Groshong catheter) is tunneled through the subcutaneous tissue in the upper chest. It is inserted into a large vein and advanced until its tip is positioned in the superior vena cava. The external end of the catheter is capped except when a chemotherapy drug is administered. An **intra-arterial catheter** is implanted in a main artery that brings blood to the organ where the cancerous tumor is located. A pump is also implanted under the skin or an externally worn portable infusion pump is used to administer regular doses of the chemotherapy drug. An **intraperitoneal catheter** is inserted into the peritoneal cavity with a capped end on the surface of the body. The chemotherapy drug is distributed by the peritoneal fluid and comes in contact with the surfaces of all the organs in the abdominopelvic cavity. An **implantable port** is a metal or plastic chamber that is placed in a subcutaneous pocket. The port is attached to a catheter that is threaded into the superior vena cava. The chemotherapy drug is given by inserting a needle through the skin and depositing the drug into a reservoir in the port which releases the drug into the blood. An Ommaya reservoir has a port beneath the scalp with the catheter in a ventricle in the brain, and the cerebrospinal fluid is used to circulate the chemotherapy drug. An **implantable wafer** is a dissolvable disk that contains a chemotherapy drug. It is implanted in an area a tumor has been excised. 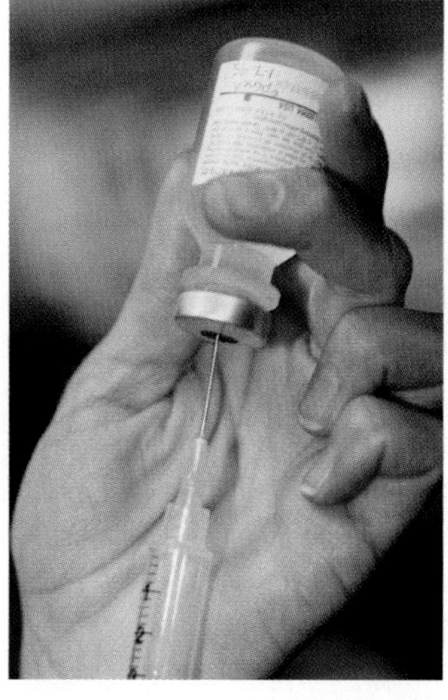 **Figure 18-12 ■ Chemotherapy.** Chemotherapy drugs specifically target cancer cells. They may be given intravenously into a vein, or into an artery, or cavity, or implanted in a wafer.

Word or Phrase	Word Part and Definition	Description
lumpectomy	**lumpectomy** (lum-PEK-toh-mee) *Lumpectomy* is a combination of the English word *lump* and the suffix *-ectomy* (surgical excision).	Surgical procedure to excise a small cancerous tumor without taking any surrounding tissue.
lymph node dissection	**dissection** (dy-SEK-shun) **dissect/o-** *to cut apart* **-ion** *action; condition*	Surgical procedure to remove several or all of the lymph nodes in a lymph node chain during extensive cancer surgery. Involved lymph nodes represent metastasis of the cancer from its original site.
percutaneous radiofrequency ablation	**percutaneous** (PER-kyoo-TAY-nee-us) **per-** *through, throughout* **cutane/o-** *skin* **-ous** *pertaining to* **ablation** (ah-BLAY-shun) **ablat/o-** *to take away; destroy* **-ion** *action; condition*	Surgical procedure in which a needle electrode or metal prong electrodes are placed through the skin and into a cancerous tumor less than 2 inches in diameter. High-frequency radiowaves (similar to microwaves) heat and kill the cancerous cells.
radical resection	**radical** (RAD-ih-kal) **radic/o-** *all parts including the root* **-al** *pertaining to*	Surgical procedure to excise the tumor as well as nearby lymph nodes, soft tissues, muscles, and even bones.
transarterial chemoembolization (TACE)	**transarterial** (TRANS-ar-TEE-ree-al) **trans-** *across, through* **arteri/o-** *artery* **-al** *pertaining to* **chemoembolization** (KEE-moh-EM-bol-ih-ZAY-shun) **chem/o-** *chemical, drug* **embol/o-** *embolus (occluding plug)* **-ization** *the process of making, creating, or inserting*	Surgical procedure in which an intra-arterial catheter is threaded through the femoral artery, aorta, and into the hepatic artery to deliver a one-time dose of chemotherapy. After the drug, an inert substance is injected to block the flow of blood and keep the drug concentrated at the site of the cancerous tumor.
Radiation Therapy		
brachytherapy	**brachytherapy** (BRAK-ee-THAIR-ah-pee) **brachy-** *short* **-therapy** *treatment* Add words to make a correct and complete definition of *brachytherapy: treatment [that originates a] short [distance from the tumor].*	Category that includes internal, interstitial, and intracavitary radiotherapy in which a radioactive substance is placed in or a short distance from the tumor.
fractionation	**fractionation** (FRAK-shun-AA-shun) *Fractionation* is a combination of the English word *fraction* and the suffix *-ation* (a process; being or having).	The total dose of external beam radiation to be given is divided into smaller doses that are given each day to decrease the occurrence of side effects.

Word or Phrase	Word Part and Definition	Description
radiotherapy	**radiotherapy** (RAY-dee-oh-THAIR-ah-pee) **radi/o-** *radius (forearm bone); x-ray; radiation* **-therapy** *treatment* Some word parts have more than one definition. The best definition of *radiotherapy* is *treatment [using] radiation.* **radiosensitive** (RAY-dee-oh-SEN-sih-tiv) **radi/o-** *radius (forearm bone); x-ray; radiation* **sensit/o-** *affected by, sensitive to* **-ive** *pertaining to* **radioresistant** (RAY-dee-oh-ree-ZIS-tant) **radi/o-** *radius (forearm bone); x-ray; radiation* **resist/o-** *withstand the effect of* **-ant** *pertaining to* **radiation** (RAY-dee-AA-shun) **radi/o-** *radius (forearm bone); x-ray; radiation* **-ation** *a process; being or having*	Treatment that uses one of several types of radiation to disrupt the atoms in the DNA in cancer cells to keep them from dividing. The radiation is in the form of waves (x-rays and gamma rays) or particles (electrons, neutrons, and protons). Radiotherapy destroys both cancerous and normal cells, but enough normal cells remain to divide and repair the damaged tissue. Side effects include alopecia, swelling at the site of the radiation, nausea, and fatigue. Radiotherapy is used to treat solid tumors. It is also used to treat leukemia and lymphoma by radiating the bone marrow. Radiotherapy can be delivered from outside the body or with implants from inside the body. Cancerous tumors that are readily destroyed by radiation therapy are said to be **radiosensitive.** Cancerous tumors that are not adversely affected by radiation therapy are said to be **radioresistant.** Also known as **radiation therapy.**
conformal radiotherapy	**conformal** (con-FOR-mal) **conform/o-** *having the same scale or angle* **-al** *pertaining to*	Uses a computer to map the location of the tumor and create a three-dimensional image of the tumor. The external beam radiation is then matched to conform to the exact shape of the tumor to protect nearby vital organs.
external beam radiotherapy	**external** (eks-TER-nal) **extern/o-** *outside* **-al** *pertaining to*	Beams of radiation are generated by a machine outside the body and directed at the patient (see Figure 18-13■). Linear accelerators are used to increase the energy of the radiation so that it can penetrate more deeply into the body. 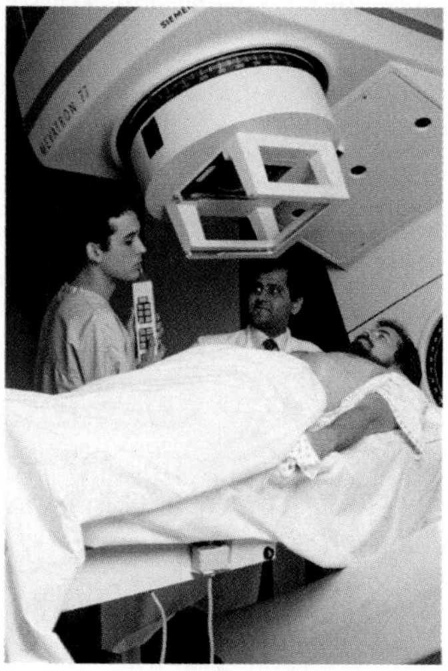 **Figure 18-13 ■ External beam radiation.** This patient is being prepared to receive external radiation therapy. The external beam of radiation is generated by the equipment over his head. Not all tumors can be treated with radiation therapy.

Word or Phrase	Word Part and Definition	Description
internal radiotherapy	**internal** (in-TER-nal) **intern/o-** *inside* **-al** *pertaining to*	An implant that contains a radioactive substance (such as cesium, iridium, iodine, phosphorus, or palladium) that emits radiation and is implanted near the tumor.
interstitial radiotherapy	**interstitial** (IN-ter-STISH-al) **interstiti/o-** *spaces within tissue* **-al** *pertaining to*	Radioactive implants (needles, wires, capsules, or pellets [seeds]) are inserted into the tumor or into the tissue around the tumor.
intracavitary radiotherapy	**intracavitary** (IN-trah-KAV-ih-tair-ee) **intra-** *within* **cavit/o-** *hollow space* **-ary** *pertaining to*	Radioactive implants are inserted into a body cavity near the tumor.
intravenous radiotherapy	**intravenous** (IN-trah-VEE-nus) **intra-** *within* **ven/o-** *vein* **-ous** *pertaining to*	Radioactive iodine is given intravenously. It concentrates in the thyroid gland and releases radiation to kill cancerous cells of the thyroid gland.

Drug Categories

Several different categories of chemotherapy drugs are used to treat cancer. The most common drugs in each category are listed.

Category	Word Part and Definition	Description	Examples
alkylating drugs	**alkylating** (AL-kih-lay-ting) Alkylation is a chemical reaction in which an alkyl group is substituted for a hydrogen molecule.	Break DNA strands in the cancerous cell by substituting an alkyl group for a hydrogen molecule in the DNA.	Cytoxan, Emcyt, Myleran, Neosar
antiemetic drugs	**antiemetic** (AN-tee-ee-MET-ik) **anti-** *against* **emet/o-** *to vomit* **-ic** *pertaining to*	Not a chemotherapy drug. Treat nausea and vomiting, side effects of chemotherapy.	Compazine, Phenergan
antimetabolite drugs	**antimetabolite** (AN-tee-meh-TAB-oh-lite) **anti-** *against* **metabol/o-** *change, transformation* **-ite** *thing that pertains to*	Block folic acid, a B vitamin required for the synthesis of some amino acids in the DNA of the cancerous cell. Other antimetabolite drugs directly block DNA from using certain amino acids.	fluorouracil (5-FU), Gemzar, methotrexate, Xeloda
chemotherapy antibiotic drugs	**chemotherapy** (KEE-moh-THAIR-ah-pee) **chem/o-** *chemical, drug* **-therapy** *treatment* **antibiotic** (AN-tee-by-AWT-ik) **anti-** *against* **bi/o-** *life; living organisms; living tissue* **-tic** *pertaining to*	Bind to DNA strands and inhibit an enzyme that must split each DNA strand for cell division to proceed.	Adriamycin, bleomycin, daunorubicin, doxorubicin

Did You Know?

Chemotherapy antibiotics are not used to treat infections like regular antibiotic drugs are. Antibiotic drugs act on the cell wall of bacteria. Human cells do not have a cell wall and are not affected by antibiotic drugs. Chemotherapy antibiotics are a special class of antibiotics that do affect human cells that are normal or cancerous.

Category	Word Part and Definition	Description	Examples
chemotherapy enzyme drugs		Break down the amino acid asparagine. Normal body cells can synthesize their own supply of asparagine, but cancerous cells cannot.	Elspar, Oncaspar

Connections

protocol (PROH-toh-kawl)

adjuvant (AD-joo-vant)
adjuv/o- *giving help or assistance*
-ant *pertaining to*

Pharmacology. Chemotherapy protocols use a combination of several different chemotherapy drugs that are administered together. This increases their effectiveness against cancerous cells while minimizing the side effects caused by large doses of just one drug. A **protocol** is a written plan of treatment for a particular type of cancerous tumor. A protocol details which chemotherapy drugs should be given, in what order they should be given, and in what dosages. Protocols are named by combining the first letter of each drug name. The ABVD chemotherapy protocol for treating Hodgkin's lymphoma consists of the chemotherapy drugs Adriamycin, bleomycin, vinblastine, and dacarbazine.

Adjuvant therapy is the use of chemotherapy drugs after another type of therapy (surgery, radiation therapy) has been used as the primary treatment.

Category	Word Part and Definition	Description	Examples
hormonal drugs	**hormonal** (hor-MOH-nal) **hormon/o-** *hormone* **-al** *pertaining to*	Produce an opposite hormonal environment from the one that the cancer needs to reproduce. For example, estrogen (a female hormone) is given to men with prostate cancer.	Arimidex, Femara, Lupron, Megace, Nolvadex, tamoxifen, Zoladex
mitosis inhibitor drugs	**inhibitor** (in-HIB-ih-tor) **inhibit/o-** *block; hold back* **-or** *person or thing that produces or does*	Cause DNA strands in the cancerous cell to break during the early stages of cell division.	Camptosar, Hycamtin, VePesid
monoclonal antibodies	**monoclonal** (MAWN-oh-KLOH-nal) **mon/o-** *one, single* **clon/o-** *identical group derived from one* **-al** *pertaining to* **antibody** (AN-tih-BAWD-ee) *Antibody* is a combination of the prefix *anti-* (against) and the English word *body* (a structure or thing).	Bind to specific antigens on the surface of a cancerous cell and destroy the cell. Monoclonal antibodies are created using recombinant DNA technology. A human antibody is modified so that it will bind to a specific antigen on a cancerous cell.	Campath, Herceptin
platinum drugs	**platinum** (PLAT-ih-num)	Create crosslinks in the DNA strands that prevent the cancerous cell from dividing. These drugs actually contain the precious metal platinum.	cisplatin, Platinol-AQ

Abbreviations

AFP	alpha fetoprotein
ALL	acute lymphocytic leukemia
AML	acute myelogenous leukemia
BMT	bone marrow transplantation
BRCA	breast cancer (gene)
Bx	biopsy
Ca	carcinoma, cancer
CEA	carcinoembryonic antigen
chemo	chemotherapy (slang)
CIN	cervical intraepithelial neoplasia
CLL	chronic lymphocytic leukemia
CML	chronic myelogenous leukemia
CRT	certified radiation therapist
CTR	certified tumor registrar
DNA	deoxyribonucleic acid
ER	estrogen receptor
FIGO	Federation Internationale de Gynécologie et Obstétrique
5-HIAA	5-hydroxyindoleacetic acid
HCG	human chorionic gonadotropin
mets	metastases (slang)
NK	natural killer (cells)
PICC	peripherally inserted central catheter
PR	progesterone receptor
PSA	prostate-specific antigen
RNA	ribonucleic acid
TACE	transarterial chemoembolization
TNM	tumor, nodes, metastases
VMA	vanillylmandelic acid

Word Alert

MEDICAL ABBREVIATIONS

Abbreviations are commonly used in all types of medical documents; however, they can mean different things to different people and their meaning can be misinterpreted. Always verify the meaning of an abbreviation.

Ca stands for *carcinoma* or *cancer,* but it also stands for *calcium.*

ER stands for *estrogen receptor,* but it also stands for *emergency room.*

Mets stands for *metastases,* but it also stands for a unit of measurement that is used during cardiac treadmill stress tests to measure metabolic rate and oxygen consumption.

Career Focus

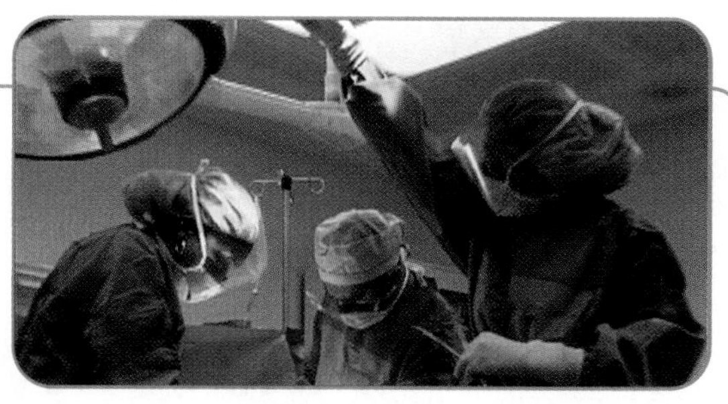

Meet Shah, a surgical assistant.

"I'm a surgical assistant. I help the doctor from the beginnning to the end of the surgery. The very best part is assisting during cesarean sections. I like that part because sometimes there's a really sick baby or baby and mom, and after cesarean section, the baby's okay and the mom is okay. For a cesarean section, we have 50 different instruments. Each doctor uses different ways and different instruments. I keep track of the instruments and buy new instruments."

Surgical assistants are allied health professionals who assist surgeons in the operating room. They position and drape the patient and prepare the patient's surgical site by shaving and prepping the skin. Using sterile technique, they assist the surgeon during the operation by holding retractors, clamping or cutting tissues, and placing sutures.

Medical oncologists are physicians who specialize in treating patients with cancer. After the patient's cancer has been diagnosed, a medical oncologist assigns a grade and stage to the cancer and prescribes chemotherapy, radiation therapy, surgery, or a combination of all three, depending on the type of cancer and how advanced it is. Medical oncologists calculate the dosage of the chemotherapy drugs based on the patient's body weight.

Radiation oncologists are physicians who have received additional training in using radiation therapy to treat cancer. They select the type of radiation and the most effective radiation technique for the type of cancer. They calculate the total dosage of radiation to be given and then divide the dosage into fractional amounts to be given each week.

surgical (SER-jih-kal)
surg/o- *operative procedure*
-ical *pertaining to*

medical (MED-ih-kal)
medic/o- *physician; medicine*
-al *pertaining to*

oncologist (ong-KAWL-oh-jist)
onc/o- *tumor, mass*
log/o- *the study of*
-ist *one who specializes in*

radiation (RAY-dee-AA-shun)
radi/o- *radius (forearm bone); x-rays; radiation*
-ation *a process; being or having*

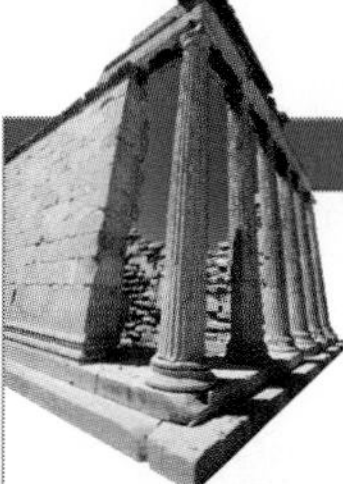

It's Greek to Me!

Did you notice that some oncology words have two different combining forms? Combining forms from both Greek and Latin languages remain a part of medical language today.

English Word	Greek	Latin	Examples of Medical Words
cancer	carcin/o-	cancer/o-	carcinogen, cancerous
cell	cyt/o-	cellul/o-	cytoplasm, cellular
embryonic	blast/o- embryon/o-	germin/o-	neuroblastoma, dysgerminoma embryonal cell carcinoma
nucleus	kary/o-	nucle/o-	karyotype, nuclear membrane

CHAPTER REVIEW EXERCISES

Review all the material in this chapter by completing the review exercises in this section. Use the Answer Key at the end of the book to check your answers.

Anatomy and Physiology

Matching Exercise

Match each numbered word or phrase to its description.

1. chromosome	____ Intracellular gel-like substance
2. cytoplasm	____ Makes lysosomes and digestive enzymes
3. gene	____ Produces energy for cell's activities
4. Golgi apparatus	____ Area on a chromosome with information to build one protein molecule
5. lysosome	____ Site of protein synthesis
6. mitochondrion	____ 23 pairs
7. ribosome	____ Inhibits mitosis
8. suppressor gene	____ Becomes active when a pathogen enters the cell

True or False

Indicate whether each statement is true or false by writing T or F on the line.

1. ____ The nucleolus is an expanded type of nucleus seen during cell division.
2. ____ An organelle is an intracellular structure embedded in the cytoplasm.
3. ____ The endoplasmic reticulum regulates mitosis.
4. ____ The gene p53 is an important suppressor gene.
5. ____ A cell has 23 pairs of chromosomes plus two sex chromosomes.
6. ____ RNA is in the shape of a double helix.

Circle Exercise

Circle the correct word from the choices given.

1. Epithelial tissues contains (**cancer, Schwann, squamous**) cells.
2. Messenger RNA carries information from the nucleus to the (**cell membrane, mitochondrion, ribosome**).
3. Loss of unique, differentiated cellular structure is known as (**anaplasia, apoptysis, mitosis**).
4. (**Astrocyte, Dermis, Mucous membrane**) is a type of nerve cell that can be affected by cancer.
5. (**Apoptosis, Mitosis, Translocation**) is the process by which a cell duplicates itself.

Medical Language Word Parts

Name That Word Part

Identify each of the word parts given here by writing in the correct letter (P, C, or S) on the line beside it. Then write the definition of the word part on the blank line. The first one has been done for you.

Prefix = P **Combining Form = C** **Suffix = S**

	Word Part	Definition		Word Part	Definition
1. -al	S	pertaining to	36. conform/o-	______	______
2. ablat/o-	______	______	37. cry/o-	______	______
3. -able	______	______	38. cutane/o-	______	______
4. aden/o-	______	______	39. cyt/o-	______	______
5. adjuv/o-	______	______	40. dendr/o-	______	______
6. ana-	______	______	41. dessic/o-	______	______
7. angi/o-	______	______	42. differentiat/o-	______	______
8. -ant	______	______	43. dissect/o-	______	______
9. anti-	______	______	44. duct/o-	______	______
10. apo-	______	______	45. dys-	______	______
11. -ar	______	______	46. -ed	______	______
12. arteri/o-	______	______	47. electr/o-	______	______
13. -ary	______	______	48. -elle	______	______
14. aspir/o-	______	______	49. embryon/o-	______	______
15. astr/o-	______	______	50. embol/o-	______	______
16. -ated	______	______	51. emet/o-	______	______
17. -ation	______	______	52. -emia	______	______
18. bas/o-	______	______	53. en-	______	______
19. bi/o-	______	______	54. endo-	______	______
20. blast/o-	______	______	55. enter/o-	______	______
21. brachy-	______	______	56. -ery	______	______
22. bronch/o-	______	______	57. -esis	______	______
23. cancer/o-	______	______	58. ex-	______	______
24. capsul/o-	______	______	59. excis/o-	______	______
25. carcin/o-	______	______	60. explorat/o-	______	______
26. cavit/o-	______	______	61. extern/o-	______	______
27. cellul/o-	______	______	62. fibr/o-	______	______
28. chem/o-	______	______	63. fulgur/o-	______	______
29. cholangi/o-	______	______	64. -gen	______	______
30. chondri/o-	______	______	65. -gene	______	______
31. chondr/o-	______	______	66. gene/o-	______	______
32. chori/o-	______	______	67. gen/o-	______	______
33. chorion/o-	______	______	68. gli/o-	______	______
34. chrom/o-	______	______	69. gonad/o-	______	______
35. clon/o-	______	______	70. -gram	______	______

	Word Part	Definition
71. -graphy	______	________________
72. hepat/o-	______	________________
73. hered/o-	______	________________
74. hormon/o-	______	________________
75. -ia	______	________________
76. -ial	______	________________
77. -ic	______	________________
78. -ical	______	________________
79. implant/o-	______	________________
80. -in	______	________________
81. incis/o-	______	________________
82. inhibit/o-	______	________________
83. intern/o-	______	________________
84. interstit/o-	______	________________
85. intra-	______	________________
86. invas/o-	______	________________
87. -ion	______	________________
88. -ist	______	________________
89. -ite	______	________________
90. -ity	______	________________
91. -ive	______	________________
92. -ization	______	________________
93. -ize	______	________________
94. kary/o-	______	________________
95. lapar/o-	______	________________
96. lei/o-	______	________________
97. leuk/o-	______	________________
98. lip/o-	______	________________
99. locat/o-	______	________________
100. log/o-	______	________________
101. -logy	______	________________
102. lymph/o-	______	________________
103. lys/o-	______	________________
104. magnet/o-	______	________________
105. malign/o-	______	________________
106. mamm/o-	______	________________
107. medic/o-	______	________________
108. melan/o-	______	________________
109. meta-	______	________________
110. metabol/o-	______	________________
111. metri/o-	______	________________
112. mit/o-	______	________________

	Word Part	Definition
113. mono-	______	________________
114. mutat/o-	______	________________
115. myel/o-	______	________________
116. my/o-	______	________________
117. necr/o-	______	________________
118. ne/o-	______	________________
119. nephr/o-	______	________________
120. neur/o-	______	________________
121. nucle/o-	______	________________
122. nucleol/o-	______	________________
123. -oid	______	________________
124. olig/o-	______	________________
125. -oma	______	________________
126. onc/o-	______	________________
127. -opsy	______	________________
128. -or	______	________________
129. -ory	______	________________
130. organ/o-	______	________________
131. -osis	______	________________
132. oste/o-	______	________________
133. -ous	______	________________
134. -pathy	______	________________
135. per-	______	________________
136. peripher/o-	______	________________
137. peritone/o-	______	________________
138. -plasm	______	________________
139. plasm/o-	______	________________
140. plas/o-	______	________________
141. -ptosis	______	________________
142. radic/o-	______	________________
143. radicul/o-	______	________________
144. radi/o-	______	________________
145. recept/o-	______	________________
146. remiss/o-	______	________________
147. resect/o-	______	________________
148. resist/o-	______	________________
149. retin/o-	______	________________
150. rhabd/o-	______	________________
151. rib/o-	______	________________
152. sarc/o-	______	________________
153. scint/i-	______	________________
154. -scopy	______	________________

		Word Part	Definition			Word Part	Definition
155.	semin/o-	______	______________	169.	thec/o-	______	______________
156.	sensit/o-	______	______________	170.	-therapy	______	______________
157.	-some	______	______________	171.	-tic	______	______________
158.	som/o-	______	______________	172.	tom/o-	______	______________
159.	son/o-	______	______________	173.	-tomy	______	______________
160.	squam/o-	______	______________	174.	trans-	______	______________
161.	-stasis	______	______________	175.	transit/o-	______	______________
162.	stas/o-	______	______________	176.	transplant/o-	______	______________
163.	stat/o-	______	______________	177.	trop/o-	______	______________
164.	stere/o-	______	______________	178.	-type	______	______________
165.	suppress/o-	______	______________	179.	ultra-	______	______________
166.	surg/o-	______	______________	180.	un-	______	______________
167.	tact/o-	______	______________	181.	ven/o-	______	______________
168.	terat/o-	______	______________	182.	vesic/o-	______	______________

Word-Building Exercise

Use the combining forms, prefixes, and suffixes given here to build oncology words that match the definitions given. Write the word that you build on the blank line. Some word parts may be used more than once. The first one has been done for you.

Word Parts

carcin/o- (cancer)	hered/o- (genetic inheritance)	lapar/o- (abdomen)	mutat/o- (to change)
differentiat/o- (being distinct or specialized)	invas/o- (to go into)	-logy (the study of)	-oma (tumor, mass)
-gen (that which produces)	-ion (action; condition)	lymph/o- (lymph; lymphatic system)	-tic (pertaining to)
gene/o- (gene)	-ity (state; condition)	onc/o- (tumor, mass)	-tomy (process of cutting or making an incision)
hepat/o- (liver)	-ive (pertaining to)		

1. Pertaining to the genes (You think *gene/o-* + *-tic*). You write genetic.
2. The study of tumors and masses ______________________
3. Action to change ______________________
4. Process of making an incision into the abdomen ______________________
5. Tumor in the liver ______________________
6. Cancerous tumor ______________________
7. That which produces cancer ______________________
8. Condition of being distinct or specialized ______________________
9. State of genetic inheritance ______________________
10. Pertaining to going into ______________________
11. Tumor of the lymphatic system ______________________

Symptoms, Signs, and Types of Cancer

True or False

Indicate whether each statement is true or false by writing T or F on the line.

1. ____ Peau d' orange is a dimpling seen in cancer of the uterus.
2. ____ Carcinomatosis shows cancerous tumors in multiple places in the body.
3. ____ A carcinoid tumor is the most serious type of cancer.
4. ____ Neoplasms are always malignant cancers.
5. ____ Carcinomas arise from connective tissues.
6. ____ Sarcomas grow rapidly and show anaplasia.
7. ____ A chondrosarcoma is a cancer of the cartilage.
8. ____ Kaposi's sarcoma most often affects patients with AIDS.
9. ____ Leukemia can be acute or chronic.
10. ____ A seminoma is an embryonal cell cancer of the breast.

Matching Exercise

Match each numbered word or phrase to its definition.

1. adenocarcinoma	____ Cancer of the muscle
2. astrocytoma	____ Enlarged lymph nodes
3. cholangiocarcinoma	____ Cancer of the smooth muscle of the uterus
4. sentinal node	____ Tumor
5. Hodgkin's lymphoma	____ First to receive lymphatic drainage from cancer site
6. leiomyosarcoma	____ Type of cancer in the brain
7. lymphadenopathy	____ Cancer of the ducts of the gallbladder
8. malignant melanoma	____ Opposite of remission
9. myosarcoma	____ Cancer of a gland
10. neoplasm	____ Shows Reed-Sternberg cells
11. relapse	____ Cancer of a melanocyte

Memory Exercise

1. Ways in which early cancer can present itself. What does this acronym stand for?

C ______________________________

A ______________________________

U ______________________________

T ______________________________

I ______________________________

O ______________________________

N ______________________________

2. Define and match each abbreviation to its definition.

a. AFP	____________	____ Can be excisional or incisional
b. Bx	____________	____ Messenger is a type
c. CML	____________	____ Normally present in a fetus
d. ER	____________	____ Type of leukemia
e. RNA	____________	____ Tells how far a tumor has spread
f. TNM	____________	____ Numbers of these effect the prognosis of breast cancer

Laboratory, Radiology, Surgery, and Drugs

Matching Exercise

Match each numbered word or phrase to its description.

1. Bence Jones protein ______ Way to stage tumor, nodes, and metastases
2. BRCA1 ______ Pap smear is an example
3. exfoliative cytology ______ Radiation therapy
4. frozen section ______ Performed while surgery is going on
5. Jewett classification ______ Used to stage bladder carcinoma
6. radiotherapy ______ Mutated gene related to breast cancer in families
7. scintigraphy ______ Protein in the urine of patients with multiple myeloma
8. TNM ______ Radioactive whole body bone scan to look for metastases

True or False

Indicate whether each statement is true or false by writing T or F on the line.

1. ____ A bone marrow aspiration is used to diagnose breast cancer.
2. ____ A karyotype is an x-ray that shows bony metastases.
3. ____ ER and PR tell whether the tumor is hormone dependent.
4. ____ PSA is performed to check for colon cancer.
5. ____ Grading is done to shave a smooth slice from a tumor.
6. ____ A colonoscopy is done to examine the colon for tumors.
7. ____ A tumor that is radioresistant will die if treated with radiation therapy.
8. ____ Brachytherapy includes internal, interstitial, and intracavitary radiotherapy.

Matching Exercise

Match each numbered word or phrase to its description.

1. cryosurgery ______ Implantable, dissolvable way to deliver chemotherapy to a site
2. excisional biopsy ______ Uses special forceps to remove a cylindrical tissue specimen
3. exenteration ______ Surgery performed through a large abdominal incision
4. exploratory laparotomy ______ Uses cold to freeze tumors
5. intrathecal catheter ______ Surgical removal of tumor, organs, and surrounding tissues and muscles
6. punch biopsy ______ Diagnostic procedure that removes the entire tumor
7. stereotactic biopsy ______ Delivers a chemotherapy drug into the spinal canal
8. wafer ______ Uses a CT scan to pinpoint the tumor location

Circle Exercise

Circle the correct word from the choices given.

1. (**Adjuvant therapy, Chemotherapy protocol, Endoscopy**) is the use of chemotherapy after radiation or surgery has been used as the primary treatment.
2. (**Endoscopy, Intravesical chemotherapy, Lymph node dissection**) is looking into a body cavity and using instruments to perform a biopsy.
3. En bloc resection means (**debulking part of a large tumor, excising the tumor and surrounding structures as one block of tissue, widening an area blocked by tumor**).
4. An (**alkylating drug, antibiotic drug, antimetabolite drug**) is one that blocks the DNA in a cancerous cell from using a vitamin or amino acid.

Abbreviations

Matching Exercise

Match each numbered abbreviation to its description.

1.	AML	_____ A cancer staging system
2.	BMT	_____ Surgical procedure to remove a tissue specimen
3.	Bx	_____ Treatment for leukemia
4.	ER	_____ Determines if breast cancer can be treated with hormones
5.	NK	_____ A way to give chemotherapy
6.	PICC	_____ Cells that attack cancer cells
7.	TNM	_____ A type of leukemia

Applied Skills

Analysis of a Medical Report

This exercise contains two pathology reports. The first is the gross description and the second is the microscopic description of the same tissue specimen. Read the reports and answer the questions.

PATHOLOGY REPORT

PATIENT NAME: FOSTER, VIRGINIA

HOSPITAL NUMBER 564-542-8763

DATE OF SURGERY: November 19, 20xx

GROSS DESCRIPTION

CLINICAL HISTORY: This is a 49-year-old white female with a right breast mass. She performs occasional self-examination of her breasts. While performing this procedure 2 days ago, she noted a lump in her right breast. She was seen by her primary care physician and referred for a mammogram. Mammography and subsequent ultrasound showed a solid rather than cystic mass. She was immediately scheduled for a biopsy. She has no family history of cancer.

PREOPERATIVE DIAGNOSIS: Rule out carcinoma of the breast.

OPERATION: Needle biopsy of right breast mass.

TISSUE SPECIMEN: Right breast mass. Specimen labeled "needle biopsy, right breast," is received in gauze for frozen section. It consists of a single piece of tissue measuring $1.0 \times 0.1 \times 0.1$ cm, that is cylindrical, tannish, soft, and pliable. It is submitted in its entirety.

Alfredo P. Martinez, M.D.

Alfredo P. Martinez, M.D.

APM:rrg
D: 11/19/xx
T: 11/19/xx

PATHOLOGY REPORT

PATIENT NAME: FOSTER, VIRGINIA

HOSPITAL NUMBER 564-542-8763

DATE OF SURGERY: November 24, 20xx

MICROSCOPIC DESCRIPTION

CLINICAL HISTORY: This is a 49-year-old white female who presented to her primary care physician with a right breast mass. Subsequent needle biopsy on 11-19-xx revealed carcinoma of the breast. She was scheduled for a right mastectomy and axillary lymph node dissection.

PREOPERATIVE DIAGNOSIS: Carcinoma of the breast.

OPERATION: Right mastectomy and axillary lymph node dissection.

TISSUE SPECIMENS: Tumor and 28 axillary lymph nodes.

MICROSCOPIC COMMENTS: Sections of the tumor reveal an invasive tumor composed of irregular nests of pleomorphic, anaplastic cells having prominent nucleoli. Some of the larger nests show central areas of necrosis. The tumor extends to an ulcerated skin surface. The margins of resection are free of tumor. A section of the nipple demonstrates tumor extending along the large ducts. A total of 28 lymph nodes are submitted. Ten are positive for metastasis. The largest positive lymph node is 2.0 cm.

DIAGNOSIS: Infiltrating ductal carcinoma, grade 3, with ulceration of the overlying skin. Metastatic carcinoma involving 10 of 28 axillary lymph nodes.

Alfredo P. Martinez, M.D.

Alfredo P. Martinez, M.D.

APM:rrg
D: 11/19/xx
T: 11/19/xx

WORD ANALYSIS QUESTIONS

1. The patient had metastasis to 10 lymph nodes. If you wanted to use the adjective form of *metastasis,* you would say, "She had cancer that was ____________________."
2. Divide *biopsy* into its two word parts and define each word part.

Word Part	**Definition**
____________	________________________________
____________	________________________________

3. Divide *dissection* into its two word parts and define each word part.

Word Part	**Definition**
____________	________________________________
____________	________________________________

4. Divide *carcinoma* into its two word parts and define each word part.

Word Part	**Definition**
____________	________________________________
____________	________________________________

FACT FINDING QUESTIONS

1. How did the patient discover her breast mass?

   ____

2. What was the first test that the doctor ordered for her to have?

   ____

3. What operative procedure was performed after the mammography?

   ____

4. How many of the patient's lymph nodes showed signs of cancer?

   ____

5. What is anaplasia?

   ____

CRITICAL THINKING QUESTIONS

1. Why is it important to know that the patient has no history of cancer in her family?

   ____

2. What is a frozen section and when is it performed?

   ____

3. A tumor that extends into the tissue near it is said to be ______________.

   a. metastatic
   b. invasive
   c. carcinoma
   d. embryonic

4. What sentence tells you that all of the tumor was removed?

   ____

Pronunciation Checklist

Read each word and its pronunciation. Practice pronouncing each word. Verify your pronunciation by listening to the Pronunciation List on the CD-ROM. Check the box next to the word after you master its pronunciation.

- ❑ adenocarcinoma (AD-eh-noh-KAR-sih-NOH-mah)
- ❑ adjuvant therapy (AD-joo-vant THAIR-ah-pee)
- ❑ alkylating chemotherapy drug (AL-kih-lay-ting KEE-moh-THAIR-ah-pee DRUHG)
- ❑ alpha fetoprotein (AL-fah FEE-toh-PRO-teen)
- ❑ anaplasia (AN-ah-PLAY-zee-ah) (AN-ah-PLAY-zha)
- ❑ angiogenesis (AN-jee-oh-JEN-eh-sis)
- ❑ angiosarcoma (AN-jee-oh-sar-KOH-mah)
- ❑ antimetabolite chemotherapy drug (AN-tee-meh-TAB-oh-lite KEE-moh-THAIR-ah-pee DRUHG)
- ❑ apoptosis (AP-awp-TOH-sis)
- ❑ aspiration biopsy (AS-pih-RAY-shun BY-awp-see)
- ❑ astrocytoma (AS-troh-sy-TOH-mah)
- ❑ basal cell carcinoma (BAY-sal SEL KAR-sih-NOH-mah)
- ❑ benign (bee-NINE)
- ❑ biopsy (BY-awp-see)
- ❑ bone marrow aspiration (BOHN MAIR-oh AS-pih-RAY-shun)
- ❑ bone marrow transplantation (BOHN MAIR-oh TRANS-plan-TAY-shun)
- ❑ brachytherapy (BRAK-ee-THAIR-ah-pee)
- ❑ bronchogenic carcinoma (BRONG-koh-JEN-ik KAR-sih-NOH-mah)
- ❑ cancer (KAN-ser)
- ❑ cancerous (KAN-ser-us)
- ❑ carcinoembryonic antigen (KAR-sih-noh-EM-bree-AW-nik AN-tih-jen)
- ❑ carcinogen (KAR-SIN-oh-jen)
- ❑ carcinoid syndrome (KAR-sih-noyd SIN-drohm)
- ❑ carcinoid tumor (KAR-sih-noyd TOO-mor)
- ❑ carcinoma (KAR-sih-NOH-mah)
- ❑ carcinomatosis (KAR-sih-NOH-mah-TOH-sis)
- ❑ cell (SEL)
- ❑ cellular (SEL-yoo-lar)
- ❑ central venous catheter (SEN-tral VEE-nus KATH-eh-ter)
- ❑ chemoembolization (KEE-moh-EM-bol-ih-ZAY-shun)
- ❑ chemotherapy (KEE-moh-THAIR-ah-pee)
- ❑ chemotherapy antibiotic drug (KEE-moh-THAIR-ah-pee AN-tee-by-AWT-ik DRUHG)
- ❑ chemotherapy drug (KEE-moh-THAIR-ah-pee DRUHG)
- ❑ chemotherapy protocol (KEE-moh-THAIR-ah-pee PROH-toh-kawl)
- ❑ cholangiocarcinoma (koh-LAN-jee-oh-KAR-sih-NOH-mah)
- ❑ chondrosarcoma (CON-droh-sar-KOH-mah)
- ❑ choriocarcinoma (KOH-ree-oh-KAR-sih-NOH-mah)
- ❑ chromosomal (KROH-moh-SOH-mal)
- ❑ chromosome (KROH-moh-sohm)
- ❑ conformal radiotherapy (con-FOR-mal RAY-dee-oh-THAIR-ah-pee)
- ❑ cryosurgery (KRY-oh-SER-jer-ee)
- ❑ cystectomy (sis-TEK-toh-mee)
- ❑ cytoplasm (SY-toh-plazm)
- ❑ debulk (dee-BULK)
- ❑ deoxyribonucleic acid (dee-AWK-see-RY-boh-noo-KLEE-ik AS-id)
- ❑ differentiation (DIF-er-EN-shee-AA-shun)
- ❑ dysgerminoma (DIS-jer-mih-NOH-mah)
- ❑ dysplasia (dis-PLAY-zee-ah) (dis-PLAY-zha)
- ❑ dysplastic (dis-PLAS-tik)
- ❑ electrosurgery (ee-LEK-troh-SER-jer-ee)
- ❑ embryonal cell cancer (EM-bree-oh-nal SEL KAN-ser)
- ❑ en bloc resection (en BLAWK ree-SEK-shun)
- ❑ encapsulated tumor (en-KAP-soo-lay-ted TOO-mor)
- ❑ endometrial carcinoma (EN-doh-MEE-tree-al KAR-sih-NOH-mah)
- ❑ endoplasmic reticulum (EN-doh-PLAS-mik reh-TIK-yoo-lum)
- ❑ endoscopy (en-DAWS-koh-pee)
- ❑ Ewing's sarcoma (YOO-ingz sar-KOH-mah)
- ❑ excision (ek-SIZH-un)
- ❑ excisional biopsy (ek-SIZH-un-al BY-awp-see)
- ❑ exenteration (eks-EN-ter-AA-shun)
- ❑ exfoliative cytology (eks-FOH-lee-ah-tiv sy-TAWL-oh-jee)
- ❑ exploratory laparotomy (eks-PLOR-ah-TOHR-ee LAP-ah-ROT-ah-mee)
- ❑ external beam radiotherapy (eks-TER-nal BEEM RAY-dee-oh-THAIR-ah-pee)
- ❑ fibrosarcoma (FY-broh-sar-KOH-mah)
- ❑ fractionation (FRAK-shun-AA-shun)
- ❑ gene (JEEN)
- ❑ genetic (jeh-NET-ik)
- ❑ glioblastoma multiforme (GLY-oh-blas-TOH-mah mul-tih-FOR-may)
- ❑ Golgi apparatus (GOHL-jee AP-ah-RAT-us)
- ❑ hepatoblastoma (HEP-ah-toh-blas-TOH-mah)
- ❑ hepatocellular carcinoma (HEP-ah-to-SEL-yoo-lar KAR-sih-NOH-mah)
- ❑ heredity (heh-RED-ih-tee)
- ❑ Hodgkin's lymphoma (HAWJ-kinz lim-FOH-mah)
- ❑ hormonal chemotherapy drug (hor-MOH-nal KEE-moh-THAIR-ah-pee DRUHG)
- ❑ human chorionic gonadotropin (HYOO-man KOH-ree-ON-ik GOH-nad-oh-TROH-pin)
- ❑ implantable port (im-PLANT-ah-bl PORT)
- ❑ in situ (in SY-too)
- ❑ incisional biopsy (in-SIZH-un-al BY-awp-see)
- ❑ internal radiotherapy (in-TER-nal RAY-dee-oh-THAIR-ah-pee)
- ❑ interstitial radiotherapy (IN-ter-STISH-al RAY-dee-oh-THAIR-ah-pee)
- ❑ intra-arterial catheter (IN-trah-ar-TEE-ree-al KATH-eh-ter)
- ❑ intracavitary radiotherapy (IN-trah-KAV-ih-tair-ee RAY-dee-oh-THAIR-ah-pee)
- ❑ intracellular (IN-trah-SEL-yoo-lar)
- ❑ intraperitoneal catheter (IN-trah-PAIR-ih-toh-NEE-al KATH-eh-ter)
- ❑ intrathecal catheter (IN-trah-THEE-kal KATH-eh-ter)

- ❑ intrathecal chemotherapy (IN-trah-THEE-kal KEE-moh-THAIR-ah-pee)
- ❑ intravenous radiotherapy (IN-trah-VEE-nus RAY-dee-oh-THAIR-ah-pee)
- ❑ intravesical chemotherapy (IN-trah-VES-ih-kal KEE-moh-THAIR-ah-pee)
- ❑ invasive (in-VAY-siv)
- ❑ Kaposi's sarcoma (KAH-poh-seez sar-KOH-mah)
- ❑ karyotype (KAIR-ee-oh-type)
- ❑ leiomyosarcoma (LIE-oh-MY-oh-sar-KOH-mah)
- ❑ leukemia (loo-KEE-mee-ah)
- ❑ liposarcoma (LY-poh-sar-KOH-mah)
- ❑ lobectomy (loh-BEK-toh-mee)
- ❑ lumpectomy (lum-PEK-toh-mee)
- ❑ lymph node dissection (LIMF NOHD dy-SEK-shun)
- ❑ lymphadenopathy (LIM-fad-eh-NAWP-ah-thee)
- ❑ lymphangiography (lim-FAN-jee-AWG-rah-fee)
- ❑ lymphocytic leukemia (LIM-foh-SIT-ik loo-KEE-mee-ah)
- ❑ lymphoma (lim-FOH-mah)
- ❑ lysosome (LY-soh-sohm)
- ❑ malignant (mah-LIG-nant)
- ❑ malignant melanoma (mah-LIG-nant MEL-ah-NOH-mah)
- ❑ mammography (mah-MAWG-rah-fee)
- ❑ medical oncologist (MED-ih-kal ong-KAWL-oh-jist)
- ❑ metastases (meh-TAS-tah-seez)
- ❑ metastasis (meh-TAS-tah-sis)
- ❑ metastasize (meh-TAS-tah-size)
- ❑ metastatic (MET-ah-STAT-ik)
- ❑ mitochondria (MY-toh-CON-dree-ah)
- ❑ mitochondrial (MY-toh-CON-dree-al)
- ❑ mitochondrion (MY-toh-CON-dree-on)
- ❑ mitosis (my-TOH-sis)
- ❑ mitosis inhibitor drug (my-TOH-sis in-HIB-ih-tor DRUHG)
- ❑ mitotic (my-TAWT-ik)
- ❑ monoclonal antibody (MAWN-oh-KLOH-nal AN-tee-BAWD-ee)
- ❑ multiple myeloma (MUL-tih-pl MY-eh-LOH-mah)
- ❑ mutation (myoo-TAY-shun)
- ❑ myelogenous leukemia (MY-eh-LAWJ-eh-nus loo-KEE-mee-ah)
- ❑ myosarcoma (MY-oh-sar-KOH-mah)
- ❑ neoplasia (NEE-oh-PLAY-zee-ah)
- ❑ neoplasm (NEE-oh-plazm)
- ❑ nephroblastoma (NEF-roh-blas-TOH-mah)
- ❑ neuroblastoma (NYOOR-oh-blas-TOH-mah)
- ❑ neurofibrosarcoma (NYOOR-oh-FY-broh-sar-KOH-mah)
- ❑ nuclear (NYOO-klee-ar)
- ❑ nuclei (NYOO-klee-eye)
- ❑ nucleolar (nyoo-KLEE-oh-lar)
- ❑ nucleoli (nyoo-KLEE-oh-lie)
- ❑ nucleolus (nyoo-KLEE-oh-lus)
- ❑ nucleus (NYOO-klee-us)
- ❑ oligodendroglioma (OHL-ih-goh-DEN-droh-glee-OH-mah)
- ❑ oncogene (AWNG-koh-jeen)
- ❑ oncologist (ong-KAWL-oh-jist)
- ❑ oncology (ong-KAWL-oh-jee)
- ❑ organelle (OR-gah-NEL) (OR-gah-nel)
- ❑ osteosarcoma (AWS-tee-oh-sar-KOH-mah)
- ❑ percutaneous radiofrequency ablation (PER-kyoo-TAY-nee-us RAY-dee-oh-FREE-kwen-see ah-BLAY-shun)
- ❑ peripheral (peh-RIF-eh-ral)
- ❑ platinum chemotherapy drug (PLAT-ih-num KEE-moh-THAIR-ah-pee DRUHG)
- ❑ radiation (RAY-dee-AA-shun)
- ❑ radiation oncologist (RAY-dee-AA-shun ong-KAWL-oh-jist)
- ❑ radical resection (RAD-ih-kal re-SEK-shun)
- ❑ radioresistant (RAY-dee-oh-ree-ZIS-tant)
- ❑ radiosensitive (RAY-dee-oh-SEN-sih-tiv)
- ❑ radiotherapy (RAY-dee-oh-THAIR-ah-pee)
- ❑ receptor assay (ree-SEP-tor AS-say)
- ❑ relapse (REE-laps)
- ❑ remission (ree-MISH-un)
- ❑ resection (ree-SEK-shun)
- ❑ retinoblastoma (RET-ih-noh-blas-TOH-mah)
- ❑ rhabdomyosarcoma (RAB-doh-MY-oh-sar-KOH-mah)
- ❑ ribonucleic acid (RY-boh-nyoo-KLEE-ik AS-id)
- ❑ ribosome (RY-boh-sohm)
- ❑ sarcoma (sar-KOH-mah)
- ❑ scintigraphy (sin-TIG-rah-fee)
- ❑ seminoma (SEM-ih-NOH-mah)
- ❑ sentinel lymph node (SEN-tih-nal LIMF NOHD)
- ❑ sentinel node biopsy (SEN-tih-nal NOHD BY-awp-see)
- ❑ squamous cell carcinoma (SKWAY-mus SEL KAR-sih-NOH-mah)
- ❑ stereotactic biopsy (STAIR-ee-oh-TAK-tik BY-awp-see)
- ❑ suppressor gene (soo-PRES-or JEEN)
- ❑ surgical technologist (SER-jih-kal tek-NAWL-oh-jist)
- ❑ teratoma (TER-ah-TOH-mah)
- ❑ tomography (toh-MAWG-rah-fee)
- ❑ transarterial chemoembolization (TRANS-ar-TEE-ree-al KEE-moh-EM-bol-ih-ZAY-shun)
- ❑ transitional cell carcinoma (trans-ZISH-un-al SEL KAR-sih-NOH-mah)
- ❑ translocation (TRANS-loh-KAY-shun)
- ❑ tumor (TOO-mor)
- ❑ tumor necrosis factor (TOO-mor neh-KROH-sis FAK-tor)
- ❑ ultrasonography (UL-trah-soh-NAWG-rah-fee)
- ❑ undifferentiated (un-DIF-er-EN-shee-aa-ted)
- ❑ urinalysis (YOO-rih-NAL-ih-sis)
- ❑ Wilms' tumor (WILMZ TOO-mor)

Experience Multimedia

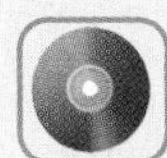

CD-ROM Learning Activities Checklist

Check off the box as you complete each learning activity.

- ❑ **CD-ROM Learning Activity 18.1: *ANATOMY WORD PARTS FLASHCARDS***
  Use flashcards to help you memorize word parts. Make your own flashcards or print out prepared flashcards. Also see the electronic flashcard game. Time: 20 minutes.
- ❑ **CD-ROM Learning Activity 18.2: *DISEASE AND OTHER WORD PARTS FLASHCARDS***
  A continuation of the flashcard learning activity. Time: 20 minutes.
- ❑ **CD-ROM Learning Activity 18.3: *MEMORY AIDS***
  Use memory aids to help you memorize medical words and meanings. Time: 5 minutes.
- ❑ **CD-ROM Learning Activity 18.4: *MEDICAL LANGUAGE SPOKEN HERE***
  Listen to actual medical reports and spell the missing medical words. Time: 10 minutes.
- ❑ **CD-ROM Learning Activity 18.5: *SPELLING CHALLENGE***
  Listen to a pronounced medical word and then spell it. Time: 5 minutes.
- ❑ **CD-ROM Learning Activity 18.6: *MEDICAL LANGUAGE PRONUNCIATION***
  Listen to a pronounced medical word and then practice pronouncing it. Time: 30 minutes.
- ❑ **CD-ROM Learning Activity 18.7: *EDUCATIONAL FUN AND GAMES***
  Enjoy these fun activities while reinforcing your knowledge. Time: 15 minutes.

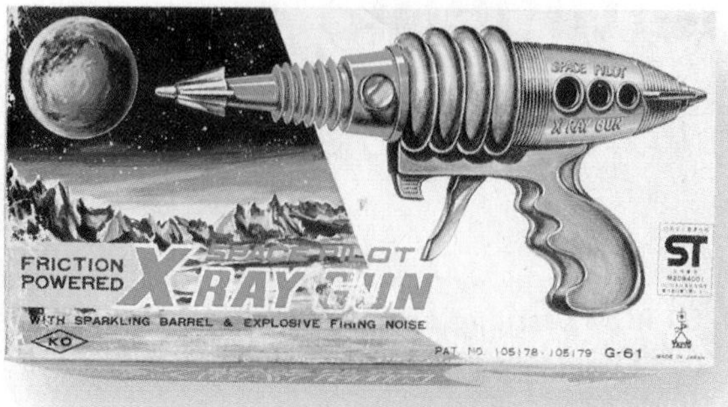

While it may seem like science fiction, X-ray technology is real, and it's not kid stuff.

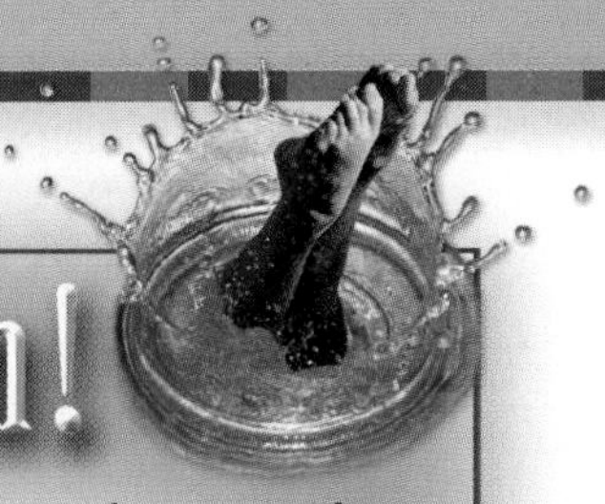

Dive In!

- The X-ray got its name because when it was discovered it was an unknown type of radiation—therefore called "X"
- Ultrasound often provides a clearer picture in space because low gravity allows sound waves to move with less distortion.
- If you think this is interesting, keep scanning. In this chapter we'll explore the language that describes the various processes of diagnostic imaging.
- You'll see the whole picture once you master the language of radiology!

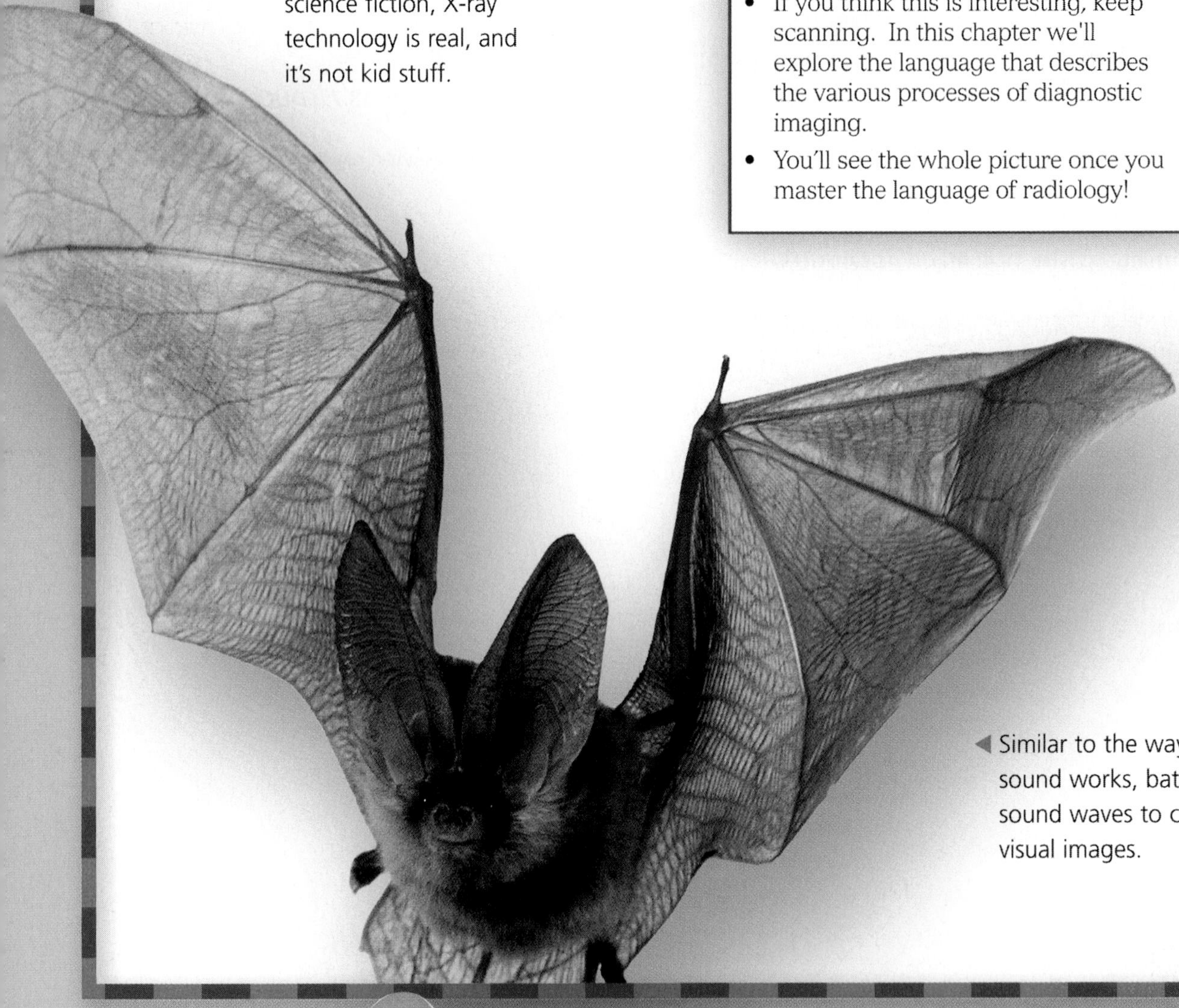

Similar to the way ultrasound works, bats use sound waves to create visual images.

Medicine Through HISTORY

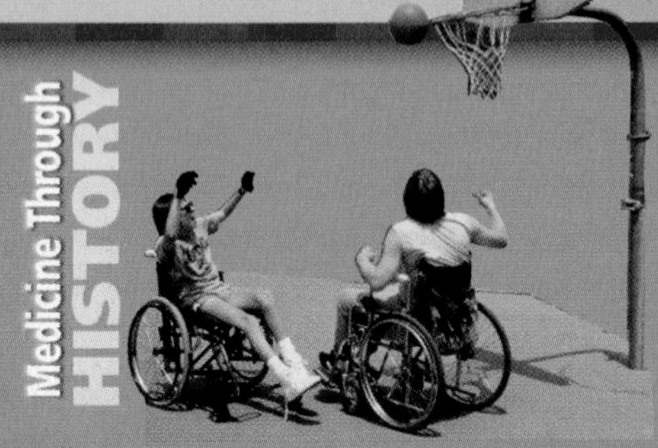

1990

The Americans with Disabilities Act (ADA) prohibits discrimination against handicapped persons

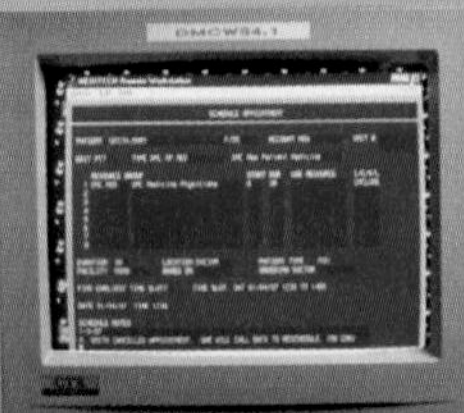

1996

The Healthcare Insurance Portability & Accountability Act (HIPAA) requires that a patient's medical information be kept secure and only released to others who are caring for the patient

CHAPTER 19
Radiology and Nuclear Medicine

Radiology (RAY-dee-AWL-oh-jee) is the medical specialty that combines study of anatomy and physiology, energy (x-rays, a magnetic field, sound waves), and radiation and uses technology to create images of the internal structures of the body. Nuclear medicine is the medical specialty that uses radioactive substances to create images of internal structures of the body for the purpose of diagnosis.

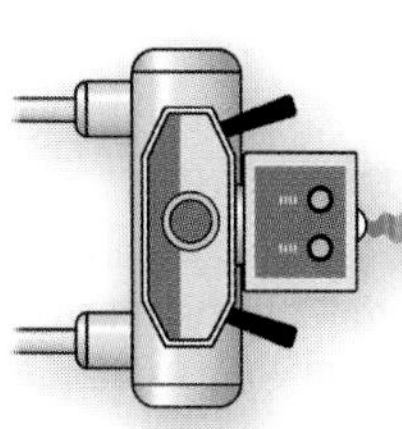

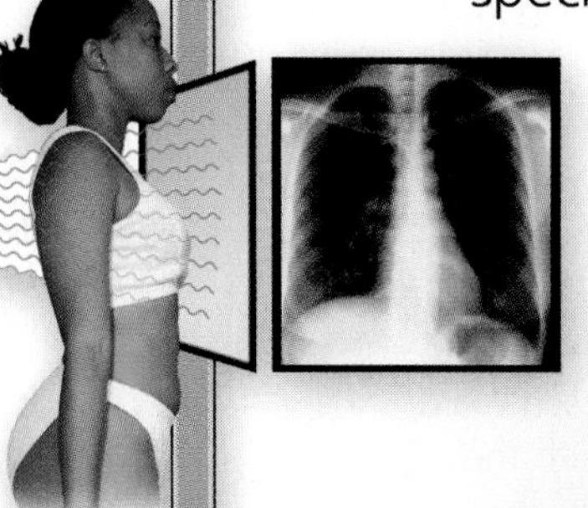

▲ X-rays travel from the machine through the body to the plate which creates the image.

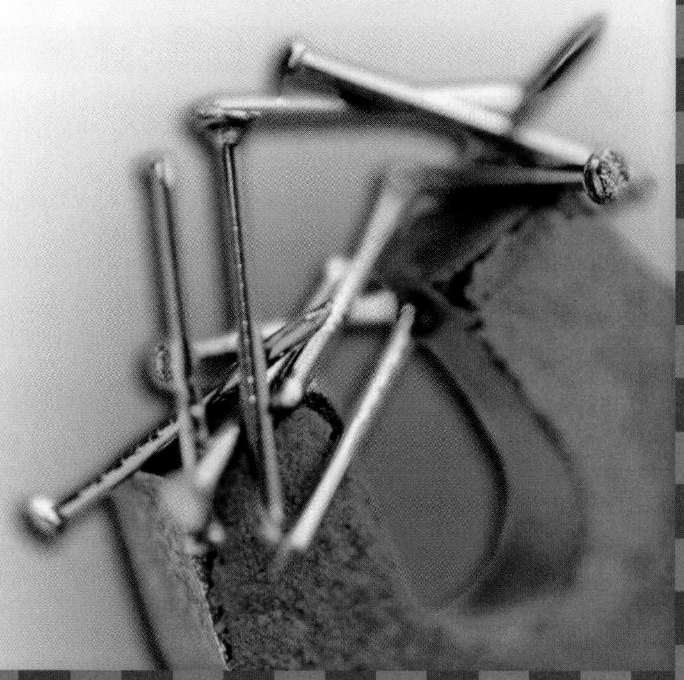

▶ Magnetic fields are used to construct diagnostic images via MRI technology.

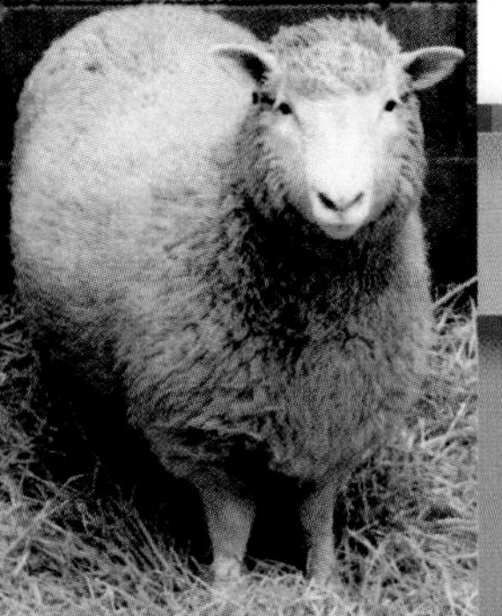

1996

Dolly the sheep becomes the first animal to be cloned from the cells of another animal

2000

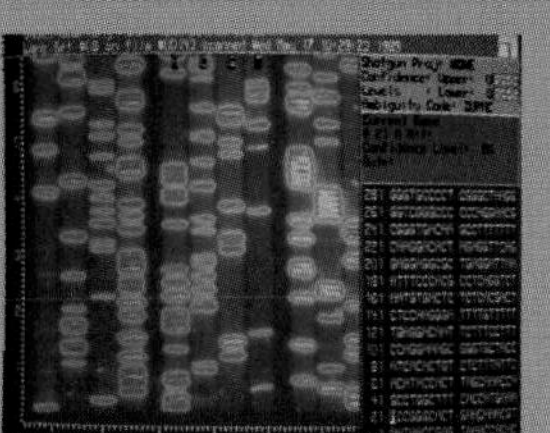

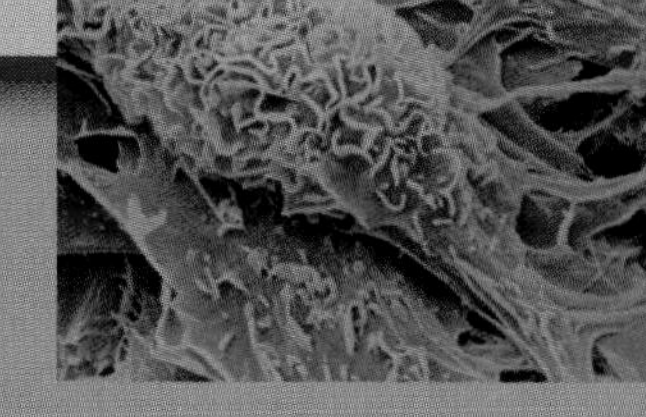

The map of the human genome is completed

2001

The first embryonic stem cell is made into a mature blood cell. This ignited a controversy over the use of embryos in stem cell research

Measure Your Progress: Learning Objectives

After you study this chapter, you should be able to

1. Describe five radiologic procedures that use x-rays.
2. Describe common roentgen views and patient positions.
3. Identify common radiologic procedures that use iodinated contrast dye.
4. Describe the radiologic procedure that uses a magnetic field.
5. Describe five nuclear medicine procedures that use gamma rays or positrons.
6. Build radiology and nuclear medicine words from combining forms, prefixes, and suffixes.
7. Define common radiology and nuclear medicine abbreviations.
8. Correctly spell and pronounce radiology and nuclear medicine words.
9. Apply your skills by analyzing a radiology report.
10. Test your knowledge of radiology and nuclear medicine by completing review exercises at the end of the chapter and learning activities on the CD-ROM.

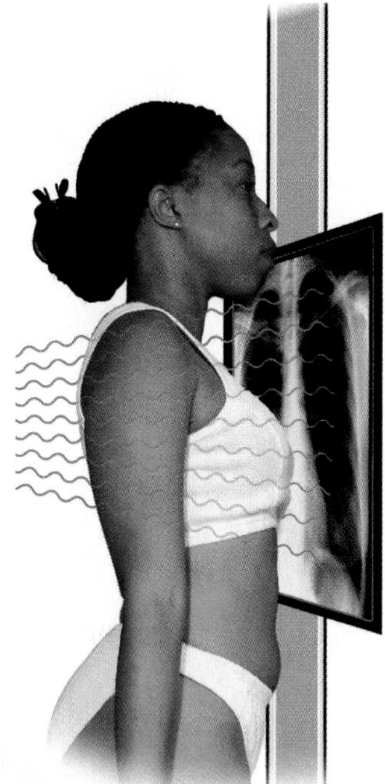

Figure 19-1 ■ Radiology and nuclear medicine.

Radiology and nuclear medicine allow us to view the internal structures and functions of the human body.

Medical Language Key

To unlock the meaning of a medical word, first define each word part. Then put the word part definitions in order, beginning with the suffix, followed by the first word part.

	Word Part	Word Part Definition
SUFFIX	-logy	*the study of*
COMBINING FORM	radi/o-	*radius (forearm bone); x-rays; radiation*

Radiology: ***The study of x-rays and radiation.***

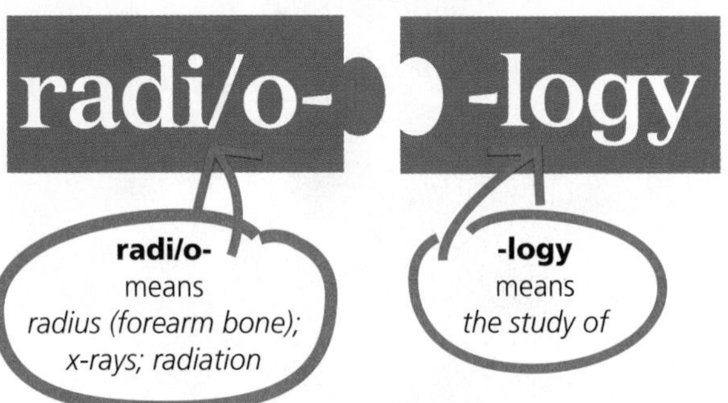

www.prenhall.com/turley

For interactive flashcards, real-life video clips, games, exercises, and audio pronunciations please explore the companion CD-ROM in the back of the book. Click on the companion website for bonus chapters, additional resources, and links to on-line learning.

Anatomy and Physiology

The anatomy and physiology of the body can be seen in a whole new way in radiology and nuclear medicine. X-rays, sound waves, and other forms of energy penetrate the body and allow us to view parts that are otherwise only accessible during surgery (see Figure 19-1■). Other radiologic procedures show the metabolic processes that make up the physiology of the body.

Radiology

Radiologic Procedures That Use X-Rays

X-rays are a type of invisible ionizing **radiation.** They have a very short wavelength and contain so much energy that they are able to pass through the body. X-rays are produced when a positively charged metal plate inside a vacuum tube is bombarded with a stream of electrons. X-rays are used in the following types of radiologic tests: roentgenography, fluoroscopy, computerized axial tomography, and mammography.

Roentgenography During **roentgenography,** the patient is placed between the x-ray beam and an x-ray plate (a large, flat, silver plate). The x-rays from the x-ray machine travel through the patient's body to the x-ray plate (see Figure 19-2■). The image is in various shades of black, white, and gray that correspond to the density of various tissues. Air (in a body cavity or the lungs) has a low density, and x-rays

x-ray (EKS-ray)
X-ray is derived from the German phrase *x-strahl,* where *x* (an unknown number) is combined with *strah* (beam, ray).

radiation (RAY-dee-AA-shun)
radi/o- *radius (forearm bone); x-rays; radiation*
-ation *a process; being or having*
Some word parts have more than one definition. The best definition of *radiation* is *being or having x-rays.*

roentgenography (RENT-geh-NAWG-rah-fee)
roentgen/o- *x-ray; radiation*
-graphy *process of recording*
The word was coined by Wilhelm Roentgen (1845–1923), a German physicist. This is an example of an eponym: a person from whom something takes its name.

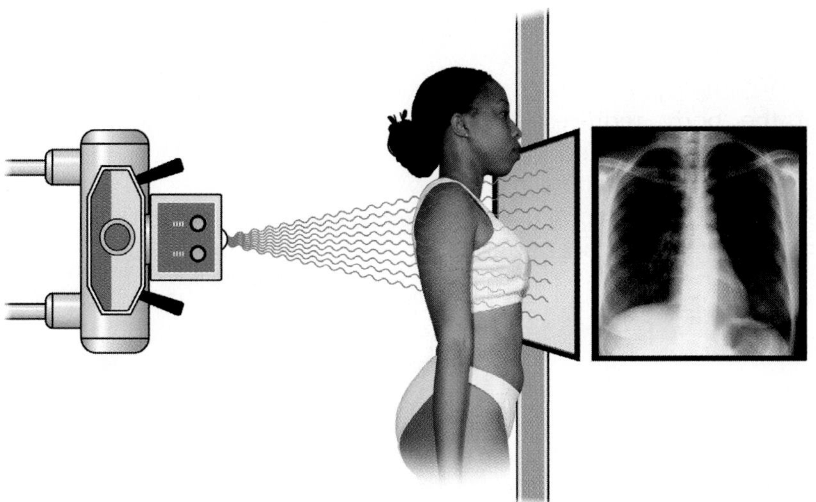

Figure 19-2 ■ Roentgenography.

This patient is having a PA (posteroanterior) chest x-ray. The x-ray machine projects a set of crossed lines onto the patient's back to help the technologist center the x-ray beam. The patient is asked to remain still so that the radiograph will not show motion artifact (a blurred image). The x-rays penetrate the patient's posterior chest. They exit through the the patient's anterior chest, enter an x-ray plate, and create an image.

pass through it, creating a nearly black area on the x-ray plate. Areas of low density are said to be **radiolucent.** A bone or body organ has a high density, and x-rays are absorbed by it, creating a white area on the x-ray plate (see Figure 19-2). Areas of high density are said to be **radiopaque.** Areas of intermediate density create various shades of gray.

The image on the x-ray plate is like the negative that is created when photographic film is exposed to light. The x-ray plate is developed with chemicals, and the positive image is printed on flexible plastic film. The radiologist views or reads the x-ray film by placing it in front of a light box (see Figure 19-3 ■) and then dictating the findings. The film image is known as a **roentgenogram** or a **radiograph.**

radiolucent (RAY-dee-oh-LOO-sent)
radi/o- *radius (forearm bone); x-rays; radiation*
luc/o- *clear and shining*
-ent *pertaining to*

radiopaque (RAY-dee-oh-PAYK)
Radiopaque is a combination of the combining form *radi/o-* and the word *opaque* (not transparent).

roentgenogram (RENT-gen-oh-gram)
roentgen/o- *x-ray; radiation*
-gram *a record or picture*
Roentgen is the unit of measurement for x-rays or gamma rays. It was named for Wilhelm Roentgen.

radiograph (RAY-dee-oh-graf)
radi/o- *radius (forearm bone); x-rays; radiation*
-graph *instrument used to record*
As commonly used in medicine, the word *radiograph* is a misnomer because it refers to the x-ray image, which does not follow the traditional meaning of the suffix *-graph* (instrument used to record).

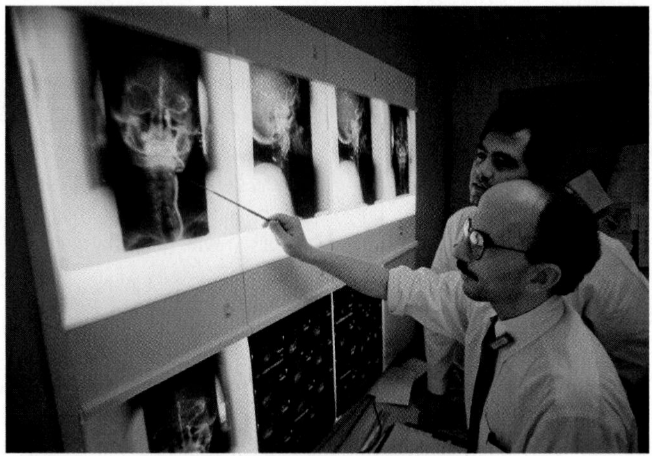

Figure 19-3 ■ Reading an x-ray.
This radiologist is viewing and reading the patient's x-ray (a cerebral arteriogram) in consultation with another radiologist. The intense light of the light box illuminates fine details on the x-ray film. After the radiologist dictates his findings, a medical transcriptionist transcribes the dictation and creates a formatted radiology report for the patient's medical record. The actual x-ray film is kept in the radiology department, not in the patient's medical record.

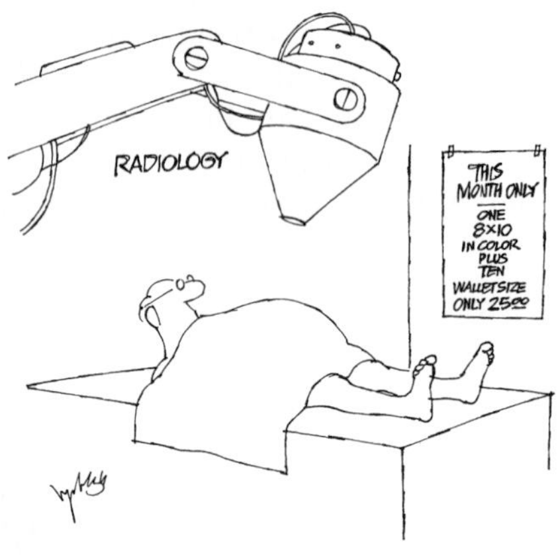

Roentgenography of different parts of the body requires the patient to be placed in different positions. These standardized positions of the angle of the patient in relation the x-ray machine are known as **projections** or views (see Table 19-1). Roentgenography uses specialized terminology to refer to other commonly used procedures and equipment (see Table 19-2).

projection (proh-JEK-shun)
project/o- *throw forward*
-ion *action; condition*

Table 19-1 Roentgen Projections

Projection	Description	Word Part and Definition
PA chest x-ray (posteroanterior)	The x-ray beam enters patient's upper back, penetrates the upper body, exits through the anterior chest, and enters the x-ray plate. Position: The patient is in a standing position with the chest next to the x-ray plate. Comment: This is the standard position and most common type of chest x-ray (see Figure 19-2).	**posteroanterior** (POHS-ter-oh-an-TEER-ee-or) **poster/o-** *back part* **anter/o-** *before; front part* **-ior** *pertaining to*
AP chest x-ray (anteroposterior)	The x-ray beam enters patient's anterior chest, penetrates the upper body, exits through the upper back, and enters the x-ray plate. Position: The patient is in a standing or lying position with the upper back next to the x-ray plate. Comment: This position is used for portable chest x-rays taken at the bedside.	**anteroposterior** (AN-ter-oh-pohs-TEER-ee-or) **anter/o-** *before; front part* **poster/o-** *back part* **-ior** *pertaining to*
lateral chest x-ray	The x-ray beam enters the patient's chest from the side, penetrates the upper body, and exits through the other side. Position: The patient is in a standing or lying position. In a left lateral x-ray, the left side of the body is beside the x-ray plate. Comment: Also known as a lateral view or side view.	**lateral** (LAT-er-al) **later/o-** *side* **-al** *pertaining to*
oblique x-ray	The x-ray beam enters the body from an oblique angle, midway between anterior and lateral. Position: The patient can be standing or lying.	**oblique** (awb-LEEK) *Oblique* is derived from a Latin word meaning *slanted.*
cross-table lateral x-ray	The x-ray beam enters the patient's chest and abdomen from the side. Position: The patient is lying on the x-ray table; the x-ray plate is on one side, and the x-ray machine is on the other. Comment: The x-ray beam travels across the x-ray table.	
lateral decubitus x-ray	The x-ray beam enters the patient's chest and abdomen from the side. Position: The patient is lying on his/her side on the x-ray table, and the x-ray plate is inside the table beneath the patient. Comment: For a left lateral decubitus film, the patient is lying on his/her left side.	**decubitus** (dee-KYOO-bih-tus) *Decubitus* is a Latin word meaning *lying down.*
flat plate of the abdomen	The x-ray beam enters the patient's abdomen, exits through the back, and enters the x-ray plate. Position: The patient is lying on the x-ray table, and the x-ray plate is inside the table beneath the patient. Comment: *Flat plate* refers to the fact that the patient is lying down flat.	
KUB	The x-ray beam enters the patient's chest and abdomen, exits through the back, and enters the x-ray plate. Position: The patient is lying on the x-ray table, and the x-ray plate is inside the table beneath the patient. KUB stands for kidneys, ureters, and bladder, the organs that are x-rayed.	

Table 19-2 Additional Roentgenography Terminology

Word or Phrase	Description	Word Part and Definition
film badge	A badge worn by all healthcare professionals who work in the radiology and nuclear medicine department. The badge contains a clear, unexposed piece of x-ray film that becomes progressively more opaque with cumulative exposure to radiation (x-rays, gamma rays from radioactive substances). Radiation exposure is measured in **rems. Dosimetry** is the process of measuring the amount of radiation exposure as detected by a film badge and measured by a **dosimeter.**	**rem** (REM) *Rem* is an abbreviation for *roentgen-equivalent man.* **dosimetry** (doh-SIM-eh-tree) **dos/i-** *dose* **-metry** *process of measuring* **dosimeter** (doh-SIM-eh-ter) **dos/i-** *dose* **-meter** *instrument used to measure*
lead apron	Lead is an extremely dense substance that does not permit x-rays to pass through it. Lead aprons are used to shield parts of the patient's body that are not being x-rayed; they are also worn by the radiology department staff if they must be in the room with the patient while the procedure is being performed.	
plain film	Any radiograph that is taken without the use of a contrast dye.	
portable film	Radiograph taken at the bedside or in the emergency department when the patient cannot be transported to the radiology department.	
scout film	Preliminary radiograph that is taken to provide an initial view of an area before a radiopaque contrast dye is administered.	

Connections

Obstetrics (Chapter 13). Pregnant woman are generally advised to avoid x-rays. However, sometimes x-rays are necessary to evaluate the mother's health. Although an exposure of 5000 rems has been shown to cause a risk of fetal deformity, most x-rays involve significantly less exposure, as shown below. The abbreviation mrem stands for microrem (one-thousandth of a rem).

dental x-ray	1 mrem
mammogram	2 mrem
chest x-ray (2 views)	8 mrem
CT scan	1000 mrem

Radiologic Procedures That Use Contrast Dye

The details on roentgenographic images and fluoroscopic images (described in the next section) can be enhanced by using barium or **iodinated contrast dyes** to outline anatomic structures.

iodinated (EYE-oh-dih-NAY-ted)
iodin/o- *iodine*
-ated *pertaining to a condition; composed of*

Word or Phrase	Word Part and Definition	Description
angiography	**angiography** (AN-jee-AWG-rah-fee) angi/o- *blood vessel; lymphatic vessel* -graphy *process of recording* **angiogram** (AN-jee-oh-gram) angi/o- *blood vessel; lymphatic vessel* -gram *a record or picture* **arteriography** (ar-TEER-ee-AWG-rah-fee) arteri/o- *artery* -graphy *process of recording* **arteriogram** (ar-TEER-ee-oh-gram) arteri/o- *artery* -gram *a record or picture* **venography** (vee-NAWG-rah-fee) ven/o- *vein* -graphy *process of recording* **venogram** (VEE-noh-gram) ven/o- *vein* -gram *a record or picture* **aortography** (AA-or-TAWG-rah-fee) aort/o- *aorta* -graphy *process of recording* **aortogram** (aa-OR-toh-gram) aort/o- *aorta* -gram *a record or picture* **rotational** (roh-TAY-shun-al) rotat/o- *rotate* -ion *action; condition* -al *pertaining to*	Contrast dye is injected to outline a blood vessel. In **arteriography,** it is injected into an artery to show blockage, narrowed areas, or aneuryms (see Figure 19-4 ■). In **venography,** it is injected into a vein to show weakened valves and dilated walls. The x-ray image is known as an **angiogram** or specifically an **arteriogram** or **venogram. Coronary angiography** uses contrast dye injected during a cardiac catheterization procedure to show narrowing or blockage of the coronary arteries. **Aortography** uses contrast dye in the aorta to show stenosis or an aneurysm. In **digital subtraction angiography (DSA),** two x-ray images are obtained, first without contrast and then after contrast has been injected. A computer compares the two images and digitally "subtracts" or removes the images of the soft tissues, bones, and muscles, leaving just the image of the arteries. In **rotational angiography,** the x-ray machine moves around the area to be examined and multiple x-rays are taken after contrast is injected. Over 100 separate images can be taken in about one minute. The computer then creates a three-dimensional image that can be rotated and viewed from all angles. This technique is particularly helpful in documenting tortuous arteries or areas where the normal anatomy is distorted. **Figure 19-4 ■ Arteriogram of the left carotid artery and cerebral arteries.** This procedure is also known as a cerebral angiography or carotid arteriography. The injected dye clearly outlines the carotid artery and its many smaller branches within the cranial cavity. There is no evidence of carotid artery plaques or cerebral aneurysm.

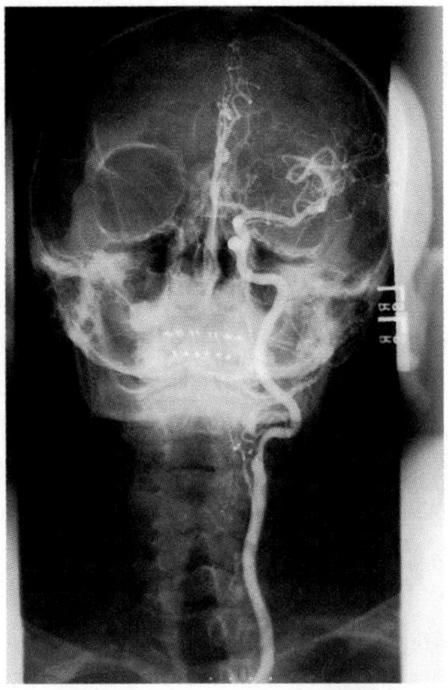

Word or Phrase	Word Part and Definition	Description
arthrography	**arthrography** (ar-THRAWG-rah-fee) **arthr/o-** *joint* **-graphy** *process of recording* **arthrogram** (AR-throh-gram) **arthr/o-** *joint* **-gram** *a record or picture*	Contrast dye is injected into the joint. It outlines the bones, capsule, and soft tissue structures of the joint. The image is known as an **arthrogram.**
barium enema	**barium** (BAIR-ee-um) **enema** (EN-eh-mah)	Barium contrast dye is instilled into the rectum. It outlines the colon and rectum and shows tumors, polyps, diverticula, and abnormalities in the bowel wall (see Figure 3-21). For a **double contrast (air contrast) enema,** the barium is removed and then air is instilled as a second contrast. Fluoroscopy and individual radiographs are done to document the results of the procedure.
cholangiography, intravenous (IVC)	**cholangiography** (KOH-lan-jee-AWG-rah-fee) **chol/o-** *bile, gall* **angi/o-** *blood vessel; lymphatic vessel* **-graphy** *process of recording* **intravenous** (IN-trah-VEE-nus) **intra-** *with* **ven/o-** *vein* **-ous** *pertaining to* **cholangiogram** (koh-LAN-jee-oh-gram) **chol/o-** *bile, gall* **angi/o-** *blood vessel; lymphatic vessel* **-gram** *a record or picture*	Contrast dye is injected intravenously. It travels through the blood to the liver and is then excreted with bile into the gallbladder. It outlines the gallbladder and shows thickening of the gallbladder wall and gallstones. The x-ray image is known as a **cholangiogram.**
cholecystography, oral (OCG)	**cholecystography** (KOH-lee-sis-TAWG-rah-fee) **chol/e-** *bile, gall* **cyst/o-** *bladder; fluid-filled sac; semisolid cyst* **-graphy** *process of recording* **cholecystogram** (KOH-lee-SIS-toh-gram) **chol/e-** *bile, gall* **cyst/o-** *bladder; fluid-filled sac; semisolid cyst* **-gram** *a record or picture*	Contrast dye in tablet form is taken orally. From the small intestine, it enters the blood, is processed by the liver, and then excreted with bile into the gallbladder. It outlines the gallbladder and shows thickening of the gallbladder wall and gallstones. The contrast dye can also be injected intravenously to perform intravenous cholecystography. The x-ray image is known as a **cholecystogram.**

Word or Phrase	Word Part and Definition	Description
hysterosalpingo-graphy	**hysterosalpingography** (HIS-ter-oh-SAL-pin-GAWG-rah-fee) **hyster/o-** *uterus* **salping/o-** *fallopian tube* **-graphy** *process of recording* **hysterosalpingogram** (HIS-ter-oh-sal-PING-oh-gram) **hyster/o-** *uterus* **salping/o-** *fallopian tube* **-gram** *a record or picture*	Contrast dye is inserted through a catheter into the vagina and then into the uterus and fallopian tubes. It outlines the walls of the uterus and fallopian tubes and shows narrowing, scarring, and blockage. The x-ray image is known as a **hysterosalpingogram.**
lymphangiography	**lymphangiography** (lim-FAN-jee-AWG-rah-fee) **lymph/o-** *lymph; lymphatic system* **angi/o-** *blood vessel; lymphatic vessel* **-graphy** *process of recording* **lymphangiogram** (lim-FAN-jee-oh-gram) **lymph/o-** *lymph; lymphatic system* **angi/o-** *blood vessel; lymphatic vessel* **-gram** *a record or picture*	Contrast dye is injected into a lymphatic vessel. It outlines several lymphatic vessels and shows enlarged lymph nodes, lymphomas, and blockages of lymphatic drainage. The x-ray image is known as a **lymphangiogram.**
myelography	**myelography** (MY-eh-LOG-rah-fee) **myel/o-** *bone marrow; spinal cord; myelin* **-graphy** *process of recording* **myelogram** (MY-eh-loh-gram) **myel/o-** *bone marrow; spinal cord; myelin* **-gram** *a record or picture*	Contrast dye is injected into the subarachnoid space at the level of the L3 and L4 vertebrae. It outlines the spinal cavity, spinal nerves, nerve roots, intervertebral disks, and shows tumors and herniated disks. The x-ray image is known as a **myelogram.** Because myelograms can have the side effect of severe headache, a CT scan or MRI scan of the spine is often performed instead.
pyelography	**pyelography** (PY-eh-LOG-rah-fee) **pyel/o-** *renal pelvis* **-graphy** *process of recording* **pyelogram** (PY-eh-loh-gram) **pyel/o-** *renal pelvis* **-gram** *a record or picture* **excretory** (EKS-kree-toh-ree) **excret/o-** *removing from the body* **-ory** *having the function of* **urography** (yoo-RAWG-rah-fee) **ur/o-** *urine; urinary system* **-graphy** *process of recording*	Contrast dye is injected intravenously. It travels through the blood and is excreted in the urine by the kidneys. It outlines the urinary tract and shows narrowing, blockage, and stones (see Figure 11-19). This procedure is known as **intravenous pyelography** or **excretory urography.** In **retrograde pyelography,** a cystoscopy is performed, and contrast dye is injected via a catheter into each ureter. The x-ray image is known as a **pyelogram** or **urogram.** *(continued)*

Word or Phrase	Word Part and Definition	Description
pyelography *(continued)*	**retrograde** (RET-roh-grayd) **retro-** *behind, backward* **-grade** *going* Every medical word must contain a combining form. The suffix of *retrograde* contains the combining form *grad/o-*. **urogram** (YOO-roh-gram) **ur/o-** *urine; urinary system* **-gram** *a record or picture*	
upper gastrointestinal series (UGI)	**gastrointestinal** (GAS-troh-in-TES-tin-al) **gastr/o-** *stomach* **intestin/o-** *intestine* **-al** *pertaining to*	Liquid barium contrast is swallowed. It outlines the esophagus and stomach to show ulcers or areas of blockage. Also known as a **barium swallow.** A **small-bowel follow-through** follows the contrast dye as it outlines the small intestine. To evaluate a patient's swallowing ability, liquid barium is mixed with crackers and swallowed (a barium meal).

Fluoroscopy **Fluoroscopy** uses a continuous x-ray beam to capture motion of the internal organs as it occurs. The x-ray beam passes through the patient's body to a fluorescent screen that transforms invisible x-rays into long wavelengths of light that the eye can see as they are displayed on a TV monitor. Fluoroscopy is used to follow the movement of contrast dye during a cardiac catheterization or upper GI series (see Figure 19-5■). Individual roentgenograms are taken to capture the most important aspects of the procedure. The entire fluoroscopy can be recorded on videotape, a procedure known as **cineradiography.**

fluoroscopy (floor-AWS-koh-pee)
fluor/o- *fluorescence*
-scopy *process of using an instrument to examine*

cineradiography (SIN-eh-RAY-dee-AWG-rah-fee)
cin/e- *movement*
radi/o- *radius (forearm bone); x-rays; radiation*
-graphy *process of recording*

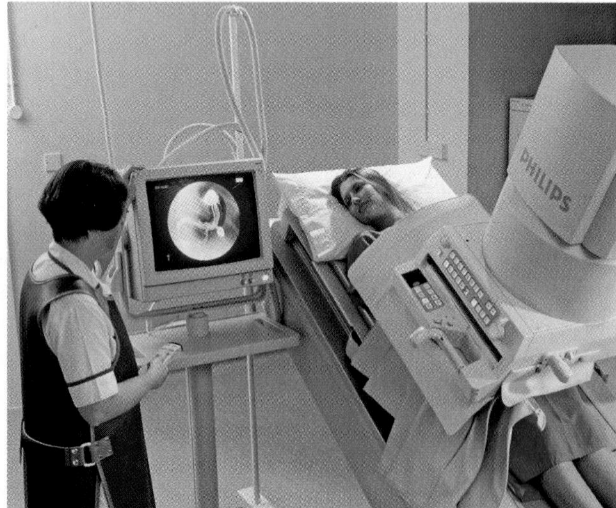

Figure 19-5 ■ Fluoroscopy.

This patient swallowed the contrast dye barium, and the tilted table allows the barium to flow through the stomach and intestine, coating and outlining them to make them visible during fluoroscopy. The radiologist has a hand-held device that allows her to create selected still roentgenograms from the continuously moving images on the fluoroscopy screen. The radiologist is wearing a lead apron to protect her from exposure to x-rays.

Mammography

Mammography uses an x-ray beam to create an image of the breast. The breast is compressed to lessen its thickness and improve the quality of the image. Mammography is used to detect areas of microcalcifications, infection, cysts, and tumors, many of which cannot be felt on a breast examination. The breast image is known as a **mammogram** (see Figure 13-26). **Xeromammography** uses a special plate processed with dry chemicals, and its image, a **xeromammogram** is printed on paper rather than x-ray film.

Bone Density Test

A bone density test uses an x-ray beam to measure bone mineral density (BMD) and determine if demineralization (from osteoporosis) has occurred. This test is also known as **bone densitometry.** The heel or wrist bone can be tested, but the hip and spine bones give the most accurate results.

There are two types of bone density tests: DEXA (or DXA) scan and quantitative computerized tomography (QCT). A **DEXA scan** uses two x-ray beams with different energy levels to create a two-dimensional image. This scan can detect as little as a 1 percent loss of bone. *DEXA* stands for dual-energy x-ray absorptiometry. Dual energy refers to the use of the two different x-ray beams. **Quantitative computerized tomography (QCT)** uses an x-ray beam and a CT scan (described in the next section) to create a three-dimensional image. QCT is able to take separate density measurements for the trabecular and cortical areas within a bone.

Computerized Axial Tomography (CAT, CT)

Computerized axial tomography (CAT), also known as **computerized tomography (CT),** uses an x-ray beam that is controlled by a computer. The patient lies on a narrow bed inside the CT scanner. The x-ray emitter moves in a circle around the patient, while the x-ray detector moves along the opposite side of the circle. The path of the x-ray emitter and detector is oriented along one of the imaginary planes of the body: coronal, sagittal, or transverse (see Figure 19-6 ■). The x-ray emitter makes one complete circle around the patient, and then the computer analyzes and creates a two-dimensional image or "slice" of that part of the body. Then the x-ray emitter moves a short distance (about 20 mm) and begins the process again to create another image or "slice." The radiologist views each of these individual images, which together make up a three-dimensional view of the area. Computerized tomography shows all types of tissues, but bony structures are particularly clear. Computerized tomography is also known as a scan because the machine scans (moves across) the body. A multidetector-row CT scanner (MDCT) has an area, not just a row, of x-ray detectors and can

---

mammography (mah-MAWG-rah-fee)
mamm/o- *breast*
-graphy *process of recording*

mammogram (MAM-oh-gram)
mamm/o- *breast*
-gram *a picture or record*

xeromammography (ZEER-oh-mah-MAWG-rah-fee)
xer/o- *dry*
mamm/o- *breast*
-graphy *process of recording*

xeromammogram (ZEER-oh-MAM-oh-gram)
xer/o- *dry*
mamm/o- *breast*
-gram *a picture or record*

densitometry (DEN-sih-TAWM-eh-tree)
densit/o- *density*
-metry *process of measuring*

DEXA (DEK-sah)

quantitative (KWAN-tih-TAY-tiv)
quantitat/o- *quantity or amount*
-ive *pertaining to*

axial (AK-see-al)
axi/o- *axis*
-al *pertaining to*
Axial refers to the axis or midline of the body. The x-ray emitter and detector rotate around the axis of the body.

tomography (toh-MAWG-rah-fee)
tom/o- *a cut, slice, or layer*
-graphy *process of recording*

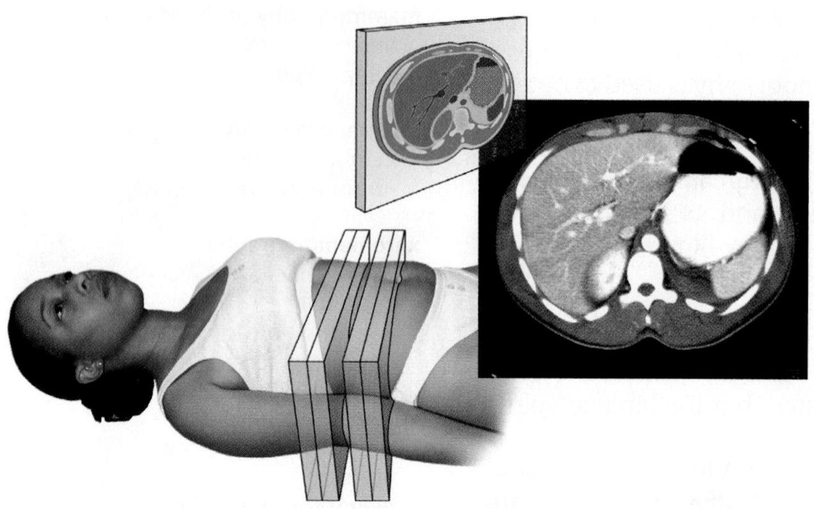

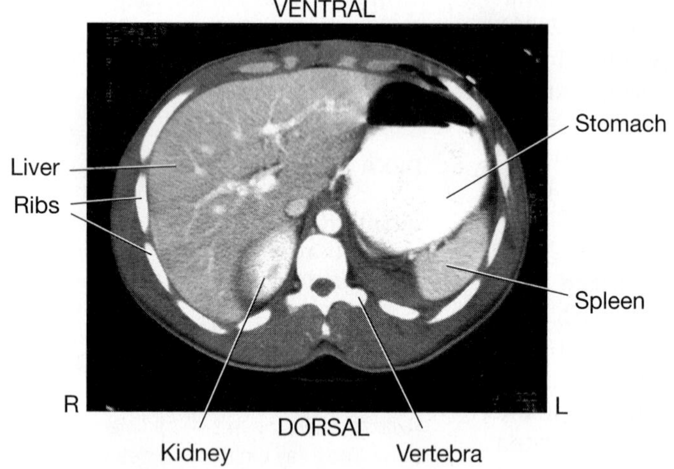

Figure 19-6 ■ Computerized axial tomography (CAT) of the abdomen taken in the transverse plane.

The radiologist reads a CT scan image as if he were standing at the patient's feet while she is lying in the scanner. This CT scan image shows the liver on the left, which is actually the patient's right side when viewed from her feet. Only one kidney is visible in this slice because the other kidney is positioned lower in the body (a normal occurrence) and will appear in subsequent slices.

quickly scan multiple "slices" simultaneously. A **spiral** or **helical CT scan** moves the patient's bed through the scanner as the x-ray emitter rotates around the patient. This produces a spiral image 10 times faster than a conventional CT scan. When a CT scan is used to guide the insertion of a needle (for a biopsy), this is known as **interventional radiology.**

An iodinated radiopaque contrast dye can be injected intravenously or into a body cavity to produce an enhanced image. A CT that uses no contrast medium is said to be unenhanced. Often two sets of images are obtained, one set before iodinated contrast dye is given and another after iodinated contrast dye is given. These are known as precontrast and postcontrast images.

spiral (SPY-ral)
spir/o- *a coil*
-al *pertaining to*

helical (HEL-ih-kal)
helic/o- *a coil*
-al *pertaining to*
Spir/o- is derived from a Latin word meaning *a coil* and *helic/o-* is derived from a Greek word meaning *a coil.*

interventional (IN-ter-VEN-shun-al)
inter- *between*
vent/o- *a coming*
-ion *action; condition*
-al *pertaining to*

Radiologic Procedure That Uses a Magnetic Field and Radiowaves

Magnetic resonance imaging (MRI) uses a strong magnetic field inside a scanner (see Figure 19-7■) to align protons in the atoms of the patient's body. Then high-frequency radiowaves are sent through the patient's body. The protons absorb the radiowaves and then emit signals. The signals, which vary according to the type of tissue, are used to construct an image. The patient lies in a scanner and an emitter and detector rotate in a circle around the patient. The computer creates a two-dimensional image (see Figure 19-8■). Like a CT scan, magnetic resonance imaging is a type of tomography that creates many individual "slice" images. The computer can combine these into a three-dimensional image. An MRI scan does not use x-rays so the patient is not exposed to any radiation. Magnetic resonance imaging is best able to show soft tissues, blood vessels, intervertebral disks, muscles, nerves, organs, tumors, and areas of infection. **Gadolinium,** a metallic element that responds to a magnetic field, can be injected intravenously for magnetic resonance angiography (MRA) or into a body cavity to produce an enhanced MRI image. An unenhanced MRI uses no gadolinium. An open MRI is performed on a modified MRI scanner that is not enclosed on all sides. Open MRI is ideal for pediatric, elderly, claustrophobic, anxious, or extremely obese patients.

magnetic (mag-NET-ik)
magnet/o- *magnet*
-ic *pertaining to*

gadolinium (GAD-oh-LIN-ee-um)

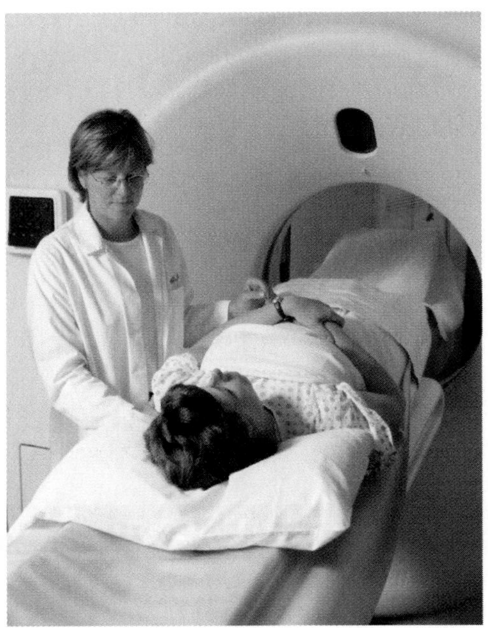

Figure 19-7 ■ MRI scan.

This radiologic technologist is positioning the patient before the bed slides into the MRI scanner. During the scan, the technician is in contact with the patient via an intercom inside the scanner.

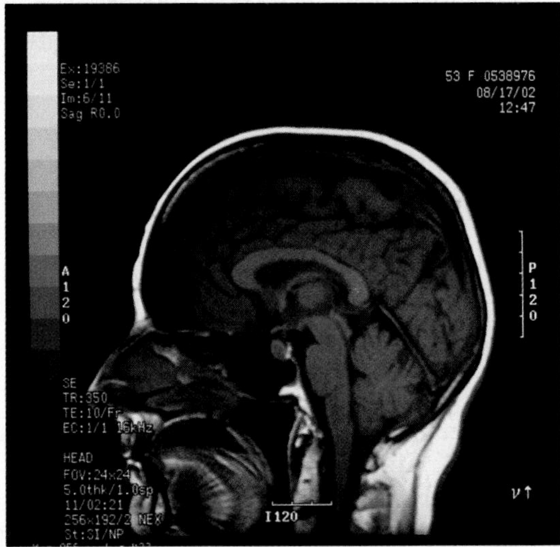

Figure 19-8 ■ Magnetic resonance imaging (MRI) of the brain.

This MRI image was created along the sagittal plane. This is just one of many thin slices that were individually imaged. The computer can merge the individual images into a three-dimensional image.

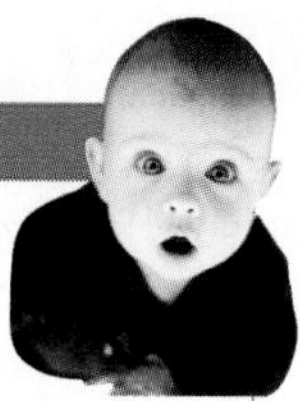

Did You Know?

Patients who undergo an MRI scan must sign a consent form that describes what types of metal items can or cannot be subjected to the magnetic field produced by the MRI scanner. You might be surprised to see which things are contraindicated and which things are allowed.

Contraindicated

- All metal objects that are not permanently attached to the body, such as glasses, watches, jewelry, hairpins, metal false teeth, artificial limbs, and clothing with metal zippers, buttons, or snaps. These objects respond to the magnetic field and can be forcefully pulled into the scanner, causing damage to the scanner.
- Nose rings, lip rings, tongue studs, pierced earrings, and other piercings must be removed or they could be forcefully pulled into the scanner, causing damage to the patient's tissues.
- Implanted devices like pacemakers, pacing wires, some heart valves, cerebral artery aneurysm clips, cochlear implants, some penile implants, artificial eyes, and some intrauterine devices may be moved by the magnetic field, causing internal tissue damage.
- Hearing aids, some pacemakers, TENS units, and insulin pumps can have their working parts damaged by the magnetic field.
- Metal workers and gunshot victims are presumed to have metal fragments in their tissues and should not undergo MRI scans. A piece of shrapnel may or may not cause a problem, depending on the location.
- Transdermal patches that deliver heart, pain, contraceptive, or stop smoking medication must be removed because some contain a small metal wire that can cause burns to the skin.
- Metallic eye shadow may cause the eyelids to flutter as they are pulled and then released by the magnetic field.

Allowed

- Permanent metal dental work like crowns are allowed because they will not detach, although they may cause artifacts on the MRI image.
- Artificial metal or ceramic joint prostheses and orthopedic hardware (screws, nails, plates, and rods).

Radiologic Procedure That Uses an Electron Beam

Electron beam tomography (EBT) uses a beam of electrons to create an image. This is known as a full body scan, although only the area from the shoulders to the upper legs is actually scanned. These scans are being marketed directly to consumers and do not need to be ordered by a physician. They are considered screening tests, not diagnostic tests. The Virtual Physical and the Virtual Colonoscopy use a spiral CT scan combined with an EBT scan to produce a detailed three-dimensional image. The Virtual Physical is able to reveal small areas of plaque in the coronary arteries, the early changes of emphysema in the lungs, and early stages of cancer. The Virtual Colonoscopy produces results that are as reliable as those of a colonoscopy but costs only about one-third as much.

electron (ee-LEK-tron)
electr/o- *electricity*
-on *substance; structure*

Radiologic Procedures That Use Sound Waves

Ultrasonography **Ultrasonography** or **sonography** uses pulses of inaudible, ultra high-frequency sound waves to create images of the internal structures of the body. A hand-held **ultrasound transducer** that emits sound waves is held against the skin over the organ or structure to be imaged. A conducting gel on the skin optimizes transmission of the sound waves. The transducer is moved back and forth to view the organ or structure from different angles. Alternately, an **ultrasound probe** can be placed inside a body cavity. Sound waves from the transducer or probe are reflected from internal structures as echoes. The echoes are changed into electrical signals and analyzed by a computer. The strongest echoes produce the brightest areas on the ultrasound image. The ultrasound image, which is viewed on a TV monitor or as individual still images, is known as a **sonogram** (see Table 19-3). When ultrasonography is used to guide the insertion of a needle (for a biopsy or for amniocentesis), this is known as interventional radiology.

Ultrasonography is used to differentiate solid tumors and stones from fluid-filled cysts of the breast, gallbladder, kidney, ovary, or uterus. It can be used to assess the internal structures of the eye. It can provide images of a fetus in the uterus (see Figure 13-27), and the fetal parts can be measured to estimate the gestational age and the mother's due date.

ultrasonography (UL-trah-soh-NAWG-rah-fee)
ultra- *beyond; higher*
son/o- *sound*
-graphy *process of recording*

sonography (soh-NAWG-rah-fee)
son/o- *sound*
-graphy *process of recording*

ultrasound (UL-trah-sound)
Ultrasound is a combination of the prefix *ultra-* (beyond, higher) and the word *sound.*

transducer (trans-DOO-ser)
trans- *across, through*
duc/o- *bring or move*
-er *person or thing that produces or does*

sonogram (SAWN-oh-gram)
son/o- *sound*
-gram *a record or picture*

Table 19-3 Ultrasonography

Type	Description
Two-dimensional	Provides a two-dimensional image in various shades of gray. Also known as a grayscale ultrasonography or B scan.
Three-dimensional	Provides a three-dimensional image. In addition to signals sent by the transducer or probe, a position sensor relays information that the computer uses to generate an image in three dimensions. The computer also colorizes the image in shades of brown.
Four-dimensional	Provides a three-dimensional, computer-colorized image that is continuously moving. The computer updates the ultrasound image on the screen at the same rate that it receives new signals from the transducer or probe and position sensor. Also known as real-time ultrasonography.

Echocardiography **Echocardiography** uses ultra high-frequency sound waves to show real-time, moving images of the heart during contraction and relaxation. The ultrasound image, which is viewed on a TV monitor or as individual still images, is known as an **echocardiogram** (see Figure 19-9 ■). **Transesophageal echocardiography (TEE)** may be ordered when a standard echocardiogram cannot produce a good-quality image. During a TEE, the patient swallows an endoscopic tube that contains a tiny sound wave-emitting transducer at its tip. The tip is positioned in the esophagus so that it is directly behind the heart.

echocardiography (EK-oh-KAR-dee-AWG-rah-fee)
ech/o- *echo (sound wave)*
cardi/o- *heart*
-graphy *process of recording*

echocardiogram (EK-oh-KAR-dee-oh-gram)
ech/o- *echo (sound wave)*
cardi/o- *heart*
-gram *a record or picture*

transesophageal (trans-ee-SAWF-ah-JEE-al)
trans- *across, through*
esophag/o- *esophagus*
-eal *pertaining to*

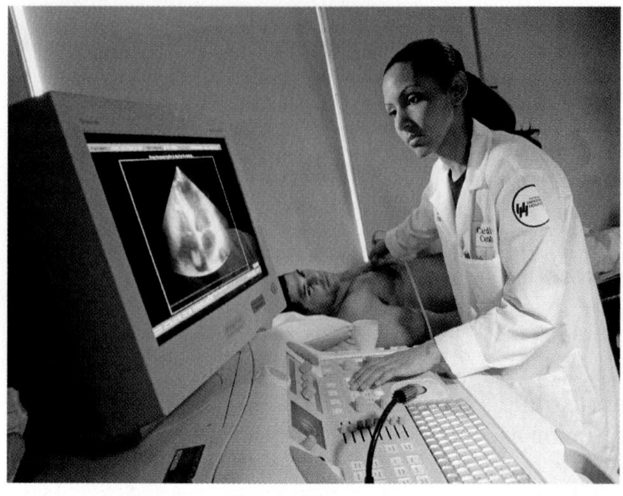

Figure 19-9 ■ Echocardiography.
This patient is having echocardiography. The technician is holding a transducer that produces sound waves. These bounce off the structures of the heart as echoes that the computer displays on the monitor screen.

Doppler Ultrasonography **Doppler ultrasonography** uses ultra high-frequency sound waves and Doppler technology to produce the audible sound of blood flowing through an artery. The transducer emits and then collects reflected sound waves. If the artery is patent, a loud "swish . . . swish . . . swish" will be heard as the blood is pumped through the artery. If the artery is blocked, little or no sound will be heard. Doppler technology is also used in automatic blood pressure machines that give a digital readout of the blood pressure and in fetal monitors that, when placed on the mother's abdomen, make the heart beat of the fetus audible.

Color flow duplex ultrasonography combines a two-dimensional ultrasound image and Doppler technology to create an ultrasound image that shows anatomy as well as colors according to the velocity, direction, and turbulence of the blood flow in that area. Used to image the coronary arteries, carotid arteries, or arteries of the legs.

Unlike many types of radiologic procedures, ultrasonography does not expose the patient to harmful radiation (see Table 19-4).

Doppler (DAWP-ler)
The Doppler effect was discovered by Christian Doppler (1803–1853), an Austrian physicist. It states that a sound wave generated by an object will change pitch as the object moves toward or away from the observer. The pitch of a train whistle gradually becomes higher as the train approaches you and then gradually becomes lower as the train moves away from you.

duplex (DOO-pleks)
du/o- *two*
-plex *parts*

Table 19-4 Radiologic Procedures and Exposure to Radiation

Source	Radiologic Procedure	Exposure to Radiation
x-rays	roentgenography fluoroscopy computerized axial tomography (CAT scan) computerized tomography (CT scan) mammography, xeroradiography	Yes Yes Yes Yes Yes
electron beam	electron beam tomography (usually coupled with CT scan)	Yes
radiowaves and magnetic field	magnetic resonance imaging (MRI scan)	No
ultra high-frequency sound waves	ultrasonography echocardiography Doppler ultrasonography	No No No

Nuclear Medicine

Nuclear medicine is the medical specialty that uses **radioactive** substances to create images of internal structures of the body. When a radioactive substance decays, it can produce alpha particles, beta particles, positrons, gamma rays, as well as other subatomic particles that are a form of radiation. Radioactive substances that produce gamma rays or positrons are used for nuclear medicine imaging. Radioactive substances that produce alpha and beta particles are used in radiation therapy to destroy cancerous cells. Radiation therapy has already been discussed in Oncology (Chapter 18).

nuclear (NYOO-klee-er)
nucle/o- *nucleus*
-ar *pertaining to*

radioactive (RAY-dee-oh-AK-tiv)
radi/o- *radius (forearm bone); x-rays; radiation*
act/o- *action*
-ive *pertaining to*

A Closer Look

Radioactive substances are composed of atoms that are unstable because there are too many protons in their nuclei. To become stable, a nucleus captures a negatively charged electron (orbiting around the nucleus) and fuses it with a positively charged proton. This produces a neutron (that stays in the nucleus) and a single gamma ray (also known as a photon) that is ejected from the atom as radiation.

Every radioactive substance is in a constant state of decay (changing from being unstable to being stable). The length of time it takes for half of the atoms in an amount of a radioactive substance to decay and become stable is known as the **half-life.**

Radiopharmaceuticals are man-made or naturally occurring radioactive substances (**radionuclides**) that have been processed and measured so that they can be given as a drug dose. They are administered intravenously, except for radioactive gases, which are administered by inhalation. Radiopharmaceuticals are also known as **tracers** because their presence in a particular area of the body can be traced by the gamma rays they produce. The radiopharmaceuticals used in nuclear medicine imaging have short half-lives of a few hours to a few days. This means that the patient is only exposed to minimal amounts of radiation.

radiopharmaceutical (RAY-dee-oh-FAR-mah-SOO-tik-al)
radi/o- *radius (forearm bone); x-rays; radiation*
pharmaceutic/o- *medicine, drug*
-al *pertaining to*

radionuclide (RAY-dee-oh-NYOO-klide)
radi/o- *radius (forearm bone); x-rays; radiation*
nucle/o- *nucleus*
-ide *chemically modified structure*
The e in *nucle/o-* has been deleted from this word.

tracer (TRAY-ser)
trac/o- *visible path*
-er *person or thing that produces or does*

Nuclear Medicine Procedures That Use Gamma Rays

Nuclear medicine radiopharmaceuticals that emit gamma rays include gallium-67, indium-111, iodine-123, krypton-81m, technetium-99m, thallium-201, and xenon-133 (Table 19-5).

Table 19-5 Radiopharmaceuticals That Emit Gamma Rays

Radiopharmaceutical	Pronunciation	Description
gallium-67	**gallium** (GAL-ee-um) *Gallium* is a combination of a Latin word meaning *Gallic, French* plus the suffix *-ium* (a chemical element). Its discoverer, Lecoq de Boisbaudran (1838–1912), a French chemist, named this chemical element after his native country and also after himself because *gallium* is derived from a Latin word meaning *rooster,* and his first name (Lecoq) means *rooster (the cock)* in French.	Given intravenously for nuclear medicine imaging of many different areas of the body to detect inflammation, infection, and benign and cancerous tumors. Commercially, gallium is used in semiconductor technology. Gallium is a soft, silvery metal that is a liquid at room temperature.
indium-111	**indium** (IN-dee-um) *Indium* is a combination of a Latin word meaning *blue* (indigo) plus the suffix *-ium.* It emits bright blue light on spectrographic analysis.	Given intravenously for nuclear medicine imaging of many different areas of the body to look for cancerous tumors. Indium-111 is combined with a hormone that is attracted to cancerous cells of the endocrine system. Indium-111 can also be combined with a monoclonal antibody that is attracted to cancerous cells of the ovary or colon. Commericially, indium is used in LCDs (liquid crystal displays). Indium is a soft, silvery metal.
iodine-123	**iodine** (EYE-oh-dine) *Iodine* is a combination of a Greek word meaning *violet* plus the suffix *-ine* (pertaining to).	Given intravenously for nuclear medicine imaging of the thyroid gland. Iodine is a purple-black, shiny crystalline solid that is a trace element in the soil. The body uses iodine to produce thyroid hormones.
krypton-81m	**krypton** (KRIP-tawn) *Krypton* is a combination of a Greek word meaning *hidden* plus the suffix *-on* (substance; structure).	A gas that is inhaled for nuclear medicine imaging of the lung. Commercially, it is one of the gases used in fluorescent lights. It is also used in krypton lasers in surgery. Until 1983, the wavelength of light from krypton was the basis of the international definition of the length of a meter. Krypton is a colorless, odorless gas that is present in trace amounts in the atmosphere.
technetium-99m	**technetium** (tek-NEE-shee-um) *Technetium* is a combination of a Greek word meaning *artificial* plus the suffix *-ium* (a chemical element).	Given intravenously for nuclear medicine imaging of many different areas of the body. It is the most common radiopharmaceutical used in nuclear imaging. Technetium, a rare silvery gray metal, is used commercially to prevent corrosion in steel.

Table 19-5 *(continued)*

Radiopharmaceutical	Pronunciation	Description
thallium-201	**thallium** (THAL-ee-um) *Thallium* is a combination of a Greek word meaning *green twig* plus the suffix *-ium* (a chemical element). It emits bright green light on spectrographic analysis.	Given intravenously for nuclear medicine imaging of the heart. Commercially, thallium is used in photocells to detect infrared light. Thallium is a gray metal that is so soft it can be cut with a knife.
xenon-133	**xenon** (ZEE-nawn) *Xenon* is a combination of a Greek word *a stranger* plus the suffix *-on* (substance; structure).	A gas that is inhaled for nuclear medicine imaging of the lungs. Commercially, xenon gas is used in strobe lights. Xenon is a colorless, odorless gas that is present in trace amounts in the atmosphere.

After a radiopharmaceutical is administered, a **gamma scintillation camera** is positioned over the organ to be scanned. When a gamma ray enters the scintillation camera, it strikes a crystal structure, the crystal emits a flash of visible light (a photon), and a computer compiles the flashes of light into a two-dimensional image. Areas of increased uptake are known as hot spots, and areas of decreased uptake are known as cold spots. When the blood flow to an organ (perfusion) is being studied, areas of decreased uptake are known as filling defects. The nuclear medicine procedure is known as **scintigraphy** and the image is known as a **scintigram.** The image is also known as a **scintiscan** because the scintillation camera moves back and forth (scanning) across the body.

Bone scintigraphy is used to detect areas of increased uptake ("hot spots") related to arthritis, fracture (with resulting area of new bone growth) osteomyelitis, cancerous tumors of the bone, or areas of bony metastasis.

Cholescintigraphy or HIDA scan is used to detect areas of decreased uptake related to cystic duct obstruction and acute cholecystitis. *HIDA* stands for hydroxyiminodiacetic acid, a molecule that carries the radiopharmaceutical to the liver.

A liver-spleen scan is used to detect areas of decreased uptake that indicate nonfunctioning tissue due to inflammation, infection, benign tumors, or cancer in the liver or spleen.

A **MUGA (multiple-gated acquisition) scan** is used to detect how well the heart walls move during a contraction. It also calculates the ejection fraction (how much blood the ventricle can eject in one heartbeat). The ejection fraction is the most accurate predictor of overall heart function. The gamma camera is coordinated (gated) with the patient's EKG so that images of the heart are taken at multiple times during the cardiac cycle of contraction and relaxation. This procedure is also known as a **nuclear ventriculogram** or a radionuclide ventriculogram (RNV) or gated blood pool scanning. A **SPECT (single-photon emission computed tomography) scan** is a MUGA scan of the heart in which the gamma camera moves in a circle around the patient to create individual images as slices of the heart (tomography).

scintillation (SIN-tih-LAY-shun)
scintill/o- *point of light*
-ation *a process; being or having*

scintigraphy (sin-TIG-rah-fee)
scint/i- *point of light*
-graphy *process of recording*

scintigram (SIN-tih-gram)
scint/i- *point of light*
-gram *a record or picture*

scintiscan (SIN-tih-skan)
Scintiscan is a combination of the combining form *scint/i-* (point of light) and the word *scan.*

cholescintigraphy (KOH-lee-sin-TIG-rah-fee)
chol/e- *bile, gall*
scint/i- *point of light*
-graphy *process of recording*

MUGA (MUH-gah)

ventriculogram (ven-TRIK-yoo-loh-gram)
ventricul/o- *ventricle*
-gram *a record or picture*

SPECT (SPEKT)

emission (ee-MISH-un)
emiss/o- *to send out*
-ion *action; condition*

An **OncoScint scan** is used to detect areas of increased activity that are metastases from a cancerous tumor primary site in the colon or ovary. OncoScint is the trade name for the combination of indium-111 and a monoclonal antibody that binds to receptors on those cancerous cells. A **ProstaScint scan** does the same thing for metastases from prostate cancer.

A thyroid scan is used to detect areas of increased activity ("hot spots") that indicate a hyperfunctioning, benign thyroid nodule or goiter or decreased activity ("cold spots") that indicate a cyst or cancerous tumor of the thyroid (see Figure 19-10■). Also known as radioactive iodine uptake (RAIU) and thyroid scan.

A **ventilation-perfusion scan (V/Q)** is a two-part test that uses two radionuclides, one that is inhaled and one that is given intravenously. It is used to detect areas of decreased uptake ("cold spots") that indicate poor air flow, pneumonia, atelectasis, or pleural effusion in the lungs. Areas of decreased uptake on the perfusion scan indicate poor blood flow to the lung tissues. Also known as a lung scan. The *Q* stands for quotient.

OncoScint (AWN-koh-sint)

ProstaScint (PRAW-stah-sint)

ventilation (ven-tih-LAY-shun)
ventilat/o- *movement of air*
-ion *action; condition*

perfusion (per-FYOO-zhun)
per- *through, throughout*
fus/o- *pouring*
-ion *action; condition*

Did You Know?

In 1898, while working with uranium, Polish physicist Marie Curie and her husband, French physicist, Pierre Curie, discovered radium,a radioactive chemical element, and coined the word *radioactivity.* Alexandre Becquerel, a French physicist, discovered that radioactivity was constantly emitted from within each radium atom. For these discoveries, they all were awarded the Nobel Prize in physics. This was the first time a woman had won the Nobel Prize. Marie Curie's subsequent work with radium also earned her a Nobel Prize in chemistry, making her the first person to ever receive a Nobel Prize in two disciplines. The Curies and Becquerel often incurred severe radiation burns from handling radium or carrying it their pockets. Marie Curie died in 1934, from leukemia or aplastic anemia, mostly likely from long-term exposure to radiation. Her oldest daughter, Irene Joliot-Curie, discovered how to produce radioactive elements artificially. She was awarded the Nobel Prize in chemistry one year after her mother's death.

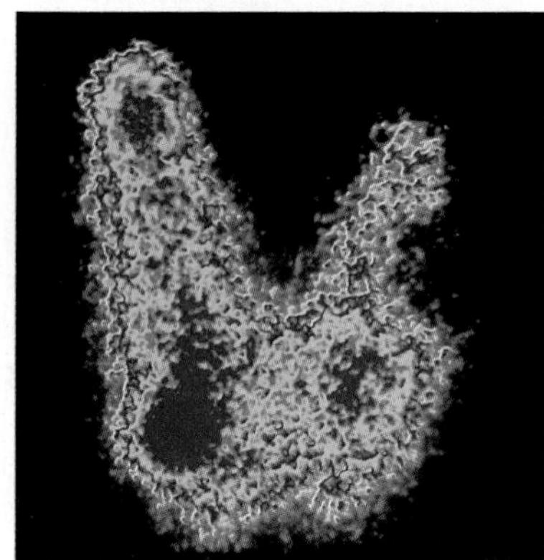

Figure 19-10 ■ Thyroid scan.
The radiopharmaceutical technetium-99m outlines the size and shape of the thyroid gland while the radiopharmaceutical iodine-123 is taken up by the thyroid gland cells. This scan shows a blue "cold spot" in the right lower lobe of the thyroid gland where the cells are not taking up iodine. This could be a cyst or a cancerous tumor. (Remember, the patient's right side is on your left when you view a scan.)

Nuclear Medicine Procedures That Use Positrons

A **positron** is a positively charged particle that has the same mass as an electron, but the opposite charge. Radioactive substances that emit positrons are used in **positron emission tomography (PET).** Like a CT scan or an MRI scan, a PET scan is a tomography that produces individual images of the body in "slices." However, unlike CT and MRI scans that produce images of the anatomy of an organ, a PET scan produces images of the physiology and metabolism of an organ.

positron (PAWZ-ih-trawn)
Positron is a shortened form of *positive* plus a shortened form of *electron*.

tomography (toh-MAWG-rah-fee)
tom/o- *a cut, slice, or layer*
-graphy *process of recording*

A Closer Look

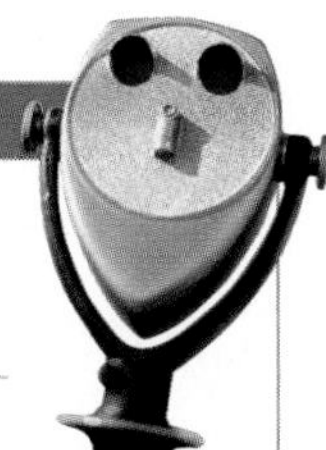

A **cyclotron** (subatomic particle accelerator) is needed to produce a radioactive substance that emits positrons. The cyclotron has a magnetic field that keeps protons going in a circular path while an alternating electrical field accelerates the protons to near the speed of light. Then the protons are used to bombard atoms and put extra protons into their nuclei. Too many protons in the nucleus make the atom unstable. To become stable again, each nucleus converts a proton to a neutron (that remains in the nucleus) and emits a positron. The half-life of radioactive substances that emit positrons is very brief (a few minutes in length). Therefore the cyclotron must be at the hospital where the PET scan is performed. A cyclotron, however, is a large, expensive piece of equipment, so PET scans are only available in the largest hospitals.

cyclotron (SY-kloh-trawn)
cycl/o- *cycle; circle*
-tron *instrument*

A positron-emitting radioactive substance is combined with glucose molecules and injected intravenously. The higher the rate of metabolism in a cell, the more glucose is consumed and the more radioactive substance that is carried into the cell. As the radioactive substance decays, it releases a positron. Almost immediately the positron collides with a nearby electron. The collision simultaneously produces two gamma rays that move in opposite directions from each other. A special circular gamma camera is set so that it only records simultaneously produced gamma rays. A computer traces the rays back to identify where they originated in an organ. This then becomes a point on the PET scan image.

PET scans are of particular value in identifying areas of cancer (because cancerous cells have a higher metabolic rate than normal cells). They also show areas of ischemia in the heart (because ischemic cells have poor blood flow and a lower metabolic rate than normal cells). PET scans also show areas of abnormally increased or decreased metabolism in the brains of patients with Alzheimer's disease (see Figure 10-16), Parkinson's disease, epilepsy, and schizophrenia.

Vocabulary Review

Now that you have studied radiology and nuclear medicine, take time to review those new words and their definitions. Memorize the combining forms and their definitions before going on to the next section.

Word or Phrase	Combining Form and Definition	Description
angiography	angi/o- *blood vessel; lymphatic vessel* rotat/o- *rotate*	Uses an x-ray beam and iodinated contrast dye injected into an artery or vein to create an image of the blood vessel. The image is known as an **angiogram.** In **digital subtraction angiography,** two images are obtained, one without and one with contrast. The computer compares the images and subtracts the soft tissues, leaving only the image of the blood vessels. In **rotational angiography,** the x-ray beam moves around the patient. In **magnetic resonance angiography (MRA),** a noniodinated contrast dye is used and an MRI scan creates the image of the blood vessels.
anteroposterior	anter/o- *before; front part* poster/o- *back part*	Pertaining to going from the front to the back
aortography	aort/o- *aorta*	Uses an x-ray beam and iodinated contrast dye to create an image of the aorta. The image is known as an **aortogram.**
arteriography	arteri/o artery	Uses an x-ray beam and iodinated contrast dye injected into an artery to create an image of the artery. The image is known as an **arteriogram.** Arteriography is one type of angiography.
arthrography	arthr/o- *joint*	Uses an x-ray beam and iodinated contrast dye injected into a joint to create an image of the joint. The image is known as an **arthrogram.** In **magnetic resonance arthrography,** a noniodinated contrast medium is used and an MRI scan creates the image of the joint.
barium		Radiopaque contrast dye made of small, chalky particles suspended in a liquid. Used for radiologic procedures of the digestive tract. It is swallowed (upper GI series, barium swallow) or instilled in the rectum and colon (barium enema).
barium enema		Uses an x-ray beam and radiopaque barium contrast dye instilled in the rectum to create an image of the colon. A **double contrast enema** uses contrast dye and then air as a second contrast medium. Images are fluoroscopy and individual radiographs.
cholangiography	chol/o- *bile, gall* angi/o- *blood vessel; lymphatic vessel*	Uses an x-ray beam and iodinated contrast dye injected intravenously to create an image of the gallbladder. The image is known as a **cholangiogram.**
cholecystography	chol/o *bile, gall* cyst/o *bladder; fluid-filled sac; cyst*	Uses an x-ray beam and iodinated contrast dye taken orally (oral cholecystography) or injected intravenously (intravenous cholecystography) to create an image of the gallbladder. The image is known as a **cholecystogram.**
cholescintigraphy	chol/e- *bile, gall* scint/i- *point of light*	Nuclear medicine procedure that uses scintigraphy and the radiopharmaceutical technetium-99m as a tracer to create an image of the gallbladder. The technetium is attached to a carrier molecule HIDA hydroxyiminodiacetic acid), Also known as a **HIDA scan.**

Word or Phrase	Combining Form and Definition	Description
computerized axial tomography (CAT)	axi/o- *axis* tom/o- *a cut, slice, or layer* spir/o- *a coil* helic/o- *a coil*	Uses an x-ray beam that is controlled by a computer and moves around the body axis of a patient inside the CT scanner. Produces individual images as "slices," as well as a composite three-dimensional view. A multidetector-row CT scanner (MDCT) has an area (not just a row) of x-ray detectors and can quickly scan multiple "slices" simultaneously. During a **spiral** or **helical CT scan,** the patient's bed moves through the scanner while the x-ray beam rotates, creating a spiral.
decubitus		Lying down position; on the back
densitometry	densit/o- *density*	Bone density test that measures the bone mineral density to diagnose osteoporosis. Two types include DEXA scan and QCT.
DEXA scan		Type of densitometry that uses two x-ray beams at two different energy levels to measure bone density. Also known as dual-energy x-ray absorptiometry or DXA scan.
Doppler ultrasonography	son/o- *sound*	Uses ultra high-frequency sound waves emitted by an ultrasound transducer placed over an artery and Doppler technology to create an audible sound of blood flow through an artery. **Color flow duplex ultrasonography** uses ultrasonography and Doppler technology to create an ultrasound image with colors that reflect the velocity, direction, and turbulence of blood in an artery or vein.
dosimetry	dos/i- *dose*	Process of measuring the amount of radiation exposure as detected by a film badge and measured by a **dosimeter**
echocardiography	ech/o- *echo (sound wave)* cardi/o- *heart*	Uses ultra high-frequency sound waves emitted by an ultrasound transducer placed on the chest. (Alternatively, a tiny transducer is swallowed and positioned in the esophagus behind the heart for **transesophageal echocardiography**). The sound waves bounce off the contracting and relaxing heart, creating echoes that are changed into an image by a computer. The image is known as an **echocardiogram.**
electron beam tomography (EBT)	electr/o- *electricity* tom/o- *a cut, slice, or layer*	Uses an electron beam and a spiral CT scan to create an image. Also known as a full body scan.
enhanced		Roentgenography, CT scan, or MRI scan that uses a contrast medium to enhance anatomic details. If no contrast medium is used, the image is said to be **unenhanced.**
film badge		Small, flat container that holds an unexposed piece of x-ray film that detects each instance of exposure to radiation or radioactive substances
fluoroscopy	fluor/o- *fluorescence* cin/e- *movement* radi/o- *radius (forearm bone); x-rays; radiation*	Uses a continuous x-ray beam to capture the motion of internal organs after the administration of a radiopaque contrast dye. A fluorescent screen acts like a TV monitor to display a series of changing images. **Cineradiography** permanently records a fluoroscopy on video tape.
gadolinium		Contrast medium used in MRI scans. It is a metallic element that responds to a magnetic field.

Word or Phrase	Combining Form and Definition	Description
gamma ray		Form of subatomic radiation emitted from a radioactive substance. Also known as a **photon.**
half-life		Length of time it takes for half of the atoms in an amount of a radioactive substance to emit gamma rays or positrons (decay) and become stable
hysterosalpingography	hyster/o- *uterus* salping/o- *fallopian tube*	Uses an x-ray beam and iodinated contrast dye inserted into the uterus to create an image of the uterus and fallopian tubes. The image is known as a **hysterosalpingogram.**
interventional radiology	vent/o- *a coming*	Uses CT, MRI, or ultrasonography to guide the insertion of a needle for a biopsy or other procedures (like an amniocentesis)
iodinated contrast dye	iodin/o- *iodine*	Radiopaque contrast dye that contains iodine, a chemical element with a high atomic weight that makes it radiopaque
lateral	later/o- *side*	Pertaining to going in from the side or going to the side
lead apron		Shielding apron worn by radiologic personnel to protect themselves from radiation exposure. A lead apron is also used to shield parts of the patient's body that are not being x-rayed.
lymphangiography	lymph/o- *lymph; lymphatic system* angi/o- *blood vessel; lymphatic vessel*	Uses an x-ray beam and iodinated contrast dye injected into a lymphatic vessel to create an image of the lymph node chains. The image is known as a **lymphangiogram.**
magnetic resonance imaging (MRI)	magnet/o- *magnet*	Uses a magnetic field and radiowaves to align the protons in atoms and then cause them to vibrate and emit energy as a signal. Produces individual images as "slices" through the body, as well as a composite three-dimensional view. The noniodinated contrast medium gadolinium can also be used to enhance the image.
mammography	mamm/o- *breast*	Uses an x-ray beam to expose an x-ray plate and create an image of the breast. The image is known as a **mammogram. Xeromammography** uses a special plate and dry chemicals to create an image on paper. This image is known as a **xeromammogram.**
motion artifact		Blurred image on a radiograph that occurs when the patient moves
multiple-gated acquisition (MUGA) scan	ventricul/o- *ventricle*	Nuclear medicine procedure that uses scintigraphy and the radiopharmaceutical technetium-99m as a tracer to create an image of the blood within the heart. The technetium is attached to the patient's red blood cells. The gamma camera is coordinated (gated) with the patient's EKG. Used to calculate the ejection fraction of the heart. Also known as a **nuclear ventriculogram,** a radionuclide ventriculogram (RNV), or a gated blood pool scan.
myelography	myel/o- *bone marrow; spinal cord; myelin*	Uses an x-ray beam and iodinated contrast dye inserted through a catheter into the subarachnoid space to create an image of the spinal cavity, spine, and spinal nerves. The image is known as a **myelogram.**
nuclear medicine	nucle/o- *nucleus*	Healthcare specialty that uses radioactive substances to create an image of the internal structures of the body

Word or Phrase	Combining Form and Definition	Description
oblique		On a slant or angle midway between anterior and lateral
OncoScint scan		Nuclear medicine procedure that uses scintigraphy and the radiopharmaceutical indium-111 as a tracer to create an image of metastases from cancer of the colon or ovary. The indium is attached to a monoclonal antibody that binds to receptors on the cancerous cells. The indium plus monoclonal antibody is the trade name drug OncoScint.
PET scan	tom/o- *a cut, slice, or layer*	Nuclear medicine procedure that uses the radiopharmaceutical fluorine-18 combined with glucose molecules. The glucose is taken up by cells with active metabolism. Radioactive fluorine-18 emits positrons that then become two gamma rays traveling in opposite directions. A circular gamma scintillation camera detects the gamma rays and creates an image that shows cellular metabolism. Also known as **positron emission tomography.**
plain film		Radiograph obtained without the use of a contrast dye
portable film		Radiograph obtained at the bedside or in the emergency department with a portable x-ray machine when the patient cannot be transported to the radiology department.
posteroanterior	poster/o- *back part* anter/o- *before; front part*	Pertaining to going from the back to the front
projection	project/o- *throw forward*	Direction in which the x-ray beam travels through the patient
ProstaScint scan		Nuclear medicine procedure that uses scintigraphy and the radiopharmaceutical indium-111 as a tracer to create an image of metastases from prostate cancer. The indium is attached to a monoclonal antibody that binds to receptors on cancerous cells. The indium plus monoclonal antibody is the trade name drug ProstaScint.
pyelography	pyel/o- *renal pelvis* excret/o- *removing from the body* ur/o- *urine; urinary system*	Uses an x-ray beam and iodinated contrast dye injected intravenously (intravenous pyelogram) or instilled into the bladder (retrograde pyelogram) to create an image of the kidneys, ureters, bladder, and urethra. Pyelography is also known as urography, and intravenous pyelography is also known as **excretory pyelography.** The image is known as a **pyelogram** or **urogram.**
quantitative computerized tomography (QCT)	tom/o- *a cut, slice, or layer*	Type of densitometry that uses an x-ray beam and a CT scan to create a three-dimensional image to measure the bone density of both trabecular and cortical bone
radiation	radi/o- *radius (forearm bone); x-rays; radiation*	The process of sending out some type of invisible ray, like x-rays or gamma rays
radioactive substance	radi/o- *radius (forearm bone); x-rays; radiation*	Substance that produces gamma rays or positrons as it decays and its atoms change from an unstable to a stable state. Used to create images in nuclear medicine.
radiology	radi/o- *radius (forearm bone); x-rays; radiation*	Healthcare specialty that uses various types of radiation and energy (x-rays, magnetic field, sound waves) to create an image of the internal structures of the body

Word or Phrase	Combining Form and Definition	Description
radiolucent	radi/o- *radius (forearm bone); x-rays; radiation* luc/o- *clear and shining*	Areas of low density in the body (like air-filled cavities) that allow x-rays to pass through and create a black area on a radiograph. Areas of high density tissue (like bone) are **radiopaque,** do not let x-rays pass through, and appear white on a radiograph.
radionuclide	radi/o- *radius (forearm bone); x-rays; radiation*	Radioactive form of a chemical element in which too many protons in the nucleus make the atom unstable
radiopharma-ceutical	pharmaceutic/o- *medicine, drug*	Naturally occurring or man-made radioactive radionuclide that has been processed and measured so that it can be given as a drug in nuclear medicine. Also known as a tracer. Radiopharmaceuticals include gallium-67, indium-111, iodine-123, krypton-81m, technetium-99m, thalium-201, and xenon-133.
rem		Unit of measurement for radiation exposure. *REM* stands for roentgen-equivalent man.
roentgenography	roentgen/o- *x-ray; radiation*	Uses an x-ray beam to expose an x-ray plate and create an image in shades of white, gray, and black. The image is known as a **roentgenogram** or **radiograph.**
scintigraphy	scint/i- *point of light*	Nuclear medicine procedure that uses a radioactive radiopharmaceutical as a tracer. It emits gamma rays that enter a gamma scintillation camera, interact with a crystal, and produce a flash of light. The procedure is also known as a **scintiscan.** The image created is known as a **scintigram.**
scout film		Radiograph obtained to provide a preliminary view of an area before contrast medium is administered
SPECT scan	tom/o- *a cut, slice, or layer*	Nuclear medicine procedure in which the gamma scintillation camera moves around the patient (a type of tomography) to create images in "slices." The computer compiles the individual images into one three-dimensional image. SPECT scans are performed during a myocardial perfusion scan or MUGA scan of the heart. SPECT stands for single-photon emission computed tomography. A photon is another name for a gamma ray.
tracer	trac/o- *visible path*	Nuclear medicine radiopharmaceutical whose presence in the body can be traced by the gamma rays it produces
ultrasonography (US)	son/o- *sound*	Uses ultra high-frequency sound waves emitted by an ultrasound transducer placed on the skin. (Alternatively, an ultrasound probe is inserted vaginally or rectally to create images of the internal pelvic organs.) The sound waves bounce off organs, creating echoes that are changed into an image by a computer. This procedure is also known as **sonography,** and the image is known as a **sonogram.** A **gray-scale ultrasonography (B scan)** creates a two-dimensional image in shades of gray. A three-dimensional ultrasound uses a position sensor to add another dimension and the computer also colorizes the image in shades of brown. **Real-time ultrasonography** creates a three-dimensional, colorized image that is updated often and shows motion.
upper gastro-intestinal (UGI) series	gastr/o- *stomach* intestin/o- *intestine*	Uses an x-ray beam and radiopaque barium contrast dye that is swallowed to create an image of the esophagus, stomach, and duodenum. Also known as a barium swallow. A **small-bowel follow-through** follows the contrast dye as it outlines the small intestine. These images are fluoroscopy and individual radiographs.

Word or Phrase	Combining Form and Definition	Description
venography	ven/o- *vein*	Uses an x-ray beam and iodinated contrast dye injected into a vein to create an image of the vein. The image is known as a **venogram.**
ventilation-perfusion (V/Q) scan	ventilat/o- *movement of air* fus/o- *pouring*	Nuclear medicine procedure that uses scintigraphy and the inhaled radiopharmaceutical to create an image of the lungs. Also known as a **lung scan.**

Building Medical Words

Combining Forms

Here are the combining forms you have learned so far. Next to each combining form, write its meaning. Use the Answer Key at the end of the book to check your answers. The first one has been done for you.

Combining Form	Medical Meaning	Combining Form	Medical Meaning
1. act/o-	action	29. later/o-	
2. angi/o-		30. luc/o-	
3. anter/o-		31. lymph/o-	
4. aort/o-		32. magnet/o-	
5. arteri/o-		33. mamm/o-	
6. arthr/o-		34. myel/o-	
7. axi/o-		35. nucle/o-	
8. cardi/o-		36. pharmaceutic/o-	
9. chol/e-		37. poster/o-	
10. col/o-		38. project/o-	
11. cin/e-		39. pyel/o-	
12. cycl/o-		40. radi/o-	
13. cyst/o-		41. roentgen/o-	
14. densit/o-		42. rotat/o-	
15. dos/i-		43. salping/o-	
16. duc/o-		44. scint/i-	
17. du/o-		45. scintill/o-	
18. ech/o-		46. son/o-	
19. electr/o-		47. spir/o-	
20. emiss/o-		48. tom/o-	
21. esophag/o-		49. trac/o-	
22. excret/o-		50. ur/o-	
23. fluor/o-		51. ven/o-	
24. fus/o-		52. ventilat/o-	
25. gastr/o-		53. vent/o-	
26. helic/o-		54. ventricul/o-	
27. hyster/o-		55. xer/o-	
28. intestin/o-			

Combining Forms and Suffixes

Read the definition hint for the medical word you are to build. Look at the combining form that is given. Write the correct suffix on the blank line. Then write the medical word. (Remember: You may need to remove the combining vowel. Always remove the hyphens and slash.) Use the Answer Key at the end of the book to check your answers. The first one has been done for you.

SUFFIX LIST

-al (pertaining to)	-gram (a record or picture)	-metry (the process of measuring)
-ation (a process; being or having)	-graphy (the process of recording)	-scopy (process of using an instrument to examine)
-er (person or thing that produces or does)	-ior (pertaining to)	

	Definition Hint	Combining Form	Suffix	Write the Medical Word
1.	Pertaining to the front part	anter/o-	-ior	anterior
2.	Process of measuring a dose	dos/i-	______	______
3.	Process of using a fluorescent instrument to examine	fluor/o-	______	______
4.	Pertaining to the side	later/o-	______	______
5.	A picture made with sound waves	son/o-	______	______
6.	Thing that makes a visible path	trac/o-	______	______
7.	Process of recording an image as a slice	tom/o-	______	______
8.	Having a point of light	scintill/o-	______	______

Combining Forms and Prefixes

Read the definition hint for the medical word you are to build. Look at the medical word or word part that is given. It already contains a combining form and a suffix. Write the correct prefix on the blank line. Then write the medical word. (Remember: You may need to remove the combining vowel. Always remove the hyphens and slash.) Use the Answer Key at the end of the book to check your answers. The first one has been done for you.

PREFIX LIST

intra- (within)	trans- (across, through)	ultra- (beyond; higher)

	Definition Hint	Prefix	Medical Word	Write the Medical Word
1.	Pertaining to within the vein	intra-	venous	intravenous
2.	Process of recording with very high sound waves	______	sonography	______
3.	Thing that makes sound move through	______	ducer	______

Drug Categories

Several different categories of drugs are used during radiologic procedures. The most common drugs in each category are listed.

Category	Word Part and Definition	Description	Examples
barium	**barium** (BAIR-ee-um)	An insoluble metallic element found in the earth. A liquid suspension of barium particles creates a white and chalky contrast dye that is radiopaque. Barium is given orally or rectally to outline the gastrointestinal system during roentgenography, fluoroscopy, and CT scans.	Baro-cat, Barosperse, Tomocat
iodinated contrast dye		Contrast dye that contains iodine. Iodine has a high atomic weight that makes it radiopaque. It is available as an oral liquid or tablet or as a liquid that is injected into a vein or artery or instilled into a body cavity. It is used during roentgenography, fluoroscopy, and CT scans.	Gastrografin, Hypaque, Isovue, Omnipaque
radiopharmaceutical drugs that emit gamma rays		Radioactive substances that are used during scintigraphy, myocardial perfusion scans, MUGA scans, thyroid scans, and ventilation-perfusion scans.	gallium-67, iodine-123, krypton-81m, technetium-99m, thallium-201, xenon-133
radiopharmaceutical indium-111 combined with monoclonal antibodies		Radioactive substances used during scintigraphy to detect cancerous cells.	ProstaScint, OncoScint

Abbreviations

AP	anteroposterior	**MUGA**	multiple-gated acquisition (scan)
Ba	barium	**PA**	posteroanterior
BE	barium enema	**PET**	positron emission tomography
CAT	computerized axial tomography	**QCT**	quantitative computerized tomography
CT	computerized tomography	**R, r**	roentgen (unit of exposure to x-rays or gamma rays)
CXR	chest x-ray	**rad**	radiation absorbed dose
DEXA, DXA	dual energy x-ray absorptiometry	**RAIU**	radioactive iodine uptake
DSA	digital subtraction angiography	**rem**	roentgen-equivalent man
EBT	electron beam tomography	**RNV**	radionuclide ventriculography
IVC	intravenous cholangiography	**RRT**	registered radiologic technologist
IVP	intravenous pyelography	**SPECT**	single-photon emission computed tomography
KUB	kidneys, ureters, bladder	**TEE**	transesophageal echocardiography
Lat	lateral	**UGI**	upper gastrointestinal (GI) series
MRA	magnetic resonance angiography	**US**	ultrasound
MRI	magnetic resonance imaging	**V/Q**	ventilation-perfusion scan

Career Focus

Meet Jennifer, a radiologic technologist.
"I became an x-ray technologist because I wanted to work in a profession where I worked with all different patients. You get to work in the emergency room; you get to work doing procedures alongside a physician, dealing with acutely ill patients. You also get to go to the operating room. We also deal with outpatients. We not only do routine x-rays, but we're also involved in minor procedures, along with assisting the radiologists during upper GIs, barium enemas, and that sort of thing. You're not in any single area all the time, and it's just very nice to see every aspect of the hospital. We use medical terminology every day in our profession. Reading the requisitions that are sent over from the doctors' offices or notifying nurses if we have questions about a patient's exam—we need to use appropriate medical terminology."

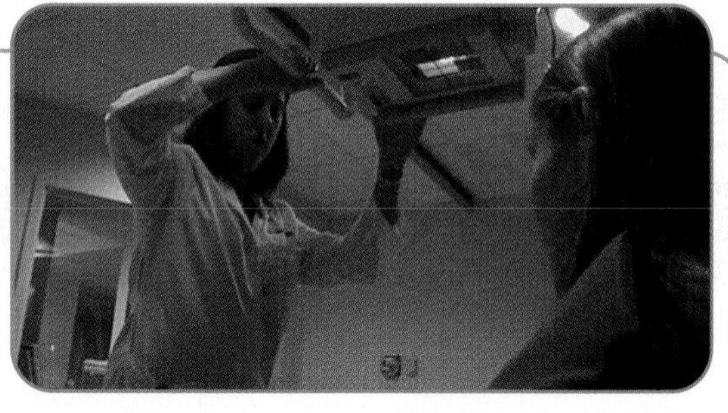

Radiologic technologists are allied health professionals who perform and document a variety of radiologic procedures and assist the physician during radiologic procedure in the hospital or radiology clinic.

Radiologists are physicians who practice in the medical specialty of radiology. They view and interpret the results of radiologic procedures to diagnose conditions of all body systems. Nuclear medicine physicians practice in the medical specialty of nuclear medicine. They view and interpret the results of nuclear medicine procedures. Radiologists and nuclear medicine physicians work in hospitals, large clinics, and ambulatory radiology centers.

radiologic (RAY-dee-oh-LAWJ-ik)
radi/o- *radius (forearm bone); x-ray; radiation*
log/o- *the study of*
-ic *pertaining to*

technologist (tek-NAWL-oh-jist)
techn/o- *technical skill*
log/o- *the study of*
-ist *one who specializes in*

radiologist (RAY-dee-AWL-oh-jist)
radi/o- *radius (forearm bone); x-rays; radiation*
log/o- *the study of*
-ist *one who specializes in*

Chapter Review Exercises

Medical Language Word Parts

Name That Word Part

Identify each of the word parts given here by writing the correct letter on the line beside it. Then write its definition on the blank line. The first one has been done for you.

Prefix = P **Combining Form = C** **Suffix = S**

		Word Part	Definition			Word Part	Definition
1.	-al	S	pertaining to	33.	gastr/o-		
2.	act/o-			34.	-grade		
3.	angi/o-			35.	-gram		
4.	anter/o-			36.	-graph		
5.	aort/o-			37.	graph/o-		
6.	-ar			38.	-graphy		
7.	arteri/o-			39.	helic/o-		
8.	arthr/o-			40.	hyster/o-		
9.	-ated			41.	-ic		
10.	-ation			42.	-ide		
11.	axi/o-			43.	inter-		
12.	cardi/o-			44.	intestin/o-		
13.	cin/e-			45.	intra-		
14.	chol/e-			46.	iodin/o-		
15.	chol/o-			47.	-ion		
16.	cycl/o-			48.	-ior		
17.	cyst/o-			49.	-ist		
18.	densit/o-			50.	-ive		
19.	detect/o-			51.	later/o-		
20.	dos/i-			52.	log/o-		
21.	duc/o-			53.	-logy		
22.	du/o-			54.	luc/o-		
23.	-eal			55.	lymph/o-		
24.	ech/o-			56.	magne/to-		
25.	electr/o-			57.	mamm/o-		
26.	emiss/o-			58.	-meter		
27.	-ent			59.	-metry		
28.	-er			60.	multi-		
29.	esophag/o-			61.	myel/o-		
30.	excret/o-			62.	nucle/o-		
31.	fluor/o-			63.	-on		
32.	fus/o-			64.	onc/o-		

		Word Part	Definition			Word Part	Definition
65.	-or	______	______	82.	scint/i-	______	______
66.	-ory	______	______	83.	scintill/o-	______	______
67.	-ous	______	______	84.	-scopy	______	______
68.	per-	______	______	85.	son/o-	______	______
69.	pharmaceutic/o-	______	______	86.	spir/o-	______	______
70.	-plex	______	______	87.	techn/o-	______	______
71.	post-	______	______	88.	tom/o-	______	______
72.	poster/o-	______	______	89.	trac/o-	______	______
73.	pre-	______	______	90.	trans-	______	______
74.	project/o-	______	______	91.	-tron	______	______
75.	pyel/o-	______	______	92.	ultra-	______	______
76.	quantitat/o-	______	______	93.	ur/o-	______	______
77.	rad/io-	______	______	94.	ven/o-	______	______
78.	retro-	______	______	95.	ventilat/o-	______	______
79.	rotat/o-	______	______	96.	vent/o-	______	______
80.	roentgen/o-	______	______	97.	ventricul/o-	______	______
81.	salping/o-	______	______	98.	xero-	______	______

Word-Building Exercise

Use the combining forms, prefixes, and suffixes given here to build medical words that match the definitions given. Write the word that you build in the blank line. The first one has been done for you.

Word Parts		
-al (pertaining to)	ech/o- (echo, sound wave)	nucle/o- (nucleus)
-ar (pertaining to)	-gram (a record or picture)	pharmaceutic/o- (medicine, drug)
arthr/o- (joint)	-graphy (process of recording)	radi/o- (x-rays; radiation)
cardi/o- (heart)	mamm/o- (breast)	scint/i- (point of light)
dos/i- (dose)	-meter (instrument used to measure)	tom/o- (a cut, slice, or layer)

1. Pertaining to the nucleus (You think *nucle/o-* + *-ar.*) You write nuclear
2. Instrument used to measure dosage of radiation exposure ______
3. Picture of an x-ray of a breast ______
4. Process of recording images that are in thin "slices" ______
5. Process of recording image of contrast dye inside a joint ______
6. Process of recording echoes of sound images of the heart ______
7. Pertaining to a radioactive substance made into a drug ______
8. Nuclear medicine picture formed by points of light from gamma rays ______

Radiology and Nuclear Medicine Procedures

Matching Exercise

Match each numbered word or phrase to its description.

1. arthrography ____ Pertaining to an area of low density on a radiograph
2. fluoroscopy ____ Uses a continuous x-ray beam
3. gamma scintillation camera ____ Uses a magnetic field and radiowaves
4. krypton-81m ____ Contrast dye is injected into a joint
5. portable film ____ Radioactive substance measured to be given as a drug dose
6. OncoScint scan ____ Radioactive gas used in nuclear medicine studies of the lungs
7. radiolucent ____ Detects gamma rays from radioactive substances
8. radiopharmaceutical ____ Used to detect metastases from colon or ovary cancer
9. MRI ____ Ventilation-perfusion scan of the lungs
10. V/Q scan ____ Radiograph done somewhere other than the radiology department

True or False

Indicate whether each statement is true or false by writing T or F on the line.

1. ____ Postcontrast images are taken after the injection of contrast dye.
2. ____ Both radiology and nuclear medicine use radioactive substances to create images of the internal structures of the body.
3. ____ The process of measuring the amount of radiation exposure is known as densitometry.
4. ____ Using a CT scan to guide the placement of a needle for biopsy is known as interventional radiology.
5. ____ Coronary angiography is done during a cardiac catheterization.
6. ____ IVC and OCG are both types of radiologic procedures that use contrast dye to view the gallbladder.
7. ____ Ultrasonography uses ultra high-frequency sound waves generated by a transducer or a probe.
8. ____ Pierre Curie coined the word *radioactivity* in the late 1800s.
9. ____ Technetium-99m is an iodinated contrast dye used during CT scans.
10. ____ A PET scan detects positrons and shows areas of cellular metabolism.
11. ____ Iodinated contrast dye contains iodine.
12. ____ The contrast dye barium is used during MRI scans.

Fill in the Blank

Fill in the blank with the correct word.

1. The radiologist uses a ________________________ to view radiographs.
2. A ________________________ chest x-ray is the most common type of chest x-ray.
3. Every person in radiology must wear a ________________________ to detect exposure to radiation or radioactive substances.
4. ________________________ is a metallic element that is used as a contrast dye in MRI scans because it responds to a magnetic field.
5. The ________________________ effect states that a sound wave generated by an object will change pitch as the object moves toward or away from the observer.
6. The ________________________ is the length of time it takes for half of the atoms in an amount of a radioactive substance to decay and become stable.
7. A subatomic particle accelerator known as a ________________________ must be used to produce radioactive substances that emit positrons.

Circle Exercise

Circle the correct word from the choices given.

1. A (**plain, portable, scout**) film is a preliminary radiograph taken before contrast dye is given.
2. A spiral or helical scan is one type of a/an (**CT, MRI, PET**) scan.
3. The Virtual Physical uses this technology: (**CAT, EBT, MRI**).
4. During all of these procedures, the patient is exposed to radiation, EXCEPT during a/an (**CT scan, mammography, MRI scan**).
5. During a (**MUGA, PET, SPECT**) scan, the patient's own red blood cells are tagged with radioactive technetium-99m.

Multiple Choice

Circle the correct answer from the choices given.

1. A roentgenogram is the same thing as a/an ______________________.
   a. IVP c. KUB
   b. radiograph d. tomography
2. All of the following procedures use an x-ray beam EXCEPT ______________________.
   a. mammography c. KUB
   b. cross-table lateral d. ultrasonography
3. Angiography is a general word that includes ______________________.
   a. arteriography and lymphangiography c. lymphangiography and myelography
   b. venography and lymphangiography d. arteriography and venography
4. When a standard echocardiogram cannot produce a good-quality image, the physician may order a/an ______________________.
   a. KUB c. MRI
   b. TEE d. DSA
5. PET scans are useful in detecting or studying ______________________.
   a. cancer c. schizophrenia
   b. epilepsy d. all of the above

Recall and List

List 10 metal items that might be on or inside a patient that should not be subjected to an MRI scan.

1. ______________________
2. ______________________
3. ______________________
4. ______________________
5. ______________________
6. ______________________
7. ______________________
8. ______________________
9. ______________________
10. ______________________

Matching Exercise

Match each numbered word or phrase to its description.

1.	barium swallow	_____ Fluoroscopy captured on video tape
2.	B scan	_____ Breast image from x-rays captured on paper rather than film
3.	bone densitometry	_____ DEXA scan and QCT
4.	cineradiography	_____ Any procedure that uses a contrast dye
5.	enhanced	_____ Urography
6.	filling defect	_____ Upper GI series
7.	HIDA scan	_____ Sonography
8.	pyelography	_____ Two-dimensional, gray-scale ultrasound
9.	radiopharmaceutical	_____ Acts as a tracer in the body
10.	ultrasonography	_____ Area of decreased uptake on a perfusion scan
11.	xeromammogram	_____ Cholescintigraphy

Abbreviation Exercise

Write the definition for each abbreviation.

1. US ______________________
2. PET ______________________
3. BE ______________________
4. CXR ______________________
5. SPECT ______________________
6. MUGA ______________________
7. CAT ______________________
8. IVP ______________________

Applied Skills

Analysis of a Medical Report

These three reports are radiologic and nuclear medicine diagnostic procedures. Read each report and answer the questions that follow.

RADIOLOGY REPORT

PATIENT NAME: BENTLEY, Jean
HOSPITAL NUMBER: 327-01-1982
DATE OF X-RAY: November 19, 20xx

PORTABLE PELVIS

Portable AP study of the right pelvis and hip in surgery shows the femoral part of the prosthesis to now be in place and in a normal relationship with the acetabular prosthesis. A total hip replacement prosthesis is also noted to be in place on the left.

Daniel P. Raddick, M.D.
Daniel P. Raddick, M.D.

DPR:apt
D: 11/19/xx
T: 11/19/xx

FACT FINDING QUESTIONS

1. What does the abbreviation AP stand for? ____________________
2. What one word and one phrase tell you that this x-ray was not taken in the radiology department?
____
3. Where did the radiologic technologist have to go to take this x-ray? ____________________
4. When this x-ray was taken, the patient was undergoing a total hip replacement in which hip? **Right** **Left**
5. Define *prosthesis:* ____________________

RADIOLOGY REPORT

PATIENT NAME: ADAMS, Bryce

HOSPITAL NUMBER: 11-98-64370

DATE OF X-RAY: November 19, 20xx

AIR CONTRAST BARIUM ENEMA

PROCEDURE

Under fluoroscopic control, the barium was allowed to flow in a retrograde manner to fill the cecum. Using a double-contrast technique, multiple films were obtained. Several small diverticula are noted. There is also some displacement of the small bowel. A soft tissue density is seen within the lower abdomen. No mucosal ulcerations or polypoid lesions are identified.

IMPRESSION

Air contrast study shows displacement of the small bowel with a tissue density. This is suggestive of a pelvic mass. No evidence of polypoid lesions is seen in the colon.

Robert C. Johnson, M.D.

Robert C. Johnson, M.D.

RCJ:smt
D: 11/19/xx
T: 11/19/xx

FACT FINDING QUESTIONS

1. What type of radiologic procedure was done?
   a. KUB
   b. flat plate of the abdomen
   c. fluoroscopy
2. Name the two types of contrast that were used for this procedure.

   ____

   ____
3. In addition to watching the procedure on a TV monitor, how many roentgenograms (films) were taken? ________________
4. Divide *fluoroscopic* into its three word parts and define each word part.

Word Part	**Definition**
________________	____
________________	____
________________	____

RADIOLOGY REPORT

PATIENT NAME: MATHESON, Latrise

HOSPITAL NUMBER: 901156-48376

DATE OF X-RAY: November 19, 20xx

RADIOACTIVE IODINE UPTAKE

The patient was given an oral capsule containing 100 microcuries of I-123, and uptake by the thyroid gland was measured at 6 hours and 24 hours. The 6-hour uptake was 5.5% (normal 4–12%). The 24-hour uptake was 14.0% (normal 7–24%).

THYROID SCAN

Fifteen minutes after the intravenous injection of 10 millicuries of technetium-99m, views of the thyroid gland were performed. The thyroid gland was in a normal position in the neck. The overall size of the gland was within normal limits, and there was uniform uptake throughout both the right and left lobes.

IMPRESSION

1. Normal thyroid radioiodine uptake.
2. Normal thyroid scan.

Victoria J. Evans, M.D.

Victoria J. Evans, M.D.

VJE:mja
D: 11/19/xx
T: 11/19/xx

FACT FINDING QUESTIONS

1. What are the names and atomic numbers of the two radiopharmaceuticals given in this procedure?

   ____

   ____

2. What are the two units of measurement for the doses of these radiopharmaceuticals?

   ____

   ____

3. What is the range of normal values for the 24-hour uptake? ______________________
4. How was the radioactive iodine administered? ______________________
5. How was the radioactive technetium-99m administered? ______________________
6. Divide *radioactive* into its three word parts and define each word part.

Word Part	**Definition**
____________	______________________
____________	______________________
____________	______________________

7. What phrase tells you that there was an equal amount of radioactive tracer present in all parts of the thyroid gland?

   ____

Pronunciation Checklist

Read each word and its pronunciation. Practice pronouncing each word. Verify your pronunciation by listening to the Pronunciation List on the CD-ROM. Check the box next to the word after you master its pronunciation.

- ❑ angiogram (AN-jee-oh-gram)
- ❑ angiography (AN-jee-AWG-rah-fee)
- ❑ anteroposterior position (AN-ter-oh-pohs-TEER-ee-or poh-SIH-shun)
- ❑ aortogram (aa-OR-toh-gram)
- ❑ aortography (AA-or-TAWG-rah-fee)
- ❑ arteriogram (ar-TEER-ee-oh-gram)
- ❑ arteriography (ar-TEER-ee-AWG-rah-fee)
- ❑ arthrogram (AR-throh-gram)
- ❑ arthrography (ar-THRAWG-rah-fee)
- ❑ artifact (AR-tih-fakt)
- ❑ barium enema (BAIR-ee-UM EN-eh-mah)
- ❑ barium swallow (BAIR-ee-UM SWAH-loh)
- ❑ cholangiogram (koh-LAN-jee-oh-gram)
- ❑ cholangiography (KOH-lan-jee-AWG-rah-fee)
- ❑ cholecystogram (KOH-lee-SIS-toh-gram)
- ❑ cholecystography (KOH-lee-sis-TAWG-rah-fee)
- ❑ cholescintigraphy (KOH-lee-sin-TIG-rah-fee)
- ❑ cineradiography (SIN-eh-RAY-dee-AWG-rah-fee)
- ❑ computerized axial tomography (com-PYOO-ter-ized AK-see-al toh-MAWG-rah-fee)
- ❑ coronary angiography (KOHR-oh-nair-ee AN-jee-AWG-rah-fee)
- ❑ cyclotron (SY-kloh-trawn)
- ❑ decubitus position (dee-KYOO-bih-tus poh-SIH-shun)
- ❑ densitometry (DEN-sih-TAWM-eh-tree)
- ❑ Doppler ultrasonography (DAWP-ler UL-trah-soh-NAWG-rah-fee)
- ❑ dosimeter (doh-SIM-eh-ter)
- ❑ dosimetry (doh-SIM-eh-tree)
- ❑ duplex ultrasonography (DOO-pleks UL-trah-soh-NAWG-rah-fee)
- ❑ echocardiogram (EK-oh-KAR-dee-oh-gram)
- ❑ echocardiography (EK-oh-KAR-dee-AWG-rah-fee)
- ❑ excretory urogram (EKS-kree-toh-ree YOOR-oh-gram)
- ❑ excretory urography (EKS-kree-toh-ree yoo-RAWG-rah-fee)
- ❑ fluoroscopy (floor-AWS-koh-pee)
- ❑ gadolinium (GAD-oh-LIN-ee-um)
- ❑ gallium (GAL-ee-um)
- ❑ helical (HEL-ih-kal)
- ❑ hysterosalpingogram (HIS-ter-oh-sal-PING-oh-gram)
- ❑ hysterosalpingography (HIS-ter-oh-SAL-pin-GAWG-rah-fee)
- ❑ interventional radiology (IN-ter-VEN-shun-al RAY-dee-AWL-oh-jee)
- ❑ intravenous cholangiography (IN-trah-VEE-nus KOH-lan-jee-AWG-rah-fee)
- ❑ intravenous pyelography (IN-trah-VEE-nus PY-eh-LOG-rah-fee)
- ❑ iodine (EYE-oh-dine)
- ❑ krypton (KRIP-tawn)
- ❑ lateral position (LAT-er-al poh-SIH-shun)
- ❑ lymphangiogram (lim-FAN-jee-oh-gram)
- ❑ lymphangiography (lim-FAN-jee-AWG-rah-fee)
- ❑ magnetic resonance imaging (mag-NET-ik REH-soh-nans IM-ah-jing)
- ❑ mammogram (MAM-oh-gram)
- ❑ mammography (mah-MAWG-rah-fee)
- ❑ MUGA scan (MUH-gah SKAN)
- ❑ multidetector (MUL-tee-dee-TEK-tor)
- ❑ myelogram (MY-eh-loh-gram)
- ❑ myelography (MY-eh-LOG-rah-fee)
- ❑ nuclear medicine (NYOO-klee-er MED-ih-sin)
- ❑ oblique position (awb-LEEK poh-SIH-shun)
- ❑ OncoScint scan (AWN-koh-sint SKAN)
- ❑ perfusion scan (per-FYOO-zhun SKAN)
- ❑ positron emission tomography (PAWZ-ih-trawn ee-MISH-un toh-MAWG-rah-fee)
- ❑ postcontrast image (pohst-KAWN-trast IM-ij)
- ❑ posteroanterior position (POHS-ter-oh-an-TEER-ee-or poh-SIH-shun)
- ❑ precontrast image (pree-KAWN-trast IM-ij)
- ❑ projection (proh-JEK-shun)
- ❑ ProstaScint scan (PRAW-stah-sint SKAN)
- ❑ pyelogram (PY-eh-loh-gram)
- ❑ pyelography (PY-eh-LOG-rah-fee)
- ❑ radioactive (RAY-dee-oh-AK-tiv)
- ❑ radiograph (RAY-dee-oh-graf)
- ❑ radiologic technologist (RAY-dee-oh-LAWJ-ik tek-NAWL-oh-jist)
- ❑ radiology (RAY-dee-AWL-oh-jee)
- ❑ radiolucent (RAY-dee-oh-LOO-sent)
- ❑ radionuclide (RAY-dee-oh-NYOO-klide)
- ❑ radiopaque (RAY-dee-oh-PAYK)
- ❑ radiopharmaceutical (RAY-dee-oh-FAR-mah-SOO-tik-al)
- ❑ retrograde pyelography (RET-roh-grayd PY-eh-LOG-rah-fee)
- ❑ roentgenogram (RENT-gen-oh-gram)
- ❑ roentgenography (RENT-geh-NAWG-rah-fee)
- ❑ rotational angiography (roh-TAY-shun-al AN-jee-AWG-rah-fee)
- ❑ scintigram (SIN-tih-gram)
- ❑ scintigraphy (sin-TIG-rah-fee)
- ❑ scintillation (SIN-tih-LAY-shun)
- ❑ scintiscan (SIN-tih-skan)
- ❑ sonogram (SAWN-oh-gram)
- ❑ sonography (soh-NAWG-rah-fee)
- ❑ SPECT scan (SPEKT SKAN)
- ❑ spiral (SPY-ral)
- ❑ technetium (tek-NEE-shee-um)
- ❑ thallium (THAL-ee-um)
- ❑ tomography (toh-MAWG-rah-fee)
- ❑ tracer (TRAY-ser)
- ❑ transducer (trans-DOO-ser)
- ❑ transesophageal echocardiogram (trans-ee-SAWF-ah-JEE-al EK-oh-KAR-dee-oh-gram)
- ❑ ultrasonography (UL-trah-soh-NAWG-rah-fee)
- ❑ ultrasound (UL-trah-sound)
- ❑ upper gastrointestinal series (UH-per GAS-troh-in-TES-tin-al SEER-ez)
- ❑ urogram (YOO-roh-gram)
- ❑ urography (yoo-RAWG-rah-fee)
- ❑ venogram (VEE-noh-gram)
- ❑ venography (vee-NAWG-rah-fee)
- ❑ ventilation-perfusion scan (ven-tih-LAY-shun per-FYOO-shun SKAN)
- ❑ xenon (ZEE-nawn)
- ❑ xeromammogram (ZEER-oh-MAM-oh-gram)
- ❑ xeromammography (ZEER-oh-mah-MAWG-rah-fee)

Experience Multimedia

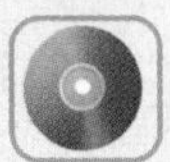

CD-ROM Learning Activities Checklist

Check off the box as you complete each learning activity.

❑ **CD-ROM Learning Activity 19.1: *FLASHCARDS***
Use flashcards to help you memorize word parts. Make your own flashcards or print out prepared flashcards. Also see the electronic flashcard game. Time: 20 minutes.

❑ **CD-ROM Learning Activity 19.2: *MEDICAL LANGUAGE PRONUNCIATION***
Listen to a pronounced medical word and then practice pronouncing it. Time: 45 minutes.

❑ **CD-ROM Learning Activity 19.3: *SPELLING CHALLENGE***
Listen to a pronounced medical word and then spell it. Time: 5 minutes.

❑ **CD-ROM Learning Activity 19.4: *EDUCATIONAL GAMES***
Enjoy these fun activities while reinforcing your knowledge. Time: 15 minutes.

Appendix A

Glossary of Medical Word Parts
Combining Forms, Prefixes, and Suffixes

A

a-	prefix	away from, without
ab-	prefix	away from
abdomin/o-	combining form	abdomen
ablat/o-	combining form	take away; destroy
-able	suffix	able to be
abort/o-	combining form	stop prematurely
abras/o-	combining form	scrape off
absorpt/o-	combining form	absorb or take in
-ac	suffix	pertaining to
access/o-	combining form	supplemental or contributing part
accommod/o-	combining form	to adapt
acetabul/o-	combining form	acetabulum (hip socket)
acid/o-	combining form	acid (low pH)
acous/o-	combining form	hearing, sound
acr/o-	combining form	extremity; highest point
acromi/o-	combining form	acromion
actin/o-	combining form	rays of the sun
act/o-	combining form	action
acu/o-	combining form	needle; sharpness
-acusis	suffix	hearing
acus/o-	combining form	the sense of hearing
ad-	prefix	toward
-ad	suffix	toward, in the direction of
addict/o-	combining form	surrender to; be controlled by
-ade	suffix	action; process
aden/o-	combining form	gland
adhes/o-	combining form	to stick to
adip/o-	combining form	fat
adjuv/o-	combining form	giving help or assistance
adnex/o-	combining form	accessory connecting parts
adolesc/o-	combining form	the beginning of being an adult
adrenal/o-	combining form	adrenal gland
adren/o-	combining form	adrenal gland
affect/o-	combining form	state of mind; mood; to have an influence on
affer/o-	combining form	bring toward the center
agglutin/o-	combining form	clumping, sticking
aggreg/o-	combining form	crowding together
ag/o-	combining form	to lead to
agon/o-	combining form	causing action
agor/a-	combining form	open area or space
-al	suffix	pertaining to
albin/o-	combining form	white
albumin/o-	combining form	albumin
alges/o-	combining form	sensation of pain
-algia	suffix	painful condition
alg/o-	combining form	pain
align/o-	combining form	arranged in a straight line
aliment/o-	combining form	food, nourishment
-alis	suffix	pertaining to
alkal/o-	combining form	base (high pH)
allerg/o-	combining form	allergy
all/o-	combining form	other; strange
alveol/o-	combining form	alveolus (air sac)
ambly/o-	combining form	dimness
ambulat/o-	combining form	walking
amnes/o-	combining form	forgetfulness
amni/o-	combining form	amnion (fetal membrane)
-amnios	suffix	amniotic fluid
amputat/o-	combining form	to cut off
amput/o-	combining form	to cut off
amygdal/o-	combining form	almond shape
amyl/o-	combining form	carbohydrate, starch
an-	prefix	without, not
-an	suffix	pertaining to
ana-	prefix	apart from; excessive
anabol/o-	combining form	building up
analy/o-	combining form	to separate
anastom/o-	combining form	unite two tubular structures
-ance	suffix	state of
ancill/o-	combining form	servant, accessory
-ancy	suffix	state of
andr/o-	combining form	male
aneurysm/o-	combining form	aneurysm (dilation)
angin/o-	combining form	angina
angi/o-	combining form	blood vessel; lymphatic vessel
anis/o-	combining form	unequal
ankyl/o-	combining form	fused together, stiff
an/o-	combining form	anus
ant-	prefix	against
-ant	suffix	pertaining to
antagon/o-	combining form	oppose or work against
ante-	prefix	forward, before

anter/o-	combining form	before; front part
anthrac/o-	combining form	coal
anti-	prefix	against
anxi/o-	combining form	fear, worry
aort/o-	combining form	aorta
apher/o-	combining form	withdrawal
aphth/o-	combining form	ulcer
apic/o-	combining form	apex (tip)
apo-	prefix	away from
appendic/o-	combining form	appendix
appendicul/o-	combining form	limb; small attached part
append/o-	combining form	small structure hanging from a larger structure; appendix
appercept/o-	combining form	fully perceived
aque/o-	combining form	watery substance
-ar	suffix	pertaining to
arachn/o-	combining form	spider, spider web
-arche	suffix	a beginning
areol/o-	combining form	small area around the nipple
-arian	suffix	pertaining to a person
-aris	suffix	pertaining to
arteri/o-	combining form	artery
arter/o-	combining form	artery
arteriol/o-	combining form	arteriole
arthr/o-	combining form	joint
articul/o-	combining form	joint
-ary	suffix	pertaining to
asbest/o-	combining form	asbestos
ascit/o-	combining form	ascites
-ase	suffix	enzyme
aspir/o-	combining form	to breathe in; to suck in
asthm/o-	combining form	asthma
astr/o-	combining form	starlike structure
-ate	suffix	composed of; pertaining to
-ated	suffix	pertaining to a condition; composed of
atel/o-	combining form	incomplete
ather/o-	combining form	soft, fatty substance
atheromat/o-	combining form	fatty deposit or mass
athet/o-	combining form	without position or place
-atic	suffix	pertaining to
-ation	suffix	a process; being or having
-ative	suffix	pertaining to
-ator	suffix	person or thing that produces or does
-atory	suffix	pertaining to
atri/o-	combining form	atrium (upper heart chamber)
attenu/o-	combining form	weakened
-ature	suffix	system composed of
audi/o-	combining form	the sense of hearing
audit/o-	combining form	the sense of hearing
augment/o-	combining form	increase in size or degree
aur/i-	combining form	ear
auricul/o-	combining form	ear
auscult/o-	combining form	listening
auto-	prefix	self
autonom/o-	combining form	independent, self-governing
axill/o-	combining form	axilla (armpit)
axi/o-	combining form	axis

B

bacteri/o-	combining form	bacterium
balan/o-	combining form	glans penis
bar/o-	combining form	weight
basil/o-	combining form	base of an organ
bas/o-	combining form	base of a structure
bas/o-	combining form	basic (alkaline)
behav/o-	combining form	activity or manner of acting
bi-	prefix	two
bil/i-	combining form	bile, gall
bilirubin/o-	combining form	bilirubin
bi/o-	combining form	life; living organisms; living tissue
-blast	suffix	immature cell
blast/o-	combining form	immature; embryonic
blephar/o-	combining form	eyelid
-body	suffix	a structure or thing
botul/o-	combining form	sausage
brachi/o-	combining form	arm
brachy-	prefix	short
brady-	prefix	slow
bronchi/o-	combining form	bronchus
bronchiol/o-	combining form	bronchiole
bronch/o-	combining form	bronchus
brux/o-	combined form	to grind the teeth
buccinat/o-	combining form	cheek
bucc/o-	combining form	cheek
bulb/o-	combining form	like a bulb
bunion/o-	combining form	bunion
burs/o-	combining form	bursa

C

cac/o-	combining form	bad, poor
calcane/o-	combining form	calcaneus (heel bone)
calcific/o-	combining form	hard from calcium
calci/o-	combining form	calcium

calc/o-	combining form	calcium
calcul/o-	combining form	stone
calic/o-	combining form	calix
cali/o-	combining form	calix
calor/o-	combining form	heat
cancell/o-	combining form	lattice structure
cancer/o-	combining form	cancer
candid/o-	combining form	Candida (a yeast)
can/o-	combining form	resembling a dog
capill/o-	combining form	hairlike structure
capn/o-	combining form	carbon dioxide
capsul/o-	combining form	capsule (enveloping structure)
carb/o-	combining form	carbon atoms
carbox/y-	combining form	carbon dioxide
carcin/o-	combining form	cancer
card/i-	combining form	heart
cardi/o-	combining form	heart
cari/o-	combining form	caries (tooth decay)
carot/o-	combining form	stupor, sleep
carp/o-	combining form	wrist
cartilagin/o-	combining form	cartilage
cata-	prefix	down
catabol/o-	combining form	breaking down
catheter/o-	combining form	catheter
caud/o-	combining form	tailbone; lower part of the body
caus/o-	combining form	burning
cavit/o-	combining form	hollow space
cav/o-	combining form	hollow space
cec/o-	combining form	cecum (first part of large intestine)
-cele	suffix	hernia
celi/o-	combining form	abdomen
cellul/o-	combining form	cell
-centesis	suffix	procedure to puncture
centr/o-	combining form	center; dominant part
cephal/o-	combining form	head
-cephalus	suffix	head
-ceps	suffix	head
-cere	suffix	waxy substance
cerebell/o-	combining form	cerebellum (posterior part of the brain)
cerebr/o-	combining form	cerebrum (largest part of the brain)
cervic/o-	combining form	neck; cervix
cheil/o-	combining form	lip
chem/o-	combining form	chemical, drug
chez/o-	combining form	to pass stool
chir/o-	combining form	hand
chlor/o-	combining form	chloride
cholangi/o-	combining form	bile duct
chol/e-	combining form	bile, gall
cholecyst/o-	combining form	gallbladder
choledoch/o-	combining form	common bile duct
cholesterol/o-	combining form	cholesterol
chol/o-	combining form	bile, gall
chondri/o-	combining form	little granule
chondr/o-	combining form	cartilage
chori/o-	combining form	chorion (fetal membrane)
chorion/o-	combining form	chorion (fetal membrane)
choroid/o-	combining form	choroid (middle layer around the eye)
chrom/o-	combining form	color
chron/o-	combining form	time
cid/o-	combining form	killing
cili/o-	combining form	hairlike structure
cin/e-	combining form	movement
circa-	prefix	about
circulat/o-	combining form	movement in an circular route
circul/o-	combining form	circle
circum-	prefix	around
cirrh/o-	combining form	yellow
cis/o-	combining form	to cut
-clast	suffix	cell that breaks down substances
claudicat/o-	combining form	limping pain
claustr/o-	combining form	enclosed space
clavicul/o-	combining form	clavicle (collar bone)
clav/o-	combining form	clavicle (collar bone)
-cle	suffix	small thing
cleid/o-	combining form	clavicle (collar bone)
clinic/o-	combining form	medicine
clon/o-	combining form	rapid contracting and relaxing
clon/o-	combining form	identical group derived from one
-clonus	suffix	condition of rapid contracting and relaxing
-cnemius	combining form	leg
coagul/o-	combining form	clotting
coarct/o-	combining form	pressed together
cocc/o-	combining form	spherical bacterium
-coccus	suffix	spherical bacterium
coccyg/o-	combining form	coccyx (tail bone)
cochle/o-	combining form	cochlea (of the inner ear)
cognit/o-	combining form	thinking
coit/o-	combining form	sexual intercourse
coll/a-	combining form	fibers that hold together

-collis	suffix	condition of the neck
col/o-	combining form	colon (part of large intestine)
colon/o-	combining form	colon (part of large intestine)
colp/o-	combining form	vagina
comat/o-	combining form	deep unconsciousness
comminut/o-	combining form	break into minute pieces
communic/o-	combining form	impart, transmit
compens/o-	combining form	counterbalance; compensate
compress/o-	combining form	press together
compromis/o-	combining form	exposed to danger
compuls/o-	combining form	drive or compel
con-	prefix	with
concept/o-	combining form	to conceive or form
concuss/o-	combining form	violent shaking or jarring
conduct/o-	combining form	carrying, conveying
conform/o-	combining form	having the same scale or angle
congenit/o-	combining form	present at birth
congest/o-	combining form	accumulation of fluid
coni/o-	combining form	dust
conjug/o-	combining form	joined together
conjunctiv/o-	combining form	conjunctiva
con/o-	combining form	cone
constip/o-	combining form	compacted stool
constrict/o-	combining form	drawn together, narrowed
construct/o-	combining form	to build
contin/o-	combining form	hold together
contra-	prefix	against
contract/o-	combining form	pull together
contus/o-	combining form	bruising
converg/o-	combining form	coming together
convuls/o-	combining form	seizure
copr/o-	combining form	feces, stool
corne/o-	combining form	cornea
cor/o-	combining form	pupil
coron/o-	combining form	encircling structure
corpor/o-	combining form	body
cortic/o-	combining form	cortex (outer region)
cosmet/o-	combining form	attractive, adorned
cost/o-	combining form	rib
crani/o-	combining form	cranium (skull)
-crasia	suffix	a mixing
-crine	suffix	a thing that secretes
crin/o-	combining form	secrete
-crit	suffix	separation of
cry/o-	combining form	cold
crypt/o-	combining form	hidden
cubit/o-	combining form	elbow
culd/o-	combining form	cul-de-sac
cusp/o-	combining form	projection, point
cutane/o-	combining form	skin
cut/i-	combining form	skin
cyan/o-	combining form	blue
cycl/o-	combining form	ciliary body of the eye; cycle
cycl/o-	combining form	cycle; circle
cyst/o-	combining form	bladder; fluid-filled sac; semisolid cyst
cyt/o-	combining form	cell
-cyte	suffix	cell

D

dacry/o-	combining form	lacrimal sac; tears
-dactyly	suffix	condition of fingers or toes
de-	prefix	reversal of; without
dec/i-	combining form	one tenth
decidu/o-	combining form	falling off
defici/o-	combining form	lacking, inadequate
degluti/o-	combining form	swallowing
delt/o-	combining form	triangle
delus/o-	combining form	false belief
dem/o-	combining form	people; population
dendr/o-	combining form	branching structure
densit/o-	combining form	density
dent/i-	combining form	tooth
dentit/o-	combining form	eruption of teeth
dent/o-	combining form	tooth
depend/o-	combining form	to hang onto
depress/o-	combining form	press down
derm/a-	combining form	skin
-derma	suffix	skin
dermat/o-	combining form	skin
derm/o-	combining form	skin
desicc/o-	combining form	to dry up
-desis	suffix	procedure to fuse together
dextr/o-	combining form	right
dextr/o-	combining form	sugar
di-	prefix	two
dia-	prefix	complete; completely through
diabet/o-	combining form	diabetes
diaphragmat/o-	combining form	diaphragm
diaphor/o-	combining form	sweating
diaphys/o-	combining form	shaft of a bone
diastol/o-	combining form	dilating
-didymis	suffix	testes (twin structures)
didym/o-	combining form	testes (twin structures)
dietet/o-	combining form	foods, diet
diet/o-	combining form	foods, diet

differentiat/o-	combining form	being distinct or specialized
different/o-	combining form	being distinct, different
digest/o-	combining form	break down food; digest
digit/o-	combining form	digit (finger or toe)
dilat/o-	combining form	dilate, widen
dipl/o-	combining form	double
dips/o-	combining form	thirst
dis-	prefix	away from
disk/o-	combining form	disk
dissect/o-	combining form	to cut apart
dissemin/o-	combining form	widely scattered throughout the body
distent/o-	combining form	distended, stretched
dist/o-	combining form	away from the center or point of origin
diverticul/o-	combining form	diverticulum
donat/o-	combining form	give as a gift
dors/o-	combining form	back; dorsum; uppermost part
-dose	suffix	measured quantity
dos/i-	combining form	dose
-drome	suffix	a running
duc/o-	combining form	bring or move
-duct	suffix	duct (tube)
duct/o-	combining form	bring or move; a duct
du/o-	combining form	two
duoden/o-	combining form	duodenum (first part of small intestine)
dur/o-	combining form	dura mater
dynam/o-	combining form	power; movement
dyn/o-	combining form	pain
dys-	prefix	painful, difficult, abnormal

E

e-	prefix	without, out
-eal	suffix	pertaining to
ec-	prefix	out, outward
ecchym/o-	combining form	blood in the tissues
ech/o-	combining form	echo (sound wave)
eclamps/o-	combining form	a seizure
-ectasis	suffix	condition of dilation
ectat/o-	combining form	dilation
ecto-	prefix	outermost, outside
ectop/o-	combining form	outside of a place
-ectomy	suffix	surgical excision
-ed	suffix	pertaining to
-edema	suffix	swelling
edentul/o-	combining form	without teeth
-ee	suffix	person who is the object of an action
efface/o-	combining form	do away with; obliterate
effer/o-	combining form	go out from the center
effus/o-	combining form	a pouring out
ejaculat/o-	combining form	to expel suddenly
electr/o-	combining form	electricity
-elasma	suffix	platelike structure
elast/o-	combining form	flexing, stretching
elimin/o-	combining form	expel, remove
-elle	suffix	little thing
em-	prefix	in
-ema	suffix	condition
emaci/o-	combining form	to make thin
embol/o-	combining form	embolus (occluding plug)
embryon/o-	combining form	embryo; immature form
-emesis	suffix	vomiting
emet/o-	combining form	to vomit
-emia	suffix	condition of the blood; substance in the blood
-emic	suffix	pertaining to blood or a substance in the blood
emiss/o-	combining form	to send out
emot/o-	combining form	moving, stirring up
emulsific/o-	combining form	droplets of fat suspended in a liquid; particles suspended in a solution
en-	prefix	in, within, inward
-ence	suffix	state of
encephal/o-	combining form	brain
-encephaly	suffix	condition of the brain
-ency	prefix	condition of being
endo-	prefix	innermost, within
-ent	suffix	pertaining to
enter/o-	combining form	intestine
-entery	suffix	condition of the intestine
enucle/o-	combining form	to remove the kernal or nucleus
enur/o-	combining form	to urinate in
-eon	suffix	one who performs
eosin/o-	combining form	eosin (acidic red dye)
ependym/o-	combining form	lining membrane
epi-	prefix	upon, above
epilept/o-	combining form	seizure
epiphys/o-	combining form	growth area on the end of a bone
episi/o-	combining form	vulva (female external genitalia)
-er	suffix	person or thing that produces or does

erect/o-	combining form	to stand up
erg/o-	combining form	activity; work
-ergy	suffix	activity; process of working
erupt/o-	combining form	breaking out
-ery	suffix	process of
erythemat/o-	combining form	redness
erythr/o-	combining form	red
-esis	suffix	condition
es/o-	combining form	inward
esophag/o-	combining form	esophagus
esthes/o-	combining form	sensation, feeling
esthet/o-	combining form	sensation, feeling
estr/a-	combining form	female
estr/o-	combining form	female
ethm/o-	combining form	sieve
-etic	suffix	pertaining to
eti/o-	combining form	cause of disease
-ety	suffix	condition, state
etym/o-	combining form	word origin
eu-	prefix	normal, good
ex-	prefix	out, away from
exacerb/o-	combining form	increase; provoke
excis/o-	combining form	to cut out
excori/o-	combining form	to take out skin
excret/o-	combining form	removing from the body
exhibit/o-	combining form	showing
exo-	prefix	away from, external, outward
explorat/o-	combining form	to search out
express/o-	combining form	communicate
extens/o-	combining form	straightening
extern/o-	combining form	outside
extra-	prefix	outside of
extrins/o-	combining form	on the outside
exud/o-	combining form	oozing fluid

F

faci/o-	combining form	face
factiti/o-	combining form	artificial, contrived
fallopi/o-	combining form	fallopian tube
fasci/o-	combining form	fascia
fec/a-	combining form	feces, stool
fec/o-	combining form	feces, stool
femor/o-	combining form	femur (thigh bone)
fer/o-	combining form	to bear
ferrit/o-	combining form	iron
ferr/o-	combining form	iron
fertil/o-	combining form	able to conceive a child
fet/o-	combining form	fetus
fibrill/o-	combining form	muscle fiber; nerve fiber
fibrin/o-	combining form	fibrin
fibr/o-	combining form	fiber
fibul/o-	combining form	fibula (lower leg bone)
filtrat/o-	combining form	filtering; straining
filtr/o-	combining form	filter
fiss/o-	combining form	splitting
fixat/o-	combining form	to make stable or still
flatul/o-	combining form	flatus
flex/o-	combining form	bending
fluor/o-	combining form	fluorescence
-flux	suffix	flow
foc/o-	combining form	point of activity
foli/o-	combining form	leaf
follicul/o-	combining form	follicle (small sac)
foramin/o-	combining form	foramen (opening into a cavity or channel)
forens/o-	combining form	court proceedings in criminal law
-form	suffix	having the form of
format/o-	combining form	structure; arrangement
fove/o-	combining form	small, depressed area
fract/o-	combining form	break up
fratern/o-	combining form	close association or relationship
-frice	suffix	thing that produces friction
front/o-	combining form	front
fruct/o-	combining form	fruit
fulgur/o-	combining form	spark of electricity
fund/o-	combining form	fundus (part farthest from the opening)
fundu/o-	combining form	fundus (part farthest from the opening)
fung/o-	combining form	fungus
fus/o-	combining form	pouring

G

galact/o-	combining form	milk
ganglion/o-	combining form	ganglion
gangren/o-	combining form	gangrene
gastr/o-	combining form	stomach
gemin/o-	combining form	twins; set or group
-gen	suffix	that which produces
-gene	suffix	gene
gene/o-	combining form	gene
gener/o-	combining form	production; creation
genit/o-	combining form	genitalia
gen/o-	combining form	arising from; produced by

germin/o-	combining form	embryonic tissue
ger/o-	combining form	old age
gest/o-	combining form	from conception to birth
gestat/o-	combining form	from conception to birth
gigant/o-	combining form	giant
gingiv/o-	combining form	gums
glandul/o-	combining form	gland
glen/o-	combining form	socket of a joint
-glia	suffix	substance that holds things together
gli/o-	combining form	substance that holds things together
glob/o-	combining form	shaped like a globe; comprehensive
globul/o-	combining form	shaped like a globe
glomerul/o-	combining form	glomerulus
gloss/o-	combining form	tongue
glott/o-	combining form	glottis (of the larynx)
gluc/o-	combining form	glucose (sugar)
glycer/o-	combining form	glycerol (sugar alcohol)
glyc/o-	combining form	glucose (sugar)
glycos/o-	combining form	glucose (sugar)
gnos/o-	combining form	knowledge
gonad/o-	combining form	gonads (ovaries and testes)
goni/o-	combining form	angle
gon/o-	combining form	seed (ovum or spermatozoon)
-grade	suffix	going
-graft	suffix	tissue for implant or transplant
-gram	suffix	a record or picture
granul/o-	combining form	granule
-graph	suffix	instrument used to record
graph/o-	combining form	record
-graphy	suffix	process of recording
-gravida	suffix	pregnancy
gustat/o-	combining form	the sense of taste
gynec/o-	combining form	female, woman

H

habilitat/o-	combining form	give ability
halit/o-	combining form	breath
hallucin/o-	combining form	imagined perception
hal/o-	combining form	breathe
hebe/o-	combining form	youth
hec/o-	combining form	habitual condition of the body
hedon/o-	combining form	pleasure
helic/o-	combining form	a coil
hemat/o-	combining form	blood
hemi-	prefix	one half
hem/o-	combining form	blood
hemoglobin/o-	combining form	hemoglobin
hemorrh/o-	combining form	a flowing of blood
hemorrhoid/o-	combining form	hemorrhoid
hepat/o-	combining form	liver
heredit/o-	combining form	genetic influence
hered/o-	combining form	genetic inheritance
herni/o-	combining form	hernia
heter/o-	combining form	other
hex/o-	combining form	habitual condition of the body
hidr/o-	combining form	sweat
hil/o-	combining form	hilum (indentation in an organ)
hirsut/o-	combining form	hairy
histi/o-	combining form	tissue
home/o-	combining form	same
hom/i-	combining form	man
horizont/o-	combining form	boundary between the earth and sky
hormon/o-	combining form	hormone
humer/o-	combining form	humerus (upper arm bone)
hyal/o-	combining form	clear glasslike substance
hydatidi/o-	combining form	fluid-filled vesicles
hydr/o-	combining form	water; fluid
hygien/o-	combining form	health
hy/o-	combining form	U-shaped structure
hyper-	prefix	above; more than normal
hypn/o-	combining form	sleep
hypo-	prefix	below; deficient
hypophys/o-	combining form	pituitary gland
hyster/o-	combining form	uterus (womb)

I

-ia	suffix	condition, state, thing
-iac	suffix	pertaining to
-ial	suffix	pertaining to
-ian	suffix	pertaining to
-ias	suffix	condition
-iasis	suffix	state of; process of
-iatic	suffix	pertaining to a state or process
iatr/o-	combining form	physician; medical treatment
-iatry	suffix	medical treatment
-ic	suffix	pertaining to
-ical	suffix	pertaining to
-ician	suffix	a skilled professional or expert
-ics	suffix	knowledge, practice

icter/o-	combining form	jaundice
ict/o-	combining form	seizure
-id	suffix	resembling; source or origin
-ide	suffix	chemically modified structure
idi/o-	combining form	unknown; individual
-ie	suffix	a thing
-il	suffix	a thing
-ile	suffix	pertaining to
ile/o-	combining form	ileum (third part of small intestine)
ili/o-	combining form	ilium (hip bone)
-ility	suffix	having the quality of
illus/o-	combining form	false perception
im-	prefix	not
-immune	suffix	immune response
immun/o-	combining form	immune response
impact/o-	combining form	wedged in
implant/o-	combining form	placed within
in-	prefix	in; within; not
-in	suffix	a substance
incarcer/o-	combining form	to imprison
incis/o-	combining form	to cut into
incud/o-	combining form	incus (anvil-shaped bone)
induct/o-	combining form	a leading in
-ine	suffix	pertaining to
infarct/o-	combining form	area of dead tissue
infect/o-	combining form	disease within
infer/o-	combining form	below
inflammat/o-	combining form	redness and warmth
infra-	prefix	below, beneath
-ing	suffix	doing
inguin/o-	combining form	groin
inhibit/o-	combining form	block; hold back
inject/o-	combining form	insert or put in
insemin/o-	combining form	plant a seed
insert/o-	combining form	to put in or introduce
inspect/o-	combining form	looking at
insulin/o-	combining form	insulin
insul/o-	combining form	island
integument/o-	combining form	skin
integu/o-	combining form	to cover
inter-	prefix	between
intern/o-	combining form	inside
interstiti/o-	combining form	spaces within tissue
intestin/o-	combining form	intestine
intra-	prefix	within
intrins/o-	combining form	on the inside
intussuscep/o-	combining form	to receive within
invas/o-	combining form	to go into
involut/o-	combining form	enlarged organ returns to normal size
iodin/o-	combining form	iodine
iod/o-	combining form	iodine
-ion	suffix	action; condition
-ior	suffix	pertaining to
-ious	suffix	pertaining to
irid/o-	combining form	iris (colored part of the eye)
ir/o-	combining form	iris (colored part of the eye)
ischi/o-	combining form	ischium (hip bone)
isch/o-	combining form	keep back; block
-ism	suffix	process; disease from a specific cause
-ist	suffix	one who specializes in
-istic	suffix	pertaining to
-istry	suffix	process related to the specialty of
-isy	suffix	condition of inflammation
-ite	suffix	thing that pertains to
-itian	suffix	a skilled professional or expert
-itic	suffix	pertaining to
-ition	suffix	a process; being or having
-itis	suffix	inflammation of
-ity	suffix	state; condition
-ium	suffix	a chemical element
-ive	suffix	pertaining to
-ix	suffix	a structure
-ization	suffix	process of making, creating, or inserting
-ize	suffix	affecting in a particular way
-izer	suffix	thing that affects in a particular way

J

jejun/o-	combining form	jejunum (middle part of small intestine)
jugul/o-	combining form	jugular (throat)

K

kal/i-	combining form	potassium
kary/o-	combining form	nucleus
kel/o-	combining form	tumor
kerat/o-	combining form	cornea
kerat/o-	combining form	hard, fibrous protein
ket/o-	combining form	ketones
keton/o-	combining form	ketones
-kinesis	suffix	condition of movement
kines/o-	combining form	movement

-kine	suffix	movement
kin/o-	combining form	movement
klept/o-	combining form	to steal
kyph/o-	combining form	bent; humpbacked

L

labi/o-	combining form	lip; labium
laborat/o-	combining form	workplace; testing place
labyrinth/o-	combining form	labyrinth (in the inner ear)
lacer/o-	combining form	a tearing
lacrim/o-	combining form	tears
lact/i-	combining form	milk
lact/o-	combining form	milk
-lalia	suffix	condition of speech
lamin/o-	combining form	lamina (flat area on the vertebra)
lapar/o-	combining form	abdomen
laryng/o-	combining form	larynx (voice box)
later/o-	combining form	side
lei/o-	combining form	smooth
lenticul/o-	combining form	lens
lent/o-	combining form	lens of the eye
-lepsy	suffix	seizure
leuk/o-	combining form	white
levo-	prefix	left
lex/o-	combining form	word
ligament/o-	combining form	ligament
ligat/o-	combining form	to tie up or bind
limb/o-	combining form	edge, border
lingu/o-	combining form	tongue
lipid/o-	combining form	lipid (fat)
lip/o-	combining form	lipid (fat)
-listhesis		see *-olisthesis*
-lith	suffix	stone
lith/o-	combining form	stone
lob/o-	combining form	lobe of an organ
locat/o-	combining form	a place
loc/o-	combining form	in one place
log/o-	combining form	word; the study of
-logy	suffix	the study of
lord/o-	combining form	swayback
luc/o-	combining form	clear and shining
lumb/o-	combining form	lower back; area between the ribs and pelvis
lumin/o-	combining form	lumen (opening)
lun/o-	combining form	moon
-ly	suffix	going toward
lymph/o-	combining form	lymph; lymphatic system
ly/o-	combining form	break down, separate, dissolve
-lysis	suffix	abnormal condition or process of breaking down or dissolving
lys/o-	combining form	break down or dissolve
-lyte	suffix	dissolved substance

M

macr/o-	combining form	large
macul/o-	combining form	small area or spot
magnet/o-	combining form	magnet
mal-	prefix	bad, inadequate
-malacia	suffix	condition of softening
malac/o-	combining form	softening
malign/o-	combining form	intentionally causing harm; cancer
malle/o-	combining form	malleus (hammer-shaped bone)
malleol/o-	combining form	malleolus
mamm/a-	combining form	breast
mamm/o-	combining form	breast
mandibul/o-	combining form	mandible (lower jaw)
-mania	suffix	condition of frenzy
man/o-	combining form	thin
manu/o-	combining form	hand
masset/o-	combined form	chewing
mastic/o-	combining form	chewing
mast/o-	combining form	breast; mastoid process
mastoid/o-	combining form	mastoid process
matur/o-	combining form	mature
maxill/o-	combining form	maxilla (upper jaw)
mediastin/o-	combining form	mediastinum
medic/o-	combining form	physician; medicine
medi/o-	combining form	middle
medull/o-	combining form	medulla (inner region)
meg/a-	combining form	large
megal/o-	combining form	large
-megaly	suffix	enlargement
melan/o-	combining form	black
melen/o-	combining form	black
meningi/o-	combining form	meninges
mening/o-	combining form	meninges
menisc/o-	combining form	meniscus (crescent-shaped cartilage)
men/o-	combining form	month
menstru/o-	combining form	monthly discharge of blood
-ment	suffix	action; state

ment/o-	combining form	mind; chin
mesenter/o-	combining form	mesentery
mesi/o-	combining form	middle
meso-	prefix	middle
meta-	prefix	after; subsequent to; transition; change
metabol/o-	combining form	change, transformation
-meter	suffix	instrument used to measure
metri/o-	combining form	uterus (womb)
metr/o-	combining form	measurement
metr/o-	combining form	uterus (womb)
-metry	suffix	process of measuring
micr/o-	combining form	small
micr/o-	combining form	one millionth
mictur/o-	combining form	making urine
mid-	prefix	middle
-mileusis	suffix	process of carving
mineral/o-	combining form	mineral; electrolyte
mi/o-	combining form	lessening
mit/o-	combining form	threadlike structure
mitr/o-	combining form	structure like a miter (tall hat with 2 points)
mitt/o-	combining form	to send
mon/o-	combining form	one, single
morbid/o-	combining form	disease
morb/o-	combining form	disease
morph/o-	combining form	shape
mort/o-	combining form	death
mot/o-	combining form	movement
-motor	suffix	thing that produces movement
muc/o-	combining form	mucus
mucos/o-	combining form	mucous membrane
mult/i-	combining form	many
muscul/o-	combining form	muscle
mutat/o-	combining form	to change
myc/o-	combining form	fungus
mydr/o-	combining form	widening
myelin/o-	combining form	myelin
myel/o-	combining form	bone marrow; spinal cord; myelin
myring/o-	combining form	tympanic membrane (eardrum)
my/o-	combining form	muscle
myos/o-	combining form	muscle
myx/o-	combining form	mucus-like substance

N

narc/o-	combining form	stupor, sleep
nas/o-	combining form	nose
-nate	suffix	born
nat/o-	combining form	birth
nause/o-	combining form	nausea
necr/o-	combining form	death
ne/o-	combining form	new
nephr/o-	combining form	kidney; nephron
nerv/o-	combining form	nerve
neur/o-	combining form	nerve
neutr/o-	combining form	not taking part
nid/o-	combining form	nest; focus
-nine	suffix	pertaining to a single chemical substance
noct/o-	combining form	night
nod/o-	combining form	node (knob of tissue)
nodul/o-	combining form	small knobby mass
non-	prefix	not
norm/o-	combining form	normal, usual
nuch/o-	combining form	neck; nape of neck
nucle/o-	combining form	nucleus (of a cell or an atom)
nucleol/o-	combining form	nucleolus
null/i-	prefix	none
nutri/o-	combining form	nourishment
nutriti/o-	combining form	nourishment

O

obes/o-	combining form	fat
obsess/o-	combining form	besieged by thoughts
obstetr/o-	combining form	pregnancy and childbirth
obstip/o-	combining form	severe constipation
obstruct/o-	combining form	blocked by a barrier
occipit/o-	combining form	occiput (back of the head)
occlus/o-	combining form	close against
ocul/o-	combining form	eye
odont/o-	combining form	tooth
odyn/o-	combining form	pain
-oid	suffix	resembling
-ol	suffix	chemical substance
olfact/o-	combining form	the sense of smell
olig/o-	combining form	scanty
-olisthesis	suffix	abnormal condition and process of slipping
-oma	suffix	tumor, mass
-omatosis	suffix	abnormal condition of multiple tumors or masses

oment/o-	combining form	omentum
om/o-	combining form	tumor, mass
omphal/o-	combining form	umbilicus, navel
-on	suffix	substance; structure
onc/o-	combining form	tumor, mass
-one	suffix	chemical substance
onych/o-	combining form	nail
o/o-	combining form	ovum (egg)
oophor/o-	combining form	ovary
operat/o-	combining form	perform a procedure; surgery
ophid/o-	combining form	snake
ophthalm/o-	combining form	eye
-opia	suffix	condition of vision
opportun/o-	combining form	well timed, taking advantage of an opportunity
oppos/o-	combining form	forceful resistance
-opsy	suffix	process of viewing
optic/o-	combining form	lenses; properties of light
opt/o-	combining form	eye; vision
-or	suffix	person or thing that produces or does
orbicul/o-	combining form	small circle
orbit/o-	combining form	orbit (eye socket)
orchi/o-	combining form	testis
orch/o-	combining form	testis
orex/o-	combining form	appetite
organ/o-	combining form	organ
or/o-	combining form	mouth
orth/o-	combining form	straight
-ory	suffix	having the function of
-ose	suffix	full of
-osing	suffix	a condition of doing
-osis	suffix	condition; abnormal condition; process
osm/o-	combining form	the sense of smell
osse/o-	combining form	bone
ossicul/o-	combining form	ossicle (little bone)
ossificat/o-	combining form	changing into bone
oste/o-	combining form	bone
ot/o-	combining form	ear
oure/o-	combining form	urine
-ous	suffix	pertaining to
ovari/o-	combining form	ovary
ov/i-	combining form	ovum (egg)
ov/o-	combining form	ovum (egg)
ovul/o-	combining form	ovum (egg)
ox/i-	combining form	oxygen
ox/o-	combining form	oxygen
ox/y-	combining form	oxygen; quick

P

palat/o-	combining form	palate
palliat/o-	combining form	reduce the severity of
palpat/o-	combining form	touching, feeling
palpit/o-	combining form	to throb
pan-	prefix	all
pancreat/o-	combining form	pancreas
papill/o-	combining form	elevated structure
par-	prefix	beside
para-	prefix	beside, apart from; two parts of a pair; abnormal
parenchym/o-	combining form	parenchyma (functional cells of an organ
-paresis	suffix	weakness
pareun/o-	combining form	sexual intercourse
pariet/o-	combining form	wall of a cavity
par/o-	combining form	birth
paroxysm/o-	combining form	sudden, sharp attack
part/o-	combining form	childbirth
-partum	suffix	childbirth
parurit/o-	combining form	to be in labor
patell/o-	combining form	patella (kneecap)
pat/o-	combining form	to lie open
-path	suffix	disease, suffering
pathet/o-	combining form	suffering
path/o-	combining form	disease, suffering
-pathy	suffix	disease, suffering
-pause	suffix	cessation
paus/o-	combining form	cessation
pect/o-	combining form	stiff
pector/o-	combining form	chest
pedicul/o-	combining form	lice
ped/o-	combining form	child
pelv/i-	combining form	pelvis (hip bone; renal pelvis)
pelv/o-	combining form	pelvis (hip bone; renal pelvis)
pendul/o-	combining form	hanging down
-penia	suffix	condition of deficiency
pen/o-	combining form	penis
pepsin/o-	combining form	pepsin
peps/o-	combining form	digestion
peptid/o-	combining form	peptide (two amino acids)
pept/o-	combining form	digestion
per-	prefix	through, throughout
percuss/o-	combining form	tapping
perfor/o-	combining form	to have an opening
peri-	prefix	around
perine/o-	combining form	perineum
peripher/o-	combining form	outer aspects
peritone/o-	combining form	peritoneum

periton/o-	combining form	peritoneum
perone/o-	combining form	fibula (lower leg bone)
person/o-	combining form	person
petechi/o-	combining form	petechiae
-pexy	suffix	process of surgically fixing in place
phac/o-	combining form	lens of the eye
-phage	suffix	thing that eats
phag/o-	combining form	eating, swallowing
phak/o-	combining form	lens of the eye
phalang/o-	combining form	phalanx (finger or toe)
pharmaceutic/o-	combining form	medicine, drug
pharmac/o-	combining form	medicine, drug
pharyng/o-	combining form	pharynx (throat)
-pharynx	suffix	pharynx (throat)
phas/o-	combining form	speech
phe/o-	combining form	gray
-phil	suffix	attraction to, fondness for
-phile	suffix	person who is attracted to or fond of
phil/o-	combining form	attraction to, fondness for
phleb/o-	combining form	vein
phob/o-	combining form	fear or avoidance
phor/o-	combining form	to bear, to carry
phor/o-	combining form	range
phosph/o-	combining form	phosphorus
phot/o-	combining form	light
phren/o-	combining form	diaphragm; mind
phylact/o-	combining form	guarding or protecting
-phylaxis	suffix	condition of guarding or protecting
-phyma	combining form	tumor, growth
physic/o-	combining form	body
physi/o-	combining form	physical function
-physis	suffix	state of growing
phys/o-	combining form	inflate or distend; grow
-phyte	suffix	growth
pigment/o-	combining form	pigment
pil/o-	combining form	hair
pituitar/o-	combining form	pituitary gland
pituit/o-	combining form	pituitary gland
placent/o-	combining form	placenta
plak/o-	combining form	plaque
-plasm	suffix	growth; formed substance
plasm/o-	combining form	plasma; formed substance
-plant	suffix	procedure to transfer or graft
plas/o-	combining form	growth, formation
plast/o-	combining form	growth, formation
-plasty	suffix	process of reshaping by surgery
-plegia	suffix	condition of paralysis
pleg/o-	combining form	paralysis
pleur/o-	combining form	pleura (lung membrane)
-plex	suffix	parts
-pnea	suffix	breathing
pne/o-	combining form	breathing
pneum/o-	combining form	lung; air
pneumon/o-	combining form	lung; air
pod/o-	combining form	foot
-poiesis	suffix	condition of formation
-poietin	suffix	a substance that forms
poikil/o-	combining form	irregular
pol/o-	combining form	pole
polar/o-	combining form	two opposite poles
poly-	prefix	many, much
polyp/o-	combining form	polyp
poplite/o-	combining form	back of the knee
por/o-	combining form	small openings; pores
port/o-	combining form	point of entry
post-	prefix	after, behind
poster/o-	combining form	back part
potent/o-	combining form	being capable of doing
pract/o-	combining form	medical practice
pre-	prefix	before; in front of
pregn/o-	combining form	being with child
presby/o-	combining form	old age
press/o-	combining form	pressure
prevent/o-	combining form	prevent
preventat/o-	combining form	prevent
prim/i-	combining form	first
pro-	prefix	before
-probe	suffix	rodlike instrument
proct/o-	combining form	rectum and anus
product/o-	combining form	produce
project/o-	combining form	throw forward
pronat/o-	combining form	lying face down
prostat/o-	combining form	prostate gland
prosthet/o-	combining form	artificial part
protein/o-	combining form	protein
prote/o-	combining form	protein
proxim/o-	combining form	near the center or point of origin
prurit/o-	combining form	itching
psor/o-	combining form	itching
psych/o-	combining form	mind
-ptosis	suffix	state of prolapse or drooping; falling
-ptysis	suffix	abnormal condition of coughing up
puber/o-	combining form	growing up

pub/o-	combining form	pubis (hip bone)
pulmon/o-	combining form	lung
pulsat/o-	combining form	rhythmic throbbing
punct/o-	combining form	hole, perforation
pupill/o-	combining form	pupil of the eye
purul/o-	combining form	pus
pyel/o-	combining form	renal pelvis
pylor/o-	combining form	pylorus
py/o-	combining form	pus
pyret/o-	combining form	fever
pyr/o-	combining form	fire; burning

Q

quadri-	prefix	four
quantitat/o-	combining form	quantity or amount

R

radic/o-	combining form	all parts including the root
radicul/o-	combining form	spinal nerve root
radi/o-	combining form	radius (forearm bone); x-rays; radiation
rap/o-	combining form	to seize and drag away
re-	prefix	again and again; backward; unable to
react/o-	combining form	reverse movement
recept/o-	combining form	receive
recess/o-	combining form	to move back
rect/o-	combining form	rectum
recuper/o-	combining form	recover
reduct/o-	combining form	to bring back; decrease
refract/o-	combining form	bend or deflect
regurgitat/o-	combining form	flow backward
relax/o-	combining form	relax
remiss/o-	combining form	send back
ren/o-	combining form	kidney
repress/o-	combining form	press back
resect/o-	combining form	to cut out and remove
resist/o-	combining form	withstand the effect of
resuscit/o-	combining form	revive or raise up again
retard/o-	combining form	to slow down or delay
retent/o-	combining form	keep, hold back
reticul/o-	combining form	small network
retin/o-	combining form	retina (of the eye)
retro-	prefix	behind, backward
rex/o-		see *orex/o-*
rhabd/o-	combining form	rod shaped
rheumat/o-	combining form	watery discharge
rhin/o-	combining form	nose
rhiz/o-	combining form	spinal nerve root
rhytid/o-	combining form	wrinkle
rib/o-	combining form	ribonucleic acid
roentgen/o-	combining form	x-ray; radiation
rotat/o-	combining form	rotate
-rrhage	suffix	excessive flow or discharge
rrhag/o-	combining form	excessive flow or discharge
-rrhaphy	suffix	procedure of suturing
-rrhea	suffix	flow, discharge
rrhe/o-	combining form	flow, discharge
rrhythm/o-	combining form	rhythm
-rubin	suffix	red substance
rub/o-	combining form	red
rug/o-	combining form	ruga (fold)

S

sacchar/o-	combining form	sugar
sacr/o-	combining form	sacrum
sagitt/o-	combining form	going from front to back
saliv/o-	combining form	saliva
salping/o-	combining form	fallopian tube
-salpinx	suffix	fallopian tube
saphen/o-	combining form	standing
sarc/o-	combining form	connective tissue
satur/o-	combining form	filled up
scal/o-	combining form	series of graduated steps
scaph/o-	combining form	boat shaped
scapul/o-	combining form	scapula (shoulder blade)
schiz/o-	combining form	split
scient/o-	combining form	science; knowledge
scint/i-	combining form	point of light
scintill/o-	combining form	point of light
scler/o-	combining form	hard; sclera (white of the eye)
scoli/o-	combining form	curved, crooked
-scope	suffix	instrument used to examine
scop/o-	combining form	examine with an instrument
-scopy	suffix	process of using an instrument to examine
scot/o-	combining form	darkness
script/o-	combining form	write
scrot/o-	combining form	a bag; scrotum
sebace/o-	combining form	sebum (oil)
seb/o-	combining form	sebum (oil)
secret/o-	combining form	produce; secrete
sect/o-	combining form	to cut
sedat/o-	combining form	to calm agitation
semi-	prefix	half; partly

semin/i-	combining form	spermatozoon; sperm
semin/o-	combining form	spermatozoon; semen
sen/o-	combining form	old age
sensitiv/o-	combining form	affected by, sensitive to
sensit/o-	combining form	affected by , sensitive to
sens/o-	combining form	sensation
sensor/i-	combining form	sensory
septic/o-	combining form	infection
sept/o-	combining form	septum (dividing wall)
ser/o-	combining form	serum of the blood; serumlike fluid
sex/o-	combining form	sex
sial/o-	combining form	saliva; salivary gland
sigmoid/o-	combining form	sigmoid colon
sin/o-	combining form	hollow cavity; channel
sinus/o-	combining form	sinus
-sis	combining form	condition; abnormal condition
skelet/o-	combining form	skeleton
soci/o-	combining form	human beings; community
somat/o-	combining form	body
-some	suffix	a body
somn/o-	combining form	sleep
som/o-	combining form	a body
son/o-	combining form	sound
sorb/o-	combining form	to suck up
-spasm	suffix	sudden, involuntary muscle contraction
spasm/o-	combining form	spasm
spasmod/o-	combining form	spasm
spast/o-	combining form	spasm
spermat/o-	combining form	spermatozoon; sperm
sperm/o-	combining form	spermatozoon; sperm
sphen/o-	combining form	wedge shape
sphenoid/o-	combining form	sphenoid bone or sinus
-sphere	suffix	sphere or ball
spher/o-	combining form	sphere or ball
sphincter/o-	combining form	sphincter
sphygm/o-	combining form	pulse
spin/o-	combining form	spine; backbone
spir/o-	combining form	breathe
spir/o-	combining form	a coil
splen/o-	combining form	spleen
spondyl/o-	combining form	vertebra
squam/o-	combining form	scalelike cell
stal/o-	combining form	contraction
-stalsis	suffix	process of contraction
staped/o-	combining form	stapes (stirrup-shaped bone)
-stasis	suffix	condition of standing still; staying in one place
stas/o-	combining form	standing still; staying in one place
stat/o-	combining form	standing still; staying in one place
steat/o-	combining form	fat
sten/o-	combining form	narrowness, constriction
stere/o-	combining form	three dimensions
stern/o-	combining form	sternum (breast bone)
-steroid	suffix	steroid
steroid/o-	combining form	steroid
-sterol	suffix	lipid-containing compound
steth/o-	combining form	chest
sthen/o-	combining form	strength
stigmat/o-	combining form	point, mark
stimul/o-	combining form	exciting, strengthening
stom/o-	combining form	surgically created opening or mouth
stomat/o-	combining form	mouth
-stomy	suffix	surgically created opening
strangul/o-	combining form	to constrict
strept/o-	combining form	curved
stress/o-	combining form	disturbing stimulus
styl/o-	combining form	stake
sub-	prefix	below; underneath; less than
sucr/o-	combining form	sugar (cane sugar)
suct/o-	combining form	to suck
sudor/i-	combining form	sweat
su/i-	combining form	self
super-	prefix	above, beyond
superfici/o-	combining form	on or near the surface
super/o-	combining form	above
supinat/o-	combining form	lying on the back
supposit/o-	combining form	placed beneath
suppress/o-	combining form	press down
suppur/o-	combining form	pus formation
supra-	prefix	above
surg/o-	combining form	operative procedure
suspens/o-	combining form	hanging
sym-	prefix	together, with
symptomat/o-	combining form	collection of symptoms
syn-	prefix	together
syncop/o-	combining form	fainting
synovi/o-	combining form	synovium (membrane)
synov/o-	combining form	synovium (membrane)
system/o-	combining form	the body as a whole
-systole	suffix	contracting
systol/o-	combining form	contracting

T

tachy-	prefix	fast
tact/o-	combining form	touch
tampon/o-	combining form	stop up
tard/o-	combining form	late, slow
tars/o-	combining form	ankle
tax/o-	combining form	coordination
techn/o-	combining form	technical skill
tele/o-	combining form	distance
tempor/o-	combining form	temple (side of the head)
tendin/o-	combining form	tendon
tendon/o-	combining form	tendon
ten/o-	combining form	tendon
tens/o-	combining form	pressure, tension
terat/o-	combining form	bizarre form
termin/o-	combining form	end; boundary
testicul/o-	combining form	testis; testicle
tetr/a-	combining form	four
thalam/o-	combining form	thalamus
thanat/o-	combining form	death
thec/o-	combining form	sheath or layers of membranes
theli/o-	combining form	cellular layer
therapeut/o-	combining form	treatment
therap/o-	combining form	treatment
-therapy	suffix	treatment
therm/o-	combining form	heat
thorac/o-	combining form	thorax (chest)
-thorax	suffix	thorax (chest)
thromb/o-	combining form	thrombus (blood clot)
thym/o-	combining form	thymus; rage
thyr/o-	combining form	shield-shaped structure (thyroid gland)
thyroid/o-	combining form	thyroid gland
tibi/o-	combining form	tibia (shin bone)
-tic	suffix	pertaining to
till/o-	combining form	to pull out
-tion	suffix	a process; being or having
toc/o-	combining form	labor and childbirth
toler/o-	combining form	to become accustomed to
-tome	suffix	instrument used to cut; an area with distinct edges
tom/o-	combining form	a cut, slice, or layer
-tomy	suffix	process of cutting or making an incision
ton/o-	combining form	pressure; tone
tonsill/o-	combining form	tonsil
-tope	suffix	place, position
topic/o-	combining form	a specific area
tort/i-	combining form	twisted position
-tous	suffix	pertaining to
toxic/o-	combining form	poison, toxin
tox/o-	combining form	poison
trabecul/o-	combining form	trabecula (mesh)
trache/o-	combining form	trachea (windpipe)
trac/o-	combining form	visible path
tract/o-	combining form	pulling
tranquil/o-	combining form	calm
trans-	prefix	across, through
transit/o-	combining form	changing over from one thing to another
transplant/o-	combining form	move something to another place
traumat/o-	combining form	injury
tremul/o-	combining form	shaking
-tresia	suffix	opening or hole
tri-	prefix	three
trich/o-	combining form	hair
trigemin/o-	combining form	threefold
triglycerid/o-	combining form	triglyceride
-tripsy	suffix	the process of crushing
-triptor	suffix	thing that crushes
trochanter/o-	combining form	trochanter
trochle/o-	combining form	structure shaped like a pulley
-tron	suffix	instrument
troph/o-	combining form	development
-trophy	suffix	process of development
trop/o-	combining form	having an affinity for; stimulating; turning
tubercul/o-	combining form	nodule; tuberculosis
tuber/o-	combining form	nodule
tuberos/o-	combining form	knoblike projection
tub/o-	combining form	tube
tubul/o-	combining form	tube, small tube
turbin/o-	combining form	scroll-like structure; turbinate
tuss/o-	combining form	cough
-ty	suffix	quality or state
tympan/o-	combining form	tympanic membrane (eardrum)
-type	suffix	particular kind of; a model of

U

-ual	suffix	pertaining to
-ula	suffix	small thing
-ular	suffix	pertaining to something small
ulcerat/o-	combining form	ulcer
-ule	suffix	small thing

uln/o-	combining form	ulna (forearm bone)
ultra-	prefix	beyond; higher
-um	suffix	a structure
umbilic/o-	combining form	umbilicus, navel
un-	prefix	not
ungu/o-	combining form	nail
uni-	prefix	single, not paired
-ure	suffix	system; result of
ureter/o-	combining form	ureter
urethr/o-	combining form	urethra
urin/o-	combining form	urine; urinary system
ur/o-	combining form	urine; urinary system
uter/o-	combining form	uterus (womb)
uve/o-	combining form	uvea of the eye

V

vaccin/o-	combining form	giving a vaccine
vagin/o-	combining form	vagina
vag/o-	combining form	vagus nerve
valv/o-	combining form	valve
valvul/o-	combining form	valve
varic/o-	combining form	varix; varicose vein
vascul/o-	combining form	blood vessel
vas/o-	combining form	blood vessel; vas deferens
veget/o-	combining form	vegetable
vegetat/o-	combining form	growth
venere/o-	combining form	sexual intercourse
ven/i-	combining form	vein
ven/o-	combining form	vein
ventil/o-	combining form	movement of air
vent/o-	combining form	a coming
ventricul/o-	combining form	ventricle (lower heart chamber; chamber in the brain)
ventr/o-	combining form	front; abdomen
verd/o-	combining form	green
-verse	suffix	to travel; to turn
vers/o-	combining form	to travel; to turn
vertebr/o-	combining form	vertebra
vert/o-	combining form	to travel; to turn
vesic/o-	combining form	bladder; fluid-filled sac
vesicul/o-	combining form	bladder; fluid-filled sac
vestibul/o-	combining form	vestibule (entrance)
vest/o-	combining form	to dress
viril/o-	combining form	masculine
vir/o-	combining form	virus
viscer/o-	combining form	viscera (internal organs)
viscos/o-	combining form	thickness
vis/o-	combining form	sight; vision
vitre/o-	combining form	vitreous humor; transparent substance
voc/o-	combining form	voice
volunt/o-	combining form	done by one's own free will
vuls/o-	combining from	to tear away
vulv/o-	combining form	vulva

X

xanth/o-	combining form	yellow
xen/o-	combining form	foreign
xer/o-	combining form	dry
xiph/o-	combining form	sword

Z

-zoon	suffix	animal; living thing
zygomat/o-	combining form	zygoma (cheek bone)

Appendix B

Abbreviations Glossary

A

5-HIAA	5-hydroxyindoleacetic acid
A fib	atrial fibrillation
A	a blood type in the ABO blood group; assessment (heading in a SOAP note)
A&P	anatomy and physiology; auscultation and percussion
AAA	abdominal aortic aneurysm
AB	a blood type in the ABO blood group
AB, Ab	abortion
ABD	abdomen
ABG	arterial blood gases
ABR	auditory brainstem response
ACE	angiotensin-converting enzyme (inhibitor)
ACS	acute coronary syndrome
ACTH	adrenocorticotropic hormone
AD, A.D.	auris dextra (right ear)
ADA	American Diabetes Association; American Dietetic Association; Americans with Disabilities Act
ADD	attention deficit disorder
ADH	antidiuretic hormone
ADHD	attention deficit hyperactivity disorder
ADLs	activities of daily living
AED	automatic external defibrillator
AFB	acid-fast bacillus
AFP	alpha fetoprotein
AGA	appropriate for gestational age
AI	aortic insufficiency
AICD	automatic implantable cardioverter-defibrillator
AIDS	acquired immunodeficiency syndrome
AKA	above-the-knee amputation
ALL	acute lymphocytic leukemia
ALS	amyotrophic lateral sclerosis
ALT	alanine aminotransferase
AMI	acute myocardial infarction
AML	acute myelogenous leukemia
AP	anteroposterior
ARDS	adult respiratory distress syndrome; acute respiratory distress syndrome
ARF	acute renal failure
ARMD	age-related macular degeneration
AS	aortic stenosis
AS, A.S.	auris sinister (left ear)
ASC	ambulatory surgery center
ASC-H	atypical squamous cells, cannot exclude HSIL
ASC-US	atypical squamous cells of undetermined significance
ASCVD	arteriosclerotic cardiovascular disease
ASD	atrial septal defect
ASHD	arteriosclerotic heart disease
ASIS	anterior-superior iliac spine
AST	aspartate aminotransferase
AU, A.U.	auris uterque (both ears)
AV	atrioventricular
AVM	arteriovenous malformation

B

B	a blood type in the ABO blood group
Ba	barium
BAEP	brainstem auditory evoked potential
BAER	brainstem auditory evoked response
bagged	manually ventilated with an Ambu bag (slang)
basos	basophils (slang)
BBT	basal body temperature
BDI	Beck Depression Inventory
BE	barium enema
BKA	below-the-knee amputation
BM	bowel movement
BMD	bone mineral density
BMT	bone marrow transplantation
BOM	bilateral otitis media
BP	blood pressure
BPD	biparietal diameter (of fetal head)
BPH	benign prostatic hypertrophy
BPM, bpm	beats per minute
BPP	biophysical profile
BRBPR	bright red blood per rectum
BRCA	breast cancer (gene)
BS	bowel sounds; breath sounds
BSE	breast self-examination
BSO	bilateral salpingo-oophorectomy
BUN	blood urea nitrogen
Bx	biopsy

C

C&S	culture and sensitivity
C1–C7	cervical vertebrae
Ca	cancer, carcinoma
Ca, Ca^{++}	calcium
CABG	coronary artery bypass graft
CAD	coronary artery disease
CAPD	continuous ambulatory peritoneal dialysis
CAT	computerized axial tomography
cath	catheterize or catheterization (slang)
CBC	complete blood count
CBD	common bile duct
CBT	cognitive behavioral therapy
CC	chief complaint
cc	cubic centimeter (measure of volume)
CCPD	continuous cycling peritoneal dialysis
CCU	coronary care unit
CDCP	Centers for Disease Control and Prevention
CDE	certified diabetes educator
CDH	congenital dislocation of the hip
CEA	carcinoembryonic antigen
CF	cystic fibrosis
chemo	chemotherapy (slang)
CHF	congestive heart failure
CIN	cervical intraepithelial neoplasia (grading system on Pap smear)
CIS	carcinoma in situ
CK	conductive keratoplasty
CK-MB	creatine kinase-M band
CLL	chronic lymphocytic leukemia
CML	chronic myelogenous leukemia
cmm	cubic millimeter
CNM	certified nurse midwife
CNS	central nervous system
CO	carbon monoxide
CO_2	carbon dioxide
COMT	catechol-*O*-methyltransferase
COPD	chronic obstructive pulmonary disease
COTA	certified occupational therapy assistant
CP	cerebral palsy
CPAP	continuous positive airway pressure
CPD	cephalopelvic disproportion
CPK-MB	creatine phosphokinase-M band
CPK-MM	creatine phosphokinase (MM bands)
CPR	cardiopulmonary resuscitation; computerized patient record
CRF	chronic renal failure
CRNA	certified registered nurse anesthetist
CRP	C-reactive protein
CRPS	chronic regional pain syndrome
CRT	certified radiation therapist
CS	cesarean section ("C-section")
CSF	cerebrospinal fluid
CT	computerized tomography
CTD	cumulative trauma disorder
CTR	certified tumor registrar
CTS	carpal tunnel syndrome
CV	cardiovascular
CVA	cerebrovascular accident
CVS	chorionic villus sampling
CXR	chest x-ray
cysto	cystoscopy (slang)

D

D&C	dilation and curettage
dB, db	decibel
D.C.	Doctor of Chiropractic
D.D.S.	Doctor of Dental Surgery
Derm	dermatology (slang)
DEXA, DXA	dual energy x-ray absorptiometry
DI	diabetes insipidus
DIC	disseminated intravascular coagulation
diff	differential count of WBCs (slang)
DIP	distal interphalangeal (joint)
DJD	degenerative joint disease
DKA	diabetic ketoacidosis
DM	diabetes mellitus
DNA	deoxyribonucleic acid
D.O.	Doctor of Osteopathy
DOE	dyspnea on exertion
D.P.M.	Doctor of Podiatric Medicine
Dr.	doctor
DRE	digital rectal examination
DS	discharge summary
DSA	digital subtraction angiography
DT	delirium tremens
DTRs	deep tendon reflexes
DUB	dysfunctional uterine bleeding
Dx	diagnosis

E

EAC	external auditory canal
EBT	electron beam tomography

EBV	Epstein-Barr virus
ECCE	extracapsular cataract extraction
ECG	electrocardiography
echo	echocardiogram (slang)
ECT	electroconvulsive therapy
ED	emergency department; erectile dysfunction
EDB	estimated date of birth
EDC	estimated date of confinement
EEG	electroencephalography
EGA	estimated gestational age
EGD	esophagogastroduodenoscopy
EHR	electronic health record
EKG	electrocardiography
ELISA	enzyme-linked immunosorbent assay
EMB	endometrial biopsy
EMG	electromyography
END	electroneurodiagnostic (technician)
ENT	ears, nose, and throat
EOM	extraocular movements
EOMI	extraocular muscles intact
eos	eosinophils (slang)
epi	epithelial cells (in the urine specimen) (slang)
EPR	electronic patient record
ER	estrogen receptor
ERCP	endoscopic retrograde cholangiopancreatography
ESRD	end-stage renal disease
ESWL	extracorporeal shock wave lithotripsy
ESWT	extracorporeal shock wave therapy
ETOH	alcohol (liquor)
ETT	endotracheal tube

F

FBS	fasting blood sugar
FEV_1	forced expiratory volume (in one second)
FHR	fetal heart rate
fib	fibula (slang)
FIGO	Federation Internationale de Gynécologie et Obstétrique
FiO_2	fraction (percentage) of inspired oxygen
FSH	follicle-stimulating hormone
FTI	free thyroxine index
FVC	forced vital capacity
Fx	fracture

G

G	gravida
G/TPAL	see *G* and *TPAL*
GC	gonococcus (*Neisseria gonorrhoeae*)
GCS	Glasgow Coma Scale (or Score)
G-CSF	granulocyte colony-stimulating factor
GERD	gastroesophageal reflux disease
GH	growth hormone
GI	gastrointestinal
GIFT	gamete intrafallopian transfer
GM-CSF	granulocyte-macrophage colony-stimulating-factor
GTT	glucose tolerance test
GU	genitourinary; gonococcal urethritis
GVHD	graft-versus-host disease
GYN	gynecology

H

H&H	hemoglobin and hematocrit
H&P	history and physical examination
HAV	hepatitis A virus
HbA_{1C}	hemoglobin A_{1C}
HBV	hepatitis B virus
HCG, hCG	human chorionic gonadotropin
HCT	hematocrit
HCV	hepatitis C virus
HDL	high-density lipoprotein
HEENT	head, eyes, ears, nose, and throat
Hgb	hemoglobin
HIPAA	Health Insurance Portability and Accountability Act
HIV	human immunodeficiency virus
HLA	human leukocyte antigen
HMD	hyaline membrane disease
HNP	herniated nucleus pulposus
hpf	high-power field
HPI	history of present illness
HPV	human papillomavirus
HRT	hormone replacement therapy
HSG	hysterosalpingography
HSIL	high-grade squamous intraepithelial lesion
HSV	herpes simplex virus
HTN	hypertension
Hx	history
Hz	hertz

I

I&D	incision and drainage
I&O	intake and output
IBD	inflammatory bowel disease
IBS	irritable bowel syndrome
ICCE	intracapsular cataract extraction
ICP	intracranial pressure
ICSI	intracytoplasmic sperm injection
IDDM	insulin-dependent diabetes mellitus
IgA	immunoglobulin A
IgD	immunoglobulin D
IgE	immunoglobulin E
IgG	immunoglobulin G
IgM	immunoglobulin M
IM	intramuscular
IOL	intraocular lens
IOP	intraocular pressure
IRS	insulin resistance syndrome
IUGR	intrauterine growth retardation
IVC	intravenous cholangiography
IVF	*in vitro* fertilization
IVP	intravenous pyelogram; intravenous pyelography

J

JVD	jugular venous distention

K

K, K^+	potassium
KUB	kidneys, ureters, bladder

L

L&D	labor and delivery
L/S	lecithin/sphingomyelin (ratio)
L1–L5	lumbar vertebrae
LA	left atriuim
LASIK	laser-assisted *in situ* keratomileusis
Lat	lateral
LBBB	left bundle branch block
LDH	lactic dehydrogenase
LDL	low-density lipoprotein
LEEP	loop electrocautery excision procedure
LES	lower esophageal sphincter
LFTs	liver function tests
LGA	large for gestational age
LH	luteinizing hormone
LLE	left lower extremity
LLL	left lower lobe (of the lung)
LLQ	left lower quadrant
LMP	last menstrual period
LP	lumbar puncture
LPN	licensed practical nurse
LSD	lysergic acid diethylamide (a street drug)
LSIL	low-grade squamous intraepithelial lesion
LTK	laser thermal keratoplasty
LUE	left upper extremity
LUL	left upper lobe (of the lung)
LUQ	left upper quadrant
LV	left ventricle
LVAD	left ventricular assist device
LVH	left ventricular hypertrophy
lymphs	lymphocytes (slang)

M

MAO	monoamine oxidase (inhibitor drug)
MCH	mean cell hemoglobin
MCHC	mean cell hemoglobin concentration
MCP	metacarpophalangeal (joint)
MCV	mean cell volume
M.D.	Doctor of Medicine
MD	muscular dystrophy
MDI	metered-dose inhaler
mets	metastases (slang)
MI	myocardial infarction
mL	milliliter (measure of volume)
mm Hg	millimeters of mercury
mm^3	cubic millimeter
mono	mononucleosis (slang)
monos	monocytes (slang)
MR	mitral regurgitation
MRA	magnetic resonance angiography
MRI	magnetic resonance imaging
MS	multiple sclerosis
MSH	melanocyte-stimulating hormone
MUGA	multiple-gated acquisition (scan)
MVP	mitral valve prolapse

N

N&V	nausea and vomiting
Na, Na^+	sodium
NB	newborn
NG	nasogastric
NICU	neonatal intensive care unit; neurologic intensive care unit
NIDDM	non–insulin-dependent diabetes mellitus
NK	natural killer (cells)
NP	nurse practitioner
NPH	neutral protamine Hagedorn (type of insulin)
NPO (n.p.o.)	nothing by mouth (nil per os)
NSAID	nonsteroidal anti-inflammatory drug
NSR	normal sinus rhythm
NST	nonstress test
NSVD	normal spontaneous vaginal delivery

O

O	a blood type in the ABO blood group; objective (heading in a SOAP note)
O&P	ova and parasites
O_2	oxygen
OA	osteoarthritis
OB	obstetrics
OCD	obsessive-compulsive disorder
OCG	oral cholecystography
OCP	oral contraceptive pill
OD	overdose
OD, O.D.	right eye (oculus dexter)
O.D.	Doctor of Optometry
OGTT	oral glucose tolerance test
OOB	out of bed
ortho	orthopedics (slang)
OS, O.S.	left eye (oculus sinister)
OSHA	Occupational Safety and Health Administration
OT	occupational therapy/therapist
OU, O.U.	both eyes (oculus uterque)

P

P	para; phosphorus; plan (heading in a SOAP note); pulse
P.O. (p.o.)	by mouth (per os)
PA	physician's assistant; posteroanterior
PAC	premature atrial contraction
PAD	peripheral artery disease
Pap	Papanicolaou (smear or test)
PAP	prostatic acid phosphatase
PCO_2	partial pressure of carbon dioxide (also pCO_2)
PCP	phencyclidine (angel dust, a street drug); *Pneumocystis carinii* pneumonia; primary care physician
PD	prism diopter
PDA	patent ductus arteriosus
PDT	photodynamic therapy
PE	physical examination; polyethylene (tube)
PEG	percutaneous endoscopic gastrostomy
PEJ	percutaneous endoscopic jejunostomy
PERRL	pupils equal, round, and reactive to light
PERRLA	pupils equal, round, reactive to light and accommodation
PET	positron emission tomography
PFTs	pulmonary function tests
pH	potential of hydrogen (acidity or alkalinity)
Pharm.D.	Doctor of Pharmacy
PICC	peripherally inserted central catheter
PID	pelvic inflammatory disease
PIP	proximal interphalangeal (joint)
PM&R	physical medicine and rehabilitation
PMDD	premenstrual dysphoric disorder
PMI	point of maximum impulse
PMN	polymorphonucleated leukocytes
PMS	premenstrual syndrome
PND	paroxysmal noctural dyspnea; postnasal drip (or drainage)
PO_2	partial pressure of oxygen (also pO_2)
polys	polymorphonucleated leukocytes (slang)
PPD	protein purified derivative (TB test); packs per day (of cigarettes)
PR	progesterone receptor
PRBCs	packed red blood cells
PRK	photorefractive keratectomy
pro time	prothrombin time (slang)
PROM	premature rupture of membranes
PSA	prostate-specific antigen
Psy, Psych	psychiatry, psychology (slang)
PT	physical therapy/therapist
PT	prothrombin time
PTC	percutaneous transhepatic cholangiography
PTCA	percutaneous transluminal coronary angioplasty
PTSD	posttraumatic stress disorder
PTT	partial thromboplastin time
PUD	peptic ulcer disease
PUVA	psoralen drug and ultraviolet A light (therapy)

PVC	premature ventricular contraction
PVD	peripheral vascular disease

Q

QCT	quantitative computerized tomography

R

R, r	roentgen (unit of exposure to x-rays or gamma rays)
RA	rheumatoid arthritis; right atrium room air (no supplemental oxygen)
rad	radiation absorbed dose
RAIU	radioactive iodine uptake
RBBB	right bundle branch block
RBC	red blood cell
RDS	respiratory distress syndrome
rehab	rehabilitation (slang)
rem	roentgen-equivalent man
RFA	radiofrequency catheter ablation
RIA	radioimmunoassay
RIND	reversible ischemic neurological deficit
RLE	right lower extremity
RLL	right lower lobe (of the lung)
RLQ	right lower quadrant
RML	right middle lobe (of the lung)
RN	registered nurse
RNA	ribonucleic acid
RNV	radionuclide ventriculography
ROM	range of motion; rupture of membranes
ROP	retinopathy of prematurity
ROS	review of systems
RP	retinitis pigmentosa
RPR	rapid plasma reagin (test for syphilis)
RRT	registered radiologic technologist; registered respiratory therapist
RSI	repetitive strain injury
RUE	right upper extremity
RUL	right upper lobe (of the lung)
RUQ	right upper quadrant
RV	right ventricle

S

S	subjective (heading in a SOAP note)
S1	first sacral vertebra
S_1	first heart sound
S_2	second heart sound
S_3	third heart sound
S_4	fourth heart sound
SA	sinoatrial
SAB	spontaneous abortion
SAD	seasonal affective disorder
SARS	severe acute respiratory syndrome
SBE	subacute bacterial endocarditis
SCC	squamous cell carcinoma
SCI	spinal cord injury
segs	segmented neutrophils (slang)
SG, sp gr	specific gravity
SGA	small for gestational age
SGOT	serum glutamic-oxaloacetic transaminase
SGPT	serum glutamic-pyruvic transaminase
SIADH	syndrome of inappropriate ADH
SIDS	sudden infant death syndrome
SLE	systemic lupus erythematosus
SNF	skilled nursing facility
SOAP	subjective, objective, assessment, plan
SOB	shortness of breath
SOM	serous otitis media
SPECT	single photon emission computerized tomography
SQ, subcu, subQ	subcutaneous
SSEP	somatosensory evoked potential
SSER	somatosensory evoked response
SSRI	selective serotonin reuptake inhibitor
STD	sexually transmitted disease
SVT	supraventricular tachycardia
Sx	symptoms

T

T&A	tonsillectomy and adenoidectomy
T1–T12	thoracic vertebrae
T_3	triiodothyronine
T_4	thyroxine
T_7	free thyroxine index (FTI)
TAB	therapeutic abortion
TACE	transarterial chemoembolization
TAH-BSO	total abdominal hysterectomy and bilateral salpingo-oophorectomy
TAT	Thematic Apperception Test
TB	tuberculosis
TEE	transesophageal echocardiogram echocardiography
TENS	transcutaneous electrical nerve stimulation (unit)

TFTs	thyroid function tests
THR	total hip replacement
TIA	transient ischemic attack
tib	tibia (slang)
TM	tympanic membrane
TMJ	temporomandibular joint
TNF	tumor necrosis factor
TNM	tumor, nodes, metastases
TNTC	too numerous to count
TPA	tissue plasminogen activator (drug)
TPAL	term newborns, premature newborns, abortions, living children
TPR	temperature, pulse, and respiration
trach	tracheostomy (slang)
TRAM	transverse rectus abdominis muscle (flap)
TRUS	transrectal ultrasound
TSE	testicular self-examination
TSH	thyroid-stimulating hormone
TURBT	transurethral resection of bladder tumor
TURP	transurethral resection of the prostate
TVH	total vaginal hysterectomy
Tx	treatment

U

UA	urinalysis
UGI	upper gastrointestinal (GI) series
URI	upper respiratory infection
US	ultrasound
UTI	urinary tract infection

V

V fib	ventricular fibrillation
V tach	ventricular tachycardia
V/Q	ventilation-perfusion (scan)
VBAC	vaginal birth after ceserean section ("V-back")
VD	venereal disease
VDRL	Venereal Disease Research Laboratory (test for syphilis)
VEP	visual evoked potential
VER	visual evoked response
VF	visual field
VLDL	very low-density lipoprotein
VMA	vanillylmandelic acid
VSD	ventricular septal defect

W

WBC	white blood cell

Z

ZIFT	zygote intrafallopian transfer

Answer Key

Chapter 1 The Structure of Medical Language

COMBINING FORMS REVIEW (p. 8)

1. lung; air 2. appendix 3. joint 4. heart 5. skin 6. sensation, feeling 7. stomach 8. blood 9. liver 10. larynx (voice box) 11. breast; mastoid process 12. nose 13. birth 14. nerve 15. mind 16. retina (of the eye) 17. tonsil 18. trachea (windpipe) 19. urine; urinary system 20. vein

SUFFIXES REVIEW (p. 10)

1. pertaining to 2. pertaining to 3. pertaining to 4. pertaining to 5. a process; being or having 6. surgical excision 7. process of recording 8. condition, state, thing 9. medical treatment 10. a skilled professional or expert 11. action; condition 12. process; disease from a specific cause 13. inflammation of 14. the study of 15. enlargement 16. tumor, mass 17. condition; abnormal condition; process 18. pertaining to 19. disease, suffering 20. process of using an instrument to examine

BUILDING MEDICAL WORDS EXERCISE (p. 11)

1. hepatic 2. nasal 3. tonsillar 4. tracheal 5. cardiac 6. cutaneous 7. gastric 8. neural 9. urinary 10. retinal 11. venous 12. urination 13. pneumonia 14. appendicitis 15. laryngitis 16. hepatitis 17. gastritis 18. tonsillitis 19. mastitis 20. arthritis 21. hepatomegaly 22. hematoma 23. psychosis 24. retinopathy 25. neuropathy 26. appendectomy 27. mastectomy 28. tonsillectomy 29. laryngectomy 30. gastroscopy 31. arthroscopy 32. psychiatry 33. cardiology 34. hematology 35. neurology 36. psychology

ANALYZING AND DEFINING MEDICAL WORDS EXERCISE: COMBINING FORMS AND SUFFIXES (p. 12)

1.	Suffix	-itis	inflammation of
	Combining Form	laryng/o-	larynx (voice box)
	Medical Word Definition	Inflammation of the larynx	
2.	Suffix	-ac	pertaining to
	Combining Form	cardi/o-	heart
	Medical Word Definition	Pertaining to the heart	
3.	Suffix	-logy	the study of
	Combining Form	neur/o-	nerve
	Medical Word Definition	The study of the nerves	
4.	Suffix	-ectomy	surgical excision
	Combining Form	mast/o-	breast; mastoid process
	Medical Word Definition	Surgical excision of the breast	
5.	Suffix	-ar	pertaining to
	Combining Form	tonsill/o-	tonsil, tonsils
	Medical Word Definition	Pertaining to the tonsils	
6.	Suffix	-scopy	process of using an instrument to examine
	Combining Form	gastr/o-	stomach
	Medical Word Definition	The process of using an instrument to examine the stomach	
7.	Suffix	-oma	tumor, mass
	Combining Form	hemat/o-	blood
	Medical Word Definition	A mass of blood	
8.	Suffix	-ic	pertaining to
	Combining Form	hepat/o-	liver
	Medical Word Definition	Pertaining to the liver	
9.	Suffix	-logy	the study of
	Combining Form	psych/o-	mind
	Medical Word Definition	The study of the mind	
10.	Suffix	-ia	condition, state, thing
	Combining Form	pneumon/o-	lung
	Medical Word Definition	A condition of the lungs	
11.	Suffix	-ous	pertaining to
	Combining Form	ven/o-	vein
	Medical Word Definition	Pertaining to the veins	
12.	Suffix	-itis	inflammation of
	Combining Form	arthr/o-	joint
	Medical Word Definition	Inflammation of the joints	

PREFIXES REVIEW (p. 16)

1. without, not 2. against 3. slow 4. painful, difficult, abnormal 5. innermost, within 6. above; more than normal 7. below; deficient 8. within 9. around 10. many, much 11. after, behind 12. before; in front of 13. below; underneath; less than 14. fast

BUILDING MEDICAL WORDS EXERCISE (p. 17)

1. postnatal 2. peritonsillar 3. intranasal 4. anesthesia 5. antipsychotic 6. subcutaneous 7. tachycardia 8. polyneuropathy 9. endotracheal 10. intravenous

ANALYZING AND DEFINING MEDICAL WORDS: PREFIXES, COMBINING FORMS, AND SUFFIXES (p. 17)

1.	Suffix	-al	pertaining to
	Prefix	post-	after, behind
	Combining Form	nat/o-	birth
	Medical Word Definition	pertaining to after birth	
2.	Suffix	-ia	condition, state, thing
	Prefix	an-	without, not
	Combining Form	esthes/o-	sensation, feeling
	Medical Word Definition	condition of being without sensation or feeling	
3.	Suffix	-al	pertaining to
	Prefix	intra-	within
	Combining Form	nas/o-	nose
	Medical Word Definition	pertaining to within the nose	
4.	Suffix	-pathy	disease, suffering
	Prefix	poly-	many, much
	Combining Form	neur/o-	nerve
	Medical Word Definition	disease of many nerves	
5.	Suffix	-ar	pertaining to
	Prefix	peri-	around
	Combining Form	tonsil/o-	tonsil
	Medical Word Definition	pertaining to around the tonsils	
6.	Suffix	-ous	pertaining to
	Prefix	sub-	below; underneath; less than
	Combining Form	cutane/o-	skin
	Medical Word Definition	pertaining to beneath the skin	
7.	Suffix	-ia	condition, state, thing
	Prefix	tachy-	fast
	Combining Form	cardi/o-	heart
	Medical Word Definition	condition of a fast heart	
8.	Suffix	-ous	pertaining to
	Prefix	intra-	within
	Combining Form	ven/o-	vein
	Medical Word Definition	pertaining to within the vein	
9.	Suffix	-al	pertaining to
	Prefix	endo-	innermost, within
	Combining Form	trache/o-	trachea
	Medical Word Definition	pertaining to within the trachea	

CHAPTER REVIEW EXERCISES

Matching Exercise (p. 26)

2, 1, 1, 3, 2, 3, 1

Definition of Prefix Exercise (p. 26)

Definition	Prefix	Example
1. within	intra-	intranasal, intravenous
2. slow	brady-	bradycardia
3. without, not	an-	anesthesia
4. below, underneath	sub-	subcutaneous
5. many, much	poly-	polyneuropathy
6. against	anti-	antipsychotic
7. after, behind	post-	postnatal
8. innermost, within	endo-	endotracheal

True or False Exercise (p. 26)

1. F 2. F 3. F 4. T 5. F 6. T 7. F 8. T

Naming Exercise (pp. 26–27)

1. combining form, suffix, prefix 2. combining vowel 3. reading, listening, thinking and analyzing, speaking, writing

Singular and Plural Forms Exercise (p. 27)

1. atrium	atria
2. vertebra	vertebrae
3. nucleus	nuclei
4. bronchus	bronchi
5. diagnosis	diagnoses
6. scapula	scapulae

Word-Building Exercise (p. 27)

1. cardiology 2. appendectomy 3. gastroscopy 4. hepatoma 5. retinopathy 6. tonsillectomy 7. tonsillitis 8. hepatitis 9. neuropathy 10. appendicitis

Matching Exericse (p. 28)

4, 8, 12, 6, 5, 9, 2, 10, 1, 11, 3, 7

Circle Exercise (p. 28)

1. phalanx 2. testis 3. vertebrae 4. gastric 5. tonsillitis 6. bacteria 7. cardiac 8. appendectomy 9. urinary 10. anesthesia

Abbreviation Exercise (p. 28)

1. computerized patient record 2. discharge summary 3. subjective, objective, assessment, plan 4. history and physical examination 5. diagnosis 6. review of systems

Word Analysis Exercise (p. 29)

1.	Suffix	-scopy	process of using an instrument to examine
	Combining Form	gastr/o-	stomach
	Combining Form	duoden/o-	duodenum
	Medical Word Definition	The process of using an instrument to examine the stomach and duodenum	
2.	Suffix	-logy	the study of
	Combining Form	ot/o-	ear
	Combining Form	rhin/o-	nose
	Combining Form	laryng/o-	larynx (voice box)
	Medical Word Definition	The study of the ears, nose, and larynx	

Chapter 2 The Body in Health and Disease

LABELING EXERCISE (pp. 57–58)

Exercise A

1. anterior (ventral) 2. posterior (dorsal) 3. medial 4. lateral 5. proximal 6. distal

Exercise B

1. cranial cavity 2. spinal cavity 3. thoracic cavity 4. abdominal cavity 5. pelvic cavity

Exercise C

Fig. 2-20 1. cardiovascular system 2. cardiology
Fig. 2-21 1. integumentary system 2. dermatology
Fig. 2-22 1. urinary system 2. urology
Fig. 2-23 1. digestive system 2. gastroenterology

BUILDING MEDICAL WORDS

Combining Forms (p. 59)

1. back; dorsum 2. abdomen 3. before; front part 4. heart 5. tailbone; lower part of the body 6. hollow space 7. head 8. cartilage 9. encircling structure 10. cranium (skull) 11. secrete 12. tooth 13. skin 14. foods, diet 15. away from the center or point of origin 16. intestine 17. outside 18. front 19. stomach 20. genitalia 21. old age 22. female, woman 23. blood 24. boundary between the earth and sky 25. physician; medical treatment 26. ilium (hip bone) 27. immune response 28. below 29. groin 30. skin 31. inside 32. intestine 33. larynx (voice box) 34. side 35. lower back; area between the ribs and pelvis 36. lymph; lymphatic system 37. large 38. physician; medicine 39. middle 40. small 41. muscle 42. birth 43. new 44. nerve 45. nerve 46. nucleus 47. pregnancy and childbirth 48. tumor, mass 49. eye 50. straight 51. ear 52. child 53. pelvis (hip bone; renal pelvis) 54. medicine, drug 55. physical function 56. back part 57. produce 58. near the center or point of origin 59. mind 60. lung 61. radius (forearm); x-rays; radiation 62. going from front to back 63. examine with an instrument 64. skeleton 65. spine; backbone 66. breathe 67. on or near the surface 68. above 69. thorax (chest) 70. a cut, slice, or layer 71. umbilicus, navel 72. urine; urinary system 73. urine; urinary system 74. blood vessel 75. front; abdomen

Combining Forms and Suffixes (p. 60)

1. abdomino/-	-al	abdominal
2. physi/o-	-logy	physiology
3. lumb/o-	-ar	lumbar
4. cephal/o-	-ad	cephalad
5. dist/o-	-al	distal
6. thorac/o-	-ic	thoracic
7. crani/o-	-al	cranial
8. poster/o-	-ior	posterior
9. dermat/o-	-logy	dermatology
10. lymph/o-	-atic	lymphatic
11. later/o-	-al	lateral
12. intern/o-	-al	internal
13. cardi/o-	-logy	cardiology
14. obstetr/o-	-ics	obstetrics
15. ur/o-	-logy	urology
16. pulmon/o-	-logy	pulmonlogy
17. ophthalm/o-	-logy	ophthalmology
18. integument/o-	-ary	integumentary
19. gynec/o-	-logy	gynecology
20. psych/o-	-logy	psychology
21. nerv/o-	-ous	nervous
22. urin/o-	-ary	urinary
23. onc/o-	-logy	oncology

Combining Form and Prefixes (p. 61)

1. endo-	-crine	endocrine
2. ana-	tomical	anatomical
3. mid-	sagittal	midsagittal
4. hypo-	chondriac	hypochondriac
5. epi-	gastric	epigastric
6. re-	spiratory	respiratory
7. re-	productive	reproductive

BUILDING MEDICAL WORDS

Combining Forms (p. 72)

1. end; boundary 2. walking 3. servant; accessory 4. listening 5. time 6. impart, transmit 7. present at birth 8. cause of disease 9. increase; provoke 10. break up 11. production; creation 12. arising from; produced by 13. knowledge 14. give ability 15. genetic inheritance 16. physician; medical treatment 17. unknown; individual 18. disease within 19. looking at 20. word; the study of 21. physician; medicine 22. new 23. nourishment 24. reduce the severity of 25. touching, feeling 26. tapping 27. physical function 28. growth, formation 29. present 30. recover 31. send back 32. chest 33. operative procedure 34. collection of symptoms 35. technical skill 36. treatment 37. treatment

Combining Forms and Suffixes (p. 73)

1. surg/o-	-eon	surgeon
2. termin/o-	-al	terminal
3. therap/o-	-ist	therapist
4. ambulat/o-	-ory	ambulatory
5. palliat/o-	-ive	palliativee
6. techn/o-	-ician	technician
7. heredit/o-	-ary	hereditary
8. path/o-	-gen	pathogen
9. symptomat/o-	-logy	symptomatology
10. palpat/o-	-ion	palpation
11. auscult/o-	-ation	auscultation
12. infect/o-	-ious	infectious
13. therapeut/o-	-ic	therapeutic
14. surg/o-	-ery	surgery
15. percuss/o-	-ion	percussion
16. chron/o-	-ic	chronic
17. congenit/o-	-al	congenital
18. eti/o-	-logy	etiology

Prefixes and Combining Forms (p. 74)

1. dia-	gnosis	diagnosis
2. de-	generative	degenerative
3. a-	symptomatic	asymptomatic
4. pro-	gnosis	prognosis
5. re-	fractory	refractory

CHAPTER REVIEW EXERCISES

Matching Exercise (p. 76)

7, 5, 1, 9, 4, 2, 6, 8, 3

Circle Exercise (p. 76)

1. blood 2. thoracic 3. cells 4. gastroenterology 5. anatomical 6. vena cavae 7. anterior 8. thoracic 9. respiratory 10. distal

English and Medical Word Equivalents (p. 77)

1. anterior or ventral 2. posterior or dorsal 3. lateral 4. sagittal 5. supine 6. prone 7. superior 8. inferior 9. cephalad 10. caudad

True or False Exercise (p. 77)

1. T 2. F 3. F 4. T 5. F 6. T 7. T 8. T 9. T 10. F

Fill in the Blank Exercise (p. 77)

1. gynecology 2. obstetrics 3. otolaryngology 4. neurology 5. dermatology 6. pulmonology 7. neonatology 8. radiology 9. orthopedics

True or False Exercise (p. 78)

1. F 2. T 3. T 4. T 5. T 6. F 7. F 8. F

Circle Exercise (p. 78)

1. physician's office 2. etiology 3. refractory 4. remission 5. hereditary

Fill in the Blank Exercise (p. 78)

1. subacute 2. palpation 3. auscultation 4. syndrome 5. idiopathic 6. symptomatology 7. clinic

Name That Word Part (p. 79)

1.	dors/o-	C	back; dorsum; uppermost part
2.	a-	P	away from, without
3.	abdomin/o-	C	abdomen
4.	-able	S	able to be
5.	-ad	S	toward, in the direction of
6.	-al	S	pertaining to
7.	ambulat/o-	C	walking
8.	ana-	C	apart from; excessive
9.	ancill/o-	C	servant; excessive
10.	anter/o-	C	before; front part
11.	-ar	S	pertaining to
12.	-ary	S	pertaining to
13.	-atic	S	pertaining to
14.	-ation	S	a process; being or having
15.	-ative	S	pertaining to
16.	-atory	S	pertaining to
17.	auscult/o-	C	listening
18.	cardi/o-	C	heart
19.	caud/o-	C	tailbone; lower part of the body
20.	cav/o-	C	hollow space
21.	cephal/o-	C	head
22.	chondr/o-	C	cartilag
23.	chron/o-	C	time
24.	communic/o-	C	impart; transmit
25.	congenit/o-	C	present at birth
26.	coron/o-	C	encircling structure
27.	crani/o-	C	cranium (skull)
28.	-crine	S	secrete
29.	crin/o-	C	secrete
30.	de-	P	reversal of, without
31.	dent/o-	C	tooth
32.	dermat/o-	C	skin
33.	dia-	P	through, complete
34.	dietet/o-	C	foods, diet
35.	dist/o-	C	away from the center or point of origin
36.	-drome	S	a running
37.	endo-	P	innermost, within
38.	enter/o-	C	intestine
39.	-eon	S	one who performs
40.	epi-	P	upon, above
41.	-ery	S	process of
42.	eti/o-	C	cause of disease
43.	exacerb/o-	C	increase; provoke
44.	extern/o-	C	outside
45.	fract/o-	C	break up
46.	front/o-	C	front
47.	gastr/o-	C	stomach
48.	-gen	S	that which produces
49.	gener/o-	C	production; creation
50.	gen/o-	C	arising from; produced by
51.	ger/o-	C	old age
52.	gnos/o-	R	knowledge
53.	gynec/o-	C	female, woman
54.	habilitat/o-	C	give ability
55.	hemat/o-	C	blood
56.	heredit/o-	C	genetic inheritance
57.	horizont/o-	C	boundary between the earth and sky
58.	hypo-	P	below; deficient
59.	-iac	S	pertaining to
60.	iatr/o-	C	physician; medical treatment
61.	-iatry	S	medical treatment
62.	-ic	S	pertaining to
63.	-ical	S	pertaining to
64.	-ician	S	a skilled professional or expert
65.	-ics	S	knowledge, practice
66.	idi/o-	C	unknown; individual
67.	immun/o-	C	immune response
68.	infect/o-	C	disease within
69.	infer/o-	C	below
70.	inguin/o-	C	groin
71.	inspect/o-	C	looking at
72.	integument/o-	C	skin
73.	intern/o-	C	inside
74.	intestin/o-	C	intestine
75.	-ion	S	action; condition
76.	-ior	S	pertaining to
77.	-ious	S	pertaining to
78.	-ist	S	one who specializes in
79.	-istry	S	process related to the specialty of
80.	-ity	S	state; condition
81.	-ive	S	pertaining to
82.	laryng/o-	C	larynx (voice box)
83.	later/o-	C	side
84.	log/o-	C	the study of
85.	-logy	S	the study of
86.	lumb/o-	C	lower back; area between the ribs and pelvis
87.	lymph/o-	C	lymph; lymphatic system
88.	macr/o-	C	large
89.	medi/o-	C	middle
90.	medic/o-	C	physician; medicine
91.	micr/o-	C	small
92.	mid-	P	middle
93.	muscul/o-	C	muscle
94.	nat/o-	C	birth
95.	ne/o-	P	new
96.	neur/o-	C	nerve
97.	nerv/o-	C	nerve
98.	nucle/o-	C	nucleus
99.	nutri/o-	C	nourishment
100.	obstetr/o-	C	pregnancy and childbirth
101.	onc/o-	C	tumor, mass
102.	ophthalm/o-	C	eye
103.	orth/o-	C	straight
104.	-ory	S	having the function of
105.	-osis	S	condition; abnormal condition; process
106.	ot/o-	C	ear
107.	-ous	S	pertaining to
108.	palliat/o-	C	to reduce the severity of
109.	palpat/o-	C	touching, feeling
110.	path/o-	C	disease, suffering
111.	ped/o-	C	child
112.	pelv/o-	C	pelvis (hip bone; renal pelvis)
113.	percuss/o-	C	tapping
114.	pharmac/o-	C	medicines drug
115.	physic/o-	C	body
116.	plas/o-	C	growth, formation
117.	poster/o-	C	back part
118.	prevent/o-	C	prevent
119.	pro-	P	before
120.	product/o-	C	produce
121.	proxim/o-	C	near the center or point of origin
122.	psych/o-	C	mind
123.	pulmon/o-	C	lung
124.	radi/o-	C	radius (forearm bone); x-rays; radiation

125. re-	P	again and again; backward; unable to
126. recuper/o-	C	recover
127. remiss/o-	C	send back
128. sagitt/o-	C	going from front to back
129. -scope	S	instrument used to examine
130. scop/o-	C	examine with an instrument
131. skelet/o-	C	skeleton
132. spin/o-	C	spine; backbone
133. spir/o-	C	a coil
134. superfici/o-	C	on or near the surface
135. super/o-	C	above
136. surg/o-	C	operative procedure
137. symptomat/o-	C	collection of symptoms
138. syn-	P	together
139. techn/o-	C	technical skill
140. termin/o-	C	end; boundary
141. therapeut/o-	C	treatment
142. therap/o-	C	treatment
143. thorac/o-	C	thorax (chest)
144. -tic	S	pertaining to
145. -tion	S	a process; being or having
146. tom/o-	C	a cut, slice, or layer
147. -tomy	S	process of cutting or making an incision
148. trans-	P	across, through
149. umbilic/o-	C	umbilicus, navel
150. urin/o-	C	urine; urinary system
151. ur/o-	C	urine; urinary system
152. vascul/o-	C	blood vessel
153. ventr/o-	C	front; abdomen
154. -verse	S	to travel; to turn

Word-Building Exercise (p. 81)

1. neur/o-	-logy		neurology
2. anter/o-	-ior		anterior
3. micr/o-	-scope		microscope
4. abdomin/o-	-al		abdominal
5. cardi/o-	-logy		cardiology
6. trans-	-verse		transverse
7. super/o-	-ior		superior
8. thorac/o-	-ic		thoracic
9. pulmon/o-	-logy		pulmonology
10. intern/o-	-al		internal
11. gastr/o-	intestin/o-	-al	gastrointestinal
12. dermat/o-	-logy		dermatology
13. re-	product/o-	-ive	reproductive
14. ped/o-	iatr/o-	ics	pediatrics

DIVIDE AND CONQUER (p. 81)

1.	ana-	tom/o-	-ical
2.		cav/o-	-ity
3.		cephal/o-	-ad
4.	endo-	crin/o-	-logy
5.		gynec/o-	-logy
6.	mid-	sagitt/o-	-al
7.		ophthalm/o-	-logy
8.		pharmacy/o-	-logy
9.		poster/o-	-ior
10.	re-	product/o-	-ive
11.		thorac/o-	-ic
12.		urin/o-	-ary

Matching Exercise #1 (p. 82)

13, 12, 7, 9, 6, 4, 16, 10, 17, 2, 15, 11, 14, 1, 5, 8, 2

Matching Exercise #2 (p. 82)

4, 5, 6, 11, 1, 8, 2, 3, 10, 9, 7

Proofreading and Spelling Exercise (p. 82)

1. anatomical 2. posteriorly 3. thoracic 4. cavity 5. cardiovascular 6. ophthalmology 7. otolaryngology 8. pulmonology 9. gynecology 10. physiology

Chapter 3 Gastroenterology

LABELING EXERCISE (pp. 103–104)

Exercise A

1. oral cavity 2. teeth 3. tongue 4. sublingual gland 5. submandibular gland 6. parotid gland 7. pharynx 8. esophagus

Exercise B

1. esophagus 2. cardiac sphincter 3. cardia 4. fundus 5. body 6. rugae 7. antrum 8. pyloric canal 9. pyloric sphincter 10. head of pancreas 11. duodenum 12. omentum

Exercise C

1. liver 2. duodenum 3. ascending colon 4. cecum 5. appendix 6. rectum 7. anus 8. transverse colon 9. descending colon 10. sigmoid colon 11. ileum 12. stomach 13. spleen 14. jejunum

BUILDING MEDICAL WORDS

Combining Forms (p. 105)

1. water; fluid 2. abdomen 3. absorb or suck in 4. food, nourishment 5. carbohydrate, starch 6. anus 7. appendix 8. small thing hanging from a larger structure; appendix 9. bile 10. heart 11. hollow space 12. cecum 13. abdomen 14. chloride 15. bile duct 16. bile, gall 17. gallbladder 18. common bile duct 19. colon 20. bladder; fluid-filled sac; semisolid cyst 21. swallow 22. break down food; digest 23. duodenum (first part of the small intestine) 24. expel, remove 25. droplets of fat suspended in a liquid; particles suspended in a solution 26. intestine 27. esophagus 28. feces, stool 29. stomach 30. tongue 31. the sense of taste 32. liver 33. ileum 34. intestine 35. jejunum 36. movement 37. milk 38. tongue 39. lipid (fat) 40. mandible (upper jaw) 41. chewing 42. mucous membrane 43. mouth 44. ear 45. pancreas 46. pelvis (hip bone; renal pelvis) 47. pepsin 48. peptide (two amino acids) 49. digestion 50. peritoneum 51. pharynx 52. point of entry 53. protein 54. pylorus 55. rectum 56. red 57. saliva 58. green

Combining Forms and Suffixes (p. 106)

1. abdomin/o-	-al	abdominal
2. gastr/o-	-ic	gastric
3. hepat/o-	-cyte	hepatocyte
4. or/o-	-al	oral
5. saliv/o-	-ary	salivary
6. lingu/o-	-al	lingual
7. mastic/o-	-ation	mastication
8. rect/o-	-al	rectal
9. lip/o-	-ase	lipase
10. appendic/o-	-eal	appendiceal
11. append/o-	-ix	appendix
12. colon/o-	-ic	colonic
13. digest/o-	-ive	digestive
14. esophag/o-	-eal	esophageal
15. degluti/o-	-tion	deglutition
16. ile/o-	-al	ileal
17. pepsin/o-	-gen	pepsinogen
18. pancreat/o-	-ic	pancreatic
19. bil/I-	-ary	biliary
20. duoden/o-	-al	duodenal

CHAPTER REVIEW EXERCISES

Matching Exercise (p. 136)

8, 3, 2, 1, 11, 5, 13, 10, 7, 4, 6, 3, 14, 2

Circle Exercise (p. 136)

1. duodenum 2. defecation 3. cardia 4. salivary gland 5. hydrochloric acid 6. sigmoid 7. bile

True or False Exercise (p. 137)

1. T 2. T 3. F 4. T 5. F 6. T 7. F 8. T 9. F 10. T 11. T 12. T

Sequencing Exercise (p. 137)

1. oral cavity 2. pharynx 3. esophagus 4. stomach 5. duodenum 6. jejunum 7. ileum 8. cecum 9. colon 10. rectum 11. anus

Name That Word Part (p. 138)

1. -al	S	pertaining to
2. abdomin/o-	C	abdomen
3. absorpt/o-	C	absorb or suck in
4. -ac	S	pertaining to
5. aden/o-	C	gland
6. adhes/o-	C	to stick to
7. aliment/o-	C	food, nourishment
8. amyl/o-	C	carbohydrate, starch
9. an-	P	without, not
10. anastom/o-	C	to reestablish an opening
11. an/o-	C	anus
12. anti-	P	against

13. aphth/o-	C	ulcer
14. appendic/o-	C	appendix; limb
15. append/o-	C	small thing hanging from a larger structure; appendix
16. -ar	S	pertaining to
17. -ary	S	pertaining to
18. -ase	S	enzyme
19. -ated	S	pertaining to a condition; composed of
20. -ation	S	a process; being or having
21. bil/i-	C	bile
22. bi/o-	C	life; living organism; living tissue
23. carcin/o-	C	cancer
24. cav/o-	C	hollow space
25. cec/o-	C	cecum
26. -cele	S	hernia
27. celi/o-	C	abdomen
28. cellul/o-	C	cell
29. cheil/o-	C	lip
30. chez/o-	C	to pass stool
31. chlor/o-	C	chloride
32. cholangi/o-	C	bile duct
33. chol/e-	C	bile, gall
34. cholecyst/o-	C	gallbladder
35. choledoch/o-	C	common bile duct
36. cirrh/o-	C	yellow
37. col/o-	C	colon
38. colon/o-	C	colon
39. constip/o-	C	compacted stool
40. cyst/o-	C	bladder; fluid-filled sac; semisolid cyst
41. -cyte	S	cell
42. degluti/o-	C	swallow
43. dia-	P	completely through
44. digest/o-	C	break down food; digest
45. diverticul/o-	C	diverticulum
46. -drome	S	a running
47. duoden/o-	C	duodenum
48. dys-	P	painful, difficult, abnormal
49. -eal	S	pertaining to
50. -ectomy	S	surgical excision
51. elimin/o-	C	expel, remove
52. -emesis	S	vomiting
53. emet/o-	C	vomiting
54. emulsific/o-	C	droplets of fat suspended in a liquid; particles suspended in a solution
55. endo-	P	innermost, within
56. -ent	S	pertaining to
57. enter/o-	C	intestines
58. -entery	S	condition of the intestine
59. epi-	P	upon, above
60. esophag/o-	C	esophagus
61. fec/a-	C	feces, stool
62. fec/o-	C	feces, stool
63. flatul/o-	C	flatus
64. gastr/o-	C	stomach
65. -gen	S	that which produces
66. gloss/o-	C	tongue
67. -grade	S	going
68. -gram	S	a record or picture
69. -graphy	S	process of recording
70. gustat/o-	C	the sense of taste
71. hemat/o-	C	blood
72. hemorrhoid/o-	C	hemorrhoid
73. hepat/o-	C	liver
74. herni/o-	C	hernia
75. hydro-	C	water; fluid
76. hyper-	P	above; more than normal
77. -ia	S	condition, state, thing
78. -iasis	S	abnormal condition, condition
79. -ic	S	pertaining to
80. ile/o-	C	ileum
81. -in	S	substance
82. incis/o-	C	to cut into
83. inguin/o-	C	groin
84. intestin/o-	C	intestines
85. intussuscept/o-	C	to receive within
86. -ion	S	action; condition
87. -itis	S	inflammation of
88. -ity	S	state; condition
89. -ive	S	pertaining to
90. -ix	S	a thing
91. jejun/o-	C	jejunum
92. lapar/o-	C	abdomen
93. kin/o-	C	movement
94. lact/o-	C	milk
95. lingu/o-	C	tongue
96. lip/o-	C	lipid (fat)
97. -lith	S	stone
98. lith/o-	C	stone
99. -logy	S	the study of
100. mal-	P	bad, inadequate
101. mastic/o-	C	chewing
102. medic/o-	C	physician; medicine
103. -megaly	S	enlargement
104. melen/o-	C	black
105. meso-	P	middle
106. mucos/o-	C	mucous membrane
107. nause/o-	C	nausea
108. obstip/o-	C	severe constipation
109. odyn/o-	C	pain
110. -oid	S	resembling
111. -oma	S	tumor, mass
112. omphal/o-	C	umbilicus, navel
113. -opsy	S	the process of viewing
114. orex/o-	C	appetite
115. or/o-	C	mouth
116. -ory	S	having the function off
117. -osis	S	condition, abnormal condition
118. -ous	S	pertaining to
119. pancreat/o-	C	pancreas
120. par-	P	beside
121. -pathy	S	disease, suffering
122. pelv/o-	C	pelvis (hip bone; renal pelvis)
123. peps/o-	C	digestion
124. pept/o-	C	to digest
125. peri-	P	around
126. peritone/o-	C	peritoneum
127. periton/o-	C	peritoneum
128. phag/o-	C	eating, swallowing
129. pharyng/o-	C	pharynx (throat)
130. -plasty	S	process of reshaping by surgery
131. poly-	P	many, much
132. polyp/o-	C	polyp
133. port/o-	C	point of entry
134. prote/o-	C	protein
135. pylor/o-	C	pylorus
136. pyr/o-	C	fire; burning
137. rect/o-	C	rectum
138. regurgit/o-	C	flow backward
139. resect/o-	C	to cut out and remove
140. retro-	P	behind, backward
141. rotat/o-	C	rotate
142. -rrhea	S	flow, discharge
143. -rrhaphy	S	procedure of suturing
144. saliv/o-	C	saliva
145. -scope	S	instrument used to examine
146. scop/o-	C	examine with an instrument
147. -scopy	S	process of using an instrument to examine
148. sial/o-	C	saliva; salivary gland
149. -sis	S	action; process
150. son/o-	C	sound
151. splen/o-	C	spleen
152. -stasis	S	condition of contraction
153. steat/o-	C	fat
154. stomat/o-	C	mouth
155. -stomy	S	surgically created opening
156. sub-	P	below; underneath; less than
157. -tion	S	a process; being or having
158. -tomy	S	process of cutting or making an incision
159. ulcerat/o-	C	ulcer
160. umbilic/o-	C	umbilicus, navel

Word-Building Exercise (p. 140)

1. or/o- + -al — oral
2. epi- + gastr/o- + -ic — epigastric
3. an- + orex/o- + -ic — anorexic
4. dys- + phag/o- + -ia — dysphagia
5. sub- + gloss/o- + -al — subglossal
6. gastr/o- + enter/o- + -itis — gastroenteritis
7. hemat/o- + -emesis — hematemesis
8. col/o- + rect/o- + -al — colorectal
9. hemat/o- + chez/o- + -ia — hematochezia
10. hepat/o- + -megaly — hepatomegaly
11. sial/o- + -lith — sialolith
12. esophag/o- + gastr/o- + duoden/o- + -scopy — esophagogastroduodenoscopy
13. cholecyst/o- + lith/o- + -tomy — cholelithotomy
14. hepat/o- + -cyte — hepatocyte
15. peri- + an/o- + -al — perianal
16. retro- + peritone/o- + -al — retroperitoneal

True or False (p. 140)

1. T 2. F 3. T 4. F 5. F 6. F 7. F 8. T

Matching Exercise (p. 141)

13, 9, 2, 6, 7, 8, 12, 1, 11, 5, 3, 4, 10

Fill in the Blank Exercise (p. 141)

1. stoma 2. antiemetic 3. albumin 4. ova and parasites 5. cholangiography 6. sonogram 7. barium swallow 8. nasogastric tube 9. herniorrhaphy 10. laxative

Circle Exercise (p. 142)

1. organ transplantation 2. sonogram 3. cholecystectomy 4. colostomy 5. obesity 6. SGPT 7. CLO 8. laparotomy 9. gastrectomy

Matching Exercise (p. 142)

8, 5, 10, 2, 1, 11, 12, 4, 13, 6, 9, 7, 3

Plural Noun and Adjective Spelling (p. 143)

1.	abdomen		abdominal
2.	mouth		oral
3.	tongue		glossal lingual
4.	mucosa		mucosal
5.	pharynx		pharyngeal
6.	esophagus		esophageal
7.	stomach		gastric
8.	pylorus		pyloric
9.	duodenum		duodenal
10.	jejunum		jejunal
11.	ileum		ileal
12.	villus	villi	
13.	cecum		cecal
14.	appendix		appendiceal
15.	col n		colonic
16.	rectum		rectal
17.	anus		anal
18.	peritoneum		peritoneal
19.	liver		hepatic
20.	pancreas		pancreatic

Proofreading and Spelling Exercise (p. 143)

1. gastroenterology 2. pharynx 3. esophagus 4. diverticula 5. hemorrhoids 6. cholelithiasis 7. lumen 8. polyps 9. rectocele 10. albumin

English and Medical Word Equivalents (p. 144)

1. belly — abdomen
2. belly button — umbilicus, navel
3. bowel, gut — intestines
4. bowel movement — defecation, feces, stool
5. chewing — mastication
6. gas — flatus, flatulence
7. heartburn — pyrosis
8. indigestion — dyspepsia
9. mouth — oral cavity
10. piles — hemorrhoids
11. swallowing — deglutition
12. throat — pharynx
13. throwing up — emesis

Dictionary Challenge (p. 144)

1. aerophagia — abnormal swallowing of air
2. eructation — belching gas from the stomach
3. tenesmus — straining to pass stool without actually passing it
4. singultus — hiccups
5. borborygmus — rumbling, gurgling noise in the stomach

Word Analysis Questions (p. 161)

1. He had sharp **gastric** pains.
2. appendic/o- — appendix; limb
   -itis — inflammation of
3. fec/a- — feces, stool
   -lith — stone
4. The pathology specimen showed marked **mucosal** hemorrhage.
5. N&V

Fact Finding Questions (p. 162)

1. antacid drugs 2. emesis 3. colon 4. wormlike 5. appendectomy 6. acute appendicitis

Critical Thinking Questions (p. 162)

1. pyrosis 2. gastroenteritis 3. appendix 4. peritonitis 5. The patient complains of rebound tenderness if the physician presses down on the lower right abdomen and then suddenly removes the hand, releasing the pressure. 6. liver 7. pancreas

Chapter 4 Pulmonology

LABELING EXERCISE (p. 166)

Exercise A

1. nasal cavity 2. pharynx 3. larynx 4. apex 5. rib 6. mainstem bronchus 7. sternum 8. base of lung 9. trachea 10. cluster of alveoli 11. bronchioles 12. diaphragm

Exercise B

1. bronchiole 2. cluster of alveoli 3. carbon dioxide 4. oxygen 5. capillary 6. red blood cell

BUILDING MEDICAL WORDS

Combining Forms (p. 167)

1. alveolus (air sac) 2. apex (tip) 3. bronchus 4. bronchiole 5. bronchus 6. heart 7. hollow space 8. rib 9. diaphragm 10. outside 11. arising from; produced by 12. shaped like a globe; comprehensive 13. glottis (of the larynx) 14. breathe 15. blood 16. hilum (indentation in an organ) 17. inside 18. larynx (voice box) 19. lobe of an organ 20. mediastinum 21. change, transformation 22. mucus 23. mucous membrane 24. nose 25. oxygen 26. parenchyma (functional cells of an organ) 27. wall of a cavity 28. pharynx (throat) 29. diaphragm; mind 30. pleura (lung membrane) 31. breathing 32. lung 33. septum (dividing wall) 34. serum of the blood; serumlike fluid 35. breathe 36. sternum (breast bone) 37. thorax (chest) 38. trachea (windpipe) 39. scroll-like structure; turbinate 40. viscera (internal organs)

Combining Forms and Suffixes (p. 167)

1. alveol/o- + -ar — alveolar
2. nas/o- + -al — nasal
3. trache/o- + -al — tracheal
4. pulmon/o- + -ary — pulmonary
5. ser/o- + -ous — serous
6. phren/o- + -ic — phrenic
7. bronchi/o- + -ole — bronchiole
8. thorac/o- + -ic — thoracic
9. apic/o- + -al — apical
10. lob/o- + -ar — lobar
11. parenchym/o- + -al — parenchymal
12. cost/o- + -al — costal

Combining Forms and Prefixes (p. 168)

1. in- + spiration — inspiration
2. inter- + costal — intercostal
3. re- + spiration — respiration
4. epi- + glottic — epiglottic
5. ex- + halation — exhalation
6. eu- + pneic — eupneic

CHAPTER REVIEW QUESTIONS

Matching Exercise (p. 191)

6, 11, 2, 3, 5, 7, 8, 9, 1, 10, 4

Circle Exercise (p. 191)

1. apex 2. bronchi 3. hilum 4. parenchyma 5. epiglottis 6. surfactant 7. phrenic nerve

True or False (p. 191)

1. T 2. F 3. F 4. T 5. F 6. F 7. T 8. T 9. T

Sequencing Exercise (p. 192)

1. nose 2. nasal cavity 3. pharynx 4. larynx 5. trachea 6. bronchi 7. hilum 8. bronchioles 9. alveoli

Name That Word Part (p. 192)

1.	-al	S	pertaining to
2.	a-	P	away from, without
3.	aden/o-	C	gland
4.	alveol/o-	C	alveolus (air sac)
5.	an-	P	without, not
6.	-ant	S	pertaining to
7.	anti-	P	against
8.	anthrac/o-	C	coal
9.	apic/o-	C	apex (tip)
10.	-ar	S	pertaining to
11.	arteri/o-	C	artery
12.	-ary	S	pertaining to
13.	aspir/o-	C	to breathe in, to suck in
14.	asthm/o-	C	asthma
15.	-ate	S	composed of, pertaining to
16.	-ated	S	pertaining to a condition
17.	ate/o-	C	incomplete
18.	-atic	S	pertaining to
19.	-ation	S	a process; being or having
20.	-ator	S	person or thing that performs
21.	-atory	S	pertaining to
22.	auscult/o-	C	listening
23.	bacteri/o-	C	bacterium, bacteria
24.	basil/o-	C	base of an organ
25.	bi/o-	C	life; living organisms
26.	brady-	P	slow
27.	bronchi/o-	C	bronchus
28.	bronchiol/o-	C	bronchiole
29.	bronch/o-	C	bronchus
30.	capn/o-	C	carbon dioxide
31.	carbox/y-	C	carbon dioxide
32.	carcin/o-	C	cancer
33.	cardi/o-	C	heart
34.	cav/o-	C	hollow space
35.	-centesis	S	puncture
36.	chron/o-	C	time
37.	circum-	P	around
38.	cocc/o-	C	spherical bacterium
39.	coni/o-	C	dust
40.	cortic/o-	C	cortex (outer region)
41.	cost/o-	C	rib, ribs
42.	cyan/o-	C	blue
43.	cyst/o-	C	bladder; fluid-filled sac; semisolid cyst
44.	de-	P	reversal of, without
45.	diaphragmat/o-	C	diaphragm
46.	dilat/o-	C	dilate, widen
47.	dys-	P	painful, difficult, abnormal
48.	-eal	S	pertaining to
49.	-ectasis	S	dilation
50.	-ectomy	S	surgical excision
51.	effus/o-	C	a pouring out
52.	em-	P	in
53.	-ema	S	condition
54.	embol/o-	C	embolus (occluding plug)
55.	-emia	S	blood; substance in the blood
56.	endo-	P	internal, within
57.	epi-	P	upon, above
58.	eu-	P	normal, good
59.	ex-	P	out, away from
60.	extern/o-	C	outside
61.	fibr/o-	C	fiber, fibers
62.	fus/o-	C	pouring
63.	gen/o-	C	arising from; produced by
64.	glob/o-	C	shaped like a globe; comprehensive
65.	glott/o-	C	glottis
66.	-graphy	S	process of recording
67.	hal/o-	C	breathe
68.	hem/o-	C	blood
69.	hil/o-	C	hilum (indentation in an organ)
70.	hyper-	P	above; more than normal
71.	hypo-	P	below; deficient
72.	-ia	S	condition, state, thing
73.	-ic	S	pertaining to
74.	in-	P	in, within, not
75.	-in	S	substance
76.	inter-	P	between
77.	intern/o-	C	inside
78.	-ion	S	action; condition
79.	-ism	S	process; disease from a specific cause
80.	-istic	S	pertaining to
81.	-isy	S	condition of inflammation
82.	-itis	S	inflammation of
83.	-ity	S	state; condition
84.	-ive	S	pertaining to
85.	laryng/o-	C	larynx (voice box)
86.	lob/o-	C	lobe of an organ
87.	-logy	S	the study of
88.	malign/o-	C	intentionally causing harm; cancer
89.	mediastin/o-	C	mediastinum
90.	metabol/o-	C	change, transformation
91.	-meter	S	instrument used to measure
92.	-metry	S	process of measuring
93.	mucos/o-	C	mucous membrane
94.	nas/o-	C	nose
95.	obstruct/o-	C	blocked by a barrier
96.	-ole	S	little, small
97.	-oma	S	tumor, mass
98.	opportun/o-	C	well timed, taking advantage of an opportunity
99.	or/o-	C	mouth
100.	orth/o-	C	straight
101.	-or	S	person or thing that produces or does
102.	-ory	S	having the function of
103.	-osis	S	condition, abnormal condition
104.	-ous	S	pertaining to
105.	ox/I-	C	oxygen
106.	ox/o-	C	oxygen
107.	ox/y-	C	oxygen
108.	pan-	P	all
109.	parenchym/o-	C	parenchyma (functional cells of an organ)
110.	pariet/o-	C	wall of a cavity
111.	paroxysm/o-	C	sudden, sharp attack
112.	pector/o-	C	chest
113.	per-	P	through, throughout
114.	pharyng/o-	C	pharynx (throat)
115.	phren/o-	C	diaphragm; mind
116.	phys/o-	C	inflate or distend
117.	pleur/o-	C	pleura (lung membrane)
118.	-pnea	S	breathing
119.	pne/o-	C	breathing
120.	pneum/o-	C	lungs; air
121.	pneumon/o-	C	lung
122.	-ptysis	S	abnormal condition of coughing up
123.	pulmon/o-	C	lung, lungs
124.	py/o-	C	pus
125.	radi/o-	C	x-ray; radiation; radium (forearm bone)
126.	re-	P	again and again; backward; unable to
127.	resect/o-	C	to cut out and remove
128.	resuscit/o-	C	revive or raise up again
129.	-scope	S	instrument used to examine
130.	-scopy	S	process of using an instrument to examine
131.	sept/o-	C	septum (dividing wall)
132.	ser/o-	C	serum of the blood; serumlike substance
133.	-spasm	C	sudden, involuntary muscle contraction
134.	spir/o-	C	breathe
135.	steth/o-	C	chest
136.	stern/o-	C	sternum (breastbone)

137. -steroid	S	steroid
138. -stomy	S	surgically created opening
139. tachy-	P	fast
140. thorac/o-	C	thorax (chest)
141. -thorax	S	thorax (chest)
142. -tic	S	pertaining to
143. tom/o-	C	a slice, cut, or layer
144. -tomy	S	process of cutting or making an incision
145. -tor	S	person or thing that produces or does
146. -tous	S	pertaining to
147. trache/o-	C	trachea (windpipe)
148. tract/o-	C	pulling
149. tubercul/o-	C	tuberculosis
150. tub/o-	C	tube
151. turbin/o-	C	turbinate (scroll)
152. tuss/o-	C	cough
153. ventil/o-	C	movement of air
154. vir/o-	C	virus
155. viscer/o-	C	viscera (internal organs)

Combining Form Exercise (p. 194)

1. trache/o-	trachea	bronchotracheal	pertaining to the bronchi and trachea
2. auscult/o-	listening	auscultation	process of listening
3. ventil/o-	movement of air	ventilator	thing that performs movement of air
		ventilation	process of movement of air
4. cyan/o-	blue	cyanosis	condition of blueness
5. pector/o-	chest	expectorant	pertaining to out of the chest
6. steth/o-	chest	stethoscope	instrument used to examine the chest

Matching Exercise (p. 194)

3, 7, 4, 1, 5, 2, 8, 9, 6

True or False (p. 195)

1. T 2. T 3. F 4. T 5. T 6. F 7. T 8. T 9. F

Fill in the Blank Exercise (p. 195)

1. bronchopneumonia 2. status asthmaticus 3. wheezing 4. cystic fibrosis 5. tachypnea 6. Legionnaire's disease 7. carcinoma 8. pulmonary edema 9. tuberculosis

Word-Building Exercise (p. 196)

1. endotracheal 2. spirometer 3. bronchoscopy 4. oximeter 5. thoracotomy 6. antitussive

Circle Exercise (p. 196)

1. lung 2. nasal cannula 3. carboxyhemoglobin 4. productive cough

Matching Exercise (p. 196)

8, 2, 6, 4, 9, 1, 5, 7, 3

Plural Noun and Adjective Spelling (p. 197)

1. nose		nasal
2. alveolus	alveoli	alveolar
3. anoxia		anoxic
4. apex	apices	apical
5. apnea		apneic
6. asthma		asthmatic
7. atelectasis		atelectatic
8. bronchiole	bronchioles	bronchiolar
9. bronchus	bronchi	bronchial
10. cilium	cilia	
11. cyanotic		cyanotic
12. diaphragm		diaphragmatic
13. epiglottis		epiglottic
14. hilum	hila	hilar
15. hypoxia		hypoxic
16. larynx		laryngeal
17. lobe	lobes	lobar
18. lung	lungs	pulmonary
19. mediastinum		mediastinal
20. mucosa		mucosal
21. pharynx		pharyngeal
22. pleura		pleural
23. pus		purulent
24. rib	ribs	costal
25. septum		septal
26. sternum		sternal
27. tachypnea		tachypneic
28. trachea		tracheal

English and Medical Word Equivalents (p. 197)

1. throat	pharynx
2. black lung disease	anthracosis
3. breast bone	sternum
4. chest	thorax
5. collapsed lung	atelectasis
6. crib death	SIDS
7. flu	influenza
8. shortness of breath	dyspnea
9. throat	pharynx
10. voice box	larynx
11. windpipe	trachea

Dictionary Challenge (p. 197)

1. Although you can find the word *cystic* in a medical dictionary, it does not provide a definition of the disease cystic fibrosis. You must look under the main heading (noun) *fibrosis* and then the subheading (adjective) *cystic* to find the definition of *cystic fibrosis*.
2. Although *asthmaticus* seems to be the most important word in this phrase, it is not a noun. This is a Latin phrase and you can find its definition by looking under *status*.

Word Analysis Questions (p. 199)

1. SOB	
2. dyspneic	
3. dys-	painful, difficult, abnormal
pne/o-	breathing
-ic	pertaining to
4. bronch/o-	bronchus, bronchi
-scopy	process of using an instrument to examine
5. cyan/o-	blue
-osis	condition, abnormal condition

6. culture and sensitivity
cardiopulmonary resuscitation
chronic obstructive pulmonary disease
right lower lobe

Fact Finding Questions (p. 199)

1. anthracosis 2. On the extremities, specifically the fingers 3. bronchoscopy 4. appendectomy 5. atelectasis, consolidative changes, density in LLL, patchy infiltrate

Critical Thinking Questions (p. 200)

1. Fever 2. Barrel chest 3. Auscultation 4. Impression 1. Right lower lobe pneumonia 5. 44 pack-year smoking history

Chapter 5 Cardiology

LABELING EXERCISES (p. 224)

Exercise A

1. aorta 2. superior vena cava 3. pulmonary valve 4. right atrium 5. tricuspid valve 6. inferior vena cava 7. right ventricle 8. apex of the heart 9. interventricular septum 10. left ventricle 11. chordae tendinae 12. aortic valve 13. mitral valve 14. left atrium 15. pulmonary artery

Exercise B

1. atrioventricular (AV) node 2. sinoatrial (SA) node 3. bundle of His 4. right and left bundle branches 5. Purkinje fibers

Exercise C

1. aortic arch 2. ascending aorta 3. thoracic aorta 4. brachial artery 5. radial artery 6. ulnar artery 7. peroneal artery 8. anterior tibial artery 9. posterior tibial artery 10. popliteal artery 11. femoral artery 12. external iliac artery 13. internal iliac artery 14. common iliac artery 15. abdominal aorta 16. renal artery 17. coronary artery 18. axillary artery 19. subclavian artery 20. common carotid artery 21. internal carotid artery

BUILDING MEDICAL WORDS

Combining Forms (p. 226)

1. axilla (armpit) 2. aorta 3. apex (tip) 4. artery 5. arteriole 6. atrium (upper heart chamber) 7. arm 8. hairlike structure 9. heart 10. stupor, sleep 11. cell 12. movement in a circular route 13. carrying, conveying 14. drawn

together, narrowed 15. encircling structure 16. projection, point 17. dilating 18. dilate, widen 19. outside of a place 20. femur (thigh bone) 21. ilium (hip bone) 22. jugular (throat) 23. mediastinum 24. structure like a miter (tall hat with 2 points) 25. muscle 26. fibula (lower leg bone) 27. back of the knee 28. point of entry 29. lung 30. radius (forearm bone); x-rays; radiation 31. kidney 32. saphenous (standing) 33. septum (dividing wall) 34. hollow cavity; channel 35. the body as a whole 36. contracting 37. cellular layer 38. thorax (chest) 39. tibia (shin bone) 40. ulna (forearm bone) 41. valve 42. blood vessel 43. blood vessel; vas deferens 44. vein 45. ventricle (lower heart chamber; chamber in the brain)

Combining Forms and Suffixes (p. 227)

1.	thorac/o-	-ic	thoracic
2.	arteri/o-	-al	arterial
3.	valvul/o-	-ar	valvular
4.	circulat/o-	-ary	circulatory
5.	cardi/o-	-ac	cardiac
6.	capill/o-	-ary	capillary
7.	ven/o-	-ous	venous
8.	system/o-	-ic	systemic
9.	atri/o-	-al	atrial
10.	brachi/o-	-al	brachial
11.	poplit/o-	-eal	popliteal
12.	saphen/o-	-ous	saphenous
13.	aort/o-	-ic	aortic
14.	vasculo-	-ar	vascular
15.	systolo-	-ic	systolic

Two Combining Forms and a Suffix (p. 228)

1.	vas/o-	dilat/o-	-ion	vasodilation
2.	cardi/o-	pulmon/o-	-ary	cardiopulmonary
3.	cardi/o-	vascul/o-	-ar	cardiovascular
4.	sin/o-	atri/o-	-al	sinoatrial
5.	vas/o-	constrict/o-	-ion	vasoconstriction
6.	my/o-	cardi/o-	-al	myocardial
7.	atri/o-	ventricul/o-	-ar	atrioventricular

Combining Forms and Prefixes (p. 228)

1.	extra-	cellular	extracellular
2.	peri-	cardial	pericardial
3.	intra-	ventricular	intraventricular
4.	epi-	cardial	epicardial
5.	intra-	cellular	extracellular
6.	tri-	cuspid	tricuspid
7.	endo-	thelial	endothelial

CHAPTER REVIEW EXERCISES

Matching Exercise (p. 259)

9, 8, 6, 2, 4, 1, 5, 3, 7, 10

True or False (p. 259)

1. F 2. T 3. F 4. F 5. F 6. F 7. F 8. F 9. F 10. T 11. T 12. T 13. T 14. T

Circle Exercise (p. 259)

1. aorta 2. valves 3. auscultation 4. foramen ovale 5. jugular 6. SA node

Name That Word Part (p. 260)

1.	-al	S	pertaining to
2.	a-	P	away from, without
3.	ablat/o-	C	take away
4.	-ac	S	pertaining to
5.	anastom/o-	C	establish an opening
6.	aneurysm/o-	C	aneurysm (dilatation)
7.	angi/o-	C	blood vessel; lymphatic vessel
8.	anti-	P	against
9.	aort/o-	C	aorta
10.	apic/o-	C	apex (tip)
111.	-ar	S	pertaining to
12.	arteri/o-	C	artery
13.	arterio/o-	C	arteriole
14.	arter/o-	C	artery
15.	-ary	S	pertaining to
16.	-ated	S	pertaining to a condition
17.	ather/o-	C	soft, fatty substance
18.	atheromat/o-	C	fatty deposit or mass
19.	-ation	S	a process; being or having
20.	atri/o-	C	atrium (upper heart chamber)
21.	-ature	S	system composed of
22.	auscult/o-	C	listening
23.	axill/o-	C	axilla (armpit)
24.	bi-	P	two
25.	bi/o-	C	life; living organisms
26.	brachi/o-	C	arm
27.	brady-	P	slow
28.	capill/o-	C	hairlike structure
29.	card/i-	C	heart
30.	cardi/o-	C	heart
31.	carot/o-	C	carotid (stupor, sleep)
32.	cav/o-	C	hollow space
33.	cellul/o-	C	cell, cells
34.	-centesis	S	puncture
35.	cholesterol/o-	C	cholesterol
36.	circulat/o-	C	movement in a circular route
37.	claudicat/o-	C	limping pain
38.	clav/o-	C	clavicle (collarbone)
39.	coarct/o-	C	pressed together
40.	compens/o-	C	counterbalance; compensate
41.	conduct/o-	C	carrying, conveying
42.	congest/o-	C	accumulation of fluid
43.	constrict/o-	C	drawn together, narrowed
44.	contract/o-	C	pull together
45.	coron/o-	C	encircling structure
46.	cusp/o-	C	projection, point
47.	cutane/o-	C	skin
48.	de-	P	reversal of, without
49.	diastol/o-	C	dilating
50.	dilat/o-	C	dilate, widen
51.	distent/o-	C	distended, stretched
52.	dys-	P	painful, difficult, abnormal
53.	-eal	S	pertaining to
54.	ech/o-	C	echo (sound wave)
55.	-ectomy	S	surgical excision
56.	ectop/o-	C	outside of a place
57.	electr/o-	C	electricity
58.	-emia	C	blood; substance in the blood
59.	emiss/o-	C	to send out
60.	endo-	P	internal, within
61.	-ent	S	pertaining to
62.	epi-	P	above, upon
63.	esophag/o-	C	esophagus
64.	extra-	P	outside of
65.	femor/o-	C	femur (thigh bone)
66.	fibrill/o-	C	muscle fiber, nerve fiber
67.	fract/o-	C	break up
68.	fus/o-	C	pouring
69.	gemin/o-	C	twins; paired set
70.	-gram	S	a record or picture
71.	-graphy	S	process of recording
72.	hyper-	P	above; more than normal
73.	hypo-	P	below; deficient
74.	-ia	S	condition, state, thing
75.	-ian	S	pertaining to
76.	-ic	S	pertaining to
77.	-id	S	resembling; source or origin
78.	-ide	S	chemically modified
79.	ili/o-	C	ilium (hip bone)
80.	-in	S	substance
81.	-ine	S	pertaining to
82.	infarct/o-	C	area of dead tissue
83.	inter-	P	between
84.	intra-	P	within
85.	-ion	S	action; condition
86.	isch/o-	C	keep back; block
87.	-itis	S	inflammation of
88.	-ity	S	state; condition
89.	-ive	S	pertaining to
90.	-ization	S	process of making, creating, or inserting
91.	jugul/o-	C	jugular (throat)
92.	lipid/o-	C	lipid (fat)
93.	lip/o-	C	lipid (fat)
94.	log/o-	C	the study of
95.	-logy	S	the study of
96.	lumin/o-	C	lumen (opening)
97.	ly/o-	C	break down, separate, dissolve

98. man/o-	C	thin
99. -megaly	S	enlargement
100. -meter	S	instrument used to measure
101. -metry	S	process of measuring
102. mitr/o-	C	structure like a miter (tall hat with 2 points)
103. my/o-	C	muscle, muscles
104. necr/o-	C	death
105. nucle/o-	C	nucleus
106. -ole	S	little, small
107. -oma	S	tumor, mass
108. orth/o-	C	straight
109. -ory	S	having the function of
110. -ose	S	full of
111. -osis	S	condition, abnormal condition
112. -ous	S	pertaining to
113. nephr/o-	C	kidney, kidneys
114. palpit/o-	C	to throb
115. -pathy	S	disease, suffering
116. pat/o-	C	to lie open
117. per-	P	through, throughout
118. peri-	P	around
119. peripher/o-	C	outer aspects
120. perone/o-	C	fibular (lower leg bone)
121. pharmac/o-	C	medicine, drug
122. phleb/o-	C	vein
123. physi/o-	C	physical function
124. -plasty	S	process of reshaping by surgery
125. polar/o-	C	two opposite poles
126. poplit/o-	C	back of the knee
127. port/o-	C	point of entry
128. pre-	P	before, in front of
129. prosthet/o-	C	artificial part
130. pulmon/o-	C	lung, lungs
131. radi/o-	C	radius (forearm bone); x-rays; radiation
`132. re-	P	again and again; backward; unable to
133. regurgitat/o-	C	flow backward
134. ren/o-	C	kidney, kidneys
135. rheumat/o-	C	painful, inflamed joints
136. rotat/o-	C	rotate
137. rrhythm/o-	C	rhythm
138. saphen/o-	C	saphenous (standing)
139. scler/o-	C	hard; sclera (white of the eye)
140. -scope	S	instrument used to examine
141. sept/o-	C	septum (dividing wall)
142. sin/o-	C	hollow cavity; channel
143. son/o-	C	sound
144. sphygm/o-	C	pulse
145. stat/o-	C	standing still; staying in one place
146. sten/o-	C	narrowness; constriction
147. steth/o-	C	chest
148. sub-	P	below; underneath; less than
149. supra-	P	above
150. system/o-	C	the body as a whole
151. systol/o-	C	contracting
152. tachy-	P	fast
153. tele/o-	C	distant
154. tens/o-	C	pressure, tension
155. tetr/a-	C	four
156. theli/o-	C	cellular layer
157. -therapy	S	treatment
158. tibi/o-	C	tibia (shin bone)
159. thorac/o-	C	thorax (chest)
160. thromb/o-	C	thrombus (blood clot)
161. -tic	S	pertaining to
162. -tome	S	instrument used to cut; an area with distinct edges
163. tom/o-	C	a cut, slice, or layer
164. trans-	P	across, through
165. transplant/o-	C	move something to another place
166. tri-	P	three
167. triglycerid/o-	C	triglycerides
168. -trophy	S	development
169. -ule	S	small thing
170. uln/o-	C	ulna (forearm bone)
171. ultra-	P	beyond, higher
172. -um	S	a structure
173. valv/o-	C	valve
174. valvul/o-	C	valve
175. varic/o-	C	varix, varicose vein
176. vascul/o-	C	blood vessel
177. vas/o-	C	blood vessel; vas deferens
178. vegetat/o-	C	growth
179. ven/o-	C	vein
180. ventricul/o-	C	ventricle
181. vers/o-	C	to travel; to turn

Word-Building Exercise (p. 262)

1. ven/o- + -ous — venous
2. peri- + cardi/o- + -al — pericardial
3. vascul/o- + -ature — vasculature
4. my/o- + cardi/o- + -um — myocardium
5. cardi/o- + pulmon/o- + -ary — cardiopulmonary
6. sin/o- + atri/o- + -al — sinoatrial
7. system/o- + -ic — systemic
8. ven/o- + -ule — venule
9. aort/o- + -ic — aortic
10. inter- + ventricul/o- + -ar — interventricular

Matching Exercise (p. 263)

4, 10, 1, 3, 7, 9, 2, 6, 5, 8, 10

Circle Exercise (p. 263)

1. Bradycardia 2. Stenosis 3. Aneurysm 4. Patent foramen ovale

True or False (p. 263)

1. F 2. T 3. T 4. T 5. F 6. F 7. T 8. F 9. F 10. T

Laboratory Test Exercise (p. 264)

PANELS AND PROFILES			TESTS		
968T	✓	Lipid Panel	19687W		Bilirubin (Direct)
315F		Electrolyte Panel	265F		HBsAg
10256F		Hepatic Function Panel	51870R		HB Core Antibody
10165F		Basic Metabolic Panel	1012F	✓	Cardio CRP
10231A		Comprehensive Metabolic Panel	23242E		GGT
10306F		Hepatitis Panel, Acute	28852E		Protein, Total
182Aaa		Obstetric Panel	141A		CBC Hemogram
18T		Chem-Screen Panel (Basic)	21105R		hCG, Qualitative, Serum
554T		Chem-Screen Panel (Basic with HDL)	10321A		ANA
7971A		Chem-Screen Panel (Basic with HDL, TIBC)	80185	✓	Cardio CRP with Lipid Profile
TESTS			26F		PT with INR
56713E		Lead, Blood	232Aaa		UA, Dipstick
2782A		Antibody Screen	42A		CBC with Diff
3556F		Iron, TIBC	20867W	✓	HDL Cholesterol
20933E	✓	Cholesterol	31732E		PTT
3084111E		Uric Acid	34F		UA, Dipstick and Microscopic
53348W		Rubella Antibody	20396R		CEA
27771E		Phosphate	45443E		Hematocrit
2111600E		Creatinine	28571E		PSA, Total
29868W		Testosterone, Total	66902E		WBC count
9704F		Creatinine Clearance	20750E		Chloride
19752E		Bilirubin (Total)	7187W		Hemoglobin
30536Rrr		T3, Total	4259T		HIV-1 Antibody
687T		Protein Electrophoresis	45484R		Hemoglobin A1c
3563444R	✓	Digoxin	67868R		Alk Phosphatase
15214R		Glucose, 2-Hour Postprandial	24984R		Iron
30502E		T3, Uptake	28512E		Sodium
7773E		Platelet Count	17426R		ALT
39685R		Dilantin (phenytoin)	MICROBIOLOGY		
30494R	✓	Triglycerides	112680E		Group A Beta Strep Culture, Throat
26013E		Magnesium	5827W		Group B Beta Strep Culture, Genitals
15586R		Glucose, Fasting	49932E		Chlamydia, Endocervix/Urethra
30237W		T4, Free	6007W		Culture, Blood
28233E		Potassium	2692E		Culture, Genitals
19208W		AST	2649T		Culture, HSV
30163E		TSH	612A		Culture, Sputum
22764R		Ferritin	6262E		Culture, Throat
20008W		Calcium	6304R		Culture, Urine
54726F		Occult Blood, Stool	50286R		Gonococcus, Endocervix/Urethra
51839W		HAV Antibody, Total	6643E		Gram Stain
430A		Blood Group and Rh Type	STOOL PATHOGENS		
28399W		Progesterone	10045F		Culture, Stool
30262E		T4, Total	4475F		Culture, Campylobacter
20289W		Carbon Dioxide	10018T		Culture, Salmonella
1156F		RPR	86140A		E. coli Toxins
30940E		Urea Nitrogen	1099T		Ova and Parasites
17417W		Albumin	VENIPUNCTURE		
28423E		Prolactin	63180		Venipuncture

Word-Building Exercise (p. 265)

1. scler/o- + - therapy — sclerotherapy
2. angi/o- + - graphy — angiography
3. electr/o- + cardi/o- + -gram — electrocardiogram
4. ultra- +son/o- + - graphy — ultrasonography
5. aneurysm/o- + - ectomy — aneurysmectomy
6. valvul/o- + -tome — valvulotome

True or False (p. 265)

1. F 2. T 3. T 4. F 5. F

Matching Exercise (p. 266)

11, 6, 3, 7, 4, 10, 2, 8, 5, 9, 1

Plural Noun and Adjective Spelling p. 266)

1. endothelium		endothelial
2. pericardium		pericardial
3. atrium	atria	atrial

4. ventricle	ventricles	ventricular
5. septum		septal
6. myocardium		myocardial
7. valve	valves	valvular
8. aorta		aortic
9. vein	veins	venous
10. heart		cardiac
11. valve	valves	valvular

Word Analysis Questions (p. 268)

1. hypertension
2. hypertensive
3. CHF congestive heart failure
   CK-MB creatine phosphokinase M bands
   CPR cardiopulmonary resuscitation
   LVH left ventricular hypertrophy
   PMI point of maximal impulse
4. de- reversal of, without
   fibrill/o- muscle fiber, nerve fiber
   -ation a process; being or having
5. vascu/o- blood vessel
   -ar pertaining to
6. cardi/o- heart
   megaly enlargement
7. *Incoherent* means rambling and without logic, not making sense
   Stuporous means impaired consciousness with marked decrease in reaction to external stimuli
   Emergently means urgently

Fact Finding Questions (p. 269)

1. 70–80 beats per minutes 2. Smoking, obesity, and diabetes (also age and hypertension) 3. Cardiac arrest 4. Portable chest x-ray

Critical Thinking Questions (p. 269)

1. Failure of the right side of the heart 2. Failiure of the left side of the heart 3. Hypertension and congestive heart failure 4. Edema and water retention because of her increasing congestive heart failure

Chapter 6 Hematology and Immunology

LABELING EXERCISES (p. 297)

Exercise A

1. eosinophil 2. neutrophil 3. lymphocyte 4. basophil 5. monocyte

Exercise B

1. tonsils and adenoids 2. axillary lymph nodes 3. mediastinal lymph nodes 4. celiac lymph nodes 5. appendix and Peyer's patches 6. inguinal lymph nodes 7. cervical lymph nodes 8. thymus 9. spleen 10. mesenteric lymph nodes 11. red bone marrow

BUILDING MEDICAL WORDS

Combining Forms (p. 298)

1. crowding together 2. basic (alkaline) 3. clotting 4. cell 5. electricity 6. eosin (acidic red dye) 7. red 8. fibrin 9. fiber 10. shaped like a globe; comprehensive 11. shaped like a globe 12. granule 13. blood 14. blood 15. immune response 16. nucleus 17. white 18. lymph; lymphatic system 19. large 20. large 21. one, single 22. shape 23. bone marrow; spinal cord; myelin 24. not taking part 25. normal, usual 26. nucleus 27. oxygen 28. disease, suffering 29. eating, swallowing 30. being formed or shaped 31. small network 32. red 33. spleen 34. press down 35. thrombus (blood clot) 36. thymus 37. poison

Combining Forms and Suffixes (p. 299)

1. hemat/o- + -poiesis	hematopoiesis
2. leuk/o- + -cyte	leukocyte
3. coagul/o- + -ation	coagulation
4. splen/o- + -ic	splenic
5. phag/o- + -cyte	phagocyte
6. lymph/o- + -oid	lymphoid
7. hemat/o- + -logy	hematology
8. erythr/o- + -poietin	erythropoietin
9. eosin/o- + -phil	eosinophil
10. path/o- + -gen	pathogen
11. hem/o- + -stasis	hemostasis
12. thromb/o- + -cyte	thrombocyte
13. fibrin/o- + -gen	fibrinogen
14. myel/o- + blast	myeloblast
15. electr/o- + -lyte	electrolyte
16. immun/o- + -ity	immunity

Combining Forms and Prefixes (p. 299)

1. endo- + toxin	endotoxin
2. a- + granulocyte	agranulocyte
3. poly- + morphonucleated	polymorphonucleated
4. pro- + thrombin	prothrombin

CHAPTER REVIEW EXERCISES

Matching Exercise (p. 322)

6, 15, 16, 12, 9, 4, 13, 8, 5, 14, 11, 7, 3, 1, 10, 2

True or False (p. 322)

1. T 2. T 3. T 4. F 5. F 6. F 7. T 8. F 9. T 10. F

Circle Exercise (p. 323)

1. Blood 2. Red blood cells 3. Fibrin 4. Pathogens 5. Electrolytes 6. IgA 7. Heme 8. Aggregation

Multiple Choice (p. 323)

1. D 2. B 3. D 4. C

Fill in the Blank Exercise (p. 323)

1. A, B, AB, O 2. Neutrophils, eosinophils, basophils 3. polymorphonucleated leukocyte, poly, PMN, seg, segmented neutrophil 4. Spleen, thymus

Matching Exercise (p. 324)

9, 4, 3, 6, 10, 11, 8, 1, 7, 5, 2

Name That Word Part (p. 324)

1. a-	P	away from, without
2. aden/o-	C	gland
3. agglutin/o-	C	clumping, sticking
4. aggreg/o-	C	crowding together
5. -al	S	pertaining to
6. an-	P	without, not
7. angi/o-	C	blood vessel; lymphatic vessel
8. anis/o-	C	unequal
9. -ant	S	pertaining to
10. anti-	P	against
11. apher/o-	C	withdrawal
12. -ar	S	pertaining to
13. -ase	S	enzyme
14. aspir/o-	C	to breathe in, to suck in
15. -ate	S	composed of; pertaining to
16. -ated	S	pertaining to a condition; composed of
17. -atic	S	pertaining to
18. -ation	S	a process; being or having
19. attenu/o-	C	weakened
20. auto-	P	self
21. bas/o-	C	basic (alkaline)
22. bi/o-	C	life; living organisms
23. -blast	S	immature cell
24. -body	S	a substance
25. calc/o-	C	calcium
26. chrom/o-	C	color
27. coagul/o-	C	clotting
28. compromis/o-	C	exposed to danger
29. cortic/o-	C	cortex (outer area)
30. -crasia	S	a mixing
31. -cyte	S	cell
32. cyt/o-	C	cell
33. defici/o-	C	lacking, inadequate
34. different/o-	C	being distinct, different
35. dissect/o-	C	to cut apart
36. dissemin/o-	C	widely scattered throughout the body
37. dys-	P	painful, difficult, abnormal
38. -ectomy	S	surgical excision
39. -ed	S	pertaining to
40. -edema	S	swelling
41. electr/o-	C	electricity
42. embol/o-	C	embolus (occluding plug)
43. -emia	S	blood, substance in the blood
44. -ency	S	condition of being
45. endo-	P	internal, within
46. eosin/o-	C	eosin (acidic red dye)
47. erythr/o-	C	red

48.	-esis	S	condition
49.	excis/o-	C	to cut out
50.	ferrit/o-	C	iron
51.	ferr/o-	C	iron
52.	fibrin/o-	C	fibrin
53.	fibr/o-	C	fiber
54.	fus/o-	C	pouring
55.	-gen	S	that which produces
56.	gen/o-	C	that which produces
57.	glob/o-	C	shaped like a globe; comprehensive
58.	globul/o-	C	shaped like a globe
59.	-gram	C	a record or picture
60.	granul/o-	C	granule
61.	-graphy	S	the process of recording
62.	hemat/o-	C	blood
63.	hem/o-	C	blood
64.	heter/o-	C	other
65.	hyper-	P	above; more than normal
66.	hypo-	P	below; deficient
67.	-ia	S	condition, state, thing
68.	-iac	S	pertaining to
69.	-ial	S	pertaining to
70.	-ic	S	pertaining to
71.	idi/o-	C	unknown; individual
72.	-immune	S	immune response
73.	immun/o-	C	immune response
74.	-in	S	substance
75.	inhibit/o-	C	block; hold back
76.	inter-	P	between
77.	intra-	P	within
78.	-ion	S	action; condition
79.	-ism	S	process; disease from a specific cause
80.	-ist	S	one who specializes in
81.	-ity	S	state; condition
82.	-ization	S	process of making, creating, or inserting
83.	kary/o-	C	nucleus
84.	-kine	S	movement
85.	leuk/o-	C	white
86.	log/o-	C	the study of
87.	-logy	S	the study of
88.	lymph/o-	C	lymph, lymphatic system
89.	ly/o-	C	break down, separate, dissolve
90.	-lysis	S	process of breaking down or dissolving
91.	-lyte	S	dissolved substance
92.	macr/o-	C	large
93.	meg/a-	C	large
94.	megal/o-	C	large
95.	-megaly	C	enlargement
96.	micr/o-	C	small
97.	mon/o-	C	one, single
98.	morph/o-	C	shape
99.	myel/o-	C	bone marrow; spinal cord; myelin
100.	neutr/o-	C	not taking part
101.	norm/o-	C	normal, usual
102.	nucle/o-	C	nucleus
103.	-oid	S	resembling
104.	-oma	S	tumor, mass
105.	opportun/o-	C	well timed, taking advantage of
106.	-opsy	S	the process of viewing
107.	-or	S	person or thing that produces or does
108.	-osis	S	condition, abnormal condition
109.	-ous	S	pertaining to
110.	ox/y-	C	oxygen
111.	pan-	P	all
112.	path/o-	C	disease, suffering
113.	-pathy	S	disease, suffering
114.	-penia	S	deficiency
115.	peripher/o-	C	outer aspects
116.	-phage	S	thing that eats
117.	phag/o-	C	eating, swallowing
118.	-phil	S	attraction to, fondness for
119.	phil/o-	C	attraction to, fondness for
120.	phleb/o-	C	vein
121.	phor/o-	C	to bear, to carry
122.	plasm/o-	C	plasma; formed substance
123.	plast/o-	C	being formed or shaped
124.	-poiesis	S	condition of formation
125.	-poietin	S	a substance that forms
126.	poikil/o-	C	irregular
127.	poly-	P	many, much
128.	pro-	P	before
129.	prote/o-	C	protein
130.	punct/o-	C	hole, perforation
131.	reticul/o-	C	small network
132.	-rrhage	S	excessive flow or discharge
133.	rub/o-	C	red
134.	septic/o-	C	infection
135.	son/o-	C	sound
136.	splen/o-	C	spleen
137.	-stasis	S	condition of standing still, staying in one place
138.	-steroid	S	steroid
139.	suppress/o-	C	press down
140.	-therapy	S	treatment
141.	thromb/o-	C	thrombus (blood clot)
142.	thym/o-	C	thymus
143.	-tic	S	pertaining to
144.	-tomy	S	process of cutting or making an incision
145.	tox/o-	C	poison
146.	trans-	P	across, through
147.	transplant/o-	C	move something to another place
148.	ultra-	P	beyond, higher
149.	-ure	S	system; result of
150.	vaccin/o-	C	giving a vaccine
151.	vascul/o-	C	blood vessel
152.	ven/I-	C	vein
153.	viscos/o-	C	thickness

Matching Exercise (p. 327)

5, 4, 8, 11, 14, 15, 7, 6, 13, 12, 2, 1, 3, 9, 10

True or False (p. 327)

1. F 2. T 3. F 4. T 5. F 6. F 7. F 8. F 9. T 10. T

Multiple Choice (p. 328)

1. C 2. A 3. B 4. D 5. C

Word-Building Exercise (p. 328)

1.	erythr/o- + -cyte	erythrocyte
2.	hem/o- + -rrhage	hemorrhage
3.	hypo- + chrom/o- + -ic	hypochromic
4.	leuk/o- + -emia	leukemia
5.	hem/o- + -lysis	hemolysis
6.	pan- + cyt/o- + -penia	pancytopenia
7.	hem/o- + -phil/o- + -ia	hemophilia
8.	coagul/o- + -ation	coagulation
9.	leuk/o- + -cyte	leukocyte
10.	thromb/o- + cyt/o- + -penia	thrombocytopenia
11.	lymph/o- + -oma	lymphoma

Circle Exercise (p. 329)

1. ferritin level 2. iliac crest 3. MCV 4. INR 5. electrophoresis 6. CD4 count 7. antithrombolytic

Matching Exercise (p. 329)

4, 1, 7, 3, 10, 6, 8, 5, 2, 9

Abbreviation Exercise (p. 329)

5, 8, 11, 6, 1, 9, 3, 2, 7, 4, 10

Fact Finding Questions (p. 330)

1. complete blood count (CBC) 2. m/cmm 3. millions per cubic millimeter 4. platelets 5. thousand

Fact Finding Questions (p. 332)

1. B 2. oral candidiasis, *Pneumocystis carinii* pneumonia 3. acquired immunodeficiency syndrome, *Pneumocystis carinii* pneumonia 4. 500, 100 5. Epivir, Retrovir, Sustiva 6. reverse transcriptase inhibitor drugs 7. CD4 count

Critical Thinking Questions (p. 332)

1. Many years of intravenous heroin use 2. C 3. Because his CD4 count was under 200 and he had an opportunistic infection 4. Weight loss, 128 pounds, wasting of the extremities 5. C 6. In the neck (cervical lymphadenopathy)

Chapter 7 Dermatology

LABELING EXERCISES (p. 347)

Exercise A

1. hair shaft 2. pore 3. sweat gland 4. hair follicle 5. duct of sweat gland 6. vein 7. artery 8. nerve 9. sweat gland 10. epidermis 11. dermis 12. subcutaneous tissue

Exercise B

1. nail root 2. cuticle 3. lunula 4. nail plate 5. nail bed

BUILDING MEDICAL WORDS

Combining Forms (p. 348)

1.	follicu/o-	follicle (small sac)
2.	adip/o-	fat
3.	all/o-	other; strange
4.	coll/a-	fibers that hold together
5.	cutane/o-	skin
6.	cut/i-	skin
7.	derm/a-	skin
8.	dermat/o-	skin
9.	derm/o-	skin
10.	elast/o-	flexing, stretching
11.	erect/o-	to stand up
12.	integu/o-	to cover
13.	integument/o-	skin
14.	kerat/o-	hard, fibrous protein
15.	lip/o-	lipid (fat)
16.	loc/o-	in one place
17.	lun/o-	moon
18.	melan/o-	black
19.	pil/o-	hair
20.	phylact/o-	guarding or protecting
21.	sebace/o-	sebum (oil)
22.	sudor/i-	sweat
23.	system/o-	the body as a whole
24.	theli/o-	tissue layer
25.	ungu/o-	nail

Combining Forms and Suffixes (p. 348)

1.	elast/o- + -in	elastin
2.	ungu/o- + -al	ungual
3.	derm/a- + -tome	dermatome
4.	kerat/o- + -in	keratin
5.	derm/o- + -al	dermal
6.	coll/a- + -gen	collagen
7.	adip/o- + -ose	adipose
8.	melan/o- + -cyte	melanocyte
9.	cutane/o- + -ous	cutaneous
10.	subace/o- + -ous	sebaceous
11.	cut/i- + -cle	cuticle
12.	lip/o- + -cyte	lipocyte
13.	integument/o- + -ary	integumentary
14.	lun/o- + -ula	lunula
15.	integu/o- + -ment	integument

Combining Forms and Prefixes (p. 349)

1.	ex- + foliation	exfoliation
2.	epi- + dermal	epidermal
3.	sub- + cutaneous	subcutaneous
4.	epi- + thelial	epithelial
5.	per- + spiration	perspiration
6.	exo- + -crine	exocrine

CHAPTER REVIEW EXERCISES

Matching Exercise (p. 380)

6, 3, 8, 5, 4, 7, 1, 2, 9

Circle Exercise (p. 380)

1. nail bed 2. keratin 3. hair 4. exfoliation 5. dermatome 6. nail

True or False (p. 380)

1. T 2. F 3. T 4. F 5. T 6. T

Name That Word Part (p. 381)

1.	abras/o-	C	scrape off
2.	actin/o-	C	rays of the sun
3.	adip/o-	C	fat
4.	-al	S	pertaining to
5.	albin/o-	C	white
6.	all/o-	C	other; strange
7.	an-	P	without, not
8.	ana-	P	apart from; excessive
9.	-ancy	S	state
10.	angi/o-	C	blood vessel; lymphatic vessel
11.	-ant	S	pertaining to
12.	anti-	P	against
13.	-ar	S	pertaining to
14.	-ary	S	pertaining to
15.	aspir/o-	C	to breathe in, to suck in
16.	-ate	S	composed of; pertaining to
17.	-ation	S	a process; being or having
18.	auto-	P	self
19.	bas/o-	C	base of a structure
20.	bi/o-	C	life; living organisms
21.	blephar/o-	C	eyelid
22.	carcin/o-	C	cancer
23.	cellul/o-	C	cell
24.	-cere	S	waxy
25.	chem./o-	C	chemical, drug
26.	-cle	S	small
27.	coll/a-	C	fibers that hold together
28.	contus/o-	C	bruising
29.	cortic/o-	C	cortex (outer region)
30.	-crine	S	a thing that secretes
31.	crin/o-	C	secrete
32.	cry/o-	C	cold
33.	cutane/o-	C	skin
34.	cut/i-	C	skin
35.	cyan/o-	C	blue
36.	-cyte	S	cell
37.	-dactyly	S	condition of fingers or toes
38.	de-	P	reversal of, without
39.	-derma	S	skin
40.	derm/a-	C	skin
41.	dermat/o-	C	skin
42.	derm/o-	C	skin
43.	desicc/o-	C	to dry up
44.	diaphore/o-	C	sweating
45.	dynam/o-	C	power; movement
46.	dys-	P	painful, difficult, abnormal
47.	ecchym/o-	C	blood in the tissues
48.	-ectomy	S	surgical excision
49.	-elasma	S	platelike structure
50.	elast/o-	C	flexing, stretching
51.	electr/o-	C	electricity
52.	-eon	S	one who performs
53.	epi-	P	upon, above
54.	erect/o-	C	to stand up
55.	erg/o-	C	activity; work
56.	-ergy	S	activity; process of working
57.	-ery	S	process of
58.	erythemat/o-	C	redmess
59.	esthes/o-	C	sensation, feeling
60.	ex-	P	out, away from
61.	excis/o-	C	to cut out
62.	excori/o-	C	to take out skin
63.	exo-	P	away from, external, outward
64.	extra-	P	outside of
65.	exud/o-	C	oozing fluid
66.	fer/o-	C	to bear
67.	follicul/o-	C	follicle (small sac)
68.	foli/o-	C	leaf
69.	fulgur/o-	C	spark of electricity
70.	fung/o-	C	fungus
71.	gangren/o-	C	gangrene
72.	-gen	S	that which produces
73.	-graft	S	tissue for implant or transplant
74.	hemat/o-	C	blood
75.	hem/o-	C	blood
76.	hidr/o-	C	sweat
77.	hirsut/o-	C	hairy
78.	hyper-	P	above; more than normal

79. hypo-	P	below; deficient
80. -ia	S	state, condition, thing
81. -iasis	S	state of; process of
82. -iatic	S	pertaining to a state or process
83. -ic	S	pertaining to
84. icter/o-	C	jaundice
85. -ile	S	pertaining to
86. -in	S	substance
87. incis/o-	C	to cut into
88. integument/o-	R	skin
89. integu/o-	C	to cover
90. intra-	P	within
91. -ion	S	condition; action
92. -ism	S	process; disease from a specific cause
93. -ist	S	one who specializes in
94. -itis	S	inflammation of
95. -ity	S	state; condition
96. kel/o-	C	tumor
97. kerat/o-	C	hard, firm protein
98. lacer/o-	C	a tearing
99. lip/o-	C	lipid (fat)
100. loc/o-	C	in one place
101. log/o-	C	the study of
102. -logy	S	the study of
103. lun/o-	C	moon
104. malign/o-	C	intentionally causing harm; cancer
105. melan/o-	C	black
106. -ment	S	action; state
107. micr/o-	C	small
108. myc/o-	C	fungus
109. necr/o-	C	death
110. ne/o-	C	new
111. nid/o-	C	nest, focus
112. -oid	S	resembling
113. -oma	S	tumor, mass
114. onych/o-	C	nail
115. -opsy	S	the process of viewing
116. -ose	S	full of
117. -osis	S	condition, abnormal condition
118. -ous	S	pertaining to
119. papill/o-	C	nipplelike protrusion
120. par-	P	beside
121. pedicul/o-	C	lice
122. per-	P	through, throughout
123. petechi/o-	C	petechiae
124. phot/o-	C	light
125. phylact/o-	C	guarding or protecting
126. -phylaxis	S	condition of guarding or protecting
127. -phyma	S	tumor, growth
128. pigment/o-	C	pigment
129. pil/o-	C	hair
130. -plasm	S	growth; formed substance
131. plas/o-	C	growth, formation
132. plast/o-	C	being formed or shaped
133. -plasty	S	process of reshaping by surgery
134. poly-	P	many, much
135. pre-	P	before, in front of
136. prurit/o-	C	itching
137. psor/o-	C	itching
138. rhin/o-	C	nose
139. rhytid/o-	C	wrinkle
140. -rrhage	S	excessive flow or discharge
141. -rrhea	S	flow, discharge
142. rrhe/o-	C	flowing discharge
143. sarc/o-	C	connective tissue
144. schiz/o-	C	split
145. scler/o-	C	hard; sclera (white of the eye)
146. sebace/o-	C	sebum (oil)
147. seb/o-	C	sebum (oil)
148. sect/o-	C	to cut
149. sen/o-	C	old age
150. sensitiv/o-	C	affected by, sensitive to
151. -sis	S	condition; abnormal condition
152. spir/o-	C	breathe
153. squam/o-	C	scalelike structure
154. -steroid	S	steroid
155. sub-	P	below, underneath, less than
156. suct/o-	C	to suck
157. sudor/i-	C	sweat
158. surg/o-	C	operative procedure
159. syn-	P	together
160. system/o-	C	the body as a whole
161. theli/o-	C	tissue layer
162. -therapy	S	treatment
163. -tic	S	pertaining to
164. -tome	S	instrument used to cut; an area with distinct edges
165. topic/o-	C	a specific area
166. trans-	P	across, through
167. trich/o-	C	hair
168. -ula	S	little
169. -um	S	a structure
170. ungu/o-	C	nail
171. vas/o-	C	blood vessel; vas deferens
172. vesic/o-	C	bladder; fluid-filled sac
173. vesicul/o-	C	bladder; fluid-filled sac
174. vir/o-	C	virus
175. xanth/o-	C	yellow
176. xen/o-	C	foreign
177. xer/o-	C	dry

Circle Exercise (p. 383)

1. fissure 2. macule 3. cyst

English and Medical Word Equivalents (p. 384)

1. abrasion 2. furuncle 3. tinea 4. verruca 5. pediculosis 6. scabies 7. urticaria 8. eczema 9. nevus 10. senile lentigo 11. papilloma 12. alopecia 13. decubitus ulcer

Divide and Conquer (p. 384)

1. abrasion		abras/o-	-ion
2. anesthesia	an-	esthes/o-	-ia
3. anhidrosis	an-	hidr/o-	-osis
4. cyanosis		cyan/o-	-osis
5. dermatitis		dermat/o-	-itis
6. dysplastic	dys-	plas/o-	-tik
7. lipoma		lip/o-	-oma
8. neoplasm	ne/o-		-plasm
9. paronychia	par-	onych/o-	-ia
10. pruritic		prur/it/o-	-ic

True or False (p. 384)

1. F 2. F 3. T 4. T 5. F 6. F 7. T

Matching Exercise #1 (p. 385)

5, 9, 1, 10, 12, 3, 11, 2, 4, 6, 8, 7

Circle Exercise (p. 385)

1. flat 2. pustule 3. excoriation 4. eschar 5. trunk 6. cellulitis 7. xanthoma 8. ringworm

Matching Exercise #2 (p. 385)

5, 6, 8, 1, 7, 2, 9, 3, 4

Word-Building Exercise (p. 386)

1. par- + onych/o- + -ia	paronychia
2. an- + hidr/o- + -osis	anhidrosis
3. hemat/o- + -oma	hematoma
4. xer/o- + -derma	xeroderma
5. onych/o- + myc/o- + -osis	onychomycosis
6. seb/o- + -rrhea	seborrhea
7. melan/o- + -oma	melanoma

Matching Exercise (p. 386)

4, 5, 2, 3, 1, 7, 6

Circle Exercise (p. 386)

1. debridement 2. curettage 3. intradermal 4. rhytidectomy 5. incisional biopsy 6. incision and drainage 7. antifungal drugs

Matching Exercise (p. 387)

4, 6, 1, 3, 5, 7, 2

Plural Noun and Adjective Spelling (p. 387)

1. follicle	follicles	follicular
2. skin		cutaneous integumentary

3.	epidermis		epidermal
4.	dermis		dermal
5.	nail		ungual
6.	epithelium		epithelial
7.	vesicle	vesicles	vesicular
8.	pruritus		pruritic
9.	cyanosis		cyanotic
10.	erythema		erythematous
11.	icterus		icteric
12.	necrosis		necrotic
13.	gangrene		gangrenous
14.	verruca	verrucae	
15.	malignancy	malignancies	malignant
16.	keratosis	keratoses	
17.	psoriasis		psoriatic
18.	seborrhea		seborrheic
19.	diaphoresis		diaphoretic

Dictionary Challenge (p. 388)

1. onychophagia — Habitual biting or chewing of the nails
2. onychocryptosis — Ingrown fingernail or toenail
3. trichotillomania — Compulsive hair-pulling with bald spots on one's own head

Word Analysis Questions (p. 390)

1. cellul/o- — cell
   -itis — inflammation of
2. erythematous

Fact Finding Questions (p. 390)

1. pruritus 2. erythematous 3. itchy bumps on the scalp, wheals, hives, welts 4. erythema nodosum 5. welts 6. Integumentary system 7. drug reaction

Critical Thinking Skills (p. 390)

1. macrolide antibiotic drugs 2. erythema nodosum, cellulitis

Chapter 8 Orthopedics (Skeletal)

LABELING EXERCISES (pp. 420–421)

Exercise A

1. mandible 2. maxillary bone 3. zygomatic bone 4. lacrimal bone 5. nasal bone 6. ethmoid bone 7. sphenoid bone 8. frontal bone 9. coronal suture 10. parietal bone 11. temporal bone 12. occipital bone

Exercise B

1. glenoid fossa 2. humerus 3. medial epicondyle 4. radius 5. ulna 6. carpal bones 7. metacarpal bones 8. phalanges

Exercise C

1. femur 2. patella 3. fibula 4. lateral malleolus 5. medial malleolus 6. tibia

Exercise D

1. tarsal bones 2. metatarsal bones 3. phalanges 4. tibia 5. calcaneus

BUILDING MEDICAL WORDS

Combining Forms (p. 422)

1. muscle 2. acetabulum 3. limb; small attached part 4. joint 5. axis 6. calcaneus (heel bone) 7. lattice structure 8. enveloping structure 9. wrist 10. cartilage 11. hollow space 12. neck; cervix 13. cartilage 14. clavicle (collar bone) 15. coccyx (tail bone) 16. body (outer region) 17. rib 18. cranium (skull) 19. shaft of bone 20. growth area upon the end of a bone 21. sieve 22. face 23. femur 24. fibula 25. front 26. socket of a joint 27. humerus (upper arm bone) 28. U-shaped structure 29. ilium (hip bone) 30. ischium (hip bone) 31. tears 32. side 33. ligament 34. lower back; area between the ribs and pelvis 35. malleolus 36. mandible (lower jaw) 37. breast; mastoid process 38. maxilla (upper jaw) 39. middle 40. medulla (inner region) 41. meniscus (crescent-shaped cartilage) 42. nose 43. occipital (back of the head) 44. straight 45. bone 46. ossicle (small bone) 47. changing into bone 48. bone 49. palate 50. wall of a cavity 51. patella (kneecap) 52. child 53. pelvis (hip bone; renal pelvis) 54. fibula (lower leg bone) 55. phalanx (finger or toe) 56. back of the knee 57. pubis (hip bone) 58. radius (forearm bone); x-rays; radiation 59. sacrum 60. scapula (shoulder blade) 61. skeleton 62. wedge shape 63. spine; backbone 64. sternum (breast bone) 65. stake 66. synovium (membrane) 67. ankle 68. temple (side of the head) 69. thorax (chest) 70. tibia (shin bone) 71. trochanter 72. scroll-like structure; turbinate 73. ulna (forearm) 74. vertebra 75. sword 76. zygoma (cheek bone)

Combining Forms and Suffixes (p. 423)

1.	crani/o- + -al	cranial
2.	thorac/o- + -ic	thoracic
3.	cost/o- + -al	costal
4.	mandibul/o- + -ar	mandibular
5.	tars/o- + -al	tarsal
6.	oste/o- + -cyte	osteocyte
7.	ligament/o- + -ous	ligamentous
8.	pelv/o- + -ic	pelvic
9.	phalang/o- + -eal	phalangeal
10.	osse/o- + -ous	osseous
11.	calcane/o- + -al	calcaneal
12.	oste/o- + -clast	osteoclast
13.	vertebr/o- + -a;	vertebral
14.	lumb/o- + -ar	lumbar

CHAPTER REVIEW EXERCISES

Matching Exercise (p. 444)

12, 4, 11, 9, 18, 17, 15, 8, 7, 13, 3, 14, 1, 4, 10, 2, 16, 5, 6

Circle Exercise (p. 444)

1. humerus 2. ossification 3. ilium 4. osteocytes 5. ankle 6. medial epicondyle 7. elbow 8. popliteal 9. clavicle

True or False (p. 445)

1. T 2. T 3. T 4. F 5. T 6. T 7. T

Name That Word Part (p. 445)

1.	-al	S	pertaining to
2.	a-	P	away from, without
3.	-ac	S	pertaining to
4.	acetabul/o-	C	acetabulum (hip socket)
5.	acromi/o-	C	acromion
6.	alg/o-	C	sensation of pain
7.	alges/o-	C	pain
8.	align/o-	C	arranging in a straight line
9.	all/o-	C	other; strange
10.	amputat/o-	C	to cut off
11.	amput/o-	C	to cut off
12.	an-	P	without, not
13.	ankyl/o-	C	fused together
14.	anti-	P	against
15.	appendicul/o-	C	limb; small attached part
16.	-ar	S	pertaining to
17.	arthr/o-	C	joint
18.	articul/o-	C	joint
19.	-ary	S	pertaining to
20.	-ate	S	composed of; pertaining to
21.	-ation	S	a process; being or having
22.	-ative	S	pertaining to
23.	auto-	P	self
24.	axi/o-	C	axis
25.	-blast	S	immature cell
26.	bunion/o-	C	bunion
27.	calcane/o-	C	calcaneus (heel bone)
28.	cancell/o-	C	lattice structure
29.	capsul/o-	C	enveloping structure
30.	carp/o-	C	wrist
31.	cartilagin/o-	C	cartilage
32.	cav/o-	C	hollow space
33.	-centesis	S	procedure to puncture
34.	cervic/o-	C	neck; cervix
35.	chem/o-	C	chemical, drug
36.	chondr/o-	C	cartilage
37.	-clast	S	cell that breaks down substances
38.	clavicu/o-	C	clavicle (collar bone)
39.	coccyg/o-	C	tail bone
40.	comminut/o-	C	break into minute pieces
41.	compress/o-	C	press together
42.	congenit/o-	C	present at birth
43.	coron/o-	C	encircling structure
44.	corpor/o-	C	body
45.	cortic/o-	C	cortex (outer region)
46.	cost/o-	C	rib
47.	crani/o-	C	cranium (skull)
48.	-cyte	S	cell
49.	de-	P	reversal of; without

50. densit/o- C density
51. depress/o- C press down
52. -desis S procedure to fuse together
53. dextro- P right
54. diaphys/o- C shaft of the bone
55. dis- P away from
56. disk/o- C disk
57. -eal S pertaining to
58. -ectomy S surgical excision
59. -ed S pertaining to
60. -ee S person who is the object of an action
61. epiphys/o- C growth area upon the end of a bone
62. ethm/o- C sieve
63. extern/o- C outside
64. extra- P outside of
65. faci/o- C face
66. femor/o- C femur (thigh bone)
67. fibul/o- C fibula (lower leg bone)
68. fixat/o- C to make stable or still
69. fract/o- C break up
70. front/o- C front
71. gener/o- C production; creation
72. gen/o- C arising from; produced by
73. glen/o- C socket of a joint
74. goni/o- C angle
75. -graft S tissue for implant or transplant
76. -gram S a record or picture
77. -graphy S the process of recording
78. hem/o- C blood
79. humer/o- C humerus (upper arm bone)
80. hy/o- C U-shaped structure
81. -ia S condition, state, thing
82. -ial S pertaining to
83. -ic S pertaining to
84. -ics S knowledge, practice
85. ili/o- C ilium (hip bone)
86. -ine S pertaining to
87. inflammat/o- C redness and warmth
88. inject/o- C to throw in
89. inter- P between
90. intra- P within
91. -ion S condition; action
92. ischi/o- C ischium (hip bone)
93. -ist S one who specializes in
94. -itis S inflammation of
95. -ity S state; condition
96. -ization S process of making, creating, or inserting
97. kyph/o- C bent; humpbacked
98. lacrim/o- C tears
99. later/o- C side
100. lev/o- P left
101. ligament/o- C ligament
102. locat/o- C a placing
103. log/o- C the study of
104. lord/o- C swayback
105. lumb/o- C lower back between the ribs and pelvis
106. mal- P bad; inadequate
107. malac/o- C softening
108. malleol/o- C malleolus
109. mandibul/o- C mandible (lower jaw)
110. maxill/o- C maxilla (upper jaw)
111. medi/o- C middle
112. medull/o- C medulla; inner region
113. menisc/o- C meniscus (crescent-shaped cartilage)
114. -ment S action; state
115. meta- P after; subsequent to; transition; change
116. -meter S instrument used to measure
117. -metry S process of measuring
118. mineral/o- C mineral; calcium
119. muscul/o- C muscle
120. myel/o- C bone marrow; spinal cord; myelin
121. nas/o- C nose
122. necr/o- C death
123. non- P not
124. occipit/o- C occiptal (back of the head)
125. -oid S resembling
126. olisthe/o- C slipping
127. -olisthesis S abnormal condition and process of slipping
128. -oma S tumor, mass
129. orth/o- C straight
130. -ory S having the function of
131. -osis S condition, abnormal condition
132. osse/o- C bone
133. ossicul/o- C ossicle (little bone)
134. ossificat/o- C changing into bone
135. oste/o- C bone
136. -ous S pertaining to
137. palat/o- C palate
138. pariet/o- C wall of a cavity
139. patell/o- C patella (kneecap)
140. path/o- C disease, suffering
141. -pathy S disease, suffering
142. ped/o- C child
143. pelv/o- C pelvis (hip bone; renal pelvis)
144. peri- P around
145. perone/o- C fibula (lower leg bone)
146. phalang/o- C phalanx (finger or toe)
147. physic/o- C physical science
148. -physis S growth
149. -phyte S growth
150. -plasty S process of reshaping by surgery
151. poplite/o- C back of the knee
152. por/o- C small openings; pores
153. prosthet/o- C artificial part
154. pub/o- C pubis (hip bone)
155. radi/o- C radius (forearm bone); x-rays; radiation
156. re- P again and again; backward; unable to
157. reduct/o- C to bring back
158. rheumat/o- C painful, inflamed condition
159. sacr/o- C sacrum
160. sagitt/o- C going from front to back
161. sarc/o- C connective tissue
162. scapul/o- C scapula (shoulder blade)
163. scint/i- C point of light
164. scoli/o- C curved, crooked
165. -scope S instrument used to examine
166. scop/o- C examine with an instrument
167. -scopy S process of using an instrument to examine
168. skelet/o- C skeleton
169. sorb/o- C to suck up
170. sphen/o- C wedge shape
171. spin/o- C spine; backbone
172. spir/o- C a coil
173. spondyl/o- C vertebra
174. stern/o- C sternum (breast bone)
175. -steroid S steroid
176. steroid/o- C steroid
177. sym- P together, with
178. synov/o- C synovium (membrane)
179. tars/o- C ankle
180. tempor/o- C temple (side of the head)
181. therap/o- C treatment
182. -therapy C treatment
183. thorac/o- C thorax (chest)
184. tibi/o- C tibia (shin bone)
185. -tic S pertaining to
186. -tion S a process; being or having
187. -tome S instrument used to cut; area with distinct edges
188. tom/o- C a cut, slice, or layer
189. tract/o- C a pulling
190. trans- P across, through
191. transplant/o- C move something to another place
192. trochanter/o- C trochanter
193. turbin/o- C turbinate (scroll)
194. uln/o- C ulna (forearm bone)
195. -ure S system; result of
196. vascul/o- C blood vessel
197. -verse S to travel; to turn
198. vertebr/o- C vertebra
199. xiph/o- C sword
200. zygomat/o- C zygoma (cheek bone)

True or False (p. 448)

1. T 2. T 3. F 4. F 5. T 6. F 7. T 8. F 9. F

Matching Exercise (p. 448)

6, 8, 7, 2, 9, 1, 5, 3, 4

Word-Building Exercise (p. 448)

1. arthr/o- + -pathy	arthropathy
2. arthr/o- + -algia	arthralgia
3. poly- + -dactyly	polydactyly
4. chondr/o- + -oma	chondroma
5. kyph/o- + -osis	kyphosis
6. chondr/o- + -malacia	chondroma
7. oste/o- + arthr/o- + -itis	osteoarthritis

Circle Exercise (p. 448)

1. osteomyelitis 2. avascular necrosis 3. demineralization 4. hemarthrosis 5. pectus excavatum 6. vertebrae 7. comminuted

Circle Exercise (p. 449)

1. goniometer 2. prosthesis 3. arthrodesis 4. rheumatoid arthritis 5. a blood test 6. bone densitometry 7. arthrography 8. orthosis 9. allograft 10. rheumatoid factor

Matching Exercise (p. 449)

3, 6, 5, 2, 7, 1, 4

Plural Noun and Adjective Spelling (p. 450)

1. cranium		cranial
2. mandible		mandibular
3. zygoma	zygomas	zygomatic
4. thorax		thoracic
5. rib	ribs	costal
6. vertebra	vertebrae	vertebral
7. clavicle	clavicles	clavicular
8. phalanx	phalanges	phalangeal
9. ilium		iliac
10. fibula	fibulas	fibular
11. patella	patellae, patellas	patellar
12. scapula	scapulae	scapular

English and Medical Word Equivalents (p. 450)

1. cranium 2. zygoma 3. fontanel, fontanelle 4. maxilla 5. mandible 6. scapula 7. sternum 8. clavicle 9. olecranon 10. phalanx 11. coccyx 2. femur 13. patella 14. tibia 15. calcaneus 16. kyphosis 17. lordosis 18. genu valgum 19. genu varum 20. talipes equinovarus 21. osteophyte 22. hallux

Dictionary Challenge (p. 450)

Answers will vary depending on which medical dictionary you use.

Word Analysis Questions (p. 451)

1. dextr/o-	right
scoli/o-	curved, crooked
-osis	condition; abnormal condition; process
2. True	
3. orth/o-	straight
ped/o-	child
-ist	one who specializes in

Fact Finding Questions (p. 452)

1. tibia 2. right leg 3. vertebrae 4. L 5. anterior-superior iliac spine

Critical Thinking Questions (p. 452)

1. to the right 2. nonsteroidal anti-inflammatory drugs (NSAIDs). Suppress inflammation and decrease pain 3. the degrees of the curvature

Chapter 9 Orthopedics (Muscular)

LABELING EXERCISES (p. 478)

Exercise A

1. slight flexion 2. abduction extension 3. flexion 4. rotation 5. flexion and adduction

Exercise B

1. frontalis muscle 2. temporalis muscle 3. masseter muscle 4. sternocleidomastoid muscle 5. trapezius muscle 6. deltoid muscle 7. triceps brachii muscle 8. biceps brachii muscle 9. brachioradialis muscle 10. latissimus dorsi muscle 11. gluteus maximus muscle 12. gastrocnemius muscle 13 tibialis anterior muscle 14. peroneus longus muscle 15. pectoralis major muscle 16. rectus abdominis muscle 17. rectus femoris muscle

BUILDING MEDICAL WORDS

Combining Forms (p. 480)

1. volunt/o-	done by one's own free will
2. anter/o-	before; front part
3. brachi/o-	arm
4. buccinat/o-	cheek
5. burs/o-	bursa
6. cleid/o-	clavicle (collar bone)
7. contract/o-	pull together
8. cost/o-	rib
9. delt/o-	triangle
10. duct/o-	bring or move; a duct
11. extens/o-	straightening
12. extern/o-	outside
13. fasci/o-	fascia
14. fibr/o-	fiber
15. flex/o-	bending
16. front/o-	front
17. gastr/o-	stomach
18. insert/o-	to put in or introduce
19. intern/o-	inside
20. masset/o-	chewing
21. mast/o-	breast; mastoid bone
22. mitt/o-	to send
23. muscul/o-	muscle
24. my/o-	muscle
25. neur/o-	nerve
26. nucle/o-	nucleus
27. orbicul/o-	small circle
28. pector/o-	chest
29. perone/o-	fibula (lower leg bone)
30. pronat/o-	lying face down
31. radi/o-	radius (lower arm bone); x-rays; radiation
32. recept/o-	receive
33. rotat/o-	rotate
34. stern/o-	sternum (breast bone)
35. supinat/o-	lying on the back
36. tempor/o-	temple (side of the head)
37. tendin/o-	tendon
38. tibi/o-	tibia (shin bone)
39. troph/o-	development
40. vers/o-	to travel; to turn
41. vert/o-	to travel; to turn

Combining Forms and Suffixes (p. 481)

1. rotat/o-	-or	rotator
2. tendin/o-	-ous	tendinous
3. muscul/o-	-ar	muscular
4. flex/o-	-ion	flexion
5. fasci/o-	-al	fascial
6. musculat/o-	-ure	musculature
7. delt/o-	-oid	deltoid
8. volunt/o-	-ary	voluntary
9. masset/o-	-er	masseter
10. orbicul/o-	-aris	obicularis
11. pector/o-	-alis	pectoralis
12. recept/o-	-or	receptor
13. supinat/o-	-ion	supination

CHAPTER REVIEW EXERCISES

Matching Exercise (p. 497)

6, 10; 1, 5; 11; 12; 13; 2; 9; 3, 4, 7, 8

Circle Exercise (p. 497)

1. origin 2. aponeurosis 3. musculature 4. striated 5. thin and thick filaments 6. big toe 7. deltoid 8. tri-

Matching Exercise #1 (p. 498)

5, 3, 7, 4, 8, 2, 6, 1

Recall and Describe (p. 498)

1. The arm is moved away from the midline of the body 2. The upper leg and lower leg are straightened. 3. The palm of the hand is turned downwards toward the floor 4. The head makes a "no" movement from side to

side 5. The lower leg is bent posteriorly. 6. The foot is raised with the top coming closer to the lower leg

Matching Exercise #2 (p. 498)

3, 6, 7, 1, 2, 8, 4, 5, 2

Name That Word Part (p. 499)

1. a- P away from, without
2. ab- P away from
3. ad- P toward
4. -al S pertaining to
5. alges/o- C pain
6. alg/o- C pain
7. -alis S pertaining to
8. an- P without, not
9. -ancy S state
10. -ant S pertaining to
11. anter/o- C before; front part
12. anti- P against
13. -ar S pertaining to
14. -aris S pertaining to
15. -ary S pertaining to
16. -ated S pertaining to a condition; composed of
17. athet/o- C without position or place
18. -ature S system composed of
19. bi- P two
20. bi/o- C life; living organisms; living tissue
21. -body S a structure or thing
22. brachi/o- C arm
23. brady- P slow
24. buccinat/o- C cheek
25. burs/o- C bursa
26. -ceps S head
27. chem/o- C chemical, drug
28. chir/o- C hand
29. cleid/o- C clavicle (collar bone)
30. -clonus S rapid contracting and relaxing of muscles
31. -cnemius S leg
32. -collis S of the neck
33. contract/o- C pull together
34. contus/o- C bruising
35. cortic/o- C cortex (outer region)
36. cost/o- C rib
37. delt/o- C triangle
38. dermat/o- C skin
39. duct/o- C bring or move
40. dys- P painful, difficult, abnormal
41. e- P without, out
42. -ectomy S surgical excision
44. -er S person or thing that produces or does
45. extens/o- C straightening
46. extern/o- C outside
47. fasci/o- C fascia
48. fibr/o- C fiber
49. flex/o- C bending
50. front/o- C front
51. ganglion/o- C ganglion
52. gastr/o- C stomach
53. -gram S record or picture
54. -graphy S process of recording
55. habilitat/o- C give ability
56. hyper- P above; more than normal
57. -ia S condition, state, thing
58. iatr/o- C physician; medical treatment
59. -iatry C medical treatment
60. -ic S pertaining to
61. -ics S knowledge, practice
62. -il S a thing
63. in- P in; within; not
64. incis/o- C to cut into
65. inflammat/o- C redness and warmth
66. inject/o- C insert or put in
67. insert/o- C to put in or introduce
68. inter- P between
69. intern/o- C inside
70. intra- P within
71. -ion S action; condition
72. -ior S pertaining to
73. -itis S inflammation of
74. -kinesis S movement
75. kines/o- C movement
76. malign/o- C intentionally causing harm; cancer
77. masset/o- C chewing
78. mast/o- C breast; mastoid bone
79. mitt/o- C to send
80. mot/o- C movement
81. multi- P many
82. muscul/o- C muscle
83. my/o- C muscle
84. myos/o- C muscle
85. neur/o- C nerve
86. non- P not
87. nucle/o- C nucleus
88. -oid S resembling
89. -oma S tumor, mass
90. -opsy S the process of viewing
91. -or S person or thing that produces or does
92. -ory S having the function of
93. orbicul/o- C small circle
94. orth/o- C straight
95. oste/o- C bone
96. -ous S pertaining to
97. -path S disease, suffering
98. -pathy S disease; suffering
99. pector/o- C chest
100. ped/o- C child
101. perone/o- C fibula (lower leg bone)
102. physi/o- C physical function
103. pod/o- C foot
104. poly- P many, much
105. pract/o- C medical practice
106. pronat/o- C lying face down
107. quadri- P four
108. radi/o- C radius (forearm bone); x-rays; radiation
109. re- P again and again; backward; unable to
110. recept/o- C receive
111. relax/o- C relax
112. rhabd/o- C rod shaped
113. rotat/o- C rotate
114. -rrhaphy S procedure of suturing
115. sarc/o- C connective tissue
116. skelet/o- C skeleton
117. sthen/o- C strength
118. stern/o- C sternum (breast bone)
119. -steroid S steroid
120. steroid/o- C steroid
121. supinat/o- C lying on the back
122. synov/o- C synovium (membrane)
123. tax/o- C movement
124. tempor/o- C temple (side of the head)
125. tendin/o- C tendon
126. tendon/o- C tendon
127. ten/o- C tendon
128. therap/o- C treatment
129. -therapy S treatment
130. thym/o- C thymus
131. tibi/o- C tibia (shin bone)
132. -tic S pertaining to
133. -tomy S process of cutting or making an incision
134. tort/i- C twisted position
135. trans- P across, through
136. tremul/o- C shaking
137. tri- P three
138. troph/o- C development
139. -trophy S development
140. vers/o- C to travel; to turn
141. vert/o- C to travel; to turn
142. volunt/o- C done by one's own free will
143. vuls/o- C to tear away

Word-Building Exercise (p. 501)

1. muscu/o- + -ature musculature
2. flex/o- + -ion flexion
3. tendin/o- + -ous tendinous

4. delt/o- + -oid deltoid
5. perone/o- + -al peroneal
6. pronat/o- + -ion pronation
7. a- + tax/o- + -ic ataxic
8. a- + trophy atrophy
9. my/o- + -pathy myopathy
10. burs/o- + -itis bursitis

Matching Exercise (p. 501)

4, 3, 1, 7, 6, 5, 2, 8, 9

True or False (p. 502)

1. T 2. F 3. F 4. T 5. F 6. F 7. T 8. T 9. T 10. F

Circle Exercise (p. 502)

1. ataxia 2. tendon 3. athetoid 4. avulsion 5. Dupuytren's 6. rhabdomyosarcoma

Multiple Choice (p. 502)

1. a 2. c 3. a 4. b 5. b

Circle Exercise (p. 503)

1. fibromyalgia 2. passive 3. thymectomy 4. incisional biopsy

Define and Match Exercise (p. 503)

1. EMG	electromyography	1	stimulates a muscle with electricity
2. ADLs	activities of daily living	4	an arm
3. NSAID	nonsteroidal anti-inflammatory drug	5	does strengthening exercises and assistive devices
4. RUE	right upper extremity	6	Progressive muscle weakness beginning in childhood
5. OT	occupational therapist	2	tasks at home and on the job
6. MD	muscular dystrophy	7	a drug route
7. IM	intramuscular	3	a drug for muscle pain and inflammation

Plural Noun and Adjective Spelling p. 503)

Singular Noun	Plural Noun	Adjective
1. muscle	muscles	muscular
2. fascia		fascial
3. tendon	tendons	tendinous
4. bursa	bursae	bursal

English and Medical Word Equivalent (p. 503)

1. bruise contusion
2. muscle wasting atrophy
3. wryneck torticollis
4. muscle cramp spasm
5. whiplash hyperflexion-hyperextension injury OR acceleration-deceleration injury

Dictionary Challenge

1. Answers will vary. Some medical dictionaries have the full definition and description under *muscle.* Other medical dictionaries have the full definition and description under *musculus.* 2. A tendon can also be named for the muscle to which it is attached.

Word Analysis Questions (p. 505)

1. my/o	muscle
-pathy	disease of the
2. eti/o-	cause of a disease
-logy	study of the
3. bi/o-	life; living organisms; living tissue
-opsy	process of viewing
4. glutaraldehyde	a liquid tissue fixative or preservative
protocol	a standard written plan

Fact Finding Questions (p. 506)

1. muscle biopsy 2. quadriceps muscle group 3. In the upper leg 4. 3 5. Difficulty climbing stairs; difficulty getting up from a chair or bed 6. red-tan 7. myopathy of undetermined etiology

Critical Thinking Skills

1. b 2. b

Chapter 10 Neurology

LABELING EXERCISES (pp. 531–532)

Exercise A

1. frontal lobe 2. parietal lobe 3. cerebrum 4. occipital lobe 5. cerebellum 6. temporal lobe

Exercise B

1. cranium 2. dura mater 3. arachnoid 4. subarachnoid space 5. pia mater 6. gray matter of the cerebrum (cortex) 7. white matter of the cerebrum

Exercise C

1. cerebrum 2. corpus callosum 3. midbrain 4. cerebellum 5. fourth ventricle 6. medulla oblongata 7. pons 8. hypothalamus 9. thalamus 10. lateral ventricle 11. gyrus 12. sulcus

BUILDING MEDICAL WORDS

Combining Forms (p. 533)

1. gemin/o-	twins; set or group
2. access/o-	supplemental or contributing part
3. affer/o-	bring toward the center
4. arachn/o-	spider, spider web
5. astr/o-	starlike structure
6. audit/o-	the sense of hearing
7. autonom/o-	independent, self-governing
8. cav/o-	hollow space
9. centr/o-	center; dominant part
10. cerebell/o-	cerebellum (posterior part of the brain)
11. cerebr/o-	cerebrum (largest part of the brain)
12. cortic/o-	cortex (outer region)
13. crani/o-	cranium (skull)
14. dendr/o-	branching structure
15. dors/o-	back, dorsum
16. dur/o-	dura mater
17. effer/o-	go out from the center
18. ependym/o-	lining membrane
19. faci/o-	face
20. fiss/o-	splitting
21. front/o-	front
22. gloss/o-	tongue
23. gustat/o-	the sense of taste
24. mening/o-	meninges
25. micr/o-	small
26. mitt/o-	to send
27. mot/o-	movement
28. muscul/o-	muscle
29. myelin/o-	myelin
30. nerv/o-	nerve
31. neur/o-	nerve
32. occipit/o-	occiput (back of the head)
33. ocul/o-	eye
34. olfact/o-	the sense of smell
35. olig/o-	scanty
36. opt/o-	eye, vision
37. parenchym/o-	parenchyma (functional cells of an organ)
38. pariet/o-	wall of a cavity
39. pathet/o-	suffering
40. peripher/o-	outer aspects
41. pharyng/o-	pharynx (throat)
42. recept/o-	receive
43. sens/o-	sensation
44. somat/o-	body
45. spin/o-	spine; backbone
46. tempor/o-	temple (side of head)
47. thalam/o-	thalamus
48. trochle/o-	structure shaped like a pulley
49. ventricul/o-	ventricle (lower heart chamber; chamber in the brain)
50. ventr/o-	front, abdomen
51. vis/o-	sight, vision

Combining Forms and Suffixes (p. 534)

1. cerebr/o-	-al	cerebral
2. neur/o-	-logy	neurology
3. crani/o-	-al	cranial
4. nerv/o-	-ous	nervous
5. audit/o-	-ory	auditory
6. ventricul/o-	-ar	ventricular
7. arachn/o-	-oid	arachnoid
8. mening/o-	-eal	meningeal
9. astr/o-	-cyte	astrocyte
10. spin/o-	-al	spinal
11. dendr/o-	-ite	dendrite
12. effer/o-	-ant	efferent
13. fiss/o-	-ure	fissure

14.	peripher/o-	-al	peripheral
15.	thalam/o-	-ic	thalamic
16.	sens/o-	-ory	sensory

Combining Forms and Prefixes (p. 535)

1.	sym- + pathetic	sympathetic
2.	hypo- + thalamus	hypothalamus
3.	epi- + dural	epidural
4.	sub- + arachnoid	subarachnoid
5.	hemi- + sphere	hemisphere
6.	tri- + geminal	trigeminal

CHAPTER REVIEW EXERCISES

Matching Exercise (p. 564)

7, 15, 9, 11, 12, 4, 2, 1, 14, 13, 8, 6, 5, 10, 3

Circle Exercise (p. 564)

1. cerebrum 2. nose 3. pia mater 4. neuron 5. left hemisphere of the cerebrum 6. below 7. oculomotor 8. acetylcholine

True or False (p. 565)

1. F 2. T 3. F 4. T 5. T 6. T 7. T 8. T

Recall and Relate (p. 565)

1. dura mater, arachnoid, pia mater 2. gyri, sulci 3. hemisphere 4. ependymal 5. hypothalamus 6. hypothalamus

Multiple Choice (p. 565)

1. c 2. b 3. a 4. d

Name That Word Part (p. 566)

1.	-al	S	pertaining to
2.	a-	P	away from, without
3.	access/o-	C	supplemental or contributing part
4.	affer/o-	R	bring toward the center
5.	alges/o-	C	sensation of pain
6.	alg/o-	C	pain
7.	an-	P	without, not
8.	angi/o-	C	blood vessel; lymphatic vessel
9.	-ant	S	pertaining to
10.	anti-	P	against
11.	-ar	S	pertaining to
12.	arachn/o-	C	spider, spider web
13.	arteri/o-	C	artery
14.	arter/o-	C	artery
15.	-ary	S	pertaining to
16.	astr/o-	C	star
17.	-ated	S	pertaining to a condition; composed of
18.	-ation	S	a process; being or having
19.	audit/o-	C	the sense of hearing
20.	autonom/o-	C	independent, self-governing
21.	axi/o-	C	axis
22.	bi/o-	C	life; living organisms; living tissue
23.	blast/o-	C	immature
24.	carp/o-	C	wrist
25.	caus/o-	C	burning
26.	cav/o-	C	hollow space
27.	-cele	S	hernia
28.	centr/o-	C	center; dominant part
29.	cephal/o-	C	head
30.	-cephalus	S	head
31.	cerebell/o-	C	cerebellum
32.	cerebr/o-	C	cerebrum (largest part of the brain)
33.	chem/o-	C	chemical, drug
34.	clon/o-	C	rapid contracting and relaxing of muscles
35.	comat/o-	C	deep unconsciousness
36.	concuss/o-	C	violent shaking or jarring
37.	conduct/o-	C	carrying, conveying
38.	contus/o-	C	bruising
39.	convuls/o-	C	seizure
40.	cortic/o-	C	cortex (outer region)
41.	crani/o-	C	cranium (skull)
42.	cutane/o-	C	skin
43.	-cyte	S	cell
44.	cyt/o-	C	cell
45.	de-	P	reversal of, without
46.	dendr/o-	C	branching structure
47.	diabet/o-	C	diabetes
48.	disk/o-	C	disk
49.	dors/o-	C	back; dorsum
50.	dur/o-	C	dura mater
51.	dys-	P	painful, difficult, abnormal
52.	-eal	S	pertaining to
53.	-ectomy	S	surgical excision
54.	effer/o-	C	go out from the center
55.	electr/o-	C	electricity
56.	-emia	S	blood; substance in the blood
57.	-emic	S	pertaining to blood or a substance in the blood
58.	emiss/o-	C	to send out
59.	encephal/o-	C	brain
60.	-encephaly	S	condition of the brain
61.	endo-	P	innermost, within
62.	-ent	S	pertaining to
63.	-eon	S	one who performs
64.	ependym/o-	C	lining membrane
65.	epi-	P	upon, above
66.	epilept/o-	C	seizure
67.	-er	S	person or thing that does or produces
68.	-ery	S	process of
69.	esthes/o-	C	sensation, feeling
70.	excis/o-	C	to cut out
71.	express/o-	C	communicate
72.	faci/o-	C	face
73.	fibrill/o-	C	muscle fiber, nerve fiber
74.	fibr/o-	C	fiber
75.	fiss/o-	C	splitting
76.	foc/o-	C	point of activity
77.	format/o-	C	structure, arrangement
78.	front/o-	C	front
79.	gemin/o-	C	twins; set or group
80.	-glia	S	substance that holds things together
81.	gli/o-	C	substance that holds things together
82.	glob/o-	C	shaped like a globe; comprehensive
83.	gloss/o-	C	tongue
84.	-gram	S	a record or picture
85.	-graph	S	instrument used to record
86.	-graphy	S	process of recording
87.	gustat/o-	C	the sense of taste
88.	hemat/o-	C	blood
89.	hemi-	P	one half
90.	herni/o-	C	hernia
91.	hydr/o-	C	water; fluid
92.	hyper-	P	above; more than normal
93.	hypo-	P	below; deficient
94.	-ia	S	condition, state, thing
95.	-ic	S	pertaining to
96.	ict/o-	C	seizure
97.	-ile	S	pertaining to
98.	infarct/o-	C	area of dead tissue
99.	inhibit/o-	C	block; hold back
100.	intra-	P	within
101.	-ion	S	action; condition
102.	isch/o-	C	keep back; block
103.	-ist	S	one who specialize in
104.	-ite	S	thing that pertains to
105.	-itis	S	inflammation of
106.	-ity	S	state; condition
107.	-ive	S	pertaining to
108.	kines/o-	C	movement
109.	lamin/o-	C	lamina (flat area on the vertebra)
110.	-lepsy	S	seizure
111.	lex/o-	C	word
112.	log/o-	C	the study of
113.	-logy	S	the study of
114.	lumb/o-	C	lower back between the ribs and pelvis
115.	lymph/o-	C	lymph, lymphatic system
116.	-lysis	S	abnormal condition or process of breaking down or dissolving
117.	magnet/o-	C	magnet
118.	mal-	P	bad, inadequate
119.	malign/o-	C	intentionally causing harm; cancer
120.	meningi/o-	C	meninges
121.	mening/o-	C	meninges
122.	ment/o-	C	mind; chin
123.	micr/o-	C	small
124.	mitt/o-	C	to send

125. mot/o- C movement
126. muscul/o- C muscle
127. myelin/o- C myelin
128. myel/o- C bone marrow; spinal cord; myelin
129. my/o- C muscle
130. narc/o- C sleep, stupor
131. nerv/o- C nerve
132. neur/o- C nerve
133. nuch/o- C neck; nape of neck
134. occipit/o- C occiput (back of the head)
135. ocul/o- C eye
136. -oid S resembling
137. olfact/o- C the sense of smell
138. olig/o- C scanty
139. -oma S tumor, mass
140. -omatosis S abnormal condition of multiple tumors or masses
141. -opsy S the process of viewing
142. opt/o- C eye, vision
143. -or S person or thing that does or produces
144. -ory S having the function of
145. -ose S full of
146. -osis S condition, abnormal condition
147. -ous S pertaining to
148. para- P beside, apart from; two parts of a pair; abnormal
149. parenchym/o- C parenchyma (functional cells of an organ)
150. -paresis S weakness
151. pariet/o- C wall of a cavity
152. pathet/o- C suffering
153. -pathy S disease; suffering
154. peripher/o- C outer aspects
155. peritone/o- C peritoneum
156. pharyng/o- C pharynx (throat)
157. phas/o- C speech
158. phob/o- C fear or avoidance of
159. phot/o- C light
160. pleg/o- C paralysis
161. poly- P many, much
162. potent/o- C being capable of doing
163. pre- P before, in front of
164. psych/o- C mind
165. punct/o- C hole, perforation
166. quadri- P four
167. radicul/o- C spinal nerve root
168. recept/o- C receive
169. retard/o- C to slow down or delay
170. rhiz/o- C spinal nerve root
171. scler/o- C hard; white of the eye
172. sect/o- C to cut
173. sen/o- C old age
174. sens/o- C sensation
175. somat/o- C body
176. somn/o- C sleep
177. spast/o- C spasm
178. -sphere S sphere or ball
179. spin/o- C spine; backbone
180. stere/o- C three dimensions
181. -steroid S steroid
182. sub- P below; underneath; less than
183. surg/o- C operative procedure
184. sym- P together, with
185. syncop/o- C fainting
186. tact/o- C touch
187. tard/o- C late, slow
188. tempor/o- C temple (side of the head)
189. thalam/o- C thalamus
190. -therapy S treatment
191. -tic S pertaining to
192. tom/o- C a cut, slice, or layer
193. -tomy S process of cutting or making an incision
194. ton/o- C pressure, tone
195. tract/o- C pulling
196. trans- P across, through
197. tri- P three
198. trochle/o- C structure shaped like a pulley
199. troph/o- C development
200. -ure S system; result of
201. vascul/o- C blood vessel
202. ven/o- C vein
203. ventricul/o- C ventricle (lower heart chamber; chamber in the brain)
204. ventr/o- C front; abdomen
205. vis/o- C sight, vision

True or False (p. 568)

1. T 2. F 3. F 4. T 5. T 6. F 7. T 8. T

Circle Exercise (p. 569)

1. Shingles 2. Aura 3. Subdural hematoma 4. Parkinson's disease
5. Paresthesias

Matching Exercise (p. 569)

6, 3, 7, 4, 10, 1, 9, 5, 8, 2, 11

Multiple Choice (p. 569)

1. b 2. d 3. d 4. c

Word-Building Exercise (p. 570)

1. intra- + crani/o- + -al intracranial
2. astr/o- + cyt/o- + -oma astrocytoma
3. cephal/o- + alg/o- + -ia cephalgia
4. hemi- + pleg/o- + -ia hemiplegia
5. comat/o- + -ose comatose
6. contus/o- + -ion contusion
7. quadri- + pleg/o- + -ia quadriplegia
8. de- + ment/o- + -ia dementia
9. concuss/o- + -ion concussion
10. neur/o- + -oma neuroma
11. hemat/o- + -oma hematoma
12. mening/o- + -itis meningitis
13. hydr/o- + cephal/o- + -ic hydrocephalic
14. neur/o- + alg/o- + -ia neuralgia
15. neur/o- + -pathy neuropathy

True or False (p. 571)

1. T 2. T 3. F 4. F

Matching Exercise #1 (p. 571)

9, 2, 7, 1, 3, 4, 5, 8, 6

Matching Exercise #2 (p. 571)

7, 3, 5, 8, 2, 4, 6, 1

Matching Exercise (p. 572)

6, 2, 1, 8, 7, 3, 5, 1

Plural Noun and Adjective Spelling (p. 572)

1. thalamus		thalamic
2. astrocyte	astrocytes	
3. cerebellum		cerebellar
4. cerebrum		cerebral
5. cortex	cortices	cortical
6. cranium		cranial
7. gyrus	gyri	gyral
8. meninx	meninges	meningeal
9. nerve	nerves	nervous
10. spine		spinal
11. sulcus	sulci	sulcal
12. ventricle	ventricles	ventricular

Word Analysis Questions (p. 574)

1. neur/o- nerve
   log/o- the study of
   -ic pertaining to
2. para- beside, apart from; two parts of a pair; abnormal
   esthes/o- sensation, feeling
   -ia condidtion, state, thing
3. VER
4. arteri/o- artery
   -graphy process of recording

Fact Finding Questions (p. 575)

1. Paresthesias in her fingers.
2. MS (multiple sclerosis)
   TIA (transient ischemic attack)
   CFS (cerebrospinal fluid)
3. Sensory examination included light touch, pinprick, vibration, position, and 2-point discrimination.

4. Mental status examination included naming current and past presidents, orientation to time, person, and place; and counting backwards by serial 7s.
5. Romberg's sign
6. Paresthesias
7. Blockage of an artery
8. Cerebrospinal fluid

Critical Thinking Questions (p. 575)

1. b 2. Lumbar puncture (spinal tap) 3. Coordination 4. Alteration in memory 5. Multiple sclerosis

Chapter 11 Urology

LABELING EXERCISES (pp. 594–595)

Exercise A

1. renal capsule 2. hilum 3. ureter 4. renal pelvis 5. renal cortex 6. minor calix 7. major calix 8. renal pyramid

Exercise B

1. kidney 2. rectum 3. prostate gland 4. anus 5. urethral meatus 6. urethra 7. penis 8. pubic bone 9. urinary bladder 10. ureter

Exercise C

1. Bowman's capsule 2. glomerulus 3. branch of renal artery 4. distal convoluted tubule 5. collecting duct 6. proximal convoluted tubule 7. loop of Henle

BUILDING MEDICAL WORDS

Combining Forms (p. 595)

1. absorpt/o-	absorb or take in
2. calic/o-	calix
3. cortic/o-	cortex (outer region)
4. dist/o-	away from the center or point of origin
5. electr/o-	electricity
6. erythr/o-	red
7. excret/o-	removing from the body
8. extern/o-	outside
9. filtrat/o-	filtering; straining
10. filtr/o-	filter
11. genit/o-	genitalia
12. glomerul/o-	glomerulus
13. hil/o-	hilum (indentation in an organ)
14. medull/o-	medulla (inner region)
15. mictur/o-	making urine
16. mucos/o-	mucous membrane
17. pelv/o-	pelvis (hip bone; renal pelvis)
18. pen/o-	penis
19. peritone/o-	peritoneum
20. prostat/o-	prostate gland
21. proxim/o-	near the center or point of origin
22. ren/o-	kidney
23. rug/o-	ruga (fold)
24. tub/o-	tube
25. tubul/o-	tube, small tube
26. ureter/o-	ureter
27. urethr/o-	urethra
28. urin/o-	urine; urinary system
29. ur/o-	urine; urinary system
30. vesic/o-	bladder; fluid-filled sac

Combining Form and Suffixes (p. 596)

1. hil/o- + -ar	hilar
2. medull/lo- + -ary	medullary
3. urin/o- + -ation	urination
4. calic/o- + -eal	caliceal
5. ren/o- + -al	renal
6. vesic/o- + -al	vesical
7. prostat/o- + -ic	prostatic
8. glomerul/o- + -ar	glomerular
9. tub/o- + -ule	tubule
10. excret/o- + -ory	excretory
11. filtr/o- + -ate	filtrate

CHAPTER REVIEW EXERCISES

Unscramble, Define, and Match (p. 621)

1. bladder	11	tube from renal pelvis to bladder
2. kidneys	4	proximal and convoluted tubule
3. hilum	9	triangular area in bladder
4. tubule	13	contains renal pyramids
5. sphincter	7	ball of twine
6. rugae	2	paired organs shaped like beans
7. glomerulus	5	ring of muscles around tube
8. capsule	14	tube from bladder to outside of body
9. trigone	1	holds urine
10. prostate	10	male gland around urethra
11. ureter	13	major and minor
12. calix	8	fibrous layer around kidney
13. medulla	3	indentation in an organ
14. urethra	6	fold in the bladder mucosa

Sequencing Exercise (p. 621)

1. renal artery 2. glomerulus 3. Bowman's capsule 4. proximal convoluted tubule 5. loop of Henle 6. distal convoluted tubule 7. collecting duct 8. calix 9. renal pelvis 10. ureter 11. bladder 12. urethra 13. urethral meatus

Name That Word Part (p. 621)

1. -al	S	pertaining to
2. absorpt/o-	C	absorb or take in
3. acid/o-	C	acid (low pH)
4. albumin/o-	C	albumin
5. alges/o-	C	sensation of pain
6. alkal/o-	C	base (high pH)
7. ambulat/o-	C	walking
8. an-	P	without, not
9. angi/o-	C	blood vessel; lymphatic vessel
10. anti-	P	against
11. -ar	S	pertaining to
12. arteri/o-	C	artery
13. -ary	C	pertaining to
14. -ate	S	composed of; pertaining to
15. -ation	S	a process; being or having
16. bacteri/o-	C	bacterium
17. bi/o-	C	life; living organisms; living tissue
18. blast/o-	C	immature; embryonic
19. calcul/o-	C	stone
20. calic/o-	C	calix
21. cali/o-	C	calix
22. cancer/o-	C	cancer
23. carcin/o-	C	cancer
24. catheter/o-	C	catheter
25. -cele	S	hernia
26. chem/o-	C	chemical, drug
27. chron/o-	C	time
28. col/o-	C	colon
29. congenit/o-	C	present at birth
30. contin/o-	C	hold together
31. corpor/o-	C	body
32. cortic/o-	C	cortex (outer region)
33. cutane/o-	C	skin
34. cyst/o-	C	bladder; fluid-filled sac; semisolid cyst
35. -cyte	S	cell
36. dia-	P	complete; completely through
37. diabet/o-	C	diabetes
38. dist/o-	C	away from the center or point of origin
39. dys-	P	painful, difficult, abnormal
40. -eal	S	pertaining to
41. -ectasis	S	dilatation
42. -ectomy	S	surgical excision
43. electr/o-	C	electricity
44. -emia	S	condition of the blood; substance in the blood
45. -emic	S	pertaining to blood or a substance in the blood
46. -ence	S	state of
47. enur/o-	C	to urinate in
48. epi-	P	upon, above
49. erythr/o-	C	red
50. -esis	S	condition
51. -etic	S	pertaining to
52. excret/o-	C	removing from the body
53. extern/o-	C	outside
54. extra-	P	outside of

55. filtrat/o-	C	filtering; straining
56. filtr/o-	C	filter
57. genit/o-	C	genitalia
58. gen/o-	C	arising from; produced by
59. glomerul/o-	C	glomerulus
60. glycos/o-	C	glucose
61. -grade	S	going
62. -gram	S	a record or picture
63. -graphy	S	process of recording
64. hemat/o-	C	blood
65. hem/o-	C	blood
66. hemoglobin/o-	C	hemoglobin
67. hil/o-	C	hilum (indentation in an organ)
68. hyal/o-	C	clear glasslike substance
69. hydr/o-	C	water
70. hypo-	P	below; deficient
71. -ia	S	condition, state, thing
72. -iasis	S	abnormal condition, condition
73. -ic	S	pertaining to
74. -ile	S	pertaining to
75. in-	P	in; within; not
76. -ine	S	pertaining to
77. infect/o-	C	disease within
78. interstiti/o-	C	spaces within a tissue
79. intra-	P	within
80. -ion	S	action; condition
81. -ist	S	one who specializes in
82. -ition	S	a process; being or having
83. -itis	S	inflammation of
84. -ity	S	state; condition
85. -zation	S	process of making, creating, or inserting
86. kal/i-	C	potassium
87. keton/o-	C	ketones
88. leuk/o-	C	white
89. lith/o-	C	stone
90. log/o-	C	the study of
91. -logy	C	the study of
92. -lysis	S	process of breaking down or dissolving
93. lys/o-	C	breaking down or dissolving
94. -lyte	S	dissolved substance
95. medull/o-	C	medulla (inner region)
96. -meter	S	instrument used to measure
97. metr/o-	C	measurement
98. -metry	S	process of measuring
99. micro-	P	small
100. micturi/o-	C	making urine
101. mucos/o-	C	mucous membrane
102. necr/o-	C	death
103. nephr/o-	C	kidney
104. neur/o-	C	nerve
105. noct/o-	C	night
106. olig/o-	C	scanty
107. -oma	S	tumor, mass
108. -opsy	S	process of viewing
109. -ory	S	having the function of
110. -osis	S	condition; abnormal condition; process
111. -ous	S	pertaining to
112. -pathy	S	disease, suffering
113. pelv/o-	C	pelvis (hip bone; renal pelvis)
114. pen/o-	C	penis
115. per-	P	through, throughout
116. peri-	P	around
117. peritone/o-	C	peritoneum
118. -pexy	S	process of surgically fixing in place
119. -plasty	S	process of reshaping by surgery
120. -poietin	S	substance that forms
121. poly-	P	many, much
122. post-	P	after, behind
123. prostat/o-	C	prostate gland
124. protein/o-	C	protein
125. proxim/o-	C	near the center or point of origin
126. -ptosis	S	state of prolapse or drooping; falling
127. pub/o-	C	pubis (hip bone)
128. pyel/o-	C	renal pelvis
129. py/o-	C	pus
130. radic/o-	C	all parts including the root
131. radi/o-	C	radius (forearm bone); x-rays; radiation
132. re-	P	again and again; backward; unable to
133. refract/o-	C	bend or deflect
134. ren/o-	C	kidney
135. resect/o-	C	to cut out and remove
136. retent/o-	C	hold, keep back
137. retro-	P	behind, backward
138. scler/o-	C	sclera; white of the eye
139. -scope	S	instrument used to examine
140. scop/o-	C	examine with an instrument
141. -scopy	S	process of using an instrument to examine
142. sensitiv/o-	C	sensitive to; affected by
143. son/o-	C	sound
144. spasmod/o-	C	spasm
145. -stalsis	S	contraction
146. supra-	P	above
147. suspens/o-	C	hanging
148. -therapy	S	treatment
149. -tic	S	pertaining to
150. tom/o-	C	a cut, slice, or layer
151. -tomy	S	process of cutting or making an incision
152. tox/o-	C	poison
153. trans-	P	across, through
154. transplant/o-	C	move something to another place
155. -tripsy	S	the process of crushing
156. -triptor	S	thing that crushes
157. tub/o-	C	tube
158. tubul/o-	C	tube, small tube
159. -ule	S	small thing
160. ultra-	P	beyond; higher
161. ureter/o-	C	ureter
162. urethr/o-	C	urethra
163. urin/o-	C	urine; urinary system
164. ur/o-	C	urine; urinary system
165. vagin/o-	C	vagina
166. ven/o-	C	vein
167. vesic/o-	C	bladder

Word-Building Exercise (p. 624)

1. urin/o- + -ary	urinary
2. hemat/o- + ur/o- + -ia	hematuria
3. glomerul/o- + scler/o- + -osis	glomerulosclerosis
4. cyst/o- + -cele	cystocele
5. dys- + ur/o- + -ia	dysuria
6. cyst/o- + -it is	cystitis
7. poly- + ur/o- + -ia	polyuria
8. cyst/o- + -scope	cystoscope
9. nephr/o- + lith/o- + -iasis	nephrolithiasis
10. lith/o- + -tripsy	lithotripsy
11. nephr/o- + -tomy	nephrotomy
12. py/o- + ur/o- + ia	pyuria

Matching Exercise (p. 625)

3, 8, 2, 6, 9, 1, 4, 10, 7, 5

Antonyms Exercise (p. 625)

1. chronic 2. polyuria 3. hypospadias 4. microscopic blood 5. incontinence

Synonyms Exercise (p. 625)

1. proteinuria 2. vesicocele 3. bedwetting 4. frank blood 5. Wilms' tumor

True or False (p. 625)

1. T 2. T 3. F 4. F 5. F 6. T 7. F 8. F 9. T 10. T 11. T

Laboratory Test Exercise (p. 626)

PANELS AND PROFILES		
968T		Lipid Panel
315F		Electrolyte Panel
10256F		Hepatic Function Panel
10165F		Basic Metabolic Panel
10231A		Comprehensive Metabolic Panel
10306F		Hepatitis Panel, Acute
182Aaa		Obstetric Panel
18T		Chem-Screen Panel (Basic)
554T		Chem-Screen Panel (Basic with HDL)
7971A		Chem-Screen Panel (Basic with HDL, TIBC)
TESTS		
56713E		Lead, Blood
2782A		Antibody Screen
3556F		Iron, TIBC
20933E		Cholesterol
3084111E	✓	Uric Acid
53348W		Rubella Antibody
27771E		Phosphate
2111600E	✓	Creatinine
29868W		Testosterone, Total
9704F	✓	Creatinine Clearance
19752E		Bilirubin (Total)
30536Rrr		T3, Total
687T		Protein Electrophoresis
3563444R		Digoxin
15214R		Glucose, 2-Hour Postprandial
30502E		T3, Uptake
7773E		Platelet Count
39685R		Dilantin (phenytoin)
30494R		Triglycerides
26013E		Magnesium
15586R		Glucose, Fasting
30237W		T4, Free
28233E		Potassium
19208W		AST
30163E		TSH
22764R		Ferritin
20008W		Calcium
54726F		Occult Blood, Stool
51839W		HAV Antibody, Total
430A		Blood Group and Rh Type
28399W		Progesterone
30262E		T4, Total
20289W		Carbon Dioxide
1156F		RPR
30940E	✓	Urea Nitrogen
17417W	✓	Albumin
28423E		Prolactin

TESTS		
19687W		Bilirubin (Direct)
265F		HBsAg
51870R		HB Core Antibody
1012F		Cardio CRP
23242E		GGT
28852E		Protein, Total
141A		CBC Hemogram
21105R		hCG, Qualitative, Serum
10321A		ANA
80185		Cardio CRP with Lipid Profile
26F		PT with INR
232Aaa		UA, Dipstick
42A		CBC with Diff
20867W		HDL Cholesterol
31732E		PTT
34F	✓	UA, Dipstick and Microscopic
20396R		CEA
45443E		Hematocrit
28571E		PSA, Total
66902E		WBC count
20750E		Chloride
7187W		Hemoglobin
4259T		HIV-1 Antibody
45484R		Hemoglobin A1c
67868R		Alk Phosphatase
24984R		Iron
28512E		Sodium
17426R		ALT
MICROBIOLOGY		
112680E		Group A Beta Strep Culture, Throat
5827W		Group B Beta Strep Culture, Genitals
49932E		Chlamydia, Endocervix/Urethra
6007W		Culture, Blood
2692E		Culture, Genitals
2649T		Culture, HSV
612A		Culture, Sputum
6262E		Culture, Throat
6304R	✓	Culture, Urine
50286R	✓	Gonococcus, Endocervix/Urethra
6643E		Gram Stain
STOOL PATHOGENS		
10045F		Culture, Stool
4475F		Culture, Campylobacter
10018T		Culture, Salmonella
86140A		E. coli Toxins
1099T		Ova and Parasites
VENIPUNCTURE		
63180		Venipuncture

Circle Exercise (p. 627)

1. sound waves 2. IVP 3. nephrectomy 4. shunt 5. UA 6. dialysis 7. contrast dye

Multiple Choice (p. 627)

1. c 2. d 3. a

Define and Match Exercise (p. 627)

1. blood urea nitrogen	7 x-ray after injection of dye
2. cubic centimeter	4 test to determine what is causing an infection and how to treat it
3. chronic renal failure	3 long-term decrease in renal function
4. culture and sensitivity	12 presence in urine means infection
5. extracorporeal shock wave lithotripsy	9 x-ray of the kidneys, ureters, and bladder
6. intake and output	2 unit of measurement of volume of liquid
7. intravenous pyelogram	10 test result reported on a urinalysis
8. potassium	1 blood test that measures kidney function
9. kidneys, ureters, bladder	6 measures consumption and excretion of fluids
10. too numerous to count	11 multiple tests done on 1one urine specimen
11. urinalysis	8 an electrolyte
12. white blood cells	5 shock waves dissolve kidney stone

Plural Noun and Adjective Spelling (p. 628)

1. cortex	cortices	cortical
2. glomerulus	glomeruli	glomerular
3. hilum	hila	hilar
4. kidney	kidneys	renal
5. medulla	medullae	medullary
6. pelvis	pelves	pelvic
7. tubule	tubules	tubular
8. ureter	ureters	ureteral
9. urethra		urethral
10. urine		urinary

Dictionary Challenge (p. 628)

Strangury: Difficulty in urination with pain as the urine comes out drop by drop.

Word Analysis Questions (p. 630)

1. ur/o-	urine; urinary system
log/o-	the study of
-ist	one who specializes in
2. supra-	above
pub/o-	pubis (hip bone)
-ic	pertaining to
3. hemat/o-	blood
ur/o-	urine; urinary system
-ia	condition, state, thing
4. anti-	against
bi/o-	life; living organisms; living tissue
-tic	pertaining to

5. kidneys, ureters, bladder
   intravenous
6. UTI

Fact Finding Questions (p. 630)

1. Clean-caught urine specimen
2. To acidify the urine and decrease the growth of bacteria
3. Renal colic: Severe pain due to spasm of the smooth muscle of the ureter, bladder, or urethra when a stone scrapes the mucosa.
   Suprapubic pain: Pain in the center of the abdomen directly above the pubic bone.
4. Catheterized urine specimen
5. To strain her urine and collect the kidney stone for analysis

Critical Thinking Skills (p. 630)

1. To show that the abdominal pain, nausea, and vomiting could not be from appendicitis. 2. To show that the abdominal pain, nausea, and vomiting was not from pregnancy or an ectopic pregnancy. The patient is in the range of childbearing years. The fact that the husband had a vasectomy and the patient has no other sexual partners (monogamous relationship) rules out a pregnancy or an ectopic pregnancy. 3. Pulse, respirations, and blood pressure are elevated at times of stress and pain. Temperature is only elevated in response to an infectious agent. (Temperature is elevated with strenuous exercise, but there is no indication of this in the patient's history.) 4. No tenderness or vaginal discharge with the vaginal examination rules out the possibility of a cervical or uterine infection. 5. The microscopic hematuria was due to the kidney stone scraping the mucosa of the urinary tract.

Chapter 12 Male Genital and Reproductive Medicine

Labeling Exercises (p. 646)

1. ureter 2. urinary bladder 3. abdominal wall muscles 4. inguinal canal 5. vas deferens 6. pubic bone 7. penis 8. corpus cavernosum 9. corpus spongiosum 10. urethra 11. glans penis 12. urethral meatus 13. testis 14. epididymis 15. scrotum 16. perineum 17. anus 18. bulbourethral gland 19. prostate gland 20. ejaculatory duct 21. seminal vesicles 22. rectum

BUILDING MEDICAL WORDS

Combining Forms (p. 647)

1. adolesc/o-	the beginning of being an adult
2. bulb/o-	bulb
3. didym/o-	testes (twin structures)
4. ejaculat/o-	to expel suddenly
5. erect/o-	to stand up
6. extern/o-	outside
7. fer/o-	to bear
8. genit/o-	genitalia
9. gen/o-	arising from; produced by
10. gon/o-	seed (ovum or spermatozoon)
11. inguin/o-	groin
12. intern/o-	inside
13. interstiti/o-	space within a tissue
14. mit/o-	thread
15. mot/o-	movement
16. pen/o-	penis
17. perine/o-	perineum
18. product/o-	produce
19. prostat/o-	prostate gland
20. puber/o-	growing up
21. scrot/o-	a bag; scrotum
22. semin/i-	spermatozoon; sperm
23. semin/o-	spermatozoon; sperm
24. spermat/o-	spermatozoon; sperm
25. testicul/o-	testis; testicle
26. tub/o-	tube
27. urethr/o-	urethra
28. urin/o-	urine; urinary system

Combining Forms and Suffixes (p. 648)

1. pelv/o- + -ic pelvic
2. scroto- + -al scrotal
3. puber/o- + -ty puberty
4. spermat/o- + -cyte spermatocyte
5. tub/o- + -ule tubule
6. erect/o- + -ion erection
7. adolesc/o- + -ence adolescence
8. genit/o- + -al genital
9. testicul/o- + -ar testicular
10. pen/o- + -ile penile
11. prostat/o- + -ic prostatic
12. ejaculat/o- + -ory ejaculatory
13. mot/o- + -ile motile
14. inguin/o- + -al inguinal

CHAPTER REVIEW EXERCISES

Matching Exercise (p. 660)

14, 5, 15, 8, 7, 11, 3, 6, 12, 13, 4, 16, 1, 2, 10, 9

True or False (p. 660)

1. T 2. F 3. T 4. F 5. F 6. T 7. T 8. T 9. F

Circle Exercise (p. 661)

1. scrotum 2. epididymis 3. seminiferous tubules 4. ejaculatory duct 5. meiosis

Sequencing Exercise (p. 661)

1. seminiferous tubules 2. epididymis 3. vas deferens 4. ejaculatory duct 5. prostatic urethra 6. urethra in the penis 7. urethral meatus

Name That Word Part (p. 661)

1. -al S pertaining to
2. a- P away from, without
3. adolesc/o- C the beginning of being an adult
4. -ad S toward, in the direction of
5. -ancy S state
6. andr/o- C male
7. anti- P against
8. -ar S pertaining to
9. -ary S pertaining to
10. aspir/o- C to breathe in; to suck in
11. -ation S a process; being or having
12. balan/o- C glans penis
13. bi/o- C life; living organisms; living tissue
14. bulb/o- C bulb
15. cancer/o- C cancer
16. -cele S hernia
17. chem/o- C chemical, drug
18. circum- P around
19. cis/o- C to cut
20. clinic/o- C medicine
21. coit/o- C sexual intercourse
22. crypt/o- C hidden
23. -cyte S cell
24. defici/o- C lacking, inadequate
25. didym/o- C testes (twin structures)
26. -didymis S testes (twin structures)
27. digit/o- C digit (finger or toe)
28. dys- P painful, difficult, abnormal
29. -ectomy S surgical excision
30. ejaculat/o- C to expel suddenly
31. -ence S state of
32. -ency S condition of being
33. epi- P upon, above
34. erect/o- C to stand up
35. -esis S condition
36. extern/o- C outside
37. fer/o- C to bear
38. fertil/o- C able to conceive a child
39. -gen S that which produces
40. genit/o- C genitalia
41. gen/o- C arising from; produced by
42. gon/o- C seed (ovum or spermatozoon)
43. -gram S a record or picture
44. -graphy S process of recording
45. gynec/o- C female, woman
46. hyper- P above, more than normal
47. -ia S condition, state, thing
48. -ic S pertaining to
49. -ile S pertaining to
50. -ility S having the quality of
51. immun/o- C immune response
52. in- P in, within, not
53. incis/o- C to cut into
54. inguin/o- C groin
55. intern/o- C inside
56. interstiti/o- C space within a tissue
57. -ion S action; condition
58. -ism S process; disease from a specific cause
59. -ist S one who specializes in
60. -itis S inflammation of
61. -ity S state; condition
62. -ive S pertaining to
63. laborat/o- C workplace; testing place
64. -logy S the study of
65. malign/o- C intentionally causing harm; cancer
66. mast/o- C breast; mastoid bone
67. mit/o- C threadlike structure
68. morph/o- C shape
69. mot/o- C movement
70. olig/o- C scanty
71. -oma S tumor, mass
72. -opsy S the process of viewing
73. orchi/o- C testis
74. orch/o- C testis
75. -ory S having the function of
76. -osis S condition, abnormal condition, process
77. -ous S pertaining to
78. pareun/o- C sexual intercourse
79. pen/o- C penis
80. perine/o- C perineum
81. -pexy S process of surgically fixing in place
82. post- P after, behind
83. pre- P before, in front of
84. product/o- C produce
85. prostat/o- C prostate gland
86. puber/o- C growing up
87. re- P again and again; backward; unable to
88. rect/o- C rectum
89. resect/o- C to cut out and remove
90. -rrhea S flow, discharge
91. scient/o- C knowledge; science
92. -scope S instrument used to examine
93. scrot/o- C a bag; scrotum
94. semin/i- C spermatozoon, sperm
95. semin/o- C spermatozoon, semen
96. son/o- C sound
97. spermat/o- C spermatozoon, sperm
98. sperm/o- C spermatozoon, sperm
99. -stomy S surgically created opening
100. testicul/o- C testis, testicle
101. -therapy S treatment
102. -tic S pertaining to
103. trans- P across, through
104. -trophy S process of development
105. tub/o- C tube
106. -ty S quality or state
107. -ule S small thing
108. ultra- P beyond, higher
109. urethr/o- C urethra
110. urin/o- C urine; urinary system
111. ur/o- C urine; urinary system
112. varic/o- C varix, varicose vein
113. vas/o- C blood vessel; vas deferens
114. venere/o- C sexual intercourse
115. vir/o- C virus
116. -zoon S animal; living thing

Word-Building Skills (p. 663)

1. varicocele 2. genitourinary 3. cryptorchism 4. gynecomastia 5. dyspareunia 6. oligospermia 7. epididymitis 8. spermatogenesis

Circle Exercise (p. 664)

1. breasts 2. balanitis 3. oligospermia 4. dyspareunia 5. syphilis 6. retrovirus 7. phimosis 8. sexual intercourse 9. phimosis 10. human immunodeficiency virus

Matching Exercise (p. 664)

12, 9, 7, 10, 11, 4, 1, 2, 5, 3, 8, 6

Circle Exercise (p. 665)

1. sperm count 2. testicular self-examination 3. orchiopexy 4. gonorrhea 5. erectile dysfunction 6. estrogen

Fill in the Blank Exercise (p. 665)

1. varicocelectomy 2. morphology 3. acid phosphatase 4. ultrasonography 5. digital rectal examination 6. resectoscope 7. vasovasostomy 8. circumcision

Definition Exercise (p. 665)

1. benign prostatic hypertrophy 2. erectile dysfunction 3. gonococcal (gonorrhea) 4. herpes simplex virus 5. prostate-specific antigen 6. sexually transmitted disease 7. transurethral resection of the prostate 8. venereal disease

Plural Noun and Adjective Spelling (p. 666)

1. tubule	tubules	tubular
2. testis	testes	testicular
3. perineum		perineal
4. spermatozoon	spermatozoa	
5. epididymis	epididymides	epididymal
6. prostate		prostatic
7. penis		penile

Proofreading and Spelling Exercise (p. 666)

1. male 2. urethra 3. glans 4. perineal 5. scrotum 6. spermatozoa 7. inguinal 8. epididymis 9. gamete 10. vas deferens 11. seminal 12. prostate 13. reproductive

English and Medical Word Equivalents (p. 666)

1. seminoma 2. dyspareunia 3. erectile dysfunction 4. venereal disease 5. cryptorchism 6. condylomata acuminata 7. benign prostatic hypertrophy

Word Analysis Questions (p. 669)

1. orchi/o- testis
   -pexy process of surgically fixing in place
2. c

Fact Finding Questions (p. 669)

1. back 2. scrotum, testis, epididymis, penis, urethra 3. Transverse incision in the suprapubic skin fold, a scrotal incision 4. True 5. under the skin 6. orchiopexy

Critical Thinking Questions (p. 669)

1. before 2. spermatic cord

Chapter 13 Gynecology and Obstetrics

LABELING EXERCISES (p. 697)

Exercise A

1. labia majora 2. mons pubis 3. clitoris 4. urethral meatus 5. vaginal introitus 6. labia minora 7. anus 8. perineum 9. vulva

Exercise B

1. fallopian tube lumen 2. corpus of uterus 3. uterine cervix 4. vagina 5. cervical os 6. cervical canal 7. broad ligament 8. myometrium 9. endometrium 10. intrauterine cavity 11. corpus luteum 12. fimbriae 13. ovary 14. follicle at time of ovulation 15. fallopian tube 16. uterine fundus

BUILDING MEDICAL WORDS

Combining Forms (p. 698)

1. gon/o-	seed (ovum or spermatozoon)
2. acr/o-	extremity; highest point
3. adnex/o-	accessory connecting parts
4. amni/o-	amnion (fetal membrane)
5. andr/o-	male
6. areol/o-	areola
7. cav/o-	hollow space
8. cephal/o-	head
9. cervic/o-	neck; cervix
10. chorion/o-	chorion (fetal membrane)
11. concept/o-	to conceive or form
12. contract/o-	pull together
13. cyan/o-	blue
14. dilat/o-	dilate, widen
15. efface/o-	do away with; obliterate
16. embryon/o-	embryo; immature form
17. estr/a-	female, woman
18. extern/o-	outside
19. fallopi/o-	fallopian tube
20. fer/o-	to bear
21. fertil/o-	able to conceive and bear a child
22. fet/o-	fetus
23. flex/o-	a bending
24. fratern/o-	close association or relationship
25. fund/o-	fundus (part farthest from the opening)
26. genit/o-	genitalia (internal and external reproductive organs)
27. gen/o-	arising from; produced by
28. gestat/o-	from conception to birth
29. gonad/o-	gonads (ovaries and testes)
30. gynec/o-	female, woman
31. intern/o-	inside
32. involut/o-	enlarged organ returns to normal size
33. isch/o-	keep back; block
34. labi/o-	lip; labium
35. lact/i-	milk
36. lact/o-	milk
37. lob/o-	lobe of an organ
38. mamm/o-	breast
39. men/o-	month
40. menstru/o-	monthly discharge of blood
41. metri/o-	uterus
42. my/o-	muscle
43. nat/o-	birth
44. ne/o-	new
45. obstetr/o-	pregnancy and childbirth
46. o/o-	ovum (egg)
47. ovari/o-	ovary
48. ov/i-	ovum (egg)
49. ovul/o-	ovum (egg)
50. ox/y-	oxygen; quick
51. parturit/o-	to be in labor
52. perine/o-	perineum
53. placent/o-	placenta
54. pregn/o-	being with child
55. product/o-	produce
56. pub/o-	pubis (hip bone)
57. secret/o-	produce; secrete
58. toc/o-	childbirth; labor
59. trop/o-	development
60. umbilic/o-	umbilicus
61. urethr/o-	urethra
62. uter/o-	uterus
63. vagin/o-	vagina
64. vulv/o-	vulva

Combining Forms and Suffixes (p. 699)

1. vagin/o- + -al	vaginal
2. mamm/o- + -ary	mammary
3. uter/o- + -ine	uterine
4. o/o- + -cyte	oocyte
5. ovari/o- + -an	ovarian
6. areol/o- + -ar	areolar
7. ovul/o- + -ation	ovulation
8. men/o- + -arche	menarche
9. cervic/o- + -al	cervical
10. menstru/o- + -ation	menstruation
11. amni/o- + -tic	amniotic
12. lact/o- + -ation	lactation
13. efface/o- + -ment	effacement
14. fet/o- + -al	fetal
15. contract/o- + -ion	contraction
16. obstetr/o- + -ics	obstetrics
17. umbilic/o- + -al	umbilical
18. ov/i- + -duct	oviduct
19. cav/o- + -ity	cavity
20. labi/o- + -al	labial

Two Combining Forms and Suffixes (p. 700)

1. lact/i- + fer/o- + -ous lactiferous
2. my/o- + metr/o- + ial myometrial
3. o/o- + gen/o- + -esis oogenesis
4. ne/o- + nat/o- + -al neonatal
5. ox/y- + toc/o- -in oxytocin
6. acr/o- + cyan/o- + -osis acrocyanosis

Combining Forms and Prefixes (p. 700)

1. re- + productive reproductive
2. post- + natal postnatal
3. intra- + uterine intrauterine
4. endo- + metrial endometrial
5. ante- + flexion anteflexion
6. infra- + mammary inframammary
7. peri- + stalsis peristalsis
8. pre- + natal prenatal
9. tri- + mester trimester

CHAPTER REVIEW EXERCISES

Matching Exercise #1 (p. 734)

4, 2, 4, 1, 8, 3, 2, 3, 6, 7, 4, 6, 1, 5, 2

Matching Exercise #2 (p. 734)

13, 5, 1, 7, 9, 12, 2, 6, 8, 11, 10, 3, 4

Matching Exercise (p. 735)

7, 4, 9, 8, 5, 3, 6, 1, 2

Sequencing Exercise (p. 735)

1. engagement 2. dilation and effacement 3. epidural anesthesia 4. crowning 5. birth of the newborn 6. placenta delivered 7. involution 8. newborn becomes an infant

True or False (p. 735)

1. T 2. F 3. T 4. T 5. T 6. F 7. T 8. F 9. F 10. F 11. F 12. T 13. T

Name That Word Part (p. 736)

1. al S pertaining to
2. a- P away from, without
3. ablat/o- C take away
4. abort/o- C stop prematurely
5. acr/o- C peripheral body parts (head, hands, feet)
6. -ad S toward, in the direction of
7. aden/o- C gland
8. adnex/o- C accessory connecting parts
9. amni/o- C amnion (fetal membrane)
10. -amnios S amnion (fetal membrane)
11. an- P without, not
12. -an S pertaining to
13. anastom/o- C unite two tubular structures
14. -ancy S state
15. andr/o- C male
16. -ant S pertaining to
17. ante- P forward, before
18. anti- P againsdt
19. -ar S pertaining to
20. -arche S beginning
21. areol/o- C small area around the nipple
22. -ary S pertaining to
23. aspir/o- C to breathe in, to suck in
24. -ate S composed of; pertaining to
25. -ation S process; being or having
26. -atory S pertaining to
27. augment/o- C increase in size or degree
28. bi- P two
29. bilirubin/o- C bilirubin
30. bi/o- C life; living organism; living tissue
31. -body S a structure or thing
32. cancer/o- C cancer
33. candid/o- C Candida (a yeast)
34. carcin/o- C cancer
35. cav/o- C hollow space
36. -cele S hernia
37. -centesis S procedure to puncture
38. cephal/o- C head
39. cervic/o- C neck; cervix
40. chem/o- C medicine, drug
41. chol/o- C bile, gall
42. chorion/o- C chorion (fetal membrane)
43. chrom/o- C color
44. colp/o- C vagina
45. concept/o- C to conceive or form
46. con/o- C cone
47. construct/o- C to build
48. contra- P against
49. contract/o- C pull together
50. cry/o- C cold
51. culd/o- C cul-de-sac
52. cyan/o- C blue
53. cyst/o- C bladder; fluid-filled sac; semisolid cyst
54. -cyte S cell
55. cyt/o- C cell
56. depress/o- C press down
57. di- P two
58. dilat/o- C dilate, widen
59. dissect/o- C to cut apart
60. dors/o- C back; dorsum
61. -duct S duct (tube)
62. dur/o- C dura mater
63. dys- P painful, difficult, abnormal
64. eclamps/o- C a seizure
65. ecto- P outside, outermost
66. -ectomy S surgical excision
67. ectop/o- C outside of a place
68. efface/o- C do away with; obliterate
69. embol/o- C embolus (occluding plug)
70. embryon/o- C embryo; immature form
71. -emesis S vomiting
72. -emia S blood; substance in the blood
73. -emic S pertaining to blood or a substance in the blood
74. endo- P innermost, within
75. epi- P upon, above
76. epsi/o- C vulva (female external genitalia)
77. -ery S process of
78. -esis S condition
79. esthes/o- C sensation, feeling
80. estr/a- C female
81. estr/o- C female
82. excis/o- C to cut out
83. extern/o- C outside
84. fallopi/o- C fallopian tube
85. fer/o- C to bear
86. fertil/o- C able to conceive and bear a child
87. fet/o- C fetus
88. fibr/o- C fiber
89. flex/o- C bending
90. -form S having the form of
91. fratern/o- C close association or relationship
92. fund/o- C fundus
93. galact/o- C milk
94. -gen S that which produces
95. gene/o- C gene
96. genit/o- C genitalia
97. gen/o- C arising from; produced by
98. gestat/o- C from conception to birth
99. gest/o- C from conception to birth
100. gonad/o- C gonads (ovaries and testes)
101. gon/o- C seed (ovum or spermatozoon)
102. -gram S a record or picture
103. -graphy S process of recording
104. -gravida S pregnancy
105. gynec/o- C female, woman
106. hem/o- C blood
107. hydratidi/o- C fluid-filled vesicles
108. hydr/o- C water
109. hyper- P above; more than normal
110. hyster/o- C uterus
111. -ia S condition, state, thing
112. -iasis S abnormal condition, condition
113. iatr/o- C physician; medical treatment
114. -ic S pertaining to
115. -ician S a skilled professional or expert
116. -ics S knowledge, practice

117.	-in	S	substance
118.	incis/o-	C	to cut into
119.	induct/o-	C	a leading in
120.	-ine	S	pertaining to
121.	inflammat/o-	C	redness and warmth
122.	infra-	P	below, beneath
123.	inject/o-	C	insert or put in
124.	insemin/o-	C	plant a seed
125.	intern/o-	C	inside
126.	intra-	P	within
127.	involut/o-	C	enlarged organ returns to normal size
128.	-ion	S	action; condition
129.	isch/o-	C	keep back; block
130.	-ist	S	one who specializes in
131.	-itis	S	inflammation of
132.	-ity	S	state; condition
133.	-ive	S	pertaining to
134.	-ization	S	process of making, creating, or inserting
135.	labi/o-	C	lip; labium
136.	lact/i-	C	milk
137.	lact/o-	C	milk
138.	lapar/o-	C	abdomen
139.	later/o-	C	side
140.	lei/o-	C	smooth
141.	leuk/o-	C	white
142.	ligat/o-	C	to tie up or bind
143.	lith/o-	C	stone
144.	lob/o-	C	lobe of an organ
145.	log/o-	C	the study of
146.	-logy	S	the study of
147.	ly/o-	C	break down, separate, dissolve
148.	mal-	P	bad, inadequate
149.	malign/o-	C	intentionally causing harm; cancer
150.	mamm/a-	C	breast
151.	mamm/o-	C	breast
152.	manu/o-	C	hand
153.	mast/o-	C	breast; mastoid process
154.	melan/o-	C	black
155.	men/o-	C	month
156.	menstru/o-	C	monthly discharge of blood
157.	-ment	S	action; state
158.	metri/o-	C	uterus (womb)
159.	metr/o-	C	uterus (womb)
160.	-metry	S	process of measuring
161.	mult/i-	C	many
162.	my/o-	C	muscle
163.	-nate	S	born
164.	nat/o-	C	birth
165.	ne/o-	C	new
166.	nuch/o-	C	neck; nape of neck
167.	null/i-	C	none
168.	obstetr/o-	C	pregnancy and childbirth
169.	-ol	S	chemical substance
170.	olig/o-	C	scanty
171.	-oma	S	tumor, mass
172.	om/o-	C	tumor, mass
173.	o/o-	C	ovum (egg)
174.	oophor/o-	C	ovary
175.	-opsy	S	the process of viewing
176.	-or	S	person or thing that does or produces
177.	-ory	S	having the function of
178.	-osis	S	condition, abnormal condition, process
179.	-ous	S	pertaining to
180.	ovari/o-	C	ovary
181.	ov/i-	C	ovum (egg)
182.	ovul/o-	C	ovum (egg)
183.	ox/y-	C	oxygen; quick
184.	pareun/o-	C	sexual intercourse
185.	pariet/o-	C	wall of a cavity
186.	par/o-	C	birth
187.	-partum	S	childbirth
188.	parturit/o-	C	to be in labor
189.	-pause	S	cessation
190.	paus/o-	C	cessation
191.	ped/o-	C	child
192.	pelv/i-	C	pelvis (hip bone; renal pelvis)
193.	pelv/o-	C	pelvis (hip bone; renal pelvis)
194.	pendul/o-	C	hanging down
195.	peri-	P	around
196.	perine/o-	C	perineum
197.	-pexy	S	process of surgically fixing in place
198.	phor/o-	C	to bear, to carry
199.	phot/o-	C	light
200.	phylact/o-	C	guarding or protecting
201.	physic/o-	C	body
202.	placent/o-	C	placenta
203.	plasm/o-	C	plasma; formed substance
204.	plas/o-	C	growth; formation
205.	-plasty	S	process of reshaping by surgery
206.	-pnea	S	breathing
207.	pne/o-	C	breathing
208.	poly-	P	many, much
209.	post-	P	after, behind
210.	pre-	P	before, in front of
211.	pregn/o-	C	being with child
212.	prim/i-	C	first
213.	pro-	P	before
214.	-probe	S	rodlike instrument
215.	product/o-	C	produce
216.	pub/o-	C	pubis (hip bone)
217.	py/o-	C	pus
218.	radic/o-	C	all parts including the root
219.	re-	P	again and again; backward; unable to
220.	recept/o-	C	receive
221.	rect/o-	C	rectum
222.	reduct/o-	C	to bring back; decrease
223.	retro-	P	behind, backward
224.	-rrhage	S	excessive flow or discharge
225.	rrhag/o-	C	excessive flow or discharge
226.	-rrhaphy	S	process of suturing
227.	-rrhea	S	flow, discharge
228.	salping/o-	C	fallopian tube
229.	-salpinx	S	fallopian tube
230.	sarc/o-	C	connective tissue
231.	-scope	S	instrument used to examine
232.	-scopy	S	process of using an instrument to examine
233.	secret/o-	C	produce; secrete
234.	-some	S	a body
235.	son/o-	C	sound
236.	spir/o-	C	a coil
237.	-stasis-	S	process of contracting
238.	stere/o-	C	three dimensions
239.	surg/o-	C	operative procedure
240.	suspens/o-	C	hanging
241.	tact/o-	C	touch
242.	therapeut/o-	C	treatment
243.	-therapy	S	treatment
244.	-tic	S	pertaining to
245.	toc/o-	C	childbirth; labor
246.	-tomy	S	process of cutting or making an incision
247.	tox/o-	C	poison
248.	trans-	P	across
249.	trop/o-	C	having an affinity for; stimulating; turning
250.	tub/o-	C	tube
251.	-ule	S	small thing
252.	ultra-	P	beyond, higher
253.	umbilic/o-	C	umbilicus
254.	urethr/o-	C	urethra
255.	uter/o-	C	uterus
256.	vagin/o-	C	vagina
257.	-verse	S	to travel; to turn
258.	vers/o-	C	to travel; to turn
259.	vulv/o-	C	vulva
260.	xer/o-	C	dry

Matching Exercise (p. 739)

5, 9, 1, 8, 6, 3, 2, 4, 7

Circle Exercise (p. 739)

1. breasts 2. Amenorrhea 3. Ovarian 4. endometriosis 5. candidiasis 6. Myometritis 7. hemosalpinx 8. breast 9. Prolapsed cord 10. jaundice 11. dyspareunia

Matching Exercise (p. 740)

1, 3, 5, 8, 4, 7, 6, 2

Word-Building Exercise (p. 740)

1.	dys- + men/o- + -rrhea	dysmenorrhea
2.	perrri- + men/o- + paus/o- + -al	perimenopausal
3.	poly- + cyst/o- + -ic	polycystic
4.	an- + -ovul/o- + -ation	anovulation
5.	lei/o- + my/o- + -oma	leiomyoma
6.	retro- + flex/o- + -ion	retroflexion
7.	leuk/o- + -rrhea	leukorrhea
8.	rect/o- + -cele	rectocele
9.	fibr/o- + aden/o- + -oma	fibroadenoma
10.	a- + men/o- + -rrhea	amenorrhea
11.	dys- + plas/o- + -ia	dysplasia
12.	vagin/o- + -itis	vaginitis
13.	ectop/o- + -ic	ectopic

True or False (p. 741)

1. F 2. F 3. F 4. T 5. T 6. F 7. F 8. T 9. T 10. T

Matching Exercise (p. 741)

8, 2, 5, 1, 4, 7, 6, 10, 3, 9

Multiple Choice (p. 742)

1. d 2. d 3. b 4. a

Matching Exercise (p. 742)

5, 10, 8, 12, 11, 13, 3, 7, 9, 8, 4, 6, 1, 12, 14, 2

Plural Noun and Adjective Spelling (p. 743)

1.	areola	areolae	areolar
2.	amnion		amniotic
3.	breast	breasts	mammary
4.	cervix		cervical
5.	fetus	fetuses	fetal
6.	fundus		fundal
7.	gonad	gonads	gonadal
8.	ovary	ovaries	ovarian
9.	ovum	ova	
10.	perineum		perineal
11.	placenta		placental
12.	umbilicus		umbilical
13.	uterus		uterine
14.	vagina		vaginal

English and Medical Word Equivalents (p. 743)

1. mammary glands 2. placenta 3. newborn, neonate 4. amniotic sac 5. Braxton Hicks contractions 6. tubal ligation 7. fontanel 8. uterus 9. nausea (hyperemesis gravidarum)

Word Analysis Questions (p. 745)

1. a. Appropriate for gestational age
   b. estimated date of birth
   c. estimated gestational age
   d. neonatal intensive care unit
   e. spontaneous abortion
2. gestational
3. gestat/o- from conception to birth
   -ion action; condition
   -al pertaining to
4. amniot/o- amnion (fetal membrane)
   -ic pertaining to
5. pre- before, in front of
   nat/o- birth
   -al pertaining to
6. NSVD

Fact Finding Questions (p. 745)

1. Breech presentation 2. version 3. No term deliveries, no premature deliveries, 1 abortion, no living children 4. Molding 5. Yes 6. Anterior fontanel is on the top of the head. Posterior fontanel is at the back of the head

Critical Thinking Questions (p. 745)

1. Intramuscularly 2. Temperature 101.2, possible pneumonia 3. Fetal distress

Chapter 14 Endocrinology

LABELING EXERCISES (p. 768)

Exercise A

1. thyroid gland 2. parathyroid glands 3. pineal body 4. hypothalamus 5. pintuitary gland 6. thymus 7. pancreas 8. adrenal glands 9. ovaries 10. testes

Exercise B

1. thyroid cartilage 2. isthmus of thyroid gland 3. right lobe of thyroid gland 4. trachea 5. tracheal cartilage 6. parathyroid glands 7. left lobe of thyroid gland

BUILDING MEDICAL WORDS

Combining Forms (p. 769)

1.	ovari/o-	ovary
2.	aden/o-	gland
3.	adren/o-	adrenal gland
4.	ag/o-	to lead to
5.	andr/o-	male
6.	antagon/o-	oppose or work against
7.	anter/o-	before; front part
8.	calc/i-	calcium
9.	cortic/o-	cortex (outer region)
10.	crin/o-	secrete
11.	erg/o-	work
12.	estr/a-	female
13.	glandul/o-	gland
14.	gluc/o-	glucose
15.	glyc/o-	glucose
16.	gonad/o-	gonads (ovaries and testes)
17.	home/o-	same
18.	hormon/o-	hormone
19.	inhibit/o-	inhibit; hold back
20.	insul/o-	island
21.	iod/o-	iodine
22.	lact/o-	milk
23.	medull/o-	medulla (inner region)
24.	melan/o-	black
25.	mineral/o-	mineral; calcium; electrolyte
26.	neur/o-	nerve
27.	ox/y-	oxygen; quick
28.	pancreat/o-	pancreas
29.	pituit/o-	pituitary gland
30.	poster/o-	back part
31.	recept/o-	receive
32.	ren/o-	kidney
33.	somat/o-	body
34.	stat/o-	standing still; staying in one place
35.	stimul/o-	exciting, strengthening
36.	testicul/o-	testis, testicle
37.	thalam/o-	thalamus
38.	thym/o-	thymus
39.	thyr/o-	shield-shaped structure (thyroid gland)
40.	thyroid/o-	thyroid gland
41.	toc/o-	childbirth; labor
42.	ton/o-	pressure, tone
43.	trop/o-	having an affinity for or stimulating

Combining Forms and Suffixes (p. 770)

1.	thym/o- + -ic	thymic
2.	hormon/o- + -al	hormonal
3.	andr/o- + -gen	androgen
4.	medull/o- + -ary	medullary
5.	ovari/o- + -an	ovarian
6.	home/o- + -stasis	homeostasis
7.	stimul/o- + -ation	stimulation
8.	thyr/o- + -oid	thyroid
9.	pancreat/o- + -ic	pancreatic
10.	testicul/o- + -ar	testicular

Combining Forms and Prefixes (p. 770)

1.	hypo- + physial	hypophysial
2.	eu- + thyroidism	euthyroidism
3.	para- + thyroid	parathyroid
4.	hypo- + thalamic	hypothalamic

5. pro- + lactin prolactin
6. syn- +ergism synergism

CHAPTER REVIEW EXERCISES

Location Exercise (p. 791)

1. In the brain below the third ventricle; in the cranial cavity 2. In the bony sella turcica; in the cranial cavity 3. Posterior to the hypothalamus; in the cranial cavity 4. In the anterior neck 5. In the anterior neck; on the lobes of the thyroid gland 6. Thoracic cavity behind the sternum 7. In the abdominal cavity behind the stomach 8. In the retroperitoneal cavity on top of the kidneys 9. In the abdominal cavity 10. In the scrotum

Unscramble and Match (p. 791)

1.	insulin	3, 5, 10	anterior pituitary gland
2.	aldosterone	4, 7	posterior pituitary gland
3.	TSH	11	pineal gland
4.	oxytocin	13	thyroid gland
5.	ACTH	1, 6	pancreas
6.	glucagon	2	adrenal cortex
7.	ADH	8	adrenal medulla
8.	epinephrine	12	ovaries
9.	testosterone	9	testes
10.	prolactin		
11.	melatonin		
12.	estradiol		
13.	thyroxine		

Circle Exercise (p. 791)

1. testis 2. ovary 3. parathyroid glands 4. adrenal glands 5. thymus

Name That Word Part (p. 792)

1.	-al	S	pertaining to
2.	acid/o-	C	acid
3.	acr/o-	C	peripheral body parts (head, hands, feet)
4.	act/o-	C	active
5.	aden/o-	C	gland
6.	ad-	P	toward
7.	adrenal/o-	C	adrenal gland
8.	adren/o-	C	adrenal gland
9.	affect/o-	C	to have an influence on
10.	ag/o-	C	to lead to
11.	-an	S	pertaining to
12.	-ance	S	state
13.	andr/o-	C	male
14.	antagon/o-	C	fight against
15.	anter/o-	C	before; front part
16.	anti-	P	against
17.	-ar	S	pertaining to
18.	-ary	S	pertaining to
19.	-ate	S	composed of, pertaining to
20.	-ation	S	a process; being or having
21.	bi/o-	C	life; living organism
22.	-body	S	a structure or thing
23.	calc/i-	C	calcium
24.	calc/o-	C	calcium
25.	carcin/o-	C	cancer
26.	chrom/o-	C	color
27.	congenit/o-	C	present at birth
28.	corti/co-	C	cortex (outer region)
29.	-crine	S	secrete
30.	crin/o-	C	secrete
31.	-cyte	S	cell
32.	cyt/o-	C	cell
33.	dem/o-	C	people; population
34.	dextr/o-	C	sugar
35.	di-	P	two
36.	dia-	P	complete; completely through
37.	diabet/o-	C	diabetes
38.	dips/o-	C	thirst
39.	-drome	S	a running together
40.	-ectomy	S	surgical excision
41.	-edema	S	swelling
42.	-emia	S	blood; substance in the blood
43.	en-	P	in
44.	endo-	P	innermost, within
45.	erg/o-	C	activity; work
46.	estr/a-	C	female
47.	eu-	P	normal; good
48.	fertil/o-	C	able to conceive and bear a child
49.	galact/o-	C	milk
50.	-gen	S	that which produces
51.	genit/o-	C	genitalia (internal and external sex organs)
52.	gestat/o-	C	from conception to birth
53.	gest/o-	C	from conception to birth
54.	gigant/o-	C	giant
55.	globul/o-	C	shaped like a globe
56.	gluc/o-	C	glucose
57.	glyc/o-	C	glucose
58.	glycos/o-	C	glucose
59.	gonad/o-	C	gonads (ovaries and testes)
60.	gynec/o-	C	female, woman
61.	hirsut/o-	C	hairy
62.	home/o-	C	same
63.	hormon/o-	C	hormone
64.	hyper-	P	above; more than normal
65.	hypo-	P	below, deficient
66.	hypophys/o-	C	pituitary gland
67.	-ia	S	condition, state, thing
68.	-ial	S	pertaining to
69.	-ic	S	pertaining to
70.	in-	P	in, without, not
71.	-in	S	a substance
72.	-ine	S	pertaining to
73.	inhibit/o-	C	block; hold back
74.	insulin/o-	C	insulin
75.	insul/o-	C	island
76.	iod/o-	C	iodine
77.	-ion	S	action; condition
78.	-ior	S	pertaining to
79.	-ism	S	process; disease from a specific cause
80.	-ist	S	one who specializes in
81.	-itis	S	inflammation of
82.	-ity	S	state; condition
83.	-ive	S	pertaining to
84.	ket/o-	C	ketones
85.	lact/o-	C	milk
86.	lob/o-	C	lobe
87.	logo-	C	the study of
88.	-logy	S	the study of
89.	mast/o-	C	breast; mastoid bone
90.	medull/o-	C	medulla (inner region)
91.	-megaly	S	enlargement
92.	melan/o-	C	black
93.	men/o-	C	month
94.	mineral/o-	C	mineral; electrolyte
95.	mult/i-	C	many
96.	myx/o-	C	mucus-like substance
97.	nephr/o-	C	kidney; nephron
98.	neur/o-	C	nerve
99.	-nine	S	pertaining to a single chemical structure
100.	nod/o-	C	node (knob of tissue)
101.	non-	P	not
102.	-oid	S	resembling
103.	-ol	S	chemical substance
104.	-oma	S	tumor, mass
105.	-on	S	a substance
106.	-opsy	S	the process of viewing
107.	-or	S	person or thing that produces or does
108.	-ose	S	full of
109.	-osis	S	condition, abnormal condition
110.	oure/o-	C	urine
111.	ovari/o-	C	ovary
112.	ox/y-	C	oxygen; quick
113.	pan-	P	all
114.	pancreat/o-	C	pancreas
115.	para-	P	beside, apart from; two parts of a pair; abnormal
116.	-pathy	S	disease, suffering
117.	-pause	S	cessation
118.	phag/o-	C	eating, swallowing
119.	phe/o-	P	gray
120.	-physis	S	state of growing
121.	pituitar/o-	C	pituitary gland
122.	pituit/o-	C	pituitary gland

123. poly- P many, much
124. poster/o- C back part
125. pro- P before
126. radi/o- C radius (forearm bone); x-rays; radiation
127. recept/o- C receive
128. ren/o- C kidney
129. resist/o- C withstand the effect of
130. retin/o- C retina (of the eye)
131. -rrhea S flow, discharge
132. secret/o- C produce; secrete
133. somat/o- C body
134. sphenoid/o- C sphenoid bone or sinus
135. -stasis S condition of standing still; staying in one place
136. stat/o- C standing still (without growth)
137. -steroid C steroid
138. stimul/o- C exciting, strengthening
139. syn- P together
140. testicul/o- C testis, testicle
141. thalam/o- C thalamus
142. thym/o- C thymus; rage
143. thyr/o- C shield-shaped structure (thyroid gland)
144. thyroid/o- C thyroid gland
145. -tic S pertaining to
146. toc/o- C childbirth; labor
147. ton/o- C pressure, tone
148. -tous S pertaining to
149. toxic/o- C poison; toxin
150. tox/o- C poison
151. trans- P across, through
152. tri- P three
153. trop/o- C having an affinity for; stimulating; turning
154. -ular S pertaining to something small
155. -ule S small
156. ur/o- C urine; urinary system
157. uter/o- C uterus
158. viril/o- C masculine

Matching Exercise (p. 794)

4, 8, 2, 7, 9, 3, 5, 1, 6

True or False (p. 794)

1. T 2. F 3. F 4. F 5. F 6. T 7. F

Divide and Conquer (p. 795)

1. biopsy		bi/o-	-opsy
2. hyperthyroidism	hyper-	thyroid/o-	-ism
3. polydipsia	poly-	dips/o-	-ia
4. thyroidectomy		thyroid/o-	-ectomy
5. thyroiditis		thyroid/o-	-itis
6. adenoma		aden/o-	-oma
7. glycosuria		glycos/o-	-uria
8. endocrinology	endo-	crin/o-	-logy

Word-Building Exercise (p. 795)

1. hyper- + para- + thyroid/o- + -ism hyperparathyroidism
2. poly- + ur/o- + -ia polyuria
3. galact/o- + -rrhea galactorrhea
4. acr/o- + -megaly acromegaly
5. aden/o- + -oma adenoma
6. thyr/o- + -megaly thyromegaly
7. hyper- + glyc/o- + -emia hyperglycemia
8. poly- + dips/o- + -ia polydipsia
9. gynec/o- + mast/o- + -ia gynecomastia
10. aden/o- + -oma + -tous adenomatous

Circle Exercise (p. 796)

1. virilism 2. thyroid scan 3. diabetes insipidus 4. glycosylated hemoglobin 5. thyroid gland 6. calcium 7. estradiol

Matching Exercise (p. 796)

6, 4, 1, 2, 3, 5

Laboratory Test Exercise (p. 797)

PANELS AND PROFILES			TESTS		
968T		Lipid Panel	19687W		Bilirubin (Direct)
315F	✓	Electrolyte Panel	265F		HBsAg
10256F		Hepatic Function Panel	51870R		HB Core Antibody
10165F		Basic Metabolic Panel	1012F		Cardio CRP
10231A		Comprehensive Metabolic Panel	23242E	✓	GGT
10306F		Hepatitis Panel, Acute	28852E		Protein, Total
182Aaa		Obstetric Panel	141A		CBC Hemogram
18T		Chem-Screen Panel (Basic)	21105R		hCG, Qualitative, Serum
554T		Chem-Screen Panel (Basic with HDL)	10321A		ANA
7971A		Chem-Screen Panel (Basic with HDL, TIBC)	80185		Cardio CRP with Lipid Profile
TESTS			26F		PT with INR
56713E		Lead, Blood	232Aaa		UA, Dipstick
2782A		Antibody Screen	42A		CBC with Diff
3556F		Iron, TIBC	20867W		HDL Cholesterol
20933E		Cholesterol	31732E		PTT
3084111E		Uric Acid	34F		UA, Dipstick and Microscopic
53348W		Rubella Antibody	20396R		CEA
27771E		Phosphate	45443E		Hematocrit
2111600E		Creatinine	28571E		PSA, Total
29868W		Testosterone, Total	66902E		WBC count
9704F		Creatinine Clearance	20750E		Chloride
19752E		Bilirubin (Total)	7187W		Hemoglobin
30536Rrr	✓	T3, Total	4259T		HIV-1 Antibody
687T		Protein Electrophoresis	45484R		Hemoglobin A1c
3563444R		Digoxin	67868R		Alk Phosphatase
15214R		Glucose, 2-Hour Postprandial	24984R		Iron
30502E		T3, Uptake	28512E	✓	Sodium
7773E		Platelet Count	17426R		ALT
39685R		Dilantin (phenytoin)	MICROBIOLOGY		
30494R		Triglycerides	112680E		Group A Beta Strep Culture, Throat
26013E		Magnesium	5827W		Group B Beta Strep Culture, Genitals
15586R	✓	Glucose, Fasting	49932E		Chlamydia, Endocervix/Urethra
30237W		T4, Free	6007W		Culture, Blood
28233E	✓	Potassium	2692E		Culture, Genitals
19208W		AST	2649T		Culture, HSV
30163E	✓	TSH	612A		Culture, Sputum
22764R		Ferritin	6262E		Culture, Throat
20008W		Calcium	6304R		Culture, Urine
54726F		Occult Blood, Stool	50286R		Gonococcus, Endocervix/Urethra
51839W		HAV Antibody, Total	6643E		Gram Stain
430A		Blood Group and Rh Type	STOOL PATHOGENS		
28399W		Progesterone	10045F		Culture, Stool
30262E	✓	T4, Total	4475F		Culture, Campylobacter
20289W		Carbon Dioxide	10018T		Culture, Salmonella
1156F		RPR	86140A		E. coli Toxins
30940E		Urea Nitrogen	1099T		Ova and Parasites
17417W		Albumin	VENIPUNCTURE		
28423E	✓	Prolactin	63180		Venipuncture

Abbreviation Exercise (p. 798)

1. IDDM 2. TFTs 3. FBS 4. DKA 5. ADA 6. HgA_{1C} 7. SAD 8. CDE 9. IRS 10. T_3

Plural Noun and Adjective Spelling (p. 798)

Singular Noun	Plural Noun	Adjective
1. hypophysis		hypophysial
2. adenoma	adenomata adenomas	adenomatous
3. cortex	cortices	cortical
4. gland	glands	glandular
5. hormone	hormones	hormonal
6. hypothalamus		hypothalamic
7. medulla	medullae	medullary
8. ovary	ovaries	ovarian
9. pancreas		pancreatic
10. testis	testes	testicular
11. thymus		thymic

Word Analysis Questions (p. 799)

1. endo- innermost, within
   crin/o- secrete
   log/o- the study of
   -ist one who specializes in
2. hypo- below; deficient
   pituitar/o- pituitary gland
   -ism process; disease from a specific cause
3. TSH

Fact Finding Questions (p. 800)

1. Ophthalmologist, endocrinologist
2. Testosterone (patch), thyroid hormone (Synthroid)
3. adrenocorticotropic hormone
   follicle-stimulating hormone
   luteinizing hormone
4. hypothyroidism

Critical Thinking Questions (p. 800)

1. MRI of the brain 2. pituitary gland 3. thyroid hormone replacement (Synthroid) 4. A SOAP note format stands for Subjective (S), Objective (O), Assessment (A), and Plan (P).

Chapter 15 Ophthalmology

LABELING EXERCISES (p. 818)

Exercise A

1. sclera 2. lacrimal gland and ducts 3. iris 4. pupil 5. limbus 6. caruncle 7. lacrimal sac 8. nasolacrimal duct

Exercise B

1. iris 2. lens 3. pupil 4. cornea 5. conjunctivae 6. ciliary body 7. sclera 8. choroids 9. retina 10. fovea 11. macula 12. optic disk 13. optic nerve 14. posterior cavity

BUILDING MEDICAL WORDS

Combining Forms (p. 819)

1. anter/o-	before; front part
2. aque/o-	watery substance
3. capsul/o-	capsule (enveloping structure)
4. cav/o-	hollow space
5. choroid/o-	choroid (middle layer around the eye)
6. cili/o-	hairlike structure
7. conjunctiv/o-	conjunctiva
8. corne/o-	cornea
9. fove/o-	small hollowed-out area
10. fund/o-	fundus (part farthest from the opening)
11. infer/o-	below
12. irid/o-	iris (colored part of the eye)
13. lacrim/o-	tears
14. later/o-	side
15. lenticul/o-	lens
16. limb/o-	edge, border
17. macul/o-	small area or spot
18. medi/o-	middle
19. mi/o-	lessening
20. mydr/o-	widening
21. nas/o-	nose
22. ocul/o-	eye
23. ophthalm/o-	eye
24. opt/o-	eye, vision
25. orbit/o-	orbit (eye socket)
26. poster/o-	back part
27. pupill/o-	pupil
28. retin/o-	retina
29. scler/o-	hard; sclera (white of the eye)
30. scop/o-	examine with an instrument
31. sebace/o-	sebum (oil)
32. stere/o-	three dimensions
33. super/o-	above
34. trabecul/o-	trabecula (mesh)
35. uve/o-	uvea of the eye
36. vis/o-	sight, vision
37. vitre/o-	vitreous humor, transparent substance

Combining Forms and Suffixes (p. 820)

1. corne/o- + -al	corneal
2. retino- + -al	retinal
3. poster/o- + -ior	posterior
4. pupill/o- + -ary	pupillary
5. scler/o- + -al	scleral
6. mydr/o- + -iasis	mydriasis
7. opt/o- + -ic	optic
8. orbit/o- + -al	orbital
9. lenticul/o- + -ar	lenticular
10. aque/o- + -ous	aqueous
11. cav/o- + -ity	cavity
12. vis/o- + -ion	vision
13. vis/o- + -ual	visual

CHAPTER REVIEW EXERCISES

Matching Exercise (p. 841)

8, 3, 9, 11, 5, 7, 0, 4, 12, 1, 2, 6

Circle Exercise (p. 841)

1. iris 2. caruncle 3. sclera 4. optic disk 5. cones 6. II

True or False (p. 841)

1. F 2. F 3. T 4. F 5. T 6. F 7. T

Sequencing Exercise (p. 842)

1. Light rays from object 2. Conjunctiva 3. Cornea 4. Aqueous humor 5. Pupil 6. Vitreous humor 7. Fovea 8. Optic nerve

Name That Word Part (p. 842)

1. -al	S	pertaining to
2. a-	P	away from, without
3. abras/o-	C	scrape off
4. accommod/o-	C	to adapt
5. acu/o-	C	needle; sharpness
6. ambly/o-	C	dimness
7. an-	P	without, not
8. angi/o-	C	blood vessel; lymphatic vessel
9. anis/o-	C	unequal
10. anter/o-	C	before; front part
11. anti-	P	against
12. aque/o-	C	watery substance
13. -ar	S	pertaining to
14. -ary	S	pertaining to
15. -ate	S	composed of; pertaining to
16. -ation	S	a process; being or having
17. bi/o-	C	life; living organisms; living tissue
18. blast/o-	C	immature; embryonic
19. blephar/o-	C	eyelid
20. capsul/o-	C	capsule (enveloping structure)
21. cav/o-	C	hollow space
22. chem/o-	C	chemical, drug
23. choroid/o-	C	choroids (middle layer around the eye)
24. cili/o-	C	hairlike structure
25. coagul/o-	C	clotting
26. conduct/o-	C	carrying, conveying
27. conjug/o-	C	joined together
28. conjunctiv/o-	C	conjunctiva
29. converg/o-	C	coming together
30. corne/o-	C	cornea
31. cor/o-	C	pupil
32. cortic/o-	C	cortex (outer region)
33. cry/o-	C	cold
34. cycl/o-	C	cycle; circle
35. cyst/o-	C	bladder; fluid-filled sac; semisolid cyst
36. dacry/o-	C	lacrimal sac; tears
37. de-	P	reveral of, without
38. diabet/o-	C	diabetes
39. dipl/o-	C	double
40. dys-	P	painful, difficult, abnormal
41. ec-	P	out, outward
42. -ectomy	S	surgical excision
43. -edema	C	swelling
44. emulsific/o-	C	particles suspended in a solution
45. en-	P	in, within, inward
46. -ence	S	state of
47. enucle/o-	C	to remove the kernal or nucleus
48. es/o-	C	inward
49. ex-	P	out, away from
50. ex/o-	C	away from, external, outward
51. extra-	P	outside of
52. fibr/o-	C	fiber
53. fove/o-	C	small, hollowed-out area
54. fund/o-	C	fundus (part farthest from the opening)
55. fundu/o-	C	fundus (part farthest from the opening)
56. gener/o-	C	production; creation
57. goni/o-	C	angle
58. -gram	S	a record or picture
59. -graphy	S	process of recording
60. hemi-	P	one half
61. hyper-	P	above; more than normal
62. -ia	S	condition, state, thing
63. -iasis	S	state of; process of
64. -iatic	S	pertaining to a process or state
65. -ic	S	pertaining to
66. -ician	S	a skilled professional or expert
67. icter/o-	C	jaundice
68. infer/o-	C	below
69. intra-	P	within
70. -ion	S	action; condition
71. -ior	S	pertaining to
72. irid/o-	C	iris (colored part of the eye)
73. ir/o-	C	iris (colored part of the eye)
74. -ism	S	process; disease from a specific cause
75. -ist	S	one who specializes in
76. -itis	S	inflammation of
77. -ity	S	state; condition
78. -ive	S	pertaining to

79. kerat/o- C cornea
80. lacrim/o- C tears
81. later/o- C side
82. lenticul/o- C lens
83. lent/o- C lens
84. limb/o- C edge, border
85. log/o- C the study of
86. -logy S the study of
87. macul/o- C small area or spot
88. matur/o- C mature
89. medi/o- C middle
90. -meter S instrument used to measure
91. metr/o- C measurement
92. -metry S process of measuring
93. micr/o- C small
94. -mileusis S carving procedure
95. mi/o- C lessening
96. mydr/o- C widening
97. nas/o- C nose
98. ocul/o- C eye
99. -oma S tumor, mass
100. ophthalm/o- C eye
101. -opia S vision
102. opt/o- C eye, vision
103. orbit/o- C orbit (eye socket)
104. -osis S condition; abnormal condition; process
105. -ous S pertaining to
106. papill/o- C elevated structure
107. -pathy S disease, suffering
108. peripher/o- C outer aspects
109. -pexy S process of surgically fixing in place
110. phac/o- C lens
111. phak/o- C lens
112. phob/o- C fear or avoidance
113. phor/o- C range
114. phot/o- C light
115. plas/o- C growth, formation
116. -plasty S process of reshaping by surgery
117. pleg/o- C paralysis
118. poster/o- C back part
119. pre- P before, in front of
120. presby/o- C old age
121. -ptosis S state of prolapse or drooping; falling
122. pupill/o- C pupil
123. recess/o- C to move back
124. refract/o- C bend or deflect
125. resect/o- C to cut out and remove
126. retin/o- C retina
127. retro- P behind, backward
128. scler/o- C hard; sclera (white of the eye)
129. -scope S instrument used to examine
130. scop/o- C examine with an instrument
131. -scopy S process of using an instrument to examine
132. scot/o- C darkness
133. sebace/o- C sebum (oil)
134. son/o- C sound
135. stere/o- C three dimensions
136. -steroid S steroid
137. stigmat/o- C point, mark
138. super/o- C above
139. -therapy S treatment
140. therm/o- C heat
141. -tic S pertaining to
142. -tome S instrument used to cut; an area with distinct edges
143. -tomy S process of cutting or making an incision
144. ton/o- C pressure, tone
145. trabecul/o- C trabecula (meshwork)
146. tract/o- C pulling
147. transplant/o- C move something to another place
148. trop/o- C having an affinity for; stimulating; turning
149. -ual S pertaining to
150. ulcerat/o- C ulcer
151. ultra- P beyond; higher
152. uve/o- C urea of the eye
153. vir/o- C virus
154. vis/o- C sight, vision
155. vitre/o- C vitreous humor, transparent substance
156. xer/o- C dry

Word-Building Exercise (p. 844)

1. conjunctiv/o- + -itis — conjunctivitis
2. hyper- + -opia — hyperopia
3. blephar/o- + -itis — blepharitis
4. phot/o- + phob/o- + -ia — photophobia
5. presby/o- + -opia — presbyopia
6. ophthalm/o- + -logy — ophthalmology
7. dipl/o- + -opia — diplopia
8. xer/o- + ophthalm/o- + -ia — xerophthalmia
9. ir/o- + -itis — iritis
10. blephar/o- + -ptosis — blepharoptosis
11. blephar/o- + -plasty — blepharoplasty

Circle Exercise (p. 845)

1. nystagmus 2. hyperthyroidism 3. glaucoma 4. floaters 5. hyperopia

Matching Exercise (p. 845)

10, 7, 5, 2, 3, 4, 11, 6, 1, 9, 8

True or False (p. 845)

1. T 2. F 3. T 4. T 5. F

Matching Exercise #1 (p. 846)

4, 6, 5, 3, 2, 1, 14, 11, 12, 10, 7, 8, 15, 13, 9

Matching Exercise #2 (p. 846)

7, 6, 1, 8, 3, 2, 4, 5

Plural Noun and Adjective Spelling (p. 846)

1.	sclera	sclerae	scleral
2.	iris	irides	iridal
3.	pupil	pupils	pupillary
4.	conjunctiva	conjunctivae	conjunctival
5.	cornea	corneas	corneal
6.	retina	retinas	retinal
7.	macula	maculae	macular
8.	fundus	fundi	fundal

Word Analysis Questions (p. 848)

1. funduscopic
2. intra- — within
   ocul/o- — eye
   -ar — pertaining to
3. an- — without, not
   icter/o- — jaundice
   -ic — pertaining to

Fact Finding Questions (p. 848)

1. Funduscopy examines the fundus, the part farthest from the opening (the pupil). 2. Myopia 3. Scintillating scotomas and temporary visual field defect of a gray curtain coming down. 4. Glaucoma 5. False 6. Pupils equal, round, and reactive to light. 7. OD

Critical Thinking Questions (p. 848)

1. diagnosis #4: blepharitis 2. the sclerae, because they are white and without jaundice 3. pronounced exophthalmia bilaterally

Chapter 16 Otolaryngology

LABELING EXERCISES (p. 868)

Exercise A

1. temporal bone 2. malleus 3. incus 4. stapes 5. oval window 6. semicircular canals 7. vestibular branch of auditory nerve 8. cochlear branch of auditory nerve 9. cochlea 10. vestibule 11. pharynx 12. eustachian tube 13. round window 14. tympanic membrane 15. external auditory canal

Exercise B

1. frontal sinus 2. turbinates 3. nasal cavity 4. hard palate 5. mandible 6. tongue 7. oral cavity 8. larynx 9. hypopharynx 10. epiglottis 11. oropharynx 12. lingual tonsil 13. palatine tonsil 14. nasopharynx 15. soft palate 16. adenoids 17. entrance to eustachian tube 18. sphenoid sinus

BUILDING MEDICAL WORDS

Combining Forms (p. 869)

1. aden/o- — gland

2. audit/o-	the sense of hearing
3. aur/i-	ear
4. auricul/o-	ear
5. bucc/o-	cheek
6. cav/o-	hollow space
7. cochle/o-	cochlea (of the inner ear)
8. dors/o-	back; dorsum; uppermost part
9. ethm/o-	sieve
10. extern/o-	outside
11. front/o-	front
12. gloss/o-	tongue
13. glott/o-	glottis (in the larynx)
14. incud/o-	incus (anvil-shaped bone)
15. infer/o-	below
16. labi/o-	lip; labium
17. laryng/o-	larynx (voice box)
18. lingu/o-	tongue
19. malle/o-	malleus (hammer-shaped bone)
20. mandibul/o-	mandible (lower jaw)
21. mast/o-	breast; mastoid process
22. maxill/o-	maxilla (upper jaw)
23. ment/o-	mind; chin
24. mucos/o-	mucous membrane
25. nas/o-	nose
26. or/o-	mouth
27. ossicul/o-	ossicle (little bone)
28. palat/o-	palate
29. pharyng/o-	pharynx, throat
30. sept/o-	septum (dividing wall)
31. sphen/o-	wedge shape
32. staped/o-	stapes (stirrup-shaped bone)
33. super/o-	above
34. tempor/o-	temple (side of the head)
35. tonsill/o-	tonsil
36. turbin/o-	turbinate (scroll-like structure)
37. tympan/o-	tympanic membrane (eardrum)
38. vestibul/o-	vestibule (entrance)
39. voc/o-	voice

Combining Forms and Suffixes (p. 870)

1. aur/i-	-cle	auricle
2. nas/o-	-al	nasal
3. audito-	-ory	auditory
4. tympano-	-ic	tympanic
5. septo-	-al	septal
6. turbino-	-ate	turbinate
7. tonsillo-	-ar	tonsillar
8. bucc/o-	-al	buccal
9. staped/o-	-ial	stapedial
10. ethm/o-	-oid	ethmoid
11. pharyng/o-	-eal	pharyngeal
12. gloss/o-	-al	glossal
13. palat/o-	-ine	palatine

CHAPTER REVIEW EXERCISES

Matching Exercise (p. 889)

5, 13, 17; 6, 7, 15, 20; 3, 11, 14; 2, 8, 12; 4, 9, 18; 19; 0; 1, 10, 16

True or False (p. 889)

1. T 2. F 3. T 4. T 5. T 6. F 7. F 8. T

Sequencing Exercise (p. 890)

1. External auditory canal 2. tympanic membrane 3. malleus 4. incus 5. stapes 6. oval window 7. vestibule 8. cochlea 9. auditory nerve 10. auditory cortex of brain

Name That Word Part (p. 890)

1. -al	S	pertaining to
2. acous/o-	C	hearing, sound
3. -acusis	S	hearing
4. aden/o-	C	gland
5. alg/o-	C	pain
6. allerg/o-	C	allergy
7. an-	P	without, not
8. -ant	S	pertaining to
9. anti-	P	against
10. -ar	S	pertaining to
11. -ary	S	pertaining to
12. -ate	S	composed of; pertaining to
13. -ative	S	pertaining to
14. audi/o-	C	the sense of hearing
15. audit/o-	C	the sense of hearing
16. aur/i-	C	ear
17. auricul/o-	C	ear
18. bi-	P	two
19. bi/o-	C	life; living organisms; living tissue
20. bucc/o-	C	cheek
21. carcin/o-	C	cancer
22. cav/o-	C	hollow space
23. cervic/o-	C	neck; cervix
24. cheil/o-	C	lip
25. chem/o-	C	chemical, drug
26. -cle	S	small
27. -coccus	S	spherical bacterium
28. cochle/o-	C	cochlea (of the inner ear)
29. conduct/o-	C	carrying, conveying
30. congest/o-	C	accumulation of fluid
31. cortic/o-	C	cortex (outer area)
32. de-	P	reversal of, without
33. dissect/o-	C	to cut apart
34. dors/o-	C	back; dorsum; uppermost part
35. -drome	S	a running
36. -eal	S	pertaining to
37. -ectomy	S	surgical excision
38. effus/o-	C	a pouring out
39. endo-	P	innermost, within
40. epi-	P	upon, above
41. ethm/o-	C	sieve
42. extern/o-	C	outside
43. faci/o-	C	face
44. front/o-	C	front
45. gloss/o-	C	tongue
46. glott/o-	C	glottis (in the larynx)
47. -gram	S	a record or picture
48. hyper-	P	above; more than normal
49. hypo-	P	below; deficient
50. -ia	S	condition, state, thing
51. -ial	S	pertaining to
52. -ic	S	pertaining to
53. impact/o-	C	wedged in
54. incud/o-	C	incus (anvil-shaped bone)
55. -ine	S	pertaining to
56. -ion	S	action; condition
57. -ist	S	one who specializes in
58. -itis	S	inflammation of
59. -ity	S	state; condition
60. -ive	S	pertaining to
61. labi/o-	C	lip; labium
62. labyrinth/o-	C	labyrinth (in the inner ear)
63. laryng/o-	C	larynx (voice box)
64. later/o-	C	side
65. leuk/o-	C	white
66. lingu/o-	C	tongue
67. log/o-	C	the study of
68. -logy	S	the study of
69. lymph/o-	C	lymph; lymphatic system
70. malign/o-	C	intentionally causing harm; cancer
71. malle/o-	C	malleus (hammer-shaped bone)
72. mandibul/o-	C	mandible (lower jaw)
73. mast/o-	C	breast; mastoid process
74. mastoid/o-	C	mastoid process
75. maxill/o-	C	maxilla (upper jaw)
76. ment/o-	C	mind; chin
77. -meter	S	instrument used to measure
78. -metry	S	process of measuring
79. mucos/o-	C	mucous membrane
80. myring/o-	C	tympanic membrane (eardrum)
81. nas/o-	C	nose
82. neur/o-	C	nerve
83. -oid	S	resembling
84. -oma	S	tumor, mass
85. or/o-	C	mouth
86. -ory	S	having the function of

87.	osm/o-	C	the sense of smell
88.	-ous	S	pertaining to
89.	-osis	S	condition; abnormal condition; process
90.	ossicul/o-	C	ossicle (little bone)
91.	ot/o-	C	ear
92.	palat/o-	C	palate
93.	pan-	P	all
94.	para-	P	beside; apart from; two parts of a pair; abnormal
95.	-pathy	S	disease, suffering
96.	pharyng/o-	C	pharynx (throat)
97.	-pharynx	S	pharynx (throat)
98.	-phyma	S	tumor, growth
99.	plak/o-	C	plaque
100.	-plasty	S	process of reshaping by surgery
101.	polyp/o-	C	polyp
102.	post-	P	after, behind
103.	presby/o-	C	old age
104.	radicul/o-	C	all parts including the root
105.	rhin/o-	C	nose
106.	-rrhea	S	flow, discharge
107.	scler/o-	C	hard; sclera (white of the eye)
108.	-scope	S	instrument used to examine
109.	scop/o-	C	examine with an instrument
110.	-scopy	S	process of using an instrument to examine
111.	sensitiv/o-	C	affected by, sensitive to
112.	sensor/i-	C	sensory
113.	sept/o-	C	septum (dividing wall)
114.	ser/o-	C	serum of the blood; serumlike
115.	sinus/o-	C	sinus
116.	sphen/o-	C	wedge shape
117.	staped/o-	C	stapes (stirrup-shaped bone)
118.	-steroid	S	steroid
119.	-stomy	S	surgically created opening
120.	strept/o-	C	curved
121.	sub-	P	below; underneath; less than
122.	suppur/o-	C	pus formation
123.	syn-	P	together
124.	tempor/o-	C	temple (side of the head)
125.	-therapy	S	treatment
126.	-tic	S	pertaining to
127.	-tome	S	instrument used to cut; an area with distinct edges
128.	-tomy	S	process of cutting or making an incision
129.	tonsill/o-	C	tonsil
130.	toxic/o-	C	poison, toxin
131.	-trophy	S	process of development
132.	turbin/o-	C	turbinate (scroll-like structure)
133.	tuss/o-	C	cough
134.	tympan/o-	C	tympanic membrane (eardrum)
135.	uni-	P	single, not paired
136.	vestibul/o-	C	vestibule (entrance)
137.	voc/o-	C	voice

Word-Building Exercise (p. 892)

1. audit/o- + -ory — auditory
2. myring/o- + -tomy — myringotomy
3. endo- + -scope — endoscope
4. presby/o- + -acusis — presbyacusis
5. ot/o- + -itis — otitis
6. an- + -acusis — anacusis
7. ot/o- + -rrhea — otorrhea
8. sinus/o- + -itis — sinusitis
9. tympan/o- + -metry — tympanometry
10. ot/o- + -scope — otoscope

True or False (p. 892)

1. F 2. T 3. T 4. F 5. F 6. T 7. F 8. F 9. T

Matching Exercise #1 (p. 893)

1, 9, 8, 7, 4, 3, 5, 2, 10, 6

Matching Exercise #2 (p. 893)

10, 2, 7, 9, 6, 8, 1, 3, 5, 4

Matching Exercise #3 (p. 893)

6, 7, 5, 2, 4, 1, 3

English and Medical Word Equivalents (p. 894)

1. ear canal — external auditory canal
2. eardrum — tympanic membrane
3. earwax — cerumen
4. hammer-shaped bone — malleus
5. anvil-shaped bone — incus
6. stirrup-shaped bone — stapes
7. nostril — naris
8. throat — pharynx
9. voice box, Adam's apple — larynx
10. seasonal allergies — allergic rhinitis
11. common cold — upper respiratory infection
12. total deafness — anacusis
13. nosebleed — epistaxis
14. earache — otalgia
15. sore throat — pharyngitis
16. ringing in the ears — tinnitus

Dictionary Challenge (p. 894)

rhinitis medicamentosa: Inflammation of the mucous membranes of the nose because of excessive use of topical medication, specifically decongestant nasal spray. Note: Afrin decongestant nasal spray is specifically mentioned as a drug this patient was using.

Word Analysis Questions (p. 895)

1. sinus/o- — sinus
   -itis — inflammation of
2. bi- — two
   later/o- — side
   -al — pertaining to
3. Tympanic membranes

Fact Finding Questions (p. 896)

1. severe pain and pressure over her right cheekbone and right forehead 2. palpation 3. sinusitis 4. amoxicillin

Critical Thinking Question (p. 896)

1. A: (Assessment) 2. frontal sinuses, maxillary sinuses 3. AU, A.U. 4. return or increase of any of these symptoms: fever, sore throat, head cold, pain and pressure over the cheekbones or forehead, fatigue, dizziness, or pain in the ears.

Chapter 17 Psychiatry

BUILDING MEDICAL WORDS

Combining Forms (p. 907)

1. amygdal/o- — almond shape
2. affect/o- — state of mind; to have an influence on
3. emot/o- — moving, stirring up
4. limb/o- — edge, border
5. neur/o- — nerve
6. mitt/o- — to send

Combining Forms and Suffixes (p. 907)

1. amygdal/o- + -oid — amygdaloid
2. limb/o- + -ic — limbic
3. emot/o- + -ion — emotion
4. affect/o- + -ive — affective

CHAPTER REVIEW EXERCISES

Matching Exercise (p. 929)

2, 4, 1, 5, 1, 4, 4, 1, 2, 3, 1

True or False (p. 929)

1. F 2. T 3. F 4. T 5. F 6. T 7. T

Matching Exercise (p. 929)

1, 4, 5; 3; 2; 1; 2; 1

Name That Word Part (p. 930)

1.	-al	S	pertaining to
2.	a-	P	away from, without
3.	acr/o-	C	extremity; highest point
4.	addict/o-	C	surrender to; be controlled by
5.	affect/o-	C	state of mind; mood
6.	agor/a-	C	open area or space
7.	amygdal/o-	C	almond shape
8.	amnes/o-	C	forgetfulness

9.	an-	P	without, not
10.	analy/o-	C	to separate
11.	-ance	S	state of
12.	-ant	S	pertaining to
13.	anter/o-	C	before; front part
14.	anti-	P	against
15.	anxi/o-	C	fear, worry
16.	appercept/o-	C	fully perceived
17.	-ar	S	pertaining to
18.	arachn/o-	C	spider, spider web
19.	-ation	S	a process; being or having
20.	-ative	S	pertaining to
21.	aut/o-	C	self
22.	behav/o-	C	activity or manner of acting
23.	bi-	P	two
24.	cata-	P	down
25.	chondr/o-	C	cartilage
26.	cid/o-	C	kill
27.	claustr/o-	C	enclosed space
28.	cognit/o-	C	thinking
29.	compuls/o-	C	drive or compel
30.	con-	P	with
31.	convuls/o-	C	seizure
32.	copr/o-	C	feces, stool
33.	cycl/o-	C	cycle; circle
34.	de-	P	reversal of, without
35.	delus/o-	C	false belief
36.	depend/o-	C	to hang onto
37.	depress/o-	C	press down
38.	dis-	P	away from
39.	dys-	P	painful, difficult, abnormal
40.	ech/o-	C	echo (sound wave)
41.	electr/o-	C	electricity
42.	emot/o-	C	moving, stirring
43.	en-	P	in, within, inward
44.	-ence	S	state of
45.	-ent	S	pertaining to
46.	-er	S	person or thing that does or produces
47.	-esis	S	condition
48.	-eu	P	normal, good
49.	-ety	S	condition, state
50.	exhibit/o-	C	showing
51.	factit/o-	C	artificial, contrived
52.	-form	S	having the form of
53.	-gen	S	that which produces
54.	glob/o-	C	shaped like a globe; comprehensive
55.	-grade	S	going
56.	hallucin/o-	C	imagined perception
57.	hebe/o-	C	youth
58.	hedon/o-	C	pleasure
59.	hom/i-	C	man
60.	hypn/o-	C	sleep
61.	hypo-	P	below; deficient
62.	-ia	S	condition, state, thing
63.	-iasis	S	state of; process of
64.	iatr/o-	C	physician; medical treatment
65.	-iatry	S	medical treatment
66.	-ic	S	pertaining to
67.	-ical	S	pertaining to
68.	-ion	S	action; condition
69.	-ior	S	pertaining to
70.	-ism	S	process; disease from a specific cause
71.	-ist	S	one who specializes in
72.	-ition	S	condition of having
73.	-ity	S	state; condition
74.	-ive	S	pertaining to
75.	-ization	S	process of making, creating, or inserting
76.	-izer	S	a thing that affects in a particular way
77.	kines/o-	C	movement
78.	klept/o-	C	to steal
79.	-lalia	S	speech
80.	-lepsy	S	seizure
81.	limb/o-	C	edge, border
82.	log/o-	C	word; the study of
83.	-logy	C	the study of
84.	ly/o-	C	break down, separate, dissolve
85.	-mania	S	frenzy
86.	menstru/o-	C	montly discharge of blood
87.	ment/o-	C	mind; chin
88.	micr/o-	C	small
89.	mitt/o-	C	to send
90.	morph/o-	C	shape
91.	ne/o-	C	new
92.	neur/o-	C	nerve
93.	obsess/o-	C	besieged by thoughts
94.	-oid	S	resembling
95.	ophidi/o-	C	snake
96.	oppos/o-	C	forceful resistance
97.	-or	S	person or thing that produces or does
98.	orex/o-	C	appetite
99.	-osis	S	condition; abnormal condition; process
100.	-ous	S	pertaining to
101.	path/o-	C	disease, suffering
102.	-pathy	S	disease, suffering
103.	ped/o-	C	child
104.	person/o-	C	person
105.	-phile	S	person who is attracted to or fond of
106.	phil/o-	C	attraction to, fondness for
107.	phob/o-	C	fear
108.	phor/o-	C	range; to bear; to carry
109.	phren/o-	C	mind
110.	pol/o-	C	pole
111.	post-	P	after, behind
112.	pre-	P	before, in front of
113.	psych/o-	C	mind
114.	pyr/o-	C	fire
115.	rap/o-	C	to seize and drag away
116.	react/o-	C	reverse movement
117.	repress/o-	C	press back
118.	retro-	P	behind, backward
119.	sex/o-	C	sex
120.	schiz/o-	C	split
121.	sensit/o-	C	affected by, sensitive to
122.	soci/o-	C	human beings; community
123.	somat/o-	C	body
124.	stress/o-	C	disturbing stimulus
125.	su/i-	C	self
126.	tard/o-	C	late, slow
127.	thanat/o-	C	death
128.	therapeut/o-	C	treatment
129.	-therapy	C	treatment
130.	thym/o-	C	thymus; rage
131.	-tic	S	pertaining to
132.	till/o-	C	to pull out
133.	toler/o-	C	to become accustomed to
134.	ton/o-	C	pressure; tone
135.	toxic/o-	C	poison, toxin
136.	tranquil/o-	C	calm
137.	trans-	P	across, through
138.	traumat/o-	C	injury
139.	trich/o-	C	hair
140.	-ual	S	pertaining to
141.	vers/o-	C	to turn; to travel
142.	vest/o-	C	to dress
143.	xen/o-	C	foreign

Word-Building Exercise (p. 932)

1.	ment/o- + -al	mental
2.	compuls/o- + -ion	compulsion
3.	acr/o- + phob/o- + ia	acrophobia
4.	cognit/o- + -ive	cognitive
5.	klept/o- + -mania	kleptomania
6.	emot/o- + -ion	emotion
7.	de- + ment/o- + -ia	dementia

Circle Exercise (p. 932)

1. Panic 2. Bulimia 3. Delirium tremens 4. before 5. echolalia 6. mood disorders 7. depression 8. nipolar disorder 9. Munchausen by proxy 10. histrionic

Matching Exercise (p. 933)

6, 10, 1, 11, 5, 12, 13, 8, 4, 2, 3, 7, 9, 15, 14

True or False (p. 933)

1. T 2. F 3. F 4. T 5. F 6. F 7. T 8. T

Divide and Conquer (p. 934)

1.	anorexia	an-	orex/o-	-ia
2.	anxiety		anxi/o-	-ety
3.	autism		aut/o-	-ism
4.	bipolar	bi-	pol/o-	-ar
5.	dementia	de-	ment/o-	-ia
6.	dysmorphic	dys-	morph/o-	-ic
7.	hallucination		hallucin/o-	-ation
8.	hypochondriasis	hypo-	chondr/i-	-asis
9.	mental		ment/o-	-al
10.	microphobia	micro-	phob/o-	-ia
11.	neologism	ne/o-	log/o-	-ism
12.	pedophile		ped/o-	-phile
13.	phobic		phob/o-	-ic
14.	posttraumatic	post-	traumat/o-	-ic

Matching Exercise (p. 934)

4, 8, 5, 7, 3, 2, 1, 6

True or False (p. 935)

1. T 2. F 3. T 4. T 5. F 6. F 7. F 8. T 9. T 10. T 11. T

Matching Exercise (p. 935)

7, 3, 2, 5, 4, 1, 6

Matching Exercise (p. 936)

5, 4, 3, 1, 10, 6, 8, 7, 9, 2

Proofreading and Spelling Exercise (p. 936)

1. psychiatry 2. affect 3. dopamine 4. serotonin 5. dysthymia 6. suicide 7. homicidal 8. schizophrenic 9. personality 10. paranoia 11. narcissistic 12. addiction 13. therapeutic 14. milieu

Word Analysis Questions (p. 938)

1.	psych/o-	mind
	soci/o-	human beings; community
	-al	pertaining to
2.	factiti/o-	artificial, contrived
	-ous	pertaining to
3.	hom/I-	man
	cid/o-	killing
	-al	pertaining to
4.	suicidal	

Fact Finding Questions (p. 938)

1. Characterized by physical and/or psychological symptoms that are consciously made up (fabricated) by the patient, which the patient knows are not real. Patients pretend to be sick (often with symptoms that are difficult to evaluate) or even make themselves sick because of a desire to be cared for. They are intelligent and knowledgeable about medicine, but they are experienced liars who often fool several physicians. 2. Family problems: Little contact with her ex-husband, caring for 2 children. Oldest son recently in trouble for speeding. Financial problems: Has worked part-time but not currently working now, causing financial difficulties.

Critical Thinking Questions (p. 938)

1. bipolar disorder 2. Delusions are continued, fixed, and unchanging false beliefs about events of everyday life despite the efforts of others to persuade or evidence showing otherwise. Hallucinations are false impressions of vision, smell, sound, taste, or touch. 3. paranoia

Chapter 18 Oncology

LABELING EXERCISE (P. 953)

1. nuclear membrane
2. nucleus
3. nucleolus
4. mitochondrion
5. cytoplasm
6. Golgi apparatus
7. endoplasmic reticulum
8. ribosomes
9. cell membrane
10. lysosome
11. chromosome

BUILDING MEDICAL WORDS

Combining Forms (p. 953)

1.	differentiat/o-	being distinct or specialized
2.	angi/o-	blood vessel; lymphatic vessel
3.	cancer/o-	cancer
4.	capsul/o-	enveloping structure
5.	carcin/o-	cancer
6.	cellul/o-	cell
7.	chondri/o-	little granule
8.	chrom/o-	color
9.	cyt/o-	cell
10.	gene/o-	gene
11.	gen/o-	arising from; produced by
12.	hered/o-	genetic inheritance
13.	invas/o-	to go into
14.	locat/o-	a place
15.	lys/o-	break apart
16.	mit/o-	threadlike structure
17.	mutat/o-	a changing
18.	necr/o-	death
19.	nucle/o-	nucleus
20.	nucleol/o-	nucleolus
21.	onc/o-	tumor, mass
22.	organ/o-	organ
23.	plasm/o-	plasma; formed substance
24.	rib/o-	ribonucleic acid
25.	som/o-	a body
26.	stas/o-	standing still; staying in one place
27.	stat/o-	standing still; staying in one place
28.	suppress/o-	press down

Combining Forms and Suffixes (p. 954)

1.	rib/o- + -some	ribosome
2.	cancer/o- + -ous	cancerous
3.	necr/o- + -osis	necrosis
4.	invas/o- + -ive	invasive
5.	gene/o- + -tic	genetic
6.	cyt/o- + -plasm	cytoplasm
7.	organ/o- + -elle	organelle
8.	cellul/o- + -ar	cellular
9.	lys/o- + -some	lysosome
10.	carcin/o- + -gen	carcinogen
11.	onc/o- + -gene	oncogene
12.	hered/o- + -ity	heredity
13.	nucle/o- + -ar	nuclear
14.	chrom/o- + -some	chromosome
15.	mutat/o- + -ion	mutation

CHAPTER REVIEW EXERCISES

Matching Exercise (p. 978)

2, 4, 6, 3, 7, 1, 8, 5

True or False (p. 978)

1. F 2. T 3. F 4. T 5. F 6. F

Circle Exercise (p. 978)

1. squamous
2. ribosome
3. anaplasia
4. astrocyte
5. mitosis

Name That Word Part (p. 979)

1.	-al	S	pertaining to
2.	ablat/o-	C	take away
3.	-able	S	able to be
4.	aden/o-	C	gland
5.	adjuv/o-	C	giving help or assistance
6.	ana-	P	apart from; through; up
7.	angi/o-	C	blood vessel; lymphatic vessel
8.	-ant	S	pertaining to
9.	anti-	P	against
10.	apo-	C	away from
11.	-ar	S	pertaining to
12.	arteri/o-	C	artery
13.	-ary	S	pertaining to
14.	aspir/o-	C	to breathe in, to suck in
15.	astr/o-	C	starlike structure
16.	-ated	S	pertaining to a condition; composed of
17.	-ation	S	a process; being or having
18.	bas/o-	C	base of a structure

19. bi/o-	C	life; living organism; living tissue
20. blast/o-	C	immature; embryonic
21. brachy-	P	short
22. bronch/o-	C	bronchus
23. cancer/o-	C	cancer
24. capsul/o-	C	capsule (enveloping structure)
25. carcin/o-	C	cancer
26. cavit/o-	C	hollow space
27. cellul/o-	C	cell
28. chem/o-	C	chemical, drug
29. cholangi/o-	C	bile duct
30. chondri/o-	C	little granule
31. chondr/o-	C	cartilage
32. chori/o-	C	chorion (fetal membrane)
33. chorion/o-	C	chorion (fetal membrane)
34. chrom/o-	C	color
35. clon/o-	C	identical group derived from one
36. conform/o-	C	having the same scale or angle
37. cry/o-	C	cold
38. cutane/o-	C	skin
39. cyt/o-	C	cell
40. dendr/o-	C	branching structure
41. dessic/o-	C	to dry up
42. differentiat/o-	C	being distinct or specialized
43. dissect/o-	C	to cut apart
44. duct/o-	C	bring or move; a duct
45. dys-	P	painful, difficult, abnormal
46. -ed	S	pertaining to
47. electr/o-	C	electricity
48. -elle	S	little
49. embryon/o-	C	embryo; immature form
50. embol/o-	C	embolus (occluding plug)
51. emet/o-	C	to vomit
52. -emia	S	condition of the blood; substance in the blood
53. en-	P	in, within, inward
54. endo-	P	innermost, within
55. enter/o-	C	intestine
56. -ery	S	process of
57. -esis	S	condition
58. ex-	P	out, away from
59. excis/o-	C	to cut out
60. explorat/o-	C	to search out
61. extern/o-	C	outside
62. fibr/o-	C	fiber
63. fulgur/o-	C	spark of electricity
64. -gen	S	that which produces
65. -gene	S	gene
66. gene/o-	C	gene
67. gen/o-	C	arising from; produced by
68. gli/o-	C	substance that holds things together
69. gonad/o-	C	gonads (ovaries and testes)
70. -gram	C	a record or picture
71. -graphy	S	process of recording
72. hepat/o-	C	liver
73. hered/o-	C	genetic inheritance
74. hormon/o-	C	hormone
75. -ia	S	condition, state, thing
76. -ial	S	pertaining to
77. -ic	S	pertaining to
78. -ical	S	pertaining to
79. implant/o-	C	placed within
80. -in	S	substance
81. incis/o-	C	to cut out
82. nhibit/o-	C	block; hold back
83. intern/o-	C	inside
84. interstit/o-	C	spaces within tissue
85. intra-	P	within
86. invas/o-	C	to go into
87. -ion	S	action; condition
88. -ist	S	one who specializes in
89. -ite	S	thing that pertains to
90. -ity	S	state; conditino
91. -ive	S	pertaining
92. -ization	S	process of making, creating, or inserting
93. -ize	S	affecting in a particular way
94. kary/o-	C	nucleus
95. lapar/o-	C	abdomen
96. lei/o-	C	smooth
97. leuk/o-	C	white
98. lip/o-	C	lipid (fat)
99. locat/o-	C	a place
100. log/o-	C	the study of
101. -logy	S	the study of
102. lymph/o-	C	lymph; lymphatic system
103. lys/o-	C	break down or dissolve
104. magnet/o-	C	magnet
105. malign/o-	C	intentionally causing harm; cancer
106. mamm/o-	C	breast
107. medic/o-	C	physician; medicine
108. melan/o-	C	black
109. meta-	P	subsequent to
110. metabol/o-	C	change, transformation
111. metri/o-	C	uterus (womb)
112. mit/o-	C	thread
113. mono-	P	one, single
114. mutat/o-	C	a changing
115. myel/o-	C	bone marrow; spinal cord; myelin
116. my/o-	C	muscle
117. necr/o-	C	death
118. ne/o-	C	new
119. nephr/o-	C	kidney
120. neur/o-	C	nerve
121. nucle/o-	C	nucleus
122. nucleol/o-	C	nucleolus
123. -oid	S	resembling
124. olig/o-	S	scanty
125. -oma	S	tumor, mass
126. onc/o-	C	tumor, mass
127. -opsy	S	process of viewing
128. -or	S	person or thing that produces or does
129. -ory	S	having the function of
130. organ/o-	C	organ
131. -osis	S	condition, abnormal condition
132. oste/o-	C	bone
133. -ous	S	pertaining to
134. -pathy	S	disease, suffering
135. per-	P	through, throughout
136. peripher/o-	C	outer aspects
137. peritone/o-	C	peritoneum
138. -plasm	S	formed substance
139. plasm/o-	C	plasma; formed substance
140. plas/o-	C	growth, formation
141. -ptosis	S	state of prolapse or drooping; falling
142. radic/o-	C	all parts including the root
143. radicul/o-	C	spinal nerve root
144. radi/o-	C	radius (forearm bone); x-rays; radiation
145. recept/o-	C	receive
146. remiss/o-	C	send back
147. resect/o-	C	to cut out and remove
148. resist/o-	C	withstand the effect of
149. retin/o-	C	retina (of the eye)
150. rhabd/o-	C	rod shaped
151. rib/o-	C	ribonucleic acid
152. sarc/o-	C	connective tissue
153. scint/i-	C	point of light
154. -scopy	S	process of using an instrument to examine
155. semin/o-	C	spermatozoon; semen
156. sensit/o-	C	affected by; sensitive to
157. -some	S	a body
158. som/o-	C	a body
159. son/o-	C	sound
160. squam/o-	C	scalelike structure
161. -stasis	S	condition of standing still or staying in one place
162. stas/o-	C	standing still; staying in one place
163. stat/o-	C	standing still; staying in one place
164. stere/o-	C	three dimensions
165. suppress/o-	C	press down
166. surg/o-	C	operative procedure
167. tact/o-	C	touch
168. terat/o-	C	bizarre form
169. thec/o-	C	sheath or layers of membranes
170. -therapy	S	treatment

171. -tic S pertaining to
172. tom/o- C a cut, slice, or layer
173. -tomy S process of cutting or making an incision
174. trans- P across, through
175. transit/o- C changing over from one thing to another
176. transplant/o- C move something to another place
177. trop/o- C having an affinity for; stimulating; turning
178. -type S particular kind of; a model of
179. ultra- P beyond; higher
180. un- P not
181. ven/o- C vein
182. vesic/o- C bladder; fluid-filled sac

Word-Building Exercise (p. 981)

1. gene/o- + -tic genetic
2. onc/o- + -logy oncology
3. mutat/o- + -ion mutation
4. lapar/o- + -tomy laparotomy
5. hepat/o- + -oma hepatoma
6. carcin/o- + -oma carcinoma
7. carcin/o- + -gen carcinogen
8. differentiat/o- + -ion differentiation
9. hered/o- + -ity heredity
10. invas/o- + -ive invasive
11. lymph/o- + -oma lymphoma

True or False (p. 982)

1. F 2. T 3. F 4. F 5. F 6. T 7. T 8. T 9. T 10. F

Matching Exercise (p. 982)

9, 7, 6, 10, 4, 2, 3, 11, 1, 5, 8

Memory Exercise (p. 982)

1. C Change in bowel or bladder habits
   A A sore that does not heal
   U Unusual bleeding or discharge
   T Thickening or lump
   I Indigestion or trouble swallowing
   O Obvious changes in a wart or mole
   N Nagging cough or hoarseness
2. alpha fetoprotein b
   biopsy e
   chronic myelogenous leukemia a
   estrogen receptor c
   ribonucleic acid f
   tumor, nodes, metastases d

Matching Exercise #1 (p. 983)

8, 3, 6, 4, 5, 2, 1, 7

True or False (p. 983)

1. F 2. F 3. T 4. F 5. F 6. T 7. F 8. T

MATCHING EXERCISE #2 (p. 983)

8, 6, 4, 1, 3, 2, 5, 7

Circle Exercise (p. 983)

1. adjuvant therapy
2. endoscopy
3. excising the tumor and surrounding structures as one block of tissue
4. antimetabolite drug

Matching Exercise (p. 984)

7, 3, 2, 4, 6, 5, 1

Word Analysis Questions (p. 985)

1. metastatic
2. bi/o- life; living organisms; living tissue
   -opsy process of viewing
3. dissect/o- to cut apart
   -ion action; condition
4. carcin/o- cancer
   -oma tumor, mass

Fact Finding Questions (p. 986)

1. Self-examination of her breasts
2. Mammography (or mammogram)
3. Needle biopsy of the right breast mass
4. The patient had 10 out of 28 axillary lymph nodes positive for carcinoma.
5. Anaplasia is the loss of the unique, differentiated cellular structure that is seen in normal, mature cells.

Critical Thinking Questions (p. 986)

1. Several genes associated with breast cancer are inherited mutations and so it would be important to know if the patient had any family members with breast cancer.
2. A frozen section is a procedure that takes a tissue specimen from a biopsy and freezes it. The specimen is then sliced into thin slices that are put on a slide, stained, and examined under the microscope. This procedure is done during surgery so that the surgeon knows immediately whether the tumor is cancerous or not.
3. Invasive
4. "The margins of resection are free of tumor."

Chapter 19 Radiology

BUILDING MEDICAL WORDS

Combining Forms (p. 1017)

1. act/o- action
2. angi/o- blood vessel; lymphatic vessel
3. anter/o- before; front part
4. aort/o- aorta
5. arteri/o- artery
6. arthr/o- joint
7. axi/o- axis
8. cardi/o- heart
9. chol/e- bile, gall
10. col/o- colon (part of large intestine)
11. cine/- movement
12. cycl/o- cycle; circle
13. cyst/o- bladder; fluid-filled sac; semisolid cyst
14. densit/o- density
15. dos/i- dose
16. duc/o- bring or move
17. du/o- two
18. ech/o- echo (sound wave)
19. electr/o- electricity
20. emiss/o- to send out
21. esophag/o- esophagus
22. excret/o- removing from the body
23. fluor/o- fluorescence
24. fus/o- pouring
25. gastr/o- stomach
26. helic/o- a coil
27. hyster/o- uterus
28. intestin/o- intestines
29. later/o- side
30. luc/o- clear and shining
31. lymph/o- lymph; lymphatic vessel
32. magnet/o- magnet
33. mamm/o- breast
34. myel/o- bone marrow; spinal cord; myelin
35. nucle/o- nucleus
36. pharmaceutic/o- medicines, drugs
37. poster/o- back part
38. project/o- throw forward
39. pyel/o- renal pelvis
40. radi/o- x-rays; radiation
41. roentgen/o- x-rays; radiation
42. rotat/o- rotate
43. salping/o- fallopian tube
44. scint/i- point of light
45. scintill/o- flash of light
46. son/o- sound
47. spir/o- a coil
48. tom/o- a cut, slice, or layer
49. trac/o- visible path
50. ur/o- urine; urinary system
51. ven/o- vein
52. ventilat/o- movement of air
53. vent/o- a coming
54. ventricul/o- ventricle (lower heart chamber; chamber in the brain)
55. xer/o- dry

Combining Forms and Suffixes (p. 1018)

1. anter/o- + -ior anterior
2. dos/i- + -metry dosimetry
3. fluor/o- + -scopy fluoroscopy

4. later/o- + -al lateral
5. son/o- + -gram sonogram
6. trac/o- + -er tracer
7. tom/o- + -graphy tomography
8. scintill/o- + -ation scintillation

Combining Forms and Prefixes (p. 1018)

1. intra- + venous intravenous
2. ultra- + sonography ultrasonography
3. trans- + ducer transducer

CHAPTER REVIEW EXERCISES

Name That Word Part (p. 1021)

1. -al S pertaining to
2. act/o- C action
3. angi/o- C blood vessel; lymphatic vessel
4. anter/o- C before; front part
5. aort/o- C aorta
6. -ar S pertaining to
7. arteri/o- C artery
8. arthr/o- C joint
9. -ated S pertaining to a condition; composed of
10. -ation S a process; being or having
11. axi/o- C axis
12. cardi/o- C heart
13. cin/e C movement
14. chol/e- C bile, gall
15. chol/o- C bile, gall
16. cycl/o- C cycle; circle
17. cyst/o- C bladder; fluid-filled sac; semisolid cyst
18. densit/o- C density
19. detect/o- C identify or detect
20. dos/i- C dose
21. duc/o- C bring or move
22. du/o- C two
23. -eal S pertaining to
24. ech/o- C echo (sound wave)
25. electr/o- C electricity
26. emiss/o- C to send out
27. -ent S pertaining to
28. -er S person or thing that makes or performs
29. esophag/o- C esophagus
30. excret/o- C removing from the body
31. fluor/o- C fluorescence
32. fus/o- C pouring
33. gastr/o- C stomach
34. -grade C going
35. -gram S a picture or record
36. -graph S instrument used to record
37. graph/o- C record
38. -graphy S process of recording
39. helic/o- C a coil
40. hyster/o- C uterus
41. -ic S pertaining to
42. -ide S chemically modified
43. inter- P between
44. intestin/o- C intestines
45. intra- P within
46. iodin/o- C iodine
47. -ion S action; condition
48. -ior S pertaining to
49. -ist S one who specializes in
50. -ive S pertaining to
51. later/o- C side
52. log/o- C the study of
53. -logy S the study of
54. luc/o- C clear and shining
55. lymph/o- C lymph; lymphatic vessel
56. magne/to- C magnet
57. mamm/o- C breast
58. -meter S instrument used to measure
59. -metry S process of measuring
60. multi- P many
61. myel/o- C bone marrow; spinal cord; myelin
62. nucle/o- C nucleus
63. -on S substance; structure
64. onc/o- C tumor, mass
65. -or S person or thing that produces or does something
66. -ory S having the function of
67. -ous S pertaining to
68. per- P through, throughout
69. pharmaceutic/o- C medicines, drugs
70. -plex S parts
71. post- P after, behind
72. poster/o- C back part
73. pre- P before, in front of
74. project/o- C throw forward
75. pyel/o- C renal pelvis
76. quantitat/o- C quantity or amount
77. rad/io- C x-rays; radiation
78. retro- P behind, backward
79. rotat/o- C rotate
80. roentgen/o- C x-ray; radiation
81. salping/o- C fallopian tube
82. scint/i- C point of light
83. scintill/o- C flash of light
84. -scopy S process of using an instrument to examine
85. son/o- C sound
86. spir/o- C a coil
87. techn/o- C technical skill
88. tom/o- C a cut, slice, or layer
89. trac/o- C visible path
90. trans- P across, through
91. -tron S instrument
92. ultra- P beyond, higher
93. ur/o- C urine; urinary system
94. ven/o- C vein
95. ventilat/o- C movement of air
96. vent/o- C a coming
97. ventricul/o- C ventricle (lower heart chamber; chamber in the brain)
98. xero- P dry

Word-Building Exercise (p. 1022)

1. nucle/o- + -ar nuclear
2. dos/i- + -meter dosimeter
3. mamm/o- + -gram mammogram
4. tom/o- + -graphy tomography
5. arthr/o- + -graphy arthrography
6. ech/o- + cardi/o- + -graphy echocardiography
7. radi/o- + pharmaceutic/o- + -al radiopharmaceutical
8. scint/i- + -gram scintigram

Matching Exercise (p. 1023)

7, 2, 9, 1, 8, 4, 3, 6, 10, 5

True or False (p. 1023)

1. T 2. F 3. F 4. T 5. T 6. T 7. T 8. T 9. F 10. T 11. T 12. F

Fill in the Blank Exercise (p. 1023)

1. light box 2. PA (posteroanterior) 3. film badge 4. gadolinium 5. Doppler 6. half-life 7. cyclotron

Circle Exercise (p. 1024)

1. scout 2. CT 3. EBT 4. MRI 5. MUGA

Multiple Choice (p. 1024)

1. b 2. d 3. a 4. b 5. d

Recall and List (p. 1025)

Any of these items are correct answers: metal zipper, metal glasses, watches, jewelry, hairpins, metal false teeth, artificial limbs, clothing with metal buttons or snaps. Nose rings, lip rings, tongue studs, pierced earrings. Implanted pacemakers, pacing wires, some heart valves, cerebral artery aneurysm clips, cochlear implants, some penile implants, artificial eyes, some intrauterine devices. Hearing aids, TENS units, insulin pumps. Patients who are metal workers or gunshot victims. Some transdermal patches. Metallic eye shadow.

Matching Exercise (p. 1025)

4, 11, 3, 5, 8, 1, 10, 2, 9, 6, 7

Abbreviation Exercise (p. 1025)

1. ultrasound 2. positron emission tomography 3. barium enema 4. chest x-ray 5. single photon emission computed tomography 6. multiple-gated acquisition (scan) 7. computerized axial tomography 8. intravenous pyelography

Fact Finding Questions (p. 1026)

1. posteroanterior 2. portable, in surgery 3. to the operating room 4. right The left total hip prosthesis was already in place from a previous operation. 5. prosthesis: an orthopedic device like an artificial hip joint or an artificial limb that replaces the patient's damaged joint or missing limb.

Fact Finding Questions (p. 1027)

1. c
2. barium and air
3. multiple
4. fluor/o- fluorescence
   scop/o- examine with an instrument
   -ic pertaining to

Fact Finding Questions (p. 1028)

1. I-123, technetium-99m
2. microcuries, millicuries
3. 7–24%
4. in an oral capsule (swallowed)
5. intravenous injection
6. radi/o- radius (forearm); x-rays; radiation
   act/o- action
   -ive pertaining to
7. uniform uptake throughout both the right and left lobes

Photo Credits

p. 2: *medical records folder labels:* Getty Images—Photodisc; *paramedic with radio:* Getty Images—Photodisc; *Chinese boy:* Dover Publications, Inc.; *Hippocrates:* Dover Publications, Inc.; *Black Death:* Prentice Hall School Division; **p. 3:** *doctor and child:* Brand X Pictures; *puzzle pieces:* EyeWire Collection/Getty Images—Photodisc; *girl brushing teeth:* Getty Images—Photodisc; *Ambroïse Paré:* Brian Warling/International Museum of Surgical Science; **p. 4:** EyeWire Collection/Getty Images—Photodisc; **p. 5:** Getty Images—Photodisc; **p. 22:** Michael Donne/Photo Researchers, Inc.

p. 32: *woman with saw:* Donna Day/Getty Images Inc.—Stone Allstock; *man looking in microscope:* Getty Images—Photodisc; *Andreas Vesalius:* Dover Publications, Inc.; **p. 33:** *hospital sign:* Getty Images—Photodisc; *kiwifruit:* Ian O'Leary/Dorling Kindersley Media Library; *foxglove plant:* Dover Publications, Inc.; *child with thermometer:* Jim Corwin/The Stock Connection; *William Harvey:* Dover Publications, Inc.; **p. 38:** *MRI:* DR Unique/Custom Medical Stock Photo, Inc.; **p. 45:** Custom Medical Stock Photo, Inc.; **p. 64:** *doctor examining woman:* S. O'brien/Custom Medical Stock Photo, Inc.; *nurse examining child:* Corbis Royalty Free

p. 86: *apple:* Getty Images, Inc.—Foodpix; *orange:* Getty Images—Photodisc; *Benjamin Franklin:* Corbis/Bettmann; **p. 87:** *baby:* Nancy Ney/Getty Images/Digital Vision; *Edward Jenner:* Mary Evans Picture Library/Photo Researchers, Inc.; *poppy:* Dorling Kindersley Media Library; **p. 96:** Nettis/Photo Researchers, Inc.; **p. 110:** David M. Martin, M.D./Photo Researchers, Inc.; **p. 112:** Dr. Larpent/CNRI/Photo Researchers, Inc.; **p. 114:** Staats/Custom Medical Stock Photo, Inc.; **p. 117:** English/Custom Medical Stock Photo, Inc.; **p. 118:** Science Heritage/Custom Medical Stock Photo, Inc.; **p. 120:** Dr. M.A. Ansary/Photo Researchers, Inc.; **p. 121:** *gallbladder:* Custom Medical Stock Photo, Inc.; **p. 124:** Custom Medical Stock Photo, Inc.; **p. 128:** Slaven/Custom Medical Stock Photo, Inc.

p. 152: *bubbles:* Lawrence Lawry/Getty Images, Inc.—Photodisc; *stethoscope:* Getty Images—Photodisc; *blood transfusion:* Dover Publications, Inc.; **p. 153:** *boy with balloon:* Omni-Photo Communications, Inc.; *woman behind bars:* Dover Publications, Inc.; *early anesthesia:* Dover Publications, Inc.; *AMA symbol:* US Army photo; **p. 160:** Jim Corwin/Photo Researchers, Inc.; **p. 174:** *left:* Dick Luria/Photo Researchers, Inc.; *right:* Custom Medical Stock Photo, Inc.; **p. 181:** *pulse oximeter:* O'Brien/Custom Medical Stock Photo, Inc.; *culture and sensitivity:* Science Heritage/Custom Medical Stock Photo, Inc.; **p. 186:** © Jenny Thomas/Pearson Education; **p. 187:** Custom Medical Stock Photo, Inc.

p. 204: *Wizard of Oz:* Picture Desk, Inc./Kobal Collection; *water pump:* Omni-Photo Communications, Inc.; *valentine:* EyeWire Collection/Getty Images—Photodisc; *handwashing:* Brian Warling/International Museum of Surgical Science; *Women's Medical College:* EMG Education Management Group; *Pfizer:* Courtesy Pfizer Inc.; **p. 205:** *eye exam:* Getty Images—Photodisc; *syringe:* Dover Publications, Inc.; **p. 218:** John Garrett/Dorling Kindersley Media Library; **p. 232:** Abrahas/Custom Medical Stock Photo, Inc.; **p. 236:** English/Custom Medical Stock Photo, Inc.; **p. 237:** SIU BioMed/Custom Medical Stock Photo, Inc.; **p. 240:** SPL/Photo Researchers, Inc.; **p. 242:** Brand X Pictures; **p. 247:** Custom Medical Stock Photo, Inc.; **p. 252:** English/Custom Medical Stock Photo, Inc.; **p. 255:** Art Resource, N.Y.

p. 274: *mosquito:* Noah Poritz/Photo Researchers, Inc.; *microorganisms:* Courtesy of the CDC; *Red Cross wagon:* Dorling Kindersley Media Library; **p. 275:** *highway:* Kimball Andrew Schmidt/The Stock Connection; *peas:* Dorling Kindersley Media Library; *horse-drawn ambulance:* Dorling Kindersley Media Library; **p. 278:** Custom Medical Stock Photo, Inc.; **p. 285:** Shout Pictures/Custom Medical Stock Photo, Inc.; **p. 302:** Peres/Custom Medical Stock Photo, Inc.; **p. 303:** Eye of Science/Photo Researchers, Inc.; **p. 305:** Caliendo/Custom Medical Stock Photo, Inc.; **p. 306:** Peres/Custom Medical Stock Photo, Inc.; **p. 309:** Custom Medical Stock Photo, Inc.; **p. 312:** Brand X Pictures; **p. 315:** Getty Images—Photodisc

p. 336: *Red Cross poster:* Eileen Tweedy/Picture Desk, Inc./Kobal Collection; *Louis Pasteur:* The Bridgeman Art Library International; **p. 337:** *Indian holy man:* Anthony Cassidy/Getty Images Inc.—Stone Allstock; *henna-painted hand:* Colin Anderson/Getty Images—Photodisc; *"The Starry Night":* Art Resource, N.Y.; *Johns Hopkins University Hospital:* Ron Solomon/The Stock Connection; **p. 353:** Meyer/Custom Medical Stock Photo, Inc.; **p. 354:** Custom Medical Stock Photo, Inc.; **p. 355:** Custom Medical Stock Photo, Inc.; **p. 356:** *keloid:* Custom Medical Stock Photo, Inc.; *decubitus ulcer:* Courtesy of Sandra Quigley, Children's Hospital, Boston, MA; **p. 358:** Gill/Custom Medical Stock Photo, Inc.; **p. 359:** SCIENCE PHOTO LIBRARY/Custom Medical Stock Photo, Inc.; **p. 361:** Custom Medical Stock Photo, Inc.; **p. 363:** Courtesy of Jason L. Smith, M.D.; **p. 365:** *Clinical Dermatology: A Color Guide to Diagnosis and Therapy,* 2nd ed., by T.P. Habif, 1990, St. Louis: Mosby-Year Book, p. 113; **p. 368:** Logical Images/Custom Medical Stock Photo, Inc.; **p. 369:** Southern Illinois/Visuals Unlimited; **p. 372:** AJ Photo/Photo Researchers, Inc.

p. 394: *house frame:* Don Farrall, Light-Works Studio/Getty Images, Inc.—PhotoDisc; *dynamite factory:* Science Photo Library/Photo Researchers, Inc.; *Sigmund Freud:* Image Works/Mary Evans Picture Library Ltd; **p. 395:** *boy with cast:* SW Productions/Getty Images, Inc.—PhotoDisc; *Marie Curie:* The Granger Collection; *aspirin:* Getty Images—Photodisc; *ambulance carriage:* Dover Publications, Inc.; **p. 400:** Elsevier; **p. 404:** *lumbar vertebra:* Elsevier; *Vesalius skeleton:* Dover Publications, Inc.; **p. 407:** © David W. Harbaugh; **p. 425:** Scott Camazine/Photo Researchers, Inc.; **p. 428:** ESRF-CREATIS/Photo Researchers, Inc.; **p. 430:** NMSB/Custom Medical Stock Photo, Inc.; **p. 432:** *osteoarthritis:* Custom Medical Stock Photo, Inc.; **p. 433:** NMSB/Custom Medical Stock Photo, Inc.; **p. 434:** Shea, MD/Custom Medical Stock Photo, Inc.; **p. 436:** *arm cast:* Steinmark/Custom Medical Stock Photo, Inc.; *leg cast:* Getty Images, Inc.—PhotoDisc; **p. 437:** Brand X Pictures; **p. 438:** Custom Medical Stock Photo, Inc.; **p. 440:** *hip prostheses:* James Cavallini/Photo Researchers, Inc.; *orthopedic plate and screws:* Mauro Fermariello/Photo Researchers, Inc.

p. 456: *man balancing on one arm:* Robert Daly/Getty Images Inc.—Stone Allstock; *sphygmomanometer:* Getty Images—Photodisc; *mosquito:* Noah Poritz/Photo Researchers, Inc.; **p. 457:** *blue yarn:* Pearson Learning Photo Studio; *apple:* Dover Publications, Inc.; *sickle cells:* Eye of Science/Photo Researchers, Inc.; *elixir:* Dover Publications, Inc.; **p. 463:** *boy doing split in the air:* Rubberball/Getty Images Inc—Rubberball Royalty Free; *girl with ponytail:* Mark Andersen/Getty Images Inc—Rubberball Royalty Free; *woman in lotus position:* Anthony Saint James/Getty Images—Photodisc; **p. 468:** Elsevier; **p. 478:** Glaser & Associates/Custom Medical Stock Photo, Inc.; **p. 487:** Dr. P. Marazzi/Photo Researchers, Inc.; **p. 490:** Glaser & Associates/Custom Medical Stock Photo, Inc.; **p. 492:** Brand X Pictures; **p. 494:** © Elena Dorfman/Pearson Education

p. 510: *carrots:* Dover Publications, Inc.; *mirror showing surgical suite:* Brand X Pictures; *chest x-ray:* Dick Luria/Photo Researchers, Inc.; **p. 511:** *motherboard:* Ryan McVay/Photodisc Green/Getty Images; *Steven Hawking:* The Scotsman/Corbis/Sygma; *police officer wearing mask:* Getty Images, Inc.—Hulton Archive Photos; *Band-Aid:* Getty Images—Photodisc; **p. 515:** Elsevier; **p. 516:** *brain:* Elsevier; *woman at blackboard:* Getty Images/Digital Vision; **p. 532:** Elsevier; **p. 537:** Simon Fraser/Photo Researchers, Inc.; **p. 541:** Science Photo Library/Custom Medical Stock Photo, Inc.; **p. 542:** PhotoLink/Getty Images—Photodisc; **p. 543:** Phanie/Photo Researchers, Inc.; **p. 544:** SIU/Custom Medical Stock Photo, Inc.; **p. 545:** Shout Pictures/Custom Medical Stock Photo, Inc.; **p. 547:** JPD/Custom Medical Stock Photo, Inc.; **p. 553:** Corbis Royalty Free; **p. 557:** Peres/Custom Medical Stock Photo, Inc.; **p. 558:** Vanstrum/Custom Medical Stock Photo, Inc.

p. 580: *asparagus:* Ian O'Leary/Dorling Kindersley Media Library; *FDR:* The Granger Collection; **p. 581:** *garden hose:* Ryan McVay/Getty Images—Photodisc;; *insulin:* Getty Images—Photodisc; *braces:* Getty Images—Photodisc; **p. 583:** Elsevier; **p. 584:** Elsevier; **p. 594:** Elsevier; **p. 597:** Custom Medical Stock Photo, Inc.; **p. 598:** Dr. E. Walker/Photo Researchers, Inc.; **p. 599:** Custom Medical Stock Photo, Inc.; **p. 601:** http://www.med.cmu.ac.th/student/patho/kamthorn/315.jpg; **p. 606:** Birn/Custom Medical Stock Photo, Inc.; **p. 607:** Faye Norman/Photo Researchers, Inc.; **p. 609:** CRNI/Photo Researchers, Inc.; **p. 616:** Visuals Unlimited

p. 634: *sperm and egg;* Getty Images Inc.—Stone Allstock; *contact lens;* Getty Images—Photodisc; *March of Dimes poster:* March of Dimes Birth Defects Foundation; **p. 635:** *rooster:* DON HEBERT/Getty Images, Inc.—Taxi; *monkey:* AP Wide World Photos; *penicillin:* Andrew McClenaghan/Photo Researchers, Inc.; *drawing blood:* Getty Images—Photodisc; **p. 652:** Biophoto Associates/Photo Researchers, Inc.; © Kenneth Greer/Visuals Unlimited; **p. 654:** Biophoto Associates/Photo Researchers, Inc.

p. 672: *sprout:* STEFAN MOKRZECKI/Photolibrary.com; *George Papanicolau:* Corbis/Bettmann; *tuberculosis poster:* The Art Archive; *nurse with newborn:* Getty Images—Photodisc; **p. 673:** *chicken egg:* BananaStock/Robert Harding World Imagery; *cigarette ad:* The Granger Collection; *two boys drinking from fountain:* Silver Image Photo Agency, Inc.; *prescription:* Getty Images—Photodisc; **p. 685:** SIU BioMed/Custom Medical Stock Photo, Inc.; **p. 686:** *A Child is Born,* by L. Nilsson, 1990, New York: Dell Publishing; **p. 702:** Z. Binor/Custom Medical Stock Photo, Inc.; **p. 703:** CNRI/Photo Researchers, Inc.; **p. 706:** SPL/Photo Researchers, Inc.; **p. 717:** Yoav Levy/Phototake NYC; **p. 718:** Getty Images—Photodisc; **p. 719:** Custom Medical Stock Photo Inc., **p. 723:** Zephyr/Photo Researchers, Inc.; **p. 727:** Getty Images—Photodisc

p. 750: *Sugar Ray Robinson:* Culver Pictures, Inc.; *John F. Kennedy:* Ted Streshinsky/Corbis/Bettmann; *Gail Devers:* Koji Sasahara/AP Wide World Photos; *control panel:* Jeff Sherman/Getty Images, Inc.—Taxi; *pacemaker:* English/Custom Medical Stock Photo, Inc.; *heart-lung machine:* Maximilian Stock Ltd./Photo Researchers, Inc.; *Jonas Salk Time magazine cover:* Getty Images/Time Life Pictures; **p. 751:** *roller coaster:* Alan Thornton/Getty Images Inc.—Stone Allstock; *CPR:* Corbis Royalty Free; *karyotype:* L. Willatt/East Anglian/Photo Researchers, Inc.; **p. 754:** Elsevier; **p. 760:** Elsevier; **p. 772:** NMSB/Custom Medical Stock Photo, Inc.; **p. 774:** Marka/Custom Medical Stock Photo, Inc.; **p. 775:** *exophthalmos:* NMSB/Custom Medical Stock Photo, Inc.; **p. 778:** © David W. Harbaugh; **p. 786:** Custom Medical Stock Photo, Inc.; **p. 788:** *injecting insulin:* Custom Medical Stock Photo, Inc.; *insulin bottle and syringe:* SIU BioMed/Custom Medical Stock Photo, Inc.

p. 804: *contact lenses:* JOHN WILKES/Getty Images, Inc.—Taxi; *birth control pills:* Dorling Kindersley Media Library; *breast implant:* Getty Images—Photodisc; *DNA double helix:* Getty Images—Photodisc; **p. 805:** *camera:* Dorling Kindersley Media Library; *young couple kissing:* Charles Gatewood/Pearson Education/PH College; *elderly couple walking:* Corbis Royalty Free; **p. 821:** Science Photo Library/Photo Researchers, Inc.; **p. 823:** James Stevenson/Photo Researchers, Inc.; **p. 824:** NMSB/Custom Medical Stock Photo, Inc.; **p. 830:** Marka/Custom Medical Stock Photo, Inc.; **p. 833:** *phorometer:* Custom Medical Stock Photo, Inc.; *pupillary response:* Custom Medical Stock Photo, Inc.; **p. 836:** Courtesy of National Eye Institute

p. 852: *skunk:* Digital Zoo/Getty Images/Digital Vision; *aspartame:* Martin Bond/Photo Researchers, Inc.; *cigarettes:* Jonathan A. Meyers/The Stock Connection; *Christiaan Barnard:* Getty Images Inc. - Hulton Archive Photos; **p. 853:** *drums:* Silver Burdett Ginn; *phone:* Getty Images—Photodisc; *med-evac helicopter:* Getty Images—Photodisc; *mammogram:* Getty Images—Photodisc; **p. 876:** Courtesy of Dr. Elizabeth Peterson, Spokane, WA; **p. 877:** *Atlas of Pediatric Physical Diagnosis,* 3rd ed., B. J. Zitelli, & H.W. Davis (Eds.), 1997, St. Louis: Mosby, Inc., p. 104; **p. 878:** Dr P. Marazzi/Science Photo Library/Custom Medical Stock Photo, Inc.; **p. 882:** *cartoon:* ©David W. Harbaugh; *otoscopy:* O'Brien/Custom Medical Stock Photo, Inc.

p. 900: *spiral staircase:* Peter Adams/Index Stock Imagery, Inc.; *valium tablets:* Getty Images—Digital Vision; **p. 901:** *cartoon:* The Cartoon Bank; *MRI:* Brand X Pictures; *Louise Brown:* Getty Images Inc.—Hulton Archive Photos; *transdermal patch:* Corbis Royalty Free; **p. 912:** NMSB/Custom Medical Stock Photo, Inc.; **p. 925:** Kramer/Custom Medical Stock Photo, Inc.

p. 942: *tomatoes:* Ian O'Leary/Dorling Kindersley Media Library; *artificial heart:* Hank Morgan/Photo Researchers, Inc.; *AIDS quilt:* Corbis Digital Stock; *safety cap:* Getty Images—Photodisc; **p. 943:** *Lance Armstrong:* Peter Dejong/AP Wide World Photos; *AIDS "cocktail":* Jana Birchum; *cataract surgery:* Joe McNally Photography; **p. 950:** *liver cancer:* CNRI/Photo Researchers, Inc.; **p. 957:** *basal cell carcinoma:* Logical Images/Custom Medical Stock Photo, Inc.; **p. 960:** Zeva Oelbaum/Peter Arnold, Inc.; **p. 961:** Siebert/Custom Medical Stock Photo, Inc.; **p. 964:** Cavallini/Custom Medical Stock Photo, Inc.; **p. 966:** Zephyr/Photo Researchers, Inc.; **p. 971:** Getty Images—Photodisc; **p. 973:** Custom Medical Stock Photo, Inc.

p. 990: *x-ray gun:* Dorling Kindersley Media Library; *bat:* Frank Greenaway/Dorling Kindersley Media Library; *wheelchair basketball:* Getty Images—Photodisc; *computer screen:* Brian Warling/Pearson Education/PH College; **p. 991:** *magnet:* AGE Fotostock America, Inc.; *Dolly the sheep:* AP Wide World Photos; *human genome:* PETER MENZEL/Stock Boston; *embryonic stem cell:* Dr. Yorgos Nikas/Photo Researchers, Inc.; **p. 994:** *doctors examining x-rays:* Corbis Royalty Free; *cartoon:* © David W. Harbaugh; **p. 997:** *arteriogram:* Corbis Royalty Free; **p. 1000:** *fluoroscopy:* Geoff Tompkinson/Photo Researchers, Inc.; **p. 1003:** *MRI machine:* Brand X Pictures; *MRI image:* DR Unique/Custom Medical Stock Photo, Inc.; **p. 1006:** Yoav Levy/Phototake NYC; **p. 1010:** Custom Medical Stock Photo, Inc.

Index

A

Abbreviations, listed. see also individual specialties
- A, 25
- AS, 257
- A, 320
- 5-HIAA, 976
- A&P, 74, 189
- AAA, 257
- AB, 320
- AB, Ab, 731
- ABD, 134
- ABG, 189
- ABR, 887
- ACE, 257
- ACS, 257
- ACTH, 789
- AD, A.D., 887
- ADA, 495, 789
- ADD, 927
- ADH, 789
- ADHD, 927
- ADLs, 495
- AED, 257
- AFB, 189
- AFP, 562, 731, 976
- AGA, 731
- AI, 257
- AICD, 257
- AIDS, 320, 658
- AKA, 442
- ALL, 320, 976
- ALS, 562
- ALT, 134
- AMI, 257
- AML, 320, 976
- AP, 36, 189, 442, 1020
- ARDS, 189
- ARF, 619
- ARMD, 839
- ASC, 74
- ASC-H, 731
- ASC-US, 731
- ASCVD, 257
- ASD, 257
- ASHD, 257
- ASIS, 442
- AST, 134
- AU, A.U., 887
- AV, 257
- AVM, 562
- B, 320
- Ba, 1020
- BAEP, 562
- BAER, 562, 887
- bagged, 189
- basos, 320
- BBT, 731
- BDI, 927
- BE, 134, 1020
- BKA, 442
- BM, 134
- BMD, 442
- BMT, 320, 976
- BOM, 887
- BP, 257
- BPD, 731
- BPH, 658
- BPM (bpm), 257
- BPP, 731
- BRBPR, 134
- BRCA, 731, 976
- BS, 134, 189
- BSE, 731
- BSO, 731
- BUN, 619
- Bx, 377, 731, 976
- C&S, 189, 619, 887
- C1-C7, 442
- Ca, 377, 442, 731, 976
- Ca, Ca^{++}, 789
- CABG, 257
- CAD, 257
- CAPD, 619
- CAT, 1020
- cath, 257, 619
- CBC, 320
- CBD, 134
- CBT, 927
- CC, 25
- cc, 619
- CCPD, 619
- CCU, 257
- CDCP, 658
- CDE, 789
- CDH, 442
- CEA, 976
- CF, 189
- chemo, 976
- CHF, 257
- CIN, 731, 976
- CIS, 731
- CK, 839
- CK-MB, 257
- CLL, 320, 976
- CML, 320, 976
- cmm, 320
- CNM, 74, 731
- CNS, 562, 927
- CO, 189
- CO_2, 189
- COMT, 562
- COPD, 189
- COTA, 495
- CP, 562
- CPAP, 189
- CPD, 731
- CPK-MB, 257
- CPK-MM, 495
- CPR, 25, 189, 257
- CRF, 619
- CRNA, 74
- CRP, 257
- CRPS, 562
- CRT, 976
- CS, 731
- CSF, 562
- CT, 562, 1020
- CTD, 495
- CTR, 976
- CTS, 562
- CV, 74, 257
- CVA, 562
- CVS, 731
- CXR, 189, 1020
- cysto, 619
- D&C, 731
- dB, db, 887
- D.C., 74
- D.D.S., 74
- Derm, 377
- DEXA, 1020
- DEXA or DXA, 442
- DI, 789
- DIC, 320
- diff, 320
- DIP, 442
- DJD, 442
- DKA, 789
- DM, 789
- DNA, 976
- D.O, 74
- DOE, 189
- D.P.M., 74
- Dr., 74
- DRE, 658
- DS, 25
- DSA, 257, 1020
- DT, 927
- DTRs, 495
- DUB, 731
- Dx, 25
- DXA, 1020
- EAC, 887
- EBT, 1020
- EBV, 320
- ECCE, 839
- ECG, 257
- echo, 257
- ECT, 927
- ED, 74, 658
- EDB, 731
- EDC, 731
- EEG, 562
- EGA, 731
- EGD, 134
- EKG, 257
- ELISA, 320
- EMB, 731
- EMG, 495
- END, 562
- ENT, 74, 887
- EOM, 839
- EOMI, 839
- eos, 320
- epi, 619
- EPR, 25
- ER, 976
- ERCP, 134
- ESRD, 619
- ESWL, 619
- ESWT, 442
- ETOH, 927
- ETT, 189
- FBS, 789
- FEV_1, 189
- FHR, 731
- A fib, 257
- fib, 442
- FIGO, 976
- FiO_2, 189
- FSH, 658, 731, 789
- FTI, 789
- FVC, 189
- Fx, 442
- G, 731
- GC, 658
- GCS, 562
- G-CSF, 320
- GERD, 134
- GH, 789
- GI, 74
- GIFT, 731
- GM-CSF, 320
- G/TPAL, 731
- GTT, 789
- GU, 619, 658
- GVHD, 320
- GYN, 74, 731
- H&H, 320
- H&P, 25
- HAV, 134
- HbA_{1C}, 789
- HBV, 134
- HCG, 976
- HCG, hCG, 731
- HCT, 320
- HCV, 134
- HDL, 257
- HEENT, 839, 887
- Hgb, 320
- HIPAA, 25
- HIV, 320, 658
- HLA, 320
- HMD, 189
- HNP, 562
- hpf, 619
- HPI, 25
- HPV, 658, 731
- HRT, 731
- HSG, 731
- HSIL, 731
- HSV, 377, 658
- HTN, 257
- Hx, 74
- Hz, 887
- I&D, 377
- I&O, 619
- IBD, 134
- IBS, 134
- ICCE, 839
- ICP, 562
- ICSI, 731
- IDDM, 789
- IgA, 320
- IgD, 320
- IgE, 320
- IgG, 320
- IgM, 320
- IM, 495
- IOL, 839
- IOP, 839
- IRS, 789
- IUGR, 732
- IVC, 134, 1020
- IVF, 732
- IVP, 619, 1020
- JVD, 257
- K, K^+, 789
- K or K^+, 619
- KUB, 619, 1020

L&D, 732
L1-L5, 442
LASIK, 839
Lat, 1020
LBBB, 257
LDH, 257
LDL, 257
LEEP, 732
LES, 134
LFTs, 134
LGA, 732
LH, 658, 732, 789
LLE, 442, 495
LLL, 189
LLQ, 43, 44*f*
LMP, 732
LP, 562
LPN, 74
L/S, 732
LSD, 927
LSIL, 732
LTK, 839
LUE, 442, 495
LUQ, 43, 44*f*
LV, 257
LVAD, 257
LVH, 257
lymphs, 320
MAO, 927
MCH, 320
MCP, 442
MCV, 320
M.D., 74
MD, 495
MDI, 189
mets, 976
MI, 257
mL, 619
mm Hg, 257
mm^3, 320
mono, 320
monos, 320
MR, 257
MRA, 1020
MRI, 38*f*, 182, 562, 1020
MS, 562
MSH, 789
MUGA, 257, 1020
MVP, 257
N&V, 134
Na, Na^+, 789
NB, 732
NG, 134
NICU, 562, 732
NIDDM, 789
NK, 976
NP, 74
NPH, 789
NPO (n.p.o), 134
NSAID, 442, 495
NSR, 257
NST, 732
NSVD, 732
O, 25, 320
O&P, 134
O_2, 189
OA, 442
OB, 74, 732
OCD, 927
OCG, 134
OCP, 732
OD, 74
O.D., 839
OD, 927
OD, O.D., 839
OGTT, 789
OOB, 495
ortho, 442, 495
OS, O.S., 839
OSHA, 495
OU, O.U., 839
P, 25, 257, 442, 732
PA, 36, 37*f*, 74, 189, 1020
PAC, 257
PAD, 257
PAP, 658
Pap, 732
PCO_2, 189
PCP, 74, 189, 927
PD, 839
PDA, 257
PDT, 377
PE, 25, 887
PEG, 134
PEJ, 134
PERRL, 839
PERRLA, 839
PET, 562, 1020
PFTs, 189
pH, 619
Pharm.D, 74
PICC, 976
PID, 732
PIP, 442
PM&R, 495
PMDD, 732, 927
PMI, 257
PMN, 320
PMS, 732
PND, 189, 887
P.O. (p.o.), 134
PO_2, 189
polys, 320
PPD, 189
PR, 976
PRBCs, 320
PRK, 839
pro time, 320
PROM, 732
PSA, 658, 976
Psy, 927
Psych, 927
PT, 74, 320, 442, 495
PTC, 134
PTCA, 257
PTSD, 927
PTT, 320
PUD, 134
PUVA, 377
PVC, 257
PVD, 134, 257
QCT, 442, 1020
R, r, 1020
RA, 189, 442
rad, 1020
RAIU, 789, 1020
RBBB, 257
RBC, 320, 619
RDS, 189
rehab, 495
rem, 1020
RFA, 257
RIA, 789
RIND, 562
RLE, 442, 495
RLL, 189
RLQ, 43, 44*f*
RML, 189
RN, 74
RNA, 976
RNV, 257, 1020
ROM, 442, 495, 732
ROP, 839
ROS, 25
RP, 839
RPR, 658
RRT, 189, 1020
RSI, 495
RUE, 442, 495
RUL, 189
RUQ, 43, 44*f*
S, 25
S1, 442
S_1, S_2, S_3, and S_4, 257
SA, 257
SAB, 732
SAD, 789, 927
SARS, 189
SBE, 257
SCC, 732
SCI, 562
segmenters, 320
segs, 320
SG, 619
SGA, 732
SGOT, 134
SGPT, 134
SIADH, 789
SIDS, 189
SLE, 377
SNF, 74
SOAP, 25
SOB, 189
SOM, 887
sp gr, 619
SPECT, 257, 1020
SQ, 377
SSEP, 562
SSER, 562
SSRI, 927
STD, 658, 732
subcu, 377
subQ, 377
SVT, 257
Sx, 74
T&A, 887
T1-T12, 442
T_3, 789
T4, 789
T_7, 789
TAB, 732
TACE, 976
TAH-BSO, 732
TAT, 927
TB, 189
TEE, 257, 1020
TENS, 562
TFTs, 789
THR, 442
TIA, 562
tib, 442
TM, 887
TMJ, 887
TNF, 320
TNM, 976
TNTC, 619
TPA, 320
TPAL, 732
TPR, 189, 257
trach, 189
TRAM, 732
TRUS, 658
TSE, 658
TSH, 789
TURBT, 619
TURP, 658
TVH, 732
Tx, 74
UA, 619
UGI, 134, 1020
URI, 189, 887
US, 1020
UTI, 619
V fib, 257
V tach, 257
VBAC, 732
VD, 658
VDRL, 658
VEP, 562
VER, 562
VF, 839
VLDL, 257
VMA, 619, 789, 976
V/Q, 189, 1020
VSD, 257
WBC, 320, 619
ZIFT, 732
Abdominal aorta, 212
Abdominal aortic aneurysm (AAA), 236
Abdominal cavity, 42, 116–17
Abdominis, 462
Abdominopelvic cavity, 42–43, 94
Abducens, 519
Abducens nerve, 519
Abduction, 464
Abductor, 464
Ablation, 249, 724
Abnormal breath sounds, 170
Abnormal presentation of the fetus, 708
Abnormal red blood cell morphology, 300
ABO blood group, 285
Abortion (AB, Ab), 711, 722, 723
Abrasion, 354
Abruptio placentae, 708
Abscess, 357
Absence, 544
Absence seizures, 544
Absorption, 97
Accessory, 519
Accessory nerve, 519
Acetabular, 408
Acetabulum, 408
Acetaminophen, 172
Acetylcholine, 218, 472, 525
Achilles tendon, 471
Achondroplasia, 773
Acid phosphatase, 653
Acid-fast bacillus (AFB), 176
Acidic, 117, 607
Acne rosacea, 366
Acne vulgaris, 365, 366*t*
Acoustic, 871
Acoustic neuroma, 871
Acquired immunodeficiency syndrome (AIDS), 175, 304–05, 652
Acrocyanosis, 690
Acromegaly, 772
Acromion, 405
Acrophobia, 909
Actinic, 360
Actinic keratoses, 360
Active immunity, 291
Acuity, 831
Acute, 64–65
Acute lymphocytic leukemia (ALL), 305, 306*f*, 961
Acute myelogenous leukemia (AML), 305, 961
Acute renal failure (ARF), 600
Acute tubular necrosis, 600

ADA (American Diabetes Association) diet, 786
Adaptive devices, 490
Addiction, 917
Addison, Thomas, 782
Addison's disease, 782
Adduction, 464
Adductor, 464
Adenocarcinoma, 110, 111, 122, 173, 707, 957
Adenohypophysis, 755
Adenoids, 861
Adenoma, 771, 774
Adenomata, 771
Adenomatous, 775
Adenomatous goiter, 774
Adhesions, 116
Adipocere, 342
Adipose, 341
Adipose tissue, 341, 342
Adjuvant, 975
Adjuvant therapy, 975
Adnexa, 678, 679
Adnexal, 679
Adolescence, 642
Adrenal, 760
Adrenal cortex, 760–61
Adrenal glands
  cortex
    aldosterone, 760, 761
    androgens, 760
    cortisol, 760
  medulla
    epinephrine, 761
    norepinephrine, 761
Adrenalectomy, 786
Adrenocorticotropic, 756
Adrenocorticotropic hormone (ACTH), 756
Adrenogenital, 782
Adrenogenital syndrome, 782
Adult respiratory distress syndrome (ARDS), 170
Affect, 905
Affective, 774, 906
Affective or mood disorders, 917–19
Afferent, 521
Afferent nerves, 521
Age spots, 362
Agglutination, 310
Aggregation, 286
Aging
  benign prostatic hypertrophy (BPH), 649
  bone breakdown, 414
  constipation, 115
  decubitus ulcers, 356
  and exercise, 471
  floaters, 825
  food, smell and taste of, 90
  hair, graying of, 342
  incontinence, 604
  kidney function, decrease in, 589
  menopause, 705
  night blindness, 825
  nocturia, 605
  pernicious anemia, 302
  presbyacusis, 872
  presbyopia, 825
  pulmonary function, decrease in, 162
  senile lentigo (age spots), 362
  skin, 344
  uterine prolapse, 704
Agoraphobia, 909
AIDS. *see* Acquired immunodeficiency syndrome (AIDS)
Ala, 858
Alae, 858
Albinism, 352
Albino, 352
Albumen, 285
Albumin, 123, 284, 285
Albuminuria, 603
Aldosterone, 760, 761
Alimentary canal. *see* Gastrointestinal system
Alkaline, 607
Alkaline phosphatase, 123
Alkylating drugs, 974
Allergens, 344
Allergic, 344, 874
Allergic reactions, 344, 360
Allergic rhinitis, 874
Allergy, 344
Allergy skin testing, 369
Allied health professionals, 67
Allogeneic, 317
Allogeneic transplants, 317
Allograft, 374, 439
Alopecia, 367
Alpha cells, 759
Alpha fetoprotein (AFP), 553, 717, 965
Alveoli, 158, 162
Alveolus, 158
Alveolar, 158
Alzheimer, Alois, 542
Alzheimer's disease, 541*f*, 542, 561, 905
Amblyopia, 828
Ambu bag, 185
Ambulatory, 68, 613
Ambulatory surgery centers (ASCs), 68
Amenorrhea, 704
American Diabetes Association (ADA), 786
American Psychiatric Association, 923
Americans with Disabilities Act (ADA) of 1990, 490
Aminoglycoside antibiotic drugs, 618
Amnesia, 536, 910
Amnestic, 910
Amniocentesis, 717
Amnion, 686
Amniotic, 686
Amniotic cavity, 686
Amniotic fluid, 686, 687
Amniotomy, 721
Amputation, 438
Amputee, 438
Amygdaloid bodies, 904, 905
Amylase, 97
Amyotrophic, 549
Amyotrophic lateral sclerosis (ALS), 549
Anacusis, 872
Anal sphincter, 93
Analgesic, 440, 493, 560
Anaphylactic, 344
Anaphylactic shock, 344
Anaphylaxis, 344
Anaplasia, 955
Anastomosis, 128, 251, 726
Anatomical position, 35, 35*f*
Anatomy, 44. see also individual systems
Ancillary departments, 67
Androgen, 657, 677, 678*f*, 760, 761
Anemia, 301
Anemias, types listed, 301–03
Anemic, 301
Anencephaly, 536
Anesthesia, 355, 549, 721
Anesthetic, 549, 561
Anesthetic drugs, 549
Aneurysmal, 236
Aneurysmal dilation, 236
Aneurysmectomy, 251
Aneurysms, 236
Angina, 229
Angina pectoris, 229
Anginal, 229
Angiogenesis, 950
Angiogram, 245, 553, 997
Angiography, 245, 553, 610, 997
Angioplasty, 252
Angiosarcoma, 959
Anhedonia, 918
Anhidrosis, 367
Anicteric, 823
Anisocoria, 823
Anisocytosis, 300
Ankylosing, 429
Ankylosing spondylitis, 429
Anorexia, 107
Anorexia nervosa, 107, 912
Anorexic, 107
Anosmia, 875
Anovulation, 701
Anoxia, 179
Anoxic, 179
Antacid drugs, 133
Anteflexion, 679
Antepartum, 687
Anterior, 36
Anterior chamber of the eye, 811
Anterior fontanel, 690
Anterior pituitary gland, 755–56. *see also* Pituitary gland
Anterior section, 36
Anteriorly (anterior direction), 36, 37*f*
Anterograde, 910
Anterograde amnesia, 910
Anteroposterior (AP), 36
Anthracosis, 174
Antianxiety drugs, 926
Antiarrhythmic drugs, 256
Antibiotic drugs, 133, 187, 254, 376, 618, 657, 729, 838, 885
Antibodies, 290, 489
Anticoagulant drugs, 318
Anticonvulsant drugs, 560
Antidepressant drugs, 926
Antidiabetic drugs, 787
Antidiarrheal drugs, 133
Antidiuretic drugs, 756
Antidiuretic hormone (ADH), 754, 756
Antiemetic drugs, 133, 974
Antiepileptic drugs, 560
Antifungal drugs, 376
Antigens, 285, 290, 653
Antihistamine drugs, 885
Antihypertensive drugs, 256
Anti-inflammatory drugs, 441
Antimetabolite drugs, 974
Antipruritic drugs, 376
Antipsychotic drugs, 927
Antiretroviral drugs, 320
Antisocial, 921
Antisocial personality, 921
Antispasmodic drugs, 619
Antisperm antibody test, 716
Antithyroglobulin, 784
Antithyroid drugs, 787
Antitubercular drugs, 187
Antitussive drugs, 187, 886
Antiviral drugs, 376, 657, 838
Antiyeast drugs, 886
Antrum of stomach, 91
Anuria, 603
Anus, 93
Anxiety, 908
Anxiety disorders, 908–10
Anxiolytic drugs, 926
Aorta, 94, 212, 233
Aortic, 208, 212
Aortic arch, 212
Aortic valve, 208
Aortogram, 245, 997
Aortography, 245, 997
Apathy, 918
Apex, 158
Apex of the heart, 208
Apex of the lung, 158
Apgar score, 721
Apgar, Virginia, 721
Aphakia, 824
Aphakic, 824
Aphasia, 536
Aphasic, 536
Apheresis, 316
Aphthous stomatitis, 107
Apical, 158, 208
Apical pulse, 250
Apices, 158
Aplastic anemia, 301
Apnea, 177, 712
Apneic, 177
Aponeurosis, 461
Apoptosis, 947
Appendectomy, 127
Appendicitis, 111
Appendicular, 397
Appendicular skeleton, 397
Appendix, 93, 94, 288
Apperception, 923
Appropriate for gestational age (AGA), 713
Aqueous humor, 811
Arachnoid, 518
Arachnophobia, 909
Areola, 682
Areolae, 682
Areolar, 682
Arrest of labor, 708
Arrhythmia, 233
Art therapy, 924
Arterial, 180
Arteries. *see* under Blood vessels
Arteriogram, 245, 553
Arteriography, 245, 553, 610, 997
Arteriolar, 211
Arterioles, 211
Arteriosclerosis, 237–38
Arteriosclerotic, 237
Arteriosclerotic cardiovascular disease (ASCVD), 237
Arteriovenous, 537
Arteriovenous malformation (AVM), 537
Artery, 20
Athetoid, 486
Athetoid movements, 486
Arthralgia, 431
Arthritis, 431
Arthrocentesis, 438
Arthrodesis, 438
Arthrogram, 434, 998
Arthrography, 434, 998

Arthropathy, 431
Arthroplasty, 439
Arthroscope, 438
Arthroscopic, 438
Arthroscopy, 438
Articular, 411
Articular cartilage, 411
Articulations, 410–11
Asbestosis, 174
Ascending aorta, 212
Ascites, 117, 599
Ascitic fluid, 117
Aspermia, 654
Asphyxia, 179
Aspiration, 315, 373, 655, 713
Aspiration pneumonia, 174
Aspirin, 172
Assay, 714, 784
Assisted reproduction, 723
Asthma, 169
Asthmatic, 169
Astigmatism, 827
Astrocytes, 522
Astrocytoma, 538, 959
Asymptomatic, 63
Asystole, 234
Ataxia, 486
Ataxic, 486
Atelectasis, 170
Atelectatic, 170
Arteriogram, 997
Atheroma, 237
Atheromatous, 237
Atheromatous plaque, 237, 238
Atherosclerosis, 229, 237
Athetosis, 545
Atlas (C1), 403
Atria, 208
Atrial, 208
Atrial septal defect (ASD), 233
Atrioventricular node (AV node), 217
Atrium, 208
Atrophic, 482
Atrophy, 482
Attending physician, 66
Attention-deficit hyperactivity disorder (ADHD), 911
Attenuated, 316
Audiogram, 879
Audiologist, 888
Audiometer, 879
Audiometry, 879
Auditory, 515
Auditory cortex, 515, 864
Auditory nerve, 519, 864
Augmentation, 727
Aura, 543
Auricle, 855
Auricular, 855
Auscultation, 64, 182, 248
Autism, 911
Autograft, 374, 439
Autoimmune, 310
Autoimmune disorders, 310, 354, 364–65
Autologous, 317
Autologous blood transfusion, 317
Autologous transplants, 317
Automatic external defibrillator (AED), 248
Automatic implantable cardioverter/defibrillator (AICD), 248
Automatisms, 544
Autonomic, 522
Autonomic nervous system, 522
AV (atrioventricular) node, 219
Avascular, 424
Avascular necrosis, 424
Aversion, 924
Aversion therapy, 924
Avoidant personality, 921
Avulsion, 482
Axial, 397, 554
Axial skeleton, 397
Axillary artery, 213
Axis (C2), 403
Axons, 524

B

B cells, 290
Babinski, Joseph, 556
Babinski's sign, 556
Bacterial vaginosis, 706
Bacteria
  Acid-fast bacilli (AFB), 176
  Chlamydia trachomatis, 602, 651
  Clostridium botulinum, 370
  Escherichia coli (E. coli), 605
  Gardnerella vaginalis, 706
  Helicobacter pylori, 110, 123
  in large intestine, 98
  Legionella pneumophilia, 173
  Mycobacterium tuberculosis, 176, 182
  Mycoplasma pneumoniae, 175
  Neisseria gonorrhoeae, 602, 652
  Staphylococcus aureus, 357, 707, 709
  Streptococcus pneumoniae, 175
  Treponema pallidum, 652
Bacterial pneumonia, 174
Bacteriuria, 603
Balanitis, 650
Ball-and-socket synovial joints, 411
Balloon angioplasty, 252
Barium, 124, 998
Barium enema, 998
Barré, Jean, 550
Barrel chest, 171
Bartholin, Casper, 681
Bartholin's glands, 681
Basal, 340, 684, 957
Basal (baseline) body temperature, 684
Basal cell carcinoma, 363, 957
Basal layer of skin, 340
Basophils, 281, 289–90
Beck Depression Inventory (BDI), 922
Becker's muscular dystrophy, 483
Behavioral, 924
Bell, Alexander Graham, 879
Bell, Charles, 550
Bell's palsy, 550
Bence Jones, Henry, 314
Bence Jones protein, 314
Benign, 114, 352, 361
Benign familial polyposis, 114
Benign prostatic hypertrophy (BPH), 649, 657
Beta cells, 759
Bethesda System
  abnormal Pap smear, 716
  normal Pap smear, 716
  Pap smear results, reporting, 715–16
  specimen adequacy, 716
Biceps, 462
Biceps brachii, 461f, 462, 468
Biceps femoris, 470, 471
Bicuspid, 208
Bicuspid valve, 208
Bigeminal, 235
Bigeminy, 235
Bilateral, 725
Bilateral clubfeet, 434
Bilateral oophorectomy, 725
Bilateral salpingo-oophorectomy (BSO), 726
Bile, 94, 97
Bile ducts, 94–95, 121
Biliary colic, 121
Biliary tree, 95
Bilirubin, 94, 123, 279
Biliverdin, 94
Bimanual, 720
Bimanual examination, 720
Biophysical, 722
Biophysical profile (BPP), 722
Biopsy (Bx), 127, 373. *see also under* Surgical procedures
Biparietal, 719
Biparietal diameter (BPD), 719
Bipolar, 917
Bipolar disorder, 917–18
Bladder, 20, 585, 601–02
Bladder cancer, 601
Blepharitis, 821
Blepharoplasty, 374
Blepharoptosis, 821
Blindness, 828
Blister, 354
Blood. *see also* Hematology
  anatomy of
    electrolytes, 284
    erythrocytes, 278–79
    hematopoiesis, 279
    leukocytes, 280–83. *see also* Leukocytes
    plasma, 277
    substances in, 284
    thrombocytes (platelets), 284
  blood type
    ABO blood group, 285
    Rh blood group, 285
    transfusion reaction, 304
    type and crossmatch, 310
  circulation of, 215f
    pulmonary circulation, 215, 216
    systemic circulation, 215, 216
  defined, 46f, 277
  donation and transfusion procedures, 316–17
  lymphatic system, interdependency with, 287
  pH, 590
Blood cell tests. *see* under Diagnostic procedures
Blood chemistries, 312–13
Blood chemistry analyzer, 312f
Blood clotting, physiology of, 286
Blood dyscrasia, 300
Blood pressure, 250–51, 590
Blood tests. *see under* Diagnostic procedures
Blood vessels
  arteries
    of abdomen, 213
    aorta, 212
    of arms, 213
    arterioles, 211
    of body, 212f
    characteristics and functions, 210
    of head and chest, 212–13
    of hips and legs, 213
    pulse, 211
    vasoconstriction, 211
    vasodilation, 211
  capillaries, 214
  defined, 210
  intima, 210
  lumen, 210
  symptoms, signs, and diseases, 236–41
  vasculature, 210
  veins
    characteristics and functions, 214
    venules, 214
Body cavities
  abdominal, 42
  abdominopelvic, 42–43, 94
  cranial, 42
  and diaphragm, 42
  and mediastinum, 42
  pelvic, 42
  spinal (spinal canal), 42
  thoracic, 42
  viscera, 43
Body directions
  anterior/anteriorly, 36, 37f
  anteroposterior (AP), 36
  caudad, 40
  cephalad, 40
  deep, 41
  distal/distally, 41
  external, 41
  inferior/inferiorly, 40
  internal, 41
  lateral/laterally, 38, 39f
  medial/medially, 38, 39f
  posterior/posteriorly, 36, 37f
  posteroanterior (PA), 36, 37f
  proximal/proximally, 41
  superficial, 41
  superior/superiorly, 40
Body dysmorphic disorder, 913
Body of stomach, 91
Body planes. *see* Coronal plane; Midsagittal plane; Transverse plane
Body systems, listed, 45, 46–50f. *see also individual systems*
Body temperature, basal (baseline), 684
Bone densitometry, 1001
Bone density tests, 435, 1001
Bone growth, 413–14
Bone marrow, 411–12
Bone marrow aspiration, 963
Bone marrow transplantation (BMT), 317
Bone tumors, 424
Bones. *see also* Fractures; Orthopedics; Skeletal system
  ankle, foot, and toes
    calcaneus, 410
    metatarsal bones, 410
    phalanges, 410
    tarsal bones, 410
  arms, upper and lower
    humerus, 406
    olecranon, 406
    radius, 406
    ulna, 406
  chest
    costal cartilage, 402
    costochondral joint, 402
    manubrium, 401
    ribs, 401–02
    sternum, 401
    thoracic cavity, 401

thorax, 401
xiphoid process, 401
head. *see also* Cranium; Facial bones
hyoid bone, 401
ossicles, 401
ossicular chain, 401
hips
acetabulum, 408
iliac crest, 408
iliac spine, 408
ilium, 408
ischium, 408
obturator foramen, 408
pelvis, 408
pubic bone, 408
pubic symphysis, 408
pubis, 408
legs, upper and lower
femur, 409
fibula, 409
lateral malleolus, 409
medial malleolus, 409
patella, 410
tibia, 409
trochanters, 409
neck and back
atlas (C1), 403
axis (C2), 403
cervical vertebrae (C1-C7), 403
coccyx, 403
intervertebral disks, 404
lumbar vertebrae (L1-L5), 403, 404*f*
nucleus pulposis, 404
sacrum, 403
spinal column, 402
spine, 402
spinous process, 404
thoracic vertebrae (T1-T12), 403
transverse processes, 404
vertebral column, 402
vertebral foramen, 404
shoulders
acromion, 405
clavicle, 405
coracoid process, 405
glenoid fossa, 405
scapula, 405
structure of, 411, 412*f*
symptoms, signs, and diseases, 424–28
wrist, hand, and fingers
carpal bones, 406*f*, 407
distal phalanx, 407
metacarpal bones, 406*f*, 407
phalangeal bones, 407
phalanges, 406*f*, 407
Bony, 397
Borderline personality, 921
Botox, 370
Bowel, 92
Bowleg, 433
Bowman's capsule, 588
Braces, 490
Brachial artery, 213
Brachii, 462
Brachioradialis, 462, 468
Bradycardia, 234
Bradycardic, 234
Bradykinesia, 486
Bradypnea, 177
Brain
brainstem
defined, 517
medulla oblongata, 517
midbrain, 517
pons, 517
substantia nigra, 517
cerebellum, 517
cerebrum
auditory cortex, 515
cerebral cortex, 515
corpus callosum, 516
defined, 514
frontal lobe, 514
gray matter, 515
gustatory cortex, 514
gyri, 515
hemispheres, 516
left-brain thinking, 516
lobes, 514
occipital lobe, 514
olfactory cortex, 515
parietal lobe, 514
right-brain thinking, 516
sulci, 515
temporal lobe, 515
visual cortex, 514
white matter, 515
cranial cavity, 513
cranium, 513
defined, 513
hypothalamus, 517
meninges
arachnoid, 518
dura mater, 518
pia mater, 518
subarachnoid space, 518
symptoms, signs, and diseases, 536–46
thalamus, 517
ventricles
cerebrospinal fluid (CSF), 517
defined, 517
Brain attack, 539
Brain death, 540
Brain tumors, 537, 538
Brainstem, 517
Braxton Hicks contractions, 687
Braxton Hicks, John, 687
BRCA1 or BRCA2 gene, 714
Breast cancer, 707
Breast implant, 727
Breast self-examination (BSE), 721
Breasts, 682, 721, 726–28
Breath, 162
Breathe, 162
Breech, 708
Breech presentation, 708
Brevis, 462
Broad ligament, 676, 679
Bronchi, 157, 169
Bronchial, 157
Bronchial tree, 157
Bronchiectasis, 169
Bronchiolar, 157
Bronchiole, 157
Bronchioles, 169
Bronchitis, 169
Bronchodilator drugs, 187
Bronchogenic, 958
Bronchogenic carcinoma, 958
Bronchopneumonia, 175
Bronchopulmonary, 157
Bronchoscope, 185
Bronchoscopy, 185
Bronchospasm, 169
Bronchus, 157
Bruit, 238
Buccal, 861
Buccal mucosa, 861
Buccinator, 466
Buffalo hump, 781
Bulbourethral, 640
Bulbourethral glands, 640
Bulimia, 912
Bulla, 355
Bullae, 355
Bundle branch block, right or left, 235
Bundle branches, 217
Bundle of His, 217
Bunionectomy, 439
Bunions, 433
Burns, 355
Bursa, 461
Bursae, 461
Bursal, 461
Bursitis, 487

C

Calcaneal, 410
Calcaneal tendon, 471
Calcaneus, 410, 471
Calcitonin, 414, 758
Calcium ions (Ca^{++}), 218, 284, 472
Calculi, 597–98
Calculogenesis, 598
Calculus, 597–98
Caliber, 604
Caliceal, 584
Calices, 584
Caliectasis, 597
Calix, 584
Callus, 355
Canal, 639, 680, 856
Cancellous, 412
Cancellous bone, 411, 412*f*
Cancer. *see also* Oncology
defined, 955
warning signs of, 956
Cancerous, 600, 955
Candida albicans, 706, 877
Candidiasis, 305, 706, 877
Canker sores, 107
Cannula, 184
Capillaries, 214
Capillary, 214
Capitis, 358
Capsular, 411
Capsule, 411, 584
Carbaminohemoglobin, 162
Carbon dioxide (CO_2), 161, 162, 179
Carbon monoxide (CO), 179, 279
Carboxyhemoglobin, 180
Carbuncle, 357
Carcinoembryonic, 965
Carcinoembryonic antigen (CEA), 965
Carcinogens, 948
Carcinoid, 955
Carcinoid syndrome, 955
Carcinoid tumor, 955
Carcinoma, 120, 173, 363, 776, 875, 957–58
Carcinoma in situ (CIS), 705
Carcinomatosis, 955
Cardia of stomach, 91, 223
Cardiac, 11, 223
Cardiac arrest, 234
Cardiac cycle, 218
Cardiac muscles, 459, 460*f*
Cardiac risk factors, 238
Cardiac sphincter, 91, 108, 223
Cardiac tamponade, 231
Cardiac valve, 223
Cardiologist, 258
Cardiology. *see also* Cardiovascular system
abbreviations, 257
defined, 11, 206
diagnostic procedures
blood tests, 241–42
heart related, 242–44
radiology and nuclear medicine procedures, 245–47
drug categories, 254–56
medical procedures, 248–51
surgical procedures, 251–54
symptoms, signs, and diseases
blood vessels, 236–41
conduction system, 233–36
heart valves and layers of the heart, 231–33
myocardium, 229–30
Cardiomegaly, 229
Cardiomyopathy, 229
Cardiopulmonary, 160, 183, 215, 251
Cardiopulmonary resuscitation (CPR), 25, 183
Cardiothoracic, 210
Cardiothoracic surgeon, 190, 258
Cardiovascular surgeon, 258
Cardiovascular system. *see also* Blood
anatomy of
blood vessels, 210–14. *see also* Blood vessels
heart, 207–10. *see also* Heart
thoracic cavity and mediastinum, 210
circulation of blood
pulmonary circulation, 215, 216
systemic circulation, 215, 216
defined, 46*f*, 206*f*, 207
heartbeat, physiology of
conduction system, 217, 233–36
heart rate, increasing, 218
on molecular level, 218
Cardioversion, 248
Carotid arteries, 213
Carpal, 407, 550
Carpal bones, 406*f*, 407
Carpal tunnel syndrome (CTS), 550
Cartilage, 402, 424–28
Cartilaginous, 402
Caruncle, 807, 808*f*
Casts, 436
Catalepsy, 920
Catatonic, 920
Cataract, 824
Cataract extraction. *see under* Surgical procedures
Catatonia, 920
Catheter, 612
Catheterization, 242, 612
Cauda equina, 520
Caudad direction, 40
Causalgia, 551
Cavities, defined, 42. *see also* Body cavities
Cavity, 159
CD4 cells, 290
Cecum, 93
Celiac disease, 113
Celiac trunk of the aorta, 94
Cell, 20
Cell membrane, 945
Cells
cell membrane, 945
cytoplasm, 945
defined, 945
intracellular contents, 945

Cells (*continued*)
- nucleolus, 947
- organelles
  - chromosomes, 946
  - defined, 946
  - endoplasmic reticulum, 946
  - Golgi apparatus, 946
  - lysosomes, 946
  - messenger RNA, 946
  - mitochondria, 946
  - nucleus, 947
  - ribosomes, 947
- structures of, 945

Cellular, 945
Cellular differentiation, 949
Cellular division and cancer
- angiogenesis, 950
- apoptosis, 947
- cell and tumor characteristics, 949–50
- contributing factors
  - carcinogens, 948
  - heredity, 949
  - oncogenes, 948
  - pathogens, 948
- genetic mutations, 948
- metastasis, 950
- mitosis, 947
- mitotic rate, 947
- suppressor genes, 947
- translocation, 948
- tumor necrosis factor (TNF), 949
- undifferentiated appearance, 949

Cellulitis, 357
Central, 513
Central nervous system (CNS), 513
Cephalad direction, 40
Cephalalgia, 537
Cephalic, 687
Cephalic presentation, 687
Cephalopelvic, 709
Cephalopelvic disproportion (CPD), 709
Cerclage, 729
Cerebellar, 517
Cerebellum, 517
Cerebral, 515
Cerebral cortex, 515
Cerebral palsy (CP), 486, 537
Cerebrospinal, 517
Cerebrospinal fluid (CSF), 517
Cerebrospinal fluid (CSF) examination, 553
Cerebrovascular, 539
Cerebrovascular accident (CVA), 539–40
Cerebrum, 514
Cerumen, 856
Cerumen impaction, 871
Cervical, 403, 680
Cervical broom, 715
Cervical canal, 680
Cervical cancer, 705
Cervical dysplasia, 706
Cervical lymphadenopathy, 876
Cervical os, 680
Cervical ripening, 687
Cervical vertebrae (C1-C7), 403
Cervix, 680, 705–06, 724
Cesarean section, 729
Chalazion, 821
Chancre, 652
Cheilitis, 107
Cheiloplasty, 883
Chemoembolization, 972
Chemotherapy antibiotic drugs, 974
Chemotherapy drugs, 133, 187, 318, 376, 440, 493, 560, 618, 657, 729, 838, 886
Chemotherapy drugs, insertion of administration devices. *see* Medical procedures; Surgical procedures
Chemotherapy enzyme drugs, 975
Chemotherapy protocols, 975
Chest x-ray, 174*f*, 182
Chiasm, 815
Chin, 860
Chiropractic, 496
Chiropractor, 496
Chlamydia, 651
Chlamydia trachomatis, 602, 651
Chloasma, 354
Chocolate cysts, 702
Cholangiocarcinoma, 958
Cholangiogram, 125
Cholangiography, 125, 998
Cholangiopancreatography, 125
Cholangitis, 121
Cholecystectomy, 128
Cholecystitis, 121
Cholecystogram, 126
Cholecystography, 126
Cholecystography, oral (OCG), 998
Cholecystokinin, 97
Choledocholithiasis, 121
Cholelithiasis, 121
Cholesteatoma, 871
Cholesterol, 237
Chondroma, 424
Chondromalacia, 424
Chondromalacia patellae, 424
Chondrosarcoma, 959
Chordae tendineae, 208–09
Chordee, 650
Chorea, 545
Choriocarcinoma, 962
Choroidal, 810
Chorion, 686
Chorionic, 686
Chorionic villus sampling (CVS), 717
Choroid, 810
Choroiditis, 824
Chromosomal, 946
Chromosome studies, 717
Chromosomes, 717, 946
Chronic, 65
Chronic bronchitis, 169, 171
Chronic lymphocytic leukemia (CLL), 305, 961
Chronic myelogenous leukemia (CML), 305, 961
Chronic obstructive pulmonary disease (COPD), 169, 171
Chronic renal failure (CRF), 600
Chyme, 92
Cicatrix (scar), 356
Cilia, 157, 158, 678
Ciliary, 810
Ciliary body, 810
Cilium, 157
Cineradiology, 1000
Cingulate, 903
Cingulate gyrus, 903
Circadian rhythm, 757
Circulation, 215
Circulation of blood, 215–16
Circulatory, 215
Circulatory system. *see* Cardiovascular system
Circumcision, 656
Circumoral cyanosis, 179
Cirrhosis, 118
Cirrhotic, 118
Claudication, 239
Claustrophobia, 909
Clavicle, 405
Clavicular, 405
Cleft, 876
Cleft lip and palate, 876
Client, 68
Climacteric, 704, 705
Clinical laboratory scientist, 659
Clinic, 68
Clitoris, 681
CLO (Campylobacter-like organism), 123
Clonic, 544
Clostridium botulinum, 370
Clotting factors, 286
Clubbing, 171, 369
Clubfoot, 434
Coagulation, 286, 307
Coagulation tests, 312
Coagulopathy, 307
Coarctation, 233
Coarctation of the aorta, 233
Coccygeal, 403
Coccyx, 403
Cochlea, 858
Cochleae, 858
Cochlear, 858
Cockroaches, 169
Coffee-grounds emesis, 108
Cognitive, 910
Cognitive disorders, 910
Cognitive function, 910
Cognitive-behavioral therapy (CBT), 924
Cold sores, 876
Colic, 111, 598
Colitis, 113
Collagen, 340
Collapsed lung, 170
Colon, 93
Colon cancer, 111
Colonic polyps, 114
Colonoscope, 130
Colonoscopy, 130
Color blindness, 825
Color blindness testing, 829
Color flow duplex ultrasonography, 1006
Colorectal adenocarcinoma, 111
Colostrum, 689
Colporrhaphy, 724
Colposcopy, 720
Coma, 540
Comatose, 540
Combining forms. *see also* Medical words
- characteristics of, 7
- combining vowel, 7
- from Greek and Latin, 75, 135, 190, 258, 321, 379, 443, 495, 563, 620, 659, 733, 790, 840, 888, 927, 977
- joining two, 19
- prefixes, joining to, 16
- root, 7
- suffixes, joining to, 11

Combining forms, listed
- abdomin/o-, 42
- ablat/o-, 724
- abort/o-, 711
- abras/o-, 354
- absorpt/o-, 97
- access/o-, 519
- accommod/o-, 831
- acetabul/o-, 408
- acid/o-, 780
- acous/o-, 871
- acr/o-, 690
- actin/o-, 360
- act/o-, 786
- acu/o-, 831
- addict/o-, 917
- aden/o-, 110
- adhes/o-, 116
- adip/o-, 341
- adjuv/o-, 975
- adnex/o-, 679
- adolesc/o-, 642
- adrenal/o-, 786
- adren/o-, 756
- affer/o-, 521
- agglutin/o-, 310
- aggreg/o-, 286
- ag/o-, 759
- agor/a-, 909
- albin/o-, 352
- albumin/o-, 603
- alges/o-, 440
- alg/o-, 431
- align/o-, 425
- aliment/o-, 93
- all/o-, 317
- alveol/o-, 158
- ambly/o-, 828
- ambulat/o-, 68
- amnes/o-, 910
- amni/o-, 686
- amputat/o-, 438
- amput/o-, 438
- amygdal/o-, 904
- amyl/o-, 97
- analy/o-, 925
- anastom/o-, 128
- ancill/o-, 67
- andr/o-, 657
- aneurysm/o-, 236
- angin/o, 229
- angi/o-, 245
- anis/o-, 300
- ankyl/o-, 429
- an/o-, 93
- antagon/o-, 763
- anter/o-, 36
- anthrac/o-, 174
- anxi/o-, 908
- aort/o-, 208
- apher/o-, 317
- aphth/o-, 107
- apic/o-, 158
- appendic/o-, 8
- appendicul/o-, 397
- append/o-, 93
- appercept/o-, 923
- aque/o-, 811
- arachn/o-, 518
- areol/o-, 682
- arteri/o-, 180
- arteriol/o-, 211
- arthr/o-, 8
- articul/o-, 410
- asbest/o-, 174
- ascit/o-, 117
- aspir/o-, 174
- asthm/o-, 169
- astr/o-, 522
- atel/o-, 170
- ather/o-, 237
- atheromat/o-, 237
- athet/o-, 486

atri/o-, 208
attenu/o-, 316
audi/o-, 879
audit/o-, 515
augment/o-, 727
aur/i, 855
auricul/o-, 855
auscult/o-, 64
aut/o-, 911
autonom/o-, 522
axill/o-, 213
axi/o-, 554
ax/o-, 397
bacteri/o-, 174
balan/o-, 650
bas/o-, 281
behav/o-, 924
bil/i-, 94
bilirubin/o-, 713
blast/o-, 538
blephar/o-, 374
brachi/o-, 213
bronchi/o-, 157
bronchiol/o-, 157
bronch/o-, 157
buccinat/o-, 466
bucc/o-, 861
bulb/o-, 640
bunion/o-, 439
burs/o-, 487
calcane/o-, 410
calc/i-, 758
calc/o-, 306
calcul/o-, 598
calic/o-, 584
cali/o-, 597
cancell/o-, 412
cancer/o-, 600
capill/o-, 214
capn/o-, 179
capsul/o-, 411
carbox/y, 180
carcin/o-, 110
card/i-, 231
cardi/o-, 7
carot/o-, 213
carp/o-, 407
cartilagin/o-, 402
catheter/o-, 242
caud/o-, 40
cavit/o-, 974
cav/o-, 42
cec/o-, 93
celi/o-, 94
cellul/o-, 120
centr/o-, 513
cephal/o-, 40
cerebell/o-, 517
cerebr/o-, 515
cervic/o-, 680
cheil/o-, 107
chem/o-, 133
chez/o-, 115
chir/o-, 496
chlor/o-, 97
cholangi/o-, 121
chol/e-, 95
cholecyst/o-, 97
choledoch/o-, 121
cholesterol/o-, 241
chol/o-, 712
chondri/o-, 946
chondr/o-, 43
chori/o-, 962
chorion/o-, 686
choroid/o-, 810
chrom/o-, 301
chron/o-, 65
cid/o-, 916
cili/o-, 810
cin/e-, 1000
circulat/o-, 215
cirrh/o-, 118
claudicat/o-, 239
claustr/o-, 909
clavicul/o-, 405
clav/o-, 213
cleid/o-, 466
clinic/o-, 659
clon/o-, 544
coagul/o-, 286
coarct/o-, 233
cocc/o-, 175
coccyg/o-, 403
cognit/o-, 910
coit/o-, 650
coll/a-, 340
col/o-, 111, 129
colon/o-, 93
colp/o-, 720
comat/o-, 540
comminut/o-, 426
communic/o-, 63
compens/o-, 230
compress/o-, 426
compromis/o-, 304
compuls/o-, 908
concept/o-, 685
concuss/o-, 540
conduct/o-, 217
conform/o-, 973
congenit/o-, 62
congest/o-, 229
coni/o-, 174
conjug/o-, 832
conjunctiv/o-, 807
con/o-, 724
constip/o-, 115
constrict/o-, 211
construct/o-, 727
contine/o-, 115
contin/o-, 604
contract/o-, 235
contus/o-, 350
converg/o-, 831
convuls/o-, 560
copr/o-, 911
corne/o-, 808
coron/o-, 35
corpor/o-, 437
cortic/o-, 188
cost/o-, 159
crani/o-, 42
crin/o-, 50
cry/o-, 370
crypt/o-, 649
culd/o-, 724
cusp/o-, 208
cutane/o-, 8
cut/i-, 343
cyan/o-, 179
cycl/o-, 832
cyst/o-, 95
cyt/o-, 280
dacry/o-, 822
defici/o-, 304
degluti/o-, 90
delt/o-, 467
delus/o-, 919
dem/o-, 774
dendr/o-, 522
densit/o-, 435
dent/o-, 51
depend/o-, 917
depress/o-, 426
derm/a-, 340
dermat/o-, 47
derm/o-, 339
desicc/o-, 371
dextr/o-, 430
diabet/o-, 552
diaphor/o-, 367
diaphragm/o-, 159
diaphys/o-, 411
diastol/o-, 217
didym/o-, 639
dietet/o-, 51
differentiat/o-, 949
different/o-, 311
digest/o-, 96
digit/o-, 655
dilat/o-, 187
dipl/o-, 828
dips/o-, 773
disk/o-, 559
dissect/o-, 236
dissemin/o-, 307
distent/o-, 230
dist/o-, 41
diverticul/o-, 112
donat/o-, 316
dors/o-, 36
dos/i-, 996
duc/o-, 1005
duct/o-, 957
du/o-, 1006
duoden/o-, 92
dur/o-, 518
dynam/o-, 377
ecchym/o-, 350
ech/o-, 247
eclamps/o-, 711
ectop/o-, 217
efface/o-, 687
effer/o-, 521
effus/o-, 177
ejaculat/o-, 640
elast/o-, 340
electr/o-, 242
elimin/o-, 98
embol/o-, 176
embryon/o-, 686
emet/o-, 133
emiss/o-, 554
emulsific/o-, 97
encephal/o-, 543
enter/o-, 46
enucle/o-, 835
enur/o-, 603
eosin/o-, 281
ependym/o-, 522
epilept/o-, 543
epiphys/o-, 412
episi/o-, 729
equin/o-, 434
erect/o-, 342
erg/o-, 344
erythemat/o-, 353
erythr/o-, 278
es/o-, 826
esophag/o-, 91
espress/o-, 536
esthes/o-, 8
esthet/o-, 549
estr/a-, 677
estr/o-, 730
ethm/o-, 399
eti/o-, 62
exacerb/o-, 65
excis/o-, 318
excori/o-, 357
excret/o-, 587
exhibit/o-, 914
ex/o-, 826
extens/o-, 462
extern/o-, 41
exud/o-, 369
faci/o-, 398
fallopi/o-, 678
fasci/o-, 492
fec/a-, 115
fec/o-, 98
femor/o-, 213
fer/o-, 342
ferrit/o-, 313
ferr/o-, 313
fertil/o-, 649
fet/o-, 686
fibrill/o-, 234
fibrin/o-, 286
fibr/o-, 171
fibul/o-, 409
fiss/o-, 351
fixat/o-, 439
flatul/o-, 115
flex/o-, 462
fluor/o-, 1000
foc/o-, 544
foli/o-, 340
follicul/o-, 342
format/o-, 537
fove/o-, 812
fract/o-, 65
fratern/o-, 685
front/o-, 35
fulgur/o-, 371
fund/o-, 679
fundu/o-, 832
fung/o-, 376
fus/o-, 182
galact/o-, 707
ganglion/o-, 492
gangren/o-, 353
gastr/o-, 8
gemin/o-, 235
gene/o-, 317
gener/o-, 62
genit/o-, 49
gen/o-, 62
germin/o-, 962
ger/o-, 51
gestat/o-, 686
gest/o-, 730
gigant/o-, 772
glandul/o-, 753
glen/o-, 405
gli/o-, 538
glob/o-, 161
globul/o-, 290
glomerul/o-, 588
gloss/o-, 89
glott/o-, 156
gluc/o-, 759
glyc/o-, 759
glycos/o-, 603
gnos/o-, 64
gonad/o-, 686
goni/o-, 437
gon/o-, 638
granul/o-, 280
gustat/o-, 514
gynec/o-, 49
habilitat/o-, 68
hallucin/o-, 917

Combining forms, listed (*continued*)
hal/o-, 160
hebe/o-, 920
hedon/o-, 918
helic/o-, 1002
hemat/o-, 8
hem/o-, 161
hemoglobin/o-, 604
hemorrh/o-, 114
hemorrhoid/o-, 132
hepat/o-, 8
heredit/o-, 62
hered/o-, 949
herni/o-, 132
heter/o-, 313
hidr/o-, 367
hil/o-, 158
hirsut/o-, 368
home/o-, 753
hom/i-, 916
horizont/o-, 39
hormon/o-, 753
humer/o-, 406
hyal/o-, 608
hydr/o-, 97
hy/o-, 401
hypn/o-, 925
hypophys/o-, 787
hyster/o-, 718
iatr/o-, 62
icter/o-, 353
ict/o-, 543
idi/o-, 62
ile/o-, 92
ili/o-, 43
immun/o-, 47
impact/o-, 871
implant/o-, 971
incarcer/o-, 116
incis/o-, 116
incud/o-, 856
induct/o-, 721
infarct/o-, 230
infect/o-, 62
infer/o-, 39
inflammat/o-, 113
inguin/o-, 43
inhibit/o-, 319
inject/o-, 436
insemin/o-, 723
insert/o-, 460
inspect/o-, 64
insulin/o-, 778
insul/o-, 759
integument/o-, 47
integu/o-, 339
intern/o-, 41
interstiti/o-, 601
intestin/o-, 46
intussuscep/o-, 111
invas/o-, 950
involut/o-, 689
iod/o-, 758
irid/o-, 808
ir/o-, 824
ischi/o-, 408
isch/o-, 229
jejun/o-, 92
jugul/o-, 214
kal/i-, 604
kary/o-, 284
kel/o-, 356
kerat/o-, 339
ket/o-, 780
kines/o-, 486
kin/o-, 97
klept/o-, 916
kyph/o-, 429
labi/o-, 681
laborat/o-, 659
labyrinth/o-, 872
lacer/o-, 357
lacrim/o-, 809
lact/i-, 682
lact/o-, 97
lamin/o-, 559
lapar/o-, 128
laryng/o-, 8
later/o-, 38
lei/o-, 703
lenticul/o-, 810
lent/o-, 826
leuk/o-, 280
lev/o-, 430
lex/o-, 543
ligament/o-, 411
ligat/o-, 726
limb/o-, 808
lingu/o-, 89
lipid/o-, 241
lip/o-, 97
lith/o-, 107
lob/o-, 158
locat/o-, 431
loc/o-, 344
log/o-, 67
lord/o-, 429
luc/o-, 993
lumb/o-, 43
lumin/o-, 252
lun/o-, 343
lymph/o-, 47
ly/o-, 256
lys/o-, 613
macr/o-, 282
macul/o-, 812
magnet/o-, 126
malac/o-, 424
malign/o-, 173
malle/o-, 856
malleol/o-, 409
mamm/a-, 727
mamm/o-, 682
mandibul/o-, 90
man/o-, 250
manu/o-, 720
masset/o-, 466
mastic/o-, 90
mast/o-, 8
mastoid/o-, 873
matur/o-, 826
maxill/o-, 401
mediastin/o-, 159
medic/o-, 46
medi/o-, 38
medull/o-, 412
meg/a-, 284
megal/o-, 302
melan/o-, 340
melen/o-, 116
meningi/o-, 538
mening/o-, 518
menisc/o-, 411
men/o-, 683
menstru/o-, 683
ment/o-, 910
metabol/o-, 162
metri/o-, 680
metr/o-, 611
micr/o-, 45
mictur/o-, 589
mineral/o-, 428
mi/o-, 809
mit/o-, 643
mitr/o-, 208
mitt/o-, 472
mon/o-, 279
morph/o-, 280
mot/o-, 491
muc/o-, 156
mucos/o-, 89
mult/i-, 722
muscul/o-, 48
mutat/o-, 948
myc/o-, 368
mydr/o-, 809
myelin/o-, 524
myel/o-, 280
my/o-, 209
myop/o-, 827
myos/o-, 484
myring/o-, 873
myx/o-, 776
narc/o-, 546
nas/o-, 8
nat/o-, 8
nause/o-, 109
necr/o-, 230
ne/o-, 352
nephr/o-, 597
nerv/o-, 48
neur/o-, 8
neutr/o-, 280
nid/o-, 368
nod/o-, 775
norm/o-, 279
nuch/o-, 546
nucle/o-, 246
nucleol/o-, 947
null/i-, 722
nutri/o-, 63
obsess/o-, 908
obstetr/o-, 49
obstip/o-, 115
obstructo/o-, 120
occipit/o-, 398
ocul/o-, 519
odyn/o-, 107
olfact/o-, 515
olig/o-, 522
om/o-, 725
omphal/o-, 116
onc/o-, 51
onych/o-, 368
o/o-, 683
oophor/o-, 725
operat/o-, 110
ophidi/o-, 909
ophthalm/o-, 50
opportun/o-, 175
oppos/o-, 911
opt/o-, 519
orbicul/o-, 466
orch/o-, 649
orex/o-, 107
organ/o-, 946
or/o-, 89
orth/o-, 47
osm/o-, 875
osse/o-, 411
ossicul/o-, 401
ossificat/o-, 413
oste/o-, 411
ot/o-, 50
oure/o-, 756
ovari/o-, 676
ov/i-, 679
ovul/o-, 683
ox/i-, 181
ox/o-, 179
ox/y-, 161
palat/o-, 401
palliat/o-, 68
palpat/o-, 64
palpit/o-, 235
pancreat/o-, 96
papill/o-, 362
parenchym/o-, 158
pareun/o-, 650
pariet/o-, 159
par/o-, 722
paroxysm/o-, 178
parturit/o-, 687
patell/o-, 410
pathet/o-, 523
path/o-, 62
pat/o-, 233
pector/o-, 178
pedicul/o-, 359
ped/o-, 47
pelv/i-, 722
pelv/o-, 42
pendul/o-, 727
pen/o-, 586
pepsin/o-, 97
peps/o-, 97
peptid/o-, 97
pept/o-, 110
percuss/o-, 64
perfor/o-, 114
perine/o-, 637
peripher/o-, 230
peritone/o-, 94
periton/o-, 117
perone/o-, 213
person/o-, 921
petechi/o-, 350
phac/o-, 835
phag/o-, 107
phak/o-, 824
phalang/o-, 407
pharmaceutic/o-, 1007
pharmac/o-, 51
pharyng/o-, 90
phas/o-, 536
phe/o-, 782
phil/o-, 173
phleb/o-, 240
phob/o-, 546
phor/o-, 313, 833
phot/o-, 377
phren/o-, 161
phylact/o-, 344
physic/o-, 66
physi/o-, 44
phys/o-, 171
pigment/o-, 354
pil/o-, 342
pituitar/o-, 771
pituit/o-, 755
placent/o-, 686
plak/o-, 876
plasm/o-, 317
plas/o-, 63
plast/o-, 286
pleg/o-, 540
pleur/o-, 159
pne/o-, 161
pneum/o-, 173
pneumon/o-, 8
pod/o-, 496
poikil/o-, 301
polar/o-, 218
pol/o-, 917

polyp/o-, 114
poplite/o-, 213
por/o-, 428
port/o-, 97
poster/o-, 36
potent/o-, 555
pract/o-, 496
pregn/o-, 685
presby/o-, 825
prevent/o-, 62
prim/i-, 722
product/o-, 49
project/o-, 994
pronat/o-, 465
prostat/o-, 586
prosthet/o-, 254
protein/o-, 603
prote/o-, 97
proxim/o-, 41
prurit/o-, 352
psor/o-, 364
psych/o-, 8
puber/o-, 642
pub/o-, 408
pulmon/o-, 46
punct/o-, 315
pupill/o-, 808
purul/o-, 172
pyel/o-, 600
pylor/o-, 92
py/o-, 172
pyr/o-, 108
quantitat/o-, 1001
radic/o-, 614
radicul/o-, 548
radi/o-, 51
rap/o-, 915
react/o-, 911
recept/o-, 472
recess/o-, 837
rect/o-, 93
recuper/o-, 65
reduct/o-, 436
refract/o-, 608
regurgitat/o-, 109
relax/o-, 493
remiss/o-, 65
ren/o-, 213
repress/o-, 914
resect/o-, 128
resist/o-, 778
resuscit/o-, 183
retard/o-, 542
reticul/o-, 279
retin/o-, 8
rhabd/o-, 485
rheumat/o-, 232
rhin/o-, 366
rhiz/o-, 559
rhytid/o-, 374
rib/o-, 947
roentgen/o-, 993
rotat/o-, 111
rrhag/o-, 705
rrhe/o-, 133
rrhythm/o-, 233
rub/o-, 95
sacr/o-, 403
sagitt/o-, 38
saliv/o-, 90
salping/o-, 701
saphen/o-, 214
sarc/o-, 364
scapul/o-, 405
schiz/o-, 368
scient/o-, 659
scint/i-, 435
scler/o-, 237
scoli/o-, 429
scop/o-, 45
scot/o-, 828
scrot/o-, 637
sebace/o-, 342
seb/o-, 367
secret/o-, 684
sect/o-, 371
semin/i-, 638
semin/o-, 640
sen/o-, 362
sensitiv/o-, 124
sensit/o-, 973
sens/o-, 514
sensor/i-, 872
septic/o-, 300
sept/o-, 155
ser/o-, 159
sex/o-, 915
sial/o-, 107
sigmoid/o-, 130
sin/o-, 217
sinus/o-, 875
skelet/o-, 47
soci/o-, 909
somat/o-, 522
somn/o-, 555
som/o-, 946
son/o-, 126
sorb/o-, 441
spasmod/o-, 619
spast/o-, 113
spermat/o-, 638
sperm/o-, 649
sphen/o-, 399
sphenoid/o-, 787
sphygm/o-, 250
spin/o-, 42
spir/o-, 46
splen/o-, 119
spondyl/o-, 429
squam/o-, 363
staped/o-, 857
stas/o-, 950
stat/o-, 239
steat/o-, 116
sten/o-, 232
stere/o-, 559
stern/o-, 159
steroid/o-, 441
steth/o-, 64
sthen/o-, 484
stigmat/o-, 827
stimul/o-, 756
stomat/o-, 107
strept/o-, 877
styl/o-, 399
suct/o-, 374
sudor/i-, 342
su/i-, 918
superfici/o-, 41
super/o-, 39
supinat/o-, 465
supposit/o-, 133
suppress/o-, 290
suppur/o-, 873
surg/o-, 65
suspens/o-, 614
symptomat/o-, 63
syncop/o-, 546
synov/o-, 411
system/o-, 215
systol/o-, 217
tact/o-, 559
tampon/o-, 231
tars/o-, 410
tax/o-, 486
techn/o-, 67
tele/o-, 244
tempor/o-, 399
tendon/o-, 488
ten/o-, 488
tens/o-, 117
termin/o-, 65
testicul/o-, 638
tetr/a-, 233
thalam/o-, 517
thanat/o-, 909
thec/o-, 968
theli/o-, 210
therapeut/o-, 65
therap/o-, 67
therm/o-, 836
thorac/o-, 42
thromb/o-, 240
thym/o-, 310
thyr/o-, 758
thyroid/o-, 758
tibi/o-, 213
till/o-, 916
toc/o-, 687
toler/o-, 917
tom/o-, 35
ton/o-, 544
tonsill/o-, 8
topic/o-, 377
tort/i-, 485
toxic/o-, 776
tox/o-, 290
trabecul/o-, 811
trache/o-, 8
trac/o-, 1007
tract/o-, 176
tranquil/o-, 926
transit/o-, 958
transplant/o-, 132
traumat/o-, 910
tremul/o-, 486
trich/o-, 368
triglycerid/o-, 241
trochanter/o-, 409
trochle/o-, 519
troph/o-, 230
trop/o-, 686
tubercul/o-, 176
tuber/o-, 176
tub/o-, 183
turbin/o-, 155
tuss/o-, 187
tympan/o-, 880
ulcerat/o-, 113
uln/o-, 213
umbilic/o-, 43
ungu/o-, 343
ureter/o-, 584
urethr/o-, 602
urin/o-, 8
ur/o-, 48
uter/o-, 679
uve/o-, 810
vaccin/o-, 316
vagin/o-, 602
valv/o-, 253
valvul/o-, 208
varic/o-, 240
vascul/o-, 46
vas/o-, 211
vegetat/o-, 232
ven/i-, 315
ven/o-, 8
ventilat/o-, 184
ventil/o-, 182
vent/o-, 1002
ventricul/o-, 208
ventr/o-, 36
verd/o-, 95
vers/o-, 248
vertebr/o-, 402
vert/o-, 465
vesic/o-, 585
vesicul/o-, 351
vest/o-, 915
viril/o-, 782
vir/o-, 175
viscer/o-, 159
viscos/o-, 303
vis/o-, 514
vitre/o-, 812
voc/o-, 863
volunt/o-, 459
vuls/o-, 482
vulv/o-, 681
xanth/o-, 362
xen/o-, 254
xer/o-, 352
xiph/o-, 401
Comedo, 365
Comminuted, 426
Common bile duct, 95, 121
Common carotid arteries, 213
Common hepatic artery, 213
Common iliac arteries, 213
Communicable diseases, 62
Compartment syndrome, 482
Compensated, 230
Compensated heart failure, 229
Complement, 291
Complement proteins, 291
Complete blood count (CBC) with differential, 311
Complex partial seizures, 544
Complex regional pain syndrome (CRPS), 551
Compression, 426
Compulsion, 908
Compulsive, 908
Computerized axial tomography (CAT, CT scan), 125, 182, 554, 609, 966, 1001–02
Computerized patient records (CPRs), 22, 25
Conception
amnion, 686
amniotic cavity, 686
amniotic fluid, 686, 687
antepartum, 687
chorion, 686
embryo, 686
fertilization, 685
fetus, 686
gestation, 686
human chorionic gonadotropin (HCG), 686
placenta, 686
pregnancy, 685
prenatal period, 687
trimesters, 686
umbilical cord, 686
zygote, 685
Concha, 156
Conchae, 156
Concussion, 540
Condom, 612
Condom catheter, 612
Conduct disorder, 911
Conduction, 555

Conduction system, 217, 233–36
Conductive, 836, 872
Conductive hearing loss, 872
Condylomata acuminata, 652
Cones, 814
Conformal, 973
Congenital, 431
Congenital diseases, 62, 599
Congenital dislocation of the hip (CDH), 431
Congenital heart abnormalities, 233
Congenital hypothyroidism, 776
Congestive, 229
Congestive heart failure (CHF), 229–30
Conization, 724
Conjugate gaze, 832
Conjunctiva, 807, 822, 823
Conjunctivae, 807
Conjunctival, 807
Conjunctivitis, 822
Consent to treatment form, 23
Constipation, 115
Contact dermatitis, 360
Contraceptives, 731
Contraction, 472, 482, 687
Contracture, 482
Contusion, 350, 483, 540
Conversion, 913
Conversion disorder, 913
Convoluted, 589
Convulsions. *see* Epilepsy
Coprolalia, 911
Cor pulmonale, 230
Coracoid, 405
Coracoid process, 405
Cord, 520
Cornea, 808, 822
Corneae, 808
Corneal, 808
Corneal abrasion, 822
Corneal transplantation, 835
Corneal ulcer, 822
Corns, 355
Coronal, 398
Coronal plane
  anterior direction (anteriorly), 36, 37*f*
  anterior section, 36
  anteroposterior (AP), 36
  coronal suture of the skull, 35, 37*f*
  defined, 35
  dorsal section, 36
  dorsal supine position, 36
  posterior direction (posteriorly), 36, 37*f*
  posterior section, 36
  posteroanterior (PA), 36, 37*f*
  prone position, 36
  ventral section, 36
Coronal suture of the skull, 35, 37*f*, 398
Coronary, 212
Coronary angiography, 997
Coronary arteries, 212
Coronary artery disease (CAD), 238
Corpora cavernosa, 641
Corporis, 358
Corpus, 679
Corpus callosum, 516
Corpus luteum, 684
Corpus of the uterus, 679–80
Corpus spongiosum, 641
Cortex, 515, 584, 760, 864
Cortical, 412, 584
Cortices, 584, 760
Corticosteroid, 319
Corticosteroid drugs, 188, 319, 376, 441, 493, 561, 788, 838, 886
Cortisol, 760, 761
Cortisone, 436
Costal, 159
Costal cartilage, 402
Costochondral, 402
Costochondral joint, 402
Cough, 178
Couplets, 235
Course, 64–65
Cowper's glands, 640
Cradle cap, 367
Cranial, 398
Cranial cavity, 42, 398, 513
Cranial nerves
  abducens (VI), 519
  accessory (XI), 519
  auditory (VIII), 519, 864
  defined, 518
  facial (VII), 519
  glossopharyngeal (IX), 519
  hypoglossal (XII), 519
  oculomotor (III), 519
  olfactory (I), 519
  optic (II), 519, 814–15
  sensory and motor, 518
  trigeminal (V), 519
  trochlear (IV), 519
  vagus (X), 519
Craniotomy, 559
Cranium
  brain, housing for, 513
  coronal and midsagittal sutures, 37*f*, 398
  defined, 398
  ethmoid bone, 399
  fontanels, 400
  foramen magnum, 399
  frontal bone, 398
  mastoid process, 399
  occipital bone, 398–99
  parietal bones, 398
  sphenoid bone, 399
  styloid process, 399
  temporal bones, 399
Creatine kinase (CK), 241
Creatine phosphokinase (CPK), 241
Creatine phosphokinase (CPK-MM), 489
Creatinine, 588, 606
Crepitus, 432
Cretinism, 776
Creutzfeldt, Hans, 541
Creutzfeldt-Jakob disease, 541
Crohn's disease, 113
Cruris, 359
Cryoprobe, 720
Cryosurgery, 370, 720
Cryotherapy, 837
Cryptorchism, 649
Cubic centimeter (CC), 25
Culdoscopy, 724
Culture, 606
Cumulative trauma disorder (CTD), 484
Curet, 371, 724
Curettage, 371
Curie, Marie, 1010
Currettage, 724
Cushing, Harvey, 781
Cushing's syndrome, 781
Cusps, 208
Cutaneous, 339
Cuticle, 343
Cyanosis, 171*f*, 179, 353
Cyanotic, 179, 353
Cycloplegia, 832
Cyclothymia, 918
Cyclotron, 1011
Cystectomy, 614
Cystic, 171
Cystic duct, 95, 121
Cystic fibrosis (CF), 171–72, 369
Cystitis, 601
Cystocele, 601, 706
Cystometer, 611
Cystometrogram (CMG), 611
Cystometry, 611
Cystoscope, 615
Cystoscopy, 615
Cystourethrogram, 611
Cystourethrography, 611
Cysts, 351
Cytobrush, 715
Cytokines, 289
Cytology, 715
Cytoplasm, 945
Cytotoxic, 290
Cytotoxic T cells, 290

D

Dacryocystitis, 822
De Humani Corporis Fabrica (The Structure of the Human Body)(Vesalius), 404
Debulk, 970
Decibels (dB), 879
Decompensated, 230
Decompensated heart failure, 229
Decongestant drugs, 886
Decubitus, 356
Decubitus ulcers, 356
Deep structures, 41
Deep tendon reflexes (DTR), 491
Deep venous thrombosis (DVT), 307
Defecation, 98, 115–16
Defibrillator, 248
Deficit, 539
Degeneration, 825
Degenerative, 432
Degenerative diseases, 62
Degenerative joint disease (DJD), 432
Deglutition, 90, 96
Delirium, 910
Delirium tremens (DT), 910
Delta (Δ), 119
Delta cells, 759
Delta hepatitis, 119
Deltoid, 467
Delusion, 919
Delusional, 919
Delusional disorder, 919
Dementia, 115, 541–42, 910
Demineralization, 428
Dendrites, 524
Densitometry, 435
Dentistry, 51
Deoxygenated, 162
Deoxygenated blood, 162
Deoxyribonucleic acid (DNA), 946
Dependence, 917
Dependent, 921
Dependent personality, 921
Depersonalization, 912
Depigmentation, 354
Depolarization, 218
Depressed, 426
Depression, 712, 918
Depressive, 918
Dermabrasion, 372
Dermal, 340
Dermatitis, 350, 360, 367
Dermatologist, 378
Dermatology. *see also* Integumentary system; Skin
  abbreviations, 377
  defined, 338
  diagnostic procedures, 369–70
  drug categories, 376–77
  medical procedures, 370–73
  surgical procedures, 373–75
  symptoms, signs, and diseases
    allergic conditions, 360
    autoimmune diseases, 354, 364–65
    benign skin markings and neoplasms, 360–62
    color, 352–54
    general, 350–52
    hair, 367–68
    herpes, 358
    infections, 357–59
    infestations, 359
    injuries, 354–57
    malignant neoplasms, 363–64
    nails, 368–69
    sebaceous glands, 365–67
    skin lesions, types of, 351*f*
    sweat glands, 367
    tinea, 358–59
Dermatome, 374, 375
Dermatomes, 340, 341*f*, 375, 521
Dermatomyositis, 484
Dermatoplasty, 374
Dermis, 339*f*, 340
Descensus, 704
Desensitization, 926
Detachment, 825
Detoxication, 924
DEXA scan, 435, 1001
Dextroscoliosis, 430
Dextrose, 785
Diabetes, 709, 773, 778
Diabetes educator, 790
Diabetes insipidus (DI), 773, 779
Diabetes mellitus (DM)
  complications, 780
  gestational, 779
  type 1, 778, 779*t*
  type 2, 779
Diabetic, 552, 778
Diabetic ketoacidosis, 780
Diabetic nephropathy, 598, 780
Diabetic neuropathy, 552, 780
Diabetic retinopathy, 780, 825
Diabetologist, 790
Diagnosis, 64
Diagnostic and Statistical Manual of Mental Disorders, fourth edition (DSM-IV), 923
Diagnostic procedures. see also individual specialties
  allergy skin testing, 369
  alpha fetoprotein (AFP), 553
  blood cell tests
    complete blood count (CBC) with differential, 311
    hematocrit (HCT), 311
    peripheral blood smear, 312
    shift to the left, 311
    type and crossmatch, 310

blood tests
acetylcholine receptor antibodies, 489
acid phosphatase, 653
albumin, 123
alkaline phosphatase, 123
alpha fetoprotein (AFP), 965
ALT (alanine transaminase), 123
antithyroglobulin antibodies, 784
arterial blood gases (ABG), 180
AST (aspartate transaminase), 123
bilirubin levels, 123
blood smear, 965
blood urea nitrogen (BUN), 606
BRCA1 or BRCA2 gene, 965
calcium, 784
carboxyhemoglobin, 180
carcinoembryonic antigen (CEA), 965
cardiac enzymes, 241
chemistries, 312–13
conjugated bilirubin, 123
cortisol level, 784
creatine phosphokinase (CPK), 241
creatine phosphokinase (CPK-MM), 489
creatinine, 606
C-reactive protein (CRP), 241
direct bilirubin, 123
drug level, 922
fasting blood sugar (FBS), 784
ferritin, 313
FSH assay and LH assay, 784
GGT/GGTP (gamma-glutamyl transpeptidase), 123
glucose self-testing, 784
glucose tolerance test (GTT), 785
glycohemoglobin, 785
glycosylated hemoglobin, 785
growth hormone, 785
hemoglobin A_{1C} (HbA_{1C}), 785
hormone testing, 653
human chorionic gonadotropin (HCG), 965
indirect bilirubin, 123
lactate dehydrogenase (LDH), 241
lipid profile, 242
liver function tests (LFTs), 123
oral glucose tolerance test (OGTT), 785
prostate-specific antigen (PSA), 653, 965
RAST, 370
rheumatoid factor, 434
SGPT and SGOT, 123
testosterone, 785
thyroid function tests (TFTs), 785
total bilirubin, 123
total iron binding capacity (TIBC), 313
troponin, 242
tumor markers, 965
unconjugated bilirubin, 123
uric acid, 434
cerebrospinal fluid (CSF) examination, 553
coagulation tests
activated clotting time (ACT), 312
international normalized ratio (INR), 312
partial thromboplastin time (PTT), 312
prothrombin time (PT), 312
culture and sensitivity (C&S), 124, 181, 369, 606, 881
cystometry, 611
cytology tests
bone marrow aspiration, 963
exfoliative cytology, 963
frozen section, 963
Her2/neu, 963
karyotype, 963
receptor assays, 963
electroencephalography (EEG), 554–55
evoked potential testing
brainstem auditory evoked potential (BAEP), 555
brainstem auditory evoked response (BAER), 555, 879
somatosensory evoked potential (SSEP), 555
somatosensory evoked response (SSER), 555
visual evoked potential (VEP), 555
visual evoked response (VER), 555
eye tests
color blindness testing, 829
fluorescein angiography, 829
fluorescein staining, 830
gonioscopy, 830
slit-lamp examination, 830
tonometry, 830
visual acuity testing, 831
gastric and stool specimen tests
CLO (Campylobacter-like organism), 123
fecal occult blood, 123–24
gastric analysis, 124
ova and parasites (O&P), 124
stool culture and sensitivity (C&S), 124
gynecologic
BRCA1 or BRCA2 gene, 714
estrogen receptor assay, 714
Pap smear, 715–16
wet mount, 716
hearing tests
audiometry, 879
auditory brainstem response (ABR), 879
brainstem auditory evoked response (BAER), 555, 879
Rinne and Weber hearing tests, 880
speech audiometry, 879
tympanometry, 880
heart related, 242–44
cardiac catherization, 242
cardiac exercise stress test, 244
elctrophysiologic study (EPS), 244
electrocardiography (ECG, EKG), 242–43
Holter monitor, 244
telemetry, 244
infertility tests
antisperm antibody test, 716
hormone testing, 716
muscle tests
electromyography (EMG), 489
Tensilon test, 489
nerve conduction studies, 555
nuclear medicine procedures
bone scintigraphy, 435
Cardiolite stress test, 246
gated blood pool scan, 246
lung scan, 182
multiple-gated acquisition (MUGA) scan, 246
myocardial perfusion scan, 246
positron emission tomography (PET) scan, 554, 922
ProstaScint scan, 654
radioactive iodine uptake (RAIU) and thyroid scan, 786
radionuclide ventriculography (RNV), 246
renal scan, 610
scintigraphy, 435, 967
single-photon emission computed tomography (SPECT) scan, 246
thallium stress test, 246
ventilation-perfusion (V/Q) scan, 182
polysomnography, 555
pregnancy and neonatal
alpha fetoprotein (AFP), 717
amniocentesis, 717
chorionic villus sampling (CVS), 717
chromosome studies, 717
L/S (lecithin/sphingomyelin) ratio, 717
pregnancy test, 717
psychiatric procedures and tests
Beck Depression Inventory (BDI), 922
Holmes Social Readjustment Rating Scale, 922
intelligence testing, 922
psychiatric diagnosis, 923
psychiatric interview, 923
Rorschach test, 923
Thematic Apperception Test (TAT), 923
pulmonary function tests (PFTs), 180
pulse oximetry, 181
radiologic procedures
angiography, 245
aortography, 245
arteriography, 245
arthrography, 434
barium enema, 124
barium swallow, 126
bone densitometry, 435
carotid duplex scan, 553
cerebral angiography, 553
chest x-ray (CXR), 174*f*, 182
cholangiography/cholangiogram, 125
cholecystogram, 126
color flow duplex ultrasonography, 247, 314
computerized axial tomography (CAT, CT scan), 125, 182, 554, 922, 966
DEXA (DXA) scan, 435
Doppler ultrasonography, 247
echocardiography, 247
endoscopic retrograde cholangiopancreatography (ERCP), 125
excretory urography, 609
flat plate of the abdomen, 125
gallbladder sonogram, 126
gallbladder ultrasound, 126
hysterosalpingography, 718
intravenous cholangiography (IVC), 125
intravenous pyelography (IVP), 609
kidneys, ureters, bladder (KUB) x-ray, 609
lymphangiography, 314, 966
magnetic resonance imaging (MRI) scan, 126, 182, 554, 966
mammography, 718, 966
myelography, 554
nephrotomography, 609
oral cholecystography (OCG), 126
percutaneous transhepatic cholangiography (PTC), 125
quantitative computerized tomography (QCT), 435
renal angiography, 610
renal arteriography, 610
retrograde pyelography, 609
sinus series, 881
skull x-ray, 554
small-bowel follow-through, 126
transesophageal echocardiogram (TEE), 247
transrectal ultrasonography (TRUS), 654
transvaginal ultrasound, 719
two-dimensional echocardiography (2-D echo), 247
ultrasonography, 610, 719, 831, 967
upper gastrointestinal series (UGI), 126
venography, 245
voiding cystourethrography (VCUG), 611
xeromammography, 718
x-rays, 435
rapid strep test, 881
saliva tests, 313
scratch test, 369
semen tests
acid phosphatase, 653
DNA analysis, 653
motility and morphology, 654
semen analysis, 654
sperm count, 654
serum tests
CD4 count, 313
electrophoresis, 313
ELISA, 313
heterophil antibody test, 313
human immunodeficiency virus (HIV) tests, 313
MonoSpot test, 313
p24 antigen test, 313
viral load test, 313
Western blot, 313
skin scraping, 370
sputum culture and sensitivity (C&S), 181
throat swab, 881
tuberculosis tests
Mantoux test, 182
tine test, 182
Tzanck test, 370
urine tests
5-HIAA, 608
17-hydroxycorticosteroids, 784
24-hour creatinine clearance, 607
ADH stimulation test, 785
Bence Jones protein, 314, 608
color, 607

Diagnostic procedures.(*continued*)
urine tests (*continued*)
culture and sensitivity (C&S), 606
drug screening, 606
for drugs, 922
estradiol, 785
glucose, 607
ketones, 608
leukocyte esterase, 606
odor, 607
pH, 607
protein, 607
red blood cells (RBCs), 608
Schilling test, 314
sediment, 608
specific gravity (SG), 608
urinalysis, 607–08, 966
vanillylmandelic acid (VMA), 608, 785
water deprivation test, 785
white blood cells (WBCs), 608
Wood's lamp of light, 370
Diagnostic tests, 64
Dialysate, 613
Dialysis, 613
Dialysis nurse, 620
Diaphoresis, 229, 367
Diaphoretic, 367
Diaphragm, 42, 159
Diaphragmatic, 159
Diaphyses, 411
Diaphysial, 411
Diarrhea, 115
Diastole, 217
Diastolic pressure, 251
Dietetics, 51
Differential, 311
Differentiation, 949
Diffuse toxic goiter, 775
Digestion
absorption, 97
chemical, 97
elimination, 98
mechanical, 96, 97
Digestive tract/system. *see* Gastrointestinal system
Digital subtraction angiography (DSA), 997
Digitalis, 255
Digitorum, 462
Digits, 407
Dilated cardiomyopathy, 229
Dilation, 687, 688*f*, 724
Dilation and curettage (D&C), 724
Diplopia, 828
Directions. *see* Body directions
Disability, 65
Discharge, 67
Disease
categories, 62–63
defined, 62
etiology, 62
onset, course, and outcome
course, 64–65
diagnosis, 64
onset, 63
outcome, 65
patient history, 63
physical examination, 63–64
treatment, 65
preventive medicine, 62
Diskectomy, 559
Disks, 404
Dislocation, 431
Displaced, 425
Disproportion, 709
Dissecting aneurysms, 236
Dissection, 318, 728
Disseminated, 307
Disseminated intravascular coagulation (DIC), 307
Dissociative, 912
Dissociative disorders, 912–13
Dissociative process, 912
Distal, 41
Distal convoluted tubule, 589
Distal direction (distally), 41
Distal interphalangeal (DIP) joint, 407
Distal phalanx, 407
Distension, 230
Diuretic drugs, 256, 618
Diverticula, 112
Diverticular disease, 112
Diverticulitis, 112
Diverticulosis, 112
Diverticulum, 112
Doctor, 66
Donation, 316
Donor, 132, 251
Dopamine, 525, 906
Doppler, 247, 314, 1006
Doppler, Christian, 1006
Doppler ultrasonography, 1006
Dorsal, 36, 720
Dorsal lithotomy position, 720
Dorsal nerve roots, 521
Dorsal section, 36
Dorsal supine position, 36
Dorsi, 467
Dorsum, 858
Dosimeter, 996
Dosimetry, 996
Double contrast (air contrast) barium enema, 998
Double pneumonia, 175
Down, John, 542
Down syndrome, 542
Drug, 20
Drug categories. see also individual specialties
ACE (angiotensin-converting enzyme) inhibitor drugs, 254
alcoholism, drugs for, 927
alkylating drugs, 974
Alzheimer's disease, drugs for, 561
amenorrhea and abnormal uterine bleeding, drugs for, 729
aminoglycoside antibiotic drugs, 618
analgesic drugs, 440, 493, 560
androgen drugs, 657
antacid drugs, 133
antianxiety drugs, 926
antiarrhythmic drugs, 256
antibiotic drugs, 133, 187, 254, 376, 618, 657, 729, 838, 885
anticoagulant drugs, 318
anticonvulsant drugs, 560
antidepressant drugs, 926
antidiabetic drugs, 787
antidiarrheal drugs, 133
antiemetic drugs, 133, 974
antiepileptic drugs, 560
antifungal drugs, 376
antihistamine drugs, 885
antihypertensive drugs, 256
antimetabolite drugs, 974
antipruritic drugs, 376
antipsychotic drugs, 927
antiretroviral drugs, 320
antispasmodic drugs, 619
antithyroid drugs, 787
antitubercular drugs, 187
antitussive drugs, 187, 886
antiviral drugs, 376, 657, 838
antiyeast drugs, 886
anxiolytic drugs, 926
aspirin, 254
barium, 1019
benign prostatic hypertrophy (BPH), drugs for, 657
beta-blocker drugs, 254, 493
bone resorption inhibitor drugs, 441
bronchodilator drugs, 187
calcium channel blocker drugs, 254
cardiac arrest, drugs for, 256
cervical dilation, drugs for, 730
chemotherapy antibiotic drugs, 974
chemotherapy drugs, 133, 187, 318, 376, 440, 493, 560, 618, 657, 729, 838, 886
chemotherapy enzyme drugs, 975
coal tar drugs, 376
colony-stimulating factor (CSF) drugs, 319
COMT inhibitor drugs, 561
contraceptives, 731
corticosteroid drugs, 188, 319, 376, 441, 493, 561, 788, 838, 886
decongestant drugs, 886
digitalis drugs, 255
diuretic drugs, 618
dysmenorrhea, 730
endometriosis, drugs for, 730
erection producing, 657
erythropoietin, 319
expectorant drugs, 188
general anesthetic drugs, 561
glaucoma, drugs for, 838
gold compound drugs, 441
growth hormone drugs, 788
H_2 blocker drugs, 133
hormonal drugs, 975
hormone replacement therapy (HRT), 730
hyperlipidemia, drugs for, 256
immunosuppressant drugs, 319
infestations, drugs for, 376
insulin, 788
iodinated contrast dye, 1019
labor inducing, 730
laxative drugs, 133
leukotriene receptor blockers, 188
mania, 927
mast cell stabilizer drugs, 188
mitosis inhibitor drugs, 975
monoclonal antibodies, 975
muscle relaxant drugs, 493
myasthenia gravis, drugs for, 561
mydriatic drugs drugs for, 838
neuromuscular blocker drugs, 494
nitrate drugs, 255
nonsteroidal anti-inflammatory drugs (NSAIDs), 441, 494
ovulation-stimulating drugs, 731
Parkinson's disease, drugs for, 561
photodynamic therapy (PDT), 377
platelet aggregation inhibitor drugs, 319
platinum drugs, 975
potassium supplements, 618
premature labor, drugs for, 730
premenstrual dysphoric disorder (PMDD), drugs for, 730
premenstrual syndrome (PMS), drugs for, 730
protease inhibitor drugs, 319
proton pump inhibitor drugs, 133
psoralen, 377
radioactive sodium iodide 131 (I-131), 788
radiopharmaceutical drugs that emit gamma rays, 1019
radiopharmaceutical indium-111 combined with monoclonal antibodies, 1019
reverse transcriptase inhibitor drugs, 319
suppositories, 133
thrombolytic drugs, 256
thrombolytic enzyme drugs, 319
thyroid supplement drugs, 788
tissue plasminogen activator (TPA) drugs, 319
tocolytic drugs, 730
topical drugs, 377
tranquilizer drugs, 926
urinary analgesic drugs, 619
vaginal yeast infections, drugs for, 730
vertigo and motion sickness, drugs for, 886
vitamin A-type drugs, 377
vitamin B_{12} drugs, 319
Drug screening, 606
Drug testing, 922
Duchenne, Guillaume, 483
Duchenne's muscular dystrophy, 483
Duct, 809
Ductal, 957
Ductal cell carcinoma, 957
Ductus, 640
Ductus arteriosus, 216, 233
Ductus deferens, 640
Duodenal ulcer, 110, 117*f*
Duodenum, 92
Duplex, 247
Dupuytren, Guillaume, 487
Dupuytren's contracture, 487
Dura mater, 518
Dural, 518
Dwarfism, 773
Diaphysis, 411, 412*f*
Dysplastic, 955
Dysconjugate gaze, 832
Dyscrasia, 300
Dysentery, 113
Dysequilibrium, 872
Dysfunction, 650
Dysfunctional, 704
Dysfunctional uterine bleeding (DUB), 704
Dysgerminoma, 962
Dyskinesia, 486, 561
Dyslexia, 543
Dysmenorrhea, 704
Dysmorphic, 913
Dyspareunia, 650, 706
Dyspepsia, 108
Dysphagia, 107
Dysphasia, 536
Dysphoric, 705
Dysplasia, 706, 955
Dysplastic, 361
Dysplastic nevus, 361
Dyspnea, 171, 178
Dyspneic, 178
Dysrrhythmia, 233
Dysthymia, 918
Dystocia, 709

Dystrophy, 483
Dysuria, 603

E

Ears, nose, and throat (ENT) system. *see also* Otolaryngology
anatomy of
external ear, 855–56
external mouth and chin, 860
external nose, 858
inner ear, 858
larynx, 863
middle ear, 856–57
nasal cavity, 859
oral cavity, 861
pharynx, 861–62
sinuses, 860
defined, 50*f*, 854*f*, 855
hearing, physiology of, 864
Eating disorders, 912
Ecchymoses, 350
Ecchymosis, 308, 350
Ecchymotic, 350
Echocardiogram, 247
Echocardiography, 247, 1005
Echolalia, 911
Eclampsia, 711
Ectocervical, 715
Ectocervical cells, 715
Ectopic, 217, 709
Ectopic pregnancy, 709
Ectopic sites, 217
Ectropion, 821
Eczema, 367
Edema, 175, 230, 350
Effacement, 687, 688*f*
Efferent, 521
Efferent nerves, 521
Effusion, 873
Ejaculation, 643
Ejaculatory, 640
Ejaculatory duct, 640
Elastin, 340
Elective, 723
Elective abortion, 723
Electrocardiographic (ECG) technician, 258
Electrocardiography (ECG, EKG), 242–43
Electrocardiography (EKG) tracings, 234*f*, 243*f*
Electroconvulsive, 924
Electroconvulsive therapy (ECT), 924
Electrodesiccation, 371
Electroencephalogram, 554, 555
Electroencephalograph, 554, 555
Electroencephalography (EEG), 543, 554–55
Electrolytes, 284, 588–89
Electromyogram, 489
Electromyography (EMG), 489
Electron beam tomography (EBT), 1004
Electronic patient record (EPR), 22, 25
Electrophoresis, 313
Electrophysiologic, 244
Electrosection, 371
Electrosurgery, 371
Elimination, 98
Embolism, 176, 307
Embolization, 726
Embolus, 176, 307
Embryo, 686
Embryonal, 962
Embryonal cell cancer, 962
Embryonic, 686
Emesis, 109
Emission, 554
Emotions, 905
Emphysema, 171, 172
Empyema, 172
Emulsification, 97
En bloc, 970
En bloc resection, 970
Encapsulated, 950
Encephalitis, 543
Encopresis, 911
Endarterectomy, 251
Endemic, 774
Endemic goiter, 774
Endocardial, 209
Endocarditis, 231
Endocardium, 209
Endocervical, 715
Endocervical cells, 715
Endocrine, 753
Endocrine system. *see also* Adrenal glands; Hormone response and feedback; Pancreas; Pituitary gland; Thyroid gland
anatomy of
adrenal glands, 760–61
hypothalamus, 754
ovaries, 761
pancreas, 759
parathyroid glands, 758
pineal body, 757
pituitary gland, 755–56
testes, 762
thymus gland, 758
thyroid gland, 757–58
bone growth, 414
defined, 50*f*, 752*f*, 753
function of, 753
hormone response and feedback, 762–63
Endocrinologist, 790
Endocrinology. *see also* Endocrine system
abbreviations, 789
defined, 752
diagnostic procedures
blood tests, 784–85
nuclear medicine tests, 786
urine tests, 785
drug categories, 787–88
medical procedures, 786
surgical procedures, 786–87
symptoms, signs, and diseases, 763
adrenal cortex: aldosterone, 781
adrenal cortex: androgens, 782
adrenal cortex: cortisol, 781–82
adrenal medulla: epinephrine and norepinephrine, 782
anterior pituitary gland: all hormones, 771
anterior pituitary gland: growth hormone, 772–73
anterior pituitary gland: prolactin, 772
ovaries: estradiol and progesterone, 783
pancreas: insulin, 778–80
parathyroid glands: parathyroid hormone, 777
pineal gland: melatonin, 774
posterior pituitary gland: antidiuretic hormone (ADH), 773
posterior pituitary gland: oxytocin, 773–74
testes: testosterone, 783
thyroid gland: T_3 and T_4 thyroid hormones, 774–77
Endometrial, 680
Endometrial ablation, 724
Endometrial carcinoma, 701, 958
Endometriosis, 702
Endometrium, 680
Endoplasmic, 946
Endoplasmic reticulum, 946
Endorphins, 525
Endoscope, 130
Endoscopic, 125, 130, 131, 883
Endoscopic sinus surgery, 883
Endoscopy, 130
Endothelial, 211
Endothelium, 210
Endotoxins, 290
Endotracheal, 183
Endotracheal tube (ETT), 183
End-stage renal disease (ESRD), 600
Enema, 124, 998
Engagement, 687
Enteritis, 113
Enteropathy, 113
Entropion, 821
Enuresis, 603
Environmental diseases, 62
Enzymes, 97
Eosinophils, 281, 289
Ependymal, 522
Ependymal cells, 522
Ependymoma, 538
Epicardial, 209
Epicardium, 209
Epidermal, 339
Epidermis, 339–40
Epididymal, 639
Epididymides, 639
Epididymis, 639, 649
Epididymitis, 649
Epidural, 520
Epidural anesthesia, 721
Epidural space, 520
Epigastric region, 43, 44*f*
Epiglottic, 156
Epiglottis, 89*f*, 100, 156, 863
Epilepsy
aura, 543
defined, 543
postictal state, 543
seizures, types of
absence (petit mal), 544
complex partial (psychomotor), 544
simple partial (focal motor), 544
tonic-clonic (grand mal), 544
status epilepticus, 543
Epileptic, 543
Epinephrine, 218, 523, 525, 761, 905
Epiphyses, 411, 412*f*
Epiphysial, 412
Epiphysial plates, 411, 412*f*
Epiphysis, 412
Episiotomy, 729
Epistaxis, 875
Epithelial, 339
Epithelial tissue, 339
Epithelium, 339
Eponyms, 173, 183, 217, 240
Epstein-Barr virus (EBV), 306
Erectile, 641
Erectile dysfunction (ED), 650
Erectile tissue, 641
Erection, 641
Erythema, 353
Erythematous, 353
Erythroblasts, 279
Erythrocytes, 97, 278–79, 300–304
Erythropoietin, 279, 319, 590
Eschar, 355
Escherichia coli (*E. coli*), 605
Esophageal ulcer, 110
Esophageal varices, 108, 240
Esophagitis, 108
Esophagogastroduodenoscopy, 130
Esophagoscopy, 130
Esophagus, 91
Esotropia, 826
Epispadias, 602
Essential hypertension, 238–39
Estimated date of birth (EDB), 722
Estimated date of confinement (EDC), 722
Estradiol, 677, 678*f*, 761
Estrogen, 414, 730
Estrogen receptor (ER) assay, 714, 963
Estrogen receptors, 714
Ethmoid, 399
Ethmoid bone, 399
Ethmoid sinuses, 860
Etiology, 62
Etymology, 20
Euphoria, 917
Eupnea, 161
Eustachian, 857
Eustachian tube, 857
Eustachio, Bartolommeo, 857
Euthyroidism, 758
Eversion, 465
Evertor, 465
Evoked, 555
Evoked potential testing, 555
Ewing, James, 424
Ewing's sarcoma, 424, 959
Exacerbation, 65
Excision, 970
Excisional, 318
Excisional biopsy, 318, 373
Excoriation, 357
Excretory, 587
Excretory system. *see* Urinary system
Excretory urography, 999
Exenteration, 970
Exercise, 471
Exfoliation, 340
Exfoliative, 715
Exfoliative cytology, 715, 963
Exhalation, 160
Exhibitionism, 914
Exocrine, 342, 753
Exocrine glands, 342
Exophthalmos, 775, 823
Exotropia, 826
Expectorant drugs, 188
Expectoration, 178
Expiration, 160
Expressive, 536
Expressive aphasia, 536
Extension, 464
Extensor, 462
Extensor digitorum, 462
External, 439
External auditory canal (EAC), 855
External auditory meatus, 855
External ear, 855–56
External iliac artery, 213
External mouth, 860
External oblique, 469
External respiration, 161
External structures, 41

External urethral sphincter, 586
Extracapsular, 835
Extracellular, 218
Extracellular fluid, 218
Extracorporeal, 437
Extraction, 835
Extraocular, 813
Extraocular eye muscles
 inferior oblique, 813
 inferior rectus, 813
 lateral rectus, 813
 medial rectus, 813
 superior oblique, 813
 superior rectus, 813
 symptoms, signs, and diseases, 826
Extrasystole, 235
Extravasation, 350
Extremity, 406
Exudate, 369
Eye color, 809
Eye patching, 832
Eye tests, 829–31
Eyeglasses prescription, 834
Eyelid, 807, 821
Eyes
 anatomy of
  anterior and posterior chambers, 811
  choroid and ciliary body, 810
  extraocular muscles, 813
  eyelid and conjunctiva, 807
  internal structures, 810*f*
  iris and pupil, 808–09
  lacrimal glands, 809
  lens, 810
  posterior cavity, 812
  retina, 812
  sclera and cornea, 808
 defined, 50*f*, 806*f*, 807
 optic globe, 807
 orbit, 807
 socket, 807
 vision, physiology of, 814–15

F

Facial, 398
Facial bones
 defined, 398, 399*f*
 inferior nasal turbinates, 400
 lacrimal bones, 400
 mandible, 400
 maxilla, 400
 nasal bones, 400
 palatine bones, 400
 vomer, 400
 zygoma (zygomatic bone), 400
Facial nerve, 519
Factitious, 913
Factitious disorders, 913
Fallopian, 678
Fallopian tubes, 678–79, 701
Fallopius, Gabriele, 678
Fallot, Ètienne-Louis, 233
Family therapy, 924
Fascia, 461
Fascial, 461
Fascicles, 472
Fasciectomy, 492
Fasciotomy, 492
Fasting blood sugar (FBS), 784
Fecalith, 115
Feces, 98, 115, 116
Female genital and reproductive system. *see also* Conception; Labor and delivery; Menstruation
 anatomy of
  breasts, 682
  external genitalia, 675–76, 681
  fallopian tubes, 678–79
  internal genitalia, 675, 676*f*
  ovaries, 676–77
  uterus, 679–80
  vagina, 676f, 679f, 680
 conception, 685–87
 defined, 49*f*, 675–76
 functions of, 676
 labor and delivery, 687–89
 menstruation, 683–85
Female hormones, 676–77, 678*f*
Femora, 409
Femoral, 409
Femoral artery, 213
Femoris, 470
Femur, 409
Ferritin, 313
Fertilization. *see* Conception
Fetal, 686
Fetal distress, 712
Fetishism, 914
Fetus, 686
 birth asphyxia, 179
 cartilaginous bones, 413
 congenital heart abnormalities, 233
 fontanels, 400
 heart structures
  ductus arteriosus, 216
  foramen ovale, 216
 meconium, formation of, 98
 oxygen, receipt via placenta, 162
 passive immunity, 291
 testes, 639
 urine production, 589
Fiber, 112
Fibrillation, 234
Fibrin, 286
Fibrinogen, 286
Fibrocystic, 707
Fibrocystic disease, 707
Fibromyalgia, 482
Fibroplasia, 826
Fibrosarcoma, 959
Fibrosis, 171
Fibula, 409
Fibulae, 409
Fibular, 409
Fight or flight response, 218, 523, 761, 904
Filtrate, 589
Filtration, 589
Fimbriae, 678
Fingerprints, 342
First stage of labor, 687
First-degree burn, 355
First-degree heart block, 235
Fissure, 351, 516
Fistula, 368, 602
Fixation, 439
Flaccid, 549
Flaccid paralysis, 548
Flagellum, 643
Flank, 583
Flatus, 98, 115
Flexion, 464
Flexor, 462
Flexor hallucis brevis, 462
Floaters and flashers, 825
Fluorescein, 829
Fluoroscopy, 1000
Flutter, 234
Focal, 544
Focal motor seizures, 544
Foley catheter, 612
Folic acid, 547, 712
Folic acid deficiency anemia, 302
Follicle, 342, 642
Follicles, 676, 677
Follicle-stimulating hormone (FSH), 642, 683, 756
Follicular, 342
Folliculitis, 367
Fontanels, 400, 690
Food and Drug Administration (FDA), 316
Foramen, 408
Foramen magnum, 399
Foramen ovale, 216, 233
Forensic science
 adipocere, 342
 carbon dioxide (CO_2) versus carbon monoxide (CO) blood levels, 179
 fingerprints, 342
 hair, testing of, 342
 nails and arsenic poisoning, 342
 rigor mortis, 485
Foreskin, 641
Fornix, 680, 904
Fossa, 405
Fovea, 812
Foveae, 812
Foveal, 812
Fractures
 closed, 425
 Colles', 426
 comminuted, 426
 compound, 425
 compression, 426
 defined, 425
 depressed, 426
 displaced, 425
 greenstick, 426
 hairline, 427
 malalignment of fragments, 425
 nondisplaced, 425
 oblique, 427
 open, 425
 pathologic, 425
 spiral, 427
 transverse, 427
Fraternal, 685
Fraternal twins, 685, 708
Freckle, 361
Frequency of urination, 603
Frontal, 398
Frontal bone, 398
Frontal lobe, 514, 905
Frontal plane. *see* Coronal plane
Frontal sinuses, 860
Frontalis, 466
Frostbite, 353*f*
Frozen section, 963
Fugue, 913
Fulguration, 371
Full-thickness burn, 355
Fundal, 679
Fundal height, 721
Fundi, 812
Fundus
 bladder, 585
 retina, 812
 stomach, 91
 uterus, 679
Funduscope, 832
Funduscopy, 832
Funny bone, 406
Furuncle, 357

G

GABA (gamma-amino butyric acid), 906
Gadolinium, 1003
Galactorrhea, 707, 772
Gallbladder, 95, 97, 121
Gallstones, 121
Gamete intrafallopian transfer (GIFT), 723
Gametes, 643
Gamma scintillation camera, 1009
Ganglion, 487
Ganglionectomy, 492
Gangrene, 353
Gangrenous, 353
Gardnerella vaginalis, 706
Gastrectomy, 131
Gastric adenocarcinoma, 110
Gastric and stool specimen tests. *see under* Diagnostic procedures
Gastric mucosa, 91
Gastric ulcer, 110
Gastric varices, 108, 240
Gastrin, 97
Gastritis, 108
Gastrocnemius, 470, 471
Gastroenteritis, 108
Gastroenterologist, 135
Gastroenterology. *see also* Digestion; Gastrointestinal system
 abbreviations, 134
 defined, 88
 diagnostic procedures
  blood tests, 123
  gastric and stool specimen tests, 123–24
  radiologic procedures, 124–26
 drug categories, 133
 medical procedures, 127
 surgical procedures, 127–32
 symptoms, signs, and diseases
  abdominal wall and abdominal cavity, 116–17
  cecum and colon, 111–14
  defecation and feces, disorders of, 115–16
  duodenum, jejunum, and ileum, 110–11
  eating, 107
  esophagus and stomach, 108–10
  gallbladder and bile ducts, 121
  liver, 117–20
  mouth and lips, 107
  pancreas, 122
  rectum and anus, 114
Gastroesophageal reflux disease (GERD), 108
Gastrointestinal system. *see also* Digestion; Gastroenterology
 anatomy of
  abdominopelvic cavity, 94
  esophagus, 91
  gallbladder, 95
  large intestine, 92*f*, 93
  liver, 94, 95*f*
  oral cavity and pharynx, 89–90
  pancreas, 95*f*, 96
  small intestine/bowel, 92
  stomach, 91–92, 97
 defined, 46*f*, 88*f*, 89
 immune response, 94

organization of, 96*f*
Gastroplasty, 132
Gastroscopy, 130
Gastrostomy, 131
Gastrostomy tube, 131
Gaze testing, 832
Gene, 714
Generalized anxiety disorder, 908
Genes, 946
Genetic, 714
Genetic mutations, 948
Genital, 637
Genital herpes, 651
Genital organs, male. *see* Male genitourinary system
Genital warts, 652
Genitalia, 637, 675–76, 721
Genitourinary, 587, 637
Genitourinary (GU) system. *see* Urinary system
Genu valgu, 433
Genu varum, 433
Geriatrics, 51
Germ cell tumor, 962
Gestation, 686
Gestational, 709
Gestational diabetes mellitus, 709, 779
Gigantism, 772
Glands, 342, 753
Glandular, 753
Glans penis, 641
Glasgow Coma Scale (GCS), 556
Glaucoma, 823
Glenoid, 405
Glenoid fossa, 405
Glioblastoma multiforme, 538, 959
Glioma, 537*f*, 538
Global, 536
Global amnesia, 910
Global aphasia, 536
Globins, 278, 291
Globulin, 291
Glomerular, 588
Glomerulonephritis, 597
Glomerulosclerosis, 598
Glomerulus, 588
Glossal, 861
Glossitis, 876
Glossopharyngeal, 519
Glossopharyngeal nerve, 519
Glottis, 863
Glucagon, 759
Glucocorticoid, 761
Glucocorticoid hormones, 760
Glucola, 785
Glucose, 759
Glucose self-testing, 784
Glucose tolerance test (GTT), 785
Gluten, 113
Gluten enteropathy, 113
Gluteus, 462
Gluteus maximus, 462, 470
Glycogen, 97, 759
Glycosuria, 603, 778, 779
Goiter
  adenomatous, 774
  causes of
    adenomata or nodules, 774
    autoimmune disease, 774
    iodine, lack of, 774
  diffuse toxic, 775
  endemic, 774
  multinodular, 774
  nodular, 774
  nontoxic, 774
  simple, 774
  thyromegaly, 774
Golfer's elbow, 487
Golgi apparatus, 946
Golgi, Camillo, 946
Glomeruli, 588
Gonadotropins, 686, 756
Gonads, 638, 676
Goniometer, 437
Goniometry, 437
Gonorrhea, 602, 652
Gout, 431
Gouty, 431
Gouty arthritis, 431
Graft, 439
Graft-versus-host disease (GVHD), 309
Grand mal seizures, 544
Graves' disease, 774, 775
Graves, Robert, 775
Gravida (G), 722
Gravidarum, 109
Gray matter, 515, 525
Greek
  combining forms, 75, 135, 190, 258, 321, 379, 443, 495, 563, 620, 659, 733, 790, 840, 888, 927, 977
  medical words, origins of, 20, 243
  nouns, singular and plural endings, 21
Greenstick, 426
Group therapy, 925
Growth abnormalities, 713
Growth hormone (GH), 414, 756
Guaiac, 123–24
Guillain-Barré syndrome, 550
Guillian, George, 550
Gustatory, 514
Gustatory cortex, 514
Gynecologic, 720
Gynecologic examination, 720
Gynecologist, 733
Gynecology and obstetrics, 722. *see also* Conception; Female genital and reproductive system; Labor and delivery; Menstruation; Newborn infants
  abbreviations, 731–32
  defined, 674
  diagnostic procedures
    gynecologic, 714–16
    infertility, 716
    pregnancy and neonatal, 717–19
  drug categories, 729–31
  medical procedures
    breast, 721
    internal genitalia, 720
    obstetrics, 721–23
  radiologic procedures, 718–19
  surgical procedures
    breast, 726–28
    cervix and vagina, 724
    obstetrics, 729
    uterus, fallopian tube, and ovaries, 724–26
  symptoms, signs, and diseases
    breasts, 707
    cervix, 705–06
    fetus and neonate, 712–13
    menstrual disorders, 704–05
    ovaries and fallopian tubes, 701
    uterus, 701–04
    vagina and perineum, 706–07
Gynecomastia, 653, 783
Gyri, 515
Gyrus, 515, 903

H

H_2 blocker drugs, 133
Hair, 342, 367–68
Half-life, 1007
Hallucinations, 920
Hallucinogens, 917
Hallucis, 462
Hallux, 410
Hallux valgus, 433
Hamstrings, 471
Hard palate, 89, 861
Hashimoto, Hakaru, 777
Hashimoto's thyroiditis, 774, 777
Haustra, 93
Health information administrators, 75
Health records
  computerized patient records (CPRs), 22
  documents in
    consent to treatment forms, 23
    informed consent, 23
    surgical consent, 23
  electronic patient records (EPRs), 22
  HIPAA (the Health Insurance Portability and Accountability Act of 1996), 23
  hospital documents
    commonly used, 24
    standard headings, 24
  medical language skills needed, 22
  paper, 22
  SOAP format, 23
Healthcare professionals
  allied health professionals, 67
  physician extenders, 66
  physicians, 66
Healthcare settings
  ambulatory surgery centers (ASCs), 68
  clinics, 68
  home health agencies, 68
  hospices, 68
  hospitals, 67
  long-term care facilities, 68
  physicians' offices, 67
Hearing loss, 872
Hearing, physiology of, 864
Heart. *see also* Cardiology; Cardiovascular system
  chambers, 207–08
  conduction system, 217
  congenital abnormalities, 233
  defined, 20, 207
  diagnostic procedures, 242–44
  layers and membranes, 209
  muscle, 209–10
  normal rates, 216
  valves, 207*f*, 208–09
Heart block, 235
Heart murmurs, 231
Heart surgeon, 258
Heart transplant, 230, 251
Heartbeat. *see* under Cardiovascular system
Heartburn, 108
Hebephrenia, 920
Heimlich, Harry, 183
Heimlich maneuver, 183
Helical, 1002
Helical CT scan, 1002
Helicobacter pylori, 110, 123
Helix, 855
Helper T cells, 290
Hemangioma, 361
Hemarthrosis, 431
Hematemesis, 108
Hematochezia, 115
Hematocrit (HCT), 311
Hematologist, 321
Hematology. *see also* Blood; Immunology
  abbreviations, 320
  blood donation and transfusion procedures, 316–17
  defined, 276
  diagnostic procedures
    blood cell tests, 310–12
    blood tests, 312–13
    coagulation tests, 312
    radiologic procedures, 314
    urine tests, 314
  drug categories, 318–19
  medical procedures, 315
  symptoms, signs, and diseases
    blood, 300
    erythrocytes, 300–304
    leukocytes, 304–06
    thrombocytes (platelets), 307–08
Hematoma, 350, 545
Hematopoiesis, 279
Hematuria, 604
Heme, 278
Hemianopia, 828
Hemiparesis, 539–40
Hemiplegia, 540
Hemiplegic, 540
Hemispheres, 516
Hemodialysis, 613
Hemoglobin, 278
Hemoglobinuria, 604
Hemolysis, 304
Hemolytic, 304
Hemolytic reaction, 304
Hemophilia, 308
Hemophiliac, 308
Hemoptysis, 176
Hemorrhage, 300, 350, 711
Hemorrhoidectomy, 132
Hemorrhoids, 114, 240
Hemosalpinx, 709
Hemostasis, 286
Hemothorax, 177
Hemotympanum, 872
Henle, Friedrich, 589
Hepatic ducts, 94
Hepatic flexure, 92*f*
Hepatitis, 118–19
Hepatitis A, 118
Hepatitis A virus (HAV), 118
Hepatitis B, 118–19
Hepatitis B virus (HBV), 118
Hepatitis C, 119
Hepatitis C virus (HCV), 119
Hepatitis D, 119
Hepatitis E, 119
Hepatoblastoma, 962
Hepatocellular, 120
Hepatocellular carcinoma, 120, 958
Hepatocytes, 94
Hepatoma, 120, 958
Hepatomegaly, 119
Hepatosplenomegaly, 119
Hereditary diseases, 62
Heredity, 948
Hernia, 109, 116

Herniated nucleus pulposus (HNP), 25, 548
Herniorrhaphy, 132
Herpes, 358
Herpes simplex, 876
Herpes simplex virus (HSV) type 1, 358, 876
Herpes simplex virus (HSV) type 2, 358, 651
Herpes varicella-zoster, 358
Herpes whitlow, 358
Hertz (Hz), 879
Hertz, Heinrick, 879
Hesitancy, 604
Heterophil, 313
Heterophil antibodies, 313
Hiatal hernia, 109
Hiatus, 109
Hiatus hernia, 109
High-density lipoprotein (HDL), 237
High-frequency hearing loss, 872
Hila, 158, 583
Hilar, 158, 583
Hilum, 158, 583
Hinge-type synovial joints, 411
HIPAA (the Health Insurance Portability and Accountability Act of 1996), 23
Hippocampus, 904, 905
Hirsutism, 368, 782
Histamine, 155, 289
Histrionic, 921
Hives, 360
Hodgkin, Thomas, 309, 962
Hodgkin's disease, 309
Hodgkin's lymphoma, 309, 962
Holmes Social Readjustment Rating Scale, 922
Home health agencies, 68
Homeostasis, 753, 763
Homicidal, 916
Homicidal ideation, 916
Hordeolum, 821
Horizontal plane. *see* Transverse plane
Hormonal, 753
Hormonal drugs, 975
Hormone replacement therapy (HRT), 730
Hormone response and feedback
- antagonism, 763
- chain reaction, 762
- homeostasis, maintenance of, 763
- inhibition, 762
- receptors, 762
- stimulation, 762
- synergism, 763

Hormone testing, 653, 716
Hormones, 653, 676–77, 753
Hospice facilities, 68
Hospital documents, 24
Hospital, 67
Human body. *see also* Disease
- anatomy, defined, 44
- body cavities, 42–43
- cavities. *see also* Body cavities
- microscopic-to-macroscopic study of, 45
- physiology, defined, 44
- planes and body directions, 35–41. *see also* Body directions; Coronal plane; Midsagittal plane; Transverse plane
- quadrants, 43, 44*f*
- systems, 45–50*f*

Human chorionic gonadotropin (HCG), 686
Human immunodeficiency virus (HIV), 304, 313, 652
Human papillomavirus (HPV), 652
Humeral, 406, 407
Humeri, 406
Humerus, 406, 407
Humoral, 407
Humorous, 407
Humpback, 429
Hunchback, 429
Huntington, George, 545
Huntington's chorea, 545
Hyaline, 608
Hyaline casts, 608
Hyaline membrane disease (HMD), 176, 713
Hydatidiform, 702
Hydatidiform mole, 702
Hydrocephalic, 545
Hydrocephalus, 545
Hydrochloric acid, 97
Hydronephrosis, 597
Hydroureter, 597
Hydroxycorticosteroids, 784
Hymen, 680
Hyoid, 401
Hyoid bone, 401
Hyperaldosteronism, 781
Hyperbilirubinemia, 713
Hypercalcemia, 306, 777
Hypercapnia, 179
Hypercholesterolemia, 241
Hyperemesis, 109
Hyperemesis gravidarum, 109, 710
Hyperesthesia, 550
Hyperextension, 483
Hyperextension-hyperflexion injury, 483
Hyperflexion, 483
Hyperglycemia, 778
Hyperinsulinism, 778
Hyperkinesis, 486
Hyperlipidemia, 241
Hyperopia, 827
Hyperopia surgery, 836
Hyperparathyroidism, 777
Hyperpituitarism, 771
Hypersecretion, 771
Hypersensitivity, 344
Hypertension, 117
Hypertension (HTN), 238–39
Hypertensive, 238
Hyperthyroidism, 776
Hypertriglyceridemia, 241
Hypertrophic, 230
Hypertrophy, 229, 473
Hyphema, 824
Hypnosis, 925
Hypoaldosteronism, 781
Hypocalcemia, 777
Hypochondriac, 43
Hypochondriac regions, 43, 44*f*
Hypochondriasis, 913
Hypochromic, 302
Hypodermic, 377
Hypogastric region, 43, 44*f*
Hypoglossal, 519
Hypoglossal nerve, 519
Hypoglycemia, 780
Hypokalemia, 604
Hypoparathyroidism, 777
Hypopharyngeal, 862
Hypopharynx, 862
Hypophysectomy, 787
Hypophysis. *see* Pituitary gland
Hypopituitarism, 771
Hyposalpinx, 701
Hypospadias, 602
Hypotension, 239
Hypotensive, 239
Hypothalamic, 517, 754
Hypothalamus, 517, 754, 904, 905
Hypothyroidism, 776
Hypoxemia, 180
Hypoxia, 180
Hypoxic, 180
Hysterectomy, 724
Hysteropexy, 726
Hysterosalpingogram, 718
Hysterosalpingography, 718, 999

I

Iatrogenic diseases, 62
Icteric, 353
Icterus, 353, 823
Ideation, 916
Identical twins, 685
Identity disorder, 913
Idiopathic, 229, 308
Idiopathic cardiomyopathy, 229
Idiopathic diseases, 62
Idiopathic thrombocytopenia purpura, 308
IgA, 291
IgD, 291
IgE, 291
IgG, 291
IgM, 291
Ileum, 92, 408
Ileus, 110, 408
Iliac, 408
Iliac crest, 408
Iliac regions, 43
Iliac spine, 408
Iliad (Homer), 471
Ilium, 408
Immune, 289
Immune response
- antibodies, 290
- basophils, 289–90
- complement proteins, 291
- cytokines, 289
- defined, 289
- endotoxins, 290
- eosinophils, 289
- gastrointestinal system and, 94, 288
- histamine, 289
- immune response chemicals
  - interferon, 290
  - interleukin, 290
  - tumor necrosis factor (TNF), 290
- immunoglobulins, 290
- lymphocytes
  - B cells, 290
  - CD4 cells, 290
  - cytotoxic T cells, 290
  - helper T cells, 290
  - memory T cells, 290
  - NK (natural killer) cells, 290
  - suppressor T cells, 290
  - T cells, 290
- monocytes (macrophages), 290
- neutrophils, 289
- pathogens, 289

Immunity, 291
Immunizations, 291, 316
Immunocompromised, 304
Immunodeficiency, 304
Immunoglobulins, 290, 291
Immunologist, 321
Immunology. *see also* Hematology; Immune response; Lymphatic system
- abbreviations, 320
- autoimmune diseases, 310
- defined, 276
- diagnostic procedures
  - radiologic procedures, 314
  - saliva test, 313
  - serum tests, 313
- drug categories, 318–19
- medical procedures, 316
- surgical procedures, 318

Immunosuppressant drugs, 319
Impaction, 871
Impedance, 880
Imperforate, 114
Imperforate anus, 114
Implantable, 971
Impotence, 650
Impulse control disorders, 916
In situ, 705, 956
In utero, 710
In vitro, 723
In vitro fertilization (IVF), 723
Incarcerated, 116
Incarcerated hernia, 116
Incision, 371
Incisional, 116, 373, 492
Incisional biopsy, 373
Incisional hernia, 116
Incompetent, 706
Incompetent cervix, 706
Incontinence, 115, 604
Incontinent, 115
Incudal, 856
Incudes, 856
Incus, 856, 857
Index, 311
Indices, 311
Indigestion, 108
Indirect inguinal hernia, 639
Induction, 721
Inertia, 711
Infarct, 539
Infarction, 230
Infection, 605
Infectious, 118
Infectious diseases, 62
Infectious hepatitis, 118
Inferior, 813
Inferior nasal turbinates, 400
Inferior oblique muscle, 813
Inferior rectus muscle, 813
Inferior section, 39
Inferior vena cava, 40*f*, 214
Inferiorly (inferior direction), 40
Infertility, 649, 783
Inflammation, 429, 483
Inflammatory, 113
Inflammatory bowel disease (IBD), 113
Influenza, 172
Informed consent, 23
Inframammary, 682
Inframammary crease, 682
Infundibulum, 678
Inguinal, 116, 639
Inguinal canal, 639
Inguinal hernia, 116
Inguinal regions, 43, 44*f*
Inhalation, 160
Inhibition, 763

Inhibitor, 319
Injections, 436, 494
Inner ear, 858
Inpatient, 67
Insemination, 723
Insertion, 460
Insipidus, 773
Inspection, 64
Inspiration, 160
Insulin, 759, 788
Insulin resistance syndrome (IRS), 778
Integument. *see* Skin
Integumentary, 339
Integumentary system. *see also* Dermatology
  allergic reactions
    anaphylactic shock, 344
    anaphylaxis, 344
    local reaction, 344
    systemic reaction, 344
  anatomy of
    adipose tissue, 341
    hair, 342
    nails, 343
    sebaceous and sweat glands, 342
    skin, 339–41. *see also* Skin
    subcutaneous tissue, 341
  defined, 47*f*, 338*f*, 339
  disease and injury, defense against, 339
Intelligence testing, 922
Intramuscular (IM) injection, 494
Interatrial, 208
Intercostal retractions, 176
Intercostals, 467
Interferon, 290
Interleukin, 290
Intermittent explosive disorder, 916
Internal, 162
Internal iliac artery, 213
Internal oblique, 469
Internal respiration, 162
Internal structures, 41
Interstitial, 601
Interstitial cells, 638
Interstitial cystitis, 601
Interventional radiology, 1002
Interventricular, 208
Intervertebral, 404
Intervertebral disks, 404
Intestines, small and large, 92–93, 94
Intima, 210
Intra-arterial, 971
Intra-articular, 436
Intra-atrial, 208
Intracapsular, 835
Intracardiac, 16
Intracavitary, 974
Intracellular, 218, 945
Intracellular contents, 945
Intracellular fluid, 218
Intracranial, 537
Intracranial pressure (ICP), 537
Intracytoplasmic, 723
Intracytoplasmic sperm injection (ICSI), 723
Intradermal, 369, 377
Intrafallopian, 723
Intramuscular, 494
Intraocular, 823
Intraocular pressure (IOP), 823
Intraperitoneal, 971
Intrathecal, 968
Intrauterine, 680
Intrauterine cavity, 680
Intrauterine growth retardation (IUGR), 713
Intrauterine insemination, 723
Intravascular, 307
Intravenous, 125
Intravenous cholangiography (IVC), 998
Intravenous pyelography (IVP), 609, 999
Intraventricular, 208, 545
Intraventricular hematoma, 545
Intravesical, 618
Intrinsic factor, 97, 302, 314
Introitus, 680
Intubation, 183
Intussusception of the intestine, 111
Invasive, 950
Inversion, 465
Invertor, 465
Involution, 689, 712
Involutional melancholia, 712
Iodinated, 997
Iodine, 774, 786
Ion, 218
Iridal, 808
Irides, 808
Iris, 808
Iritis, 824
Iron deficiency anemia, 302
Irreducible hernia, 116
Irritable bowel syndrome (IBS), 113
Ischemia, 229
Ischemic, 539, 685
Ischemic phase, 685
Ischial, 408
Ischium, 408
Ishihara color plate, 829*f*
Islets of Langerhans, 759
Isthmus, 757

J

Jakob, Alfons, 541
Jaundice, 120, 353, 713, 823
Jejunostomy, 132
Jejunostomy tube, 132
Jejunum, 92
Jenner, Edward, 316
Joint capsule, 411
Joints, 410–11, 431–33
Jugular, 214
Jugular veins, 214
Jugular venous distention, 230

K

Kaposi, Moritz, 364
Kaposi's sarcoma, 305, 364, 960
Karyotype, 963
Kegel exercises, 604
Keloids, 356
Keratectomy, 837
Keratin, 339, 343
Keratitis, 822
Keratomileusis, 837
Keratoplasty, 836
Keratoses, 360
Keratosis, 360
Ketones, 780
Ketonuria, 605, 608
Kidney stones, 597–98
Kidney transplantation, 615
Kidneys
  defined, 583
  functions of
    blood pressure, 590
    erythropoietin, secretion of, 590
    pH of blood, 590
  hilum, 583
  major calix, 584
  minor calix, 584
  poles, upper and lower, 583
  renal capsule, 584
  renal cortex, 584
  renal medulla, 584
  renal pelvis, 584
  renal pyramids, 584
  symptoms, signs, and diseases, 597–600
Kleptomania, 916
Knee jerk, 491
Knock-knee, 433
Kwashiorkor, 599
Kyphoscoliosis, 429
Kyphosis, 429
Kyphotic, 429
Kyphotic curvature, 429

L

Labia majora, 681
Labia minora, 681
Labial, 681
Labor and delivery
  arrest of, 708
  assisted delivery, 721
  Braxton Hicks contractions, 687
  cephalic presentation, 687
  cervical ripening, 687
  colostrum, 689
  engagement, 687
  first stage of labor, 687
    dilation, 687, 688*f*
    effacement, 687, 688*f*
    rupture of membranes (ROM), 687
  induction of labor, 721
  involution, 689
  lactation, 689
  lochia, 689
  oxytocin, 687
  postnatal period, 689
  postpartum, 689
  second stage of labor
    crowning, 688
    umbilical cord, cutting of, 688
  symptoms, signs, and diseases, 708–12
  third stage of labor, 689
  vertex presentation, 687
Labyrinthitis, 872
Lacerations, 357
Lacrimal, 400, 809
Lacrimal bones, 400
Lacrimal ducts, 809
Lacrimal glands, 809, 822
Lacrimal sac, 809
Lactase, 97
Lactate dehydrogenase (LDH), 241
Lactation, 689
Lactation, failure of, 707, 772
Lactiferous, 682
Lactiferous lobules, 682
Laminectomy, 559
Landsteiner, Karl, 285
Language skills, 6, 22
Laparoscope, 128
Laparoscopic, 128
Laparoscopy, 725
Laparotomy, 131
Laparoscopic cholecystectomy, 128
Large for gestational age (LGA), 713
Large intestine, 92*f*, 93, 98, 111–14
Laryngeal, 156
Laryngeal prominence, 863
Laryngitis, 876
Laryngoscope, 183
Larynx, 156, 863
Laser, 371
Lateral, 409
Lateral malleolus, 409
Lateral rectus muscle, 813
Laterally (lateral direction), 38, 39*f*
Latin
  combining forms, 75, 135, 190, 258, 321, 379, 443, 495, 563, 620, 659, 733, 790, 840, 888, 927, 977
  medical words, origins of, 20
  nouns, singular and plural endings, 21
Latissimus, 467
Latissimus dorsi, 467
Laxative drugs, 133
Leaflets, 208
Lecithin, 717
Left bundle branch block, 235
Left heart catheterization, 242
Left lower quadrant (LLQ), 43, 44*f*
Left upper quadrant (LUQ), 43, 44*f*
Left ventricular assist device (LVAD), 230, 251
Left-brain thinking, 516
Left-sided congestive heart failure, 230
Legionella pneumophilia, 173
Legionnaire's disease, 173
Leiomyoma, 703
Leiomyomata, 703
Leiomyosarcoma, 703, 960
Lens, 810, 824–25
Lens capsule, 810
Lenses, 810
Lenticular, 810
Lentigo, 362
Lesion, 351
Let-down reflex, 756
Leukemia, 305–06, 961
Leukocyte esterase, 606
Leukocytes
  agranulocytes, 280
  basophils, 281
  eosinophils, 281
  granulocytes, 280
  lymphocytes, 282
  monocytes, 282
  neutrophils, 280
  symptoms, signs, and diseases, 304–06
  types and characteristics, listed, 283*t*
Leukoplakia, 876
Leukorrhea, 706
Leukotriene receptor blockers, 188
Levoscoliosis, 430
Ligamentous, 411
Ligaments, 411, 431–33, 676
Ligation, 726
Limbic, 808
Limbic lobe, 903
Limbic system, 903
Limbus, 808
Linea nigra, 354
Lingual, 862
Lingual tonsils, 862
Lipase, 97
Lipectomy, 374

Lipid, 242
Lipocytes, 341
Lipoma, 361
Lipoproteins, 237
Liposarcoma, 960
Liposuction, 374
Liquid cytology, 715
Lithogenesis, 598
Lithotomy, 720
Lithotripsy, 616
Lithotriptor, 616
Liver, 94, 95*f*, 97, 117–20
Liver cancer, 120
Liver spots, 362
Lobar, 158, 175
Lobar pneumonia, 175
Lobectomy, 186, 787
Lobes
  brain, 514
  lungs, 158
  thyroid gland, 757
Lobules, 682
Local, 344
Local allergic reaction, 344
Lochia, 689
Long-term care facility, 68
Longus, 470
Loop of Henle, 589
Lordosis, 429
Lordotic, 429
Lordotic curvature, 429
Low-density lipoprotein (LDL), 237
Lower esophageal sphincter (LES), 91, 108
Low-frequency hearing loss, 872
L/S (lecithin/sphingomyelin) ratio, 717
Lubb-dupp (S_1 and S_2), 208
Lumbar, 403
Lumbar puncture (LP), 557
Lumbar region, 43, 44*f*
Lumbar vertebrae (L1-L5), 403, 404*f*
Lumen
  blood vessels, 210
  bronchi and bronchioles, 157
  fallopian tubes, 678
  intestine, 92
  seminiferous tubules, 638
Lumpectomy, 726, 972
Lung cancer, 173
Lung scan, 182
Lungs, 157*f*, 158, 170–76
Lunula, 343
Lupus erythematosus, 364
Luteinizing hormone (LH), 642, 683, 756
Lyme disease, 431
Lymph, 287, 288
Lymph nodes, 287
Lymphadenopathy, 309, 876, 955
Lymphangiogram, 314, 966
Lymphangiography, 314, 966, 999
Lymphatic system. *see also* Immune response
  anatomy of
    lymph, 287
    lymph nodes, 287
    lymphatic vessels, 287
    lymphoid organs, 288–89
    lymphoid tissues, 288
  blood, interdependency with, 287
  defined, 47*f*, 276*f*, 277, 288*f*
  symptoms, signs, and diseases, 309–10
Lymphatic vessels, 287
Lymphedema, 309
Lymphoblasts, 282
Lymphocytes, 282, 290
Lymphocytic, 305
Lymphoid, 288
Lymphoid organs, 288–89
Lymphoid tissues, 288
Lymphoma, 309, 538, 962
Lymphs, 282, 288
Lysosomes, 946

M

Macrocyte, 300
Macrophages, 282, 290
Macroscopic, 45
Macula, 812, 813
Maculae, 812
Macular, 812
Macular degeneration, 825
Macules, 351, 813
Mad cow disease, 316, 541
Magnetic, 126
Magnetic resonance angiography (MRA), 1003
Magnetic resonance imaging (MRI) scan, 38*f*, 182, 537*f*, 554, 1003–04
Major depression, 918
Malalignment, 425
Male genitourinary system. *see also* Male reproductive medicine
  anatomy of
    bulbourethral glands, 640
    penis, 641
    prostate gland, 640
    scrotum, 637
    seminal vesicles and ejaculatory duct, 640
    testis and epididymis, 638–39
    vas deferens, 640
  defined, 49*f*, 636*f*, 637
  ejaculation, 643
  genitalia, external and internal, 637, 638*f*
  spermatogenesis, 642–43
Male pattern baldness, 367
Male reproductive medicine. *see also* Male genitourinary system; Sexually transmitted diseases (STDs)
  abbreviations, 658
  defined, 636
  diagnostic procedures
    blood tests, 653
    radiology and nuclear medicine procedures, 654
    semen tests, 653–54
  drug categories, 657
  medical procedures, 655
  surgical procedures, 655–56
  symptoms, signs, and diseases
    male breast, 653
    penis, 650–51
    prostate, 649–50
    sexually transmitted diseases, 651–52
    testis and epididymis, 649
Malformation, 537
Malignancy, 363, 485
Malignant, 173, 352
Malignant melanoma, 363, 958
Malingering, 913
Mallear, 856
Mallei, 856
Malleolar, 409
Malleoli, 409
Malleolus, 409, 856–57
Malleus, 856
Malpresentation, 708
Malpresentation of the fetus, 708
Malrotation, 111
Mammaplasty, 727. *see also under* Surgical Procedures
Mammary, 682
Mammary glands, 682
Mammogram, 718
Mammography, 718, 966, 1001
Mammoplasty, 727
Mandible, 400, 401
Mandibular, 401
Mania, 917
Manic, 917
Manic-depressive disorder, 917
Manometer, 557
Mantoux test, 182
Manubrium, 401
Marquis de Sade, 915
Masochism, 914
Massage therapist, 496
Masseter, 466
Mast cells, 155
Mast cell stabilizer drugs, 188
Mastectomy, 728. *see also under* Surgical Procedures
Mastication, 90, 96
Mastitis, 709, 873
Mastoid, 399, 856
Mastoid process, 399, 856
Mastoidectomy, 883
Mastoiditis, 873
Mastopexy, 727
Maxilla, 400
Maxillary, 401
Maxillary sinuses, 860
Maximus, 462
Mean, 311
Meati, 855
Meatus, 586, 855
Mechanical digestion, 96, 97
Meconium, 98, 690
Meconium aspiration, 713
Medial, 409
Medial malleolus, 409
Medial rectus muscle, 813
Medially (medial direction), 38, 39*f*
Mediastinal, 159
Mediastinum, 42, 159, 210
Medical assistant, 135
Medical illustrations, 404
Medical language
  benefits of learning, 5
  communication, 6
  five language skills, 6
  origins, 20
Medical oncologist, 977
Medical procedures. see also individual specialties
  accommodation, 831
  ADA (American Diabetes Association) diet, 786
  amniotomy, 721
  Apgar score, 721
  assisted delivery, 721
  assisted reproduction
    gamete intrafallopian transfer (GIFT), 723
    intracytoplasmic sperm injection (ICSI), 723
    intrauterine insemination, 723
    in vitro fertilization (IVF), 723
    zygote intrafallopian transfer (ZIFT), 723
  auscultation, 182, 248
  Babinski's sign, 556
  biophysical profile (BPP), 722
  blood donation and transfusion
    apheresis, 316
    autologous blood transfusion, 317
    donation, 316
    packed red blood cells (PRBCs), 317
    plasmapheresis, 317
    stem cell transplantation, 317
    transfusion, 317
  bone marrow aspiration, 315
  bone marrow transplantation (BMT)
    allogeneic transplants, 317
    autologous transplants, 317
    stem cell transplantation, 967
  Botox injections, 370
  braces and adaptive devices, 490
  breast self-examination (BSE), 721
  cardiopulmonary resuscitation (CPR), 183
  cardioversion, 248
  casting/casts, 436
  catheterization
    condom catheter, 612
    Foley catheter, 612
    suprapubic catheter, 612
  chemical peel, 372
  chemotherapy drugs, insertion of devices to administer
    intrathecal catheter, 968
    intravenous line, 968
    intravesical chemotherapy, 968, 969
    peripherally inserted central catheter (PICC), 968
  closed reduction, 436
  collagen injections, 370
  colposcopy, 720
  convergence, 831
  cortisone injections, 436
  cryosurgery, 370, 720, 968
  curettage, 371
  debridement, 371
  deep tendon reflexes (DTR)
    knee jerk, 491
    patellar reflex, 491
  dermabrasion, 372
  dialysis
    continuous ambulatory peritoneal (CAPD), 613
    continuous cycling peritoneal (CCPD), 613
    hemodialysis, 613
    peritoneal, 613
  digital rectal examination (DRE), 655
  dilated funduscopy, 832
  elective abortion, 723
  electrosurgery
    electrodesiccation, 371, 968
    electrosection, 371
    fulguration, 371, 968
  endotracheal intubation, 183
  epidural anesthesia, 721
  extracorporeal shock wave therapy (ESWT), 437
  eye patching, 832
  eyeglasses prescription
    axis, 834
    cylinder, 834
    sphere, 834
  fundal height, 721

gaze testing, 832
Glasgow Coma Scale (GCS), 556
goniometry, 437
grading, 968
gynecologic examination, 720
Heimlich maneuver, 183
incentive spirometry, 184
incision and drainage (I&D), 371
induction of labor, 721
intake and output (I&O), 614
intra-articular injection, 436
laser skin resurfacing, 372
laser surgery, 371
lumbar puncture (LP), 557
microdermabrasion, 372
mini mental status examination (MMSE), 557
muscle strength test, 491
Nägele's rule, 722
nasogastric tube, insertion of, 127
neurologic examination, 558
newborn genital examination, 655
nonstress test (NST), 722
nose, sinus, mouth, and throat examination, 882
obstetrical history
gravida (G), para (P), and abortion (A), 722
G/TPAL system, 722
orthosis, 437
otoscopy, 882–83
oxygen therapy
Ambu bag, 185
nasal cannula, 184
ventilator (respirator), 184–85
pelvimetry, 722
peripheral vision, 833
phlebotomy, 315
phorometry, 833
physical therapy, 437
prosthesis, 437
pupillary response, 833
radiofrequency catheter ablation, 249
radiofrequency catheter occlusion, 249
rehabilitation exercises, 492
Romberg test, 558
Romberg's sign, 883
sclerotherapy, 249
skin examination, 372
skin resurfacing, 372
spinal traction, 558
staging, 969
suturing, 373
Tanner staging, 721
testicular self-examination (TSE), 655
therapeutic abortion (TAB), 723
traction, 438
transcutaneous electrical nerve stimulation (TENS) unit, 558
trigger point injections, 492
urine specimens, obtaining, 614
vaccination, 316
venipuncture, 315
version, 723
vital signs (TPR and BP)
blood pressure, 250–51
pulse, 249–50
respiration, 185
Medical specialties, listed, 46–50*f*, 51. *see also individual specialties*
Medical words
analyzing and defining
combining forms and suffixes, 12
prefixes, combining forms, and suffixes, 17
building
combining forms and suffixes, 11
prefixes, combining forms, and suffixes, 16
nouns, singular and plural endings, 21
origins, 20
pronouncing, 14, 19
word parts, 7–19
combining forms, 7–8, 19. *see also* Combining forms; Combining forms, listed
prefixes, 15–16. *see also* Prefixes; Prefixes, listed
suffixes, 9–10, 19. *see also* Suffixes; Suffixes, listed
Medulla, 584
Medulla oblongata, 517
Medullae, 584
Medullary, 412, 584
Medullary cavity, 411, 412*f*
Megakaryoblasts, 284
Megakaryocytes, 284
Megaloblasts, 302
Meibom, Heinrich, 807
Meibomian glands, 807
Meiosis, 643
Melancholia, 712
Melanin, 340, 342, 757
Melanocytes, 340, 342, 756
Melanocyte-stimulating hormone (MSH), 756
Melanoma, 363
Melatonin, 757
Melena, 116
Melenic, 116
Mellitus, 709
Memory T cells, 290
Menarche, 683
Ménière, Prosper, 872
Ménière's disease, 872
Meningeal. *see also* Cranial nerves
Meninges. *see also* Cranial nerves
Meningioma, 538
Meningitis, 546
Meningocele, 547
Meningomyelocele, 547
Meniscal, 411
Menisci, 411
Meniscus, 411, 433
Menopause, 704–05, 783
Menorrhagia, 705
Menses, 683
Menstrual, 683
Menstrual cycle. *see under* Menstruation
Menstrual phase, 683
Menstruation
cycle phases
ischemic, 685
menstrual, 683
ovulation, 684
proliferative, 684
secretory, 684
follicle-stimulating hormone (FSH), 683
luteinizing hormone (LH), 683
menarche, 683
menses, 683
onset, 683
oocytes, 683
oogenesis, 683
ovulation, 683
symptoms, signs, and diseases, 704–05
Mental, 542, 860
Mental retardation, 542
Mentum, 860
Mesentery, 94
Messenger RNA, 946
Metabolic, 162
Metabolism, 162
Metacarpal, 407
Metacarpal bones, 406*f*, 407
Metacarpophalangeal (MCP) joint, 407
Metastases, 950
Metastasis, 950
Metastasize, 950
Metastatic, 950
Metatarsal, 410
Metatarsal bones, 410
Metered-dose inhaler (MDI), 187
Methadone clinic, 68
Metrorrhagia, 705
Microcyte, 300
Microcytic, 302
Microdermabrasion, 372
Microglia, 522
Microkeratome, 837
Microphobia, 909
Microscope, 45
Microscopic, 45, 604
Micturition, 589
Midbrain, 517
Middle ear, 856–57
Midsagittal plane
defined, 38
lateral direction (laterally), 38, 39*f*
medial direction (medially), 38, 39*f*
sagittal suture of the skull, 37*f*, 38, 398
Migraine, 546
Migraine headache, 546
Milieu, 926
Mineralocorticoid, 760
Mineralocorticoid hormones, 760
Miosis, 809
Miscarriage, 711
Mitochondria, 946
Mitochondrial, 946
Mitochondrion, 946
Mitosis, 643, 947
Mitosis inhibitor drugs, 975
Mitotic, 947
Mitotic rate, 947
Mitral, 208
Mitral valve, 208
Mitral valve prolapse (MVP), 233
Mixed hearing loss, 872
Mohs, Frederic, 374
Molding of head, 690
Mole, 702
Moles, 361
Monoblasts, 282
Monoclonal antibodies, 975
Monocytes, 282, 290
Mononucleosis, 306
Mons pubis, 681
Mood, 905
Moon face, 781
Morning sickness, 710
Morphology, 300, 654
Morton's neuroma, 552
Motile, 639
Motility, 654
Motion sickness, 872
Motor, 518
Motor strength, 491
Movement disorders, 486–87
Mucosa, 89, 91, 92, 155, 156, 162, 585, 859
Mucosal, 156, 585
Mucous, 156, 162
Mucous colitis, 113
Mucous membrane, 155
Mucus, 155, 156, 162, 859
Multigravida, 722
Multi-infarct dementia, 541
Multinodular, 775
Multinodular goiter, 774
Multinucleated, 472
Multinucleated muscle fibers, 472
Multiparous, 722
Multiple myeloma, 306, 962
Multiple sclerosis (MS), 550
Munchausen by proxy, 913
Munchausen, Karl, 913
Munchausen syndrome, 913
Murmur, 231
Muscle, 20, 459
Muscle biopsy, 492
Muscle contraction
acetylcholine, 472
calcium ions (Ca^{++}), 472
fascicles, 472
multinucleated muscle fibers, 472
myofibrils, 472
neuromuscular junction, 472
neurotransmitters, 472
receptors, 472
Muscle contusion, 483
Muscle hypertrophy, 473
Muscle spasm, 483
Muscle strain, 483
Muscles. *see also* Muscle contraction; Muscular system
abdomen
external oblique, 469
internal oblique, 469
rectus abdominis, 469
arms and hands
biceps brachii, 468
brachioradialis, 468
thenar, 468
triceps brachii, 468
extraocular eye
inferior oblique, 813
inferior rectus, 813
lateral rectus, 813
medial rectus, 813
superior oblique, 813
superior rectus, 813
head and neck
buccinator, 466
frontalis, 466
masseter, 466
orbicularis oculi, 466
orbicularis oris, 466
platysma, 466
sternocleidomastoid, 466
temporalis, 466
hypertrophy, 473
legs and buttocks
biceps femoris, 470, 471
gastrocnemius, 470, 471
gluteus maximus, 470
hamstrings, 471
peroneus longus, 470
quadriceps femoris, 470, 471
rectus femoris, 470, 471

Muscles. *see also* Muscle contraction; Muscular system (*continued*)
  sartorius, 470
  semimembranosus, 471
  semitendinosus, 471
  tibialis anterior, 470
  vastus intermedius, 471
  vastus lateralis, 471
  vastus medialis, 471
 movement, types of
  abduction, 464
  adduction, 464
  eversion, 465
  explained, 463
  extension, 464
  flexion, 464
  inversion, 465
  pronation, 465
  rotation, 465
  supination, 465
 names and their meanings
  biceps brachii, 461*f*, 462
  brachioradialis, 462
  extensor digitorum, 462
  flexor hallucis brevis, 462
  gluteus maximus, 462
  recognizing, 461
  rectus abdominis, 462
  temporalis, 462
  triceps brachii, 462
 origins, insertions, and related structures
  aponeurosis, 461
  bursa, 461
  fascia, 461
  insertion point, 460
  origin, 460
  retinaculum, 461
  tendons, 461
 shoulders, chest, and back
  deltoid, 467
  intercostals, 467
  latissimus dorsi, 467
  pectoralis major, 467
  trapezius, 467
 strength and size, 473
 symptoms, signs, and diseases, 482–87
 types of
  cardiac, 459, 460*f*
  skeletal, 459, 460*f*
  smooth, 459, 460*f*
  striated, 459
  voluntary, 459
Muscular, 459
Muscular dystrophy, 483
Muscular system. *see also* Muscle contraction; Muscles
 anatomy of
  abdomen, 469
  arms and hands, 468
  head and neck, 466
  legs and buttocks, 470–71
  movement, types of, 463–65
  muscle types, 459, 460*f*
  names and their meanings, 461–62
  origins, insertions, and related structures, 460–61
  shoulders, chest, and back, 467
 defined, 48*f*, 458*f*, 459
 musculature, 459
Musculature, 459
Musculoskeletal, 397, 459
Musculoskeletal system. *see* Muscular system; Skeletal system
Mutation, 948
Myalgia, 484
Myasthenia gravis, 484, 561
Mycobacterium tuberculosis, 176, 182
Mycoplasma pneumoniae, 175
Mydriasis, 809
Mydriatic, 832
Mydriatic drugs, 832, 838
Myelin, 524, 525
Myelinated, 524, 525
Myeloblasts, 280
Myelocytes, 280
Myelogenous, 305
Myelogram, 554
Myelography, 554, 999
Myeloma, 306, 962
Myelomeningocele, 547
Myocardial, 209
Myocardial infarction (MI), 230
Myocardium, 209–10, 229–30
Myoclonus, 486
Myofibrils, 472
Myomectomy, 725
Myometrial, 680
Myometritis, 703
Myometrium, 680
Myopathy, 484
Myopia, 827
Myopia surgery, 837
Myorrhaphy, 493
Myosarcoma, 960
Myositis, 484
Myringitis, 873
Myringotome, 884
Myringotomy, 884
Myxedema, 776

N

Nägele, Franz, 722
Nägele's rule, 722
Nail bed, 343
Nail plate, 343
Nail root, 343
Nails, 343, 368–69
Narcissism, 921
Narcissistic personality, 921
Narcolepsy, 546
Narcotic, 560
Nares, 858
Naris, 858
Nasal, 400
Nasal bones, 400
Nasal cannula, 184–85
Nasal cavity, 155, 156*f*, 859
Nasal conchae, 155, 859
Nasal dorsum, 858
Nasal mucosa, 155, 859
Nasal polyp, 875
Nasal septum, 858
Nasogastric, 127
Nasolabial, 860
Nasolabial fold, 860
Nasolacrimal, 809
Nasolacrimal duct, 809
Nasopharyngeal, 861
Nasopharynx, 861
Nausea, 109
Nausea and vomiting (N&V), 109
Nauseated, 109
Necrosis, 230, 353, 424, 949
Necrotic, 239, 353
Neisseria gonorrhoeae, 602, 652
Neologisms, 920
Neonatal, 690
Neonate, 690, 712–13, 717. *see also* Newborn infants
Neonatologist, 733
Neonatology, 51
Neoplasms, 352, 956
Neoplastic, 956
Neoplastic diseases, 63
Nephrectomy, 616
Nephritis, 600
Nephroblastoma, 600, 963
Nephrolithiasis, 597–98
Nephrolithotomy, 616
Nephrologist, 620
Nephron, 588
Nephropathy, 598
Nephropexy, 616
Nephroptosis, 599
Nephrotic, 599
Nephrotic syndrome, 599
Nephrotomography, 609
Nephrotoxic, 618
Nerve conduction studies, 555
Nerve transmission
 gray matter, 525
 neuron, parts of
  axon, 524
  cell body, 524
  dendrites, 524
  myelin, 524, 525
  nucleus (of cell body), 524
 neurotransmitters
  acetylcholine, 525
  dopamine, 525
  endorphins, 525
  epinephrine, 525
  norepinephrine, 525
  role of, 524
  serotonin, 525
 receptors, 524
 synapse, 524
 white matter, 525
Nerves, 521, 549–52
Nervous, 513
Nervous system. *see also* Brain; Cranial nerves; Neuroglia
 anatomy of
  brain, 513–18
  central nervous system (CNS), 513
  cranial nerves, 518–19
  neurons and neurolgia, 521–22
  peripheral nervous system, 513
  spinal cord, 520
  spinal nerves, 521
 autonomic, 522
 defined, 48*f*, 512*f*, 513
 divisions of, 523*f*
 parasympathetic, 523
 somatic, 522
 sympathetic, 523
Neural, 547
Neural tube defects, 547, 712
Neuralgia, 551
Neuritis, 551
Neuroblastoma, 962
Neurofibrillary, 542
Neurofibrillary tangles, 542
Neurofibroma, 552
Neurofibromata, 552
Neurofibromatosis, 552
Neurofibrosarcoma, 960
Neurogenic bladder, 601
Neuroglia
 astrocytes, 522
 defined, 521
 ependymal cells, 522
 microglia, 522
 oligodendroglia, 522
 Schwann cells, 522
Neurohypophysis, 755
Neurologic, 539
Neurologic examination, 558
Neurologist, 563
Neurology. *see also* Nervous system
 abbreviations, 562
 defined, 512
 diagnostic procedures
  electroencephalography (EEG), 554–55
  evoked potential testing, 555
  laboratory tests, 553
  nerve conduction studies, 555
  radiology and nuclear medicine procedures, 553–54
  sleep studies (polysomnography), 555
 drug categories, 560–61
 medical procedures, 556–58
 surgical procedures, 559–60
 symptoms, signs, and diseases
  brain, 536–46
  nerves, 549–52
  spinal cord, 547–49
Neuroma, 552, 871
Neuromuscular, 472
Neuromuscular junction, 472
Neuromuscular system. *see* Nervous system
Neurons, 521, 524
Neuropathy, 552
Neurosurgeon, 563
Neurosurgery, 559
Neurotransmitters, 472, 524, 525, 905–06
Neutrophils, 280, 289
Nevus, 361
Newborn infants
 acrocyanosis, 690
 anterior fontanel, 690
 clavicle, fracture during birth, 405
 colostrum, 689
 congenital dislocation of the hip (CDH), 431
 congenital heart abnormalities, 233
 conjunctivitis, 822
 cradle cap, 367
 eye color, 809
 fontanels, 400, 690
 genital examination, 655
 heart rate, 216
 kneecaps, absence of, 409
 meconium, 690
 molding of head, 690
 passive immunity, 291, 689
 premature, 690
 respiratory rate, 162
 term neonate, 690
 vernix caseosa, 690
Night blindness, 825
Nitroglycerin, 255
NK (natural killer) cells, 290
Nocturia, 605
Node, 287
Nodular, 775
Nodular goiter, 774
Nodule, 775, 777, 878
Non-Hodgkin's lymphoma, 309, 962

Nonmedical departments, 67
Nonsteroidal, 441
Nonstress test (NST), 722
Nontoxic, 774
Nontoxic goiter, 774
Norepinephrine, 761, 905–06
Norepinephrine, 523, 525
Normal sinus rhythm (NSR), 218
Normoblasts, 279
Normochromic, 301
Normocytic, 301
Nose, 155, 156*f*
Nosocomial diseases, 63
Nuchal, 546, 713
Nuchal cord, 713
Nuchal rigidity, 546
Nuclear, 947
Nuclear medicine. *see also* Radiology
  cyclotron, 1011
  defined, 1007
  gamma ray procedures
    cholescintigraphy, 1009
    MUGA (multiple-gated acquisition) scan, 1009
    nuclear ventriculogram, 1009
    OncoScint scan, 1010
    ProstaScint scan, 1010
    radiopharmaceuticals, listed, 1008–09
    SPECT (single-photon emission computed tomogaphy) scan, 1009
    ventilation-perfusion (V/Q) scan, 1010
  positron emission tomography (PET) scan, 1011
Nuclear medicine procedures. *see* under Diagnostic procedures
Nuclei, 947
Nucleolar, 947
Nucleoli, 947
Nucleolus, 947
Nucleus (of a cell), 20, 524, 947
Nucleus pulposis, 404, 548
Nulligravida, 722
Nurse midwife, 733
Nurse, 67
Nursing unit, 67
Nutritional diseases, 63
Nystagmus, 826

O

Oblique, 427
Obsession, 908
Obsessive, 908
Obsessive-compulsive disorder, 908, 921
Obstetrical history, 722
Obstetrician, 733
Obstetrics
  chloasma, 354
  hyperemesis gravidarum, 109
  linea nigra, 354
  medical procedures, 721
  striae, 354
  surgical procedures, 729
Obstipated, 115
Obstipation, 115
Obstructive, 120
Obstructive jaundice, 120
Obstructive sleep apnea, 177
Obturator, 408
Obturator foramen, 408
Occipital, 398
Occipital bone, 398–99
Occipital lobe, 514
Occlusion, 249
Occult, 123
Occult blood, 123, 608
Occupational lung diseases, 174
Occupational Safety and Health Administration (OSHA), 484
Oculi, 466
Oculomotor, 519
Oculomotor nerve, 519
Odynophagia, 107
Olecranon, 406
Olfactory, 515
Olfactory cortex, 515
Oligodendroglia, 522
Oligodendroglioma, 538, 960
Oligohydramnios, 710
Oligomenorrhea, 705
Oligospermia, 649
Oliguria, 605
Omentum, 91*f,* 94
Omphalocele, 116
Oncogenes, 948
Oncologist, 135
Oncology. *see also* Cells; Cellular division and cancer; Radiation therapy
  abbreviations, 976
  anatomy related to, 945–50
  defined, 944
  diagnostic procedures
    blood tests, 965
    cytology tests, 963–64
  drug categories, 974–75
  medical procedures, 967–69
  radiation therapy, 972–74
  surgical procedures, 969–72
  symptoms, signs and types of cancer
    blood and lymphatic system, 961–62
    carcinomas, 957–58
    embryonal cell cancer, 962–63
    general, 955–56
    sarcomas, 959–61
OncoScint scan, 1010
Onset, 63
Onychomycosis, 368
Oocytes, 683
Oogenesis, 683
Oophorectomy, 725
Ophidiophobia, 909
Ophthalmologist, 840
Ophthalmology
  abbreviations, 839
  defined, 806
  diagnostic procedures
    eye tests, 829–31
    radiologic procedures, 831
  drug categories, 838
  medical procedures, 831–34
  surgical procedures, 835–38
  symptoms, signs, and diseases
    brain and visual cortex conditions, 828
    extraocular muscles, 826
    eyelid, 821
    iris, pupil, and anterior chamber, 823–24
    lacrimal gland, 822
    lens, 824–25
    posterior cavity and retina, 825–26
    refractive disorders, 827
    sclera, cornea, and conjunctiva, 822–23
Opportunistic, 175
Opportunistic infection, 175, 305
Oppositional, 911
Oppositional defiant disorder, 911
Ophthalmoscope, 832
Optic, 519, 807, 812
Optic chiasm, 815
Optic disk, 812
Optic globe, 807
Optic nerve, 519, 812, 814–15
Optician, 840
Optometrist, 840
Optometry, 840
Oral, 861
Oral and maxillofacial surgeon, 888
Oral candidiasis, 877
Oral cavity, 89, 107, 861
Oral mucosa, 861
Orbicularis, 466
Orbicularis oculi, 466
Orbicularis oris, 466
Orbit, 807
Orbital, 807
Orchiectomy, 656
Orchiopexy, 656
Orchitis, 649
Orifice, 584
Origin, 460
Oris, 466
Oropharyngeal, 862
Oropharynx, 862
Orthopedic plate and screws, 440*f*
Orthopedics. *see also* Fractures; Muscular system; Skeletal system
  abbreviations, 442, 495
  defined, 396, 458
  diagnostic procedures
    blood tests, 489
    laboratory tests, 434
    muscle tests, 489
    radiology and nuclear medicine procedures, 434–35
  drug categories, 440–41, 493–94
  medical procedures, 436–38, 490–92
  surgical procedures, 438–40, 492–93
  symptoms, signs, and diseases
    bones and cartilage, 424–28
    bony thorax, 433
    joints and ligaments, 431–33
    legs and feet, bones of, 433
    movement disorders, 486–87
    muscles, 482–87
    tendon, bursa, or fascia, 487–88
    vertebrae, 429–30
Orthopedist, 443
Orthopnea, 178
Orthopneic, 178
Orthosis, 437
Orthostatic hypotension, 239
Os, 680
Osseous, 411
Osseous tissue, 411
Ossicles, 401, 856, 857
Ossicular, 401, 857
Ossicular chain, 401, 856–57
Ossification, 413
Osteoarthritis, 432
Osteoblasts, 414
Osteoclasts, 414
Osteocytes, 414
Osteogenic, 424
Osteogenic sarcoma, 424, 961
Osteoma, 424
Osteomalacia, 428
Osteomyelitis, 428
Osteopaths, 496
Osteopathy, 496
Osteophyte, 432
Osteoporosis, 428
Osteoporotic, 428
Osteosarcoma, 424, 961
Osteotome, 440
Otalgia, 873
Otitis externa, 873
Otitis media, 873
Otolaryngologist, 888
Otolaryngology. *see also* Ears, nose, and throat (ENT) system
  abbreviations, 887
  defined, 854
  diagnostic procedures
    hearing tests, 879–80
    laboratory and radiologic tests, 881
  drug categories, 885–86
  medical procedures, 882–83
  surgical procedures, 883–85
  symptoms, signs, and diseases
    ears, 871–74
    mouth, throat, and neck, 875–78
    nose and sinuses, 874–75
Otorhinolaryngologist, 888
Otorrhea, 874
Otosclerosis, 874
Otoscope, 883
Otoscopy, 882–83
Ototoxicity, 886
Outcome, 65
Outpatient, 68
Ova, 124, 676, 677
Oval window, 857
Ovarian, 676
Ovarian cancer, 701
Ovaries, 676–77, 701, 761
Overactive bladder, 602
Oviduct, 678, 679
Ovulation, 683, 684
Ovum, 124, 677, 685
Oximeter, 181
Oximetry, 181
Oxygen, 161–62
Oxygen therapy, 184–85
Oxygenated, 161
Oxygenated blood, 161
Oxyhemoglobin, 161, 278
Oxytocin, 687, 754, 756

P

Packed red blood cells (PRBCs), 317
Pack-years, 169
Palatine, 401
Palatine bones, 400
Palatal, 861
Palates, hard and soft, 90, 861
Palatine, 862
Palatine tonsils, 862
Palliative care, 68
Pallor, 353*f,* 354
Palpation, 64
Palpitations, 235
Palsy, 537
Pancreas, 95*f,* 96, 97, 122
  alpha cells, 759
  beta cells, 759
  delta cells, 759
  glucose, 759
  glycogen, 759
  hormones secreted

Pancreas (*continued*)
glucagon, 759
insulin, 759
somatostatin, 759
islets of Langerhans, 759
Pancreatic, 122
Pancreatic cancer, 122
Pancreatic duct, 95*f*, 96
Pancreatitis, 122
Pancytopenia, 300
Panhypopituitarism, 771
Panic, 908
Panic disorder, 908
Panlobar, 175
Panlobar pneumonia, 175
Pansinusitis, 875
Pap smear, 715–16
Papanicolaou, George, 715
PAPette, 715
Papilledema, 825
Papilloma, 362
Papules, 351
Para (P), 722
Paralysis, 548
Paramedic, 24
Paranasal, 860
Paranasal sinuses, 860
Paranoia, 919
Paraplegia, 548
Paraplegic, 548, 549
Parasites, 124
Parasympathetic, 523
Parasympathetic nervous system, 523
Parathyroid, 758
Parathyroid glands, 758
Parathyroid hormone, 414, 758
Parathyroidectomy, 787
Parenchyma, 158, 521, 588
Parenchymal, 158
Paresthesias, 550, 552
Parietal, 159
Parietal bones, 398
Parietal lobe, 514
Parietal pleura, 159
Parkinson, James, 546
Parkinson's disease, 546, 561
Paronychia, 369
Parotid glands, 90
Paroxysmal, 178
Paroxysmal nocturnal dyspnea (PND), 178
Paroxysmal tachycardia, 236
Parturition. *see* Labor and delivery
Passive immunity, 291
Patella, 410
Patellae, 410, 424
Patellar, 410
Patellar reflex, 491
Patent, 114, 233
Patent ductus arteriosus (PDA), 233
Patent foramen ovale, 233
Pathogens, 62, 289
Pathologic, 425
Pathological, 916
Pathological gambling, 916
Patient, 63
Patient history, 63
Peau d'orange, 707, 957
Pectoralis, 467
Pectoralis major, 467
Pectoris, 229
Pectus excavatum, 177, 433
Pediatrician, 733
Pediatrics
bone growth, 413, 414
childhood immunizations, 291
defined, 51
intramuscular (IM) injection site, 494
skin, 344
sudden infant death syndrome (SIDS), 178
urine production, 589
Pediculosis, 359
Pedis, 359
Pedophile, 915
Pedophilia, 915
Peduncle, 114
Pedunculated polyps, 112*f*, 114
PEG (percutaneous endoscopic gastrostomy) tube, 131
PEJ (percutaneous endoscopic jejunostomy) tube, 132
Pelves, 584
Pelvic, 408, 584
Pelvic cavity, 42
Pelvic inflammatory disease (PID), 703
Pelvimetry, 722
Pelvis, 20, 408, 584
Pendulous, 727
Penile, 586, 641
Penile implant, 656
Penile urethra, 586
Penis, 586, 641
Pepsin, 97
Pepsinogen, 97
Peptic, 110
Peptic ulcer disease (PUD), 110
Peptidase, 97
Percussion, 64
Percutaneous, 125, 131, 252, 616
Perforated duodenal ulcer, 117*f*
Perfusion, 182, 239, 246
Pericardial, 209
Pericardial fluid, 209
Pericardial sac, 209
Pericardiocentesis, 253
Pericarditis, 231
Pericardium, 209
Perimenopausal, 704
Perimenopausal period, 704
Perineal, 637
Perineum, 637, 681
Periosteal, 411
Periosteum, 411, 412*f*
Peripheral, 230, 312
Peripheral artery disease (PAD), 239
Peripheral edema, 230
Peripheral nervous system, 513
Peripheral vascular disease (PVD), 239
Peripheral vision testing, 833
Peristalsis, 91, 96, 584, 678, 679
Peritoneal, 94
Peritoneal dialysis, 613
Peritoneal fluid, 94
Peritoneum, 94
Peritonitis, 111, 117
Pernicious, 302
Pernicious anemia, 97, 302, 314
Peroneal, 409–10
Peroneal artery, 213
Peroneus, 470
Peroneus longus, 470
Personality, 921
Personality disorders, 921
Perspiration, 342
Petechia, 350
Petechiae, 308, 350
Petechial, 350
Petit mal seizures, 544
Peyer's patches, 94, 288
pH
acidic, 607
alkaline, 607
blood, 590
urine, 607
Phacoemulsification, 835
Phagocytes, 280
Phagocytosis, 280
Phalangeal, 407
Phalangeal bones, 407
Phalanges, 406*f*, 407, 410
Phalanx, 407
Pharmacologic, 244
Pharmacologic stress test, 244
Pharmacology, 51
Pharmacy technician, 563
Pharyngeal, 156
Pharyngitis, 877
Pharynx, 90, 156, 861–62
Pheochromocytoma, 782
Philtrum, 860
Phimosia, 651
Phlebitis, 240
Phlebotomist, 321
Phlebotomy, 315
Phobia, 20
Phobias, 908–09
Phobic, 908
Phorometer, 833
Phorometry, 833
Photodynamic, 377
Photophobia, 546, 824
Photorefractive, 837
Phototherapy, 713
Phrenic nerve, 161
Physiatrist, 496
Physiatry, 496
Physical, 437
Physical examination, 63–64
Physical medicine and rehabilitation (PM&R), 496
Physical therapist, 443
Physical therapy, 437
Physician extender, 66
Physician, 20, 66
Physician's assistant, 378
Physicians' offices, 67
Physiology
defined, 44
digestion, 96–98
respiration, 160–62
Pia mater, 518
Pica, 712
Piles, 114
Piloerection, 342
Pilonidal sinus, 368
Pineal, 757
Pineal body, 757
Pinna, 855
Pinnae, 855
Pitting edema, 230
Pituitary, 755
Pituitary gland
anterior pituitary gland (adenohypophysis)
adrenocorticotropic hormone (ACTH), 756
follicle-stimulating hormone (FSH), 756
growth hormone (GH), 756
hormones secreted, 755*f*, 756
luteinizing hormone (LH), 756
melanocyte-stimulating hormone (MSH), 756
prolactin, 756
thyroid-stimulating hormone (TSH), 756
posterior pituitary gland (neurohypophysis)
antidiuretic hormone (ADH), 756
hormones secreted, 755*f*, 756
oxytocin, 756
sella turcica, 755
Placenta, 686
Placenta previa, 710
Placental, 686
Planes. *see* Body planes
Plaque, 237, 238, 542
Plasma, 277
Plasmapheresis, 317
Plasminogen, 319
Plastic surgeon, 378
Platelet aggregation, 286
Platelets, 284, 307–08
Platinum drugs, 975
Platysma, 466
Play therapy, 925
Pleura, 159, 177
Pleural, 159
Pleural effusion, 177
Pleural fluid, 159
Pleural friction rub, 177
Pleurisy, 177
Pleuritic, 177
Pleuritis, 177
Pneumococcal, 175
Pneumococcal pneumonia, 175
Pneumoconiosis, 174
Pneumocystis carinii pneumonia (PCP), 175, 305
Pneumonectomy, 186
Pneumonia, defined, 174
Pneumonias, 174–75
Pneumophilia, 173
Pneumothorax, 177
Podiatric medicine, 496
Podiatrist, 496
Podiatry, 496
Poikilocytosis, 301
Polycystic, 599
Polycystic kidney disease, 599
Polycystic ovary syndrome, 701
Polycythemia vera, 303
Polydactyly, 362
Polydipsia, 773, 778, 779
Polyhydramnios, 710
Polymorphonucleated, 280
Polymorphonucleated leukocyte (PMN), 280
Polymyalgia, 484
Polymyositis, 484
Polyneuritis, 551
Polypectomy, 114, 132
Polyphagia, 107, 778, 779
Polyposis, 112*f*, 114
Polyps, 114, 875
Polysomnography, 555
Polyuria, 605, 773, 778, 779
Pons, 517
Popliteal, 410
Popliteal artery, 213
Popliteal space, 410
Port, 971
Porta hepatis, 214
Portal, 117
Portal hypertension, 117
Portal vein, 97, 117, 214
Port-wine stains, 361
Positron, 1011
Positron emission tomography (PET) scan, 541*f*, 554, 1011

Postcoital, 650
Posterior, 36
Posterior cavity of the eye, 812
Posterior chamber of the eye, 811
Posterior pituitary gland, 755*f*, 756. *see also* Pituitary gland
Posterior section, 36
Posteriorly (posterior direction), 36, 37*f*
Posteroanterior (PA), 36, 37*f*
Postictal, 543
Postictal state, 543
Postnasal, 874
Postnasal drip (PND), 874
Postnatal period, 689
Postoperative, 110
Postoperative ileus, 110
Postpartum, 689
Postpartum depression, 712
Postpartum hemorrhage, 711, 773
Posttraumatic, 910
Posttraumatic stress disorder (PTSD), 910
Postvoid, 602
Postvoid residual, 602
Potassium (K^+), 218, 284
Potassium supplements, 618
Potential, 555
Precocious, 783
Precocious puberty, 783
Preeclampsia, 711
Prefixes. *see also* Medical words
  amount, describing, 15
  characteristics, describing, 16
  characteristics of, 15
  combining forms with suffixes, joining to, 16
  location/direction, describing, 15
  size, describing, 15
  time/speed, describing, 16
Prefixes, listed
  a-, 63
  ab-, 464
  ad-, 464
  an-, 15
  ana-, 35
  ante-, 679
  anti-, 16
  apo-, 947
  auto-, 310
  bi-, 208
  brachy-, 972
  brady-, 16
  cata-, 920
  circum-, 179
  con-, 914
  de-, 62
  di-, 677
  dia-, 64
  dis-, 431
  dys-, 16
  e-, 465
  ec-, 821
  ecto-, 715
  em-, 171
  en-, 774
  endo-, 15
  epi-, 43
  eu-, 161
  ex-, 160
  exo-, 342
  extra-, 350
  hemi-, 516
  hyper-, 15
  hypo-, 15
  im-, 114
  in-, 108
  infra-, 682
  inter-, 176
  intra-, 15
  kilo-, 311
  macro-, 45
  mal-, 111
  meso-, 94
  meta-, 407
  mid-, 38
  multi-, 472
  non-, 441
  pan-, 175
  par-, 90
  para-, 523
  per-, 125
  peri-, 15
  poly-, 15
  post-, 16
  pre-, 16
  pro-, 65
  quadri-, 470
  re-, 46
  retro-, 125
  sub-, 15
  supra-, 236
  sym-, 408
  syn-, 63
  tachy-, 16
  trans-, 39
  tri-, 208
  ultra-, 247
  un-, 949
  uni-, 876
Pregnancy, 685
Pregnancy test, 717
Pregnant, 685
Prehypertension, 238
Premalignant, 361
Premalignant skin lesions, 361
Premature, 651
Premature atrial contractions (PACs), 235
Premature contractions, 235
Premature ejaculation, 651
Premature infants
  gestation period of, 690
  respiratory distress syndrome (RDS), 176
  retrolental fibroplasia, 826
Premature labor, 711
Premature rupture of membranes (PROM), 711
Premature ventricular contractions (PVCs), 235
Prematurity, 826
Premenstrual, 705
Premenstrual dysphoric disorder (PMDD), 705, 918
Premenstrual syndrome (PMS), 705
Prenatal period, 687
Prepuce, 641
Presbyacusis, 872
Presbyopia, 825
Presenile, 542
Presenile dementia, 542
Pressure sores, 356
Preventive medicine, 62
Priapism, 651
Primary care physician (PCP), 66
Primary site, 956
Primigravida, 722
Process, 399, 404
Progesterone, 677, 678*f*, 761
Progesterone receptor (PR) assay, 963
Progestin, 730
Prognosis, 65
Projections, 994–95. *see also* Roentgenography
Prolactin, 756
Prolapse, 233, 704, 711
Prolapsed cord, 711
Proliferative, 684
Proliferative phase, 684
Pronation, 465
Pronator, 465
Prone position, 36
Prophylactic, 728
Proprioception, 558
Prostaglandin, 704
ProstaScint scan, 1010
Prostate, 640, 649–50
Prostate gland, 586, 640
Prostate gland, cancer of, 650
Prostatectomy, 656
Prostatic, 586
Prostatic fluid, 640
Prostatic urethra, 586
Prostatitis, 650
Prosthesis, 437, 656, 727
Prosthetic, 254, 437
Prosthetic device, 437
Protease, 97, 319
Proteinuria, 603
Prothrombin, 286
Protocol, 975
Proton pump inhibitor drugs, 133
Proximal, 41
Proximal convoluted tubule, 589
Proximal direction (proximally), 41
Proxy, 913
Pruritic, 352
Pruritus, 352
Psoralen, 377
Psoriasis, 364
Psoriatic, 364
Psychiatric, 923
Psychiatric diagnosis, 923
Psychiatric interview, 923
Psychiatrist, 927
Psychiatry
  abbreviations, 927
  anatomy related to
    amygdaloid bodies, 904
    fornix, 904
    hippocampus, 904
    hypothalamus, 904
    limbic lobe and limbic system, 903
    thalamus, 904
  defined, 902
  diagnostic procedures
    blood and urine tests, 922
    psychiatric procedures and tests, 922–23
    radiologic procedures, 922
  drug categories, 926–27
  emotion and behavior, physiology of
    affect, 905
    amygdaloid bodies, 905
    dopamine, 906
    emotions, 905
    epinephrine, 905
    frontal lobe, 905
    GABA (gamma-amino butyric acid), 906
    hippocampus, 905
    hypothalamus, 905
    mood, 905
    neurotransmitters, 905–06
    norepinephrine, 905–06
    serotonin, 906
  symptoms, signs and mental disorders
    affective or mood disorders, 917–19
    anxiety disorders, 908–10
    childhood disorders, 911
    cognitive disorders, 910
    dissociative disorders, 912–13
    eating disorders, 912
    factitious disorders, 913
    impulse control disorders, 916
    personality disorders, 921
    psychosis, 919–20
    sexual and gender identity disorders, 914–15
    somatoform disorders, 913–14
    substance-related disorders, 917
  therapies
    art therapy, 924
    aversion therapy, 924
    cognitive-behavioral therapy (CBT), 924
    detoxication, 924
    electroconvulsive therapy (ECT), 924
    family therapy, 924
    group therapy, 925
    hypnosis, 925
    play therapy, 925
    psychoanalysis, 925
    psychotherapy, 925
    systematic desensitization, 926
    therapeutic milieu, 926
Psychoanalysis, 925
Psychologist, 927
Psychology, 927
Psychomotor, 544
Psychomotor seizures, 544
Psychosis, 919–20
Psychotherapy, 925
Psychiatric therapies. *see under* Psychiatry
Ptosis, 484
Puberty, 642
Pubic, 408, 681
Pubic bone, 408, 681
Pubic symphysis, 408
Pubis, 408
Pulmonary, 158, 208
Pulmonary arteries, 213
Pulmonary artery, 158
Pulmonary circulation, 215, 216
Pulmonary edema, 175, 230
Pulmonary embolism, 176
Pulmonary parenchyma, 158
Pulmonary valve, 208
Pulmonary vein, 158
Pulmonologist, 190
Pulmonology. *see also* Respiration; Respiratory system
  abbreviations, 189
  defined, 154
  diagnostic procedures, 180–82
  drug categories, 187–88
  medical procedures, 182–85
  radiology and nuclear medicine procedures, |182
  surgical procedures, 185–86
  symptoms, signs, and diseases
    bronchi and bronchioles, 169
    lungs, 170–76
    oxygen and carbon dioxide levels, 179–80
    pleura and thorax, 177
    respiration, 177–78

Pulse, 211, 249–50
Pulse oximetry, 181
Pulse points, 249–50
Puncture, 557
Pupil, 808
Pupillary, 808
Pupillary response, 833
Purkinje fibers, 217
Purkinje, Johannes, 217
Purpura, 308
Purulent material (pus), 172
Pus, 172
Pustules, 351
Pyelogram, 609
Pyelography, 609, 999–1000
Pyelonephritis, 600
Pyloric sphincter, 92
Pylorus, 91
Pyometritis, 703
Pyosalpinx, 701
Pyothorax, 172
Pyromania, 916
Pyrosis, 108
Pyuria, 605

Q

Quadrants of abdominopelvic area, 43, 44*f*
Quadriceps, 470
Quadriceps femoris, 470, 471
Quadriplegia, 548, 549
Quadriplegic, 548, 549
Quantitative computerized tomography (QCT), 1001
Quantitative, 1001

R

Radial, 406
Radial artery, 213
Radial pulse, 249
Radiation, 601, 993
Radiation cystitis, 601
Radiation oncologist, 977
Radiation therapy
  brachytherapy, 972
  fractionation, 972
  radiotherapy
    conformal, 973
    external beam, 973
    internal, 974
    interstitial, 974
    intracavitary, 974
    intravenous, 974
Radical, 614
Radiculopathy, 548
Radii, 406
Radioactive, 786
Radioactive iodine uptake (RAIU) and thyroid scan, 786
Radioactive substances, 1007
Radiography, 182
Radiologic procedures. *see under* Diagnostic procedures
Radiologic technologist, 1020
Radiologist, 1020
Radiology. *see also* Nuclear medicine
  abbreviations, 1020
  bone density tests, 1001
  cineradiology, 1000
  computerized axial tomography (CAT, CT scan), 1001
  contrast dyes, 997–1002
  defined, 992
  drug categories, 1019
  electron beam, 1004
  fluoroscopy, 1000
  magnetic fields and radiowaves, 1003–04
  mammography, 1001
  sound waves, 1005–06
  x-rays, 993–96
Radionuclide, 246
Radionuclides, 1007
Radiopharmaceuticals, 1007
Radioresistant cancerous tumors, 973
Radiosensitive cancerous tumors, 973
Radiotherapy, 973–74
Radius, 406
Rales, 170
Rape, 915
Rapist, 915
Rash, 352
Raynaud, Maurice, 240
Raynaud's disease, 240
Rays, 407, 410
Reabsorption, 589
Reactive, 911
Reactive airway disease, 169
Reactive attachment disorder, 911
Receptive, 536
Receptive aphasia, 536
Receptor assays, 963
Receptors, 472, 524, 763
Recession, 837
Reconstructive, 727
Reconstructive breast surgery, 727, 728
Rectocele, 114, 707
Rectum, 93, 469
Rectus, 462, 469
Rectus abdominis, 462, 469
Rectus femoris, 470, 471
Recuperation, 65
Red blood cells (RBCs), 97, 278–79
Red bone marrow, 411–12
Red corpuscles. *see* Erythrocytes
Reducible hernia, 116
Reduction, 440
Reflex, 491, 521
Reflux, 108, 491
Refractive disorders, 827
Refractometer, 608
Refractory, 65, 218
Refractory period, 218
Regional enteritis, 113
Regions of the abdominopelvic area, 43, 44*f*
Regurgitation, 109, 233
Rehabilitation, 492
Rehabilitation exercises, 492
Rehabilitation services, 68
Relapse, 65, 956
Remission, 65, 956
Rems, 996
Renal, 583. *see also* Kidneys
Renal angiography, 610
Renal arteries, 213, 583
Renal arteriography, 610
Renal cell cancer, 600
Renal colic, 598
Renal failure, 600
Renal parenchyma, 588
Renal vein, 583
Repetitive strain injury (RSI), 484
Repolarization, 218
Repression, 913
Reproductive medicine physician, 659
Resection, 128, 186, 837
Resectoscope, 617, 656
Resident, 68
Resistance, 778
Resorption, 441
Respiration. *see also* Pulmonology; Respiratory system
  accessory muscles of, 159
  defined, 160
  exhalation (expiration), 160
  external, 161
  functions of, 160
  gas exchange, 161, 162, 179–80
  inhalation (inspiration), 160
  internal, 162
  involuntary process of, 161
  metabolism, 162
  symptoms, signs, and diseases, 177–78
Respirator, 184–85
Respiratory, 46
Respiratory distress syndrome (RDS), 176, 713
Respiratory rate, 162
Respiratory system. *see also* Ears, nose, and throat (ENT) system; Pulmonology; Respiration
  anatomy of
    bronchi, 157
    larynx, 156
    lungs, 157*f*, 158
    nose and nasal cavity, 155, 156*f*
    pharynx, 156
    thoracic cavity, 159
    trachea, 157
  upper and lower, defined, 46*f*, 154*f*, 155
Respiratory therapist, 190
Respiratory tract. *see* Respiratory system
Restless legs syndrome, 487
Resuscitation, 183
Retardation, 542
Reticulocytes, 279
Reticulum, 946
Retina, 812
Retinaculum, 461
Retinal, 812
Retinal detachment, 825
Retinitis pigmentosa (RP), 825
Retinoblastoma, 826, 963
Retinopathy, 825
Retinopathy of prematurity, 826
Retroflexion, 703
Retroflexion of the uterus, 703
Retrograde, 125
Retrograde amnesia, 910
Retrograde pyelography, 999
Retrolental, 826
Retrolental fibroplasia, 826
Retroperitoneal, 583
Retroversion, 703
Retroversion of the uterus, 703
Reverse transcriptase, 319, 320
Reversible ischemic neurologic deficit (RIND), 539
Reye's syndrome, 172
Rh blood group, 285
Rh factor, 285
Rhabdomyoma, 485
Rhabdomyosarcoma, 485, 961
Rheumatic heart disease, 232
Rheumatoid, 432
Rheumatoid arthritis, 432
Rheumatologist, 443
Rhinitis, 874
Rhinophyma, 366, 875
Rhinoplasty, 885
Rhinorrhea, 874
Rhizotomy, 559
Rhonchi, 170
Rhythm strip, 242
Rhytidectomy, 374
Ribonucleic acid (RNA), 946
Ribosomes, 947
Ribs, 401–02
Right bundle branch block, 235
Right heart catheterization, 242
Right lower quadrant (RLQ), 43, 44*f*
Right upper quadrant (RUQ), 43, 44*f*
Right-brain thinking, 516
Right-sided congestive heart failure, 230
Rigor mortis, 485
Rinne and Weber hearing tests, 880
Rinne, Friederich, 880
Rods, 814
Roentgenogram, 994
Roentgenography
  explained, 993–94
  projections
    AP chest x-ray, 995
    cross-table lateral x-ray, 995
    defined, 994
    flat plate of the abdomen, 995
    KUB, 995
    lateral chest x-ray, 995
    lateral decubitus x-ray, 995
    oblique x-ray, 995
    PA chest x-ray, 995
  radiolucent, 994
  radiopaque, 994
  rems, 996
  terminology
    film badge, 996
    lead apron, 996
    plain film, 996
    portable film, 996
    scout film, 996
Romberg, Moritz, 558, 883
Romberg test, 558
Romberg's sign, 883
Rongeur, 440
Rorschach, Hermann, 923
Rorschach test, 923
Rotation, 465
Rotational, 997
Rotational angiography, 997
Rotator, 465
Rotator cuff tear, 485
Round window, 857
Rugae, 91, 585
Rupture of membranes (ROM), 687
Ruptured tympanic membrane, 874

S

SA node, 217
Sac, 809
Sacral, 403
Sacrum, 403
Sadism, 915
Sagittal, 398
Sagittal suture of the skull, 37*f*, 38, 398
Saliva, 90
Salivary glands, 90
Salpingectomy, 726
Salpingitis, 701
Salpingo-oophorectomy, 726
Saphenous, 214
Saphenous veins, 214
Sarcoma, 364, 424, 959–61

SARS (severe acute respiratory syndrome), 176
Sartorius, 470
Scabies, 359
Scale, 351
Scapula, 405
Scapulae, 405
Scapular, 405
Scars, 356
Schizophrenia, 920
Schizophrenic, 920
Schizotrichia, 368
Schwann cells, 522
Schwann, Theodor, 522
Schwannoma, 538
Sciatica, 548
Scintigram, 435, 1009
Scintigraphy, 435, 967, 1009
Scintiscan, 1009
Sclera, 808, 823
Sclerae, 808
Scleral, 808
Scleral icterus, 823
Scleroderma, 365
Sclerosis, 549
Sclerotherapy, 249
Scoliosis, 430
Scoliotic, 430
Scoliotic curvature, 430
Scotoma, 828
Scrotal, 637
Scrotum, 637
Seasonal affective disorder (SAD), 774, 918
Sebaceous, 342
Sebaceous glands, 342, 365–67, 807
Seborrhea, 367
Seborrheic, 367
Seborrheic dermatitis, 367
Sebum, 342
Secondary hypertension, 239
Secondary site, 956
Second-degree burn, 355
Second-degree heart block, 235
Secretory, 684
Secretory phase, 684
Seizures. *see* Epilepsy
Sella turcica, 755
Semen, 640
Semen tests, 653–54
Semicircular, 858
Semicircular canals, 858
Semimembranosus, 471
Seminal, 640
Seminal fluid, 640
Seminal vesicles, 640
Seminiferous, 638
Seminiferous tubules, 638
Seminoma, 649, 963
Semitendinosus, 471
Senile, 362
Senile dementia, 541
Senile lentigo, 362
Senile plaques, 542
Sensitivity, 124, 369, 606
Sensorineural, 872
Sensorineural hearing loss, 872
Sensory, 514, 518
Septal, 208
Septal defects, 233
Septal deviation, 875
Septicemia, 300
Septum, 208, 858
Sequela, 65
Serotonin, 525, 906
Serous, 159, 873
Serous membrane, 159
Serum, 119, 277
Serum hepatitis, 119
Sessile, 114
Sessile polyps, 114
Severe acute respiratory syndrome (SARS), 176
Sex chromosomes, 685
Sexual and gender identity disorders, 914–15
Sexually transmitted diseases (STDs)
  acquired immunodeficiency syndrome (AIDS), 652
  Chlamydia, 651
  defined, 651
  genital herpes, 651
  genital warts, 652
  gonorrhea, 652
  syphilis, 652
Shaken baby syndrome, 540
Shift to the left, 311
Shin splints, 488
Shingles, 358, 551
Shunt, 560
Sialolith, 107
Sialolithiasis, 107
Sick sinus syndrome, 235
Sickle cell anemia, 303
SIDS (sudden infant death syndrome), 178
Sigmoid colon, 93
Sigmoidoscope, 130
Sigmoidoscopy, 130
Sign, 63
Simple goiter, 774
Simple partial seizures, 544
Sinoatrial node (SA node), 217
Sinus, 20, 218, 860
Sinuses, 860
Sinusitis, 875
Skeletal, 397
Skeletal muscles, 459, 460*f*
Skeletal system. *see also* Bones; Orthopedics
  anatomy of
    arms, 406–07
    axial and appendicular skeleton, 397
    bone, structure of, 411, 412*f*
    chest, 401–02
    head, 398–401. *see also* Cranium; Facial bones
    hips, 408
    joints, cartilage, and ligaments, 410–11
    legs, 409–10
    neck and back, 402–04
    shoulders, 405
  bone growth, 413–14
  defined, 47*f*, 396*f*
Skeletomuscular, 397
Skeletomuscular system. *see* Skeletal system
Skeleton. *see* Bones; Skeletal system
Skene, Alexander, 681
Skene's glands, 681
Skilled nursing facility (SNF), 68
Skin
  dermis
    collagen fibers, 340
    dermatomes, 340, 341*f*
    elastin fibers, 340
  disease and injury, defense against, 343
  epidermis
    basal layer, 340
    exfoliation, 339–40
    keratin, 339
    melanocytes, 340
    superficial layer, 339–40
Skin cancer, 363–64
Skin injuries, 354–57
Skin lesions, types of, 351*f*
Skin turgor, 352
Skull. *see* Cranium; Facial bones
Sleep studies, 555
Slipped disk. *see* Herniated nucleus pulposus (HNP)
Slit-lamp examination, 830
Small cell carcinoma, 958
Small for gestational age (SGA), 713
Small intestine/bowel, 92, 110–11
Smallpox, 316
Smegma, 651
Smoking, 158, 169, 344
Smooth muscles, 459, 460*f*
SOAP format, 23, 25
Social, 909
Social phobia, 909
Social worker, 927
Socket, 807
Sodium ions (Na^+), 218, 284
Soft palate, 89, 861
Solar, 360
Solar keratoses, 360
Somatic, 522
Somatic nervous system, 522
Somatoform, 913
Somatoform disorders, 913–14
Somatosensory, 555
Somatostatin, 759
Sonogram, 126
Sonography, 1005
Spasm, 483
Spasms, 113
Spastic, 549
Spastic colon, 113
Spastic paralysis, 548
Specialty care unit, 67
Speculum, 720, 882
Speech, 863
Sperm, 20, 638
Spermatic, 639
Spermatic cord, 639
Spermatocytes, 642
Spermatogenesis, 642–43
Spermatozoa, 638, 685
Spermatozoon, 638
Sphenoid, 399
Sphenoid bone, 399
Sphenoid sinuses, 860
Sphincter, 586
Sphingomyelin, 717
Sphygmomanometer, 250
Spina bifida, 547
Spinal, 402
Spinal canal, 42, 520
Spinal cavity, 42, 520
Spinal column, 402
Spinal cord, 520, 547–49
Spinal cord injury (SCI), 548–49
Spinal nerves, 520*f*, 521
Spinal tap, 557
Spine, 402, 408
Spinous, 404
Spinous process, 404
Spiral, 427, 1002
Spiral CT scan, 1002
Spirometer, 184
Spirometry, 180, 184
Spleen, 287, 289, 318
Splenectomy, 318
Splenic, 289, 318
Splenic capsule, 289
Splenic flexure, 92*f*
Splenomegaly, 310, 318
Spondylitis, 429
Spondylolisthesis, 430
Spontaneous abortion, 711
Sprain, 433
Sputum, 171
Squamous, 363
Squamous cell carcinoma, 363, 958
Staging, 969
Stapedes, 856
Stapedial, 857
Stapes, 856, 857
Staphylococcus aureus, 357, 707, 709
"The Starry Night" (van Gogh, 1889), 255
Stasis, 307
Status asthmaticus, 169
Status epilepticus, 543
Steatorrhea, 116
Stenosis, 232
Stent, 253
Stereoscopic, 815
Stereoscopic vision, 815
Stereotactic, 559
Stereotactic biopsy, 373
Stereotactic neurosurgery, 559
Sternal, 159
Sternal retractions, 176
Sternocleidomastoid, 466
Sternum, 159, 401
Stethoscope, 64, 182, 248
Stimulate, 756
Stimulation, 763
Stoma, 129
Stomach, 91–92, 97, 108–10, 129
Stomach cancer, 110
Stomatitis, 107, 129
Stone basketing, 617
Stool, 98, 115, 116
Strabismus, 826
Strabismus surgery, 837
Strain, 483
Strangulated hernia, 116
Strep throat, 877
Streptococcus, 877
Streptococcus pneumoniae, 175
Stress tests, 244, 246
Stressors, 922
Striae, 354
Striated, 459
Striated muscles, 459
Stridor, 170
Stroke, 539
Stress incontinence, 604
Stye, 821
Styloid, 399
Styloid process, 399
Subacute, 65
Subacute bacterial endocarditis (SBE), 231
Subarachnoid, 518
Subarachnoid space, 518
Subclavian arteries, 213
Subcutaneous, 341
Subcutaneous tissue, 341
Subdural, 545
Subdural hematoma, 545
Sublingual glands, 90
Submandibular glands, 90

Submental, 861
Submental lymph nodes, 861
Substance-related disorders, 917
Substantia nigra, 517
Sudden infant death syndrome (SIDS), 178
Sudoriferous, 342
Sudoriferous glands, 342
Suffixes. *see also* Medical words
  characteristics of, 9
  combining forms, joining to, 11
  diseases, describing, 9
  instruments, describing, 10
  joining two, 19
  medical specialties/specialists, describing, 10
  procedures, describing, 10
Suffixes, listed
  -able, 63
  -ac, 9
  -acusis, 872
  -ad, 40
  -ade, 231
  -al, 9
  -alis, 462
  -amnios, 710
  -an, 678
  -ance, 778
  -ancy, 363
  -ant, 173
  -ar, 9
  -arche, 683
  -aris, 466
  -ary, 9
  -ase, 97
  -ate, 114
  -ated, 109
  -atic, 47
  -ation, 9
  -ative, 62
  -ator, 184
  -atory, 46
  -ature, 210
  -blast, 279
  -body, 290
  -cele, 114
  -centesis, 186
  -cephalus, 545
  -ceps, 462
  -cere, 342
  -clast, 414
  -cle, 176
  -clonus, 486
  -cnemius, 471
  -coccus, 877
  -collis, 485
  -crasia, 300
  -crine, 50
  -crit, 311
  -cyte, 94
  -dactyly, 362
  -derma, 352
  -desis, 438
  -didymis, 639
  -drome, 63
  -duct, 679
  -eal, 90
  -ectasis, 169
  -ectomy, 10
  -ed, 304
  -edema, 309
  -ee, 438
  -elasma, 362
  -elle, 946
  -ema, 171
  -emesis, 108
  -emia, 180
  -emic, 301
  -ence, 115
  -encephaly, 536
  -ency, 304
  -ent, 115
  -entery, 113
  -eon, 66
  -er, 466
  -ery, 65
  -esis, 313
  -etic, 367
  -ety, 908
  -form, 914
  -gen, 63
  -gene, 948
  -glia, 521
  -grade, 125
  -graft, 254
  -gram, 125
  -graph, 555
  -graphy, 10
  -gravida, 722
  -ia, 9
  -iac, 43
  -ial, 311
  -ian, 66
  -iasis, 107
  -iatic, 364
  -iatrics, 51
  -iatry, 10
  -ic, 42
  -ical, 35
  -ician, 67
  -ics, 47
  -id, 90
  -ide, 246
  -il, 472
  -ile, 362
  -immune, 310
  -in, 95
  -ine, 62
  -ing, 236
  -ion, 9
  -ior, 36
  -ious, 62
  -ism, 9
  -ist, 67
  -istic, 175
  -istry, 51
  -isy, 177
  -ite, 524
  -itian, 10
  -itic, 177
  -ition, 588
  -itis, 9
  -ity, 89
  -ive, 49
  -ix, 93
  -ization, 218
  -ize, 950
  -kine, 289
  -kinesis, 486
  -lalia, 911
  -lepsy, 546
  -lith, 107
  -logy, 10
  -ly, 36
  -lysis, 304
  -lyte, 284
  -mania, 916
  -megaly, 9
  -ment, 339
  -meter, 181
  -metry, 180
  -mileusis, 837
  -nate, 690
  -nine, 758
  -oid, 114
  -ol, 677
  -ole, 157
  -olisthesis, 430
  -oma, 9
  -omatosis, 552
  -on, 759
  -opia, 825
  -opsy, 127
  -or, 187
  -ory, 65
  -ose, 240
  -osing, 429
  -osis, 9
  -ous, 9
  -paresis, 539
  -partum, 687
  -path, 496
  -pathy, 9
  -pause, 783
  -penia, 299
  -pexy, 616
  -phage, 282
  -pharynx, 862
  -phil, 280
  -phile, 915
  -phylaxis, 344
  -phyma, 366
  -physis, 408
  -phyte, 432
  -plasm, 352
  -plasty, 132
  -plex, 1006
  -pnea, 161
  -poiesis, 279
  -poietin, 279
  -probe, 720
  -ptosis, 599
  -ptysis, 176
  -rrhage, 300
  -rrhaphy, 132
  -rrhea, 115
  -salpinx, 701
  -scope, 45
  -scopy, 10
  -some, 717
  -spasm, 169
  -sphere, 516
  -stalsis, 91
  -stasis, 286
  -steroid, 188
  -stomy, 129
  -therapy, 133
  -thorax, 172
  -tic, 63
  -tion, 63
  -tome, 253
  -tomy, 44
  -tor, 184
  -tous, 775
  -tripsy, 616
  -triptor, 616
  -tron, 1020
  -trophy, 229
  -ty, 642
  -type, 963
  -ual, 831
  -ula, 343
  -ular, 775
  -ule, 214
  -um, 209
  -ure, 315
  -verse, 39
  -zoon, 638
Sugar diabetes, 779
Suicidal, 918
Suicidal ideation, 918
Sulci, 515
Sulcus, 515
Superficial structures, 41
Superior, 813
Superior oblique muscle, 813
Superior rectus muscle, 813
Superior section, 39
Superior vena cava, 40*f*, 214
Superiorly (superior direction), 40
Supination, 465
Supinator, 465
Supine position, 36
Suppositories, 133
Suppressor, 290, 947
Suppressor genes, 947
Suppressor T cells, 290
Suppurative, 873
Suprapubic, 612
Suprapubic catheter, 612
Supraventricular tachycardia, 236
Surfactant, 158
Surgeon, 66, 135
Surgery, 65
Surgical assistant, 977
Surgical consent, 23
Surgical procedures. see also individual specialties
  adenoidectomy, 885
  adrenalectomy, 786
  amputation, 438
  aneurysmectomy, 251
  appendectomy, 127
  arthrocentesis, 438
  arthrodesis, 438
  arthroplasty, 439
  arthroscopy, 438
  bilateral oophorectomy, 725
  bilateral salpingo-oophorectomy (BSO), 726
  biopsy (Bx)
    closed, 492
    core needle, 969
    defined, 127, 373
    excisional, 373, 559, 714, 969
    fine-needle aspiration, 655, 714, 787, 969
    incisional, 373, 492, 655, 714, 970
    muscle, 492
    open, 492
    punch, 373, 970
    renal, 617
    sentinel node, 970
    shave, 373
    stereotactic, 714, 970
    vacuum-assisted, 714, 970
  bladder neck suspension, 614
  blepharoplasty, 374, 835
  bone graft, 439
  bowel resection and anastomosis, 128
  bronchoscopy, 185
  bunionectomy, 439
  capsulotomy, 835
  cardiopulmonary bypass, 251
  carotid endarterectomy, 251, 559
  cartilage transplantation, 439
  cataract extraction
    extracapsular (ECCE), 835
    intracapsular (ICCE), 835
    phacoemulsification, 835
  cerclage, 729
  cesarean section, 729
  cheiloplasty, 883
  chemotherapy drugs, insertion of devices to administer
    central venous catheter, 971

implantable port, 971
implantable wafer, 971
intra-arterial catheter, 971
intraperitoneal catheter, 971
chest tube insertion, 185
cholecystectomy, 128
choledocholithotomy, 129
circumcision, 656
cochlear implant, 883
colonoscopy, 130
colostomy, 129
colporrhaphy, 724
conization, 724
corneal transplantation, 835
coronary artery bypass graft (CABG), 251
craniotomy, 559
culdoscopy, 724
cystectomy, 614
cystoscopy, 615
debulking, 970
dermatoplasty, 374
dilation and curettage (D&C), 724
diskectomy, 559
en bloc resection, 970
endometrial ablation, 724
endoscopic sinus surgery, 883
endoscopy, 130, 970
enucleation, 835
episiotomy, 729
esophagogastroduodenoscopy, 130
esophagoscopy, 130
exenteration, 970
exploratory laparotomy, 131, 971
external fixation, 439
fasciectomy, 492
fasciotomy, 492
ganglionectomy, 492
gastrectomy, 131
gastroplasty, 132
gastroscopy, 130
gastrostomy, 131
glossectomy, 884
heart transplantation, 251
hemorrhoidectomy, 132
herniorrhaphy, 132
hyperopia surgery
conductive keratoplasty (CK), 836
laser thermal keratoplasty (LTK), 836
hysterectomy
abdominal, 724
TAH-BSO (total abdominal hysterectomy and bilateral salpingo-oophorectomy), 724
vaginal (TVH), 724
hysteropexy, 726
ileostomy, 129
jejunostomy, 132
joint replacement surgery, 439
kidney transplantation, 615
laminectomy, 559
laparoscopic cholecystectomy, 128
laparoscopy, 725
laryngectomy, 884
laser photocoagulation, 836
lipectomy, 374
liposuction, 374
lithotripsy
extracorporeal shock wave lithotripsy (ESWL), 616
percutaneous ultrasonic lithotripsy, 616
liver transplantation, 132
lobectomy, 186
lumpectomy, 726, 972
lung resection, 186
lymph node biopsy, 318
lymph node dissection, 318, 972
mammaplasty (mammoplasty)
augmentation, 727
mastopexy, 727
reconstructive, 727
reduction, 727
mastectomy
axilary node dissection, 728
modified radical, 728
prophylactic, 728
radical, 728
simple, 728
total, 728
mastoidectomy, 883
Moh's surgery, 374
myomectomy, 725
myopia surgery
laser-assisted *in situ* keratomileusis (LASIK), 837
photorefractive keratectomy (PRK), 837
myorrhaphy, 493
myringotomy, 884
needle aspiration, 373
nephrectomy, 616
nephrolithotomy, 616
nephropexy, 616
oophorectomy, 725
open reduction and internal fixation (ORIF), 440
orchiectomy, 656
orchiopexy, 656
otoplasty, 884
pacemaker insertion, 252
parathyroidectomy, 787
penile implant, 656
percutaneous endoscopic gastrostomy (PEG), 131
percutaneous endoscopic jejunostomy (PEJ), 132
percutaneous radiofrequency ablation, 972
percutaneous transluminal angioplasty (PTCA), 252–53
pericardiocentesis, 253
pneumonectomy, 186
polypectomy, 132, 884
prostatectomy, 656
radical cystectomy, 614
radical neck dissection, 884
radical resection, 972
reconstructive breast surgery
prosthesis, use of, 728
TRAM (transverse rectus abdominis muscle) flap, 728
renal biopsy, 617
retinopexy, 837
rhinoplasty, 885
rhizotomy, 559
rhytidectomy, 374
salpingectomy, 726
salpingo-oophorectomy, 726
sigmoidoscopy, 130
skin grafting
allograft, 374
autograft, 374
synthetic, 375
xenograft, 375
splenectomy, 318
stapedectomy, 885
stereotactic neurosurgery, 559
stone basketing, 617
strabismus surgery, 837
subtotal thyroidectomy, 787
suction-assisted lipectomy, 374
tenorrhaphy, 493
thoracocentesis, 186
thoracotomy, 186
thymectomy, 318, 493, 787
thyroid lobectomy, 787
thyroidectomy, 787
tonsillectomy, 885
total hip replacement (THR), 439
trabeculoplasty, 838
tracheostomy, 186
tracheotomy, 186
transarterial chemoembolization (TACE), 972
transphenoidal hypophysectomy, 787
transurethral resection of a bladder tumor (TURBT), 617
transurethral resection of the prostate (TURP), 656
tubal anastomosis, 726
tubal ligation, 726
tumor excision, 970
tympanoplasty, 885
tympanostomy, 884
urethroplasty, 617
uterine artery embolization, 726
uterine suspension, 726
valve replacement, 254
valvoplasty, 253
valvuloplasty, 253
vasectomy, 656
vasovasostomy, 656
ventriculoperitoneal shunt, 560
vitrectomy, 836
Suspension, 614
Sutures, 373, 398, 410
Swayback, 429
Sweat glands, 342, 367
Sympathetic, 523
Sympathetic nervous system, 523
Symphysis, 408
Symptom, 63
Symptomatology, 63
Synapse, 524
Syncopal, 546
Syncopal episode, 546
Syncope, 546
Syndactyly, 362
Syndrome, 63, 113, 781, 877
Syndrome of inappropriate ADH (SIADH), 773
Synovial fluid, 411
Synovial joints, 410–11
Synovial membrane, 411
Syphilis, 652
System, 339
Systematic desensitization, 926
Systemic, 344, 364
Systemic allergic reaction, 344
Systemic circulation, 215, 216
Systemic lupus erythematosus (SLE), 364
Systems. *see* Body systems
Systole, 217
Systolic pressure, 250–51

T

T cells, 290
Tachycardia, 235–36
Tachycardic, 235, 236
Tachypnea, 178
Tachypneic, 178
Talipes equinovarus, 434
Tampons, 707
Tanner staging, 721
Tardive, 561
Tardive dyskinesia, 561, 927
Tarsal, 410
Tarsal bones, 410
Taste, 89
Tears, 809
Technician, 67
Technologist, 67
Teeth, 90
Telemetry, 244
Temporal, 399
Temporal bones, 399
Temporal lobe, 515
Temporalis, 462, 466
Temporomandibular, 861
Temporomandibular joint (TMJ), 861
Temporomandibular joint (TMJ) syndrome, 877
Tenaculum, 724
Tendinous, 461
Tendonitis, 488
Tendons, 461
Tennis elbow, 488
Tenorrhaphy, 493
Tenosynovitis, 488
Tensilon test, 489
Teratoma, 963
Term neonates, 690
Terminal illness, 65
Testes, 638, 639, 649, 762
Testicles, 638
Testicular, 638
Testicular cancer, 649
Testis, 638
Testosterone, 638, 762
Tetralogy, 233
Tetralogy of Fallot, 233
Thalamic, 517
Thalamus, 517, 815, 904
Thalassemia, 303
Thallium, 246
Thanatophobia, 909
Thematic Apperception Test (TAT), 923
Thenar, 468
Therapeutic, 65
Therapeutic abortion (TAB), 723
Therapeutic milieu, 926
Therapist, 67, 190
Therapy, 65, 437
Thermal, 836
Third stage of labor, 689
Third-degree burn, 355
Third-degree heart block, 235
Thoracic, 159
Thoracic aorta, 212
Thoracic cavity, 42, 159, 210, 401
Thoracic vertebrae (T1-T12), 403
Thoracocentesis, 186
Thoracotomy, 186
Thorax, 20, 159, 162, 177, 401, 433
Three-dimensional ultrasonography, 719*f*
Thrombi, 286
Thrombocytes, 283, 307–08
Thrombocytopenia, 308
Thrombolytic, 256, 319
Thrombophlebitis, 240
Thromboplastin, 286
Thrombosis, 307
Thrombus, 286, 307
Thrush, 877
Thymectomy, 318, 493, 787
Thymic, 288
Thymoma, 310
Thymosins, 289, 758

Thymus, 287, 288–89, 758
Thyroid, 756
Thyroid carcinoma, 776
Thyroid function tests (TFTs), 785
Thyroid gland
  hormones secreted
    calcitonin, 758
    thyroxine (T_4), 758
    triiodothyronine (T_3), 758
  isthmus, 757
  lobes, 757
Thyroid nodule, 777
Thyroid scan, 786
Thyroid storm, 776
Thyroidectomy, 787
Thyroiditis, 777
Thyroid-stimulating hormone (TSH), 756
Thyromegaly, 774
Thyrotoxicosis, 776
Thyroxine (T_4), 758
Tibia, 409
Tibiae, 409
Tibial, 409
Tibial arteries, 213
Tibialis, 470
Tibialis anterior, 470
Tic douloreux, 551
Tinea, 358–59
Tinea capitis, 358
Tinea corporis, 358
Tinea cruris, 358
Tinea pedis, 358, 359*f*
Tinnitus, 874
Tocolytic drugs, 730
Tolerance, 917
Tomography, 125, 182, 246, 435
Tone deafness, 872
Tongue, 89, 861
Tonic, 544
Tonic-clonic seizures, 544
Tonometer, 830
Tonometry, 830
Tonsillar, 862
Tonsillectomy, 878, 885
Tonsillectomy and adenoidectomy (T&A), 885
Tonsillitis, 878
Tonsils, 862, 878
Tophi, 431
Tophus, 431
Topical, 377
Torn meniscus, 433
Torticollis, 485
Tourette, Georges Gilles de la, 911
Tourette's syndrome, 911
Toxic, 707
Toxic shock syndrome, 707
Trabecular, 811
Trabecular meshwork, 811
Tracers, 1007
Trachea, 157
Tracheal, 157
Tracheobronchial, 157
Tracheobronchial tree, 157
Tracheostomy, 186
Tracheotomy, 186
Tract, 160, 810
Traction, 438, 558
Tragi, 856
Tragus, 855, 856
TRAM (transverse rectus abdominis muscle) flap, 728
Tranquilizer drugs, 926
Transarterial, 972
Transarterial chemoembolization (TACE), 972
Transcriptase, 319
Transcutaneous, 558
Transdermal, 377
Transducer, 1005
Transection, 548
Transesophageal, 247
Transesophageal echocardiography (TEE), 1005
Transferrin, 313
Transfusion, 304, 317
Transfusion reaction, 304
Transhepatic, 125
Transient ischemic attack (TIA), 539
Transitional, 958
Transitional cell carcinoma, 958
Translocation, 948
Transluminal, 252
Transphenoidal, 787
Transplantation, 132, 251, 317, 439, 615, 835
Transposition of the great vessels, 233
Transrectal, 654
Transrectal ultrasonography (TRUS), 654
Transsexualism, 915
Transurethral, 617
Transurethral resection of a bladder tumor (TURBT), 617
Transurethral resection of the prostate (TURP), 656
Transvaginal, 719
Transvaginal ultrasound, 719
Transverse, 404, 427
Transverse plane
  caudad direction, 40
  cephalad direction, 40
  defined, 39
  inferior direction (inferiorly), 40
  inferior section, 39
  superior direction (superiorly), 40
  superior section, 39
Transverse processes, 404
Transvestism, 915
Trapezius, 467
Treadmill exercise stress test, 244
Treatment, 65
Tremor, 486
Tremulous, 486
Treponema pallidum, 652
Triceps, 462
Triceps brachii, 462, 468
Trichotillomania, 916
Tricuspid, 208
Tricuspid valve, 208
Trigeminal, 235, 519, 551
Trigeminal nerve, 519
Trigeminal neuralgia, 551
Trigeminy, 235
Triglycerides, 237
Trigone, 585
Triiodothyronine (T_3), 758
Trimesters, 686
Triskaidekaphobia, 908
Trochanteric, 409
Trochanters, 409
Trochlear, 519
Trochlear nerve, 519
Troponin, 242
Tubal, 709
Tubal anastomosis, 726
Tubal ligation, 726
Tubal pregnancy, 709
Tubercles, 176
Tuberculosis (TB), 176
Tuberculosis tests, 182
Tubular, 589
Tubule, 589
Tumor, 949, 956
Tumor excision, 970
Tumor necrosis factor (TNF), 290, 949
Tumor, site of, 956
Turbid, 607
Turbinates, 155, 400, 859
Turgor, 352
Twins, 685
Tympanic, 856
Tympanic membrane (TM), 856, 874
Tympanogram, 880
Tympanometry, 880
Tympanostomy, 884
Type 1 diabetes mellitus, 778, 779*t*
Type 2 diabetes mellitus, 779
Tzanck, Arnault, 370

U

Ulcer, 110, 356
Ulcerative, 113
Ulcerative colitis, 113
Ulcerative keratitis, 822
Ulna, 406
Ulnae, 406
Ulnar, 406
Ulnar artery, 213
Ultrasonic, 616
Ultrasonography, 247, 314, 610, 654, 719, 831, 967, 1005–06
Ultrasound, 126
Ultrasound probe, 1005
Ultrasound transducer, 1005
Umbilical, 116, 686
Umbilical cord, 686, 688
Umbilical hernia, 116
Umbilical region, 43, 44*f*
Umbilicus, 43, 686
Undifferentiated cell appearance, 949
Ungual, 343
Unilateral, 876
Universal donor, 285
Upper respiratory infection (URI), 875
Urea, 588
Uremia, 600
Uremic, 600
Ureteral, 584, 586
Ureteral orifices, 584
Ureters, 584, 586, 587*f*
Urethra, 586, 587*f*, 602, 641
Urethral, 586
Urethral glands, 681
Urethral meatus, 586
Urethritis, 602
Urethroplasty, 617
Urgency, 605
Uric acid, 434, 588
Urinalysis, 607–08
Urinary, 583
Urinary analgesic drugs, 619
Urinary retention, 602
Urinary system, 590. *see also* Kidneys; Urology
  alternate names for, 587
  anatomy of
    bladder, 585
    kidneys, 583–84
    ureters, 584
    urethra, 586
  defined, 48*f*, 582*f*, 583
Urinary tract infection (UTI), 605
Urination, 589, 603–05
Urine, 589, 603–05
Urine dipstick, 607*f*, 785
Urine formation
  collecting duct, 589
  distal convoluted tubule, 589
  electrolytes, 588–89
  filtration, 589
  glomerulus, 588–89
  loop of Henle, 589
  nephrons
    Bowman's capsule, 588
    glomerulus, 588
  process of, 590*f*
  proximal convoluted tubule, 589
  reabsorption, 589
  urination, 589
  waste products
    creatinine, 588
    urea, 588
    uric acid, 588
Urinometer, 608
Urogenital, 587
Urogenital system. *see* Urinary system
Urogram, 609
Urography, 609, 999
Urologist, 620
Urology. *see also* Kidneys; Urinary system
  abbreviations, 619
  defined, 582
  diagnostic procedures
    blood tests, 606
    radiology and nuclear medicine procedures, 609–10
    urine tests, 606–08
  drug categories, 618–19
  medical procedures, 612–14
  surgical procedures, 614–17
  symptoms, signs, and diseases
    bladder, 601–02
    kidneys and ureters, 597–600
    urethra, 602
    urine and urination, 603–05
Urticaria, 360
Uterine, 679
Uterine artery embolization, 726
Uterine descensus, 704
Uterine inertia, 711, 774
Uterine prolapse, 704
Uterine suspension, 726
Uterus, 679–80, 701–04
Uvea, 810
Uveal tract, 810
Uveitis, 824
Uvula, 89, 861

V

Vaccination, 291, 316
Vaccine, 316
Vagina, 676f, 679f, 680, 706–07, 724
Vaginal, 680
Vaginal canal, 680
Vaginal introitus, 680, 681
Vaginitis, 707
Vaginosis, 706
Vagus, 519
Vagus nerve, 519
Valves, 207*f*, 208–09, 231–33
Valvoplasty, 253
Valvular, 208
Valvuloplasty, 253
Valvulotome, 253

van Gogh, Vincent, 255
Varices, 108
Varicocele, 649
Varicose, 240
Varicose veins, 240
Varix, 108
Vas deferens, 640
Vascular structures, 219
Vasculature, 210
Vasectomy, 656
Vasoconstriction, 211
Vasodilation, 211
Vasovasostomy, 656
Vastus intermedius, 471
Vastus lateralis, 471
Vastus medialis, 471
Vegetations, 232
Vein, 20
Veins, 214
Vena cava, 214
Venae cavae, 214
Venereal disease (VD). *see* Sexually transmitted diseases (STDs)
Venipuncture, 315
Venogram, 245, 997
Venography, 245, 997
Venous, 214
Venous stasis, 307
Ventilation, 182
Ventilation-perfusion (V/Q) scan, 182, 1010
Ventilator, 184–85
Ventral, 116
Ventral hernia, 116
Ventral nerve roots, 521
Ventral section, 36
Ventricle, 208
Ventricles, 517
Ventricular, 208, 517
Ventricular fibrillation, 234
Ventricular septal defect (VSD), 233
Ventriculography, 246
Ventriculoperitoneal, 560
Ventriculoperitoneal shunt, 560
Venules, 214
Vermiform appendix, 93
Vermilion, 860
Vermilion border, 860
Vernix caseosa, 690
Verruca, 359
Verrucae, 359
Version, 723
Vertebra, 402
Vertebrae, 402, 429–30
Vertebral, 402
Vertebral column, 402
Vertebral foramen, 404
Vertex, 687
Vertex presentation, 687
Vertigo, 874
Very low-density lipoprotein (VLDL), 237
Vesalius, Andreas, 404
Vesical, 585, 586
Vesicle, 351, 586, 640
Vesicovaginal, 602
Vesicovaginal fistula, 602
Vesicular, 351
Vestibular, 858
Vestibule, 858
Villi, 92, 97
Villus, 717
Viral, 175
Viral hepatitis, 118
Viral pneumonia, 175
Virchow, Rudolph, 305
Virilism, 782
Viscera, 43
Visceral, 159
Visceral pleura, 159
Viscosity, 303
Vision, 815
Vision, physiology of, 814–15
Visual, 514
Visual acuity testing, 831
Visual cortex, 514, 815
Vital signs, 185
Vitamins
  B_{12}, 97, 302, 319
  K, 98, 286
Vitiligo, 354
Vitreous humor, 812
Vocal, 863
Vocal cord nodule or polyp, 878
Vocal cords, 863
Voiding, 589
Voiding cystourethrogram, 611
Voiding cystourethrography (VCUG), 611
Voluntary muscles, 459
Volvulus, 111
Vomer, 400
Vomit/vomitus, 109
von Recklinghausen, Friedrich, 552
von Recklinghausen's disease, 552
von Sacher-Masoch, Leopold, 914
Voyeurism, 915
Vulva, 681
Vulvar, 681

W

Wadlow, Robert, 772
Walking pneumonia, 175
Warts, 359
Weber, Ernst, 880
Weightlessness, effects of, 414
Well-baby clinic, 68
Wet mount, 716
Wheal, 351
Wheezes, 170
White blood cells (WBCs). *see* Leukocytes
White corpuscles. *see* Leukocytes
White matter, 515, 525
White-coat hypertension, 239
Wilms, Max, 600
Wilms' tumor, 600, 963
Wood, Robert, 370
Wood's lamp of light, 370
Word parts. *see under* Medical words
Wound, 352
Wryneck, 485

X

Xanthelasma, 362
Xanthoma, 362
Xenograft, 254, 375
Xenophobia, 909
Xeroderma, 352
Xeromammogram, 718
Xeromammography, 718, 1001
Xerophthalmia, 822
Xiphoid, 401
Xiphoid process, 401
X-rays, 435, 993. *see also* Radiologic procedures

Y

Yellow bone marrow, 411, 412*f*

Z

Zygoma, 400
Zygomatic, 400
Zygomatic bone, 400
Zygote, 685
Zygote intrafallopian transfer (ZIFT), 723

SINGLE PC LICENSE AGREEMENT AND LIMITED WARRANTY

READ THIS LICENSE CAREFULLY BEFORE OPENING THIS PACKAGE. BY OPENING THIS PACKAGE, YOU ARE AGREEING TO THE TERMS AND CONDITIONS OF THIS LICENSE. IF YOU DO NOT AGREE, DO NOT OPEN THE PACKAGE. PROMPTLY RETURN THE UNOPENED PACKAGE AND ALL ACCOMPANYING ITEMS TO THE PLACE YOU OBTAINED THEM. ***THESE TERMS APPLY TO ALL LICENSED SOFTWARE ON THE DISK EXCEPT THAT THE TERMS FOR USE OF ANY SHAREWARE OR FREEWARE ON THE DISKETTES ARE AS SET FORTH IN THE ELECTRONIC LICENSE LOCATED ON THE DISK:***

1. GRANT OF LICENSE and OWNERSHIP: The enclosed computer programs and data ("Software") are licensed, not sold, to you by Pearson Education, Inc. ("We" or the "Company") and in consideration of your purchase or adoption of the accompanying Company textbooks and/or other materials, and your agreement to these terms. We reserve any rights not granted to you. You own only the disk(s) but we and/or our licensors own the Software itself. This license allows you to use and display your copy of the Software on a single computer (i.e., with a single CPU) at a single location for academic use only, so long as you comply with the terms of this Agreement. You may make one copy for back up, or transfer your copy to another CPU, provided that the Software is usable on only one computer

2. RESTRICTIONS: You may not transfer or distribute the Software or documentation to anyone else. Except for backup, you may not copy the documentation or the Software. You may not network the Software or otherwise use it on more than one computer or computer terminal at the same time. You may not reverse engineer, disassemble, decompile, modify, adapt, translate, or create derivative works based on the Software or the Documentation. You may be held legally responsible for any copying or copyright infringement which is caused by your failure to abide by the terms of these restrictions.

3. TERMINATION: This license is effective until terminated. This license will terminate automatically without notice from the Company if you fail to comply with any provisions or limitations of this license. Upon termination, you shall destroy the Documentation and all copies of the Software. All provisions of this Agreement as to limitation and disclaimer of warranties, limitation of liability, remedies or damages, and our ownership rights shall survive termination.

4. LIMITED WARRANTY AND DISCLAIMER OF WARRANTY: Company warrants that for a period of 60 days from the date you purchase this SOFTWARE (or purchase or adopt the accompanying textbook), the Software, when properly installed and used in accordance with the Documentation, will operate in substantial conformity with the description of the Software set forth in the Documentation, and that for a period of 30 days the disk(s) on which the Software is delivered shall be free from defects in materials and workmanship under normal use. The Company does not warrant that the Software will meet your requirements or that the operation of the Software will be uninterrupted or error-free. Your only remedy and the Company's only obligation under these limited warranties is, at the Company's option, return of the disk for a refund of any amounts paid for it by you or replacement of the disk. THIS LIMITED WARRANTY IS THE ONLY WARRANTY PROVIDED BY THE COMPANY AND ITS LICENSORS, AND THE COMPANY AND ITS LICENSORS DISCLAIM ALL OTHER WARRANTIES, EXPRESS OR IMPLIED, INCLUDING WITHOUT LIMITATION, THE IMPLIED WARRANTIES OF MERCHANTABILITY AND FITNESS FOR A PARTICULAR PURPOSE. THE COMPANY DOES NOT WARRANT, GUARANTEE OR MAKE ANY REPRESENTATION REGARDING THE ACCURACY, RELIABILITY, CURRENTNESS, USE, OR RESULTS OF USE, OF THE SOFTWARE.

5. LIMITATION OF REMEDIES AND DAMAGES: IN NO EVENT, SHALL THE COMPANY OR ITS EMPLOYEES, AGENTS, LICENSORS, OR CONTRACTORS BE LIABLE FOR ANY INCIDENTAL, INDIRECT, SPECIAL, OR CONSEQUENTIAL DAMAGES ARISING OUT OF OR IN CONNECTION WITH THIS LICENSE OR THE SOFTWARE, INCLUDING FOR LOSS OF USE, LOSS OF DATA, LOSS OF INCOME OR PROFIT, OR OTHER LOSSES, SUSTAINED AS A RESULT OF INJURY TO ANY PERSON, OR LOSS OF OR DAMAGE TO PROPERTY, OR CLAIMS OF THIRD PARTIES, EVEN IF THE COMPANY OR AN AUTHORIZED REPRESENTATIVE OF THE COMPANY HAS BEEN ADVISED OF THE POSSIBILITY OF SUCH DAMAGES. IN NO EVENT SHALL THE LIABILITY OF THE COMPANY FOR DAMAGES WITH RESPECT TO THE SOFTWARE EXCEED THE AMOUNTS ACTUALLY PAID BY YOU, IF ANY, FOR THE SOFTWARE OR THE ACCOMPANYING TEXTBOOK. BECAUSE SOME JURISDICTIONS DO NOT ALLOW THE LIMITATION OF LIABILITY IN CERTAIN CIRCUMSTANCES, THE ABOVE LIMITATIONS MAY NOT ALWAYS APPLY TO YOU.

6. GENERAL: THIS AGREEMENT SHALL BE CONSTRUED IN ACCORDANCE WITH THE LAWS OF THE UNITED STATES OF AMERICA AND THE STATE OF NEW YORK, APPLICABLE TO CONTRACTS MADE IN NEW YORK, AND SHALL BENEFIT THE COMPANY, ITS AFFILIATES AND ASSIGNEES. HIS AGREEMENT IS THE COMPLETE AND EXCLUSIVE STATEMENT OF THE AGREEMENT BETWEEN YOU AND THE COMPANY AND SUPERSEDES ALL PROPOSALS OR PRIOR AGREEMENTS, ORAL, OR WRITTEN, AND ANY OTHER COMMUNICATIONS BETWEEN YOU AND THE COMPANY OR ANY REPRESENTATIVE OF THE COMPANY RELATING TO THE SUBJECT MATTER OF THIS AGREEMENT. If you are a U.S. Government user, this Software is licensed with "restricted rights" as set forth in subparagraphs (a)-(d) of the Commercial Computer-Restricted Rights clause at FAR 52.227-19 or in subparagraphs (c)(1)(ii) of the Rights in Technical Data and Computer Software clause at DFARS 252.227-7013, and similar clauses, as applicable.

Should you have any questions concerning this agreement or if you wish to contact the Company for any reason, please contact in writing: Prentice-Hall, New Media Department, One Lake Street, Upper Saddle River, NJ 07458.